Bridget Hulsey

Contents

Maternal-Infant
Nursing Care

second edition

Maternal-Infant Nursing Care

Elizabeth Jean Dickason, RN, MA, MEd
Professor Emeritus, Queensborough Community College,
Bayside, New York;
Nurse Consultant, East Chatham, New York

Bonnie Lang Silverman, RNC, MS, NNP
School of Public Health, University of Massachusetts,
Amherst, Massachusetts

Martha Olsen Schult, RN, MA
Professor, Department of Nursing,
Queensborough Community College,
Bayside, New York

with 650 illustrations, 600 in full color

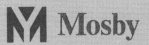 Mosby

St. Louis Baltimore Boston Chicago London Madrid Philadelphia Sydney Toronto

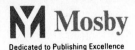

Dedicated to Publishing Excellence

Editor: Michael S. Ledbetter
Senior Developmental Editor: Teri Merchant
Associate Developmental Editor: Linda Caldwell
Design: Elizabeth Fett
Cover Design: Bert Vander Mark
Manufacturing Supervisor: Betty Richmond

A NOTE TO THE READER:

The author and publisher have made every attempt to check dosages and nursing content for accuracy. Because the science of pharmacology is continually advancing, our knowledge base continues to expand. Therefore we recommend that the reader always check product information for changes in dosage or administration before administering any medication. This is particularly important with new or rarely used drugs.

SECOND EDITION

Copyright © 1994 by Mosby–Year Book, Inc.

Previous edition copyrighted 1990

Printed in the United States of America

Composition by Carlisle Communications, Ltd.
Printing/binding by Von Hoffmann Press, Inc.

Mosby–Year Book, Inc.
11830 Westline Industrial Drive
St. Louis, Missouri 63146

Library of Congress Cataloging in Publication Data
Dickason, Elizabeth J.
    Maternal-infant nursing care / Elizabeth Jean Dickason, Bonnie
Lang Silverman, Martha Olsen Schult. — 2nd ed.
    Includes bibliographical references and index.
    ISBN 0-8016-7408-5
    1. Maternity nursing. 2. Pediatric nursing. 3. Family nursing.
I. Silverman, Bonnie Lang. II. Schult, Martha Olsen. III. Title.
    [DNLM: 1. Maternal-Child Nursing.   WY 157.3 D547m 1993]
RG951.D53   1993
610.73′678—dc20
DNLM/DLC   93-30219
for Library of Congress   CIP

94 95 96 97 98   9 8 7 6 5 4 3 2

Contributors

Martha J. Allan, RN, BSN, MA
Health Educator
Lodi, Wisconsin
Chapters 10 and 23

Carolyn D'Avanzo, DNSc, RN
Assistant Professor
Women's Health, Health Promotion Unit
School of Nursing
University of Connecticut
Storrs, Connecticut
Chapter 2

Catherine Faye, RNC, BA
University of Connecticut Health Center
John Dempsey Hospital
Farmington, Connecticut
Chapter 29

Madeline Hogan, RN, MS
Instructor
Maternal and Child Nursing
Nassau Community College
Garden City, New York
Chapters 3,4, and 17

Beth Iovanne, RNC, MSN, NNP
Neonatal Intensive Care
Lawrence and Memorial Hospital
New London, Connecticut
Chapter 28

Catherine A. McDonough-Tuccillo, RNC, BSN
University of Connecticut Health Center
John Dempsey Hospital
Farmington, Connecticut
Chapter 29

Briget Recker, RNC, MS
Clinical Coordinator
Department of Pediatrics
Maimonides Medical Center
Brooklyn, New York
Chapter 24

Mary Ann Shea, RN, JD
Attorney-at-Law
Kirkwood, Missouri
Chapter 30

Francine Stier, RN, MA
Childbirth Educator
Mt. Sinai Hospital
Hartford, Connecticut
Chapters 5 and 6

Contributors to the First Edition

Susan E. Anderson, RN, MS, EdD
School of Nursing
Salem State College
Salem, Massachusetts
Labor Process

Constance Flink Castor, RN, BS
Council of Childbirth Education Specialists, Inc.
East Lyme, Connecticut
Childbirth Preparation, Labor Nursing Care

Gloria C. Essoka, RN, MSN, PhD
Professor
Hunter–Bellevue School of Nursing
Hunter College, New York, New York
Hematologic and Respiratory Problems during Pregnancy

Janice French, RN, CNM, MS
Doctoral Student, Department of Epidemiology
University of North Carolina at Chapel Hill
Chapel Hill, North Carolina
Infectious Problems during Pregnancy

Patricia Hassid, RN, MEd
Council of Childbirth Education Specialists, Inc.
New York, New York
Preparation for Pregnancy

Madeline Hogan, RN, MS
Instructor
Maternal and Child Nursing
Nassau Community College
Garden City, New York
Anatomy and Physiology
Postpartum Nursing Care

Helen Jacobson, RN, MSN, CNM
Assistant Professor
Hunter–Bellevue School of Nursing
Hunter College, New York, New York;
Staff Midwife
Planned Parenthood of Essex County, New Jersey
Cardiovascular Problems of Pregnancy

Lutgarde Jans, RD, MS
Nutritionist
St. Luke's–Roosevelt Hospital Center;
    Faculty member, Bronx VA Dietetic Internship
New York, New York
Nutrition for Metabolic Problems

Hilda Koehler, RN, MS, CNM
Learning Center Resource Nurse
St. Luke's–Roosevelt Hospital Center
New York, New York
Metabolic Problems during Pregnancy

Cynthia S. Luke, RN, MS
Director of Nursing Programs
Area Health Education Center
Wilmington, North Carolina
Reproductive Problems during Pregnancy

James A. McGregor, MD, CM
Professor
Department of Obstetrics and Gynecology
University of Colorado
Denver, Colorado
Infectious Problems during Pregnancy

Margherita M. Modica, RN, MS
Director of Nursing
Community Family Planning Council
New York, New York
Physiologic Changes of Pregnancy

Carole Ann Moleti, RNC, CNM, MS, MPH
Women's Health Care
Weller Hospital of the Albert Einstein College of
   Medicine
Bronx Municipal Hospital Center
Bronx, New York
*Psychosocial Support of High-Risk Women and
   Adolescents*

Kathleen M. Nokes, RN, PhD
Assistant Professor
Hunter–Bellevue School of Nursing
Hunter College
New York, New York
Legal Issues in Maternity Care

Lawrence O'Donnell, MSW
Staff Therapist, Marital and Family Specialist
West Bergen Mental Health Center
Ridgewood, New Jersey
Family Care

Susan Peterson-Roberson, MS, RNC
Perinatal Nurse Practitioner
Planned Parenthood of Nassau County
Merrick, New York
Care of the Newborn Infant

Francine Stier, RN, MA
Childbirth Educator
Mt. Sinai Hospital
Hartford, Connecticut
Family Planning, Infertility

Henry O. Thompson, PhD
Adjunct Professor, Nursing/Ethics
School of Nursing
University of Pennsylvania
Philadelphia, Pennsylvania
Ethical Issues in Maternity Care

Joyce E. Thompson, CNM, DrPH, FAAN
Professor
Director, Graduate School of Nurse–Midwifery
School of Nursing
University of Pennsylvania
Ethical Issues in Maternity Care

Jane Wilson, RN
Nurse Clinician
Worksite Hypertension, Inc.
New York, New York
Lactation: Process, Nutrition, and Education

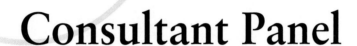

Consultant Panel

Linda Bertucci, RNC, MS
Saddleback Memorial Hospital
Laguna Hills, California

Joea E. Bierchen, RN, BSN, MSN, EdD
Professor of Nursing
St. Petersburg Junior College
St. Petersburg, Florida

Jennifer Calhoun, RN, MS
Instructor, Nursing Education Options
Guilford Technical Community College
Jamestown, North Carolina

Ruth Clark, RN, CNM
Retired
St. Luke's–Roosevelt Hospital Center
New York, New York

Dorothy S. Crowder, BSN, MS, RN, CCE
Associate Professor, Maternal Child Nursing Department
Virginia Commonwealth University—Medical College of
  Virginia
Richmond, Virginia

Alice Day, RN, BS, MS
Assistant Professor, Division of Nursing
South Georgia College
Douglas, Georgia

Noreen Esposito, NP, EdD
Assistant Professor of Nursing
College of Nursing
University of South Florida
Tampa, Florida

Nancy Jackson, MEd, RN, EdD cand
Assistant Professor, School of Nursing
The City College of New York
New York, New York

Valerie Massimo, MSW, PhD cand
Adoption Specialist
New York State Adoption Services
Albany, New York

Barbara S. Migliore, RN, BSN
Professor of Nursing
Los Angeles Pierce College
Woodland Hills, California

Roberta Paige, RN, MA
Maternal-Infant Care Coordinator
Baby Care Program
Home Life Health Care
Portsmouth, Virginia

Judy Palsgraf, RN
Coordinator, Lactation Center
North Shore University Hospital
Manhasset, New York

Toni Ross, MS, RNC, PhD cand
Maternal-Child HIV Nurse Specialist
Elmhurst Hospital Center
Elmhurst, New York

Beth M. Wagner, RN, MSN
Pediatric and Obstetric Staff Development Instructor
Pocono Medical Center
Saylorsburg, Pennsylvania

*To students of maternity and infant nursing
because you are the ones who will aspire to the goals in this text
and change maternal and infant health care*

Preface

Approach

Nursing care in the 1990s must be focused because of short hospital stays for maternity clients. The nurse must thoroughly understand the normal progression of pregnancy and childbirth to identify, plan, and intervene for the health care requirements of today's clients. To promote this understanding and to emphasize that childbearing is a normal and natural process, we first present the complete cycle of pregnancy, labor, and birth as it proceeds in most women. The student who thoroughly comprehends the normal processes and patterns is best prepared to learn to identify the complications that may occur and thus implement the appropriate nursing interventions.

Many of today's maternity clients are knowledgeable about their own health and desire to participate actively in their care. Others, unfortunately, come to the pregnancy poorly informed or misinformed. For these women, preventive health care is the key to achieving the lowest possible rates of maternal and infant morbidity and mortality. Therefore we stress the importance of promoting self-care activities and educating clients about factors that contribute to the achievement of a healthy pregnancy.

Of particular importance in maternity nursing are the impact of the client's cultural background and the involvement of the family. The nurse must be aware of cultural influences and family dynamics to identify specific needs and to develop an individualized plan of care. Cultural considerations and family interaction are examined in Chapter 2 and integrated throughout this text.

Structure and Organization

In spite of the universality of the childbearing experience and the health needs of families in our society, maternal and infant nursing often has been taught in very brief courses. The sequence of this text is structured so that it may be used in a short course. The text proceeds from women's health care through the normal, usual experiences of pregnancy, birth, and recovery. Once this foundation has been established, the student may quickly grasp the physiologic basis of complications. Thus, in an integrated curriculum, this structure facilitates the use of pregnancy complications in discussion of body system alterations within medical-surgical courses.

Traditionally, maternity texts have been locked into the time sequence of trimesters, a division derived from an outdated way of viewing care. The sequence based on body system adaptation to pregnancy or complications has more educational validity because most problems in pregnancy antedate or begin early in pregnancy. For each of the complications of pregnancy, the physiology of the body system is reviewed and rationales for alterations are explained.

The text is clinically oriented. Case studies and reality-based nursing planning and intervention engage the student in interaction with "the way things are." Frank discussion of socioeconomic risk factors of STDs, substance abuse, poverty, and powerlessness will find echoes in real life situations. The student is challenged to become involved in seeking changes in routine health care, which often misses the real needs of the high-risk client. Legal aspects are covered in specific detail, especially for accountability in documentation. The high rate of legal suits in perinatal care requires that even students understand their responsibilities for ensuring both maternal and fetal health. There are no easy answers for some ethical issues. The student is asked to consider and react to a number of troubling societal problems.

Because solutions must be sought, we have included no specific answers to issues raised within clinical decisions and self-discovery situations. Inductive learning is the basis of our philosophy of education. Thinking through facts and applying principles will result in a solution based on problem-solving skills, producing a generation of creative, problem-solving nurses.

Unifying Principles

Several main threads are woven through the text. Physical assessment is stressed consistently as the basis of data collection before planning. For instance, the many methods of assessment of fetal health, especially by means of fetal monitoring, lead into physical assessment of the neonate. Nursing process is a structural framework.

The collaborative role of nursing is recognized, and delineation of nursing and medical functions is noted, with emphasis on the nurse's role in preventive health care teaching. With short hospital stays, home care has assumed new importance. Of special note are the models in Chapter 26 of home care for the high-risk client.

Pharmacologic factors, which change during pregnancy and lactation, are discussed in detail in Chapter 16. They also are noted throughout the text and are emphasized in **Drug Profiles** that contain the most current information on medications commonly used in pregnancy and childbirth. In view of the current HIV epidemic, precautions for mother, baby, and the health care team are thoroughly detailed. Infection is recognized in Chapter 25 as a major health problem. Coverage of genetic defects and teratogenic problems in the infant is extensive.

The thread of cultural diversity is woven through the text, beginning with Chapter 2, in which three ethnic groups are discussed in detail. The client must be considered as the *person-in-environment* before any planning takes place. Unless students can learn to listen attentively—separating their own needs and biases from those of the client—their planning will be superficial. Legal aspects are described in Chapter 30, an especially comprehensive chapter, and in Chapter 13, which emphasizes accountability in monitoring labor progress.

Special Features

Our goal has been to make this book easy to teach from and, more important, easy to learn from. The text is interactive. **Test Yourself** feedback questions often follow a discussion. If the student cannot answer the questions, he or she should reread the prior section. Answers to these questions are in the Student Learning Guide.

Clinical Decisions are scattered throughout the text to help the student think through novel situations. These can be used in class or conference as open-ended discussion topics, for example, "What would you do if . . . ?" To stimulate thinking about the topic the text provides no answers to these or to the **Test Yourself** questions. The **Study Questions** at the ends of chapters, however, contain answers as a final check on learning.

Our goal is a user-friendly learning guide for students. The reader-friendly features start with easy readability. **Learning Objectives** are clearly listed at the beginning of each chapter to provide the reader with a basic guideline for the major points to be presented and learned from the chapter. **Key Terms** are defined on first use and highlighted to reinforce student learning. The **Student Resource Shelf** guides students to additional reading for in-depth mastery. Students can test their knowledge of the **Key Points** at the end of the chapter. These help the reader summarize major points, make connections, and synthesize information.

More than 600 full-color illustrations enhance understanding of anatomy and physiology, assessment, nursing skills and procedures, and birth sequences.

Teaching-Learning Package

An extensive number of ancillary products for instructors and students to use in class and clinical settings is offered.

INSTRUCTOR'S RESOURCE MANUAL

The Instructor's Resource Manual to accompany *Maternal-Infant Nursing Care* is designed to help faculty develop lectures, reinforce teaching through classroom and clinical activities, and evaluate student comprehension. This valuable resource manual follows the textbook chapter by chapter and includes lecture outlines, chapter overviews, learning activities, and enrichment activities. Each chapter includes a short-answer review quiz. A **Test Bank** containing more than 500 test items also has been provided. An answer key with correlating page numbers is included at the end of the manual.

STUDENT LEARNING GUIDE

This useful book contains suggestions for journal entries, learning activities, case studies, and quizzes to reinforce student learning. The material in this book also is included in the Instructor's Resource Manual and may be copied and distributed to students.

OVERHEAD TRANSPARENCIES

One hundred full-color transparency acetates focus on key material in the text, helping instructors to increase student understanding.

QUICK REFERENCE FOR MATERNAL-INFANT ASSESSMENT

This is a handy, pocket-sized resource that accompanies every copy of the text. The guide focuses on maternal, fetal, and newborn assessment.

MICROTEST III

Available in IBM, Computest is the computerized version of the **Test Bank** from the **Instructor's Resource Manual.** Complete with a user's guide, Computest allows instructors to edit, add, delete, or select questions on the computer.

• • •

Pregnancy and birth affect all members of the family. Nursing care is most effective when it is given with the belief that the family is the unit of care. We hope that we have helped build a foundation on which nurses can achieve comprehensive and individualized nursing care.

ELIZABETH JEAN DICKASON
BONNIE LANG SILVERMAN
MARTHA OLSEN SCHULT

To the Student

We think you will enjoy reading this text. Your maternity nursing course will be short and filled with new experiences. This is a good time to start a personal journal because these experiences will affect your own feelings about life and death and parenting. To help you get started, reflection questions called **Self-Discovery** are marked by the symbol ✸. Record your ideas, experiences, and feelings. Some students keep the last pages of their lecture notebook for their personal record; others keep a diary.

Because we want you to develop skill in making **Clinical Decisions,** a second type of question, marked with the symbol 🗲, asks for your judgment concerning a short client care situation. No answers are given, but you can discuss the situation with your classmates.

A third method is use of **Test Yourself** feedback questions, which provide no answers because the answer is in the preceding material. This format will focus your attention on what it is you have just read. At each chapter's end **Study Questions** include terminology definitions and multiple choice, true-false, or matching questions and answers. Brief descriptions of drugs, with specific applications to maternity care, are found in **Drug Profiles,** which are marked by the symbol 🗁.

At the end of each chapter you may check your understanding by reviewing the **Key Points** noted by the symbol 🔑. References of special interest for students are annotated and indicated by the symbol ✎.

Major themes are interwoven through the text. First, we live in a multicultural society and must learn how pregnancy and parenting are viewed by each cultural group with whom we will work. Look for the **Cultural Aspects of Care** marked by the symbol 🌐.

Second, assessment always precedes planning. Physical assessment of the woman, fetus, and newborn infant is emphasized. Only after learning normal parameters can you learn to detect when things go wrong. For this reason, too, the text begins with normal pregnancy and birth and then discusses how complications occur and are treated. Third, nursing process guides care planning and evaluation. Suggested diagnoses and outcomes are given for major care needs. You may use these, but the wording should be individualized for each client. For example, a care plan is specific to one case. Evaluation is achieved by means of answers to general questions.

Nursing accountability is emphasized because childbirth places two clients at risk. Legal issues and documentation of nursing activity are major aspects of the material you will be learning. For instance, fetal monitoring and assessment are involved in two thirds of the lawsuits in obstetrics; failure to monitor correctly or to document or report changes often is the basis of a legal charge against a nurse. For this reason, even while a student, you must learn the patterns that signal fetal distress. Finally, ethical issues and care of socially high-risk women will involve you in debate about "what is right" in maternity care. Our care depends on our recognition of discrimination in quality of care for the affluent and those in poverty. Nurses are learning to be advocates for their clients and to produce models of care for high-risk women that define creative solutions to chronic problems in our society.

Sometimes you may feel overwhelmed by the mass of material a textbook must include. Concentrate on learning the basic anatomy and physiology of pregnancy and newborn changes and subsequent complications. In this way you may understand clinical management and be able to plan nursing interventions. Our goal is to assist you in building the basis for competence, which is your goal. Only when you feel compe-tent in providing care can you use creative problem-solving interventions.

This is an interactive text. We want you to enjoy learning maternity nursing. We are especially interested in receiving feedback from you regarding this text, *Maternal-Infant Nursing Care.* Be kind enough to send in the attached questionnaire after you have completed the course. By doing so you will become an important part of the revision process.

ELIZABETH JEAN DICKASON
BONNIE LANG SILVERMAN
MARTHA OLSEN SCHULT

Feedback to the Authors:

In which course and semester did you use this text?_____

How many weeks was the course?_____

How did you respond to the use of interactive questions within the chapter?_____

_____

What did you like best about the text?_____

_____

_____

What could we improve for the next time?_____

_____

Send responses to:
Teri Merchant, Senior Developmental Editor,
Nursing Division
Mosby–Year Book, Inc.
11830 Westline Industrial Drive
St. Louis, MO 63146

Acknowledgments

A collaborative work depends on the efforts of many people: the authors of each section, the editors, and the production and art and design personnel. This text is indeed a result of the creative process for which there were many seed ideas and discussions.

First we particularly thank our students who shaped our teaching methods because they freely interacted with the content and with their clients. Readers of the manuscript helped clarify content because the question "What does a student of maternity and infant care need to know?" was emphasized.

Illustrations were generously shared by Fredda Diamond, St. Luke's–Roosevelt Medical Center, New York, New York; St. John's Mercy Medical Center, St. Louis, Missouri; Corometrics, Wallingford, Connecticut; PPG Medical Systems, Pleasantville, New York, March of Dimes Birth Defects Foundation, White Plains, New York; Ross Laboratories, Columbus, Ohio; Mead Johnson Company, Evansville, Indiana; Hill-Rom, Batesville, Indiana; and Community Health and Family Planning Council, New York, New York. A special thanks to Bill Schmertz and Ross Laboratories.

In many instances the publishers and authors of medical and nursing texts granted permission to use illustrations. Many illustrations are classics in the field. Derivative work is seen today, but the forefathers and foremothers shaped our thinking and we have chosen to reproduce their work. Photographers include Mark Sick, John Young, R.O. Roberson, Richard Silverman, and Marjorie Pyle of Lifecircle, Costa Mesa, California.

Work of contributors to our first edition of *Maternal-Infant Nursing Care* is reflected in this publication.

Their names are included in the Contributors to the First Edition.

The creation of a text of this complexity would not be possible without the full support of the editorial staff at Mosby. The decision to produce a full-color text created a special opportunity to search for superior illustrations, a task ably executed by Teri Merchant, Senior Developmental Editor. She walked alongside us at every step of development, and much of the credit for organization and illustrations is hers. Linda Duncan, Executive Editor, ran interference and sparked creativity in the approach to the full-color format. These editors are invaluable. Linda Caldwell, Associate Developmental Editor, gracefully accomplished the tasks of tracking down illustrations and permissions and communicating with reviewers.

We also wish to thank Nancy L. Coon, Editor-in-Chief of Nursing, for initiating the second edition; Amy Adams Squire Strongheart, Senior Production Editor, for her diligence, assistance, and interest in the project; Elizabeth Fett, Designer, for creating a fun, reader-friendly, colorful design; Nadine Sokol, medical illustrator, for many of the color charts and illustrations; and Bert Vander Mark, for the wonderful cover.

Finally, many families participated by sharing experiences and photographs. Special thanks to the Suddath, Livingstone, Hopewell, Bodden, Schult, Roberson, and Silverman families.

We are indebted to our computers and our families, who supported this endeavor to the full.

ELIZABETH JEAN DICKASON
BONNIE LANG SILVERMAN
MARTHA OLSEN SCHULT

Brief Table of Contents

Contents

xxiii

UNIT FIVE   PREGNANCY AT RISK

21   Reproductive System Alterations, 543

22   Cardiorespiratory Dysfunction, 585

23   Hematologic, Immunologic, and Neurologic Problems, 615

Maternal-Infant Nursing Care

One

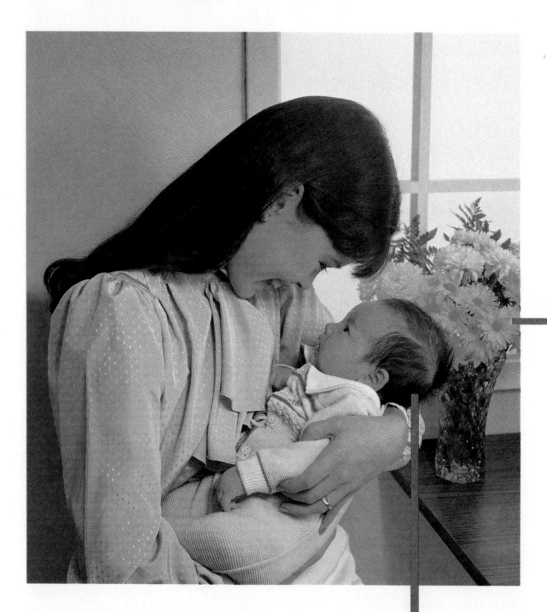

MATERNAL-INFANT NURSING

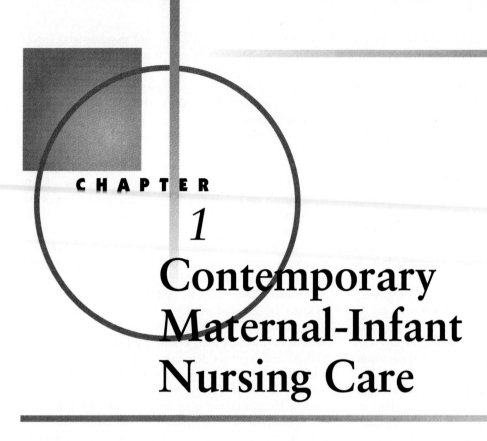

CHAPTER

1
Contemporary Maternal-Infant Nursing Care

KEY TERMS

Assault
Battery
Clinical Nurse
  Specialist
Community
  Standards of Care
Emancipated Minor
Ethics
Informed Consent
Malpractice
Morbidity
Mortality
Negligence
Noetic
Nurse Entrepreneur
Nurse Practitioner
Prenatal Abuse

Professional
  Standards of Care
Years of Potential
  Life Lost (YPLL)

LEARNING OBJECTIVES

1. Describe four trends in delivery of maternity and infant care.
2. Identify examples of community and professional standards of care.
3. Identify sources of resistance to full participation in family-centered maternity care.
4. Differentiate between independent and collaborative nursing functions.
5. Define the steps in the formation of a nursing diagnosis.
6. Discuss socioeconomic and educational factors that result in better provision of prenatal care.
7. Discuss problems contributing to maternal and infant morbidity and mortality.
8. List four components of informed consent, comparing the nurse's and physician's roles in obtaining consent.

Goal of Care

The goal of maternal and infant nursing care is the birth of a healthy infant into a family able to parent appropriately. This text assumes that childbearing is a developmental challenge for the woman and her family. The birth of a baby always changes things. Life will be different for the parents because the patterns of their relationship will change. These changes are especially felt when the first child is born.

There is a **noetic** dimension as well. With the birth of the baby, parents feel more in touch with a spiritual dimension, brought about by the wonder at new life. When things go well, there is awe and a sense of joy.

5

Because the spiritual dimension is tapped, if technologic or physiologic problems occur, fear and anxiety may seem more intense.

No one can assume that parenting is a natural skill developed through instinct. Children learn to parent by watching their own parents. When role models are inadequate, however, conflict may exist among the new parents' societal expectations, their own needs, and their memories of "how to do it." The nurse must recognize that parents may have feelings of low self-esteem and guilt because of their own ideas of what a "good parent" does. Regardless of the situation, these parents need support in their efforts to raise children.

Pregnancy and parenting can be considered a maturational crisis, presenting a challenge in learning how to cope.

Family coping will always be tested in pregnancy. There is potential for growth in relationships or the possibility of distancing from the perceived problem. Usually only the woman is seen during health care visits. Often it is not until problems arise that personnel inquire about the father's adaptation.

An individual is expected to accomplish specific tasks associated with the developmental age. If these tasks are achieved, the individual can progress to the next growth task and mature with some degree of competence and self-esteem. Application of this concept to parenthood can help the nurse to understand the ways in which parenthood conflicts with other circumstances in a person's life. For example, the adolescent mother trying to establish her own identity may have difficulty focusing on the needs of her infant. A woman in the midst of a career challenge may feel a conflict between self-actualization through her work and through parenting.

Every effort must be made to support the parent. It is said that the new mother needs to be mothered so she can mother. This statement can be extended to include both parents. Smoyak (1977) states:

Children do not become normal adults unless nurtured in some type of close continuing social unit, where norms are clearly set, where self-esteem is fostered, and where separateness/connectedness issues are worked on openly and directly. The most important work of parents as socializing agents is to get each succeeding generation to want to go on. Parents, in one way or another, have to accomplish getting their children "hooked" on the idea of continuity. Simply put, they have to make it pleasant to be alive, and further, to suggest that one's "debt" for such pleasure is to pass it on to the next person or generation.

You must not personalize your own family history in working with childbearing families. You will find that much of the content of this course may be personally meaningful. However, each family is unique. Culture and structure of the family need to be considered before plans are made by health care personnel. While learning the support role of the nurse, remember to focus on discovering the environmental and psychosocial forces intruding on families. These forces may contribute to parents' ways of reacting to stress. In addition, a number of parents do not respond in positive ways to pregnancy or to their children. The increasing incidence of elective abortion, child abuse, and child neglect must be a concern of all health professionals. Chapter 2 will introduce the family in its context.

As a maternity nurse, you can communicate and interact with families at a crucial time. Because society is culturally mixed, you will provide nursing support to people who react in different ways to children. You may meet parents who value boys above girls, for instance. You will learn to recognize that the nurse, with brief but significant contact with parents, is able to promote the infant's special characteristics, as well as the parents' acceptance of the child. It will be frustrating, however, to learn the limits of what you can do in so short a time.

Klaus and Kennell (1982) showed certain parenting behaviors toward the newborn are unrelated to gender. Fathers and mothers demonstrated these acquaintance, attachment, and bonding behaviors when getting close to their newborn infants. As a nurse, you may observe specific behaviors and plan interventions when the parent is hesitant or is frightened by the baby. Chapter 8 explains the process of bonding in detail, and Chapter 20 discusses ways of working with parents as they learn to understand their child's patterns of growth and development.

FACTORS INFLUENCING GOAL ACHIEVEMENT

To achieve the goal of supporting healthy childbearing, the following information is useful in determining if any problems interfere with a positive outcome for the pregnancy or birth:

1. Know the positive or harmful environmental factors influencing family functioning.
2. Have an idea of the state of the family's emotional and physical health.
3. Know if there are genetic or environmental factors that may harm the infant.
4. Assess whether or not the family has reasonable access to adequate health care during and after pregnancy.
5. Know if there are any complications during pregnancy that will affect maternal or fetal condition or the newborn infant.
6. Know what the mother has experienced during labor and birth and how she is recovering.
7. Have an idea of how much informed common sense about child rearing the parents bring to the process.
8. Know if there are unusual financial, social, psychologic, or physical constraints that prevent caring for the infant.

Trends in Maternal-Infant Care

Recent trends in maternal-infant care include regionalization, community standards of care, cost containment, early discharge, and family-centered care.

REGIONALIZATION

Before the birth, the mother at risk may be transported to a tertiary (large, centrally located) medical center. In this way, high-risk infants are born in an area adjacent to a neonatal intensive care unit (NICU) and do not have to be transported there after birth. This trend is called *regionalization* and has lowered infant death rates. It includes the trend for a number of small hospitals to close their maternity services because back-up care for high-risk infants and mothers was not adequate.

COMMUNITY STANDARDS OF CARE

Transport of known high-risk mothers before birth and all infants at risk when stabilized after birth is standard care for almost all community hospitals now. **Community standards of care** are criteria expected from practitioners working in a particular setting or geographic area. These standards develop over time and are subject to improvement.

Use of technology such as fetal monitoring and ultrasound is now a community standard of care. Community standards of care are always considered in legal action; therefore physicians are hesitant to omit any step in treatment of the pregnant woman. As a result, sometimes the client may be made to feel that she must comply with multiple examinations when she would prefer not to do so.

RISING CESAREAN BIRTH RATES

With the use of fetal monitoring and ultrasound for prenatal evaluation of fetal condition has come an increased rate of cesarean birth, which has the following positive aspects: distressed babies are rescued before potential injury occurs, and maternal mortality and morbidity may be prevented. Negative aspects include the potential complications of surgery and anesthesia, the high cost, and maternal discomfort from a potentially unnecessary operation. Federal health planners have called for a serious attempt to reduce the numbers of repeat cesarean births. Today, a trial of vaginal birth after cesarean (VBAC) is recommended if conditions permit.

INCREASED COST OF HIGH-TECH CARE

As the medical profession has developed increasingly sophisticated technology, costs have escalated. For example, the minimum cost for an ultrasound screening is more than $300. This exam may be repeatedly ordered, along with fetal monitoring, for a woman in the last weeks of her pregnancy if there is a question of a problem. In fact, today, maternity care is a lucrative business, and several hospitals in the same location may compete to attract clients. Hospitals will advertise, provide tours, and seek client evaluation of services (Box 1-1).

At the same time, cost containment is an important trend in health care. Early discharge with home care is becoming more common. Cost containment changes the way nurses plan care for the mother. Chapters on home care have been included in the text for this reason.

EARLY DISCHARGE

Just 40 years ago, a woman was hospitalized for 7 days after birth. Bed rest was maintained for 3 days, and physical activity was increased very gradually, over a long period. Recovery was called *confinement*. Over the years, however, health care personnel have realized that early return to normal activities is the best course for

---

BOX 1-1   Sample Ad Descriptions of Hospital Birth Settings In One City*

Setting 1: Private hospital

LDRP rooms. All rooms have TV, VCR, stereo, CD player, refrigerator, sofa bed, and private bathroom with whirlpool tub for use during labor.
Vaginal Birth: 1-day stay—$1,800 to $2,400
Cesarean Birth: 3 to 4 days stay—$5,800 to $6,800

Setting 2: HMO-run hospital

Users of HMO (only) can have normal birth in labor, delivery, and recovery room. Pastel decorated space with TV, sofa bed, maple furniture, and view of the river. After 1 day, transfer to semiprivate family-centered unit.
Vaginal Birth: $6.00 to $160
Cesarean Birth: $6.00 to $160

Setting 3: University hospital center

Spare surroundings but the place for high-risk pregnancies and births. Labor in shared rooms with TV and chair. Move to delivery room then to mother-baby unit for recovery.
Praised for expert nursing care and best neonatal intensive care (one of only two units in the city).
Vaginal Birth: 1 day stay—$1,800
                     2 day stay—$2,800
Cesarean Birth: 5 day stay—$5,900

*Hospital charges only. Obstetrician and anesthesiologist fees not included.

uncomplicated births. Until very recently, the mother was hospitalized for 3 to 4 days for normal vaginal delivery and 5 to 7 days for cesarean births (Lemmer, 1987).

Effects of Diagnostic Related Groups

These days hospital recovery time may be even shorter. Some women request early discharge because they are well prepared for self-care or because of financial constraints. Others may be discharged early because of recently developed rules of *diagnostic related groups (DRG)*. These groups assign a predetermined number of days deemed, first by federal government guidelines and now by many private insurance companies, as essential for hospital treatment of a particular condition and for which the hospital will receive payment. However, not all clients fit into these established categories, and therefore some persons may be slated for discharge before they are ready. Others are discharged early because they do not qualify for assistance and have no insurance.

Implications for Nursing Care

DRG guidelines allow 2.7 days for an uncomplicated vaginal birth and 4.3 days for a cesarean birth. Before, nurses had at least 2 days to evaluate recovery and to prepare parents as primary care givers. If women go home during critical recovery time, they must express needs, learn lessons, assimilate information, and prove comprehension by return demonstrations in a brief time (Halloran and Halloran, 1985).

Nursing personnel must develop new approaches to physical assessment, psychosocial evaluation, and teaching. Prenatal education is essential in reducing the need for formal postpartum classes. Postdelivery inclusion of the father is essential in preventing the mother from being overloaded with information and responsibilities as well as ensuring that he is not left out of the planning process.

Home Care

Early discharge with home care is becoming more common and is an effective way to follow through on immediate postbirth care. Some health care centers have developed comprehensive follow-up care; others provide visits only to adolescent mothers or those with psychosocial or medical problems. In situations when women are not supported by extended families, if they are sent home before they are fully recovered or before they understand how to care for the infant, the first few weeks at home can be very difficult. Home care is an area where **nurse entrepreneurs** are developing independent practice, since some area institutions have not yet developed good home monitoring or follow-up care.

FAMILY-CENTERED MATERNITY CARE

The postpartum unit and newborn nursery were once separate areas. Babies stayed in the nursery, except during feeding, and were cared for by neonatal nurses. Because of greater emphasis on parents' rights and their need to learn primary care of the infant, the concept of **rooming-in** was introduced. The baby stayed with the mother during some of her waking hours and was returned to the nursery during visiting hours and while the mother was asleep. Because babies were "out," the nursery nurse was better able to make rounds and offer teaching and assistance with infant care. Despite the general acceptance of this arrangement, a number of hospitals found it inconvenient and resisted it.

This concept has been revised in the philosophy of *family-centered maternity care (FCMC)*. In this framework, the mother and child are considered a unit, a *dyad,* with one nurse assigned to primary care. Within FCMC, infant assessments are performed at the bedside with maternal checks. Parents are encouraged to record feeding times and amounts and voiding and stooling patterns. In this way, although the nurse is still responsible for determining the stability of the newborn, the parents begin to see the factors involved in their child's care. They become aware of sleep patterns and are more comfortable with the newborn's behavior. Because parents have fewer nurses with whom to relate, they may be freer to ask and obtain assistance, reassurance, and instruction. Care of the mother-infant dyad has been demonstrated to be efficient and effective. Breastfeeding is enhanced in this setting (Figure 1-1).

There still is resistance to such innovation; observe the policies of the institution with which you are familiar. If FCMC is not used, why? Is the rationale client or administration centered?

Many hospitals have rebuilt or constructed new family-centered units where the partner and sometimes siblings may join the mother during all or part of the birth process. **Labor-delivery-recovery (LDR)** rooms are becoming more common. In an LDR, the woman is not moved from place to place during the labor process, but once settled in her room, completes the birth there (when all is normal) and spends a few hours of recovery in the same room with the infant at her side. Where the census of births is not too high, some units have LDRP rooms, labor-delivery-recovery and postrecovery (or postpartum) rooms in which the woman stays for the entire hospital period. This LDRP plan is not usually feasible in a unit with a high census.

Homelike Birth Settings

In a number of states, clients may choose a more homelike birth setting outside of the hospital. Certified nurse- and lay-midwives may actually monitor the birth in the woman's home. Or, with her partner, siblings, and

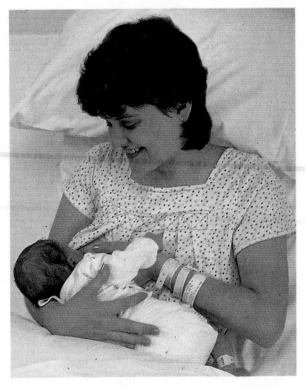

FIGURE 1-1 Breast-feeding. (Courtesy Ross Laboratories, Columbus, Ohio.)

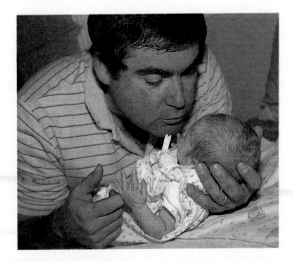

FIGURE 1-2 Father involvement is to be encouraged in family-centered maternity care. (Courtesy Marjorie Pyle, RNC, *Lifecircle*.)

friends, she may come to a birthing center to be assisted by a nurse-midwife. These freestanding centers have back-up with an adjacent hospital if problems should occur during the birth process. The client in such a center usually will go home within 12 to 24 hours. In addition, women who elect home or birthing center births are screened for potential problems before the decision is made. High-risk pregnancies need the more extensive resources of a hospital.

Fathers

Traditionally, the father was an observer during the intrapartum period. Not only was he an inactive participant in the birth event, but also he was not permitted in the delivery area. Today, the picture is very different. Most fathers choose to be a vital part of the process as coach during birth. With increased societal emphasis on shared parenting and the recognition of paternal bonding, many fathers are active in care giving and enjoy the closeness it brings.

Almost universally, hospitals have an open visiting policy for fathers. Fathers are involved in baby care classes and are instructed with the mothers.

Although many cultures encourage the father's participation in the entire birth event, many do not. For example, traditionally, it was considered improper and unac-

ceptable for Asian men to be with their wives during childbirth. Other societies see it as unmasculine to be involved in "women's business." Care must be taken to respect each person's feelings and not impose one's own values while giving encouragement and support.

The nurse who has developed rapport with a father reluctant to be in the labor or birthing area may effect significant change by being supportive. One Asian father expressed reluctance to personally witness the birth. After an explanation of the significance of his presence for his wife, he voluntarily participated. He expressed astonishment, joy, and pleasure at witnessing the birth of his son. The family-centered maternity care setting encourages the father to share the birth experience, introduces the grandchild to the grandparents, and welcomes siblings to meet the new infant (Figure 1-2).

These changes promise a richer birth experience for the family, but they also create a challenge for nurses in maternity care. Because of the focus on promoting independence for the family, the nurse has a new role.

Directions for Maternity and Infant Care

The role of nursing is changing. Naisbett (1982) described the major trends in society, including significant changes in health care. Nursing can grow as society shifts from an industrial to an information base. There is also a move toward self-help and networking in health care. Many options are presented when a care issue arises; a person no longer passively allows the first opinion to prevail. The search for alternatives has become important, and the physician no longer has absolute authority.

Health information is available to almost everyone. The distribution of information about HIV infection, for example, reached every household in the United States. The distribution of complete health information is still uneven, yet clients are more knowledgeable than ever before. You will work with couples who have some knowledge but who need additional knowledge so that they may care for their own needs.

The role of nursing in maternal and infant care is increasingly "high tech" yet needs to remain "high touch," illustrated by the nurse's role during the birth process. The nurse must determine what the family needs, participate in intensive technical monitoring, and give support. Coordination of care demands an ability to go beyond technical tasks to see the family. It will become more important to be *holistic* in maternity nursing care and not isolate the mother or infant from the rest of the family.

You must promote self-monitoring, self-care, and infant care and nurturing. It is no longer enough to get the mother through recovery; she must also be helped in her new role as nurturer of the infant. You must integrate multicultural family theory into care during the childbearing cycle and will have to find a personal balance between technical and educative-supportive care.

PUTTING THEORY INTO PRACTICE

Maternity nursing benefits from increased application of theory to practice. Nurses have a more consistent rationale for interventions. Nursing actions no longer come only from physicians' orders, although collaborative functions are often written on the order page.

A number of theoretical conceptual models are used to achieve a framework for nursing practice. "Conceptual models are ways of approaching a problem, a framework or context in which events may be viewed" (Fawcett, 1988). You will recognize these models throughout the text. Research findings also are clarifying ways of practice. For example, the work of Klaus and Kennell on bonding theory has been one of the important changes directing maternal-infant care in the last decade. In addition, use of the nursing process has become a standard of care.

PROFESSIONAL STANDARDS OF CARE

Many groups interested in maternal and child health have proposed standards of care. The American Nurses Association (ANA) has developed standards of care for nursing in each specialty area. The Association of Women's Health, Obstetric, and Neonatal Nurses (AWHONN), formerly the Nurses Association of American College of Obstetrics and Gynecology (NAA-

COG), has also detailed standards for each area. These standards are used when policies and procedures are formulated for an area of health care. Standards may be referred to as a guide for care, as well as a reference if a question of negligence arises. **Professional standards of care** are also changing, with greater demands on and accountability of the maternity nurse than ever before.

As care becomes more technologically sophisticated, nurses are required to continue updating their knowledge and skills. For example, it is unacceptable for a nurse who is hired to work with women during labor to say, "I couldn't provide the care she needed because I didn't know how to do it." If a nurse is assigned to work in a specialized area, the hospital must provide orientation, and the nurse must study how to manage care and insist on an apprentice orientation period in which she is supervised.

Nurses are *advocates for women,* often seeing that necessary referrals are done and that other personnel communicate clearly. Nurses may help smooth roadblocks in care services and ensure that treatments are fully understood while the patient's rights are respected.

PHYSICIANS, MIDWIVES, AND NURSES

In maternity care, a special emphasis must be placed on collaborative relationships between physicians, midwives, and nurses. In many settings collegial relationships have developed over the last decade. In other settings, nurses are still acting in "old ways," caught in a hierarchy that places the physician in sole authority for care. Hostility often marks relationships in these settings. As nursing theory is developed and nursing roles are clarified, there is hope that nurses will be assertive and professional in relationships with physicians and midwives so that quality care is made available to maternity clients.

LEGAL OBLIGATIONS

A nurse caring for mothers and infants has a special need to give safe and competent care. The legal obligations of care have assumed a greater importance than in earlier decades, since people are more knowledgeable and since there are two clients for whom suit may be brought. There are also many kinds of technology in use and options for care. Decisions may be made rapidly in changing situations. As a result, documentation has become increasingly important. The idea that it was not done if it was not written is the current belief in the courts. For example, the nurse who may be a primary nurse in the labor area may become involved in situations in which legal and ethical decisions will be made with little time to consider alternatives. This nurse must document actions and client responses as soon as possible.

Some important legal issues include assault and battery, emancipated minors, informed consent, negligence and malpractice, prenatal abuse, and the obligation to report child abuse (see Chapter 30).

Emancipated Minor

An emancipated minor is a person under legal age who is a parent, is in the military, lives away from home, or is self-supporting and thus has all the legal rights of an adult.

Informed Consent

To protect autonomy and to avoid duress, the client must freely give **informed consent** before any invasive treatment or procedure is performed. Each client has the right to refuse consent. She must receive a full explanation (in her primary language) of the benefits and risks to herself or the unborn child (fetus). She must be given, in language she understands, the alternative choices of treatment or nontreatment with the goals of care. Then she must sign a consent form. The consent should be obtained by the physician or nurse practitioner, and the conference and signature or merely the signature must be witnessed by another person (usually the nurse). If the signature alone is witnessed, a note to that effect should be added to the consent form. The nurse should provide time for the client to ask any questions that occur later and be aware that a client may change her mind.

Assault and Battery

To threaten to do harm to an individual is **assault**. **Battery** is to harm or touch a person without consent (except in an emergency).

It follows that any nursing procedure should be fully explained before the client is touched. Even though a formal consent is not required, to preserve a trusting nurse-client relationship, it is important to educate the client about the reasons for and results of care before initiating the procedure. Nurses must advocate for their clients, especially in clinic situations where the woman may be seen by a number of physicians and students. Remember, *touching someone without consent constitutes battery.*

Prenatal Abuse

Because it is more evident that prenatal care reduces the incidence of infant morbidity and mortality, **prenatal abuse** is becoming a legal issue. If the woman does not protect the fetus by maintaining her own health or seeking prenatal care or continues to abuse substances that may injure the fetus, she may be held liable for damages to the fetus. This is a controversial issue (Sise, 1988) discussed further in Chapter 30.

Obligation to Report Child Abuse

It is mandatory for health care professionals to report suspected child abuse. These professionals know about signs and symptoms of child abuse and therefore are responsible for informing the appropriate agency so the matter may be investigated. Failure to report may result in a fine or liability for damages. Permissive reporting is allowed for community persons who believe the child has been abused. These individuals are protected by legislation from suit when a good-faith report is given (Rhodes, 1987). Chapter 30 reviews sample cases for which legal aspects in the perinatal period must be considered.

Negligence and Malpractice

Negligence is failing to make sure a client understands a treatment or procedure, to inform the client fully regarding consequences of interventions, or to follow set protocols in a situation that could result in harm. **Malpractice** is the failure to do the reasonable or prudent practice expected by a professional in the specific situation or performing actions outside of one's area of competence that result in injury. *Negligence* may apply to any citizen. *Malpractice* is narrowed to the professional; it is professional negligent conduct. Such negligence may be further defined in the following way:

In a health care agency, a nurse has the duty to provide care for clients. This duty may be interpreted as malpractice when a *breach of duty* occurs by *omission*, for example, forgetting to check a monitor, give medication, instruct in home self-care, or failing to notify a physician of a change in client status. Or, the breach may occur by *commission*, for example, giving the wrong medication or identifying the baby incorrectly. In some way the breach of duty must *cause physical or mental injury* to the client. It must be shown that the commission or omission of an act by the nurse *resulted in physical injury or unnecessary pain and suffering.* A busy unit is not an excuse for failure to act correctly. Nurses must follow hospital policies and procedures, acting within their job descriptions and scope of practice as written in the state license.

 Self-Discovery

What do you think are the issues with prenatal abuse when it includes maternal exposure to smoking, alcohol, or drugs?

When there are legal or ethical issues presented by a case, staff members may consult the hospital risk-management team. No delay should occur before advice is sought from the risk manager. Chapter 30 details legal and ethical aspects of maternity care and discusses actual cases that have arisen in suits and in risk-management decisions.

Pregnant Patient's Bill of Rights

The Pregnant Patient's Bill of Rights develops some aspects of what is *the right thing to do* when a woman is receiving care during pregnancy, labor, birth, and recovery (see Appendix 1). This document does not have the force of a rule or regulation, but it can guide the nurse's thinking in upgrading care to be as "right" as possible in a setting.

EXPANDED CARE ROLES FOR NURSES

The roles of nursing in maternity care have been expanded, and further education may offer nurses the opportunity to participate in more independent practice. Several choices are available today. A nurse may become a clinician, such as a lactation consultant, through continuing education and concentration in an area that brings additional responsibility in the hospital. The nurse also may become certified in a specialty area, such as neonatal intensive care. In the same way, women's health practitioners offer a wider range of health care services than nurses with only a basic background. Today a number of programs offer specialization. Almost all clinical programs require a baccalaureate degree in nursing, as well as basic experience in the chosen specialty area, for a nurse to proceed to a master's degree or take a qualifying examination in a specialty.

A **nurse practitioner** is a professional licensed nurse who, with additional study, develops a specialization in maternity, neonatal, or perinatal nursing or in women's health care. This practitioner may manage care of well clients or stabilized ill clients.

A **clinical nurse specialist** is a professional licensed nurse who has completed a master's degree in a specialty area and will usually be in a role to upgrade nursing practice in client care areas.

 Clinical Decision

Note at least two situations during clinical rotation that might have become a basis for a legal suit. What was the nursing implication?

Certified Nurse-Midwife

A certified nurse-midwife (CNM) is a professional midwife who is certified according to the requirements of the National Certifying Board of the American College of Nurse-Midwives. This person is educated in nursing and midwifery. A nurse-midwife may also have a baccalaureate, master's, or doctoral degree in public health administration, nursing, or a health-related science.

International definition of *midwife*. A midwife is a person who, having been regularly admitted to a midwifery educational program fully recognized in the country in which it is located, has successfully completed the prescribed course of studies in midwifery and has the qualifications to be registered and legally licensed to practice midwifery.

Midwives must be able to give the necessary supervision, care, and advice to women during pregnancy, labor, and the postpartum period; to conduct deliveries on their own responsibility; and to care for the newborn and infant. This care includes preventive measures, detection of abnormal conditions in mother and child, procurement of medical assistance, and execution of emergency measures in the absence of medical help.

The midwife has an important task in counseling and education for clients and the family and community. The work should involve antenatal education and preparation for parenthood and extends to certain areas of gynecology, family planning, and child care (Richmond and Wise, 1986).

The CNM may practice in hospitals, clinics, health units, domiciliary wards, or any other service.

Since the 1930s, nurses have been entering nurse-midwifery. Before then, the majority of midwives had no nursing education. There is pressure on the College of Nurse-Midwives to admit lay-midwives into professional training programs. However, few states have practicing lay-midwives.

Lay-Midwife

Throughout the world, most births are attended by lay-midwives who have received some training or who, by experience, are accorded the responsibility of normal births. Several states in the United States do license lay-midwives. The Midwives Alliance of North America (MANA) is the group with which they are encouraged to affiliate.

Birth Attendant

The birth attendant is internationally recognized as a health care worker who fulfills a useful role in areas where health services are not sufficiently developed. In most countries, on-the-job orientation and working experience enable the birth attendant to assist women during childbirth and the immediate postpartum period, including newborn home care.

NURSING EDUCATION

The trend in nursing education has been to cut down to a few weeks the nursing student's experience in maternity care. Different rationales are used, none of which take into account that this area of health care touches more families than any other and contributes to the best potential for children's good beginnings. Maternal and infant care can seem simple at first glance. Dealing with healthy people, gaining rapport, teaching, guiding, and assessing take a certain level of nursing interaction. The nursing interventions that can be learned in this aspect of care are listed below. No matter what the later choice of specialization, every nurse should have a basic knowledge of the way a family functions during the childbirth cycle (Box 1-2).

What is the focus of maternity nursing? Nursing students have already studied sociology, psychology, human growth and development, and anatomy and physiology. Using this knowledge, you may best learn in this area of nursing the following functions:

1. Assessment of the impact of family structures on parenting
2. Preventive health teaching regarding risk factors in the environment
3. Teaching regarding child-spacing or infertility
4. Preventive health care during the childbearing cycle
5. Screening for risk factors for mother and infant
6. Assessment of levels of risk
7. Monitoring of pregnancy, labor, and recovery
8. Assessment of maternal adjustment to the pregnancy
9. Support of body systems if mother or baby is stressed or ill
10. Education about self-monitoring techniques during pregnancy, labor, and recovery
11. Assessment of newborn status and gestational age
12. Promotion of attachment and parent-infant bonding
13. Promotion of parents' "dependent self-care" of the infant
14. Education for support of positive nurturing

In addition, you should master the descriptions of normal anatomy and physiology for childbearing. This knowledge will benefit your understanding of *the way things work* during the childbearing cycle of a family's life.

BOX 1-2   Maternal-Infant Practice Competencies for Graduates of Nursing Programs

1. The graduate of a program in nursing will practice maternal-infant nursing based on theoretic and empiric knowledge of normal and selected abnormal patterns of biophysic and psychosocial growth and development of the pregnant woman, fetus, newborn, and family.
2. The graduate of a program in nursing uses the nursing process to assess, diagnose, implement, evaluate, and revise a safe plan of nursing care based on standards of practice to achieve mutually agreed on priorities and goals with the healthy childbearing family.
3. The graduate of a program in nursing assists families in understanding and coping with normal developmental and common situational crises during childbearing.
4. The graduate of a program in nursing promotes the maintenance and restoration of the reproductive health of individuals and families during the preconceptional and interconceptional phase and of individuals who decide not to bear or cannot bear children.
5. The graduate of a program in nursing is expected to maintain and upgrade his or her knowledge, develop proficiency in psychomotor skills, and reevaluate appropriateness of affective behaviors required for maternal-infant nursing practice.
6. The graduate of a program in nursing collaborates with nurses and others in using community resources to provide care to childbearing families.
7. The graduate of a program in nursing improves maternal-infant nursing practice through use of research findings and evaluation of current practice.

From Sherwen LN: MICC: The Maternal-Infant Core Competency Project, White Plains, NY, 1987, March of Dimes Birth Defects Foundation.

USE OF THE NURSING PROCESS

Implementation of the nursing process as a way of approaching nursing problems (health care problems for which a nurse can intervene) has developed rapidly in the last decade. The nursing process is derived from a scientific method and in its current form is similar to the methods used by other professional groups such as social workers. Although terminology may change slightly, the process has been integrated into the nursing approach. There is still some resistance to the "paperwork," but the nurse who can understand the usefulness of this method will be far ahead in the care of clients.

With this approach, the focus is on the concerns and problems of the client rather than on protocols and physicians' orders only. An example is a study that asked women after birth to identify their own health concerns. The results were quite different from the routine approach taken by nurses. If you focus on the client rather than on the routines, she will feel like she is being cared for as an individual and not just another client. As a result, her motivation to follow health care guidelines will be enhanced. In the nursing process, the client is a partner who agrees to the goals, which are detailed in the category known as *expected outcomes*.

Collaborative Approach

The beginning student may have difficulty determining the relationships among independent, interdependent, and dependent actions in the health care field. The nursing process allows you to determine independent nursing actions, actions you may initiate under the professional nursing license defined by the nurse practice act in each state. Generally, this definition includes diagnosing and treating human responses to health problems.

Much of hospital-based nursing practice includes *collaborative* or *interdependent* actions based on medical regimens and suggestions or orders from other disciplines (e.g., respiratory, dietary, or physical therapy departments) that may be involved in the client's care. Others have called this role "dependent," but that term is too restrictive because a great deal of input is required by the nurse, who coordinates care 24 hours of the day. When the problem is primarily medical, some have called it a "clinical problem" to distinguish it from nursing problems. The goals for these clinical problems are set primarily by the physician, and interventions are prescribed on the order sheet.

The nursing role increasingly includes management of care and coordinating efforts to provide holistic care. Such coordination must use the management principle of anticipating problems rather than reacting to them after they arise. These same principles are widely used in business management today.

Ideally, when collaborative problems occur, medical *and* nursing personnel should identify the goals of care because both are involved in analyzing, monitoring, recording, and evaluating the client's progress. When there is overlap, the situation is discussed under the heading of *clinical management*.

Assessment Phase: Data Collection

When you are assigned to a client with a potential health problem, you should do nothing until you collect data from a variety of sources. First, obtain the client's health history, statements about current signs and symptoms, and family situations affecting care needs. Next, perform a physical assessment to detect other problems and confirm subjective statements. The physician or midwife will order diagnostic tests to determine the medical problem. From these sources, the nurse identifies client care problems requiring nursing intervention.

Analysis Phase: Nursing Diagnosis

Problems that can be managed through nursing interventions are selected, categorized, and put in order of priority. Problems that need resolution by other health care professionals are referred to the appropriate departments. Your most difficult task will be to analyze the data and identify the nursing diagnostic statement that applies to the problem. It is important to understand the defining characteristics of the problem because some diagnoses appear to overlap.

A steady effort has been made to clarify diagnoses. Since 1973, the conference on classification of nursing diagnoses meets biannually to study and tighten classifications. This group is the North American Nursing Diagnosis Association (NANDA). This text uses the NANDA diagnostic listing released in 1992. In maternity care, problem-oriented nursing diagnoses do not always apply. Positive health behaviors, adequate coping, and knowledgeable clients do not fit the framework. It is therefore important to be aware of a new approach based on developmental tasks. Starn and Neiderhauser (1990) used Roy's adaptation model to undergird nursing diagnoses and planning. Other health-related diagnoses are in the process of development.

Each statement must be individualized by adding an etiologic component, or factors that influenced or precipitated the health problem. The second part of the diagnostic statement, "related to," are factors that can be affected by nursing activity. The diagnoses will not direct nursing care as intended if they contain causes that need medical, economic, or social services intervention. The statement should not be related to unchangeable factors. For example, "dysfunctional grieving related to death of the infant." The death is a fact; no one can intervene. Instead, this nursing diagnosis might be stated in several ways, depending on the situation of the client: "dysfunctional grieving related to unsupportive significant others in family, unrealistic expectations of self, or unresolved anger." You should not reword medical etiologies, nor be too vague in the etiologic statement of the nursing diagnosis. In this text there are suggestions for nursing diagnoses. Since every client presents different sets of data, these are only a guide for your planning.

The nurse should consider general categories of nursing diagnoses for problems during pregnancy and birth.

When a woman becomes pregnant, *ambivalence* is a major feeling during the first trimester. Depending on her delight in or anxiety about being pregnant, she will react to the discovery of potential problems in fairly consistent ways. For many women, bearing a child continues to be considered a way of expressing the feminine role. A women who does not feel successful because of losing the pregnancy or having complications may suffer from lowered self-esteem. Depending on her support system, her situation may confirm old feelings of insecurity and low self-worth. *Lowered self-esteem* is seen especially in teen pregnancies and in women who have suffered spouse abuse. It may be too complex to determine the source of the unsuccessful feelings; however, referral for additional help can be important for this person.

A degree of *fear and anxiety for self* and for the infant will always be present. In many cases, fear is well founded. Many women have read about their conditions and will have many questions. You may encourage the woman to express how she finds strength for difficult problems. If she desires, you can help her to find a chaplain or counselor to talk with further. Enlist the support of the extended family.

There is always a measure of *grieving*, even for the lost perfect child when a baby has a problem. There is usually intense grieving after intrauterine death, abortion, or neonatal defect or death. Chapter 29 suggests ways of interacting to support the grieving couple.

Family coping always will be tested by pregnancy. There is potential for growth in relationships or the possibility of distancing from the problem. Usually you see the woman only briefly during visits. You must never forget the larger context of the family. *Alteration in family coping* or *individual coping* may become one of the highest priorities in care. Referrals for support services, information, and empathetic conversation are an important part of nursing care.

Health-seeking behaviors will always need to be considered. Because self-monitoring is essential during pregnancy, information giving is a major nursing role in prenatal care. Absolutely basic to any cooperation in self-care is the understanding of what to do and why. Box 1-3 lists the major areas for which nurses plan care for women and infants.

Planning Phase: Expected Outcomes

Your statement must provide a focus for the goals of care, which are specified in the "expected outcomes" or evaluative criteria. Planning includes setting outcomes and listing summaries of interventions and precedes nursing actions. These objectives should be specific, individualized, and measurable and should list a specified amount of time for achievement. You should date and sign the plan and update, revise, reevaluate, and reanalyze it as necessary. In this text, there are suggested outcomes. Reword these and add when you are planning care.

BOX 1-3 Major Areas for Nursing Care Planning Before Birth

- Potential alteration in reproductive ability or function related to age extremes (maternal or paternal), history of genetic disease or more than two spontaneous abortions, or history of previously ill neonate
- Alteration in length of gestation related to preterm labor or pregnancy extending after term
- Alteration in fetal growth and development related to regulation of maternal and genetic factors
- Alteration in maternal metabolic processes related to regulation of diabetes mellitus or inborn errors of metabolism
- Alteration in maternal nutrition; less or more than body requirements
- Potential for transplacental infection related to protozoal infections, bacterial infection, or HIV and other viruses
- Alteration in maternal perfusion related to cardiac disease, chronic or pregnancy-induced hypertension, congenital or acquired anemia, or placental alterations (placenta previa or abruptio placentae)
- Potential for injury related to external environmental factors such as drug use or abuse, environmental toxins, or medications used during labor and delivery (anesthetics, analgesics, oxytocin, tocolytics)

- Positive adaptation to growth tasks of pregnancy and parenting
- Potential alteration in parenting or potential for ineffective coping (family or individual) related to client's response to drug abuse, poverty, single-parent household, history of child abuse or abusing parents, lack of maternal support systems, failed abortion, or marked age extremes (teenage or elderly primipara)
- Anticipatory grieving/possibly dysfunctional related to previous or current high-risk pregnancy
- Noncompliance related to psychosocial or financial factors
- Alteration in length of labor (extended or precipitous) related to primiparity, multiparity, or dystocia
- Potential for infection associated with birth related to early or premature rupture of membranes, repeated vaginal examinations, or ascending vaginal infections
- Alteration in fetal or newborn oxygenation/perfusion related to maternal hypotension or bleeding, alterations in fetoplacental circulation, or neonatal cardiorespiratory depression and resuscitation
- Potential for injury during birth related to operative delivery or fetopelvic disproportion

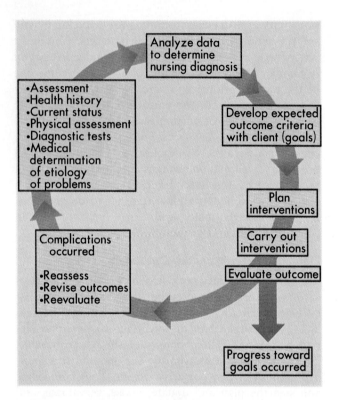

FIGURE 1-3 The circular nature of the nursing process.

Implementation Phase: Nursing Interventions

Implementation is nursing intervention. The information written on the care plan or Kardex should be formulated with the entire hospital stay of the client in mind. However, the client's condition usually changes, and these plans are updated, revised, or discontinued regularly as needed. If the nurse selects a nursing diagnosis with a formulated plan and does not intervene so that the client makes progress toward the expected outcomes, or if the client does not learn the needed self-care skills before discharge, it may be thought of as negligence by the nurse.

Nursing intervention should be related to the etiologic statement, and it is within your independent function to modify the environment to prevent hazards; to assist with activities of daily living (ADL), rest, sleep, and maintaining body functions; to guide and teach self-care and medication activities; to support, socialize with, and be an advocate for the client. These actions do not require direction from others.

In addition, nursing actions can also be collaborative, such as when you monitor progress, maintain supportive technologic equipment, carry out physicians' orders to medicate and perform treatments, or prepare the client for surgery.

Evaluation Phase

If the client has been involved with formulation of expected outcomes of care, you should be able to determine whether there has been progress toward resolution of the problem. Otherwise, you may only *hope* that the client understands and is motivated to perform self-care or keep medication intervals, for instance. It is important to validate hopes with proof. During discharge planning, special efforts must be made to ensure that the client understands self-care and infant care. If she shows that she does, documentation must reflect that fact. If she still has questions or difficulty, documentation should reflect that also. In Figure 1-3, you will see that the nursing process proceeds in sequence but in a continuous, circular manner.

In this text there are questions for evaluation. Ask questions related to the outcomes to be able to document an evaluation statement.

Evaluation of Maternal and Infant Care

The results of health care are reflected in morbidity and mortality statistics. These statistics are important in determining whether there has been progress in achieving the goals of health planning and care. Throughout this text, you will see statistics of risk. This will assist you by focusing on the frequency with which complications occur. You should be aware of the complications that carry the highest risk of morbidity and mortality and those that should be preventable with good prenatal care. This country, with its abundance of physicians and hospitals, should have much lower maternal and infant mortality and morbidity rates. Nurses must identify causes of and solutions for these problems and work toward change in the delivery of adequate care.

Although maternal mortality has been reduced, as seen in Table 1-1, the United States continues to have too high an infant mortality. This country now ranks seventeenth in relation to infant mortality statistics from other industrialized nations. A few years ago, the ranking was twelfth (Arnold, 1989). The major causes of infant mortality in the perinatal period are related to socioeconomic disadvantages affecting life-style, nutrition, and access to health care. In addition, premature birth contributes significantly to infant death and illness.

Prenatal care is the most important vehicle for providing needed services to pregnant women. It has been responsible for the significant decrease in maternal mortality seen over the last few decades. The decreased mortality also is related to the use of antibiotics and increased understanding of the processes of the maternal-fetal physiology and intervention when problems occur. The success of prenatal care is reflected in the statistics. The point in her pregnancy at which the mother seeks prenatal care is directly related to the amount of schooling she has had. Those with less schooling begin care much later (National Center for Health Statistics, 1992).

Even though the rates of death have dropped significantly in the last 50 years, black women and immigrants from Central and South America have 2.8 to 3 times the rate of death as white women (see Table 1-1 on p. 20). These statistics show a continuing discrepancy in the quality and availability of health care. Women in certain ethnic groups are more likely to seek care later in pregnancy or only when things go wrong. They may not even seek care at all, coming to the hospital or clinic during labor without having obtained previous care. Puerto Rican mothers are least likely to seek early care. Women with lower incomes who come from Central and South America are also less likely to seek early care. These women are less likely to seek care because of inability to pay, distance from care providers, and lack of money for transport or child care. Most women want care when it is available, low cost, "user-friendly," and perceived to be sympathetic (National Center for Health Statistics, 1992).

The way a woman is treated in the office or clinic setting influences her compliance, self-esteem, and preparations she will make for the birth. For example, one clinic makes a special effort to have appointments and to see each woman within 1 hour of her appointment. The social worker, nutritionist, and physician or midwife are in the same setting. In the same city, in another clinic, women come early to take numbers. They sit all day and are called at intervals to be weighed, to give a urine sample, and finally to see the midwife or physician. They are tired and hungry when they leave. The wasted time is not used to educate these women about prenatal and infant care.

There is national interest in preventing pregnancy complications and prematurity. The Surgeon General set goals for 1990 of a reduction in total infant mortality to below 9 in 1000, and a special emphasis reducing mortality for infants of poor families (see Table 1-2 on p. 22). This goal caused health care professionals to analyze deficiencies. Almost a decade later this statement by Richmond and Wise (1986) holds true:

We raise these issues because we are deeply distressed, both by these numbers and by the tone of our national debate regarding our commitment to the less advantaged in our society, and particularly to the children of the less advantaged in our society. We often hear the rationalization that we can no longer afford to assure a healthier beginning for these children. We often hear that we are entering a period of "scarce resources."

Our national budget approaches 1 trillion dollars, . . . 11% spent on health care. Resources are hardly scarce; they are merely competitive. Unfortunately, children are not competing very well for their just share of our national resources.

Let it be stated clearly that our inability to reach the Surgeon General's goals for better infant health is a reflection of our inaction and our lack of national commitment, not our lack of capability.

More than 15 years ago, the Carnegie report on the status of the nation's families suggested at least four ways that families could receive supportive help (Keniston and the Carnegie Council on Children, 1978):

1. Perhaps the simplest way is to encourage and provide better education for future parents, including the opportunity for adolescent parents to have experience with children, learning growth and development and methods of child care.
2. Day-care facilities need to encourage the participation of parents and other family members so they can continue to be primary care givers in the upbringing of their children.
3. A wider recognition by society of the important role of parenting must underlie any regulatory changes in institutions supporting the family. It is hoped that this recognition would bring more support to ease the child-care problems of working parents by allowing tax breaks, child allowances, and more flexible working hours. It would also allow a parent to stay at home to be a full-time parent if he or she chose to do so.
4. New family income and health care programs need to replace welfare payments. The stability of the poor family is in jeopardy, and such families may need dramatic supports to allow survival.

It is interesting and discouraging to consider progress since that report. In many ways, the poor family is worse off, but some advances in child care and flexible working hours have been made.

In August 1988, the National Commission to Prevent Infant Mortality repeated some of the following concerns from reports it issued during the 1970s:

1. Broaden private and public health insurance coverage for childbearing women and for infants.
2. Extend Medicaid coverage for infants and for pregnant women with incomes up to 200% of federal poverty levels.
3. Coordinate and fund public programs of family planning.
4. Simplify applicant procedures for Medicaid.
5. Increase providers of maternity care for low-income women.

 Self-Discovery

Note news reports regarding support services for women and children. Are there signs of political awareness for need for increased funding? Where in society do you see evidenced a concern for reducing risk of infant mortality?

6. Increase public awareness of the problems of morbidity and mortality.

This report was timely. Even now, Medicaid has been extended for pregnant women. Other services are available but access is there only if someone contacts the woman.

CAUSES OF PROBLEMS

Maternal Chronic Disease

For a few women, chronic disease has been recognized and treated before pregnancy. For example, the woman with preexisting diabetes will know that pregnancy places additional stress on her system and on the balance of glucose that has been achieved. She may be managing her condition skillfully, and yet her system may be thrown out of balance by the changes induced by pregnancy. However, because of her experience, she may need less care than the woman whose diabetes is first diagnosed during pregnancy. The new diabetic client will need a great deal of teaching and support to master self-monitoring (see Chapter 24).

Hypertension and cardiovascular disease are major health problems in this country. Depending on genetic inheritance, health status, and stress, a pregnant woman may already have chronic hypertension or cardiac dysfunction. Although more common in the older population, hypertension is also found in younger people. If a pregnant woman has a previously elevated diastolic BP, she can become increasingly hypertensive and may need hospitalization. Pregnancy-induced hypertension (PIH) occurs exclusively during the second part of pregnancy and may occur in those without a history of hypertension (see Chapter 22).

Cardiac dysfunction in young adults is usually a result of rheumatic fever, congenital defects, or hypertensive disease. Pregnancy places stress on the cardiovascular system and can increase cardiac problems in some women. However, today fewer cases of rheumatic fever are seen, and the incidence of cardiac disease during pregnancy has diminished.

Pregnancy-Related Problems

A high-risk pregnancy may be lost by spontaneous abortion before the fetus is viable. Approximately 20% of all pregnancies are lost in this way, many for reasons that are not traceable to any pathologic problem. Known maternal factors include poor nutrition, anemia, borderline fertility, and maternal chronic disease. In addition, about 30% of aborted conceptions are lost because of poor implantation or because of a malformed, poorly developing embryo.

After the age of viability, an abnormal outcome may result when a pregnancy ends in a stillbirth or neonatal death or results in a compromised infant with a less than optimal chance for a healthy life. The term *fetal wastage* is sometimes used for these outcomes.

Prenatal period. Problems related to the site of implantation or to the structure of the placenta make up a large group of the complications of pregnancy. The uterine structure normally accommodates itself to the growth and development of the infant, the amniotic fluid, and the placenta. If the placenta is poorly situated, early hemorrhage may result. If the placenta separates from the uterine wall, fetal hypoxia or death may result. Much of prenatal care involves assessment and diagnosis of potential problems with placental or fetal growth. Chapters 11 and 14 describe this means of evaluation.

Labor and birth. A few women have difficulty with the birth process either because of problems with the forces of labor or the mechanisms of labor. The nurse participates in monitoring and assessment and assists the physician or midwife during operative interventions. When caring for the woman needing assisted birth, be sure to identify her requirements for information and support. The experience may be frightening, and there is always a great deal of fear for the infant.

Recovery. Recovery problems may include hemorrhage, depression, and infection. Types of infection that alter maternal and fetal health are described in Chapter 25. Infection is a major focus of maternal care today. The prevalence of STDs and the ease with which the fetus may become infected have directed attention to the important issues of prevention. The importance of asepsis, universal precautions, and education will be evident to you as you care for these women and their infants.

The incidence of drug dependencies has also increased. Depending on geographic location or urban or rural settings, you may encounter women who use addictive drugs during pregnancy. Most nurses encounter women who smoke excessively or abuse alcohol. Because of the adverse effect of these substances on the fetus, every effort must be made to encourage the pregnant woman to avoid drug use during pregnancy. In some states a woman may be sued for child abuse if she continues intake of these adverse chemicals. When a newborn's test results are positive on a toxicology screen, the case will be referred to a child welfare agency, and the woman may not be able to care for her child until she receives treatment. Chapter 28 reviews care of these infants, and Chapter 26 describes the care of women at high risk because of social problems.

High-Risk Infant

Birth-associated problems. If an infant is born before its development is completed, immaturity in every body system will handicap normal growth. Immaturity and low birth weight are no longer considered the same thing; however, about two thirds of low-birth-weight infants are also born prematurely. One third of these small infants are fully developed but have poor fetal weight gain because of intrauterine stress or malnourishment. If all premature and low-birth-weight infants are included in a single group, they account for about 65% of all deaths in the first year of life.

The handicaps and long-term effects produced by intrauterine stress or malnourishment should not be underestimated. If the infant is subjected to a reduced nutritional or oxygen supply, optimal development is prevented.

The problems of preterm and postterm infants differ in degree and cause, but the same interventions are often used for both (see Chapter 28). The beginning practitioner will not do primary care in the NICU for these infants, yet should be able to recognize the signs of developing problems, the risk factors, and the ways of supporting body systems. The nurse in the NICU will need additional clinical education to function in a collaborative role in the care of these ill babies. However, the beginning practitioner who understands the signs of and the risk factors for neonatal problems can provide preventive care and support for parents.

Environmental chemicals. A number of teratogens may disturb body function or growth, and their effects on the development of the fetus have been identified. Chapter 27 identifies environmental agents that are toxic to sperm or ova before conception and those that alter structure, biochemistry, or growth of the fetus.

Many occupational health rules are circumvented in the workplace. Regulations must be enforced to prevent workplace pollution. In addition, environmental protection must be a major issue for health in the 1990s. Chemical effluents are entering the environment every day, and the list of offending chemicals is very long. Not only can there be an immediate effect from these chemicals, but also genetic defects may result from mutations and may be passed to the next generation. Nurses may be in the forefront of those who defend health by seeking changes in and compliance with environmental laws.

Genetic problems. Approximately 3% to 4% of birth defects are from traceable genetic causes. The study of genetics is rapidly developing, and many diseases of unknown etiology are now linked to a chromosomal or single gene defect (see Chapter 27).

VITAL STATISTICS

Copies of statistics from all birth certificates are sent to the National Center for Health Statistics. The birth worksheet is made out by the parents 1 or 2 days after birth and completed by a clerk and the physician. The

CONFIDENTIAL MEDICAL REPORT (Each question MUST be answered)

Only for scientific purposes approved by the Board of Health: not open to inspection or subject to subpoena

NAME OF CHILD ____________ BIRTH NO. ____________

	10. Race-White, Black, American Indian, Other *(specify)*	11. Ancestry (e.g. Afro-American, Chinese Cuban, German, Italian Puerto Rican etc.)	12. Education (Record highest Yr. completed) Elm/High School 0-12	College 1-4 5+	13. Occupation: Mother, most recent Father, usual	14. Kind of business or Industry	15. Employed During This Pregnancy
MOTHER	10a.	11a.	12a.		13a.	14a.	15a. 1 ☐ Yes 0 ☐ No
FATHER	10b.	11b.	12b.		13b.	14b.	

16. Previous Pregnancies (Complete all Sections)

Total Number of Previous Pregnancies	Born Alive		Spontaneous Terminations			Induced Terminations		
	Now Living	Now Dead	Under 13 Weeks	13 to 19 Weeks	20 Weeks or more	Under 13 Weeks	13 to 19 Weeks	20 Weeks or more
a. Number ___ None ☐	b. Number ___ None ☐	c. Number___ None ☐	d. Number ___ None ☐	e. Number ___ None ☐	f. Number ___ None ☐	g. Number ___ None ☐	h. Number ___ None ☐	i. Number ___ None ☐

17. Prior Terminations Type	Date Month Year
a. First Live Birth	
b. Last Live Birth	
c. Last Other Termination	

18. Date Last Normal Menses Began Mo. Day Year

19. Prenatal Care
a. Date First visit to any provider Month Day Year
b. Providers *(check all that apply)* 1 ☐ Hosp. 4 ☐ SHF 2 ☐ MIC 5 ☐ Pvt Phy 6 ☐ Other 3 ☐ Other Clinic
c. Total Number of visits to all providers ______ 0 ☐ NONE

20. Mother's Blood Group and Rh

21. Primary Financial Coverage this Birth
1. ☐ Medicaid
2. ☐ HMO
3. ☐ Other 3rd Party
4. ☐ Self

22. During this pregnancy, did Mother participate in:
1. ☐ WIC 4. ☐ AFDC
2. ☐ SNAP 5. ☐ Other
3. ☐ PCNP Specify ______
0 ☐ None

23. Check if Mother was
1 ☐ Private Physician's Patient
2 ☐ General Services Patient

24. Was Hospital of this Delivery a:
1 ☐ Prelabor Referral for High Risk
2 ☐ Emergency Transfer Prior to Delivery
Specify Transfer From ______
0 ☐ Neither

FIGURE 1-4 Worksheet for preparing the birth certificate.

TABLE 1-1 Maternal Death Rates*

MATERNAL MORTALITY TERMS

MATERNAL DEATH

Arises from any cause while pregnant or within 42 days of the end of pregnancy (even if abortion or ectopic pregnancy). For international comparisons, the World Health Organization (WHO) divides the postbirth period into two periods: 1 to 7 days and 8 to 42 days.

Direct maternal death

Results from obstetric complications or from interventions, omissions, or incorrect treatment during these days.

Indirect maternal death

Results from a previously existing disease or one that developed during pregnancy that was aggravated by the effects of pregnancy.

Nonmaternal death

Results from accidental or incidental causes unrelated to pregnancy or its management.

Maternal death rate

The number of all maternal deaths per 100,000 pregnancies that ended within the specific year.

Race	1950	1960	1970	1987	1990
All races	83.3	37.1	24.7	8.5	7.9
White	61.1	26.0	14.4	6.3	5.6
Nonwhite	221.6	97.9	55.9	17.6	16.5

Compiled from National Center for Health Statistics: Annual summaries of births, marriages, divorces, and deaths, United States Vital Statistics Reports.
*Per 100,000 live births.

copy sent to the Bureau of Health or the city registrar is recorded, and an official certificate is sent to the parents several weeks later.

Read the birth worksheet shown in Figure 1-4 noting the categories to be filled in by the parents. The certificate should give the full name of the infant and the father's surname as last name if the couple is married. If the mother is single, the child receives her surname unless official *paternity papers* are attached to the form and submitted with the initial certificate. Changing names later may require an appearance in court.

Race needs interpretation. "White" includes most Hispanic people such as Mexican, Mexican-American, Cuban, and Puerto Rican. "Other" includes all who are not grouped into the white or black categories, such as Asians, Native Americans, Eskimos, and Asian Indians. The country or ethnic group of parental origin (for example, Korean, Japanese, German, and Italian) should

be listed. Since 1989 the baby has been assigned the race of the mother. Because these worksheets were revised in 1989, more information will be available through this national data collection required for all birth certificates. The second part of the certificate is a confidential medical report not open to inspection or subpoena (Figure 21-1).

Maternal Mortality and Morbidity

Statistics are collected from 10% of the hospitals throughout the United States, and statistical projections are made on the basis of data from these reporting hospitals. Table 1-1 gives definitions and rates of maternal death and lists statistics that indicate the adequacy of health care (see also Box 1-4). In recent years the morbidity and mortality rates for the major pregnancy problems of hemorrhage, hypertension, and infection have been reduced through more comprehensive health care. However, as can be seen by the numbers, health care is unevenly applied to women in this society.

Although fewer women die from infection, the number of cases of infection during pregnancy is increasing. The rate of spontaneous and elective abortion is relatively unchanged. The incidence of pregnancy in adolescents remains high (see Chapter 8), and the incidence of pregnancy in older women is increasing. A woman older than 35 is considered at higher risk because she may have concurrent chronic disease and lowered fertility.

A study of maternal mortality in the United States from 1979 to 1986 (Atrash et al., 1990) has shown that

BOX 1-4 Categories of Maternal Mortality

- Complications of pregnancy, childbirth, and the puerperium
- Ectopic pregnancy
- Toxemias of pregnancy and the puerperium, except abortion with toxemia
- Hemorrhage of pregnancy and childbirth
- Abortions
  Abortions induced for legal indications
  Abortions induced for other reasons
  Spontaneous abortions
  Other and unspecified abortions
- Sepsis of childbirth and the puerperium
- All other complications of pregnancy, childbirth, and the puerperium
- Delivery without mention of complication

Maternal deaths are those assigned to complications of pregnancy, childbirth, and the puerperium, category numbers 630-676 of the *Ninth Revision International Classification of Diseases*, 1975. Rates per 100,000 live births in specified group. Beginning in 1989, race for live births is tabulated according to race of the mother instead of the father.

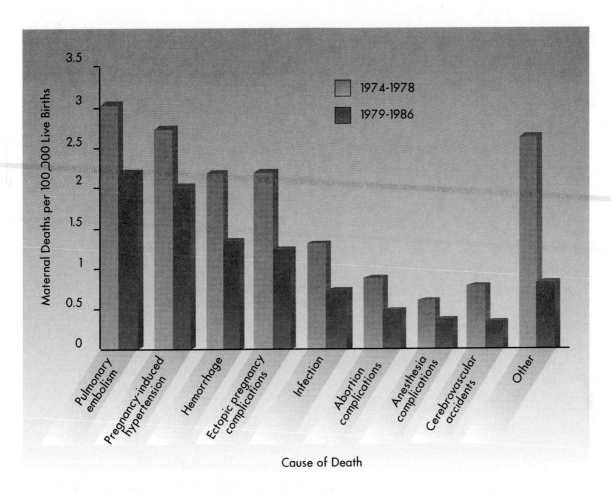

FIGURE 1-5 Causes of maternal deaths and cause-specific maternal mortality ratios, United States, 1974-1978 (Kaunitz et al.) and 1979-1986. (From Atrash HK et al.: Maternal mortality in the United States, 1979-1986, *Obstet Gynecol* 76(6):1055, 1990.)

maternal mortality may be underestimated if the traditional definitions are used. The study enlarged the definition to include deaths during or within 1 year after pregnancy if the deaths resulted from (1) complications of pregnancy, (2) a chain of events begun by the pregnancy, or (3) a chronic condition aggravated by pregnancy. When calculated this way, 11% of the deaths occurred after 42 days of birth. The leading cause of death was pulmonary embolism. See the comparison in Figure 1-5.

Infant Mortality and Morbidity

Mortality figures must account for deaths from the age of viability, gestational age 20 weeks (Figure 1-6). Few of the very tiny babies 20 to 28 weeks survive, but the potential is there. Therefore several terms are needed (Table 1-2). A baby that is more developed than 20 weeks or weighs 1 lb or more or is 16.5 cm crown-to-rump length who dies in utero is called an *intrauterine fetal death,* meaning one who is stillborn. A younger fetus is called an *abortion.* If there is no heartbeat or respiratory effort at birth, the infant is listed as a death

in utero and becomes part of the fetal and perinatal death rate. Of babies who survive birth, the neonatal period—from day 1 to 28—is crucial. Especially, premature infants or those with birth defects may die within these 28 days and are listed in the *neonatal mortality* statistics. The infant death rate includes all deaths of liveborn infants from birth through the first birthday. Box 1-5 lists the categories of causes of infant death. The tragedy of an infant or perinatal death is reflected in the potential life lost. Parental responses are discussed in Chapter 29.

Premature mortality. Premature mortality for the high-risk infant has been calculated by a formula that determines the **years of potential life lost (YPLL).** This calculation focuses on the problem of serious handicaps. Table 1-3 shows that deaths from congenital defects and from all the problems of prematurity rank fifth and sixth in the leading causes of premature mortality. Sudden infant death syndrome (SIDS), which occurs at an increased rate in those prematurely born and those affected by drug withdrawal, ranks seventh.

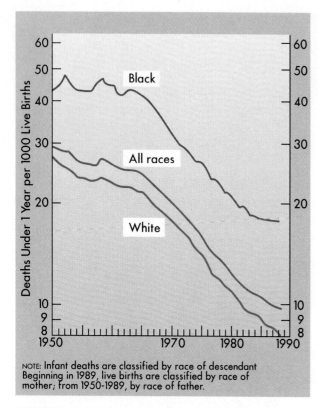

NOTE: Infant deaths are classified by race of descendant Beginning in 1989, live births are classified by race of mother; from 1950-1989, by race of father.

FIGURE 1-6 Infant mortality by race: United States, 1950-1989. (From Monthly Vital Statistics Report, National Center for Health Statistics.)

TABLE 1-2   Infant Death Rates*

INFANT DEATH RATE

The number of deaths in the first year of life, including the first 28 days.

Neonatal mortality

The number of deaths from birth through the first 28 days of life, regardless of prematurity.

Fetal mortality

The number of deaths of infants after the twentieth week of development but before the day of birth.

Perinatal mortality

A combination of fetal and neonatal mortality figures.

YEAR

RATE	1950	1960	1970	1988	1990
Infant death rate	29.2	26.0	19.8	9.9	9.0

Compiled from Morbidity and Mortality Weekly Reports, National Center for Health Statistics.
*Per 1000 live births.

BOX 1-5   Categories of Causes of Deaths of Infants under 1 Year of Age

- All causes
- Congenital anomalies
- Hyaline membrane disease/respiratory distress syndrome
- Asphyxia, anoxia, and other hypoxic conditions
- Immaturity, unqualified
- Complications of pregnancy
- Difficult labor, with and without birth injury
- Conditions of placenta and umbilical cord

TABLE 1-3   Estimated YPLL Before Age 65 and Cause-Specific Mortality (by Cause of Death): United States, 1985

CAUSE OF MORTALITY (NINTH REVISION ICD)	YPLL*
All causes (total)	11,844,475
Unintentional injuries† (E800-E949)	2,235,064
Malignant neoplasms (140-208)	1,813,245
Diseases of the heart (390-398, 402, 404-429)	1,600,265
Suicide, homicide (E950-E978)	1,241,688
Congenital anomalies (740-759)	694,715
Prematurity‡	444,931 (765,769)
SIDS (798)	313,386
Cerebrovascular disease (430-438)	253,044
Chronic liver diseases and cirrhosis (571)	235,629
Pneumonia and influenza (480-487)	168,949
AIDS	152,595
Chronic obstructive pulmonary diseases (490-496)	129,815
Diabetes mellitus (250)	128,229

Modified from CDC: Premature mortality due to congenital anomalies, *MMWR* 23(36):370, 1987.
*For details of calculation, see footnotes to Table V, *MMWR* 36:56, 1987.
†Equivalent to accidents and adverse effects.
‡Category derived from disorders relating to short gestation and respiratory distress syndrome.

Thus problems of infancy have a major impact on life expectancy.

Maternity and infant care continues to need nursing interventions. Along with changes in policies supporting health of mothers and infants, perhaps community education, parenting classes in school, and emphasis on prenatal care will all contribute to a reduction in morbidity and mortality for mothers and children.

KEY POINTS

- All maternity and family care focuses on the birth of a healthy infant. Pregnancy is a time to promote parenting skills.
- Each family is unique and brings varied cultural expectations to the perinatal period.
- Trends in care include putting high-risk women and infants into tertiary hospitals. Thus much of the day-to-day maternity care of smaller hospitals and birthing centers is for the normal healthy woman and infant.
- Increasing use of high-tech care has, however, raised the costs of care. Early discharge to reduce costs sometimes has been too early for complete assessment and interventions.
- Home care is increasingly important for women and newborn infants. This is an area for independent nursing practice.

- New hospital construction focuses on family-centered maternity facilities. Because obstetric care is financially rewarding, hospitals compete for consumer attention.
- FCMC has become widely accepted, and fathers, friends, siblings, and grandparents may have a part in supporting the woman.
- Physician, midwife, and nurse relationships must work toward being collegial rather than competitive.
- The nurse has legal obligations for care in the obstetric setting. Lawsuits are not unusual, and it is important to avoid nursing liability.
- Community and professional standards of care are considered when negligent actions are being questioned.
- Collaborative and independent care functions can be clear when using the nursing process to focus care planning.

STUDY QUESTIONS

1-1 Fill in the terms that best match the brief statements given below.
  a. Rates of death for mothers or infants._____
  b. A person under legal age living independently of her or his family._____
  c. The single most important factor in the successful outcome of a pregnancy._____
  d. The chief consideration about whether a lawsuit is possible._____
  e. Numbers of persons who fall ill because of conditions related to pregnancy._____
  f. Actions that a nurse may initiate under her professional license._____

1-2 Name four factors influencing a healthy pregnancy outcome.

  a. _____
  b. _____
  c. _____
  d. _____

1-3 Match the terms with their definitions.

  a. Death in utero before 20 weeks
  b. Rate includes fetal and neonatal death rate
  c. Death of a live-born infant
  d. Death of fetus at 32 weeks

  1. Fetal mortality
  2. Neonatal mortality
  3. Infant mortality
  4. Perinatal mortality
  5. Abortion

Answer Key

1-1 a. Mortality rate b. Emancipated minor c. Prenatal care d. Was there a breach of duty? e. Morbidity rate f. Independent functions 1-2 a. Consistent prenatal care b. Educational level of woman c. Improved standards of care d. Regionalization for high-risk care 1-3 a. 5 b. 4 c. 3 d. 1

REFERENCES

Arnold LS et al: Lessons from the past, *Matern Child Nurs J* 14(2):79, 1989.

Atrash HK et al: Maternal Mortality in the United States, 1979-1986, *Obstet/Gynecol* 76(6):1055, 1990.

Fawcett J: Conceptual models and theory development, *J Obstet Gynecol Neonatal Nurs* 15(6):400, 1988.

Halloran E, Halloran DC: Exploring the DR9/Nursing equations, *Am J Nurse* 85(10):1093, 1985.

Hughes D et al: *The health of America's children: maternal and child health data book,* Washington, DC, 1987, Children's Defense Fund.

Kenniston K, The Carnegie Council on Children: *All our children: the American family under pressure,* New York, 1978, Harcourt Brace Jovanovich.

Kaunitz AM, et al: Causes of maternal mortality in the United States, *Obstet Gynecol* 65:605, 1985.

Klaus M, Kennell J: *Parent-infant bonding,* ed 2, St. Louis, 1982, Mosby.

Lemmer CM: Early discharge: outcomes of primiparas and their infants, J Obstet Gynecol Neonatal Nurs 16(4):230, 1987.

Naisbett J: *Megatrends,* New York, 1982, Warner Books.

National Center for Health Statistics: Advance report of final natality statistic, 1989, June 1992, Monthly Vital Statistics Report.

Rhodes AM: The nurse's legal obligations for reporting child abuse, *Matern Child Nurs J* 12(5):313, 1987.

Rhodes AM: Maternal liability for fetal injury, *MCN Am J Matern Child Nurs* 15(1):41, 1990.

Richmond JB, Wise PH: Midwifery and medicine in America, *J Nurse Midwifery* 31(5):219, 1986.

Sise CB: Maternal rights versus fetal interests: an ethical issue with nursing implications, *J Prof Nurs* 4(4):262, 1988.

Smoyak SA, ed: Symposium on parenting, *Nurs Clin North Am* 12(3):4, 1977.

Starn J, Neiderhauser V: A MCN model for nursing diagnosis to focus intervention, *MCN Am J Matern Child Nurs* 15(3):180, 1990.

U.S. Institute of Medicine: *Prenatal care: reaching mothers, reaching infants,* Washington, DC, 1988, National Academy Press (edited by S Brown).

U.S. National Commission to Prevent Infant Mortality: *Death before life: the tragedy of infant mortality,* Washington, DC, 1988, The Commission.

Waxman H: Midwifery care: a political perspective, *J Nurse Midwifery* 31(5):224, 1986.

 STUDENT RESOURCE SHELF

Avant KC: Stressors on the childbearing family, *J Obstet Gynecol Neonatal Nurse* 3:179, 1988.
Identifies where stress points come in the childbearing cycle.

Halpern S: Government involvement in maternal and child health care, *J Nurse Midwifery* 32(1):33. 1987.
An annotated bibliography of basic information for the political novice confronted with various governmental agencies and programs.

Steven KA: Nursing diagnosis in wellness, *J Obstet Gynecol Neonatal Nurse* 17(5):329, 1988.
Emphasizes the well person and strengths instead of using diagnoses that are problem based.

Styles M: Challenges for nursing in this new decade, *MCN Am J Matern Child Nurs* 15(6):347, 1990.
From keynote address at MCN conference. Challenges a new style of nursing.

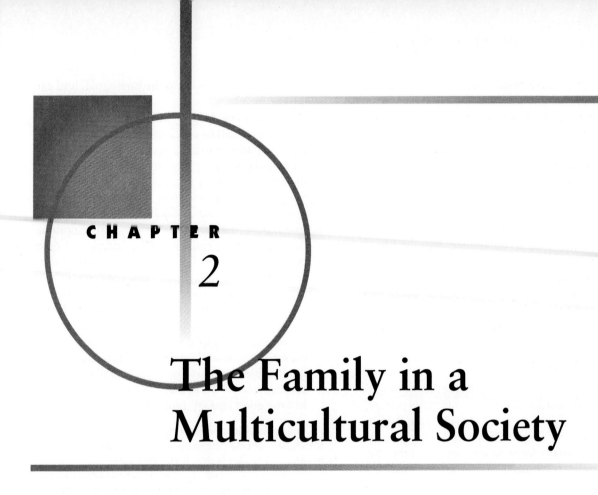

The Family in a Multicultural Society

KEY TERMS

Attachment Behavior
Blended Families
Boundary
Cohesiveness
Disengagement
Enmeshed Families
Ethnicity
Ethnocentrism
Family Genogram
Family System
Poverty Level
Reconstituted
  Families
Refueling

Remarried Family
Replenishment
Stage-Appropriate
  Task System
Transcultural Nursing

LEARNING OBJECTIVES

1. Describe the four major goals of the family.
2. State the six stages of the family, using Duvall's life-cycle descriptions.
3. Locate a specific family on a continuum regarding family developmental tasks.
4. Contrast ethnicity and family culture for specific families.
5. Describe examples of ethnic value orientations.
6. Describe the main stressors on the American family: distinguish among nuclear, single-parent, and blended families.
7. Specify stressors most prevalent in families with incomes below the poverty level.

"There is no such thing as a baby."

This startling statement, made by the pediatrician and psychoanalyst D. W. Winnicott, illustrates that when you find a baby, you find a mother. Although individuals, a mother and an infant are also a related pair located in and affected by a family. The mother comes from a biologic family, and the infant, too, has a biologic father, grandparents, and perhaps siblings.

The word *family* has a variety of meanings and applies to different groupings. Families can be defined by the nature of the bonds that tie their members together. A *biologic* family is defined by blood relationships, the relationships of parent to child and sibling to sibling. The biologic family is the fundamental, historical way in which people view a family. The **legal family** is defined by the civil or religious bonds of marriage and adoption. The **functional family** is distinguished by shared household living, responsibilities, and activities. The **ethical family** is determined by basic expectations of trust, reliability, loyalty, and long-term commitment.

Of course, all of these bonds overlap in the family. However, families are not uniform. Each is as unique as its individual members. How you interact and communicate and the values and attitudes you hold are influenced by your ethnic background and social class, by the cultural environment in which you live, and by your parents' child-rearing practices. Your individuality is shaped by your family context; actions are governed by characteristics of the family. One family might find a specific behavior acceptable and normal, whereas another family might find it unfamiliar. Family life is therefore rich and varied.

Beginning with the abstract term *family*, generalizations that apply to all families can be made. From this point, you can understand the variations of the families with whom you will interact.

Family as a System

Another word for family is **system,** the totality of objects with their mutual interactions. The family is the primary and most powerful system to which you belong (McGoldrick, 1985). The family system is the place in which infants normally learn to interact with other humans. The family is changed by the arrival of a new member, and that member is imprinted by the family's history, structure, and style. This process of imprinting on and being imprinted by the family and carrying the pattern for interaction into other areas of life is the "output" of a family system (Koman and Stechler, 1985).

GOALS AND PURPOSES

Terkelsen (1980) suggests that family members interact with intense **attachment behavior** (love, caring, affection, and loyalty). These interactions continue throughout the lifetime. Membership in the family, through birth, adoption, or marriage, is virtually permanent. The purposes of these interactions are physical survival and personal development for all members. You may assess a family's capacity to achieve these goals.

Personal development can occur only when there is security about physical survival. These goals are achieved when the family achieves the following objectives:

1. *Reproduction, recruitment, and release of family members.* Families give birth to or adopt children, rear them to maturity, and release them as self-sufficient adults to start families of their own. They also incorporate new members by marriage and establish policies by which other persons become family members.
2. *Physical maintenance.* The family meets the needs of each member for food, clothing, and shelter. These material resources are acquired and allocated by family members responsible for procuring income, managing the household, and caring for members.
3. *Socialization of children.* The family guides the individual's internalization of increasingly mature and acceptable patterns such as in controlling elimination, food intake, sexual drives, and aggression. Through the establishment of types and intensity of interactions, patterns of affection, and administration of sanctions, conformity to family norms is encouraged.
4. *Emotional maintenance.* Individual emotional development depends on the satisfaction of emotional needs. The family unit is committed to creating and sustaining the senses of being valued, cared about, and accepted, as well as the sense of permanence of affectional ties (Terkelsen, 1980). As members are rewarded for achievements, encouraged, and helped to overcome crises, a sense of satisfaction and purpose is provided. These family objectives distilled from Duvall's works are summarized by Terkelsen (1980) in his definition of "the good enough family":

A family is sufficient or good enough to the extent that it is matching specific elements of structure to specific needs. . . . The idea is this: If you give a living thing what it needs, it *grows itself up.* That is, *under conditions of need attainment,* growing up is something that the organism does for itself. The heart of the matter is that *need attainment* is the mainspring of development. And despite our complexity, we human beings share this property with the rest of the living world. The implication for our notion of sufficiency is simply this: the task of the family is to create a resource, in the form of interpersonal enactments, that matches or meets a need. When the family performs this task, each member "grows itself up."

You will deal with families that are not "good enough," families that cannot meet the needs of their members because of financial, physical, or emotional handicaps. Part of your responsibility will be to assess the sufficiency of families to carry out their purpose.

STAGES OF DEVELOPMENT

McGoldrick and Carter (1980) indicate that most people in our culture marry in their 20s and have children who start to school at age 6, throw the household into a turmoil in their teens, and move out as young adults and leave their parents to deal with each other, their own aging parents, retirement, and eventually death. This pattern suggests different stages in the family's history. By carefully examining these stages, you can learn the **stage-appropriate tasks** of the family system. In addition to understanding a model of the successful family, you will be able to identify the family's developmental stage. You will also be able to recognize how well the family accomplishes its tasks.

Each individual moves through stages of development: fetus, infant, toddler, child, adolescent, and adult. Each label denotes a stage of development. At each stage, different processes or tasks take place. Erikson (1950) outlined the maturational tasks of the individual in psychosocial terms. Growth means movement through stages of development; attainment of the ensuing stage depends on accomplishment of the tasks of the previous stage.

Duvall (1977) applied Erikson's stages of development of the individual to formulate a conceptual framework for viewing family life:

There is a predictability about family development that helps us to know what to expect of a given family at any given stage. Much as each individual who grows, develops, matures and ages, undergoes the same successive changes and readjustments from conception to senescence as every other individual, the life cycle of individual families follows a very universal sequence of family development.

The typical family's life cycle as described by Duvall is only a representative example. It does not fit every family. It applies mostly to the nuclear family, which consists of parents and their children residing together until the children achieve maturity or marry. It is less applicable to single-parent or blended families.

Table 2-1 describes a child-centered model of the family. The growth of the oldest child moves the family through the stages outlined by Duvall. Although this movement may be viewed as a limitation of the framework, it is actually one of its strengths because the family's purpose is promoting the physical, mental, emotional, and social development of each of its members. The stage of the family life cycle determines its development. Developmental tasks and growth responsibilities arise at certain stages and must be fulfilled for the family to move successfully to the next stage.

Beginning Families

In the first stage of the family life cycle, the couple establish themselves as a unit separate emotionally and financially from their families of origin. Traditionally the marriage ceremony is the rite that signals the beginning of a new family. Despite the way in which a couple validates their union, all couples must form a durable relationship capable of carrying out the tasks of the later stages. The couple's investment in their relationship is crucial. This beginning is connected to the couple's completion of tasks in their own families of origin: achieving a sufficient degree of solid personal identity and emotional independence. It is the successful completion of the *individuation-separation* process of growing up in the family that makes the successful founding of a new family possible. A marriage is not so much a beginning as a stage in a multigenerational process.

Childbearing Families

Whether the first stage is successfully negotiated or not, all couples face decisions about children: to have or not to have them, and how many to have and when to have them. From conception, the newcomer affects the relationship. The arrival of the child transforms a dyadic (two-person) system into a triadic (three-person) system, and the structure (patterns of interaction) changes profoundly. The previously childless couple must make space in their relationship for another person. The child deprives the new parents of privacy and time for each other. A triangle in which two members are close and the third is an outsider can develop. In young families the father may feel left out because the mother forms an intense alliance with "her" child. The outsider may become more involved in work and leave most of the responsibility for running the household and parenting to the mother. The challenging task of the childbearing family is to establish an interactional structure in which there is time and space for the needs of the couple as a couple, while the needs of the children are met.

Families with Young Children

A child's extremely rapid development from suckling infant requiring frequent feedings to toddler capable of crawling and climbing requires an almost constant process of readjustment on the part of the parents (Gluck, 1980). The constant readjustment to the changing needs of growing children over the years causes energy depletion and lack of privacy. Mahler (1975) speaks of "refueling" and Rhodes (1977) of "replenishment." Rhodes explains that parenting results in depletion of the ability to give and ultimately to self-absorption if replenishment is not available.

As the maternity nurse addressing the needs of the childbearing family, you should be sensitive to these tasks of system realignment and parental replenishment. You must be alert to problems that deprive the parent of replenishment. For example, the single parent lacking a spouse to meet her needs is particularly dependent on refueling sources outside the family.

Test Yourself

- Mary and Joe are 24 and are expecting their first child. They are in which stage of family development?

FAMILY PATTERNS

Repetitive patterns of interactions in the family, organized patterns in which the members interact, determine who, when, and to whom members relate. There can be

TABLE 2-1   Stages of the Family Life Cycle

FAMILY LIFE-CYCLE STAGE	EMOTIONAL PROCESS OF TRANSITION: KEY PRINCIPLES	SECOND-ORDER CHANGES IN FAMILY STATUS REQUIRED TO PROCEED DEVELOPMENTALLY
Leaving home: single young adults	Accepting emotional and financial responsibility for self	Differentiation of self in relation to family of origin Development of intimate peer relationships Establishment of self regarding work and financial independence
The joining of families through marriage: the new couple	Commitment to new system	Formation of marital system Realignment of relationships with extended families and friends to include spouse
Families with young children	Accepting new members into the system	Adjusting marital system to make space for child(ren) Joining in child rearing, financial, and household tasks Realignment of relationships with extended family to include parenting and grandparenting roles
Families with adolescents	Increasing flexibility of family boundaries to include children's independence and grandparents' frailties	Shifting of parent-child relationships to permit adolescent to move in and out of system Refocus on midlife marital and career issues Beginning shift toward joint caring for older generation
Launching children and moving on	Accepting a multitude of exits from and entries into the family system	Renegotiation of marital system as a dyad Development of adult-to-adult relationships between grown children and their parents Realignment of relationships to include in-laws and grandchildren Dealing with disabilities and death of parents (grandparents)
Families in later life	Accepting the shifting of generational roles	Maintaining own and/or couple functioning and interests in face of physiologic decline; exploration of new familial and social role options Support for a more central role of middle generation Making room in the system for the wisdom and experience of the elderly; supporting the older generation without overfunctioning for them Dealing with loss of spouse, siblings, and other peers and preparation for own death; life review and integration

From Carter EA, McGoldrick M: *The changing family life cycle: a framework for family therapy,* ed 2, New York, 1988, Gardner Press.

many patterns of interaction; the *pattern of communication* describes who says what to whom and in what way; the *pattern of power* describes who influences whom and how; the *pattern of role performance* describes who does what.

Knowledge of internal family dynamics may appear to be outside the scope of the nurse's responsibility. It is true that contact with the client does not allow a comprehensive view of the inner workings of her family. However, the individual is embedded in the family system and cannot truly be understood without attention to it. The family focus allows you to see that an individual's self-understanding, role expectations, value orientation, and motivation are not simply within her; they develop in interaction with the other members of her family system.

Boundaries

Boundaries refer to the invisible lines around individuals and groups that protect the separateness and autonomy of family members and define who participates and in what ways. The boundaries may be visible; for example, the closed door that separates the parents' bedroom from the children's room is a boundary between marital and sibling subgroups. Of course, a boundary may not be obvious. Parents may decide not to discuss certain matters in front of children. That decision becomes a family rule regulating information shared. It also identifies a boundary. Family rules that regulate information shared, the access members have to one another, and the activities in which members are permitted to participate create boundaries.

These boundaries are not fixed, like those dividing a map into political territories. Boundary-making in the family is a dynamic process that balances the comfort of members with their interaction with the outside. The purpose is to protect members from intrusive threats and to permit interchange. Thus boundaries should be flexible.

An individual's boundary preserves the right to be a separate person. However, this boundary must be flexible enough to promote interaction so the individual feels and is recognized as a family member. The person needs to be emotionally connected to other family members and able to give and receive support and affection.

Similarly, the boundary around a couple provides an area for the satisfaction of their needs without the intrusion of in-laws, children, and others. At the same time, this boundary must be flexible enough to permit contact between them and their children, their families of origin, and the external environment. The achievement of clear, firm, and flexible boundaries is a constant challenge as the family develops.

Disengagement. Minuchin (1974) characterizes the failures of adequate boundary-making as **disengagement.** When boundaries are overly rigid, they restrict contact between individuals, the family system, and outside systems. Rigid boundaries result in disengaged families, and members of these families are underresponsive to one another. The individual feels distant and isolated. The behavior of the individual seems to be of no concern to the others. In a disengaged family, distance may permit autonomy, but it may also minimize affection and deprive the individual of support. You may detect disengagement when parents display a surprising ignorance of important information about their children, for example. Or you may notice that a mother is tearful as she talks to you about her fears, but her husband sits beside her, seemingly unmoved by her distress. An absence of conflict and a lack of concern for one another's interests are signs of the disengaged family and may suggest that it may be difficult for you to connect with its members.

Enmeshed patterns. The opposite of rigid boundaries is diffuse boundaries. Whereas the rigid boundary is impermeable, the diffuse boundary is overly permeable. In the nuclear family with diffuse boundaries, the parents and siblings are overly close; individuals are dependent on one another. Minuchin (1974) calls these relationships **enmeshed.** Any action by one member triggers strong and immediate reactions from the others. In contrast to disengaged parents, enmeshed parents may spend too much time with their children and do things for them that the children could do for themselves. You can recognize the enmeshed family when its members interrupt each other, speak for each other, and argue with each other. You won't be able to finish your conversation with the mother-to-be without intrusions from other members, and you may find yourself included in a family argument.

Boundaries may vary according to cultural group. Disengagement may characterize families in certain cultural groups where the paternal authority is unquestioned. Conversely, in many groups diffuse boundaries are the norm. For example, the boundaries of a black family may function well as diffuse and more flexible. Aunts, uncles, and cousins may be involved in primary support of the mother. Kinship networks may not follow genograms of first-degree relatives as in other families. This is true also of extended families from cultures where many relatives may be involved in caring for the child. The nurse should ask who will be taking a direct care role for the newborn and providing a supporting role for the mother (Figure 2-1).

Tracing a Genogram

An understanding of family structure helps you to understand what happens when a child is born. The birth of a child calls for a radical restructuring of the family. The stages of this restructuring can be dia-

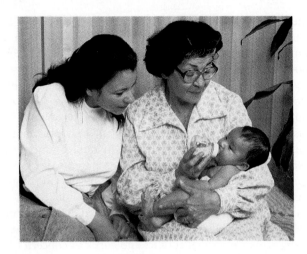

FIGURE 2-1 Family support system extends beyond parents.

 Self-Discovery

Are you able to follow your family line for more than three generations? Note your family origin to the third generation. Which cultural or ethnic patterns have entered the family? Which have remained strong influences?

gramed by the use of a **genogram** (Figures 2-2 and 2-3), a format for drawing at least a three-generation diagram of a family tree to record information about family members and relationships.

The establishment of a stable, affectionate relationship between parents and child is essential for healthy growth. However, to be effective parents, the parental couple must be a functioning marital couple. In addition to bonding to their child, they must bond to one another, meaning that they must establish firm, clear, and flexible boundaries between themselves and their child. As parents, they bear responsibility for nurturing and guiding their child, but as a couple, they must meet each other's needs. If overinvolvement as parents results in underinvolvement as spouses, either or both parents can feel isolated or unsupported.

As a nurse, you are a privileged participant during the first days of a couple's transition from childlessness to parenthood. This transition is not easily navigated, as Nichols (1984) reminds us:

All too often, husband and wife give up the space they need for supporting each other when the children are born. Husband and wife are sustained as a loving couple and enhanced as parents if they have time to be alone together—alone to talk, alone to go out to dinner occasionally, alone to fight, and alone to make love. Unhappily the demands of small children often make parents lose sight of their need to maintain a boundary.

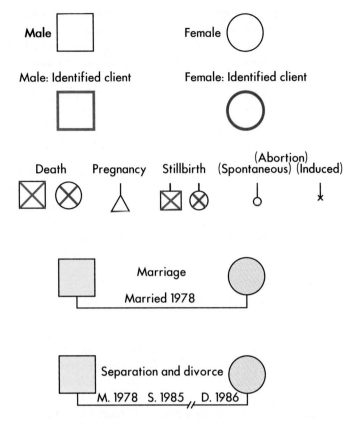

FIGURE 2-2 Genogram using the standardized symbols developed by McGoldrick.

Your understanding of the transformation of the family structure after the addition of a child will permit you to support the new parents.

CULTURE

Families do not exist in isolation. They are connected to the extended family and the families of origin (Figure 2-4). Bowen (1978) has calculated that each person is the product of 64 families of origin within six generations. In 10 generations, it is 1024 families of origin, and in 15 generations, it is 32,768. The new couple's understanding of what it means to be husband, wife, or parent is derived from their respective families. Their parents learned these understandings from their parents.

Every social or human system has a belief system, a set of beliefs, values, and rules regarding what is true and desirable. These beliefs create a sense of cohesiveness and belonging among members and thus promote the goals of the family system, and the development of individual members. Each family does not start from scratch to create its beliefs. Families do not exist in a vacuum. Each family is connected to other families by race, religion, or national or geographic origins that create a sense of commonality, which, transmitted over

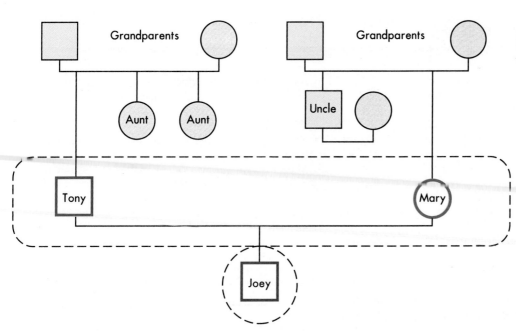

FIGURE 2-3 New genogram now includes Tony and Mary with new baby boy.

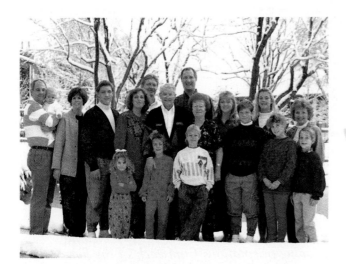

FIGURE 2-4 An extended family including grandparents, parents, and grandchildren.

generations, is called ethnicity. "Ethnicity patterns our thinking, feeling, and behavior in obvious and subtle ways. It plays a major role in determining what we eat, how we work, how we relax, how we celebrate holidays and rituals, and how we feel about life, death, and illness" (Giordano, McGoldrick, and Pearce, 1982). You must understand your client's family culture and beliefs about pregnancy, parenthood, infant care, and contraception to provide personal care.

Common ancestry, biologic descent from common ancestors, is intertwined with culture, the beliefs and values about the world and human existence, the language, foods, habits, skills, arts, architecture, and institutions of a people in a given period of time. **Ethnicity,** the particular social and cultural heritage shared by a group, is transmitted through time by the biologic descendants of people, by families. Inherited culture makes Jews Jewish, Italians Italian, and Africans African, for example, by providing a sense of identity.

In the United States, cultural groups from all over the world have coexisted for over 200 years. This coexistence has not been smooth and has not produced a "melting pot" of national homogeneity in which ethnic differences have disappeared. Rather, it has produced a "salad bowl" effect in which the uniqueness of cultural groups has been retained.

Although there is a mainstream of values that we can attribute to the middle class, not every ethnic group has been acculturated (that is, absorbed and transformed by the cultural mainstream). How affected a person may be by ethnic background may not be simple to determine. It depends on the length of time the family has lived in the country, the number of generations born after immigration, the number of intermarriages (cross-cultural marriages) that have occurred, the strength with which family tradition has maintained ethnic identity, and the degree that the family has chosen to assimilate into the larger society.

Ethnic Values

People live and are usually governed by *values*—rules that shape their attitudes, beliefs, and behaviors. Cultural groups generally have dominant ethnic value orientations that they share with other members of the group (Box 2-1). Such ethnic value orientations provide a starting point for becoming acquainted with the cultural views of other ethnic groups.

All human beings experience life on the basis of their particular cultural values and assumptions. Most of

Ethnocentrism — believing ones own ethnic culture is the only correct one

BOX 2-1 **Ethnic Value Orientations**

Time

- Attitudes about the temporal focus of human life
  Past: Values tradition
  Present: Values "now" with no sense of urgency
  Future: Values planning for the future and being on time and saving time and places importance on novelty and youth

Activity

- Attitudes about patterns of action in interpersonal relations
  Doing: Values personal accomplishments and emphasizes getting the job done
  Being: Values self-expression and spontaneous emotion
  Being-becoming: Values the development of different aspects of the person in a rounded, integrated fashion

Relational orientation

- Attitudes about relating in groups
  Individual: Values autonomy vs responsibility and emphasizes pursuit of self-interest
  Collateral: Values consensus and equal distribution of power

  Lineal: Values hierarchic organization, including authority from above and obedience from below

Man-nature orientation

- Attitudes about man's relationship to the natural (and/or supernatural) environment
  Mastery-over-Nature: Values man's power and technology to solve all problems
  Harmony-with-Nature: Values a balance between human actions and the forces and influences in the heavens and on earth
  Subjugation-to-Nature: Values human passivity and endurance in the face of uncontrollable forces

Basic nature of man

- Attitudes about the innate good or evil in human behavior
  Neutral-Mixed: Man is born neither good not evil but is a clean slate upon which parents, school, community, and nation leave their imprint
  Evil: Man is born evil but is perfectible and is thus in need of discipline, rules, and regulations
  Good: Man is born good but is corruptible and must thus avoid temptation

Modified from Spiegel J: An ecological model of ethnic families. In McGoldrick M, Pierce JK, Gordano J, eds: *Ethnicity and family therapy,* New York, 1982, The Guilford Press.

these assumptions are outside their awareness. You will also see clients through your own "cultural filter." If you have mainstream American values, you will expect the client to keep appointments punctually and to follow schedules for health care (Time: Future). You may pay more attention to what the client is doing to help herself rather than how she is (Activity: Doing). You will expect her to be confident of improvement (Man-Nature: Mastery-over-Nature) and will not expect her to connect her illness with guilt or shame (Man-Nature: Harmony-with-Nature). You may resent the "intrusiveness" of the client's family (Relational: Individual). In this case, you are judging the client by the standards of your cultural system and are guilty of **ethnocentrism,** believing that your cultural values are the "correct" ones. You must be aware of your client's values and recognize the differences from yours. You can do this if you become aware of your own values and develop a sensitivity to clients' values.

Nurses can be informed about ethnic patterns in several ways. Literature that describes ethnicity is available, but perhaps the best way to learn about ethnic beliefs is to learn from clients or from family members themselves. The maternity nurse must consider cultural

 Self-Discovery

Think about and select one of the ethnic value orientations from each of the five categories in Box 2-1 that best describes your family.

influences on the client, some of which are identified in Box 2-2.

In following chapters you will find cultural variations discussed in relation to practices during pregnancy, labor, and birth. Various patterns of family interaction will become evident to you. Stereotyping and assuming values and motivations to be true will interfere with your assessment and planning of nursing care. Therefore it is wise to learn to listen to the differences people have. Table 2-2 lists selected birth practices for different cultural groups.

Culture is not the only factor to be considered when assessing and understanding your client as a member of

BOX 2-2   Cultural Beliefs Relevant to Maternal Nursing Care

- *Fertility*: Man's virility demonstrated in having a child; woman blamed for infertility
- *Family planning*: Contraception contradicts desire for large families or religious tenets
- *Pregnancy*: Norms for activity and rest, sexual intercourse, social relations, emotional climate, touching
- *Labor and delivery*: The position assumed during delivery, the management of pain
- *Postpartal care*: Reestablishing body balances, restoring bodily purity
- *Food*: Food restrictions and preferences
- *Cause of disease*: Attribution of symptoms to social and interpersonal conflict or supernatural activity
- *Pain*: Denial or exaggeration of pain, fatalistic acceptance of pain as punishment
- *Treatment*: Reliance on folk practitioners (for example, spiritual advisors, lay midwives, herbalists)
- *Maleness and femaleness*: Attitudes and behaviors toward the sex of the child
- *Parenting*: Roles of mother and father; involvement of the extended family

a family system. Gender, social class, and economic status are also important. Choose additional reading from the Student Resource Shelf at the end of this chapter.

Nursing Responsibility for Culturally Aware Care

In the 1960s nursing educators began to recognize the need for including multicultural (or **transcultural**) concepts in the curricula of schools of nursing, and to determine what constitutes "culturally appropriate" care. This process was fostered by first gaining an understanding of factors that influence health and illness behaviors in various cultural groups (Tripp-Reimer, Brink, and Saunders, 1988). One framework for assessment of such factors (Giger and Davidhizar, 1991) focuses on six phenomena evidenced by all cultural groups: communication, space, social organization, time, environmental control, and biologic variations. Using this framework in client assessment helps clarify similarities and differences between ethnic groups and has been used as a unifying principle for the following discussion.

Providers need to give greater consideration to the interaction of culture with the health care environment, and how that influences client actions and behavior. Discomfort with providers in an antepartal clinic, for example, may cause women either not to accept services or to be noncompliant. The nurse should not dismiss cultural health beliefs or practices as unscientific or primitive without further evaluation. By defining whether such practices are *efficacious, neutral, dysfunctional,* or *uncertain* (Giger and Davidhizar, 1991), the nurse can support practices that promote health and discourage those that are harmful.

If a health practice is efficacious, it provides health benefits, even though the scientific reason may be nebulous. Home remedies such as spices, herbal teas or massage, or the use of prayer are examples of practices that may be efficacious, or they may be neutral—doing neither good nor harm.

SOUTHEAST ASIAN-AMERICANS

Communication

Perhaps nothing is more essential to the nurse-client interaction than effective communication. It is through both verbal and nonverbal communication that the client expresses her needs and desires to the nurse, and the nurse responds. Yet because communication is "culture bound," misunderstandings may arise when the nurse and client are from different cultures. The frank speech and direct gaze of the American nurse may be considered rude by an Asian client. Alternately, the nurse may perceive the passive attitude and averted gaze of the client as evidence for evasion and inability to confront problems (Sue, 1981).

When a Southeast Asian woman enters a maternity service, her unspoken goal may be to be a "good" patient and cause her to yield outwardly to the wishes of authority figures such as health providers. She may smile, nod, and answer "yes" to requests of care givers. But the smile may mask confusion, and the nod and affirmative answer may mean only that she hears, not that she understands or agrees (D'Avanzo, 1992). If English fluency is a problem, the use of translators or family members may help. Keep in mind, however, that the client may be reluctant to share intimate or confidential information in the presence of others. Because family elders often play a key role in decision making, the nurse also must be careful not to act in ways that may be interpreted as disrespectful to them, or the nurse-patient relationship will be jeopardized.

The cultural norm for Cambodian and Laotian women tends to be subservience to male authority, such as their husbands or eldest sons, but Vietnamese women are usually the prime movers in making health care decisions for their families. Subjects such as childbearing, sex, or contraception, however, may not be considered appropriate topics to discuss when men are present. It may be considered shameful to cry out during delivery in the presence of a male.

TABLE 2-2   Examples of Cultural Birth Practices

PREGNANCY/BIRTH	RECOVERY/NEWBORN
AFGHANISTAN	
Washes self and clothing immediately after birth.	Chant prayers for newborn. Husband is only visitor for 1 week.
CAMBODIA	
Childbirth is a "cold" condition. Mother must stay warm, covers even head with towel.	Woman refuses to bathe after delivery or drink iced drinks. Lying-in for 1 week. Might not hold baby right after delivery. No compliments about baby to avoid evil spirits.
DOMINICAN REPUBLIC	
Satisfy cravings during pregnancy.	Traditional women do not bathe, wash hair, or have intercourse for 40 days. Protect child from evil spirits by wearing red. May save umbilical cord.
EGYPT	
Western technology in labor. Desire high degree of pain relief. Express discomfort during labor.	Grandmother is significant other in labor and in child care. Seventh day celebration for infant.
ETHIOPIA	
Mother may turn away from newborn as symbol of rejection of pain caused by baby. Some women may have ritual circumcision.	Mother may be confined for 2 to 4 weeks. Colostrum wasted as not good for baby. Sugar water given until milk comes in.
GAMBIA	
Squatting position for birth. Father may cut umbilical cord.	Naming on eighth day with celebration, rituals. Breast-feeding only on second day, water for 24 hours.
HAITI	
Birth in squatting or semiseated position, supported by husband or close relative.	Placenta may be buried beneath doorway, or burned. Postpartum is a "hot" state; avoid "hot" foods.
INDIA	
Must satisfy cravings as these are fetal desires. Husband should not be present. Female relatives assist.	Family members care for infant for first 10 days. Mother rests. Naming rites only after 10 days or when astrologically beneficial. Boys valued more than girls, especially as firstborn.
IRAN	
Woman may shave body before birth. Husband is not present.	Baby must be protected against Evil Eye. Males circumcised at birth and up to 5 years. A naming ritual is done.
JAPAN	
Natural childbirth without anesthesia often preferred. Labor silently and eat during labor for strength.	Long recovery period, up to 3 months. Remain indoors. May not wash for a week. Children highly prized, number limited.
SOUTH KOREA	
Stoic response to labor pain. Father not allowed at birth.	Thanks offerings immediately after birth. Avoid cold, no iced drinks. Warm special postpartum foods. Only sons' births celebrated.

TABLE 2-2   Examples of Cultural Birth Practices—cont'd

PREGNANCY/BIRTH	RECOVERY/NEWBORN
LAOS Husband may or may not be welcome at birth.	Compliments about baby considered bad luck. Baby is considered 1 year old at birth. Mother stays in home for 30 days, may sit near fire to "dry up womb."
ISRAEL Woman uses regular loud verbalization combined with deep slow breaths during labor. Husband not present until wife and baby washed and dressed.	Stays in home for 6 weeks, keeps warm, and eats warm foods. Avoids bathing, exercise. Some Orthodox Jews may wish to bury placenta, and Orthodox women keep hair covered during labor and birth.
PHILIPPINES During pregnancy wash often to have a clean baby. Avoid sexual intercourse during pregnancy. Western technology in use for deliveries.	Keeps warm and rests for 10 days, without bathing. Special bath at 2 weeks.
SWEDEN Any position to deliver, even underwater. Father/siblings may stay in unit overnight and witness the birth.	Up to 12 months of paid leave for newborn care. Wide range of choices for newborn care.
THAILAND Home birth with husband holding wife's head and shoulders between his knees.	Husband buries placenta. Many rituals during postpartum month. Mother keeps very warm during recovery.

From Geissler E: *Pocket guide to cultural assessment*, St Louis, 1994, Mosby.

Nurses often communicate through touch, yet an action such as stroking the hair of a laboring Southeast Asian woman may be distressing to her. The head is considered the most sacred and honorable part of the body, and should not be touched except by close intimates. The nurse's hands on the infant's head and the removal of vernix after delivery also may be interpreted adversely.

Space

The culture in which we live, and even our geographic locations within cultures, determine our views of personal space. One's "comfort zone" relative to personal space varies within cultures and from culture to culture (Haber et al, 1992). The loss of control over personal boundaries is frequently mentioned by Southeast Asian women as a negative aspect of U.S. maternity care. Vietnamese women often prefer a female friend to be present during delivery. Chinese-Vietnamese may prefer the mother-in-law. Laotian women may prefer the husband to be present. Hospital policies that allow "fathers only" in delivery rooms may therefore be distressing to some Southeast Asian groups.

Squatting also is common for delivery in Southeast Asia, and although it may be less traumatic for both mother and infant (Paciornik, 1990), it is often viewed as primitive by U.S. care givers and may not be allowed. Many women state that they feel embarrassed because of the loss of privacy and control over their personal space during the process of labor and delivery, but this may be particularly acute for the Southeast Asian woman. The nurse should maintain a sense of acceptance regarding her client's need for modesty, such as allowing her to tie a draw sheet around her in sarong-fashion during the laboring process. The presence of female midwives, if available, also will help mitigate some of this discomfort.

Social Organization

In all cultures, children learn social behavior such as basic beliefs and common ties from their parents and others with whom they have contact (Figure 2-5, A and B). These interactions have long-standing effects regarding their attitudes and beliefs about important life events or milestones such as the childbearing process. Individuals within cultures generally embrace to some degree the concept of ethnocentrism, which maintains that one's own culture is best (and often implies that others are inferior). Variations occur within ethnic groups, but individuals within cultural groups share

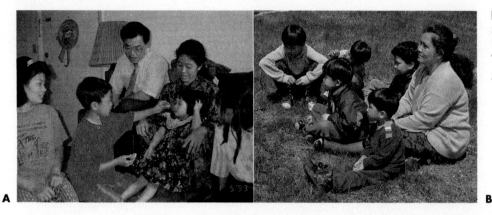

FIGURE 2-5 A and B, Southeast Asian families may be large and closely spaced. They are often a tightly knit group.

A

B

certain common traits, such as religious beliefs and food preferences. These necessarily affect health behaviors and relationships with care givers during the maternity cycle.

Religious beliefs such as Buddhism often influence how Southeast Asians react to life events and health practices. Pain or other suffering may be seen as punishment for transgressions in this or previous lives; thus help-seeking behaviors are considered inappropriate. Adherents to this teaching often appear stoic. They may smile and say they are okay even when they are experiencing postpartum pain, which makes assessment of nonverbal behavior even more important. The nurse should be aware that because of the small body size of many Asians, average medication doses for pain may be too large.

Especially prominent in Laotian hill tribe people, animism is rooted in the idea that gods, demons, and spirits control one's life. Help from a "shaman" may be sought to purge the person of maladies. Strings may be tied on the infant's wrists or ankles, or amulets may be worn to prevent "soul loss" and later illness. Removal of such items by health care professionals should be done with extreme caution, and thoroughly explained to the family.

Closely tied to religious beliefs, Chinese medical tradition rests on principles of universal balance and harmony between the equal and opposite forces of yin (hot) and yang (cold). Childbirth is seen as a critical time when women are in a "cold" state that may lead to future illness. To balance this state, Southeast Asian women may wish to eat "hot" foods in the postpartum period to "strengthen the blood": meats and soups with chili and black peppers, sweets, and wine steeped with herbs. Cold drinks such as ice water and juices may be avoided. Steamed rice is a dietary staple and is preferred with all meals.

Time

Cultural groups often differ in their perception of time, which influences their perceptions relative to past, present, or future orientations. The future orientation of most North Americans allows for greater apprecia-

tion of the benefits of preventive health care and the need to be on time for appointments. Most Southeast Asians, however, come from a system where health care is crisis oriented, with symptom relief in the present as the goal. In addition to herbal medicines from the Chinese tradition, many are used to taking facsimiles of Western drugs that are sold over the counter in Southeast Asia. On occasion this causes problems such as resistance to certain antibiotics. It is important, therefore, to determine whether herbal or other medicines are being taken during pregnancy in addition to any prescribed medications.

The present orientation of Southeast Asians also presents problems relative to our appointment system. Whatever is occurring at any given moment may take precedence over the future, including prenatal or postpartum appointments. Such time orientation, perfectly reasonable to the Southeast Asian, is usually annoying to the nurse, who believes the client is being irresponsible and "noncompliant."

Environmental Control

Most individuals prefer to maintain some control over their general surroundings or environment. Hospital settings, however, are notorious for making clients of all cultures feel they are in an alien environment where health care providers control their actions. The biomedical approach of most health care settings in the United States and Canada is often in conflict with traditional health care practices. For example, food preferences of Southeast Asian women after delivery would be considered *neutral*, provided the needs for optimal nutrition are met (Figure 2-6). Ritual disposal of the placenta by Laotian clients is another neutral practice. However, some Southeast Asian women believe they should discard colostrum as "old" milk and feed the baby rice paste or boiled sugar water for several days after delivery. This practice would constitute a *dysfunctional* traditional practice because of the benefits of colostrum in bolstering newborn immunity. The taking of potentially harmful herbs or over-the-counter medicines also constitutes a dysfunctional traditional practice. Nurses

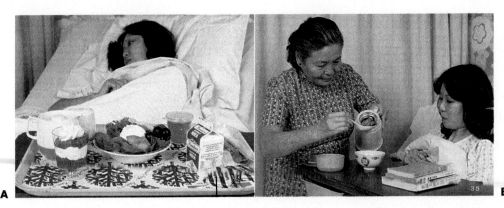

FIGURE 2-6 A, The first postpartum meal is refused by some Asian women because special foods are considered essential for recovery (**B**). (Courtesy Concept Media, Irvine, Calif.)

should seek to accept and support traditional health practices that are *neutral* or *efficacious,* while discouraging those that are dysfunctional or *uncertain.*

Biologic Variations

Most nurses are educated to standardized norms that do not include cultural variations among racial groups. Therefore significant deviations from the norm may be seen as unusual, even though they are within the norms of that cultural group. Often, such deviations are simply differences that can be attributed to being nonwhite (Overfield, 1977).

As a group Asians are generally shorter in stature and weigh less at birth than their American counterparts. Infants also differ in appearance by the epicanthic folds of the eyelids; smaller, flatter noses; larger teeth; and skin color. Mongolian spots—bluish spots that resemble bruises in the lumbosacral region—appear in about 80% of Asians (Jacob and Walton, 1976) (see Chapter 18). It is also rare to find an Rh-negative blood type in Asians.

They also may metabolize drugs differently. If a cesarean birth is required, care givers should be aware that analgesics and muscle relaxants may produce different reactions in Asians. The muscle relaxant succinylcholine, for example, may cause prolonged muscle paralysis in an Asian client (Giger and Davidhizar, 1991). It is apparent that knowledge of biologic variations among cultural groups is an essential and integral part of the process of client assessment.

AFRICAN-AMERICANS

Communication

Variations in the way standard English is spoken become evident as one travels across the United States. In African-Americans, many of these variations in grammar, syntax, and pronunciation have been traced to several West African languages and are called black English. Anglo nurses may have difficulty understanding words or phrases or may perceive these cultural variations as inferior or uneducated speech, which

serves only to decrease communication and widen the gap between provider and client.

The importance of effective nurse-client communication in improving the health of African-American women and their children cannot be overestimated. The Anglo nurse must get beyond any limitations of language that may occur, and convey a willingness to communicate.

As is true with clients who speak languages other than English, clarification of meanings of words or phrases is essential. Familiarity with health-related terms that may be used by African-Americans, such as those given by Stokes (1977) ("miseries" for pain, for example), helps nurses substitute more understandable phrases. As is true for Asian clients, nonverbal behaviors such as smiling or nodding may not indicate agreement, or that the client is attendant to what the nurse is saying (Sue, 1981).

Space

African-Americans, not unlike other ethnic groups such as Central Americans, may have a greater tolerance for physical closeness (Sue, 1981). What may seem to the nurse like too many people and too much confusion in the room may be perfectly comfortable for an African-American. If the nurse's discomfort shows, the client may misinterpret the source of the nurse's discomfort to mean she is uncomfortable with African-Americans, especially if the client has had prior experiences with health providers that made her feel inferior.

The African-American woman may prefer a female attendant during childbirth. She may request that a sister or her mother pray with her. She may feel that contact with air or wind is undesirable and wish windows and doors closed after delivery. As is true with all ethnic groups, there may be individual preferences within groups.

Lack of prenatal care is known to have an adverse effect on pregnancy outcomes. African-American women, poor women, and adolescents are most likely to receive inadequate care in the United States, with at least 15% of pregnant African-American women between the ages of 15 and 19 either initiating care in the third trimester, or receiving no care at all (Scholl et al, 1987). In contrast to white Americans, African-American infants are twice as likely to die during the first month of life. This is believed to be related to the high incidence of low-birth-weight infants (<2500 g) and increased prematurity in neonates. Researchers are attempting to determine to what extent untreated hypertension, more common in African-Americans, may contribute to this increased neonatal mortality (Geronimus, Andersen, and Bound, 1990).

The high incidence of single female–headed African-American families, accompanied by a lack of educational opportunities and low income, has been documented (Wilson, 1987). It is reported that almost 60% of African-American families are matriarchal—headed by females—compared with 23% of Hispanic and 14% of white households (Covell and Turngull, 1982).

When the African-American woman enters the maternal-child unit at the hospital, she may be the prime decision maker with regard to her health, or she may look to the family matriarch for advice (Figure 2-7). She is often a strong survivor of multiple social problems, and the "glue" that binds and strengthens her family. Like women in other ethnic groups, African-American women may feel it is unlucky to name an unborn baby, or furnish a nursery, until after the birth.

Social Organization

The description of the United States as a "melting pot" is recognized as out-of-date. The United States today more closely resembles a "salad bowl," where cultures intermingle and assimilate but retain their own cultural characteristics. As an ongoing consequence of segregation, many African-Americans have not been fully assimilated into mainstream America, and their life-styles

often are unequal in addition to being separate (Cherry and Giger, 1991).

The morals, beliefs, and attitudes of African-American culture were shaped by the destructive process of slavery that virtually obliterated family security and structure. Many traits shared within the group, however, such as food preferences and religion, serve to strengthen cultural ties and bring self-esteem and a sense of community. Most cultures have "food taboos" during pregnancy, often learned from mothers or other female family members. In the southern United States, African-Americans have reported that they believe they should avoid fresh fruits, vegetables, and acid foods during pregnancy (Kay, 1982). The incidence of pica, where substances such as clay or laundry starch are eaten, has been reported (Kay, 1982) and may be greater in African-American women than in white women.

Religion is very important in the lives of many African-Americans. Over the years it has been a source of hope and exuberant expression. Churches within black communities also serve an important social function, as the advice of the minister is sought for both social and health-related situations. Health professionals may find it helpful to enlist the support of the minister to bridge gaps between themselves and clients (Cherry and Giger, 1991).

Time

Because the majority of health professionals in the United States are from the Anglo culture, their perception of time is *future-oriented*. Many African-Americans also share this perception of the importance of time, and being on time. They may, however, hold the view that time is more flexible, and that lateness of up to an hour is acceptable (Cherry and Giger, 1991). Time also may not be valued as a function of poverty, discouragement, and the belief that things won't change for the better regardless of one's actions.

Present happenings may be more important than future events to African-Americans. This present time orientation may negate the need to be on time for appointments, take medicines on time, or practice preventive health care. Health care may become crisis-oriented (Sue, 1981). An example of how *present orientation*, expressed as a lack of concern for illness prevention, may correlate with poor pregnancy outcome in African-American women was given by Burks (1992). The most common reason given for late prenatal care in her study was lack of awareness of the pregnancy. The second most common response was denial or ambivalence. The greatest influence on their seeking services was illness or undesirable physical symptoms, i.e., crisis care. It is clear that health care providers must be flexible regarding time when clients are present oriented, yet convey the importance of seeking prenatal care before problems arise.

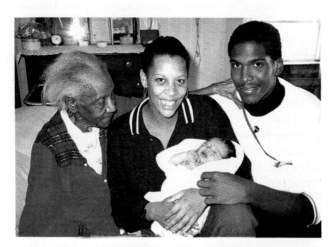

FIGURE 2-7 The extended family is important in an African-American family. Here the new infant is brought to greet great great-grandmother. (Courtesy Camille Bodden.)

Lack of future orientation is common among most teenagers. Nationally, however, unmarried black teenagers are five times more likely to give birth than white teens, and they may receive no prenatal care at all (Randolph and Gesche, 1986). There also may be other time-related impediments to care, such as the distance to the provider and the difficulties inherent in getting there. Because of rising malpractice costs, rural obstetric services are harder to obtain (Bushy, 1990). McClanahan (1992) suggests that home health care nurses could provide much-needed antenatal services to this population.

It is common for individuals in all cultures to practice some degree of self-treatment such as the use of aspirin, vitamins, or heat before seeking the aid of practitioners. When assessing African-American clients it is important to determine what specific remedies have been used, for how long, and how successful they have been in alleviating symptoms without putting value judgments on such practices.

Biologic Variations

Experienced nursery nurses say that African-American infants seem to have better muscle tone and neurologic reflexes than white children, and this has been reported (Falkner and Tanner, 1978). Compared with white infants, African-American infants at birth weigh about 240 g less, have head circumferences 0.7 cm smaller, and are 2 cm shorter in length. This seems to be true only after the thirty-fifth week of pregnancy, when gestational growth slows for African-American infants (Cherry and Giger, 1991).

Skin pigmentation is determined by the amount of melanin in the skin. *Mongolian spots*, melanocytes deep within the skin layers, are commonly found in African-American infants. These are dark blue and are frequently seen in the lumbosacral region. They also may be present in other areas and may appear to be bruises.

Because lactose intolerance is present in a large percentage of African-Americans, cow's milk formula may not be tolerated (see Chapter 27).

Some of the most difficult health and social problems confronting African-Americans today relate to substance abuse. Cocaine use has been cited as the cause of 10% of the cases of low birth weight in African-American newborns in certain communities. It is known that cocaine use is associated with increased risk of abruptio placentae (Chasnoff et al, 1985), intrauterine growth retardation, and preterm delivery. AIDS is the leading cause of death for African-American women between the ages of 14 and 44 in New York state and New Jersey. African-American and Hispanic women constitute 17% of the female population in the United States, but represent 73% of the women with AIDS (CDC, 1992). Given the woman's role within the

African-American family unit, these figures are nothing short of catastrophic.

MEXICAN-AMERICANS
Communication

As a result of high fertility rates and increased immigration, the Mexican-American (alternatively Mexicano or Chicano) population in the United States is steadily increasing. About 63% of the Hispanic population in the United States originates from Mexico (U.S. Bureau of the Census, 1990). They are a heterogeneous group socioeconomically, ranging from acculturated second- or third-generation individuals to illegal immigrants in search of better economic conditions. Many live in the Southwestern United States and travel freely back and forth across the border, thereby retaining more of their language and cultural customs than some other Hispanic groups. Most Mexican-Americans are employed in farm work or other low-paying jobs where there is little opportunity to learn English. Although Spanish is the dominant language, they may speak one of over 50 dialects (Monrroy, 1983), or may blend Spanish and English in a way that is incomprehensible to speakers of either language.

When communicating with health care providers, children are frequently relied on to complete paperwork and to translate. Communications are guided by cultural concepts. "Platica" mandates a low-keyed approach to conversation, whereas "simpatia" encourages respectful outward agreement that may mask either a lack of understanding or agreement. Small talk by the provider before interviewing is considered to be polite and necessary to acquiring desired information, whereas direct confrontation may be perceived as deliberately rude. Joking and use of idioms or colloquialisms by providers may be interpreted as disrespectful or prejudicial (Murillo, 1978).

Large families are valued, and fertility rates of Mexican-American women are markedly higher than other Hispanic groups such as Puerto Ricans and Cubans. They have the lowest rates of early sexual activity, but the highest rates of teen births, since they use contraception to prevent pregnancy less often, and infrequently have abortions if pregnancy results (Aneshensul, 1990).

Publicly supported health services are available to persons without citizenship in the United States provided that proof of identification such as income, residence, or number of dependents can be provided. Undocumented aliens without the legal right to be in the United States are therefore ineligible for public assistance such as Medicaid or Medicare. Illegal Mexican immigrant women who are pregnant frequently avoid medical facilities, which might reveal their illegal status to the authorities. A 1985 U.S. Department of Health and Human Services survey reported that 32% of persons of Hispanic origin are not covered either by private or public health insurance, compared to 12% of Anglo-Americans and 22% of African-Americans (Urrutia-Rojas and Aday, 1991).

In contrast, the prevalence of premature births is relatively higher (Mendoza et al, 1991), and the miscarriage/stillborn rate for Mexican women who are farm workers is more than double that of other population groups (Guendelman, 1985). Despite the lack of prenatal care, and poverty, it has been observed that low birth weight (LBW) is infrequent in infants of Mexican-born women. Mexican-origin women born in the United States have higher incomes, educational status, and more health care access, yet their infants have a 60% higher risk for LBW than Mexican-born women. This phenomenon is attributed to an increase in smoking and drinking, and decreased weight gain during pregnancy in U.S.-born women.

The roles of Mexican-American women are changing as they interact with American women and encounter the multiple stressors of low education, poverty, and prejudice. Divorce rates are increasing, and the number of Hispanic female heads of households is about twice that of non-Hispanic households (U.S. Bureau of the Census, 1990). When a husband is present in the household, he is more likely to be dominant in health care decision making. Recognition of this factor by the nurse will help to ensure that prenatal appointments are kept, and that the family experiences greater satisfaction with the care received.

Space

Mexican-Americans usually enjoy physical closeness and are more comfortable with smaller interpersonal distances within their family and social groups than many Anglo-Americans. As is true of many new immigrants, it is common for several related families to live together; therefore the client is used to the presence of many people. Because giving birth is a joyous event for Mexican-Americans, the client may be overwhelmed by well-wishers. Nurses who are unaccustomed to this cultural pattern should exercise patience and understanding toward visitors while ensuring that the client also receives adequate care, including rest.

Modesty is highly valued in the Mexican-American culture, and exposure of intimate body parts and touching of genitalia during labor and delivery is frequently a source of intense embarrassment. This may be expressed by the woman as "feeling hot." Female nurses and physicians who avoid undue exposure of the client are usually well accepted, whereas treatment by males may be refused for modesty's sake. The client may be wearing a *muneco,* a cord that is placed under the

breasts with a knot over the umbilicus. Because this is believed to ensure a safe delivery, the nurse should not attempt to remove it.

There is generally a strong bond of affection between Mexican-American women and their female relatives, and the cultural norm is to have one or several present during childbirth (Griffith, 1982). The nurse should be aware that abnormalities, should they occur, may be ascribed to cosmic or environmental events. For example, if the mother witnesses a lunar eclipse the infant may be born with a cleft palate; exposure to mild earthquakes may cause miscarriage or premature birth; strong earthquakes may cause breech deliveries (Clark, 1970). "Susto," or loss of the spirit, may be suspected if there are newborn abnormalities. This is thought to be related to a fright during pregnancy. The spirit may be returned by sweeping the mother with herbs as she lies outstretched on the floor.

Mexican-Americans share some of the beliefs held by both Southeast Asians and African-Americans in relation to cold and wind. Cold is to be avoided after delivery. Because water and wind are considered "cold" regardless of the temperature, the Mexican-American mother may refuse to shower and insist that the doors and windows be kept closed. Violations of these principles are believed to cause diseases such as arthritis in old age. In addition, a period of quarantine, called "la cuarentina," which includes abstention from sexual relations, may be observed by the mother (Clark, 1970).

Social Organization

The processes of adaptation and integration into mainstream American life by Mexican-Americans depend primarily on whether their presence is sanctioned, and they are given the privileges of legal status (Salgado de Snyder, 1986). Families that have been in the United States for generations are part of the mainstream and enjoy levels of economic success similar to other Americans. Cultural identity remains strong, with many immigrants consistently helping to maintain their economically less fortunate relatives in Mexico. For undocumented immigrants, there is constant fear of arrest and deportation by authorities. In addition, they may be exploited at will by employers because they have no legal rights. Such immigrants, at risk for multiple stress-related physical and emotional problems, are the least likely to seek health services. Mexican-Americans underutilize health and social services (Guendelman, 1985), and are substantially less likely to begin prenatal care early. They frequently obtain late or no prenatal care at all. Some Mexican-Americans believe that pregnancy is a "hot" state, and that they should dissipate the heat by bathing and by not ingesting "hot" foods. Acid foods and fresh fruits and vegetables also may be avoided, and the prevalence of "pica" in the form of eating clay has been reported (see Chapter 10). Conversely, after birth they are considered to be in a "cold" state, so that "cold" foods such as dairy products and chicken, and bathing, may be avoided. The concept of "compadrazgo" or coparenthood helps to maintain and protect the child. Godparents are chosen who usually have greater socioeconomic status than the parents, and are agreeable to taking coresponsibility for the child's welfare (Kemper, 1982). This is considered both an honor and a responsibility, and the godparents and child usually maintain a close relationship throughout their lives.

Although family ties are generally strong, language and other educational skills propel Mexican-American children into the mainstream faster than the parents, often causing disruption of traditional roles and relationships. The integration of women into the work force has also necessitated changes in traditional gender roles. However, the tendency to solve problems within the family and to give mutual aid generally remains. Group needs are superior to individual needs, and the dishonor or shame of an individual affects the whole family. In some families, intense emotional attachment to the family (called familism), as well as to places and things, is believed to retard both individual and collective progress (Kulpers, 1991).

Time

Most Mexican-Americans who are second or third generation have the future-oriented perception of time that is common to most Americans. Studies of students, for example, indicate that time perceptions of Mexican-American students are similar to their Anglo-American counterparts, even though they maintain strong cultural ties to the Mexican community. These acculturated Mexican-Americans can be depended on to keep prenatal appointments, take medications appropriately, and to value prevention strategies that are likely to ensure good pregnancy outcomes. They usually have the resources to obtain prenatal and postpartum care, either through private or public means.

The Mexican-American who is a newer arrival may have a present time orientation more similar to Southeast Asian clients. Such an orientation gives little credence to future possibilities, and may cause families to spend years of savings on events such as weddings or religious festivals. This lack of future orientation, combined with a sense that they are controlled by external supernatural forces, often delays upward mobility and cultural integration (Kulpers, 1991). Because they perceive time as elastic, these Mexican-Americans may be late or not appear for scheduled prenatal or postpartum appointments unless they are not feeling well. They may not follow medication schedules, and may devalue activities that focus on long-term planning or prevention. Health teaching that emphasizes the present or short-term may be best accepted. Some Mexican-Americans cannot look beyond the day-to-day struggle to survive.

Environmental Control

The nurse should make every effort to provide cultural comfort when the Mexican-American client enters a health care setting. The client's beliefs and use of health practices that are culturally appropriate for her should be assessed, so that support can be given to those that appear to be efficacious or neutral and can be an adjunct to scientific health care. If the nurse does not reject these nonharmful cultural practices, the client is more likely to be receptive to health teaching relative to those practices that appear either dysfunctional or uncertain. Health is frequently seen as either good luck or as a reward from God for a sinless life.

Although some cultural practices, such as ensuring a good weight gain during pregnancy are efficacious, certain practices most often held by new immigrants, can be dangerous. A child with symptoms of crying, diarrhea, loss of weight, and high fever may be thought to be the victim of "mal ojo," the evil eye, caused by being looked at by a person with supernatural powers. Touching the infant is believed to prevent or help cure this condition. Eggs and water may be mixed and put under the infant's bed to drive out the evil influence, rather than seeking health care. Symptoms of severe dehydration, such as a depressed anterior fontanelle, may be ascribed to an imbalance between the fontanelle and hard palate. The mother may pull hairs, apply eggs to the infant's head, or hold it in a head-down position to attempt to alleviate the depression (Ruiz, 1985) (Figure 2-8). Mexican-American women are less likely to breast-feed than Anglo-American women, and if they do they stop earlier (Rassin et al, 1984). They generally believe that a fat baby is a healthy baby, and observe that formula-fed babies are fatter. They may opt not to breast-feed, feeling that this is best for their infant.

Before seeking health care, or concurrently, the client may consult one or more folk healers within her community. Family members pass down knowledge of treating illness just as mothers and grandmothers do in the Anglo-American culture. Self-medication is also common in Mexico. Alternatively, a "yerbero" who specializes in spices and herbs may be sought. For serious physical or emotional complaints, the client may seek help from a male *"curandero"* or female *"curandera"* whose gift of healing derives from both American Indian and Roman Catholic traditions, and who usually provides care in his or her home. This traditional practitioner may pray, give herbs, massage, counsel, or use white or black magic as part of the cure. Imbalances between the person and God, and hot and cold elements, are believed to contribute to illness (Ruiz, 1985). The

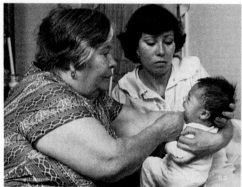
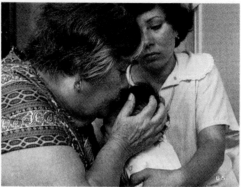

A

B

FIGURE 2-8 A and B, In some Mexican-American groups the grandmother has special rituals to perform for the new baby. (Courtesy Concept Media, Irvine, Calif.)

primary aim of treatment is to free the client of the sin that has made her sick, while restoring the balance of heat and cold. Inability to become pregnant is believed to be related to a "cold" womb and is treated with heat. A decrease in the mother's milk supply after birth is considered to be a result of "coldness," and heat, such as hot herbs, may be used to increase lactation. In some ethnic communities in the United States, curanderos/curanderas have successfully worked with health practitioners for the mutual benefit of the client.

Biologic Variations

Depending on their ethnic heritage, Mexican-Americans range from being pure Mongoloid (American Indian) to pure caucasian of Spanish descent (Salgado de Snyder, 1987) with corresponding darker to lighter skin coloring. Mongolian spots in infants are commonly found, often disappearing before school age. Mexican-Americans are at greatest risk for health problems related to communicable disease: diarrhea resulting from amebiasis or parasitosis, respiratory conditions, and skin disorders. Tuberculosis is common in Mexico and is frequently found in newly arrived immigrants and migrant workers. The leading cause of death for Mexican children is malnutrition. Gastrointestinal disease resulting from amebiasis/parasitosis and bacterial pneumonia rank second, followed by accidents and violence (Anthony-Tkach, 1981). When a Mexican-American woman seeks health care for her pregnancy, the nurse should ensure that an accurate and complete assessment, including laboratory work, is done for the woman and her family, particularly if she is a new arrival to the United States. Because of the high incidence of diabetes and hypertension, gestational diabetes mellitus (GDM) and pregnancy-induced hypertension (PIH) should be assessed for throughout the pregnancy.

Consumption of alcohol, especially for males, has become a serious health and social hazard (Arrendondo, 1987). Hispanics are also overrepresented in the number of AIDS cases in the U.S. population (Centers for Disease Control, 1992). Nurses should use both prenatal and postpartum contacts as an opportunity to educate clients

about this disease, and encourage behavioral change in persons at high risk.

Stresses on the Family System

Families do not exist by themselves; they exist in the real order, with other families and people. Our beliefs and laws spell out the way things should be, but we live and practice the way things are. For example, we say in general that marriage ought to be monogamous, that premarital sex and marital infidelity are taboo, that marriage should last until death, that children belong to parents, and that the state interferes with their socialization only under extreme circumstances, but reality is much different. The family is considered to be the economic unit for consumption, mutual property, and inheritance, and it is the residential unit until the child achieves majority. Our laws support these ideas about marriage and the family.

The actual behavior of many American families is often in direct conflict with these assumptions. The family reacts to tensions within and social stressors from without.

SOCIAL FACTORS

Contraception

The basic tension within marriage is between the desire to provide a stable family structure for rearing children and the desire to achieve a satisfying and meaningful relationship with the opposite sex. Effective contraception essentially separates reproduction and the sexual relationship. Hobbs (1970) suggests that the tension between the two aims of marriage—sexual relationship and child rearing—has changed because of an emphasis on romantic love as a basis for marriage. Mate selection on the basis of sexual compatibility may not coincide with mate selection on the basis of suitability for establishing and maintaining a family. Hobbs asks whether too much has been expected of the institution of marriage if men and women expect to find their only sexual relationship, their only partners-in-dialogue,

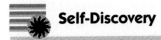

Self-Discovery

List benefits young couples receive if their families select the marriage partners.

their primary valuation and appreciation as persons, and the fulfillment of their romantic longings. Perhaps the family established by marriage has always suffered from this inner tension of romance vs reproduction, but, until the turn of the century, family behavior was more rigidly controlled by social mores, public opinion, and ecclesiastical and civil law. As the end of the twentieth century approaches, great changes in American society have removed much of the framework of external social control. The result is more and more families with alternative structures or life-styles that differ from the traditional idea. The nurse should also remember that in most societies of the world, mate selection is not primarily the choice of the two partners but is affected by extended family wishes.

Mobility

One of the most potent forces that changed the family was the shift from a primarily rural and agricultural society to an urban and industrial society. This relocation of work from farm to city disrupted extended family structures. Only the nuclear family tended to migrate, which left the extended family behind. The average American household consisted of five persons from 1890 to 1910 but shrank to four persons from 1920 to 1950; it has shrunk even further, to three persons (U.S. Bureau of the Census, 1988).

High residential mobility is still a mark of American society. Forty million Americans, 18% of the population, move every year. There is a debate about the extent of this separation from the extended family, and it is probably rare for a nuclear family to be completely isolated from the family network. However, although contact may be maintained and help obtained in extended crises, contacts are usually short and limited. Telephone calls and visits on holidays are no substitute for living in the same house or on the same street.

Therefore the parents become the sole child rearers in the geographically and socially isolated nuclear family. However, when the mother and the father become the only effective models that the children can emulate, other influences become value determiners, including schools, adolescent subculture, and the popular media. This turning away from parental values and expectations has been a source of intergenerational conflict in modern American families (Logan and Dawkins, 1986).

Marriage Rate

In the 1950s the estimated median age of women at first marriage was 20 years; one half of women marrying were less than 20. In 1984 the median age was 22.8 years. Thus women are now postponing marriage longer than their mothers did. The fact that more women are enrolled in higher education programs may partially explain the delay, reflecting the uncertainties faced by contemporary women. The possibility of remaining unmarried, being childless, or being divorced raises the need to be prepared for an income-producing occupation.

The 1,094,169 births to unmarried mothers in 1989 represented a 64% increase over those in 1980, reflecting the divorce trends and the change in cultural insistence on marriage before childbearing (MVSR, 1992).

Fertility Rate

Fertility rate varies by racial group. In 1989 the Hispanic population had a rate of 104.9 per 1000 women between 16 and 44, which was 60% higher than the rate of 65.7 per 1000 for non-Hispanic women between 16 and 44 years old (MVSR, 1992).

Today, a growing number of men and women are voluntarily sterilized after having their desired number of children. Therefore women are having fewer children and reaching the end of childbearing earlier than their mothers. This decrease in family size allows for planning the number and timing of births. In addition, having fewer children enables parents to better provide for the needs of the children they have.

Divorce Rate

The Census Bureau defines a family as two or more persons related to each other by blood, marriage, or adoption who live together. Divorce now accounts for more than 40% of single-parent families. Half of the states have adopted some form of no-fault divorce laws, which allow a couple to terminate their marriage without any expectations of punitive consequences after the negotiation of joint property settlements and arrangements for the maintenance of children and the spouse. The highest incidence of divorce occurs in families with preschool children and school-age children. Two thirds of women who divorce do so before age 30, and seven eighths of all women who divorce do so before middle age. Most children are under age 7 when their parents separate legally or divorce. As a result, many families are single-parent or remarried families.

CONSEQUENCES

Single-Parent

As previously discussed, the objectives of the family system are to establish an income, maintain a household, develop social relationships in the community, and teach children to become productive members of that community. The challenges of the family stage of development in the childbearing years are coping with energy depletion and lack of privacy. The danger of task overload can be great for the single mother with young children. When a mother divorces and seeks employment, the children experience a double loss—the loss of the father through divorce and the loss of the mother through employment. The divorced mother is often cut off emotionally from her ex-husband's extended family system. Divorced women tend to have fewer friends and belong to fewer organizations than married women. The social isolation experienced by these mothers tends to intensify the parent-child relationship. As a result these women frequently complain of being trapped in a world of children (Beal, 1980).

Although the percentage of single-parent families has doubled since 1970, it is usually a temporary arrangement for most families. Because four of every five divorced persons remarry, the single-parent family serves as a transition for the parent from one marital partner to another and between parenthood and stepparenthood.

Remarried Family

Remarried families, blended families, or reconstituted families are complex family systems that result from the remarriage of persons who have lost their first spouses through death or divorce. If these persons are already parents, the remarriage creates family relationships involving stepparents, stepchildren, stepsiblings, and stepgrandparents. If the spouses have children between them, there are also half-siblings. A child in a stepfamily can have two "mothers," three or four sets of grandparents, full siblings, half-siblings, and stepsiblings. In this case, it can be difficult to answer questions about family and the nature of family relationships.

The stepfamily is becoming more common. McGoldrick and Carter (1980) provide an important reminder to all who have to deal with stepfamilies:

> Unfortunately, the 'instant intimacy' that remarried families expect of themselves is impossible to achieve and the new relationships are all the harder to negotiate because they do not develop slowly, as intact families do, but must begin midstream, after another family's life cycle has been dislocated. Naturally, second families carry the scars of first families. Neither parents, nor children, nor grandparents can forget the relationships that went before. Children *never give up their attachment* to their first parent, no matter how negative the relationship with that parent was or is. Having the patience to tolerate the ambiguity of the situation and allowing each other the space and the time for feelings about past relationships is crucial to the process of forming a remarried family.

The challenge of forming a remarried family will increase in difficulty, depending on whether the spouses have no children from previous marriages (difficult), have grown children (more difficult), or have young or adolescent children who still require parenting (most difficult). Visher and Visher (1979) point out that adults in stepfamilies *chose* this life but that children are in stepfamilies through no choice of their own (Table 2-3).

The birth of a child to a remarried couple has many possible ramifications for the stepfamily. The couple's decision to have a child may come from a loving commitment or more problematic motivations—to assure spousal commitment, to demonstrate family solidarity, to satisfy cultural expectations, or to surpass the parenting results of the former marriage. Despite the motivations of the parents, other factors play a part in how the birth of a child affects family structure. If both spouses are parents from previous marriages or if one of the spouses has not previously had children, the birth of the new child has a different impact. The ages of stepchildren also make a difference. Young stepchildren may fear that they will be loved less than the newcomer. Conversely, the new half-brother or half-sister can serve as a link between stepsiblings, as well as between the couple, and thus bring **cohesiveness** to the stepfamily. As a nurse you can bring a special service to the new mother if you are sensitive to the emotional issues involved in such a birth.

Adolescent Parents

One segment of single-parent families that presents special needs is the teenage mother. The United States leads nearly all other developed nations in its incidence of pregnancy among teenage women.

Teenage childbearing varies by race of the mother. Births under age 20 are uncommon for Chinese (1%), Japanese (3%), and Filipino and other Asian mothers (6%). White teenage mothers had a rate of 11% in 1989. Hawaiian teenage mothers (17%) and Native American mothers (20%) approached the 23% rate for black mothers.

Even within a racial group outcomes vary depending on socioeconomic class and most recent country of origin. Of teenage Hispanic mothers of Cuban and South and Central American background, 7% to 9% were younger than 20 years old compared with 17% to 22% of mothers of Mexican and Puerto Rican background (MSVR, 1992). These statistics are general statements that point to areas where health care providers should address improved delivery of services.

With the stigma of illegitimacy largely removed, less than 5% of teenage mothers surrender their babies for adoption. Only one in five of 30,000 girls younger than 15 who become pregnant each year receive any prenatal care during the first 3 months of pregnancy. The negative medical consequences of pregnancy in adolescence are discussed in Chapter 8.

TABLE 2-3   Differences Between Traditional Nuclear Family and Stepfamily

NUCLEAR FAMILY	STEPFAMILY
This family originates with marriage of never-married persons who are childless; thus the family is born of individuals coming together in step-by-step progression from courtship to marriage through parenthood.	This family originates with remarriage of divorced or widowed persons who may or may not be childless; thus the new family is born of separation and loss (usually an unfinished process) preceding rapid entry into instant multiple roles.
First marriage joins the two families of origin of each partner.	Remarriage involves interweaving three, four, or more families whose previous life cycles had been disrupted by death or divorce (and may join spouses of differing life cycle stages [e.g., father of adolescent children and never-married wife]).
Both biologic parents are included.	One biologic parent who exists as memory (in the case of death) or as noncustodial parent outside the family circle may be excluded.
Relationship between spouses predates the relationship between parent and child.	Relationship between natural parent and child predates the relationship of the new couple.
Biologic mother has 9 months to prepare for her role as mother.	Stepmother (whether or not she has a child or children of her own) has indeterminate period of acquaintance with children to assume role of primary mother, other mother, comanager, or friend.
Natural parents have important postnatal period of bonding to develop psychologic attachment with child.	Stepparent has postmarriage period of adjustment to develop familial affection for spouse's children.
Natural parents begin parenting an infant who knows no other parent.	Stepparent begins parenting children of various ages who have lost a parent through divorce or death.
Couple bond of the natural parents (normally) takes priority over all other family relationships and provides a solid foundation for a unified household.	Natural bond between biologic parent and child can take priority over the new marital bond and can create a competitive or conflicting environment of divided loyalties. This is not an inevitable consequence but a possibility.

ECONOMICS AND THE FAMILY

Every family exists within a socioeconomic context, and there are great differences in financial security. Those who exist in an impoverished physical context (that is, those who live in substandard housing and have inadequate clothing and insufficient food) and those families who enjoy an abundance of food, clothing, and housing face different issues. The key to material abundance is regular employment that rewards the worker with an income. Many parents do not have such employment and cannot provide for their children.

Poverty is statistically defined in the United States by the government **poverty level,** which changes from year to year. Approximately 20% of all children under age 18 live in families whose income is below the poverty level. Half of these children live in households headed by women (that is, in single-parent families maintained by the mother). Thus an American child has one chance in 10 of being poor if his father is the provider; he has one chance in two of being poor if his mother is the provider. Without a legitimate, stable job role the poor adult man or woman has great difficulty functioning as

a parent. The chronic stress of surviving puts the stability of the poor family at risk.

The life cycle of poor families is drawn by Colon (1980). The young adult, thrown out of or tearing away from his family of origin, ill-equipped with the skills necessary to do well in a technologically complex society, enters an unmarried or married state. Because of limited job options, the adolescent boy frequently cannot form a supporting relationship, and the young childbearing girl emerges as the organizing force within the family. As the father becomes peripheral to the family or disengaged, the mother, who is chronically overburdened and often depressed, may be unable to respond to her children on an individual basis. The children, without attention from their mother or absent father, fail to develop the cognitive, affective, and communication skills that will enable them to benefit from a middle-class–oriented school system. These children are usually absorbed by peer culture.

Poverty can frustrate the goals of the family. Not every family living below the poverty level can be described by this "worst possible" scenario. On the other hand, to function properly as parents, people need the support of the larger economic system. The initia-

tives taken by government health services need better implementation so that the children and families may develop in healthy directions.

KEY POINTS

- A family may be defined as biologic, legal, functional, and ethical. Each family is unique in its emphasis on and configurations of these aspects.
- The overall goal is physical survival and the personal development needed to mature and pass on a secure life to the next generation.
- A "good enough" family provides basic needs for its members and provides an environment wherein each member "grows itself up."
- When basic needs cannot be met because of poverty or illness, additional means of support are sought through outside interventions.
- Individuals and families move through predictable stages of growth and development. Stressors may inhibit development from one stage to the next.
- Patterns of communication, power, and role performance demonstrate family dynamics and influence family health.

- Ethnicity patterns our thinking, feeling, and behavior in obvious and subtle ways. Nurses with mainstream American ethnicity patterns must give sensitive multicultural care to those with differing ethnic backgrounds.
- The divorce rate greatly affects the family by increasing complexity of relationships and often results in single parents, who may easily become depleted of the energy needed for parenting.
- Remarried or blended families may adjust easily or with great difficulty depending on the new spouses' previous marriages and numbers of children who still require parenting.
- Adolescent parenting rates vary from group to group, and carry psychosocial and economic problems into attempts to build a family.

STUDY QUESTIONS

Select terms described in this chapter to complete the statements below.

2-1a. America is facing a new, divorce-related social problem called the "feminization of poverty." Often, single mothers live on lower incomes that are below the ___poverty level___

b. At every stage of human development, intimacy, love, and commitment are important. These three words describe ___Attachment behaviors___

c. The Italians and Polish place great emphasis on family weddings. This statement describes ___Ethnicity___

d. A child is cast into the role of a parent and is required to care for younger children because a single parent goes to work. This is a change in _____ tasks.

e. When you look at the interactions of a family causing one member to be labeled a "black sheep," you are looking at the family ___Boundaries___

f. The primary goals of the family are ___physical survival___ and ___personal development___

2-2 The highest incidence of divorce in this decade occurs between:
   a. Couples with college-age children
   b. Middle-aged men and women
   c. Couples with preschool and schoolchildren
   d. Retired men and women

Match a term in column 1 with the descriptions below.

2-3 Number of babies born per 1000 fertile women ___b___
2-4 Family members interact well together ___c___
2-5 Family members do not share much time or feeling ___d___
   a. Marriage rate
   b. Fertility
   c. Cohesiveness
   d. Disengagement

2-6 A Vietnamese woman refuses the presence of her husband in labor, despite the urging of the nurse. This cultural difference illustrates her preference to:
   a. Be alone during childbearing
   b. Avoid her husband
   c. Be accompanied by a female friend
   d. Have her mother-in-law with her

2-7 If a Hispanic woman is not punctual for clinic appointments, she may be indicating a cultural value of
   a. Activity:Being
   b. Time:Present
   c. Man-Nature:Passivity
   d. Time:Future

2-1 a. Poverty line, b. Attachment behaviors, c. Ethnicity, d. Stage-appropriate behavior, e. Boundaries, f. Physical survival, personal development 2-2 c 2-3 b 2-4 c 2-5 d 2-6 c 2-7 b

REFERENCES

Aneshensul C et al: Onset of fertility-related events during adolescence: a prospective comparison of Mexican American and non-Hispanic white females, *Am J Public Health* 80:959, 1990.

Anthony-Tkach C: Care of the Mexican-American patient, *Nurs Health Care* 2:424, 1981.

Arrendondo R et al: Alcoholism in Mexican-Americans: intervention and treatment, *Hosp Community Psychiatry* 38:180, 1987.

Beal W: Separation, divorce and single parent families. In Carter EA, McGoldrick M, eds: *The family life cycle: a framework for family therapy,* New York, 1980, Gardner Press, Inc.

Binkin N, Rust K, Williams R: Racial differences in neonatal mortality: what causes of death explain the gap, *Am J Dis Child* 142:434, 1988.

Bowen M: *Family therapy in clinical practice,* New York, 1978, Jason Aronson.

Burks J: Factors in utilization of prenatal services by low income Black women, *Nurs Pract* 17:34, 1992.

Bushy A: Rural determinants in family health: considerations for community health, *Fam Comm Health* 12:29, 1990.

Centers for Disease Control: *US AIDS cases reported through February 1992, HIV/AIDS surveillance: March 1992.*

Chasnoff I et al: Cocaine use in pregnancy, *N Engl J Med* 313:666, 1985.

Cherry B, Giger J: Black Americans. In Gieger J, Davidhizar R, eds: *Transcultural nursing,* St Louis, 1991, Mosby–Year Book.

Chin J: Current and future dimensions of the HIV/AIDS pandemic in women and children, *Lancet* 336:221, 1990.

Clark M: Health in the Mexican-American culture: a community study, Berkeley, Calif, 1970, University of California Press.

Colon F: The family life cycle of the multiproblem poor family. In Carter EA, McGoldrick M, eds: *The family life cycle: a framework for family therapy,* New York, 1980, Gardner Press.

Covell K, Turngull W: The long term effects of father absence in childhood on male university students' sex role identity and personal adjustment, *J Genet Psychol* 141:271, 1982.

D'Avanzo C: Bridging the cultural gap with Southeast Asians, *MCN Am J Matern Child Nurs* 17:204, 1992.

Duvall EM: *Marriage and family development,* ed 5, Philadelphia, 1977, JB Lippincott.

Erikson E: *Childhood and society,* New York, 1950, WW Norton.

Falkner R, Tanner J: *Human growth I: principles and prenatal growth,* New York, 1978, Plenum Press.

Geronimus A, Andersen H, Bound J: Differences in hypertension among US black and white women of childbearing age, *Public Health Rep,* 1990.

Giger J, Davidhizar R: *Transcultural nursing,* St Louis, 1991, Mosby.

Giordano J, McGoldrick M, Pearce J, eds: *Ethnicity and family therapy,* New York, 1982, Guildford Press.

Gluck NK: Women in families. In Carter EA, McGoldrick M, eds: *The family life cycle: a framework for family therapy,* New York, 1980, Gardner Press.

Griffith S: Childbearing and the concept of culture, *J Obstet Gynecol Neonatal Nurs* 11:181, 1982.

Guendelman S: At risk: health needs of Hispanic children, *Health Soc Work* 10:183, 1985.

Haber J et al: *Comprehensive psychiatric nursing,* New York, 1992, Mosby.

Jacob A, Walton R: Incidence of birth marks in the neonate, *Pediatrics* 58:218, 1976.

Kay M, ed: *Anthropology of human birth,* Philadelphia, 1982, FA Davis.

Kemper R: The compadrazgo in urban Mexico, *Anthropol Quart* 55:17, 1982.

Koman, Stechler: Making the jump to systems. In Merlin MP, Koman SL, eds: *Handbook of adolescent and family therapy,* New York, 1985, Gardner Press.

Kulpers J: Mexican-Americans. In Giger J, Davidhizar R, eds: *Transcultural nursing,* St Louis, 1991, Mosby.

Logan BB, Dawkins CE, eds: *Family-centered nursing in the community,* Menlo Park, Calif, 1986, Addison-Wesley Publishing.

Mahler AH: *The psychological birth of the human infant,* New York, 1975, Basic Books.

McClanahan P: Improving access to pretnatal care, *J Obstet Gynecol Neonatal Nurs* 21:280, 1992.

McCormick M: The contribution of low birth weight to infant mortality and childhood morbidity, *N Engl J Med* 312:82, 1985.

McGoldrick M: Genograms in family assessment, New York, 1985, WW Norton.

McGoldrick M, Carter EA: Forming a remarried family. In *The family life cycle: a framework for family therapy,* New York, 1980, Gardner Press.

Mendoza F et al: Selected measures of health status for Mexican-American, mainland Puerto Rican and Cuban-American children, *JAMA* 265:227, 1991.

Minuchin S: Families and family therapy. Cambridge, 1974, Harvard University Press.

Monrroy L: Nursing care of Raza/Latina patients. In Orque M, Bloch G, Monrroy L, eds: *Ethnic nursing care,* St Louis, 1983, Mosby.

Monthly Vital Statistics Report (MVSR): *Advance report of final natality statistics, 1989,* National Center for Health Statistics, September 1992.

Murillo N: The Mexican American family. In Hernandexz D, Haug M, Wagner N, eds: *Chicanos: social and psychological perspectives,* St Louis, 1978, CV Mosby.

Nichols MP: Family therapy: concepts and methods, New York, 1984, Gardner Press.

Overfield T: Biological variations, *Nurs Clin North Am* 12:199, 1977.

Paciornik M: Commentary: arguments against episiotomy and in favor of squatting for birth, *Birth* 17:104, 1990.

Randolph L, Gesche M: Black adolescent pregnancy: preventions and management, *J Community Health* 11:10, 1986.

Rassin D et al: Incidence of breast feeding in low socioeconomic group of mothers in the United States: ethnic patterns, *Pediatrics* 73:132, 1984.

Rhodes SL: A developmental approach to the life cycle of the family, *Soc Casework* 15:305, 1977.

Romanczuk AN: Helping the step-parent to parent, *Matern Child Nurs J* 12(3):106, 1987.

Ruiz P: Cultural barriers to effective medical care among Hispanic-American patients, *Ann Rev Med* 36:63, 1985.

Salgado de Snyder V: Factors associated with acculturative stress and depressive symptomatology among married Mexican immigrant women, *Psych Women Quart* 11:475, 1986.

Scholl T et al: Prenatal care adequacy and the outcome of adolescent pregnancy: effects on weight gain, preterm delivery and birth weight, *Obstet Gynecol* 69:312, 1987.

Smith J: The role of the black clorgy as allied health care professionals in working with black patients. In Luckraft D, ed: *Black awareness: the implications for black care,* New York, 1976, Am J Nurs.

Stokes L: Delivering health services in a black community. In Reinhardt AM, Quinn MB, eds: *Current practice in family-centered community nursing,* vol I, St Louis, 1977, Mosby.

Sue D: *Counselling the culturally different: theory and practice,* New York 1981, Doubleday.

Terkelson KG: Toward a theory of the family life cycle. In Carter EA, McGoldrick M, eds: *The family life cycle: a framework for family therapy,* New York, 1980, Gardner Press.

Tripp-Reimer T, Brink P, Saunders J: Cultural assessment: content and process, *Nurs Outlook* 32:78, 1988.

Urrutia-Rojas C, Aday L: A framework for community assessment: designing and conducting a survey in a Hispanic immigrant and refugee community, *Public Health Nurs* 8:20, 1991.

US Bureau of the Census: *The Hispanic population in the United States: March 1989,* Current Pop Reports Series P-20, No 444, Washington, DC, 1990.

US Bureau of the Census: *Statistical abstracts of the United States,* "1988" annualed 108, Washington DC, 1988.

Visher EB, Visher JS: *Step-families: a guide to working with stepparents and stepchildren,* New York, 1979, Brunner/Mazel.

 STUDENT RESOURCE SHELF

Beckman CA: Maternal-child health in Brazil, *J Nurse Midwifery* 16:238, 1987.

Choi E: Unique aspects of Korean mothers, *J Obstet Gynecol Neonatal Nurs* 15:394, 1986.

Choi E, Hamilton R: The effects of culture on mother-infant interaction, *J Obstet Gynecol Neonatal Nurs* 15:256, 1986.

Engle N: An American's experience of childbirth in Japan, *Birth* 16:81, 1989.

Feldman P: Sexuality, birth control and childbirth in orthodox Jewish tradition, *Can Med J* 146:24, 1992.

Fong C: Ethnicity and nursing practice, *Top Clin Nurs* 7:1, 1985.

Ganong LH et al: Stereotyping by nurses and nursing students, *Res Nurs Health* 10:49, 1987.

Geissler E: *Pocket guide to cultural assessment,* St Louis, 1994, Mosby.

Harris K: Beliefs and practices among Haitian-American women in relation to childbearing, *J Nurse Midwifery* 32:149, 1987.

Harwood A: The hot and cold theory of disease, *JAMA* 216:153, 1971.

Wilson J: *The truly disadvantaged: the inner city, the underclass and public policy,* Chicago, 1987, University of Chicago Press.

Leininger M: Transcultural nursing; its progress and its future, *Nurs Health Care* 2:365, 1981.

Lightfoot-Klein H, Shaw E: Special needs of ritually circumcised women patients, *J Obstet Gynecol Neonatal Nurs* 20:102, 1991.

Kay M, ed: *Anthropology of human birth,* Philadelphia, 1982, FA Davis.

Primeau M: American Indian health care practices: a cross cultural perspective, *Nurs Clin North Am* 12:587, 1977.

Spector RE: *Cultural diversity in health and illness,* ed 2, Norwalk, Conn, 1985, Appleton & Lange.
   This is a comprehensive guide to the various ethnic groups in the United States.

Stern PN, Tilden OP, Maxwell EK: Culturally induced stress during childbearing: the Filipino-American experience, *Health Care Women Int* 6:105, 1985.

Waxman AG: Navajo childbirth in transition, *Med Anthropol* 12:187, 1990.

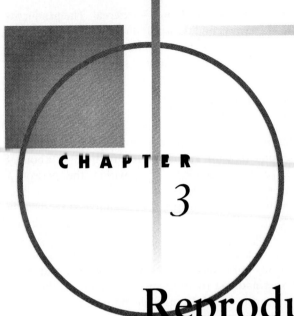

CHAPTER

3

Reproductive Anatomy and Physiology

KEY TERMS

Ampulla
Areola
Cervix
Corpus Luteum
Dysmenorrhea
Ejaculation
Endometrium
Epididymis
Estrogen
Fallopian Tubes
Fimbriae
Follicle-Stimulating
  Hormone (FSH)
Follicular Phase
Fundus
Gamete
Gender
Gonad
Graafian Follicle
Ischemic Phase
Luteal Phase
Luteinizing
  Hormone (LH)
Menarche
Menopause

Menstrual Phase
Myometrium
Oocyte
Oogenesis
Osteoporosis
Ova
Ovaries
Ovulation
Pelvic Floor
Penis
Perimetrium
Progesterone
Proliferative Phase
Prostaglandins

Prostate
Pubescence
Scrotum
Secretory Phase
Semen
Seminiferous Tubules
Spermatozoa
Spermatogenesis
Testes
Testosterone
Uterus
Vagina
Vas Deferens
Vulva

LEARNING OBJECTIVES

1. Identify major reproductive structures of men and women.
2. Describe the physiologic changes initiating puberty, menstruation, and fertility.
3. Explain feedback mechanisms of the menstrual cycle, describing hormone action in each phase.
4. Compare and contrast the decline in fertility in men and women.
5. Describe premenstrual syndrome with regard to onset and known causes to date.
6. Discuss current nursing care related to PMS and dysmenorrhea.
7. Identify the phases of the sexual excitement cycle for men and women.
8. Differentiate between the concepts of gender and sexuality.

Human reproduction is intricate and complex. Long before male and female sex cells unite to form a new infant, an internal process of development and maturation takes place. This process involves a precise harmony between several systems of the body. To understand the process of childbirth, you must first know the reproductive structures. The processes take place with relatively few mistakes. Thus a couple desiring pregnancy usually achieves it within a year, unless some preventive method is used.

Although very clearly different, male and female reproductive anatomies are initially identical (undifferentiated). There is no cellular difference until about the fifth week after conception. At that time primordial sex cells, originating in the walls of the yolk sac, begin to develop and migrate into the embryo to form the gonads, the major sex organs. At this point the sex of the embryo can be determined microscopically. External genitalia begin differentiation by the end of the eighth week, with completion by the twelfth week. Because of the common beginning, as sexual development continues there are apparent parallels in several structures and in the function of the sexual hormones.

A review of the male and female reproductive systems follows. It will help you to better understand what is necessary for successful conception, pregnancy, and delivery.

Male Reproductive Anatomy

Although it may appear that male sexual structures are more external than internal, only the bifunctional penis and the supportive scrotum are external. The productive testes, the storage and transport ducts, the accessory structures of the seminal vesicles, the prostate, and the bulbourethral glands are all internal structures (Figure 3-1).

INTERNAL STRUCTURES

The **testes** are two small, white, oval glands, about 2 inches in size and weighing about 12 g. They begin development with sexual differentiation at about 8 weeks after conception, lying within the peritoneal cavity until about the twenty-eighth week, when they begin their descent through the inguinal canal into the scrotal sac. Descent usually occurs before birth; the testes then remain outside the abdominal cavity, suspended in the external scrotum to maintain the lower-than-body temperature necessary to produce and maintain **spermatozoa** (mature sperm). Failure of the testes to descend is called cryptorchidism or may be referred to as "ectopic testes."

Each testis is protected by a fibrous tissue layer called the tunica albuginea. This membrane covers and serves as the outside layer and then extends inward as septa (dividers to create hundreds of individual lobes). The effect is similar to orange or grapefruit sections. The "fruit" of each lobe is a long mass of threadlike fibers, tightly coiled to fit in this small space. These are the **seminiferous tubules,** the site of **spermatogenesis** (sperm production). Surrounding these tubules are Sertoli's cells, which secrete nourishment for the developing spermatozoa.

Other specialized cells are contained in the interstitial tissue. Clusters of Leydig's cells, stimulated by

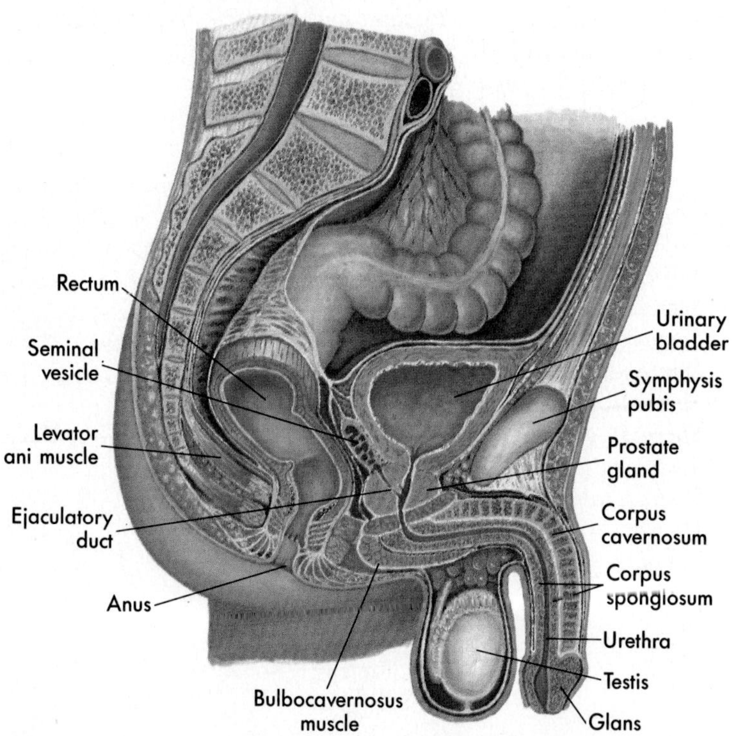

FIGURE 3-1 Male reproductive organs. Sagittal section of pelvis showing placement of male reproductive organs.

Rectum

Seminal vesicle

Levator ani muscle

Ejaculatory duct

Anus

Bulbocavernosus muscle

Urinary bladder

Symphysis pubis

Prostate gland

Corpus cavernosum

Corpus spongiosum

Urethra

Testis

Glans

hormones from the anterior pituitary gland, produce the male hormone **testosterone,** responsible for male sexual functioning and characteristics.

The ends of all the seminiferous tubules join to form a common collection area known as the rete testis, which leads to ducts that enter the **epididymis,** the storage structure located on the lateral and posterior sides of each testis. Here the sperm mature, nourished by secretions within the coiled tube, and remain until ejaculation (Figure 3-1).

Sperm exit each epididymis via a **vas deferens,** a tube about 40 cm long that connects to the prostatic urethra. It joins the spermatic cord to pass through the inguinal canal into the pelvis, where it meets with the vas from the other side. These then join with the seminal vesicles (located posterior to the bladder) at the ejaculatory ducts, receiving alkaline fluid rich in nutrition and containing prostaglandins. Although the function of these substances is not fully understood, they may enhance fertilization and aid the zygote in reaching the uterus.

The ducts enter the **prostate,** a gland below the bladder that surrounds the urethra like a balloon on a Foley catheter surrounds the catheter. Composed of numerous glands embedded in fibromuscular tissue, the prostate is pierced by the ejaculatory ducts and allows emptying into the urethra. There, the majority of the fluid for ejaculation is formed to facilitate sperm motility and protect sperm from the acidic vaginal environment. Additional fluid is produced by the bulbourethral (Cowper's) glands. These fluids, added to the sperm, create **semen,** which is emptied into the prostatic urethra and expelled by **ejaculation** (Figure 3-2).

Test Yourself

Where do these functions take place?

- Sperm production_____
- Secretion of testosterone_____
- Storage of sperm_____
- Addition of nutritional fluids to semen_____

SPERMATOGENESIS

During the fifth week of embryonic life, primitive germ cells enter the developing gonads, where they become part of the primitive sex cords that become the seminiferous tubules. There are no primordial sex cells in the gonads at birth; instead, production of them starts at puberty under the influence of gonadotropic hormones. Sperm maturation or **spermatogenesis** is stimulated by testosterone. The spermatogonia, or primitive male germ cells, begin to develop into primary spermatocytes and then undergo their first meiotic division to become secondary spermatocytes. Unlike the female, however, there is no delay in further maturation, and these cells immediately begin the final change into mature **spermatozoa.** Although mature sperm may remain in the epididymis for up to 6 weeks, depending on the frequency of ejaculation, they can only live 2 to 3 days once in the female genital tract (Figure 3-3).

During ejaculation, sperm leave the epididymis, travel through the vas deferens, and become lubricated with fluids secreted by the seminal vesicles, prostate gland, and bulbourethral glands. At this point, the fluid passes down through the urethra and out of the penis by the wavelike spasms.

Characteristics of Sperm

At any time, one portion of the seminiferous tubule may contain primary spermatocytes in meiotic division while another portion may contain secondary spermatocytes becoming spermatids (Figure 3-4). Millions of sperm are produced at the same time; in one ejaculation of semen, there may be as many as 20 to 60 million. Only one will fertilize the ovum; the others will die en route or be altered in the uterus or fallopian tubes.

The spermatozoon is made up of a head and a tail (see Figure 3-3, *D*). The acrosome, nucleus, and nuclear vacuoles make up the head. The head carries half the number of chromosomes (haploid number) needed for the new cell that will become the fetus and is the portion of the sperm that penetrates the ovum wall. The tail or flagellum is long and flexible and propels the sperm through the female genital tract. It drops off as the head enters the ovum. See Chapter 6 for discussion of sperm and infertility.

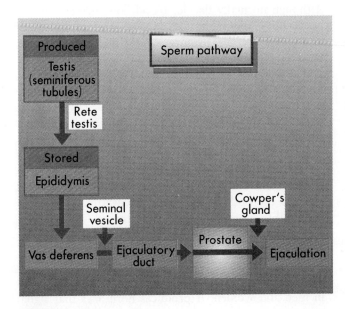

FIGURE 3-2 Sperm pathway.

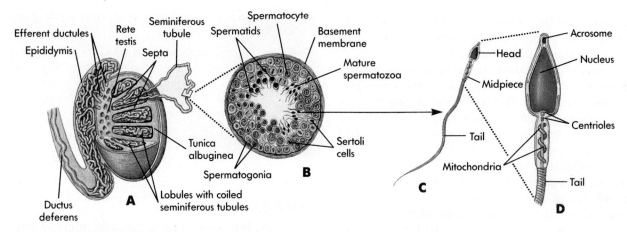

FIGURE 3-3 Histology of the testis. **A,** Gross anatomy of the testis with a section cut away to reveal internal structures. **B,** Cross-section of a seminiferous tubule. Spermatogonia are near the periphery, and mature sperm cells are near the lumen of the seminiferous tubule. **C,** Mature sperm cell. **D,** Head of a mature sperm cell. (Courtesy Bill Ober.)

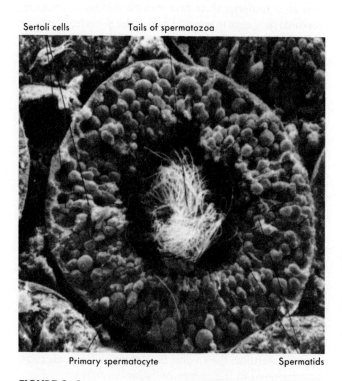

FIGURE 3-4 Scanning electron micrograph of cross-section of seminiferous tubule that shows spermatogonia, least differentiated of cells close to outer lining membrane of tubule. Primary spermatocytes, spermatids, and Sertoli's cells can also be seen in wall of tubule, and tails of spermatids undergoing transition into mature spermatozoa can be seen extending into tubule lumen. (From Kessel RG, Kardon RH: *Tissues and organs: a text-atlas of scanning electron microscopy.* ©1979, WH Freeman & Co. Reprinted with permission.)

EXTERNAL STRUCTURES

The **penis** is a long, flexible structure located in front of the scrotum and below the symphysis pubis. It is an excretory and reproductive organ because the urethra is used as a passageway for urine and semen. The penis is divided into the body, or shaft, and a rounded end known as the glans. The glans is smooth and, like its female counterpart, extremely sensitive to stimuli. At birth, it is covered by the prepuce, or foreskin, which may be surgically removed for religious, cultural, or hygienic reasons, leaving the glans exposed (Figure 3-1).

The shaft of the penis consists of three urethral layers surrounded by three longitudinal layers of tissue, including two corpora cavernosa and one corpus spongiosum. Although normally flaccid, blood flow increases in the penis with sexual excitation, and venous exit is impaired. The tissue becomes engorged, and the organ stiffens, becoming erect so it can penetrate the female vagina.

The **scrotum**, a baglike structure anterior to the anus, is suspended behind the penis. It is a supportive structure that holds the testes. The scrotum is divided by a septum (partition) of connective tissue so each testis has its own compartment. The scrotum protects its internal structures by sensitivity to touch, pain, and temperature.

Because the temperature of the testes must remain cooler than body temperature, the scrotum tightens close to the body when environmental temperature is cold and becomes looser when warm.

HORMONAL CONTROL

The hypothalamus is responsible for hormonal control in men and women. It produces hormones that signal the anterior pituitary gland to secrete gonad-stimulating hormones, including **follicle-stimulating hormone (FSH)** and **luteinizing hormone (LH).** Once they reach the gonads, production of **gametes** (sex cells) and sex hormones is initiated. Hormonal changes governing fertilization and pregnancy are described in Chapters 7 and 9.

Female Reproductive Anatomy

Female sexual anatomy is also divided into internal and external portions (Figure 3-5). Internal structures are the ovaries, fallopian tubes, uterus, and vagina. The vulva is the main external female structure. Although not directly involved in reproduction, the breasts are considered accessory sexual structures. The major controlling organs of female reproduction are the two **ovaries.** These two small organs, similar to almonds in shape and size, are located approximately 4 to 5 inches below the waist. The ovaries serve to both develop **ova,** the female sex cells or gametes, and produce hormones (**estrogen** and **progesterone**).

Production of ova, **oogenesis,** occurs in the third to fifth week of embryonic life, when primitive germ cells begin to form, migrate to the **gonads** or ovaries, and turn into oogonia (early ova). They undergo rapid mitosis (cell division), develop into primary **oocytes,** enter the first meiotic (sex cell) division, and do not complete this division until puberty. By the seventh month of fetal life, the oocytes are surrounded by tissue that later becomes follicles. Although there are 700,000 to 2 million primary oocytes at birth, the number is reduced to about 40,000 by puberty. At this time, hormones from the anterior pituitary gland stimulate ripening of one ovum and its release from the ovary. This process, called **ovulation,** leaves the once smooth ovarian surface scarred, with a characteristic bumpy appearance.

FALLOPIAN TUBES

The **fallopian tubes,** also known as oviducts, lie adjacent to the ovaries at one end and are attached to the uterus at the other end. Approximately 4 in (10 cm) in length with a rich blood supply, they serve as the passageway for the expelled ovum, with cells that secrete proteins to nourish the ovum as it travels to the uterus.

Each tube is divided into three segments: the infundibulum, the ampulla, and the isthmus. The wide, funnel-shaped infundibulum is fringed and wrapped around the ovaries but does not cover and is not attached to them. The fingerlike projections of the infundibulum, the **fimbriae,** swell at ovulation and they, the cilia that line them, and the entire tube reach out to capture the ovum as it is released from its follicle, pulling it into the tube and preventing it from being absorbed by the abdominal cavity. The ovum is propelled through the tube by the cilia and peristaltic waves influenced by estrogen and **prostaglandins.**

The infundibulum becomes the **ampulla,** the curved distal two thirds of each tube. Fertilization occurs in this section. The straight, narrow tubal isthmus attaches the tubes to the uterus between the fundus and the corpus.

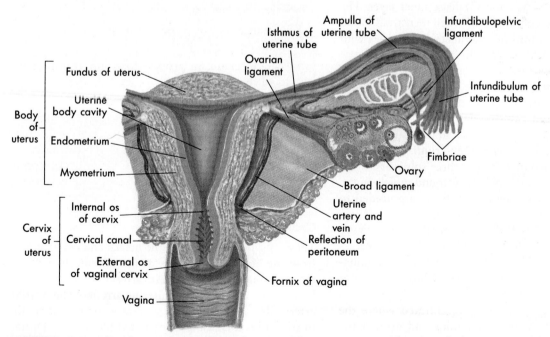

FIGURE 3-5 Female pelvic organs in a frontal section. The entire uterus is shown, with the upper portion of the vagina and the left uterine tube and ovary.

UTERUS

Commonly known as the "womb," the **uterus** lies behind the pubic bones, posterior to the bladder, and between the rectum and abdominal wall (Figure 3-5). It has the shape of an inverted pear. In its nonpregnant or nongravid state it is about the size of a fist, but it can stretch to hold even a 13-pound infant during gestation. It is normally hollow and flat; its walls almost touch each other. Ordinarily, it tilts anteriorly. The uterus provides a nourishing and protective environment for the developing embryo and fetus.

Segments of Uterus

The divisions of the uterus are the corpus and cervix. The corpus is the upper two thirds of the uterus and is further divided into the fundus, cornua, body, and uterine isthmus.

The **fundus** is the rounded, top portion of the uterus and is the easiest to palpate through the abdominal wall. It extends above the fallopian tubes. The cornua are is the wide segments where the tubal isthmus portion of the fallopian tubes enters the uterus. The body is the center segment, and the uterine isthmus, which contains the uterine canal, is the narrower, bottom segment leading to the cervix.

Uterine Layers

The walls of the uterus are made up of two distinct tissue layers and a third covering layer. All layers are suited to maintaining pregnancy and accomplishing labor and birth. The inner layer, the **endometrium,** is composed of three sublayers: (1) surface layer, (2) spongy middle layer (loose connective tissue), and (3) dense inner layer. The first and second layers slough off when menstrual blood and tissue are shed; thus the endometrium changes with the female reproductive cycle. Its mucous cells temporarily produce nutrients for the fertilized ovum.

The **myometrium** is comprised of layers of smooth muscle fibers that extend in three directions. These fibers intertwine with and connect elastic tissues and blood vessels throughout the uterine wall and also connect to the dense, inner layer of the endometrium. Like the endometrium, the myometrium has three sublayers:

1. The outer myometrial layer is found mostly in the fundus. Its long longitudinal fibers are needed to push the fetus downward at birth.
2. The middle, muscle fibers are interlaced in a figure 8 pattern, encircling large blood vessels. Contraction of this portion causes hemostasis (termination of bleeding) and control of blood loss after placental separation.
3. The inner layer is most concentrated where the fallopian tubes join the fundus and around the internal os. These muscles act as sphincters to prevent menstrual blood from ascending into the tubes and to hold the contents of the uterus during pregnancy.

By contracting, the myometrium pulls on and opens up the cervix to expel the fetus. Later, by contracting, the myometrium controls blood loss after childbirth.

The **perimetrium,** an outer, serosal covering, is an extension of the parietal peritoneum.

CERVIX

Approximately 2.5 cm in length and diameter, the cervix is composed of very elastic smooth muscle and connective tissue. When visualized on a vaginal examination, it appears doughnutlike, with its opening in the center seen as a dimpling. In reality, the cervical canal has two openings: the **internal os,** connected to uterine tissue, and the **external os,** which is the portion seen at the end of the vagina. This distinction is important when studying the changes that occur in the cervix as it prepares for delivery. The endocervical lining is characteristically pink in a nonpregnant state but turns bluish with pregnancy (see Chapter 9).

The cervix feels pressure but has few nerve endings, is lined with cells producing mucus that lubricates and cleanses the vagina, and protects the vagina against bacteria. Mucus production is altered by the menstrual cycle and pregnancy. During pregnancy, it is thick and forms a plug to seal off the uterus for gestation.

Test Yourself

Fill in the blanks.

- Secretions that nourish the ovum _____
- Substance that traps the ovum at ovulation _____
- These mechanisms provide for ovum transport down the tube _____
- Usual site of fertilization _____
- Layer of uterus that contracts during labor _____
- Vaginal lubrication is produced at this site _____

Circulation

The major blood supply to the uterus and cervix comes from the aorta as it divides at the umbilical level into the two iliac arteries. These arteries divide into the hypogastric and finally the uterine arteries. The ovarian artery also joins the uterine artery after feeding the ovaries, thus increasing oxygenated blood flow. During pregnancy the blood vessels proliferate and enter at every level of the myometrium (Figure 3-6).

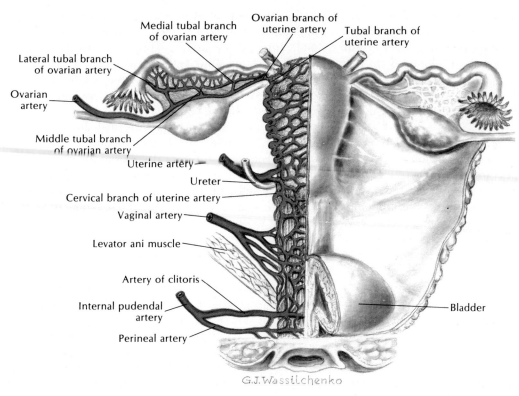

FIGURE 3-6 Blood supply to uterus and surrounding structures. (From Bobak IM, Jensen MD: *Essentials of maternity nursing: the nurse and the childbearing family,* ed 2, St Louis, 1987, Mosby.)

Innervation

Parasympathetic fibers from sacral nerves stimulate vasodilation and inhibit muscle contraction. Efferent sympathetic motor nerves (T5 through T10) reach the uterus through the uterosacral ligament ganglia, causing vasoconstriction and the ability to contract (see Chapter 13).

Although the autonomic system regulates action of the uterus, the uterus can also relax and contract on its own. Radiating pain sensations from the uterus join in the paracervical areas and proceed upward. They travel to levels T11 and T12 of the spinal cord. They also join with nerves from the ovaries and ureters.

Ligaments

The weight of a pregnant uterus requires a strong and well-developed support system within the pelvis. This system is provided by the following ligaments attached to the ovaries and uterus:

1. *Broad ligaments,* two ligaments that are double folds of the parietal peritoneum. They cover the uterus like sheets hanging on a line (Beischer and MacKay, 1986). The fallopian tubes, ovaries, blood vessels, and round and ovarian ligaments are suspended within them. They are made of loose connective tissue and help to keep the uterus in place.

2. *Cardinal ligaments,* the chief support for the uterus. These are actually the base of the broad ligament. They extend from the cervix to the pelvic walls and wrap the ureter and uterine vessels.

3. *Round ligaments,* parallel with the broad ligament. These two pieces of smooth muscle and connective tissue attach to the uterus at the cornua and pass through the inguinal canal, ending in the labia majora.

4. *Uterosacral ligaments,* two cordlike folds of peritoneum extending from the lower cervix to the fascia over the second and third sacral vertebrae, attaching on either side of the rectum. They encircle the rectum posterior to the uterus, forming Douglas' cul-de-sac behind the cervix.

5. *Ovarian ligaments,* which attach the ovaries to the cornua.

VAGINA

Commonly called the "birth canal," the **vagina** serves as the passageway from the internal reproductive organs to the external genitalia. It is a long, tubular structure, about 10.5 cm in length between the vaginal *introitus* (opening) and the uterine cervix and slants upward and slightly posterior when the woman is standing. Because it meets at a *right angle* with the cervix, its anterior wall is shorter than its posterior wall by about 1.5 cm. The distal vagina terminates in a cul-de-sac known as a *fornix,* a space surrounding the cervix. The fornix collects seminal fluid after coitus, keeping sperm near the cervix for easier entry.

The inner walls of the vagina are called *rugae,* smooth, gland-containing mucous membranes folded back on themselves. These foldings allow the marked stretching during childbirth. Vaginal membranes range from wet to dry under the influence of hormones and sexual excitation and generally maintain an acidic environment hostile to invading bacteria.

PELVIC FLOOR

The **pelvic floor,** a muscular diaphragm, closes off and supports the structures within the pelvic cavity. Its most important segments are the circumvaginal muscles, the levator ani, and the fascia that covers it. The places that this muscle does not completely cover are filled with the coccygal and piriformal muscles. Changes during pregnancy and labor are discussed in Chapters 9 and 13.

EXTERNAL STRUCTURES

Vulva

The **vulva** is the female external genitalia (Figure 3-7). The *mons,* made up of soft, fatty tissue, lies directly over the symphysis pubis and is covered with hair just before puberty. The mons divides into two "lips," the labia majora, which are covered with hair on the outside but smooth inside. When these outer labia are spread, the thin, pink inner labia minora can be seen; they are smooth, hairless, and extremely sensitive to pressure, touch, and temperature. During sexual

excitation, they swell and become darker because of additional blood flow to them. Both sets of labia cover and protect the vestibule, which contains the clitoris, urethral meatus, and vagina.

Anteriorly, the labia minora join to form a soft fold of skin or hood called the *prepuce* that partially covers the clitoris. Like the penis, the clitoris is also composed of a glans and a shaft. The glans is small and round and is filled with many nerve endings and a rich blood supply. The shaft is a cord connecting the glans to the pubic bone; within it is the major blood supply of the clitoris. Finally, the vestibular bulbs are erectile tissue along the sides of the vestibule; these blood and nerve supplies account for engorgement, swelling, and sensitivity during sexual stimulation. Sebaceous glands secrete smegma, a fatty substance with a distinct odor similar to that of the smegma from the penis.

The urethral meatus (the opening of the bladder) and then the vaginal introitus are posterior to the clitoris and are surrounded by and sometimes partially covered by a thin membrane called the *hymen.* Perivaginal or Bartholin's glands, small round buds thought to produce fluid for lubrication during intercourse, are on either side of the introitus. The fourchette, a thin membranous ridge at the back of the vestibule, is formed by the juncture of the labia majora and minora.

The perineal body is between the posterior vaginal introitus and the anus. It serves as an anchor for genital muscles and ligaments.

Breasts

The mammary glands begin to develop during the sixth week of fetal life; only the main lactiferous ducts are formed at birth. The mammary glands themselves remain undeveloped until puberty, when their growth occurs in response to circulating hormones. Finally, during pregnancy the glands complete development in preparation for lactation (see Chapter 17). Because they

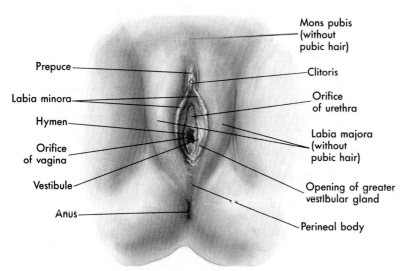

Mons pubis (without pubic hair)

Prepuce

Clitoris

Labia minora

Orifice of urethra

Hymen

Orifice of vagina

Labia majora (without pubic hair)

Vestibule

Anus

Opening of greater vestibular gland

Perineal body

FIGURE 3-7 External genitals of the female. (Courtesy David J. Mascaro & Associates.)

are not directly involved with reproduction, the breasts are secondary sex organs. They, too, are influenced by hormones.

Structure. The breasts consist of two mammary glands located on each side of the chest wall, attached by connective tissue and covered with and given shape by fatty tissue. In an adult, they extend from the second to the sixth or seventh rib and lie between the sternum and the axillary border with an axillary tail extending upward and laterally. Although size and shape vary a great deal from person to person, they are generally dome-shaped and weigh about 100 to 200 g. Symmetry between both breasts is rarely perfect, but their contours should be smooth with no dimpling, lumps, or retracted areas (Figure 3-8).

An intricate system of glandular tissue that manufactures and stores milk is inside the breast. In each breast, there are 15 to 20 lobes, each containing clusters of alveoli, which resemble tiny bunches of grapes and are richly lined with many capillaries to absorb nutrients from the blood for milk production. The smallest parts of alveoli are the acini, the saclike end of the glandular system. The acini are lined with epithelial cells that secrete colostrum and milk and the muscle layer that contracts to expel milk.

Little canals called *ductules* exit the alveoli and join to form larger canals, the lactiferous ducts. During lactation, milk flows from the alveoli, through the duct system, to balloonlike sacs known as lactiferous sinuses, where it is stored. The sinuses merge into openings on the nipple through which the infant obtains milk. The nipple is a round, pigmented portion of fibromuscular tissue and may be firm and elevated, flat, or even inverted. It is sensitive to temperature and tactile stimuli. Surrounding the nipple is the **areola,** the smooth, pigmented circle of skin containing tiny sebaceous glands (tubercles of Montgomery) that secrete fatty substances needed to lubricate and protect the nipple. Muscle fibers that tighten to create nipple erectness are also within the areola.

Test Yourself

Fill in the blanks.

• Cells that secrete colostrum _____
• Canals that carry milk _____
• Storage site of milk _____
• Glands that lubricate the nipple _____

Blood vessels and lymphatics. The breasts are highly vascular structures. The lymphatic system drains the breasts. Blood vessels enlarge during pregnancy.

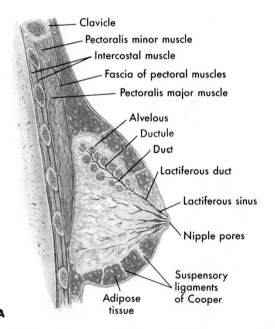

A

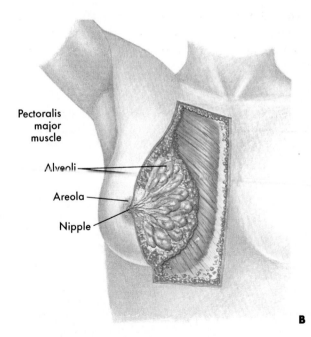

B

FIGURE 3-8 The female breast. **A,** Sagittal section of a lactating breast. Notice how the glandular structures are anchored to the overlying skin and to the pectoral muscles by the suspensory ligaments of Cooper. Each lobule of glandular tissue is drained by a lactiferous duct that eventually opens though the nipple. **B,** Anterior view of a lactating breast. Overlying skin and connective tissue have been removed from the medial side to show the internal structure of the breast and underlying skeletal muscle. In nonlactating breasts the glandular tissue is much less prominent, with adipose tissue comprising most of each breast.

Hormonal influences. Estrogen and progesterone increase vascularity in the breasts and stimulate acini and duct growth. Water and fatty secretions are increased, resulting in fullness, heaviness, and discomfort during the premenstrual period. During pregnancy, the breasts respond to estrogen and progesterone, human placental lactogen (HPL), and prolactin (PRL) to prepare and develop a fully functioning lactating system (see Chapter 17).

Pubescence and Puberty

Both males and females reach sexual maturity through a system of growth and change known as **pubescence.** Physical changes begin 1 to 2 years before puberty. Secondary sex characteristics begin with pubic and axillary hair and breast budding with gradual enlargement of the breasts. Males experience characteristic deepening of the voice, development of body hair, and enlargement of the genitalia. Secondary sex characteristics continue to develop slowly for the next few years after puberty.

The growth spurt precedes puberty by about 1 year. During pubescence, 20% to 25% of linear growth occurs. Males add 8 to 12 inches and females 2 to 8 inches to their height during these growth spurts. Hands and feet grow first and then long bones. This explains why the young grower seems so awkward. In girls linear growth is considered almost complete once menstruation starts, because of epiphyseal closure under estrogen influence. Weight also increases, up to 20 or 30 pounds during this period.

The age at which the growth spurt associated with puberty begins varies from person to person. Puberty occurs as it slows. For girls, puberty begins with the first menstrual period (**menarche**). For boys, the first noctur-

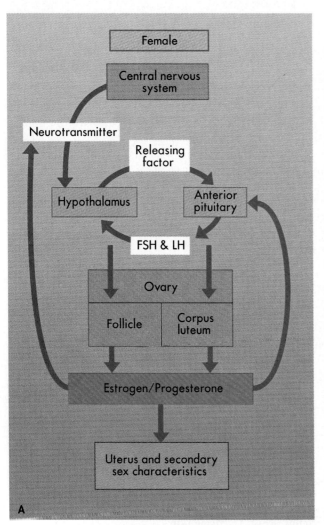
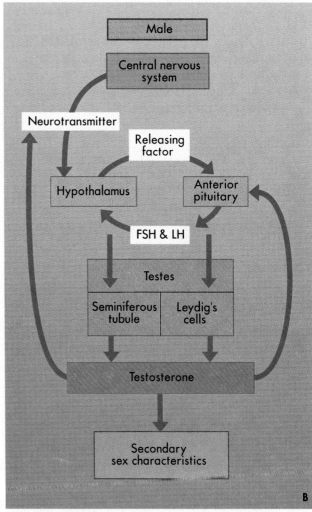

FIGURE 3-9 Feedback process in female (**A**) and male (**B**) reproductive hormone secretion. Solid line indicates positive feedback; broken lines indicate negative feedback.

nal emission (**ejaculation**) of semen begins puberty. In the United States, the average age of menarche is 12.3 years (± 1.2 years); boys mature 6 to 12 months later. However, puberty can occur at any time between 9 and 15 years of age for girls and 10 and 17 for boys.

Most children experience the changes in their bodies with interest and ambivalence; the changes are a profound and bewildering difference in physique, emotional response, and psychologic growth. Growth spurts leave the pubescent feeling unfamiliar with a new body size and shape and leads to an awkward and uncoordinated appearance. Boys and girls have heightened awareness of and interest in the opposite sex and focus on their peers as gauges for behavior.

At puberty, children move into adolescence, the time of preparation for adulthood; adolescence generally includes the ages from 13 to 19. It is often called the "period of transition" because the teenager's emotions and mind attempt to keep up with rapid physical changes.

During this time, an adolescent can become a parent before he or she is emotionally or developmentally prepared. Often, nurses involved in community education or maternity or pediatric care help these "children having children" to cope with pregnancy and successful preparation for parenthood.

ONSET OF PUBERTY

Hormonal Factors

The onset of puberty is controlled by a complex process beginning when the gonads are differentiated in the embryo. Unstimulated throughout infancy and childhood, gonadal function and maturation are dormant until, at puberty, the central nervous system triggers them (Figure 3-9).

There is a sudden surge of estrogen in girls (Figure 3-10). LH and FSH are active in the first part of the menstrual cycle. FSH stimulates the ovaries to produce the **graafian follicle,** resulting in rising estrogen levels. LH comes into play when the follicle is ripe and mature; it triggers follicular rupture and release of the ovum. For the boy, FSH and LH produce androgens necessary for spermatogenesis.

Other hormones also participate in rapid maturation during puberty, including the somatotropic (growth) hormone (STH), adrenocorticotropic hormone (ACTH), and thyroid hormone. Hormonal interplay functions on a feedback mechanism; that is, hormone levels and glandular activities are interdependent and reciprocal. This process has positive and negative influences. For instance, at times during the menstrual cycle, the presence of estrogens results in a positive feedback to enhance secretion of FSH and LH; at other times estrogens and progesterones result in negative feedback that suppresses FSH and LH secretion.

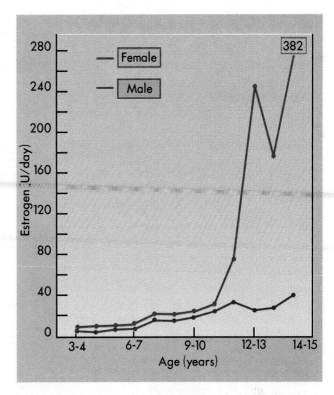

FIGURE 3-10 Excretion of estrogen in urine of children. Sudden change occurs just before puberty in girls.

Hormone levels change with the cycle. FSH activates several ovarian follicles to grow and mature each cycle. As they mature, they produce estrogens that at first stimulate additional FSH secretion. At the same time, the LH level rises, reaching its peak about 16 to 18 hours before ovulation. This peak is frequently used to study the menstrual cycle of a woman experiencing fertility problems (Figure 3-11). LH and estrogens peak immediately before ovulation. When one follicle becomes the "ripest," it ruptures and releases the mature ovum. There is only a slight drop in estrogen levels after ovulation, and then, as progesterone levels rise, FSH and LH production decreases, suppressing the maturation of another follicle while the body prepares to receive a fertilized ovum. (During pregnancy, higher levels of estrogen and progesterone also suppress follicle growth and ovulation.) The estrogenic hormones cause changes in the breasts, uterus, fallopian tubes, and vagina in preparation for pregnancy.

After ovulation, LH induces changes in the ruptured follicle. The empty follicle, now known as the **corpus luteum,** continues to function under the influence of LH and LTH. It releases progesterone, and this hormone, estrogens, and LTH prepare the uterine lining for implantation of the fertilized ovum by thickening its mucous membrane and increasing its blood supply. If the ovum is not fertilized, the levels of estrogens and progesterone begin to fall after ovulation causing lower

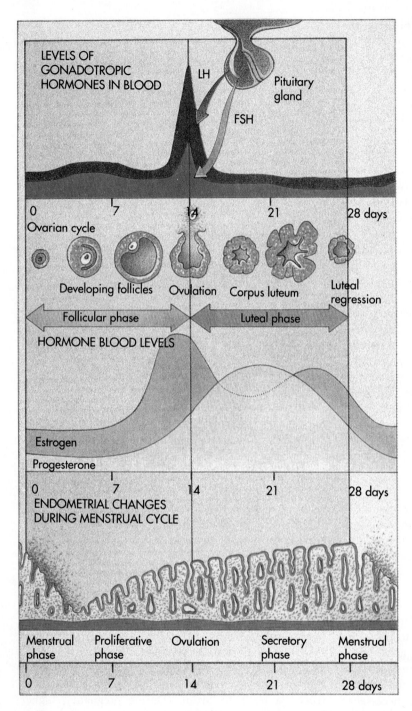

FIGURE 3-11 Events of the menstrual cycle. The various lines depict the changes in blood hormone levels, the development of the follicles, and the changes in the endometrium during the cycle. (Courtesy Kevin A. Sommerville.)

levels of these hormones in the bloodstream. The hypothalamus is no longer inhibited by estrogens and secretes the follicle-stimulating hormone-releasing factor (FSHRF), a gonadotropin-releasing factor, to the anterior pituitary, which releases FSH and restarts the cycle (Box 3-1).

Other hormones do not control the reproductive cycle but influence its function. Hormones called **prostaglandins** (PGs), produced in most organs of the body, affect smooth muscle contractility and hormonal activ-

ity during menstruation and ovulation, influence fertility, cervical mucus properties, motility of the fallopian tubes, and contractility of the uterus, and cause the onset of spontaneous abortion, as well as labor.

Menarche

The first menstrual period experienced is called the menarche, which usually occurs between 11 and 13 years of age. Although the precise mechanism is unknown, it is thought to be related to maturation of the hypothalamus.

BOX 3-1   Effects of Estrogen and Progesterone

Estrogen
- Stimulates growth of ovaries and graafian follicles
- Stimulates growth of smooth muscle and epithelium of reproductive tract
  - Fallopian tubes: Increase motility and ciliary action
  - Uterus: Increases motility and prepares endometrium for implantation
  - Cervix: Secretes clear, stretchable mucus
  - Vagina: Changes vaginal secretions by raising pH and glucose
- Stimulates secondary female characteristics
- Governs growth of external genitalia and pattern of body hair
- Governs growth of breasts, especially ducts
- Governs development of body contours
- Stimulates more sebaceous gland secretions (anti-acne)
- Closes epiphyseal layer of bone
- Affects feedback on hypothalamus and anterior pituitary
- Promotes retention of fluid during menstrual cycle and pregnancy
- Stimulates prolactin secretion during lactation
- Affects vascular system when deficiencies such as hot flashes or slight vasodilation occur

Progesterone
- Stimulates secretory effects of endometrial glands during second part of cycle
- Maintains pregnancy by inhibiting motility of fallopian tubes and uterus
- Stimulates growth of uterine muscle during pregnancy
- Changes cervical mucus to thick and sticky and thus impenetrable to sperm
- Stimulates growth of glandular tissue in breast
- Affects feedback on hypothalamus and anterior pituitary

Secreted in larger amounts, gonadatropin-stimulating hormone influences production of gonadatropins by the anterior pituitary. FSH, LH, and luteotropic hormone (LTH) influence growth of the primary follicles in the ovaries, awaiting maturation.

Menarche appears to also be triggered by attainment of a specific percentage of body fat (17%) and body weight (approximately 48 kg or 105 lb). Although secretion of estrogen by the follicles has begun a cyclical pattern 2 to 3 years earlier, the sufficient level of estrogen necessary to establish a consistent hormonal cycle does not occur until puberty.

MENSTRUAL CYCLE

It takes approximately 1 month to complete the female reproductive cycle from the start of the ripening follicle to the shedding of the uterine lining. The monthly discharge of blood, cellular material, and mucus is called **menstruation** and lasts 3 to 6 days. The length of the cycle varies among individuals and within 1 year for the same woman. Although the average cycle occurs every 28 to 30 days, the length may vary as much as 5 to 10 days. Some women have 21-day cycles, some only menstruate every 32 to 35 days. Many factors influence the length of the cycle, including illness, stress, fatigue, environmental conditions, and hormonal differences. Periodic changes can be described by phases or cycles. One of these cycles is called the ovarian cycle and is divided according to hormonal activity; another cycle is the uterine cycle, which describes the varying thicknesses of the endometrium. Both phases occur simultaneously (Figure 3-11).

Uterine Cycle

The first day of menstrual flow is the first day in the uterine cycle, which begins the **menstrual phase.** By the time this cycle ends, the endometrial lining is thin, estrogen levels are low, and the uterus is dormant. The time from cessation of menses until the beginning of ovulation is the **proliferative phase;** it is marked by enlargement of the endometrial glands in response to new estrogen stimulation. The endometrial layers become very thick and filled with blood. The cervical mucus becomes abundant, thin, and clear, and its pH changes to a more alkaline state to allow for and encourage the entry of sperm. The mucus also becomes very stretchable during ovulation, a condition known as spinnbarkheit.

After ovulation, the **secretory phase** begins. Under the influence of progesterone, the endometrial cells swell and dilate, increasing vascularity in preparation for the fertilized ovum. If fertilization and implantation do not occur, the levels of estrogen and progesterone fall and vasoconstriction occurs, causing a decreased blood supply to large areas of the endometrium; this, in turn, causes tissue breakdown, marking the final **ischemic phase.** As endometrial tissue sloughs off, capillaries break, and blood begins to escape with the tissue and mucus, as the menstrual phase begins again.

Ovarian Cycle

The ovaries also go through rhythmic, cyclical changes. The ovaries of a girl approaching puberty contain all the cells necessary for sexual reproduction. Each primary oocyte within the ovary is surrounded by several layers of cells that will become a follicle. Cells that produce estrogens surround the follicle as it matures. In each cycle, only one follicle from approximately 40,000 matures into a graafian follicle, which ruptures to liberate the ovum inside. Other follicles grow and develop simultaneously, but once one ripens and ruptures, the others decrease in size. (The exception to this rule occurs with fraternal twins, when two follicles mature and rupture and are fertilized by two different sperm.)

There are two ovarian phases. The **follicular phase** begins immediately after menses and ends in about the middle of the uterine cycle. During this phase the primordial follicle matures because of FSH from the anterior pituitary gland. The final maturation of a follicle and subsequent release of the ovum is influenced by a surge of LH from the anterior pituitary gland. The follicular phase is marked by the rapid growth and repair of the endometrial tissue after the menses. This regeneration is thought to be activated by the hormonal control of estrogen, which produces its maximum effect until ovulation occurs. Note especially in Figure 3-12 the developing follicle in relation to the growth of the endometrial tissue.

The **luteal phase** begins when the graafian follicle ruptures and the ovum is released. The precise mechanism causing rupture is not known, but the following factors contribute to it:

1. Increased pressure of fluid within the graafian follicle
2. Compression of the surrounding blood vessels because of size
3. Surge of LH from the anterior pituitary gland

After rupture, follicle walls collapse, turn yellow, and form the corpus luteum, which has a life span of 10 to 12 days unless the ovum is fertilized. During that span, it produces progesterone, a thermogenic hormone. In most cycles, the ovum is not fertilized and the corpus luteum degenerates, becoming a dry, scarred area called the *corpus albicans*. It produces no hormones, estrogen and progesterone levels drop, body temperature returns to the preovulatory range, and the spongy, edematous layer of the endometrium sloughs off.

Menstruation begins for most women 14 ± 2 days after ovulation, regardless of the length of the menstrual phase. Variation in the length of the cycle may be caused by a slower or more rapid buildup of the endometrium and follicle.

ALTERED MENSTRUAL PATTERNS

The term *cycle* implies regularity and predictability. The reproductive cycle begins with the ripening of the ovarian follicle and, if pregnancy does not occur, culminates in the shedding of the uterine lining—menstruation. Approximately 35 ml of blood, mucus, and cellular material may be accompanied by fatigue, myometrial contractions, and generalized discomfort.

For the majority of women, the menses occurs on a schedule of 28 to 32 days, lasts 3 to 7 days, and is an inconvenience. For some it is more debilitating because of the alteration in comfort and the type and amount of flow or because the regularity of menstruation is changed.

Dysmenorrhea

Dysmenorrhea is difficult or painful menses that interferes with normal functioning and requires treatment. *Primary dysmenorrhea* begins about a year after menarche and can include nausea, vomiting, diarrhea, headache, and pelvic, abdominal, and lower back pain. Prostaglandins are implicated in this condition because they are known to affect the myometrium and other smooth muscles such as the intestine. *Secondary dysmenorrhea* is usually related to pelvic pathologic conditions with a specific change in site, character, severity, or duration of menstrual discomfort. Endometriosis is found in about one half of women who are seen with secondary dysmenorrhea, and it may also be increased with the use of intrauterine contraceptive devices (IUDs) and with pelvic inflammatory disease, uterine fibroids, or endometrial polyps.

Many women experience severe cramping only on the first day of the cycle, others on more days. Pain may be relieved by nonpharmacologic methods: resting, applying heat, massage of abdomen or back, exercise as tolerated, and often relaxation techniques. Some women may require medication to alleviate pain. Current therapy includes antiprostaglandins such as ibuprofen (Motrin), naproxen (Naprosyn), and naproxen sodium (Anaprox). Some studies suggest beginning medication 2 to 3 days before expected menses. Women must be informed of side effects such as gastrointestinal upset and renal involvement. Experiments with transcutaneous electrical nerve stimulation (TENS) are promising and may be useful (Dawood and Ramos, 1990). Hormonal manipulation of the menses through use of oral contraceptives may be necessary for selected women.

May use diuretics, caffeine for diuretic effect.

Amenorrhea

Absence or changes in the cyclic regularity occur throughout the reproductive years. Theoretically, menses occurs every month, but normal ranges of 22- to 35-day intervals do occur. Both perimenarchal and perimenopausal women may notice months with shortened or lengthened cycles or an absence of menstruation. These omissions may be caused by anovulatory cycles. *Amenorrhea* is called *primary* if menarche has never occurred. Smaller or poorly nourished girls as well as athletes often delay attainment of adequate body fat to trigger menstruation. Family history is also a factor in assessing potential problems. Generally, until the girl reaches age 16, it is not considered a problem.

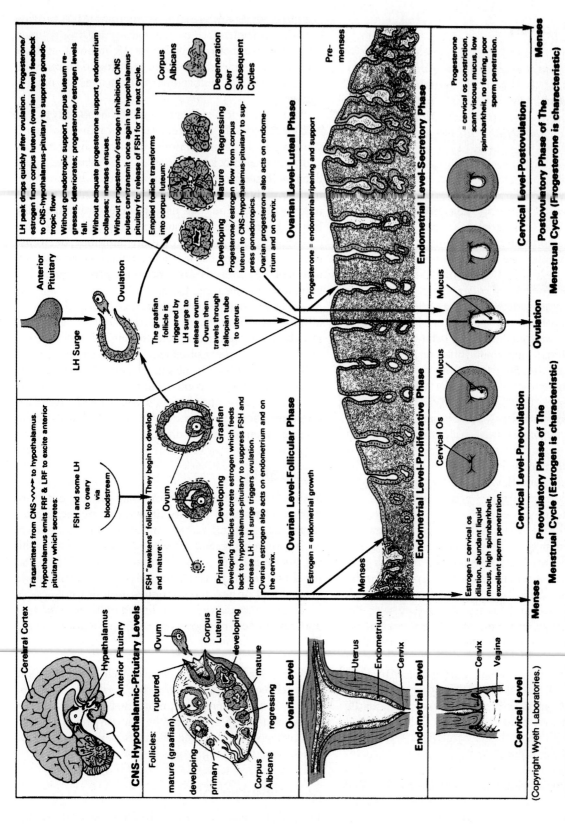

FIGURE 3-12 Menstrual cycle influences. Note mucus changes (*bottom of chart*) that correspond to changing hormonal influences. At endometrial and ovarian levels, note development of follicle in relation to growing endometrial tissue. *FRF,* Follicle-releasing factor; *LRF,* luteinizing-releasing factor. (Courtesy Wyeth Laboratories, Philadelphia, Pa.)

Self-Discovery

During the time you are studying maternity nursing, record the signs and symptoms of each menstrual cycle in yourself, a partner, or an adolescent in your family. Note if stress changes menstrual timing.

The main causes of *secondary* amenorrhea are pregnancy, use of oral contraceptives, and menopause, which are all related to hormonal feedback mechanisms or hormonal decrease.

Premenstrual Syndrome

The premenstrual syndrome (PMS) has been recognized as a significant problem only recently. PMS describes a wide variety of symptoms including behavioral, neurologic, ophthalmologic, gastrointestinal, respiratory, dermatologic, and breast alterations. The woman reports no problems for most of the cycle; symptoms are present only in the luteal phase of the cycle (5 to 11 days before menstruation). These changes must be noted in at least two consecutive cycles to be considered PMS.

It is estimated that at least 40% of women in the United States experience PMS routinely, about 70% of whom are incapacitated for a period of time by the symptoms. Epidemiology elsewhere is difficult to calculate, because cultural norms influence women's awareness of or willingness to report such difficulties. The precise triggering of PMS is unknown, although hormonal imbalance, vitamin deficiencies, prostaglandin levels, and psychologic factors have been proposed. Research has shown an increase in estrogen, with decreased progesterone, ovarian steroid hormones, endogenous opioids, and lower levels of magnesium and zinc. Lower levels of vitamins B_6, E, and A have also been linked to these symptoms (Hsia and Ling, 1990).

Because the exact cause of PMS is unknown, there is no universal treatment. Treatment approaches are based on theories. Various studies show the advantages of altering diet to decrease intake of caffeine, excess sodium, refined sugar, alcohol, and tobacco. It is recommended to increase complex carbohydrates, fiber, and protein. Supplements with vitamin B_6, A, and E either throughout the cycle or in the 10 days before menses have been found useful. Addition of magnesium, zinc, and calcium has also been beneficial for some women. Care must be taken to avoid vitamin overdose.

Stress reduction throughout the cycle appears to relieve the symptom severity. Maintaining adequate rest

avoid Chocolate

and relaxation and teaching coping strategies provide the woman some sense of control. An exercise regimen involving a minimum of 30 to 45 minutes at least three or four times a week has been found to raise the serum levels of endorphins that act as a natural analgesic.

Pharmacologic treatment should be an adjunct to diet and exercise routines. Effectiveness is individual, with some relief of symptoms noted from beta-blockers, calcium channel blockers, bromocriptine (Parlodel), and danazol (Danocrine), an androgen that inhibits endometrial development. Diuretics may be prescribed to eliminate water buildup, and use of antianxiety drugs may help decrease feelings of nervousness and panic. The action of evening primrose oil is not described, but its use has been found to be beneficial. Finally, hormonal adjustment by means of natural progesterone or gonadotropic-releasing factor (GRF) agonists may be prescribed to regain steroidal balance. Prostaglandin inhibitors have been tried with inconsistent success. Therapy should be specific for each woman, according to her needs and the results obtained.

These variations in menstrual patterns have gained serious attention at women's health centers. Especially as perimenopause approaches, a woman will have many questions about her reproductive cycle. Women's health care and menopause are discussed in Chapter 4.

Sexuality

Sexuality encompasses far more than just the gender of a person or sexual activity. It involves physical, emotional, and cultural factors and is an intrinsic part of each human being. Sexuality begins at conception, with sex determination, grows in infancy and childhood as the infant learns to relate to the people and the world around him or her, and continues until death.

The term *sexuality* is often linked only with romance and genital activity; however, sexuality is intrinsic and influences every aspect of a person's life. The product of many factors, it impinges on a person's choice of career as well as sexual partner, friends as well as interests, and both self-perception and how that person is viewed by others. Sexuality enervates, motivates, defines, and also grows and changes with the individual person. Gender identity, sexual roles, and choice of sex partner are all parts of that ongoing process.

GENDER IDENTITY

Biologically, sexuality cannot be changed after conception, but awareness and identification of one's sex can be influenced from birth. By age 3, this view of self as male or female is already formed, determined by how the child is treated and sex role models. It is also affected by the exploration and manipulation of infantile and childhood sex play, as the child discovers his or her own body and its sensations and pleasures. Play in later childhood allows for practice of sexual roles as perceived by the child, doing what is established as appropriate for men and women. Positive or negative reinforcement of identity is derived from parents' and care givers' reactions to this play.

During adolescence identity formation evolves, influenced by familial, cultural, religious, societal, and environmental factors. Traveling between childhood and adulthood, the adolescent is confused, insecure, and uncertain and expresses sexuality without care or awareness of its impact on self or others.

As the adult matures through middle age and into older age, sexual functioning may be affected by physical changes that may limit sexual activity or alter self-esteem. However, sexuality can easily remain intact as the person explores new or alternative ways to express it.

SEX ROLES

Masculine and feminine behavior is defined by society, family culture, and religion. Characteristics considered acceptable are assigned to each sex, although they are often not peculiar to one sex or the other but found in both. Traits such as determination, drive, and dominance that are traditionally considered masculine are certainly present in women, just as sensitivity, gentleness, and the tendency to be passive are integral traits of men.

Sex roles define how gender identity is expressed in and for the person's world. This expression differs from family to family and culture to culture. In some societies, there is a sharp distinction between acceptable male and female roles, actions, and basic self-worth. Men may be considered to have more rights and more value in the society in matters of finance and politics, whereas a woman's role may be subservient and evaluated in her ability to nurture within the home, caring for her husband and children. Other cultures reverse this pattern, affording more respect to women and making them the dominant force.

In Western society today, as a result of the emphasis on women's rights, abilities, and equality, traditional roles of the male as provider and the female as child-rearer and homemaker have given way to nontraditional settings. Personal choice, economic need, and new family structures have given rise to more women becoming "breadwinners" as some men assume or share homemaker tasks. Sex roles have merged, and it will be interesting to see the results in the years ahead.

Sexual behavior is also regulated by society. Freedom to engage in or prohibitions against that sexual activity are established by culture and often by religion. When norms are challenged, whether by influx of another culture or by internal culture influences such as advertising or entertainment, there can be confusion, and even guilt, as individuals struggle with the role they have been taught is acceptable and the new one they feel they "should" espouse. This is especially difficult in the adolescent stage of searching and validating sexual identity.

SEXUAL RESPONSE

Both males and females respond to any sexual stimulation by experiencing a cycle of events. Masters and Johnson (1966) are the best known in describing the four phases of *excitement, plateau, orgasm,* and *resolution*. In both sexes, these phases are characterized by vasocongestion and myotonia (muscle tension and increased contractility). Both sympathetic and parasympathetic pathways are involved, and hormones also play a part, with testosterone and serotonin/dopamine release influencing male and female responses.

Both sexes are stimulated by both physical and emotional factors. Although the genitals and breasts are the most sensitive as erogenous areas, any part of the body can cause sexual arousal, initiating the physical response cycle.

Female Responses

Sexual stimulation in the female initiates the excitement phase of her response cycle. Parasympathetic innervation increases blood flow to the vagina, vulva, and clitoris, causing enlargement of the clitoris and swelling and elongation of the vagina. The vestibular glands are stimulated to secrete introitus and vaginal lubrication. During the plateau phase, the clitoris is most sensitive, and with pelvic and vaginal congestion decreasing vaginal diameter, penile friction also stimulates receptors in the walls of the vagina, triggering orgasm. With this phase of heightened pleasure, central nervous system reflexes cause contractions of the perineum, uterus, and fallopian tubes. These rhythmic pulsations are thought to aid the sperm in entering the cervix and traveling through the rest of the reproductive tract (Figure 3-13).

The muscle spasms allow trapped blood to be drained by the venous system. Female resolution is not as complete as the male's. Because much blood may remain trapped, her erectile tissue remains engorged and sensitive, so a woman is able to achieve multiple orgasms within a short period of time. The sexual response in the breasts is illustrated in Figure 3-14.

Male Responses

In the male sexual stimulation in the excitation phase results in triggering of the central nervous system.

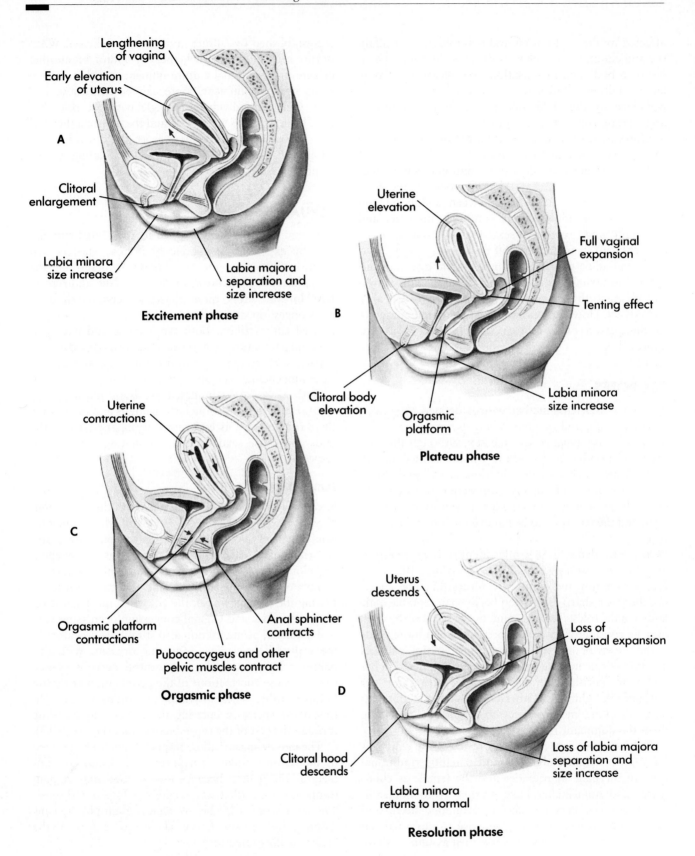

FIGURE 3-13 Major external and internal changes in the female during the female sexual response cycle. **A,** Excitement phase. **B,** Plateau phase. **C,** Orgasmic phase. **D,** Resolution phase. (Courtesy Medical and Scientific Illustration, Crozet, Va.)

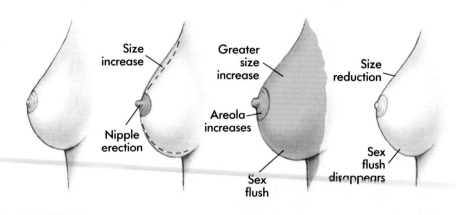

FIGURE 3-14 Changes in the breast during the female sexual response cycle. (Courtesy Medical and Scientific Illustration, Crozet, Va.)

Parasympathetic vasodilation increases blood flow into the corpora cavernosa, causing engorgement and compressing veins, which prevents venous drainage. During the plateau phase, the penis becomes erect and increases in length and diameter, and the testes are drawn up toward the abdomen.

Orgasm occurs at the peak of sexual excitement, involving intense feelings of pleasure and sensitivity. Impulses are sent via sympathetic fibers to the testes, epididymis, and the ductal system, resulting in release and transport of sperm by peristaltic waves, and secretion of fluids by the seminal vesicles, prostate, and bulbourethral glands to create seminal fluid. Pressure from the engorged penis stimulates forceful, rhythmic muscle contractions that propel semen out through the meatus (Figure 3-15).

Resolution occurs as stimuli change, causing vasodilation to allow venous drainage. As circulation returns to normal the penis returns to usual size and flaccidity.

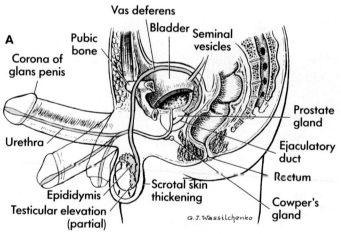

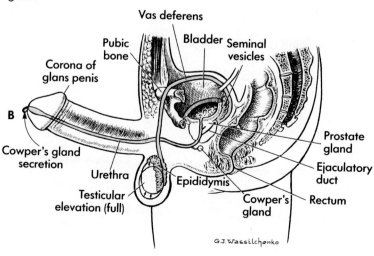

FIGURE 3-15 Major external and internal changes in the male during the male sexual response cycle. **A,** Excitement phase. **B,** Plateau phase.

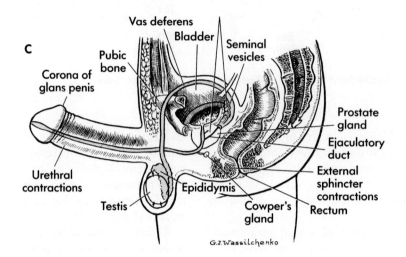

C

Corona of glans penis

Pubic bone

Vas deferens

Bladder

Seminal vesicles

Prostate gland

Ejaculatory duct

External sphincter contractions

Rectum

Urethral contractions

Testis

Epididymis

Cowper's gland

G.J.Wassilchenko

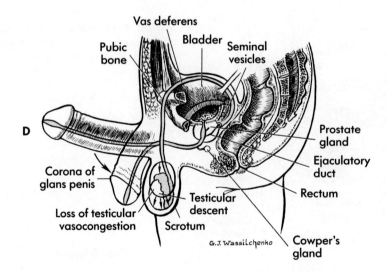

D

Pubic bone

Vas deferens

Bladder

Seminal vesicles

Prostate gland

Ejaculatory duct

Rectum

Corona of glans penis

Loss of testicular vasocongestion

Testicular descent

Scrotum

Cowper's gland

G.J.Wassilchenko

FIGURE 3-15, cont'd C, Orgasmic phase. D, Resolution phase. (Courtesy GJ Wassilchenko.)

KEY POINTS

The intricate interworking of anatomy and physiology in the human reproductive cycle will underlie the remainder of this text. When you discover you have a clear picture of "how it works," you will be able to assess and plan nursing care more readily.

- Male and female anatomy is initially identical until about the fifth week of development.
- Because of a common beginning, there are parallels in structures and function of hormones.
- The spermatozoa live 2 to 3 days after ejaculation, whereas the ovum survives only 24 hours.
- Pubescence precedes puberty by about 2 years. Gradual development of secondary sex characteristics signals the approach of puberty.

- Most girls and women are not well educated about the menstrual cycle, despite monthly experiences.
- Estrogen and progesterone can be thought of as counteracting several of each other's effects but work together for other effects.
- Premenstrual syndrome has finally been described and is being studied, and treatment is offered to the 40% of women who experience symptoms.
- Human sexuality is integral in life regardless of whether intercourse is practiced.
- Surrounded with cultural values and restrictions, adolescents try to break parental restrictions in sexual experimentation; thus clear cause-and-effect education about sex is important early in adolescence.

STUDY QUESTIONS

3-1 Which of the terms in this chapter apply to the following statements?
   a. The mobile end of the fallopian tube is the _____ .
   b. The uterine layer responsible for contractions during birth is _____ .
   c. Except for the days around ovulation, the vaginal environment is usually _____ because of its pH.
   d. _____ , a hormone found in many body tissues, is involved in uterine cramping during menstruation.
   e. The continuous process of forming the male reproductive cell is _____ .
   f. Sperm are formed first in the _____ .
   g. The term for painful menses is _____ .

3-2 Which is true of spermatogenesis?
   a. Immature sperm begin to develop in Leydig's cells.
   b. Sperm do not develop until testicular descent into the scrotum.
   c. Spermatozoa develop under the influence of hormones at puberty.
   d. Sexual excitation triggers formation of spermatozoa.

3-3 The portion of the uterus that extends above the insertion of the fallopian tubes is the:
   a. Cervix
   b. Body

   c. Isthmus
   d. Fundus

3-4 Menarche is defined as the first:
   a. Cycle of ovulation
   b. Menstrual period
   c. Development of sex characteristics
   d. Complete hormonal cycle

3-5 Symptoms of premenstrual syndrome include:
   a. Irregular periods and decreased flow
   b. Hot flashes and joint aches
   c. Retention of fluid and mood swings
   d. Heavy vaginal bleeding and cramping

3-6 Match the length of menstrual cycle with what you know of its phases.
   a. If Marie ovulated on day 20 of her cycle, when would her next menstrual period be likely to begin?
   b. If Jane ovulates on day 12 of her cycle, when would her next period begin?
      1. Day 38
      2. Day 32
      3. Day 28
      4. Day 26

3-7 Which nutritional change is recommended in the treatment of the symptoms of PMS?
   a. Increase in total calories
   b. Decrease in caffeine
   c. Increase in sucrose intake
   d. Decrease in protein

Answer Key

REFERENCES

Adams L, Swider SM: Changing factors and changing needs in women's health care, *Nurse Clin North Am* 21(1):111, 1986.

Beischer & MacKay 1986 p. 94.

Bernhard LA, Dan AJ: Redefining sexuality from women's own experience, *Nurs Clin North Am* 21(2):125, 1986.

Dawood MY, Ramos J: Transcutaneous electrical nerve stimulation (TENS) for the treatment of primary dysmenorrhea, *Obstet Gynecol* 75(4):657, 1990.

Friedman C: *Behavior and the menstrual cycle,* New York, 1982, Marcel Dekker.

Gray H: *Anatomy of the human body,* Philadelphia, 1985, Lea & Febiger.

Harrison WM, Endicott J, Nee J: Treatment of premenstrual depression with nortriptyline: a pilot study, *J Clin Psychol* 50:136, 1989.

Hsia LS, Ling MH: Premenstrual syndrome: current concepts in diagnosis and management, *J Nurs Midwifery* 35(6):351, 1990.

Mason E: Medical causes of abnormal vaginal bleeding, *NAACOG's Clinical Issues in Perinatal and Women's Health Nursing* 2(3):294, 1991.

Masters WH, Johnson VE: *Human sexual response,* Boston, 1966, Little Brown.

Mishell R, Brenner PF: *Management of common problems in obstetrics and gynecology,* Oradell, NJ, 1983, Medical Economics Books.

Mitchell ES: The elusive premenstrual syndrome, *NAACOG's Clinical Issues in Perinatal and Women's Health Nursing* 2(3):294, 1991.

Moore K: *Essentials of human embryology,* Philadelphia, 1988, BC Decker.

Phillips L: That time of the month, *Nursing Times* 87(7):3, 1991.

Speroff L, Glass RH, Kasee NG: *Clinical gynecologic endocrinology and infertility,* Baltimore, 1982, Williams & Wilkins.

Stone FB et al: Fluoxetine in the treatment of late luteal phase dysphoric disorder, *J Clin Psychol* 52:290, 1991.

STUDENT RESOURCE SHELF

Bernhard LA, Dan AJ: Redefining sexuality from women's own experience, *Nurs Clin North Am* 21:125, 1986.
Much is being learned about women and sexuality, some of which is spelled out in this article.

Hsia LS, Ling MH: Premenstrual syndrome: current concepts in diagnosis and management, *J Nurs Midwifery* 35:351, 1990.
An overview of the current understanding of PMS.

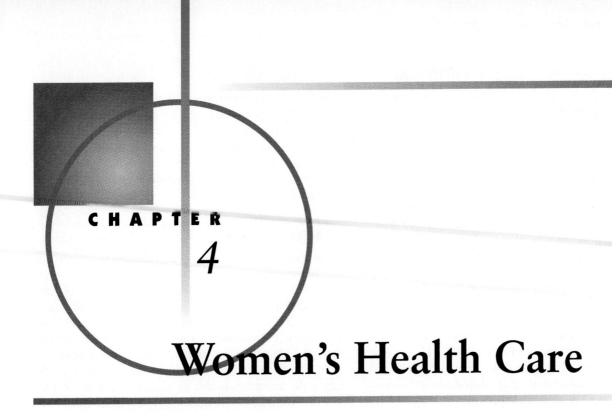

CHAPTER
4

Women's Health Care

KEY TERMS

*Breast Self-
  Examination*
Cancer Staging
Climacteric
Dyspareunia
Early Detection
Empower
*Estrogen
  Replacement
  Therapy (ERT)*
*Hormone
  Replacement
  Therapy (HRT)*
Mammography
Menopause
Osteoporosis

*Sexually Transmitted
  Diseases (STDs)*
*Toxic Shock Syndrome
  (TSS)*

LEARNING OBJECTIVES

1. *Discuss changes and current concerns in women's health care.*
2. *Identify the role of the nurse during the health visit.*
3. *Explain manual breast self-examination.*
4. *Recognize warning signs of physical, sexual, and psychologic abuse.*
5. *Develop a teaching plan for gynecologic hygiene.*
6. *Describe symptoms and prevention of toxic shock syndrome.*
7. *Identify learning needs to avoid sexually transmitted diseases.*
8. *Plan nursing care to meet the needs of the menopausal woman.*
9. *Identify risk factors for women's cancer, and develop a teaching plan for prevention, detection, and treatment.*

The birth of a new approach to women's health care today is the result of a long and complicated gestation nurtured by the feminist movement. Traditionally only reproductive issues were recognized as needing management by physicians, with general health issues often ignored, misdiagnosed, or misunderstood. Women perceived that the physician held the power, determined what needed to be done to treat any particular problem, and chose the course of therapy. Unsuccessful treatment often left the woman with the realization that her complaints were seen as vague and psychogenic and that she "would just have to live with it." Difficult menstruation, body changes after menopause, and even nongynecologic symptoms such as chest pains or abdominal discomfort all too frequently were not given appropriate attention and follow-up. Acceptance of a passive and cooperative role left a woman with little choice but simply to accept and follow instructions, whether helpful or not.

Changes in Women's Health Care

Contemporary approaches to women's health care are the result of societal trends in feminism and consumerism. Women are no longer satisfied with having only minimal input concerning their diagnoses and treatments. The focus now is to provide holistic health care that values the woman's participation and cooperation, demystifies the health care experience, and creates a more collegial environment in which the woman is the true owner and caretaker of her body. At the same time the role of physician is evolving from authoritative and hierarchic to consultative and supportive.

As the philosophy has changed, so have the settings and the providers of care. Although women's health care still is based mainly in obstetric-gynecologic settings, there is a move to develop offices or clinics that will serve as centers for women's total health management. All aspects of health needs would be included, with physical, emotional, and reproductive concerns intrinsic to helping the whole person.

Within this changing environment, nursing is able to develop more fully the role it always has played in health care. Long known as advocates, teachers, and counselors, today nurses' expanded roles as primary care givers include clinical nurse specialists, nurse practitioners, and certified nurse-midwives. Women can now receive total assessment, planning, treatment, education, counseling, and support from nurses either in collaborative practice with a physician or in their own private practices. Although some women find it difficult to accept diagnosis and prescription from someone other than a physician, many appreciate the new approach.

GOALS OF CARE

Goals for women's health have changed from treatment of problems to maintenance of wellness, which promotes self-care through education and support. The major objective is to **empower** each woman—to give back control over her body and its health by treating her as an informed and independent learner, to respect informed decisions about how she will be treated, and to encourage the sharing of information from woman to woman. Total physical, psychologic, and sexual wholeness is the expected outcome of this exciting and challenging new approach.

These goals are set for an ever-changing population—to meet needs of the young and older woman, the physically challenged and chronically ill, the sexually active heterosexual and lesbian woman, the corporate executive, and the homeless mother. Wellness for all women is the ultimate aim.

The Health Visit

A woman's first impression of the health care setting often influences her decisions to continue seeking care. The surroundings, sense of respect and privacy, and the attitude of all staff members combine to make the experience a positive and valuable one. Courtesy, an unhurried atmosphere, and sensitivity to the woman's feelings decrease anxiety and put her more at ease.

HEALTH HISTORY

After initial introductions and explanations of personnel and their roles, a careful history is taken by interview or in writing, or a combination of the two (Figure 4-1). Questions should be clear, nonthreatening, and specific. If the history is taken verbally, adequate privacy must be provided to allow for honesty without fear of embarrassment or disclosing relevant information. The history should include any area that might affect the woman's health or the maintenance of that health. Her medical, surgical, reproductive, nutritional, sexual, psychologic, social, occupational, economic, cultural, and religious status is reviewed, along with any history of substance use or abuse. Educational level is evaluated so that teaching is personalized to meet each woman's level of understanding. On completion the health history should be reviewed with the woman so that both she and the interviewer can ask questions or clarify information.

PHYSICAL ASSESSMENT

General Examination

The woman often perceives the physical examination as unpleasant and traumatic. Being inspected while undressed, having her body touched, probed, and pal-

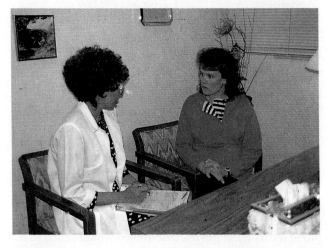

FIGURE 4-1 Each client is interviewed to identify individual concerns. (Courtesy Marjorie Pyle, RNC, Lifecircle.)

pated, and assuming uncomfortable and embarrassing positions make her feel a loss of privacy, dignity, and control. Many women avoid health care because of it. Explanations, provision of a private and secure area to change to patient gown, and not exposing body parts unnecessarily can alleviate some anxiety. In addition, allowing the woman to sit at a 30- to 45-degree angle instead of lying flat allows eye contact and communication during the genital and pelvic examination. Provision should be made to allow someone of her choosing to stay with her at all times. If the examiner is male, a female staff member should be present to guard against any misunderstanding or misinterpretation of conduct.

Examination of the woman may involve simply a reproductive assessment or a complete physical review of systems if her care is not being followed by any other practitioner. Vital signs, height, and weight always are obtained, and cardiopulmonary wellness should be ascertained. Usual laboratory work includes complete blood count; electrolytes, glucose, cholesterol, and triglyceride values. Rubella titer, blood type, and Rh status may be done.

For a woman at risk, testing for hepatitis B, syphilis, gonorrhea or toxoplasmosis and, with the woman's consent, human immunodeficiency virus (HIV) may be included. Urine is analyzed for blood, glucose, acetone, and protein, and, if indicated, a tine or purified protein derivative (PPD) test may be used to detect tuberculosis exposure. During the gynecologic examination, specimens may be obtained for culture or cytologic analysis.

Gynecologic Examination

Gynecologic assessment includes examination of the breasts, vulva, vagina, cervix, and uterus. The rectum also should be included in the evaluation.

Breasts. Breast examination is an essential part of any woman's physical examination, with explanation of the procedure and findings clearly given. The procedure should be performed in both upright and supine positions, allowing for visual inspection and palpation. The woman should be encouraged to perform breast self-examination before, along with, or after the practitioner.

Breast self-examination. The procedure for manual self-examination recommended by the American Cancer Society and may be performed either while standing or when lying down (Box 4-1). In a supine position the woman is instructed to place one arm behind her head, while examining the breast on that side. With the tips or pads of the three middle fingers, the entire breast is felt (palpated) firmly but gently. To ensure covering the entire area, the woman may choose one of the following patterns:

- In circular motion, starting at the nipple and moving outward

- In a line back and forth across the breast
- By dividing the breast into wedges and palpating each segment separately

The nurse also should teach the woman to palpate up into the axilla to examine the tail of the breast. The woman then switches sides and examines the second breast in the same manner. Many women prefer to do this in the shower, where warm soapy water eases the movement of fingers and is less irritating to the skin.

Teaching includes visual examination in front of a mirror. The woman should inspect for skin dimpling or pulling, redness or swelling, or nipple changes.

Genitalia. The genital and pelvic examination is performed with the woman supine, her head and shoulders elevated if possible. Stirrups support her feet, and she is instructed to move her buttocks to the bottom end of the table. She is draped whenever the area is not being visualized, and she is informed before she is touched. A mirror may be provided so that she is able to observe what the examiner is doing and learn about her own normal anatomy for self-examination.

For many women, being instructed and encouraged to look at, to touch, and become thoroughly familiar with their genitalia may be a natural and comfortable experience. Others, however—because of personal, cultural, or religious influences—find this difficult, embarrassing, or even distasteful. By teaching this aspect of self-care as part of total health maintenance, the nurse may alleviate anxiety and foster the woman's sense of self-mastery and control. If she does not wish to participate, she is still informed of the results of each step of the examination.

The external genitalia are first inspected for infection, lesions, or trauma. A warmed and lubricated speculum is then inserted into the vagina to visualize the vaginal vault, walls, and cervix (Figure 4-2). Secretions or drainage is noted, and specimens for the Papanicolaou smear or culture may be obtained. Once the speculum is removed, a bimanual pelvic examination is performed, with two fingers of one hand inserted into the vagina while the examiner's other hand palpates the uterus for size, position, shape, tenderness, and masses (see Figure 9-10).

There should be little or no discomfort during the vaginal and pelvic and rectal examinations. Most women tend to tense before digital or speculum insertion; some grab the table or someone's hand. Although this may seem reassuring, it actually increases the resistance the examiner encounters and causes discomfort. Preparing the woman for the sensations of pressure and assisting her with techniques such as slow, rhythmic breathing will relax vaginal and pelvic floor muscles, allowing easier access for examination.

After changing gloves, the examiner assesses the rectum by palpation with a lubricated gloved finger. A

BOX 4-1   Breast Self-Examination

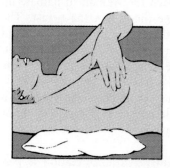

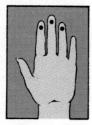

Finger Pads

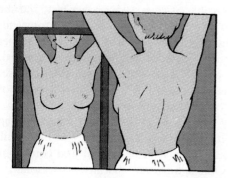

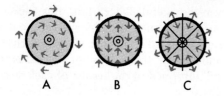

A   B   C

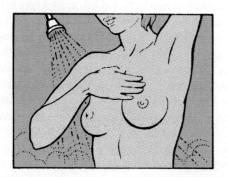

The best time to do breast self-exam is right after your period, when breasts are not tender or swollen. If you do not have regular periods or sometimes skip a month, do it on the same day every month.

1. Lie down and put a pillow under your right shoulder. Place your right arm behind your head.
2. Use the finger pads of your three middle fingers on your left hand to feel for lumps or thickening. Your finger pads are the top third of each finger.
3. Press firmly enough to know how your breast feels. If you're not sure how hard to press, ask your health care provider. Or try to copy the way your health care provider uses the finger pads during a breast exam. Learn what your breast feels like most of the time. A firm ridge in the lower curve of each breast is normal.
4. Move around the breast in a set way. You can choose either the circle (*A*), the up and down line (*B*), or the wedge (*C*). Do it the same way every time. It will help you to make sure that you've gone over the entire breast area, and to remember how your breast feels.
5. Now examine your left breast using right hand finger pads.
6. If you find any changes, see your doctor right away.

Courtesy American Cancer Society.

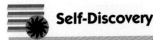

Self-Discovery

Teach yourself or a relative about breast self-examination.

specimen may be obtained at this time for a *guaiac* test (blood in the stool). Offer tissues to remove lubricant.

Safety is important when the woman returns to a sitting position. With assistance she is instructed to move up on the table and lower both legs together as the examiner supports her back.

Postexamination Discussion

Explanation and discussion of results, goal setting, and planning should take place outside the examining room, with the client fully clothed and comfortable. This is a time for clarification and collaboration, for explanation, teaching, support, and counseling. Before the woman leaves the office, she should know how to obtain the results of any tests she had, as well as with whom she can discuss the tests. If she needs a second visit, one should be scheduled at this time.

WOMEN'S HEALTH EDUCATION

Gynecologic Hygiene

General hygiene is an important part of any person's total health maintenance. In our society, cleanliness is considered extremely important, with an emphasis on eliminating, preventing, or disguising natural body secretions and odors. Perineal hygiene in particular is a major concern for most women, and products abound that promise "freshness" to their users. Although cleansing is necessary, frequent use of soap and water usually is sufficient to maintain hygiene. Over-the-counter (OTC) feminine hygiene products often contain chemicals that can alter normal flora, irritate tissues, predispose to infection, and disguise conditions that should be assessed and treated by a professional. Towelettes, deodorants, and sprays are unnecessary for most women and should be avoided.

Many women consider douching useful or even essential to ensure cleanliness. In fact, douches should be employed only if ordered as a specific treatment and then used with caution. Douches are administered by gravity, with the bag held less than 24 inches above hip level and never with the force of a bulb syringe. The nurse instructs the woman to use warm, not hot, water to prevent tissue trauma and to avoid instilling the solution under pressure, which could force the fluid or air into the uterus and out into the abdominal cavity.

Douching may be associated with ascending infection into the fallopian tubes (see Chapter 25).

Menstrual Hygiene

Menstruation is perceived as a particular problem for women. Menstrual flow with its normal musky odor is a source of embarrassment for Western women. Most often, bleeding is absorbed with use of disposable sanitary pads or napkins made of natural or synthetic absorbent materials. Culture or finances may necessitate the use of homemade fabrics such as cloth rags. Whatever the woman's choice, care must be taken to protect others from exposure to her blood by careful disposal or washing of the pads.

Many women prefer the use of internal vaginal tampons, either alone or with a sanitary pad. Made of combinations of cotton and synthetic fibers, they are small and compact for insertion with or without an applicator, and they expand as they absorb vaginal drainage. If inserted without trauma, positioned properly, and changed at least every 4 hours or sooner if saturated, they are a safe, comfortable, and effective way to eliminate the bulkiness of a pad and the chance of bleeding through or around it. Some women are unable to use tampons because of physical limitations or sensitivity to the products. Others may feel uncomfortable with genital manipulation or handling the soiled tampon. For those who wish to use tampons, correct use does not damage the hymen or affect virginity. Teenagers as well as adult women can use them.

Careful hand washing is essential with the use of tampons, both before and after insertion. Proper disposal to prevent contamination from blood also is an important consideration. Most tampons may be flushed in toilets that are connected to a sewer system, but to prevent bacterial build-up, they should not be flushed if a septic tank is used. Applicators generally are not flushable. Tampons also may be wrapped and disposed of appropriately in the garbage.

Tampons come in different absorbencies to accommodate various menstrual flow patterns. It is recommended to use the least absorbent size to guarantee changing it often enough. This is important to prevent **toxic shock syndrome (TSS)**, a condition arising from the growth of bacteria in the warm, moist, and nutritive medium that a saturated tampon provides. Although rare, TSS can cause serious illness and even death from systemic sepsis (see Box 4-2). TSS is discussed in more detail later in this chapter.

Specific Health Concerns
PSYCHOSOCIAL CONCERNS

Women are at risk for more than reproductive problems. They experience specific emotional problems in

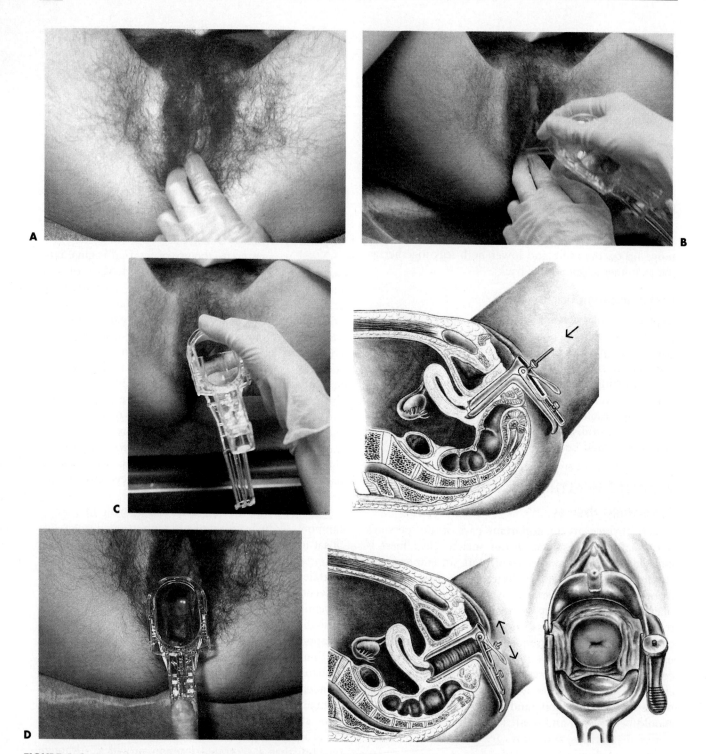

FIGURE 4-2 Vaginal examination. **A,** Preparing for insertion of speculum: applying downward pressure in posterior vaginal opening with two fingers. **B,** Inserting closed speculum over fingers. **C,** Directing speculum downward at 45-degree angle. **D,** Speculum in place, locked and stabilized. Note cervix in full view. (From Seidel HM et al: *Mosby's guide to physical examination,* ed 2, St Louis, 1991, Mosby.)

Self-Discovery

If you have had a pelvic examination, recall your own feelings. What are ways the nurse can increase client acceptance of the procedure?

higher proportion than do men, particularly with eating disorders, substance abuse, and depression. Alcohol and drug use has risen; smoking, however, is reported to be on the decrease (American Cancer Society, 1993; Horton, 1992).

An area of particular concern to women is their risk for becoming victims of physical and sexual abuse. Traditional or cultural views of the woman, particularly wife-as-property, devalue and render a woman powerless. Even though traditions are changing, domestic violence and rapes appear to be on the rise. It is suggested that simply more cases are being reported today. It has been estimated that 21% to 30% of women have been beaten by a partner at least once and that 1 in 600 women are rape victims (Horton, 1992) (for discussion of abuse see Chapter 26).

Often symptoms of abuse are hidden by the woman or overlooked by care givers. Physical examination must include careful attention to warning signs of repeated unexplained injuries, frequent emergency department visits, and bruises or scars. Building a relationship of trust, respect, and confidentiality with the woman may allow her to admit to the trauma. Collaboration with counselors trained in helping rape or abuse victims may aid these women.

Age does not protect a woman from abuse, and increasing numbers of older women are being treated and counseled as victims of abuse from spouses and children. Fear, guilt, and shame often prevent them from reporting their situations, and the health practitioner must be sensitive to all physical signs as well as verbal and nonverbal clues. (Chapter 26 discusses the nursing care of the psychosocially high-risk woman.)

PHYSICAL CONCERNS

Chronic Diseases

The number of women with chronic conditions such as hypertension, hypercholesterolemia, hyperlipidemia, and diabetes mellitus is significant, as is the rate of autoimmune disorders such as lupus erythematosus and rheumatoid arthritis (see Chapters 22, 23, and 24). Menopausal women also are at risk for osteoporosis and coronary artery disease.

SEXUALLY TRANSMITTED DISEASES

Women must be assessed for **sexually transmitted diseases (STDs)**. Syphilis, once considered under control, is now on the rise, along with gonorrhea. Chlamydia is the most frequently reported female STD today. Human papillomavirus (HPV), which causes genital warts, affects not only the woman's total health but predisposes her to other infections and increases her risk for cervical cancer. If the woman becomes pregnant, most STDs can be transmitted to the baby in utero or at birth. (See Chapter 25 for full discussion.)

Today two viruses threaten women as potentially lethal infections. Hepatitis B and the virus for acquired immunodeficiency syndrome (AIDS) can be acquired through sexual relations with an infected partner, and both are increasing in the female population. In 1991, 11% of new hepatitis cases and about 10% of reported human immunodeficiency virus (HIV) infections occurred in women (Horton, 1992). Because AIDS initially was seen as a gay men's problem, heterosexual women were considered to be safe and thus did not require education or warning about the disease.

AIDS, however, has become an increasingly severe problem for women, who are contracting the disease from sex partners infected through drug use, previous sexual activity, or exposure to contaminated blood. Education is essential in the control and treatment of AIDS in women. If it is at all possible that they have been exposed to the HIV virus, they should be taught to recognize early gender-specific indicators:

- Chronic candidal (yeast) infections, especially if they are unrelieved by local antifungal treatments
- Recurrent episodes of pelvic inflammatory disease, genital warts, and/or cervical carcinoma
- Menstrual irregularities or amenorrhea

Safe sex should be practiced with every partner, every time. If the woman is using a contraceptive method, she must understand that, although it may prevent pregnancy, it is not protective against the AIDS virus. Explanation that blood testing is important to the woman's well-being and not intended to be punitive or invade her privacy can assist in earlier diagnosis and allow treatment and follow-up care.

The total effect of AIDS on the families of the affected women and on society in general is yet to be seen, but as numbers increase, so must services, teaching, and support systems.

Vulvovaginitis

Not all vaginal infections are related to sexual activity. Many women experience irritations and infections that simply may be annoying or may lead to potential complications if left untreated (see Chapter 25).

BACTERIAL VAGINOSIS

Bacterial vaginosis (BV) has been known by many names, including *Haemophilus vaginalis* vaginitis, *Corynebacterium vaginale* vaginitis, nonspecific vaginitis, *Gardnerella vaginalis* vaginitis, and anaerobic vaginosis. This vaginal condition is not caused by one particular species of bacteria. Further, it does not induce the host inflammatory response. BV is associated with changes in the number and types of bacteria that are present in the vagina. *Lactobacillus* species and species of anaerobic bacteria are decreased in number, whereas *G. vaginalis* and possibly *Mycoplasma hominis* are greatly increased in numbers. Although BV is detected more frequently among women at risk for STDs, direct evidence of sexual transmission has not been established. BV accounts for 30% to 50% of all office visits for vaginitis; yet more than 50% of women with it have no symptoms and therefore do not seek treatment.

Signs

Most commonly experienced signs are increased thin discharge and odor. Odor may be especially noticed after intercourse because semen and vaginal secretions produced during sexual arousal increase vaginal pH, which then causes the release of gaseous amines that produce the odor. Vaginal irritation, burning or pruritus is uncommon.

Clinical Management

Diagnosis of BV can be made clinically by identifying three of the following four characteristics (Amsel et al., 1983):

- Increased, thin, homogenous, gray discharge
- Elevated vaginal pH > 4.5
- Presence of amine (fishy) odor spontaneously or with the addition of 10% KOH to the discharge
- Presence of "clue" cells on microscopic examination of a saline wet-preparation slide

Treatment for bacteria vaginosis in the absence of symptoms is not recommended at this time. If there are symptoms, ampicillin and amoxicillin are effective in 40% to 70% of women and may be used during pregnancy. Treatment of sexual partners also is not recommended. BV frequently recurs despite adequate treatment and may be frustrating to the woman and her partner.

don't have to abstain from sex but will aid healing.

TRICHOMONAL VAGINITIS

Trichomonal vaginitis is caused by the flagellated protozoan *Trichomonas vaginalis* and is responsible for approximately 25% of symptomatic vaginal infections. It is estimated that 2.5 to 3.0 million women contract trichomonal infections annually in the United States. *T. vaginalis* inhabits the urethra of men and women, in addition to the female vagina. It is transmitted primarily sexually, with an incubation period of 4 to 28 days.

Transmission by fomites, wet clothing or towels, and splashes from toilets, for example, has not been documented but is possible (Rein, 1984). Risk factors for acquisition of trichomonal infections are the same as for other STDs, with the most prominent factor being an increased number of sexual partners.

Signs

Approximately 50% of women with trichomoniasis may be symptom free. When present, the symptoms include increased gray to yellow-green, occasionally malodorous discharge, vaginal pruritus, dyspareunia, and dysuria. Examination reveals labia that may be pallid or erythematous. Discharge may be present on the vulva, and speculum examination frequently reveals excessive discharge. Vaginal walls may be erythematous. Gonorrhea cultures should be obtained for women with trichomoniasis because up to 50% of affected women may have concomitant infection with *Neisseria gonorrhoeae.*

Clinical Management

Referral of the woman's sexual partners for evaluation and treatment is recommended to prevent reinfection. A woman should be advised to abstain from intercourse or to use condoms until she and her sexual partner complete therapy.

Treatment is recommended both for symptom-free persons and those with symptomatic trichomonal infection. Oral metronidazole is the recommended treatment except during pregnancy. During the first trimester symptomatic relief may be achieved by using a *gentle,* dilute vinegar douche: 2 tablespoons of vinegar in 1 L water or a saline douche daily for 1 week and then twice weekly until beyond the first trimester. Clotrimazole antifungal cream provides symptomatic relief and has produced cure among 60% to 80% of women.

YEAST VAGINITIS

Yeast vaginitis is the second most common type of vaginitis. It is estimated that nearly three fourths of all women will have at least one episode of yeast vaginitis in their lifetime. These attacks may occur once or intermittently and may respond easily to treatment or may be recurrent, persistent, and chronic, resisting all forms of traditional therapy. Predisposing conditions that increase the risk for yeast vaginitis include pregnancy, oral contraceptive use, menstruation, obesity, antibiotics, corticosteroids, diabetes mellitus, and immunosuppression. Asymptomatic *Candida albicans* colonization occurs during pregnancy, affecting 30% to 40%. The newborn may contract the disease during birth. See Chapter 19 for treatment.

Increased glycogen stores in vaginal epithelium and increasing levels of estrogen and progesterone may provide the energy source and directly influence the virulence and growth of *Candida* organisms. In addition, the decrease in cell-mediated immunity noted during pregnancy may facilitate this process (Sobel, 1985). Women with recurrent or chronic candidal vaginitis should be screened for underlying disorders such as diabetes mellitus, hypothyroidism, and HIV infection.

Signs

Symptoms may be mild to severe. The most common symptoms are vulvovaginal itching, burning, soreness, dyspareunia, dysuria, and increased discharge often described as lumpy. Examination frequently reveals reddened vulva and vagina. Discharge often appears as white, curdlike plaques adherent to vaginal walls.

Clinical Management

Recommended treatments include a wide variety of antifungal vaginal creams, suppositories, or tablets. Vaginal therapies such as miconazole or clotrimazole require single daily dosing for 7 to 10 days. Single-dose and 3-day dosing regimens have been developed for clotrimazole but are not as effective as longer treatments in pregnant women. Even though miconazole and clotrimazole are considered safe for use during pregnancy, they should be used with caution during the first trimester. Follow-up examinations 1 to 2 weeks after completion of treatment are performed to evaluate treatment effectiveness. OTC preparations are now available but may be used ineffectively or discontinued too soon.

The lay press has recommended the use of vaginal preparations of lactobacillus for treatment of candidiasis. Such preparations have been shown to be contaminated with enteric microorganisms, including group D streptococcal enterococcus and *Clostridium* species, and are potentially hazardous to women and unborn babies (Hughes and Hillier, 1988).

Sexual partners do not require concomitant treatment. Abstinence during treatment has not been shown to improve therapeutic effectiveness or decrease recurrences.

After symptomatic infection has been detected, instruction on the method of administering medication, dosing frequency, and duration is essential. Panty liners may be desired to avoid staining of clothing with vaginal preparations. Some evidence suggests that tight clothing increases the vulval temperature and may promote candidal infection. Women often are advised to use cotton underwear and discontinue wearing pantyhose to increase air circulation in the vulval area.

A study recommends the use of a microwave on wet cotton panties to kill yeast spores because home washer and dryer temperatures are inadequate (Friedrick and Phillips, 1988). Care must be taken, however, because underwear may contain other fabrics (e.g., nylon or elastic) that may ignite in the microwave.

Clinical Decision

A client states that she douches vigorously four times a week because of a vaginal odor. What assessment questions should you ask, and which precautions should you teach?

TOXIC SHOCK SYNDROME

Toxic shock syndrome (TSS) is a severe, acute, multisystem, potentially fatal illness associated with distinctive bacterial pathogens. The exact pathogenesis of TSS remains to be understood. It generally is accepted that most cases are mediated by toxins secreted by distinct strains of *Staphylococcus aureus*. Colonization with toxin-producing *S. aureus* is not uncommon.

TSS was first described as a syndrome affecting children and adolescents in 1978 (Todd et al, 1978). After this report, TSS was noted among menstruating women and in 1980 was linked with superabsorbent tampon use.

TSS may affect women, men, and children of any age but most frequently occurs among young menstruating, white women between the ages of 10 and 30. Most cases among women (99%) are associated with the use of tampons. TSS rarely has been associated with use of contraceptive diaphragms and sponges. Nonmenstrual TSS may occur in association with puerperal sepsis, postcesarean delivery infection, mastitis, staphylococcal wound or skin infection that includes furuncles, infected abrasions, burns, or insect bites. Menstrual-associated TSS occurs annually in 6 or 7 of 100,000 women. Nonmenstrual TSS appears to have increased, whereas menstrual-associated TSS is declining.

Reasons for increased susceptibility during menstruation or after birth are unclear. *S. aureus* is more often isolated from the vagina during these times, suggesting some changes in the normal flora related to increased presence of menstrual fluid or lochia. Tampons and tampon constituents are being investigated to identify how their presence may increase toxic production of bacterial growth or cause local trauma that might facilitate systemic entrance of the toxin.

Signs

The characteristic symptoms of TSS reflect multiple system involvement. Onset may be sudden, with high fever, chills, sore throat, headache, myalgia, vomiting, diarrhea, hypotension, and a generalized sunburn-like rash (Box 4-2). Mucous membranes of the vagina and oropharynx may appear beefy red. Mucous membrane ulcerations may develop later. Generalized desquamation or sloughing and peeling of skin, including ends of

BOX 4-2   Toxic Shock Syndrome

- Sudden fever over 101° F
- Diarrhea
- Vomiting
- Muscle aching (myalgia)
- Rash similar to sunburn

fingers and toes, palms, and soles, occur 1 to 2 weeks after onset.

When death occurs, it is from cardiac arrhythmias, respiratory failure, and disseminated intravascular coagulation. Survivors may suffer prolonged sequelae, including renal failure, gangrene of fingers and toes, peripheral neuropathies, memory impairment, and the inability to concentrate.

Clinical Management

No specific diagnostic tests exist to identify TSS. The diagnosis is based on the recognition of clinical signs associated with the syndrome. Treatment depends on early recognition and requires integrated care for and support of cardiac, respiratory, renal, hepatic, metabolic, and central nervous system functions. Vigorous and persistent fluid resuscitation is uniformly required, with monitoring of blood pressure, renal function, and central venous pressure. Women should be advised of basic hygiene practices such as washing hands before and after tampon insertion. Labia should be held open with one hand while the tampon is inserted with the other hand.

Vaginal contraceptive devices should not be worn for prolonged periods and should not be used to control menstrual flow. Perhaps tampons and vaginal contraceptives should be avoided if possible *S. aureus* infections (e.g., boils) occur on other parts of the body.

Women should be advised that if they "lose" tampons or contraceptive devices, they should see a health care provider immediately so that the device may be removed promptly. Furthermore, women should be taught the symptoms of TSS and advised to seek medical attention if they occur during menstruation or the postpartum period.

Climacteric

Aging occurs in terms of reproductive capabilities. The man does not experience as dramatic a reduction in hormone production as does the woman, and therefore the male climacteric may occur more gradually and over a longer period of time. In the man the changes are more psychologic, producing a sense of the loss of youth and vigor and perhaps a realization that his life goals may not have been met. Subtle physical changes take place in the man from gradual diminution of testosterone levels (e.g., loss of skin elasticity and loss of muscle mass). Unless the man experiences a pathologic change in his reproductive anatomy, sperm production and fertility do not decrease.

For the woman, however, a definite and dramatic change in sexual functioning occurs. She experiences a period of transition, known as the climacteric, during which gonadal activity slows and ultimately ceases completely, resulting in physical and psychologic changes.

The climacteric is divided into the *premenopausal*, *menopausal*, and *postmenopausal* phases. Although menstruation may not cease until around the age of 50, premenopause may start as early as ages 36 to 42, with alteration in hormonal function. As the number of healthy ovarian follicles declines and sensitivity to gonadotropins decreases, estrogen levels fluctuate, with resultant changes in the menstrual cycle. Irregularities, as well as differences in character and duration of flow, often are noted.

PHYSIOLOGIC COMPONENTS

Menopause is defined by the last menses. Ovulatory function ceases, and estrogen levels drop, causing changes in estrogen-dependent tissues. Low estrogen levels affect stability between the hypothalamus and the autonomic nervous system and contribute to triggering the classic hot flushes or flashes experienced by 85% of menopausal women. Flushes also coincide with surges of luteinizing hormone (LH). Characteristic signs are reddening of the skin of the face, neck, and chest, along with a feeling of intense heat. Diaphoresis may occur. These episodes take place especially at night and in times of stress. It is surprising that hyperthermia does not occur; in fact, core body temperature drops during these flashes.

Breast tissue atrophy and vaginal lining thinning are related directly to decreased estrogen levels. Decreased vaginal mucus production also is universally noted.

Much attention has been paid recently to osteoporosis as a sequela of menopause. There is a loss of quantity of bone tissue, leading to increased fragility and postural changes. The mechanism involved is related to the effect of low estrogen on calcitonin levels, allowing calcium loss from the bone.

Lower levels of estrogen affect the cardiovascular system. During the premenopausal period, estrogen may lower serum low-density lipoprotein (LDL) and raise high-density lipoprotein (HDL) levels, decreasing the risk of myocardial infarction and cerebrovascular accidents.

Also included in the menopausal syndrome are symptoms with less well-defined causes. Fatigue, joint pain, dizziness, and palpitations are common. Emotional symptoms such as insomnia, nervousness, irritability, depression and abrupt mood swings are equally as common and frequently more disturbing than the physical symptoms. All too often in the past, only somatic discomforts were treated, and women were advised either to simply accept or to seek psychiatric help to deal with the emotional effects. Today more holistic care makes it easier for women to adjust to menopause and postmenopause, the years after the cessation of menstruation.

CARE DURING THE CLIMACTERIC

If the average age for menopause is 52 years, we realize that women will live approximately one third of their lives as postmenopausal persons. Many women have no difficulties adjusting to this new phase, whereas others need help to deal with problems related to hormonal changes. Nurses can help women accept menopause as a natural and nonpathologic process and realize that measures are available to ease the transition.

Nonpharmacologic Interventions

Common but noncritical symptoms such as hot flashes, flushes, atrophic vaginal changes, **dyspareunia** (pain during vaginal intercourse), urinary incontinence, insomnia, and mood swings or depression can be approached simply. Wearing layered, porous clothing, avoiding hot areas, and drinking cool liquids help lessen flash sensation. Relaxation techniques, especially slow rhythmic breathing and avoidance of stress, have been shown to increase vasomotor control, alleviating the embarrassment and discomfort that this sensation usually involves.

Kegel exercises help decrease stress incontinence. Lubrication with water-soluble jelly or oils and application of estrogen creams can compensate for vaginal dryness and tightness, making intercourse easier. Eliminating smoking is a healthy response to menopause. Adherence to a diet low in refined sugars, alcohol, caffeine, and sodium helps control body weight. Along with an exercise and relaxation regimen and stress reduction in general, these actions promote total wellness in addition to relieving individual symptoms.

Emotional and psychologic symptoms also can be affected by diet and exercise. Physical activity increases dopamine and circulating endorphin levels. Individual

 Self-Discovery

Interview a friend or relative in premenopausal, menopausal, or postmenopausal periods. Ask her to share symptoms and her reactions to these events.

or group support and counseling are of major help to the menopausal woman, offering her the opportunity to share her experiences with a professional and with other women. Often the ability to talk freely to an interested person or persons who can validate perceptions and offer practical advice may determine how easily a woman manages to cope during this time.

Prevention of Coronary Artery Disease

Decreased estrogen levels are involved with the major health problems of coronary artery disease, the leading cause of death in women. Diet modifications have an impressive effect on these conditions. Cholesterol and triglyceride levels can be lowered by limiting daily fat intake to 30% of the total calories, with no more than 10% of fat intake in saturated fats. The diet is then balanced with 20% of the calories obtained from protein and 50% to 60% from complex carbohydrates, especially those high in fiber.

Elimination of other risk factors such as smoking can make a critical difference in the severity of cardiovascular changes.

Prevention of Osteoporosis

The postmenopausal decrease in estrogen can cause osteoporosis, which predisposes the woman to fractures and their disabling sequelae. Slowing of bone resorption and increased bone mass can be accomplished by exercises that put stress on the bones, such as brisk walking, jogging, and weight lifting. Calcium and vitamin supplements, especially A and possibly K, are bone sparing as well. These preventive measures can spare the woman not only the general discomforts related to osteoporosis—such as lessening of height, kyphosis, and backache—but serious complications such as fractures related to increased bone fragility and poor healing potential, as well as respiratory compromise stemming from thoracic anatomic changes.

> **Test Yourself**
>
> List two signs in each of the following phases of the climacteric and the nonpharmacologic interventions for each sign:
> - Premenopause
> - Menopause
> - Postmenopause

Hormone replacement therapy (HRT). Although women can "learn to live" with some results of menopause, the trend is to prescribe HRT. Some are more at risk for serious cardiovascular effects and osteoporosis by heredity, physical status, or life-style. Others find that suggested changes are unsuccessful. For these women, hormone replacement therapy usually will be prescribed (Lichtman, 1991).

Much is written about the benefits and risks of taking estrogen or estrogen with progesterone to simulate premenopausal levels. Estrogen has been proved to dramatically decrease cardiovascular crises such as myocardial infarction (MI) in postmenopausal women (Philosophe and Seibel, 1991). By affecting liver metabolism, it maintains the level of HDL, preventing hypercholesterolemia, a known component of coronary heart disease. Estrogen also acts as a vasodilator and affects platelet aggregation. It has been estimated that the number of women suffering an MI is halved when estrogen replacement is given.

The concern in giving estrogen is its connection to breast and endometrial cancers, which leads to the question of whether estrogen replacement therapy (ERT) increases a woman's risk for malignancy. Many breast tumors are estrogen-receptor positive, that is, requiring and thriving on estrogen. Women with a very strong family history of breast cancer or those who have had cancer themselves generally are not considered to be candidates for ERT, although this no longer is viewed as an inviolable rule.

Estrogen is implicated in endometrial cancer because of its hyperproliferative effect on the tissue lining, causing cellular dysplasia that can become cancerous. The results of an endometrial biopsy should be considered before women who have had unexplained vaginal bleeding decide on ERT. Because estrogen is conjugated in the liver, ERT also should be withheld if the woman has active liver disease or chronic impaired liver function. Acute thrombophlebitis, a history of gallbladder disease in pregnancy, and a current pregnancy all are contraindications to ERT.

In addition to its effects on circulation and bones, estrogen replacement treats the vaginal atrophic changes, the loss of bladder control, vasomotor instability and insomnia, decreased libido, mood swings and/or depression, and memory loss related to menopause. Its benefits cannot be disputed, although its risks must be considered.

The risk of endometrial cancer can be decreased by the addition of progesterone to the hormone replacement therapy regimen. Progesterone has a protective effect related to decreasing estrogen receptor activity and breaking down estradiol. Unfortunately, progesterone does not have as positive an effect on the cardiovascular system and actually can lower HDL levels. Giving natural nonandrogenic progesterone and limiting the dose seem to alleviate this problem.

Dosage and duration appear to be factors in the relation of HRT to cancer. It generally is accepted that the smallest dose should be given for the shortest amount of time. HRT may be given as short-term therapy to alleviate symptoms during menopause, tapering off after cessation of menses, or as a long-term prophylactic measure. To achieve the desired effect on the cardiovascular and genitourinary systems and the bones, HRT may need to be taken for life. This may pose a significant problem for some women inasmuch as some studies suggest that although there is no significant increase of breast cancer when HRT is used for up to 5 years, there may be a 30% increase in rate when it is continued more than 15 years (Sitruk-Ware and Utian, 1991).

Replacement regimens should be individualized, on the basis of the woman's needs and tolerance. Doses should be adjusted to obtain the best effect from the least medication. Other risk factors actually may play a larger role in cancer formation than do the hormones. Obesity, for example, is strongly linked to both breast and endometrial cancers because estrogen is metabolized in fat cells, and levels of estrogen will be higher as fat cell mass rises. Controlling these factors may allow use of hormones with less risk.

Medication choices. Natural estrogens are used most often and are less potent than synthetic preparations. Estrogens can be taken orally, parenterally, by subcutaneous implant, suppository, vaginal ring, or in transdermal form. The oral route affects liver metabolism, therefore aiding in HDL level maintenance but possibly overloading the liver, causing gastrointestinal upset. Vaginal rings, which deliver medication well but may be irritating and cause inflammation and infection, are not as commonly used.

The easiest and most constant route is the ***transdermal patch,*** which is changed only twice a week and allows slow absorption, keeping levels constant. The Estraderm patch (estradiol) can irritate the skin but usually is well tolerated.

Dosage routine. Oral estrogen usually is given for 3 weeks and then stopped for 1 week of each month. When progesterone is given, it may be on a daily basis or as part of the cycle, added to the estrogen for at least 10 to 12 days. In the week that nothing is taken, menses will occur, which sometimes is unwelcome to the woman who has just gotten used to not menstruating. Progesterone is available in natural or synthetic form,

   Self-Discovery

After considering the risks and benefits of HRT, would you consider this therapy for menopausal symptoms?

and the nonandrogenic type usually is chosen to eliminate the hormone's effect on HDL. *Medroxyprogesterone acetate* (MPA) (Provera) commonly is used, and oral dosages vary according to form and route.

The decision to use HRT ultimately rests with each woman. She should be helped to assess her greatest risks and the options available to control them. Many women choose to use hormone therapy because they believe the benefits outweigh the potential risks. They should continue to be monitored carefully and screened meticulously according to guidelines.

Cancer in Women

Statistics published by the American Cancer Society (ACS) in 1993 describe trends in cancer death rates in the 30-year period between 1957-1959 and 1987-1989. Deaths of women from cancer of all sites increased from 120,969 to 232,843 in that time, and it is estimated that in 1993 249,000 women will die of cancer. Although the overall rate of cancer in women has not changed significantly in the last 4 years, specific sites showed dramatic increase.

LUNG CANCER

Deaths of women from lung cancer jumped from 4967 in 1959 to 48,098 in 1989—a 440% increase! Since 1987 more women have died of lung cancer than of breast cancer, making it the leading cause of cancer death in women. Smoking and exposure to secondary smoke are the major causes, with environmental pollutants and radiation also considered risk factors. Even though cigarette smoking among women has declined, cancer deaths continue because early detection is difficult. Tumors may grow for years *even after cessation of smoking* and are evident only when large enough for detection by radiograph. Consequently the overall 5-year survival rate is only 13% regardless of stage of diagnosis. Education of all women, especially teenagers and young adults, who often smoke, should include the facts about this preventable disease.

Test Yourself

- Why is lung cancer hard to detect early enough for better survival rates?

BREAST CANCER

Breast cancer continues to be a major threat to women, with the ACS estimating occurrence rates of 1 in every 9 women by age 85. Increased risk is seen in women who are older than 40 years of age, who have a personal or close family history of the disease, who never had children (nulliparity), or whose first pregnancy occurred after 30 years of age. Because current studies show an increased connection between estrogen and breast cancer, early menarche and late menopause are now being added as risk factors. High-dose or prolonged ERT may increase the chances of breast cancer in women already at risk.

Other possible links with breast cancer are alcohol use, high fat and caffeine intake, and smoking. Obesity also may increase chances of breast cancer because estrogen metabolism occurs partly in fat cells.

Screening

Probably the most common and important screening method women can use is manual breast self-examination. Every woman should know and practice breast self-examination monthly. A clinical physical examination by a professional is recommended every 3 years for 20- to 40-year-old women and every year after the age of 40 (see Figure 4-2).

Mammography is an important part of early detection. Although there is some controversy about its safety and efficacy, it still is endorsed by the ACS as a necessary part of screening. Guidelines include a baseline mammogram by age 40, repeated every 1 to 2 years between ages 40 and 49, and once a year for women older than 50. For younger women and those with denser breast tissue, examination by ultrasound (sonogram), computerized axial tomography (CAT), and magnetic resonance imaging (MRI) may prove more beneficial.

Although universal agreement on timing of specific procedures does not exist, it is known that consistency in screening affects success in diagnosis and treatment. Until mammography is readily available to all women regardless of economic status, diagnosis will be denied to many in need and mortality will increase among the poor.

Staging of Breast Cancer

Early detection is the key to successful treatment of breast cancer. In an effort to project a prognosis, a system was developed on the basis of cancer staging: primary tumor location and size (T) (Box 4-3), nodal involvement (N), and metastasis (M) (spread to other body sites). In general the lower the staging number, the better the prognosis. Treatment regimens also are based on the staging at diagnosis.

Clinical Management

Early detection and treatment by surgery, hormone manipulation, chemotherapy, or radiation therapy, or a combination, can increase the survival rate to around 90%, depending on staging at diagnosis.

BOX 4-3   Staging for Breast Cancer

Stage I	Tumor is 2 cm or less
Stage II	Tumor more than 2 cm, less than 5 cm
Stage III	Tumor more than 5 cm in greatest dimension
Stage IV	Tumor of any size with extension to chest/skin

From American Cancer Society: *Cancer facts and figures,* New York, 1993, The Society.

Surgery. Removal of all or part of the breast, muscles, and lymph nodes has been the treatment of choice for breast cancer. In early stages (stage I and even stage II), simple *lumpectomy* with axillary node removal is preferred when possible. In later stages a modified or even radical *mastectomy* may be needed. Reconstructive surgery can make it easier for the woman to adjust to a major procedure. Emotional support and practical assistance are available from self-help groups such as the ACS's Reach to Recovery.

Hormonal manipulation. After removal the tumor is tested for estrogen-receptor sensitivity. The estrogen receptor–positive tumor responds to the presence of estrogen for growth, which can be inhibited by binding the receptor sites with a drug such as tamoxifen (Nolvadex) to block estrogen uptake and prevent or slow tumor growth. Researchers are investigating the prophylactic use of this method in women with high-risk profiles.

Chemotherapy. Aggressive systemic treatment with a variety of chemotherapeutic agents is employed with or without surgical intervention. Although many women find it difficult to cope with the side effects of this therapy, advances in the management of symptoms such as severe nausea have eased treatment considerably, and results are encouraging. Autologous bone marrow transplantation also may be suggested to treat the devastating bone marrow suppression that may be caused by the chemotherapy regimen.

Radiation therapy. Whether or not tumor or breast removal is performed, the tumor may be treated locally by a course of radiotherapy. Preoperative radiation often is used to "shrink" tumors and to reduce the extent of surgery.

Most women are treated by multiple modalities, depending on staging, tumor type, estrogen assay, and general condition. Each treatment plan should be individualized and thoroughly explained so that the woman is able to make a well-informed decision.

CERVICAL CANCER

Cervical cancer has decreased 69% and uterine cancer by 52% in the past 20 years, but both are still significant risks. Women at risk for cervical cancer are those whose first intercourse occurred before the age of 18, who have multiple or promiscuous partners, and who smoke. History of infection with herpes simplex virus type 2 or human papillomavirus (genital warts) may predispose cervical cells to cancerous changes. Cervical cancer is most prevalent in African-American women and among lower socioeconomic groups, probably because they lack access to health teaching and the financial means to obtain screening services. As with breast cancer, cervical cancer is described by staging (Box 4-4).

Papanicolaou's Test

Papanicolaou's test (Pap smear) is credited as the main factor in earlier detection and treatment of cervical cancer. The ACS recommends that the first Pap test be performed when the woman becomes sexually active, or by the age of 18, and then every year with a pelvic examination. After three or more consecutive negative smear results, testing may be performed every 1 to 3 years on the basis of woman's risk status. Some experts believe that the test should be repeated once after the initial smear, and if both results are negative, the woman should have routine Pap tests every 3 years until age 35 and then every 5 years until age 60 when no further testing is necessary. Every woman exposed to diethylstilbestrol (DES) as a fetus should continue yearly testing because of the higher associated risk.

For the Pap test to be as accurate as possible, the woman should be instructed not to douche or use any vaginal products and to refrain from intercourse for 24 hours before the test. The examiner must use only water as a lubricant and follow accepted procedure for obtaining the cervical sample. Cells mistakenly taken from the vaginal walls or vault yield false negative results.

The woman also should be taught genital self-examination to detect changes on the labia and at the

---

BOX 4-4   Staging for Cervical Cancer

Stage 0	In situ, intraepithelial carcinoma
Stage I	Carcinoma confined to cervix
Stage II	Involvement of upper vagina
Stage III	Involvement of lower third of vagina/extension to pelvic side wall
Stage IV	Extension beyond the true pelvis

From American Cancer Society: *Cancer facts and figures,* New York, 1993, The Society.

vaginal introitus. Changes in color, lesions, or discharge can then be assessed early and treated.

Clinical Management

Precancerous cervical changes may be treated with *cryosurgery* (destruction of the cells by extreme cold) or by *electrocoagulation* (destruction through intense heat or electrical charges). Local surgery may remove the tumor, or more extensive surgery may be needed in later stages. Radiation therapy also is used.

UTERINE CANCER

Women most at risk for endometrial cancer generally are older, with a history of failure to ovulate, infertility, heavy or unusual periods, diabetes, obesity, and prolonged use of tamoxifen or ERT, especially without a progesterone component. Before menopausal women with a family history or other compromising factors begin ERT, an endometrial biopsy should be performed.

Signs

Uterine cancer is not always detected by the Pap smear; however, suspicious signs and symptoms include bleeding outside the menstrual cycle, unusual vaginal discharge, chronic pain, or bleeding after menopause. If cervical cancer is detected early, survival rates at 5 years can be as high as 89%, and 94% for cancer of the endometrium.

BOX 4-5   Warning Signs of Cancer

Lung
Cough, sputum streaked with blood, chest pain, back pain, and recurring lung infections

Breast
Breast changes that persist throughout the menstrual cycle, a lump, a thickening, swelling, skin dimpling, skin irritation, retraction, distortion, pain, scaliness, or nipple tenderness

Cervical and Uterine
Positive Pap smear, unusual bleeding, pain

Ovarian
Abdominal enlargement; vague digestive disturbances that persist and cannot otherwise be explained

Colorectal
Rectal bleeding, blood in the stool, a change in bowel habits

---

Clinical Management

Surgery and radiation are the usual therapies for uterine carcinoma. Hysterectomy is avoided as much as possible, especially in premenopausal women, but in later stages of the disease, hysterectomy with salpingo-oophorectomy may be indicated. Later-stage tumors also may require chemotherapy to control metastasis.

Test Yourself

- Correlate risk factors associated with each type of cancer listed in Box 4-5.

OVARIAN CANCER

Other cancers of concern to women are ovarian and colorectal. Ovarian cancer, the reproductive tract cancer that causes the most deaths, most often occurs in women older than the age of 60. Women who were never pregnant have twice the risk as those who have given birth. Early age with first pregnancy and early menopause, as well as oral contraceptive use, seem to be related to lower risk. The risk for ovarian cancer doubles in women who have had breast cancer. (See Box 4-6 for staging.)

Signs

Symptoms often are vague and not evident until late in the disease. Nausea, vomiting, abdominal bloating, discomfort, or pain commonly occur. Diagnosis is made by a pelvic, ultrasound, or laparoscopic examination. A new blood test, the Ca-125, may prove helpful in earlier discovery but is believed to produce inconsistent results at the present time. Because diagnosis often is delayed, the overall survival rate is 39% (ACS, 1993).

Clinical Management

Along with surgery, radiation therapy and chemotherapy are the common treatment modalities for women

---

BOX 4-6   Staging for Ovarian Cancer

Stage I	Tumor limited to ovaries
Stage II	Tumor involves one or both ovaries with pelvic extension
Stage III	Tumor involves one or both ovaries with peritoneal metastasis outside pelvis
Stage IV	Distant metastasis

From American Cancer Society: *Cancer facts and figures*, New York, 1993, The Society.

with ovarian cancer. In early stages, to prevent surgical menopause only the involved ovary is removed. In later stages, in addition to bilateral oophorectomy, the fallopian tubes and the uterus also may be removed, as well as any other intraabdominal lesions.

Together with traditional chemotherapy regimens, a new drug is being used with encouraging results. *Taxol,* derived from the bark of the Pacific yew tree, has been used successfully to treat ovarian cancers that were unresponsive to conventional therapy. It also is being investigated for use with breast and other cancers.

COLORECTAL CANCER

Colorectal cancer has declined since 1958, in large part probably a result of more frequent testing of stool for *occult blood.* Each woman should have this test with each physical examination, and after the age 40 a digital rectal examination should be performed every year. Survival rates have improved to 91% for colon and 85% for rectal cancers if they are detected at an early, localized stage (ACS, 1993).

Although cancer is not completely preventable, altering common risk factors of diet, smoking, and life-style may have some effect, and guidelines should be included in all health teaching (Figure 4-3).

Signs

Available screening procedures should be taught and encouraged as part of all health teaching (see Box 4-5). Analysis of a stool specimen for covert (hidden) blood by use of *guaiac* testing is a simple, effective, and inexpensive tool for spotting tumors; in addition, results can be obtained quickly. Positive results should be followed by proctoscopy or biopsy for further examination.

Clinical Management

Surgery to remove the tumor is the usual therapy, which may be accompanied or followed by radiation therapy. Surgery may involve resection (cutting out) or the

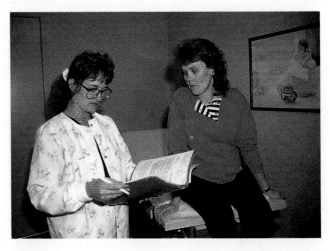

FIGURE 4-3 After the physical examination, findings should be discussed and self-care taught. (Courtesy Marjorie Pyle, RNC, *Lifecircle.*)

creation of an *ostomy,* bringing a portion of the intestine to the surface of the abdomen for evacuation stool into an external appliance. Current results using chemotherapy in the treatment of colorectal cancer are encouraging.

Test Yourself

- What does early detection mean for breast, cervical, and colorectal cancer?

Many cancers are preventable, and some are treatable or even curable with early detection and intervention. The hope is that with education and support, women will be able and willing to make necessary life-style changes to avoid becoming a cancer "victim." Nurses are working to make testing, services, and treatments available to all so that fewer women will be lost to this cruel disease.

KEY POINTS

- Woman's health care has changed dramatically in the past two decades. The hope is that less traditional settings and the change in practitioners' care and their goals to enable and empower women will improve the total quality of women's health.
- Women, who are victims of physical and sexual violence, need encouragement and education to admit their situations and to plan for protection.
- Women need teaching and counseling to avoid dangerous diseases such as sexually transmitted diseases (STDs), hepatitis B, HIV, and cancer.

- Women must be made aware of available resources and encouraged to take an active part in their own health maintenance.
- Client teaching for women clients should emphasize personal hygiene, with additional specific teaching at appropriate stages about menstruation, dysmenorrhea, premenstrual syndrome, and coping with the climacteric.
- Today the role of nursing is expanded and strengthened as specialists within the profession fill the void in women's health care.

STUDY QUESTIONS

4-1 Select key terms that describe the following statements.
a. The most important procedure in the detection of breast cancer is ___BSE___ .
b. ___TSS___ is a potential complication of the use of tampons.
c. Changes in frequency, regularity, or quality of the menstrual cycle may signal the woman in her 40s that she has begun menopause, or the ___Climacteric___ .
d. ___Osteoporosis___ is a common and potentially serious effect of postmenopausal estrogen depletion.
e. Chlamydial, gonococcal, and trichomonal infections are classified as ___STD's___ .

4-2 A client states that she is afraid of pain during a pelvic examination. The best nursing intervention is to:
a. Offer her a hand to squeeze during the procedure.
b. Position her flat to relax pelvic muscles.
c. Encourage her to breathe slowly and rhythmically.
d. Instruct her to bear down during bimanual palpation.

4-3 Women should be instructed to schedule a mammogram:
a. When they first become sexually active.
b. Every 3 years if results of the first one are negative.
c. Only when a lump is detected by self-examination.
d. Every year after age 50.

4-4 Preparatory teaching for a woman scheduled for a Pap smear should include:
a. Refraining from sex for 1 week before the test.
b. Wearing cotton underwear the day of the test.
c. Eliminating douching for 24 hours before the test.
d. Avoiding use of aspirin or ibuprofen for 24 hours before the test.

4-5 A decrease in estrogen is related to cardiovascular disease because low estrogen:
a. Predisposes to obesity.
b. Precipitates hypertension.
c. Alters HDL levels.
d. Causes fluid volume overload.

4-6 Which statement is most accurate concerning the risk of cancer related to hormone replacement therapy (HRT)?
a. Smoking, obesity, and diet increase the risk.
b. There is no significant risk with HRT.
c. HRT should never be continued for more than 2 years.
d. The benefits obviously far outweigh the risks.

Answer Key

c 4-3 d 4-4 c 4-5 c 4-6 a

4-1 a. Breast self-examination, b. Toxic shock syndrome, c. Climacteric, d. Osteoporosis, e. Sexually transmitted diseases 4-2

REFERENCES

American Cancer Society (ACS): *Cancer facts and figures,* New York, 1993, The Society.

Amsel R et al: Nonspecific vaginitis, *Am J Med* 74(91):14, 1983.

Bernhard LA, Dan A: Redefining sexuality from women's own experiences, *Nurs Clin North Am* 21(1):125, 1986.

Brucker MC, Scharbo-De Haan M: Breast disease: the role of the nurse midwife, *J Nurse Midwife* 36(1):63, 1991.

Clay LS: Midwifery assessment of the well woman, *J Nurse Midwife* 35(6):341, 1990.

Corson SL: Physiology of menopause and update on hormonal replacement therapy, *NAACOG's Clin Issues Perinat Women's Health Nurs* 2(4):483, 1991.

Cutler WB, Ramon-Garcia C: *The medical management of menopause and premenopause,* Philadelphia, 1984, JB Lippincott.

Dodds ME et al: A breast screening program in a community hospital, *J Community Health* 16(5):241, 1991.

Frank ME: Transition into midlife, *NAACOG's Clin Issues Perinat Women's Health Nurs* 2(4):421, 1991.

Franklin M: Reassessment of the metabolic effects of oral contraceptives, *J Nurse Midwife* 35(6):358, 1990.

Freedman RR, Woodward S: Behavioral treatment of menopausal hot flushes: evaluation by ambulatory monitoring, *Am J Obstet Gynecol* 167(2):436, 1992.

Friedrich E, Phillips LE: Microwave sterilization of *Candida* on underwear, *J Reprod Med* 33(2):1, 1988.

Hellberg D et al: Smoking and cervical neoplasia, *Am J Obstet Gynecol* 158(4):910, 1983.

Horton J: *The women's health data book,* New York, 1992, Elsevier.

Hughes VI, and Hillier SL: Lactobacilli from non-prescription products used for the treatment of vaginitis (Abstract No. C-218). Paper presented at the 88th Annual Meeting of American Society for Microbiology, Miami Beach, Fla, May 8-13, 1988.

Lichtman R: Perimenopausal hormone therapy—review of the literature, *J Nurse Midwife* 36(1):30, 1991.

Maddox M: Women at midlife: hormone replacement therapy, *Nurs Clin North Am* 27(4):959, 1992.

Mason E: Medical causes of abnormal vaginal bleeding, *NAACOG's Clin Issues Perinat Women's Health Nurs* 2(3):322, 1991.

McCraw R: Psychosexual changes associated with perimenopausal period, *J Nurse Midwife* 36(1):17, 1991.

Mishell DR, Brenner PF: *Management of common problems in obstetrics and gynecology,* New York, 1987, Year Book Medical Publishers.

Philosophe R, Seibel M: Menopause and cardiovascular disease, *NAACOG's Clin Issues Perinat Women's Health Nurs* 2(4):430, 1991.

Quinn AA: Menopause: plight or passage, *NAACOG's Clin Issues Perinat Women's Health Nurs* 2(3):304, 1991.

Quinn AA: A theoretical model of the perimenopausal process, *J Nurse Midwife* 36(1):25, 1991.

Rein MF: Nosocomial sexually transmitted diseases, *Infect Control* 5(3):117, 1984.

Rickert B: Estrogen replacement: making informed choices, *RN* 55(9):27, 1992.

Scharbo-De Haan M, Brucker MC: The perimenopausal period—implications for nurse-midwifery practice, *J Nurse Midwife* 36(1):9, 1991.

Sitruck-Ware R, Utian W: *The menopause and hormonal replacement therapy—facts and controversies,* New York, 1991, Marcel Dekker.

Sobel JD: Epidemiology and pathogenesis of recurrent vulvovaginitis candidiasis, *J Obstet Gynecol* 152:924, 1985.

Thomas B: Challenges for teachers of women's health, *Nurs Educ* 17(5):10, 1992.

Thorne S: Women's health studies at Queens' bring feminist perspectives to family practice, *Can Med Assoc J* 146(10):1815, 1992.

Todd JK et al: Toxic shock syndrome associated with phage-group-I staphylococci, *Lancet,* 36: 1116, Nov 25, 1978.

Videt W, Hutchinson D: New perspectives in the relationship of hormone changes to affective disorders in the perimenopause, *NAACOG's Clin Issues Perinat Women's Health Nurs* 2(4):453, 1991.

Whitman S et al: Patterns of breast and cervical cancer screening at three public health centers in inner city urban areas, *Am J Public Health* 81(12):1651, 1991.

Zapda J et al: Changes in mammography use: economic need and service factors, *Am J Public Health* 82(10):1345, 1992.

 ## STUDENT RESOURCE SHELF

Clay L: Midwifery assessment of the well woman, *J Nurse Midwife* 35(6):341, 1990. Although geared to the nurse-midwife, the information in this article is applicable to any nurse involved in the health care of women throughout the life cycle.

Maddox M: Women at midlife: hormone replacement therapy, *Nurs Clin North Am* 27(4):959, 1992. HRT is the most important topic for women to consider. Although benefit-risk ratios appear to be directed toward benefits, each woman needs to make a choice.

Women's health care: *J Nurse Midwife* 36(1), 1991. Entire issue devoted to various topics in women's health.

Women's health care: *Am J Women's Health* 1(1), 1992. Contains a number of relevant articles.

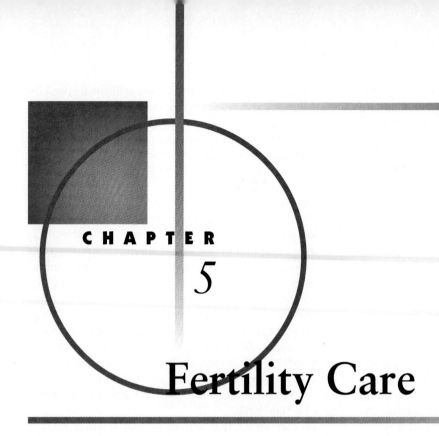

CHAPTER

5

Fertility Care

KEY TERMS

Abstinence
Amenorrhea
Basal Body
  Temperature (BBT)
Billings Method
Calendar Method
Chemical Barriers
Coitus Independent
Coitus Interruptus
Condom
Contraception
Diaphragm
Fertility Awareness
  Method
Intrauterine
  Device (IUD)

Lactation Amenorrhea
  Method (LAM)
Mechanical Barriers
Natural Family
  Planning (NFP)
Norplant Subdermal
  Implant
Oral Contraceptives
  (OC) ("The Pill")
Pelvic Inflammatory
  Disease (PID)

"Perfect Use"
Postcoital Contracep-
  tion
Sexually Transmitted
  Diseases (STDs)
Spermicidal
Spermistatic
Surgical Sterilization
Symptothermal
  Method

LEARNING OBJECTIVES

1. *Describe the advantages and disadvantages for each fertility control method.*
2. *Discuss application of the nursing process in planning care for clients seeking contraceptive assistance.*
3. *Describe the nursing role in counseling for reproduction and fertility control.*

Fertility Control

Fertility control is not a new concept; in fact, many methods have been used throughout history to prevent pregnancy. In ancient Egypt, for example, women used domes formed of hollowed lemon halves to cover the cervix. Other cultural groups have used tampons or followed elaborate rituals to prevent conception.

Today **contraception** means choosing and using a method to delay, prevent, or space pregnancy. It affords many alternatives and choices during the reproductive years. World population has doubled since the beginning of this century and is projected to reach 6 billion by the end of the century (Diczfalusy, 1991). Concern about this rapid population growth has prompted governments of many developing countries to underwrite family planning programs since the early 1960s (when an explosion in contraceptive technology began with the use of oral contraceptives and intrauterine devices). Thus family planning has become a well-recognized foundation for health care in most developing countries. Also since the 1960s it has been recognized that the health care aspect of family planning encompasses the control of sexually transmitted diseases and maternal, infant, and child well-being, as well as birth control.

In the United States the rising pregnancy rates for adolescents has engendered much concern among health care professionals in terms of prevention of sexually transmitted diseases and unwanted pregnancy. Accidental or unwanted pregnancies occur when contraception fails or when contraceptive needs remain unmet. Meeting contraceptive needs means being able to focus the interventional efforts on the "user perspective" (Diczfalusy, 1991). Understanding the user's perspective means the ability to step inside the shoes of the client and understand the cultural and socioeconomic constraints governing the choice and use of the birth control method. Often counseling is best received when a person is highly motivated to prevent pregnancy, such as after a recent birth. Many communities are placing the prevention of teenage pregnancy as a high priority for the health care of their citizens. Innovative programs of sex education and health care counseling are being proposed for the high schools, but funding for such programs is quite limited. A great deal of funding, effort, resources, and genuine interest in solving the teenage pregnancy problem are required before any real changes in the statistics can occur.

Contraceptive choices may be limited or enhanced by long-range personal or family goals, the expense of the method, feelings about sexuality, the relationship of the couple, the cultural significance of birth planning in the client's life, and religious beliefs about and psychologic importance of pregnancy (Tanis, 1977).

An ideal method of birth control follows these criteria:

1. Easy to use
2. **Coitus independent** (unrelated to the sexual act)
3. Safe
4. Inexpensive
5. 100% effective
6. No side effects
7. Acceptable to religious and cultural beliefs and practices of the users

No one method meets all these criteria. Consistency of use and persistence in using a contraceptive method are important factors in the prevention of pregnancy. Contraceptive failure, misuse, and nonuse are especially high among less educated people, adolescents, and homeless people. Moreover, the less educated and adolescent populations tend to rely on ineffective methods on the basis of hearsay or on measures that are cheaper and more readily available to them. Thus a great deal of work is needed to provide everyone with suitable contraceptive information and follow-up.

RATES OF EFFECTIVENESS

Part of the general evaluation of a method's acceptability is its rate of effectiveness. These rates, statistically projected from studies of small samples, use a percent-

age reading based on the results of use of the method by 100 women for 1 year. The phrase "per women-years of use" often is used, or a percentage based on the study of 100 women is given. If, for example, 100 women used a method and three became pregnant in that year, the effectiveness rating would be 97% or three pregnancies per 100 women per year of use.

Effectiveness rates can be misleading unless placed in careful context. For instance, the package inserts included with the contraceptive device (e.g., oral contraceptives, diaphragm, condom) often include "**perfect use**" effectiveness, which means the use of the method perfectly and consistently *every* time (e.g., taking the birth control pill every day without fail for 1 year). Also included in the package insert statistics are the average or "**typical use**" rates, which are real-world estimates of typical users. With methods that involve much user participation and responsibility, such as the diaphragm, condom, and spermicide, the gap between the perfect use effectiveness and the typical use effectiveness rates may be very large.

Another factor that affects the effectiveness rates is the age of the woman using the method. The older the woman, the more skillful, motivated, and diligent she becomes in her use of birth control. Older women also may be prone to have more predictable or planned times for intercourse, making contraceptive use easier (Gladwell, 1993). Effectiveness of contraception increases with other factors as well, such as income, education, and life-style (Mosher, 1990). It has been demonstrated in some studies that nonsmokers have better contraceptive use and effectiveness rates than do smokers, perhaps because of a less risk-taking approach to their lives (Helbig, 1987; Lethbridge, 1991). The most highly motivated contraceptive users seem to be young, single, educated women with careers. This group, perhaps the most successful users of contraception, may approach the "perfect use" statistic for any of the methods they choose. (Effectiveness rates used in this chapter are from Hatcher et al, 1990, unless otherwise indicated.)

 Self-Discovery

If you have used a family planning method, how would you describe its ease of use and side effects for you and your partner? Would you consider an alternate method? If you have not used a method, imagine a scenario in which you need a method. After you read this chapter, which one appeals to you and why?

Nonhormonal Family Planning Methods

FERTILITY AWARENESS AND NATURAL FAMILY PLANNING

The **natural family planning (NFP)** and **fertility awareness methods** are based on the events of the menstrual cycle. The ovum is viable for approximately 1 day after ovulation, and sperm are viable for approximately 2 to 3 days after being deposited in the vagina. The "unsafe" time during each menstrual cycle then is 2 days before and after the day of ovulation (minimum of 5 days). Because the variation in length of the cycle occurs before ovulation, the couple using this method must refrain from intercourse during a longer period. The partner needs to be an integral part of this method, and accurate records of the cycles must be kept. The means of calculating the woman's peak fertility follow.

Rhythm or Calendar Method

The rhythm or **calendar method** is based on a record of the woman's previous six menstrual cycles. The number of days in the shortest and longest cycles are noted. The woman then calculates the first unsafe day (the beginning of the fertile time) by subtracting 18 days from the shortest cycle. The last unsafe day is then determined by subtracting 11 days from the longest cycle. An example of the calculations follows:

Shortest cycle = 25 days	Longest cycle = 32 days
25	32
−18	−11
Day 7	Day 21

For the woman in this example, the fertile or unsafe period is calculated to be 14 days, from days 7 through 21 of each of her cycles. Using the calendar method alone, this woman must abstain from sexual intercourse for longer than she may desire. To shorten the period of abstinence the couple can use some or all of the following methods.

Basal Body Temperature

The temperature is taken every day after the woman awakens and before any physical or emotional activity occurs. She uses a basal thermometer, which measures in 0.1 calibrations rather than 0.2 increments so that small changes are easily noted. Before ovulation, the **basal body temperature (BBT)** remains low. About 24 hours before ovulation the temperature dips slightly (0.1° F to 0.2° F) and then rises sharply within 24 hours. The rise of 0.7° to 0.8° F is maintained during the life of the corpus luteum for about 12 days. The day before menstruation, it drops again to the previous low levels (Figure 5-1). This shift results from the thermogenic influences of progesterone, which is secreted in higher levels after ovulation. Therefore a temperature elevation lasting 3 days signifies an end to the need for abstinence even if the calendar count has not ended.

Many factors, including infection, stress, fatigue, alcohol use, jet lag, and alteration in normal sleep patterns, can alter the expected outcome of the temperature chart. These factors should be noted on the temperature chart.

Methods Based on Cervical Mucus Changes

The **Billings method** relies on the changes in cervical mucus secretions (Figure 5-2). After menstruation the discharge appears yellowish and viscid and is impenetrable to sperm. Two or three days before ovulation, the mucus changes to a clear, colorless liquid similar to an egg white. If this mucus were tested, the glucose levels would be increased and the pH would be more alkaline (Figure 5-3).

Interference with the natural cycle through the use of contraceptive foams, jelly, creams, or douching, and vaginal infections make any test of the mucus inaccurate. The use of nasal decongestants also may have a drying effect on the mucus.

The **symptothermal method** combines the use of the BBT with analysis of cervical mucus changes to make predictions more accurate. Individual changes also may be noted. A urine test that detects the luteinizing hormone (LH) surge that occurs before ovulation may be used at home. Because this method is not affected by illness, stress, or activity levels, it is reliable when used in combination with other fertility indicators. If used every month, however, it is costly.

Commercially available computerized devices that aid fertility control are on the market. The Bioself 110 and the Rabbit Fertility Computer are technologic versions of the calendar and symptothermal methods. An electronic device called Cue is a hand-held digital monitor that probes for cyclic changes in the estrogen levels. It has been found, however, that highly technologic fertility aids have some drawbacks. Many times the ovulation detection kits may not give enough advance warning of impending ovulation. A woman who relies solely on external monitoring devices may not become familiar enough with her own bodily changes to determine the "unsafe" times. Daily observation of cervical mucus changes is a more accurate predictor (see Figure 5-3) (Fehring, 1991).

Advantages. There is no cost involved in fertility awareness methods, except for a thermometer, charts, or the ovulation detection kits. There is no need for a physician's prescription. The method is easy to learn, and motivated couples are afforded the chance to share in mutual choices. Finally, it is the only method sanctioned by the Roman Catholic church.

Effectiveness rates are based on the use of a combination of fertility indicators. According to Hatcher

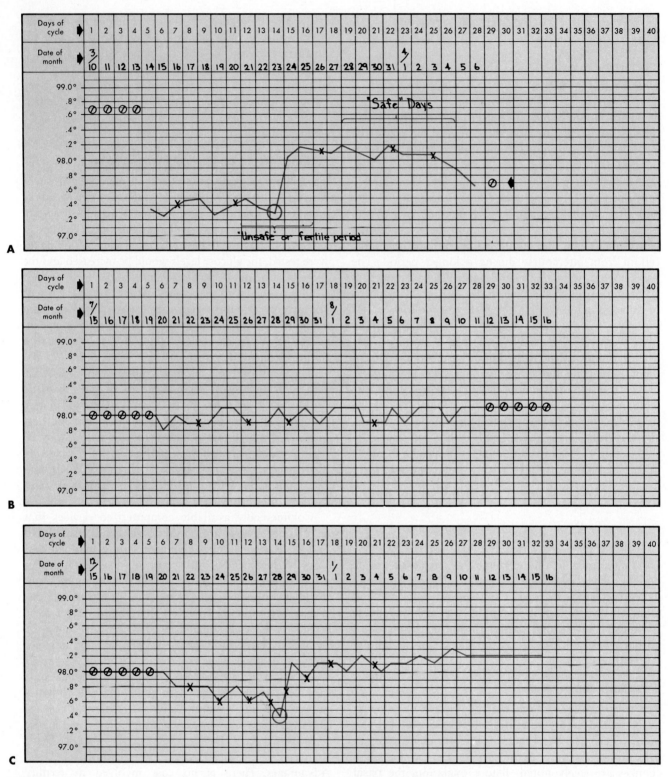

FIGURE 5-1 Charting basal body temperature (BBT). **A,** Normal cycle. **B,** Anovulatory cycle. **C,** After conception. ⌀, Menstruation; *X*, intercourse during previous 24 hours; ⊙, ovulation.

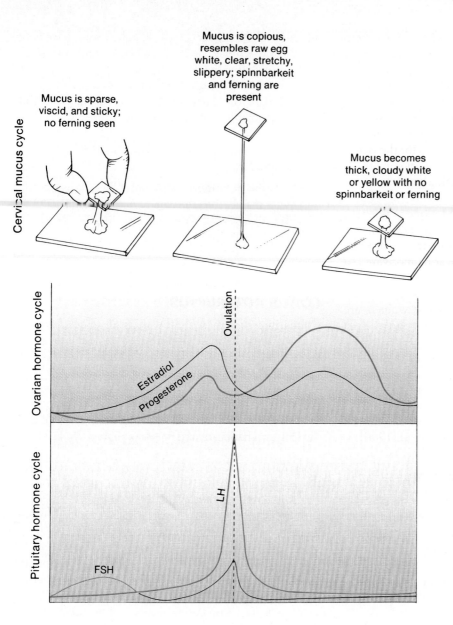

Mucus is sparse, viscid, and sticky; no ferning seen

Mucus is copious, resembles raw egg white, clear, stretchy, slippery; spinnbarkeit and ferning are present

Mucus becomes thick, cloudy white or yellow with no spinnbarkeit or ferning

Cervical mucus cycle

Ovarian hormone cycle

Estradiol

Progesterone

Ovulation

Pituitary hormone cycle

LH

FSH

FIGURE 5-2 Parameters of cervical mucus at ovulation. *Ferning* is the term for the crystalline pattern formed when the mucus is spread on a glass slide, dried, and viewed under a microscope. *Spinnbarkeit* is the term for the egg-white consistency of mucus that is more alkaline, has a higher sodium and glucose content, and is more receptive to sperm. (From Fogel CI and Woods NF: *Health care of women: a nursing perspective,* St Louis, 1981, Mosby.)

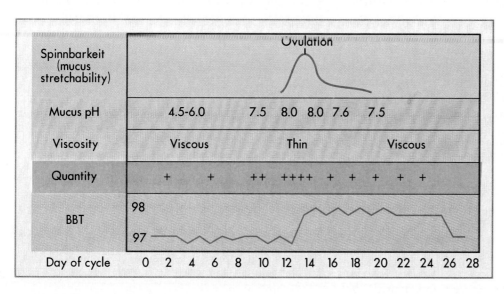

FIGURE 5-3 Comparison between qualities of cervical mucus during the menstrual cycle. Ovulation occurs when conditions are most favorable. (Redrawn from Moghiss KS. In Wallach EE, Kempers RD, editors: *Modern trends in infertility and conception control,* vol 1, Baltimore, 1979, Williams & Wilkins.)

(1989), the method is more effective when unprotected intercourse is limited to the postovulatory days only. During the first year of typical use, the method is approximately 80% effective; that is, 20% of the women will become pregnant. Hatcher goes on to predict that among perfect users of the NFP method, the accidental pregnancy rate for unprotected intercourse during the postovulatory only is about 2%, about 6% for the symptothermal method, about 8% for the ovulation method, and about 10% for the calendar method.

Disadvantages. The calendar method alone is not reliable because the time of ovulation is difficult to determine and the viability of the sperm or the ovum may vary in some persons. The couple must be motivated to pay attention to the details of the method and be vigilant about either abstaining or using another method during the unsafe period. Some women are unable to identify cervical mucus or BBT patterns even with persistent record keeping. Fertility awareness methods provide no protection against **sexually transmitted diseases (STDs)**. In fact, the use of alternative methods of sexual expression (which may be used by some couples during the fertile time) such as oral or anal sex may increase the transmission of the human immunodeficiency virus (HIV) (Hatcher et al, 1990).

LACTATION AMENORRHEA METHOD

Hoping to capitalize on the well-known phenomenon that breast-feeding women who do not menstruate rarely become pregnant, researchers are trying to establish guidelines for greater effectiveness of the **lactation amenorrhea method (LAM)**. Current suggestions include the informed use of breast-feeding by a woman who continues to be amenorrheal and who is not feeding her infant supplements.

It is believed that women who follow these guidelines will have a 2% chance of accidental pregnancy (Kennedy et al, 1992). There is a high probability that the woman who is amenorrheal while breastfeeding will be able to regulate her fertility in the first 6 months postpartum even if she introduces some supplementation to the baby's feedings. The key to the suppression of fertility is excellent breast-feeding skills, as long as amenorrhea continues. Once spotting or menses begins, other methods of contraception need to be implemented.

Advantages. The woman who uses the LAM must concern herself with birth control when she experiences her first menses or spotting. There is neither cost nor physician's visit involved.

Disadvantages. The woman needs to be extremely confident in her abilities to breast-feed and nourish the infant without reliance on supplementary feedings. Should the woman need to return to work after the birth of the baby, the levels of breast milk may diminish and menses may return. Clinical research involving this method is in the early stages; however, more flexible guidelines may be developed in the future.

> **Test Yourself**
> • Describe the differences among the following methods: rhythm, Billings, symptothermal, and BBT alone. Which method has the best "perfect use" rating?

COITUS INTERRUPTUS

Coitus interruptus (withdrawal) is an ancient method that requires the male to withdraw his penis from the vagina immediately before ejaculation. As a result, semen is not deposited in or near the vagina.

Advantages. The withdrawal method is useful to those who have no other method available. It involves no cost, devices, or chemicals and is available in any situation.

Disadvantages. This method may be extremely frustrating because both partners must maintain control. Even though ejaculation may be held back, preejaculatory fluid (which may contain semen stored in the prostate or Cowper's glands) can escape before ejaculation. A small drop of semen may contain millions of sperm. It is possible for sperm deposited near the external genitalia to reach an ovum. Thus this method is unreliable, with a failure rate of about 18%. It provides some protection, however, if no other method is available. Coitus interruptus provides no protection against HIV infection because bodily secretions mix during sexual arousal and penetration (Hatcher et al, 1990).

ABSTINENCE

The advent of acquired immunodeficiency disease (AIDS) has created more of an understanding of the option of **abstinence** among adults. Among teenagers, peer pressure and a feeling of invulnerability and risk-taking behavior may serve to inhibit the choice of abstinence as a method of birth control (Brown et al, 1992; Moore, 1991; Winter, 1991). Teenagers need help to be able to postpone a first sexual experience and to learn skills in avoiding sexual pressure. Many programs are recognizing that peer counseling in the school setting or family planning clinic may help teens "take ownership" of their bodies in sexual situations.

Sexual expression can involve a range of activities of intimacy up to and including the penis in the vagina. Touching, cuddling, dancing, massage, and many other activities, excluding coitus, are capable of meeting the need to be nurtured and loved and to give it in return. Although sexual expression without intercourse is an extremely effective contraceptive, it is not easy to accomplish. Therefore family planning counselors need to be supportive of abstinence and help establish programs for young people that enable them to choose abstinence as a method of preventing pregnancy (Hatcher et al, 1990).

CHEMICAL BARRIERS

Chemical barriers are usually **spermicidal** (sperm killing) or **spermistatic** (sperm stopping). In addition, they may have some blocking action at the cervix. Sperm thrive best at an alkaline pH of 8.5 to 9.0. Because the vagina normally is acidic until ovulation, chemical barriers are designed to keep the vaginal pH near 4.

The foam, jelly, suppository preparations, or vaginal contraceptive films (Figure 5-4) are inserted deep in the vagina. Foams and jellies are instantly effective, but suppositories or tablets and film take time to dissolve in the vaginal fluids.

After insertion the effectiveness of the chemical barrier lasts about 1 hour. All chemical agents must be used immediately before intercourse (e.g., 10 to 30 minutes) and therefore cannot be isolated from intercourse. Repeated intercourse requires reapplication. The woman should not douche for 6 hours after intercourse because it removes the chemical and may allow sperm to enter

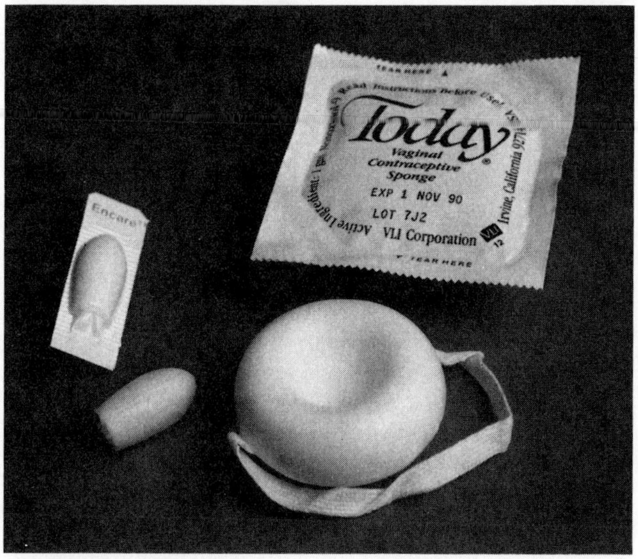

FIGURE 5-4 Chemical-barrier birth control devices available over the counter. Sponge and suppository. (Photo by Mark 6, New York.)

the uterus. If a chemical barrier is used in the weeks after childbirth, a double application is necessary until the stretched vaginal tissue returns to prepregnant size.

Advantages. Chemical contraceptives need no prescription, are less expensive and simpler to use, and may be used more often by adolescents. For the woman who forgets her birth control pill for 2 days or who has infrequent intercourse, a chemical barrier may be especially useful as a temporary measure. When used alone, chemical barriers require no special manipulative skills; insertion is much like that of a tampon. The chemical agents do not alter body physiology but increase vaginal lubrication. Because of its bacteriostatic effect, spermicides may offer increased protection against STDs, including herpes, gonorrhea, trichomoniasis, chlamydiosis, and AIDS. Greater protection, however, occurs with use of both a chemical barrier and a condom.

Disadvantages. Failure rates with "typical use" is approximately 21 pregnancies per 100 women per year of use. A small percentage of women and men experience burning from the agent. An additional major disadvantage is the amount of liquefied agent discharge. Because the method must be used immediately before intercourse, planning and forethought are involved (which may make it more difficult psychologically for adolescents who tend to romanticize the sexual act). Some women dislike the genital manipulation involved. Occasional allergy to the spermicide has been demonstrated. The use of spermicides at the point of conception or during early pregnancy may pose a risk of birth defects (Hatcher et al, 1990).

MECHANICAL BARRIERS

Sperm are prevented from entering the cervix by mechanical barriers (Figure 5-5). The condom, diaphragm, cervical cap, and sponge are widely used in the United States today. Because bacteria in semen or the vagina cannot ascend the cervical canal, the use of the mechanical with the chemical barrier may significantly reduce the risk of **pelvic inflammatory disease (PID)**. Only the condom, however, when used correctly can prevent the transmission of the HIV virus.

Diaphragm

The **diaphragm** is a curved rubber dome enclosed by a flexible metal ring that rests in the vagina and covers the cervix. Diaphragms are available in a variety of sizes; a fitting is needed and the size will need to be changed after pregnancy or weight gain or loss of 10 lb or more.

Spermicidal cream or jelly is placed in the cup portion and on the rim of the diaphragm before insertion so that the spermicide contacts the cervix. The

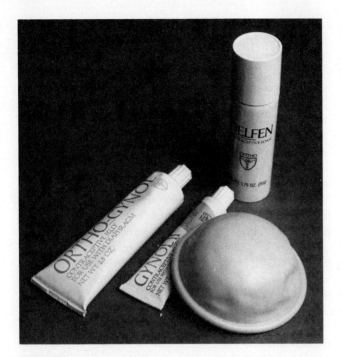

FIGURE 5-5 Mechanical- and chemical-barrier birth control devices. Diaphragm, jelly, and foam. (Photo by Mark 6, New York.)

contraceptive effect of the diaphragm is due partly to its role as a container for the spermicide.

The woman should check for proper placement by feeling for the cervix (which feels like a rounded knob or the tip of the nose). The anterior rim can be felt resting against the symphysis pubis. Once in place, the diaphragm should not be felt by either partner during intercourse. (Note Figure 5-6 for method of placement.)

The diaphragm should remain in place for at least 6 hours after intercourse but no longer than 24 hours. If coitus occurs again within 6 hours with the diaphragm still in place, an additional application of foam or jelly should be used. The woman should not douche during the 6-hour period because it may dislodge the diaphragm and force sperm into the cervix. Periodic inspection for holes or tears in the diaphragm is important.

Toxic shock syndrome (TSS) has occurred with the use of tampons and mechanical devices such as the diaphragm or sponge when left in place longer than instructed.

Toxic shock syndrome. With use of barrier methods and tampons, toxic shock syndrome (TSS) has occurred on occasion. When the method is dispensed, the nurse

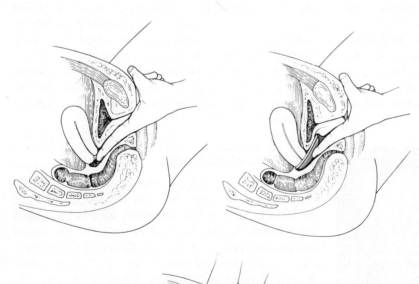

FIGURE 5-6 Proper placement of diaphragm between posterior fornix and symphysis pubis. (From Fogel CI, Woods NF: *Health care of women: a nursing perspective,* St Louis, 1981, Mosby.)

should discuss the risk factors and signs of illness (see Box 4-2). The risk of TSS may be significantly reduced if (1) the woman washes her hands with soap and water before inserting or removing a sponge, diaphragm, or cervical cap, (2) leaves the device in position for less than 24 hours, (3) does not use the device in the immediate postpartum period, (4) seeks treatment for vaginal infection before reusing a device, and (5) cares for the device, using soap, water, and careful drying.

Advantages. The effectiveness rate of "perfect use" can be as high as 98%. Manipulation is required but once learned becomes matter of fact. It neither interferes with physiologic functioning nor alters sexual sensation for most women.

Disadvantages. Typical first-year use results in an accidental pregnancy rate of up to 18%. Motivation and preplanning are required. There is an initial expense of an office or clinic visit, as well as the expense of the chemical barrier. Vaginal manipulation may be culturally unacceptable or may be distasteful to some women. The diaphragm may contribute to recurrent cystitis as a result of upward pressure of the rim against the urethra. In unusual coital positions the diaphragm may slip out of place. Sometimes a woman may experience pelvic discomfort, cramps, or pressure on the bladder or rectum. Allergy to latex or spermicides is a contraindication to its use.

Vaginal Contraceptive Sponge

The first vaginal contraceptive sponge was approved for use in the United States by the Food and Drug Administration (FDA) in 1983. It is a small, rounded, one-size-fits-all polyurethane device that has a dimple on one side so that it fits snugly over the cervix (see Figure 5-4). The other side of the sponge has a woven loop used for its removal from the vagina. The sponge is permeated with spermicide. Water is used to moisten the sponge for easier insertion. Once in place, it provides continuous protection for 24 hours. It should remain in place for at least 6 hours after intercourse. Sperm become trapped in the sponge and are then destroyed by the spermicide.

Advantages. The availability of the sponge is a benefit for many women. It may be inserted within 18 hours before intercourse. It is more convenient to use than some of the other vaginal contraceptives, and it may decrease the spread of STDs (including gonorrhea and chlamydiosis) to the uterus.

Disadvantages. Allergic reactions or irritation of the vaginal mucosa from the spermicide or the polyurethane have been reported. Some women experience difficulty in removing the sponge because care is needed not to tear it. Others have complained that the sponge absorbs too much of their vaginal secretions and thus creates excessive dryness in the vagina. The incidence of vaginal yeast infections may increase in women using the sponge. Also, use of the sponge may increase a woman's risk for TSS and should be avoided by those with a history of TSS. Typical rates for accidental pregnancy in the first year of use are 18 for nulliparas and 28 for parous women. It also is fairly expensive.

Cervical Cap

Recently approved by the FDA for use in the United States, the Prentif cervical cap is a popular mechanical device in other countries. The cap functions in much the same manner as the diaphragm but is smaller, thicker, and less flexible than the diaphragm (Figure 5-7). Made of soft rubber, the cervical cap may be left in place for as long as 24 hours. A spermicide must be used inside

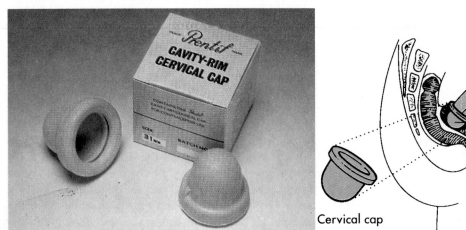
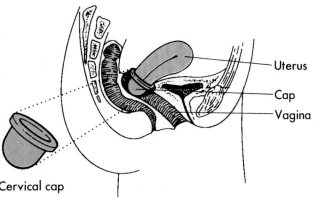

FIGURE 5-7 A, Cervical cap. **B,** Cervical cap placement.

the dome of the cap, which must not be removed for 6 hours after intercourse. Care for the cap is similar to that of the diaphragm. It needs careful fitting and is obtained through prescription.

Advantages. Similarities between the advantages of the cervical cap and the diaphragm exist. Most users express satisfaction with its use. Because it is smaller than the diaphragm, it may be less noticeable to the woman or man. There is no pressure on the bladder; thus fewer urinary tract infections are noted.

Disadvantages. The major drawbacks to use of the cap are the possible effects of long-term exposure to secretions, spermicide, and bacteria trapped inside it. Trauma to the tissues of the cervix or the vagina during insertion occurs only rarely. Fitting and teaching the woman to use the cervical cap are more time consuming than for the diaphragm. Because of its limited range of sizes, fitting, inserting, and removing the cap may present more difficulties than the diaphragm does. Allergy to latex or spermicides, PID, or repeated urinary tract infections are contraindications to its use. It is also not recommended for use for 6 to 12 weeks after a full-term delivery. Changes in Papanicolaou (Pap) test results may occur with the use of the cap, which may be a response of the cervical tissue to the irritation from a tight fit. It is strongly recommended that cervical cap users have a Pap smear before the cap fitting, 3 months subsequent to its use, and yearly thereafter (Franklin, 1990). Precautions for TSS must be observed. Failure rates range from 8% to 18% per 100 women per year of use.

Condom

The **condom** has been used since the fourteenth century. Originally designed to protect against venereal disease, it was found that the condom also prevented pregnancy. A sheath is placed over the erect penis to prevent semen from entering before any contact is made with the vulva or vagina. A small pouch of airless space should be left at the tip of the condom to catch the ejaculate and to prevent the condom from tearing (Figure 5-8). Condoms can be lubricated or nonlubricated. In 1982 a spermicidal condom (a condom with a small amount of nonoxynol 9 on its inner and outer surfaces) was introduced and was found to be highly effective in killing sperm within the condom, as well as protecting against STDs and HIV.

After ejaculation, the penis must be withdrawn from the vagina while still erect, and care must be taken to prevent the condom from slipping off to prevent semen from entering the vagina. Should the accidental leakage of sperm occur, the insertion of a dose of spermicidal foam or jelly helps (but still may not prevent pregnancy).

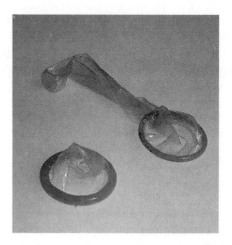

FIGURE 5-8 Condom. (Custom Medical Stock Photo.)

Advantages. The effectiveness of the condom can be as high as 96% if used exactly as directed with each coital act. Effectiveness improves with use of a spermicidal condom or with use of both a condom and vaginal foam. The condom also has been found to be effective in preventing STDs, such as AIDS, trichomoniasis, herpes, chlamydiosis, gonorrhea, and syphilis, and also protects against reinfection from vaginal infections when one partner is under treatment. Condom use encourages male participation and responsibility in the act of sexual intercourse. Condoms are inexpensive and readily available in any pharmacy and even from some vending machines in public restrooms.

Disadvantages. Typical user failure rates can be as high as 10% to 15%, depending on the study cited. Because it covers the glans, some men feel that the condom curtails some of their pleasurable sensations. Foreplay may be interrupted to apply it before vaginal penetration. In addition, a small number of persons are allergic to the latex condoms and must use the natural skin type instead; skin-type condoms do not provide protection against STDs. Sometimes in cases of allergy to latex, clinicians may recommend using the "skin" sheath underneath a latex condom to maintain protection against STDs.

Condom for Women

FDA approval has been obtained for a vaginal pouch or condom for women called the *WPC-333*. It is a soft polyurethane pouch that is lubricated with nonoxynol 9, and it has two flexible rings at either end. One ring surrounds the cervix to keep the pouch stable while the other ring remains outside the vagina (Figure 5-9). It is approximately as effective as the male condom. Theoretically it could offer excellent protection from STDs.

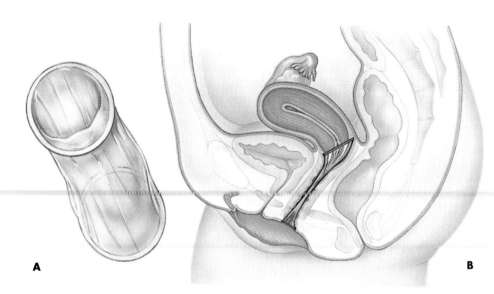

FIGURE 5-9 A, Vaginal pouch. B, Correctly inserted in vagina. The top ring covers the cervix. (Redrawn from Franklin M: *J Nurse Midwife* 35(6):371, 1990.)

INTRAUTERINE DEVICE

The **intrauterine device (IUD)** is a highly effective form of birth control. It is inserted into the uterus and left there for 1 year (Progestasert) and the new device ParaGard may be used up to 8 years. It is recommended for women who have been pregnant and are in a stable, monogamous relationship—essentially women determined to be at very low risk for STDs. Many developing countries have fostered its use because of its low cost and long action. Most IUDs have been unavailable in the United States in the recent past, however, because of lawsuits involving the Dalkon shield type of IUD. The Progestasert and, more recently, the ParaGard (Copper T 380A) currently are the two IUDs distributed in the United States (Figure 5-10).

Mode of Action

Although the exact method of preventing pregnancy is unclear, some local effects seem to create a uterine environment hostile to implantation. The metals (copper) and medications (progesterone) added to the flexible polyethylene provide time-released action in minute amounts. Current theories concerning the mechanism of change within the uterus are as follows (IUDs—a new look, 1988):

1. The IUD acts as a foreign body in the uterus, generating an inflammatory response in the endometrium, keeping it "out of phase" in the menstrual cycle. The inflammatory cells may be spermicidal or may damage the ova so that fertilization is impossible. In addition, increased local production of prostaglandins occurs, inhibiting implantation. Increased mobility of the ovum in the fallopian tubes also is noted as a result of this process.

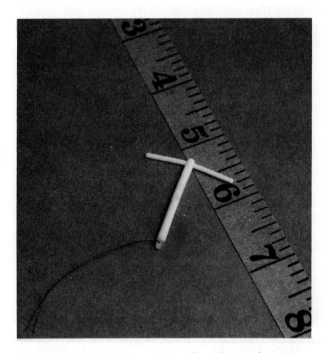

FIGURE 5-10 Progestasert IUD. (Photo by Mark 6, New York.)

2. The sperm are immobilized as they pass through the uterine cavity. Many fewer sperm are found in the fallopian tubes of IUD users.
3. The cervical mucus becomes altered in consistency and pH because of the release of progesterone on the Progestasert.
4. The copper may interfere with the intracellular metabolism within the endometrium.

Rarely, implantation may occur despite the IUD. Women who become pregnant with an IUD in place have an extremely high rate of spontaneous abortions

Self-Discovery

Visit a drug store and note the cost (per unit) of over-the-counter contraceptive methods. What do your findings suggest about compliance in using an OTC method?

(about 40 %). Because of the increased risk of infection, the clinician usually makes every effort to remove the IUD if pregnancy occurs. If the pregnancy continues to term, the IUD tends to become embedded in the maternal side of the placenta and the fetus usually is unharmed by the device. Long-range side effects of the medicated (copper or progesterone-releasing) IUDs on the fetus have not yet been determined.

Advantages. The IUD is **coitus independent.** Its cost is minimal (Pap test, insertion, instructions, and revisits) at a clinic or Planned Parenthood Center. Its effectiveness varies from 1 pregnancy per 100 women per year of use (1%) to three pregnancies per 100 women per year of use (3%). Expulsion rates and side effects such as cramping or heavy bleeding are lower for the progesterone-releasing IUDs. The Progestasert IUD releases a minimal amount of the hormone (65 µg) with virtually no systemic absorption.

The ParaGard system contains copper and can remain in the uterus for up to 8 years. This method is ideal for a woman who has completed her childbearing and desires a coitus-independent method without exposure to the hormonal effects of the birth control pill. The Progestasert method is ideal for the woman who wishes to delay pregnancy for a year or to space a pregnancy.

Most women who desire to become pregnant after the IUD is removed are able to conceive as rapidly as non-IUD users (IUDs, 1988). IUD use, however, does add to the risk of PID, which may cause tubal infertility.

Disadvantages. The inflammatory process caused by the IUD may increase uterine contractility after insertion and thus result in expulsion of the device. Because the possibility of expulsion may continue for three or four subsequent menstrual cycles, there is a need for a back-up method of contraception. Initially during menses, a woman may experience cramping, heavy bleeding, or pelvic pain. If these symptoms persist, the IUD may have to be removed. After menstruation and about once a week thereafter, the woman must check with her finger for the nylon threads that protrude into the vagina through the cervix; this action may be distasteful for some women. If there is any doubt about the position or length of the string or if a cycle is missed, the woman should contact her clinician.

The Progestasert system does not prevent ectopic pregnancy; the woman with this particular IUD has a sixfold to tenfold frequency of ectopic pregnancy compared with the woman who has a copper IUD. Because of the increased risk for repeat infections, women with a history of gonorrheal or chlamydial infections should not use the Progestasert.

PID is a serious complication; however, the risk is reduced if the woman has only one sexual partner. Should an infection develop, the IUD is removed immediately; vigorous antibiotic therapy will be prescribed.

An integral part of the information given to the woman with an IUD is the early IUD danger signals (Hatcher et al, 1990; IUDs, 1988). Hatcher et al recommend the following acronym for easier client recall:

P Period late (pregnancy suspected), abnormal spotting or bleeding
A Abdominal pain or pain with intercourse
I Infection (abnormal vaginal discharge)
N Not feeling well, fever, chills
S Strings lost, shorter or longer

Hormonal Control of Fertility
ORAL CONTRACEPTIVES

The **oral contraceptive (OC) ("the pill")** has been on the market since the early 1960s. A steady decline in the dosage of estrogens and progesterones in the pill has reduced serious estrogen-related side effects. Dosages of estrogens now range from 20 to 50 µg compared with the 50 to 150 µg range used in the 1960s. Two types of pills are on the market in the United States.

Combined Regimen

Varied combinations of estrogens and progesterone in synthetic form compose the *combined* OC, which is available in three forms. *Monophasic pills* contain synthetic estrogens and progesterones in each pill and must be taken every day for 21 days or 28 days. The 28-day pack has 21 pills with medication and 7 pills with no medication so that withdrawal bleeding occurs during the 7 days. *Biphasic pills* contain a certain level of estrogens throughout the cycle. To mimic body patterns in the 21-day pack, there is a small dose of progestins (synthetic progesterones) for 10 days and then a slightly higher dose for 11 days. *Triphasic pills* alter the levels of estrogens and progesterones continuously throughout the cycle. The total dose of hormones per cycle is less than the biphasic pills.

Mode of action. The combined regimen pill suppresses ovulation by inhibiting the hypothalamus, the pituitary, and the ovarian release of hormones. Follicle-stimulating hormone (FSH) and luteinizing hormone (LH) are suppressed; thus the two hormones required to stimulate ovulation are drastically reduced by the influence of estrogen and progesterone in the pills. Changes in the endometrium that inhibit implantation are secondary effects of the pill. The progesterone in the pill stimulates changes in the cervical mucus; it becomes thick and maintains a pH environment hostile to sperm throughout the cycle.

Advantages. The combined regimen pill, if taken correctly, is almost 100% effective. Human error may account for the failure rates of 0.1% to 0.5% per 100 women per year of use.

Coitus independence is achieved for women taking the pill, and many women experience greater satisfaction in the sexual act once the fear of pregnancy has been eliminated. Withdrawal bleeding occurs more or less predictably, with a decreased flow. Beneficial side effects of the combined-regimen pill include alleviation of symptoms of premenstrual syndrome and the reduction or elimination of dysmenorrhea, endometriosis, and menorrhagia, iron deficiency anemia (because menstrual blood flow is decreased), and ovarian cysts (Franklin, 1990). Rates of severe PID in oral contraceptive users are less than those for users of other methods of birth control. Although recent research indicates a lower rate of ovarian and endometrial cancers among combined-regimen pill users (Speroff, 1989), the risk of cervical cancer seems to be increased with prolonged use (Beral et al, 1988). Careful monitoring is necessary for susceptible women, including those whose mother or sisters have had breast, uterine, or cervical cancer.

In many women, acne often is improved while they take the pill. A reduced incidence of benign breast disease and lowered risk of ectopic pregnancy also has been found. For healthy, nonsmoking women older than the age of 40, the benefits of preventing pregnancy may outweigh the possible risks of oral contraceptive use.

Disadvantages. The main disadvantages of the combined-regimen pill lies in its side effects. Many of these side effects may be eliminated by careful selection of the ratio of estrogens to progesterone. Comparison of the different chemical formulations of progestins also is essential in choosing the correct pill because each different progestin has an estrogenic effect, an androgenic effect, and an antiestrogenic effect that must be tailored to the woman's physical needs. A physician may use an estrogen profile, which provides data on each woman's estrogen levels, to assist in the choice of an acceptable pill. The profile provides a picture of body type because the type of pill a woman will receive is based on her body build, history of menstrual cycles, libido levels, energy levels, and age. Table 5-1 compares a balanced profile (76% to 80% of all women) with a hypoestrogenic or hyperestrogenic state. For a woman with a hypoestrogenic level, a pill with a more estrogenic effect might be chosen, for instance. A woman whose profile is hyperestrogenic may benefit from a pill with antiestrogenic effects (Box 5-1).

BOX 5-1   Contraindications to the Combined Pill

- History of thromboembolic, cerebrovascular, or cardiovascular disease
- History of breast cancer or estrogen-dependent tumors
- Pregnancy, lactation, smoking
- Liver tumors, disease, or dysfunction
- Diabetes, mental depression

TABLE 5-1   Estrogen Levels

HYPERESTROGENIC, 10% TO 12%	BALANCED, 76% TO 80%	HYPOESTROGENIC, 10% TO 12%
Heavy menstrual flow	Normal menses	Scanty menses at longer intervals
Large breasts	Normal contours	Small breasts
Tendency to gain weight	Normal weight	Boyish look
Premenstrual syndrome		
Fluid retention		
Emotional lability		
Increased libido		Lower libido
Increased vaginal secretion	Normal vaginal cytology and secretions	Thinner vaginal lining
Mastalgia		More vaginitis and pruritus
Tendency toward fibroids		

Contraindications. Contraindications include migraines, hypertension, gallbladder or renal disease, lactation, age of 45 or older, elective surgery planned within the month, sickle cell disease, and acute infectious mononucleosis. Women who smoke heavily, who have a history of mental depression, who have epilepsy and are taking rifampin or phenytoin (more estrogens are required for ovulation suppression), or who have varicose veins or frequent vaginal yeast infections should not use the pill.

Side effects related to estrogens tend to mimic the unpleasant symptoms of early pregnancy; these side effects are nausea, fluid retention, headaches, melasma (chloasma), breast tenderness and fullness, and occasionally blurred vision (Table 5-2). If the woman experiences these symptoms, her physician may change the pill to one containing lower estrogen doses.

Progesterone-related side effects include fatigue, depression, acne, oily skin and scalp, weight gain, headaches, pruritus, increased low-density lipoprotein (LDL) cholesterol levels and decreased high-density lipoprotein (HDL) cholesterol levels. Breakthrough bleeding also may be a problem, occurring more often during the first two cycles of use. This signifies endometrial adjustment to the new hormone levels, but if spotting continues, the woman should see her clinician for reevaluation of the dosage.

Postpill **amenorrhea** may occur more often in the woman who begins the pill close to menarche or who had a late menarche. No relationship has been demonstrated between the length of time the pill has been taken or the type of pill and postpill amenorrhea (Hatcher et al, 1990).

There may be delay in conception among former pill users. Therefore a woman planning to become pregnant

TABLE 5-2 Results of Estrogen and Progestogen Excess

ESTROGEN	PROGESTOGEN
GASTROINTESTINAL SYSTEM	
Nausea, bloated feeling	Increased appetite, real weight gain
VASCULAR AND RENAL SYSTEMS	
Fluid retention, venous capillary engorgement	
Occasional occurrence of spider nevi	
Headaches (migraine) and perhaps some elevation of blood pressure	Depression, nervousness, fatigue
A slight chance of thromboembolism in women at high risk	
UTERUS	
Hypermenorrhea, myoma growth	Scanty menses
	Dysmenorrhea usually improved; sometimes breakthrough bleeding
VAGINA	
Leukorrhea, excess secretion	Reduction in lining thickness and secretions; more *Candida* infection, pruritus
BREASTS	
Mastalgia; possible enlargement of benign cysts	Regression of breast tissue
SKIN	
Chloasma (darkening of skin over nose and cheeks)	Possible occurrence of acne
GLUCOSE METABOLISM	
Increased levels in fasting state	
Decreased glucose tolerance, increased insulin response to glucose	

should discontinue the pill for 6 to 18 months before she would like to conceive. At least three cycles off the pill is recommended before conception. Currently no evidence exists that oral contraceptives increase the incidence of infertility (Franklin, 1990). The combined pill should be avoided by nursing mothers because the effects tend to suppress prolactin production and milk supply. Instead, progesterone–only pills are used for lactating women who wish to continue taking the pill. Finally, the pill can affect the proper metabolism of certain vitamins (especially vitamin C), and thus supplementation may be required.

Other side effects of the pill are hypertension (which frequently disappears when the pill is stopped), increased risk of gallbladder disease, alteration in certain laboratory data (aspartate aminotransferase [AST; also known as SGOT], alanine aminotransferase [ALT; also known as SGPT], and sulfobromophthalein [Bromsulphalein; BSP]) and a change in the corneal curvature in some women who wear contact lenses (which may necessitate a change in the type of lens or a switch to glasses). Drug interactions that change the potency of barbiturates, phenytoin, ampicillin, anticoagulants, antidepressants, beta blockers, vitamin C, bronchodilators, antihypertensives, and phenylbutazone occur. The use of diazepam (Valium) in long-term pill users can induce an unintended overdose because the elimination of diazepam from the liver is slowed.

Many family planning clinics and physicians require informed consent before prescribing oral contraceptives. A list of early danger signals may be included in the consent form (Hatcher et al, 1989):

A Abdominal pain—severe (may mean a gallbladder or liver problem)

C Chest pain (severe), cough, shortness of breath (may mean a blood clot)

H Headache (severe), dizziness, weakness, numbness (may mean hypertension or impending stroke)

E Eye problems—vision loss or blurring, speech problems (may mean stroke)

S Severe pain in legs, calf, or thighs (may mean blood clot)

A very important disadvantage is that the use of oral contraceptives may increase the woman's risk of becoming infected with HIV or other STDs. No physical barrier to these infections exists with the use of oral contraceptives alone. Therefore, the nurse needs to counsel teenagers to use the condom along with the pill. In addition, the cost of the pill and the time spent for follow-up care may be prohibitive.

Progesterone-Only Regimen

Progesterone-only oral contraceptives are called "minipills" because of the low dosage of synthetic progesterone. The minipills contain the same progestins

available in the combined-regimen oral contraceptive but in smaller doses. If they are taken for 21 days, ovulation is not suppressed but fertility is lowered.

Mode of action. Progesterone induces physiologic changes that interfere with the endometrial phase and the properties of cervical mucus. Thus the uterine environment becomes hostile to sperm motility, as well as to implantation, if fertilization should occur. The small doses of progesterone do not suppress ovulation but may alter the reciprocal interaction of the pituitary-ovarian hormones.

Advantages. The minipill contains no estrogens and less progesterone than the combined pill so that some progesterone-related side effects, including weight gain, candidal vaginitis, and acne, may be alleviated. When lactating women want hormonal contraception, clinicians prescribe the minipill because it does not diminish the quantity of milk or adversely affect the infant's health. The minipill may be chosen by women older than 35 and for women with a history of headaches or mild hypertension. Effectiveness rates are slightly lower when compared with the combined-regimen pill, ranging from 0.5 to 3.7 pregnancies per 100 women per year of use. Dosages of progesterone in the minipill range from a low of 0.075 mg (Ovrette) to 0.35 mg (Micronor).

Disadvantages. The major side effects of this type of oral contraceptive are the unpredictability of menses, the lack of cycle control, and the lower effectiveness rate compared with the combined-regimen pill.

PROGESTERONE SUBDERMAL IMPLANTS

FDA approval of the **Norplant subdermal implant** was given in 1991. This system provides slow release of the synthetic progestin levonorgestrel. With use of a local anesthetic, six cylindric capsules are inserted under the skin on the inside upper portion of the woman's arm. The Norplant device can remain in place for up to 5 years and then must be removed surgically (also with the woman under local anesthetic). Biodegradable implants that do not require removal currently are being tested. Removal of the Norplant system is a bit more difficult than the insertion (Figure 5-11).

The Norplant device acts in much the same manner as the progesterone-only minipill and thus has the similar advantages and disadvantages. Accidental pregnancy rates range between 0.6 and 1.5 per 100 women per year of use (Sharts-Engel, 1991; Shoupe and Mishel, 1989). The Norplant device may be a viable contraceptive method for women older than 35 years of age, women who cannot use estrogens, and women who have difficulty with other methods. The contraceptive

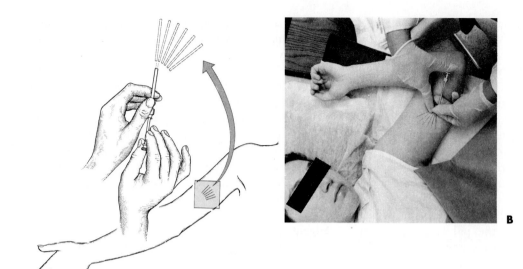

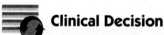

FIGURE 5-11 A, Norplant is one of the newest contraceptive devices. It contains six porous capsules of synthetic progestin. **B,** They are placed just under the skin inside the upper portion of the arm. (**A** from William C. Andrea; **B** from Joel Gordon Photography.)

benefits of the implants end soon after they are removed. Additional disadvantages of the Norplant system over the minipill are that there is a slight risk of infection and pain during the insertion and removal procedures. The implant also is initially more expensive than pills and other short-term methods, but the effects last for 5 years so that the expense can be prorated. Implants may be visible on some thin or highly muscular women. The woman cannot discontinue using the implant on her own. Women who weigh more than 70 kg (154 lb) have a higher pregnancy rate over the 5-year period (Lynn and Holdcroft, 1992).

POSTCOITAL CHOICES

"Morning after" pills are highly effective when used within 72 hours after unprotected midcycle intercourse. The drug most commonly used for postcoital contraception is Ovral, which contains progesterone and estrogen. The FDA has not approved the use of Ovral for general postcoital contraceptive purposes; yet the method is used frequently on college campuses and in many family planning clinics to treat rape victims. Postcoital contraception either prevents fertilization or stops the fertilized egg from implanting. Side effects are nausea and vomiting, which may be severe. Treatment is not recommended for women with high blood pressure, blood clots, or breast cancer.

RU 486 (a competitive antagonist of progesterone) and prostaglandins have been approved for use in early pregnancy. There is still considerable popular resistance to RU 486 in the United States because of its controversial abortifacient (abortion-inducing) effect, although it is being used successfully in Europe.

Clinical Decision

You have an opportunity to teach to a class of tenth-grade girls. The topic is "the best methods to prevent pregnancy." List your suggestions.

Menstrual extraction may be performed to induce menstruation when it is overdue (up to 2 weeks late). The procedure may be done on an outpatient basis.

Surgical Sterilization

Surgical sterilization usually is a permanent measure and should be undertaken only after a great deal of consideration. It is most desirable if both partners sign the informed consent; however, it is legal in most states when only the client signs. If the person relies on federal or state funding for the procedure, the following regulations apply: the individual must be at least 21 years of age and be mentally competent; many states require a waiting period of 30 to 90 days between the time that the consent is signed and the procedure is performed. Surgical sterilization is not considered 100% effective. Pregnancies do occur, yet the rate is quite low, depending on the surgical technique.

Psychologic implications accompany the loss of reproductive ability. Everyone choosing the option of sterilization needs to explore personal feelings. Reproductive prowess often is equated with the degree of maleness or femaleness a man or woman feels, and loss of reproductive ability may lower self-esteem. Most men and women who undergo surgical sterilization, however, are not adversely affected. With fear of unwanted pregnancy gone, many couples report improvement in their sex lives and more frequent intercourse. It should be noted that surgical sterilization does not prevent or alter the transmission of HIV or other STDs.

FEMALE STERILIZATION

Several surgical techniques exist for sterilization of women. Tubal ligation and hysterectomy are two such measures. Hysterectomy rarely is used for sterilization purpose because the complications of major surgery are far greater than for other measures. Blocking of the tubes may be performed by several methods. Most approaches make use of laparoscopy to perform a minilaparotomy, which leaves a small abdominal incision. The tubes are cut and tied in various ways (Figure 5-12).

The best time for a tubal ligation is within 24 to 48 hours after the woman has given birth, when the tubes have been displaced toward the anterior part of the abdomen and are easily visualized. Local anesthetics can be used, but many women prefer a more general anesthetic such as an epidural injection. Recovery may be delayed, but there usually are few complications.

If surgery is performed on an outpatient basis, the woman may be sent home within a few hours if she is stable. She may require a mild analgesic for postoperative pain. The woman should rest for a few days and avoid heavy lifting for a week. Side effects are minimal, and uterine function is not altered. Ovulation still occurs, but the ovum is absorbed into the peritoneal cavity.

Reversal of a tubal ligation has become more promising with the use of microsurgical techniques. Pregnancy rates after reversing female surgical sterilization, however, are only about 40% to 70% (Hatcher et al, 1990).

MALE STERILIZATION

Vas ligation or vasectomy is a popular form of surgical sterilization and can be performed in the physician's office under local anesthesia. It does not affect the production of male hormones and sperm or the ability to have an erection, nor does it alter sexual function. It should be considered permanent, although reversal can occur in 40% to 90% of cases. Fertility, however, may not be restored by rejoining the vas deferens because changes may have occurred within the testes; some men (up to 50%) develop antibodies against their own sperm after a vasectomy and may remain infertile because of the autoimmune reaction (Hatcher et al, 1990). Men who have had vasectomies are not at increased risk for cardiovascular disease. It is recommended that a man store his sperm in a sperm bank in case he might desire a child at a later time.

The vas deferens is severed during the procedure, making passage of the sperm from the testes to the urethra impossible (Figure 5-13). Postoperative care may involve the use of mild analgesics for pain, ice packs on the scrotum intermittently for swelling, and scrotal support, as well as no heavy lifting until the incision has healed. Abstinence from sexual intercourse is required only until the incision heals (approximately 3 days). Sterility is achieved when a minimum of 16 ejaculations have occurred because sperm remain in the area beyond the ligation. The couple is advised to use another method of birth control until analysis confirms that two samples are free of sperm. In addition, the man should bring a specimen of the ejaculate for a sperm count 2 to 3 months and again at 1 year after surgery.

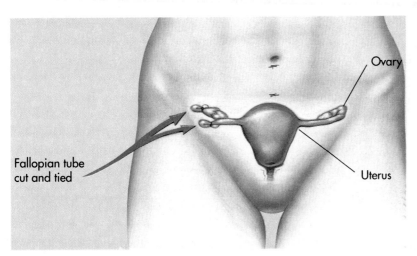

FIGURE 5-12 Tubal ligation. (Courtesy Ronald J. Ervin.)

Ovary

Uterus

Fallopian tube cut and tied

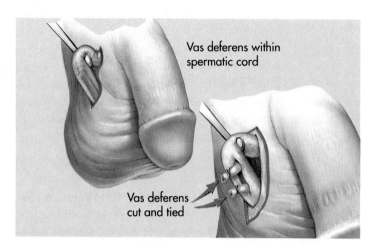

FIGURE 5-13 Vasectomy. Vas deferens has been tied off and severed. Sperm cannot enter ejaculatory duct. (Courtesy Ronald J. Ervin.)

Side effects are rare but can include infection, hematoma at the site, or small spermatic granulomas. These complications usually are not serious and are easily treated.

Research Methods

Many methods currently under investigation in the United States are being used freely in other parts of the world. In this country, stringent FDA guidelines and clinical trials require long-range study of the safety and effectiveness of all new methods.

Male contraceptive measures are being studied. Fertility-regulating drugs and a vaccine to influence the maturation and fertilizing capacity of sperm also are being investigated. The drug sulfasalazine (Azulfidine), an ulcerative colitis drug, causes decreased sperm counts and impairs sperm motility. It is being studied because it affords a quick return to fertility. Gossypol is another drug under investigation that may interfere with spermatogenesis. Reversible vasectomy devices, such as a Shug, consist of two flexible silicone plugs and are undergoing clinical trials (Franklin, 1990).

Long-acting hormonal interruption of the ovarian cycle by means of an injection, biodegradable subdermal capsules, pills, and vaginal rings are being studied. All these methods involve the use of progesterone and could cause side effects. Two vaccines are being studied: a vaccine against human chorionic gonadotropin (hCG) and a vaccine that provides immunity against luteinizing hormone–releasing hormone (LHRH), or the surface of the sperm or ova.

The use of prostaglandin as a nasal spray or vaginal suppository to induce menses is being examined. Oral abortifacients (drugs that induce abortion), postcoital drugs, and lower-dosage oral contraceptives are under study. Tests are being performed on a disposable diaphragm covered with spermicide; these devices can be compared with the condom that contains spermicide.

Inhibin is a gonadal hormone that controls FSH and may be both a male and female contraceptive. It too is currently under investigation.

Issues to Consider

Throughout history the issue of contraception has elicited much thought. When technologic advances make available new methods to women who choose to control their own fertility, these advances are applauded and encouraged by women. As a vehicle for political gain or social change, it is possible that contraceptive innovations may be used in a way that usurps the woman's control of her own fertility. For instance, issues such as mandatory sterilization for the mentally handicapped have been considered. Other issues such as enforced contraception have surfaced regarding judicial

Clinical Decision

Mrs. J. is an unemployed single parent of four dependent children. Discuss advantages and disadvantages of at least three contraceptive choices for her.

Clinical Decision

Teresa is 16, sexually active, and embarrassed to talk about it. You have a chance to counsel her. How would you begin the conversation?

punishment for the crime of child abuse (*State of California vs. Darlene Johnson* (1990); Judge Harold Broadman ordered Darlene Johnson, convicted of child abuse, to obtain a Norplant device or to face several years in jail). Similar cases of enforced or coerced contraception appear in certain states that withhold or limit public assistance for women who give birth to a large number of children. The fundamental flaw in the imposition of these policies is the assumption that contraception will somehow cure the child abuser or alleviate the problems of poverty without some form of rehabilitation (Charo, 1992).

The American Medical Association Board of Trustees has taken a strong stand against the political imposition of contraception, pointing out that the freedom to procreate, to refuse medical intervention, and to exercise personal choice in contraception are constitutional rights (Board of Trustees, AMA, 1992).

Nursing Responsibilities

Contraception has become an integral part of life for many people. Every birth control method available for use today has risks and benefits associated with its use. Each method carries responsibilities on the part of the user to learn about the side effects, advantages, and disadvantages. All education about fertility control is based on a firm understanding of the anatomy and physiology of reproduction. Using this knowledge, nurses can counsel and support individuals in their choices and in health care.

Many options exist for those who do not want a child or who want to postpone having a child. Hormonal contraception in the form of pills or subdermal implants are available. The use of intrauterine devices and barrier methods (either chemical or mechanical, or both) is widespread. Fertility awareness methods as a part of natural family planning are being used by many women whose health histories or religious or ecologic convictions preclude other methods. Surgical sterilization is considered to be a permanent method of contraception. Finally, abstinence is an effective method of birth control.

▶ ASSESSMENT

To create an accurate picture of the client's needs, the nurse needs to acquire pertinent information by observing the behavior, obtaining a sexual history to identify any dysfunction, determining whether pregnancy needs to be delayed or prevented, obtaining a marital history, and learning of religious or cultural beliefs that may affect the choice of contraceptive. Discomfort in talking about intercourse, for example, may mean that the person experiences difficulty in planning for the sexual

act; thus more success may be achieved with a coitus-independent method. (Although the subject may be embarrassing for some, the person has chosen to come to a specialist to receive help with family planning matters and after some initial discomfort may become more relaxed about discussing his or her needs.) The following factors should be considered in gathering data:

1. Client's educational level
2. Client's socioeconomic level and stress factors
3. Client's age and prior experiences with contraception
4. Cultural beliefs, myths, and misinformation
5. General physical health of the client (careful attention to allergies, e.g., latex, spermicides)
6. Motivation level and career goals
7. Menstrual and obstetric history
8. Satisfaction with current method

▶ NURSING DIAGNOSES

If a person is experienced with a particular method and is educated and motivated, the nurse may need only to provide new information about the chosen method. In this instance nursing diagnoses may include the following:

1. Health-seeking behavior regarding the chosen method, use, side effects, and expected results
2. Altered health maintenance related to the requirements of the method (e.g., the use of the pill or use of other medications while taking the pill)

In a different situation, such as for a young teenager, the nursing diagnoses may need to include more extensive counseling and preparation such as the following:

1. Health-seeking behavior regarding the menstrual cycle, times of fertility, and choices of method
2. High risk for noncompliance in contraceptive use and protection from STDs
3. High risk for infection

▶ EXPECTED OUTCOMES

As part of the process in establishing the appropriate method, the nurse needs to help the person think about why birth control is personally necessary and to determine if the preference is to prevent pregnancy permanently or merely to space the interval between children. The developmental stage of the person or the couple should be assessed. For instance, if a client is 23 years old and has four children, she may choose a different form of contraception than if she were 35 years old and newly married. The client's life-style should be evaluated—whether the person is settled or transient. The nurse needs to establish whether one person in the relationship takes responsibility for contraception, or whether both partners become involved. Some selected outcomes follow.

1. The client will develop a trusting relationship with the health care provider as evidenced by asking questions freely.
2. The client will develop knowledge of the chosen method by (a) describing or demonstrating the correct procedure for use and (b) listing the advantages, disadvantages, and risks associated with the method.
3. The client will contact the clinician should harmful side effects or questions arise about the use of the method.
4. The client will maintain health in relation to the chosen method.

▶ NURSING INTERVENTIONS

In the office or clinic, birth control choices are discussed with the client and the method of choice will be provided. Each woman undergoes a pelvic examination before the decision is made concerning the type of birth control she chooses. The nurse explains what to expect during the examination, including speculum insertion and abdominal and breast palpation, to help her establish trust and reduce anxiety. If she becomes anxious, the nurse suggests relaxation measures such as deep breathing or visual imagery. If possible, the nurse stands near her head and talks with her during the examination to alleviate stress because some persons find silence difficult. After the examination is complete, the nurse is available for the woman's questions or concerns and talks with her while she is sitting rather than lying flat on the examination table. Active participation helps to lower anxiety and facilitates learning the successful use of contraception, which requires self-monitoring.

Teaching is an integral part of nursing care for the person desiring birth control. Teaching aids are useful, and literature available from manufacturers of birth control methods should be given to the client for review at home. Information should include the correct procedure for using a particular method, the advantages, disadvantages, and risks associated with its use, and a demonstration and return demonstration of correct use, as well as discussion concerning unusual circumstances (such as missed pills or broken condoms.) (See Figure 5-14.)

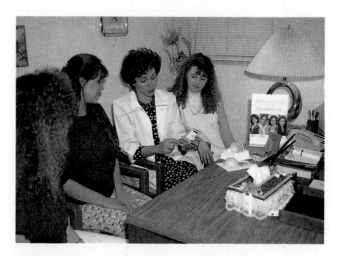

FIGURE 5-14 Personal instruction is the key to gaining compliance of teenage women. (Courtesy Marjorie Pyle, RNC, *Lifecircle.*)

▶ EVALUATION

Determining the client's achievement of outcomes is not easy in many situations. When possible, the nurse looks for the following keys.

1. Was the client able to describe the use of the chosen method?
2. Did she demonstrate correct use of the method and explain when the clinician should be notified about problems?
3. Does she know when to return to clinic or office for follow-up?

Evaluation means detecting whether the method was satisfactory to the client and determining whether the method is successful in preventing pregnancy. Life changes such as divorce, widowhood, or menopause, however, may cause clients to seek other methods of contraception. Unacceptable side effects prompt other clients to seek a change in method. When this occurs, a reassessment of client needs is required along with revision of the care plan. (See Nursing Care Plan.)

Test Yourself

- List at least six factors that should be considered before choosing a family planning method.

NURSING CARE PLAN • Family Planning

CASE: Lucille, a 26-year-old Hispanic, seeks help for family planning after having had two elective abortions. She smokes a pack of cigarettes a day. Weight is 160 pounds and height 5 feet 5 inches. There are no presenting medical problems. Her life-style is active, and she has several boyfriends.

ASSESSMENT

1. Level of understanding and prior attempts at contraception. Prior pregnancies and outcomes. Pattern of sexuality related to type of contraception. Menstrual history and description.
2. Observed level of health-seeking behavior. Use of interacting substances such as cigarettes. Assessment of understanding of side effects or adverse effects of chosen method. Nutritional assessment especially related to contraception.
3. Understanding of need for follow through if method is unsatisfactory.

NURSING DIAGNOSES

1. Health-seeking behavior regarding choices for life-style and contraception.
2. High risk for noncompliance in use of contraceptive.
3. High risk for noncompliance in changing habit of smoking.

EXPECTED OUTCOMES

1. States points to follow in use of chosen method.
2. States satisfaction with method.
3. Describes adverse effects resulting from continued overweight and smoking on use of contraceptive pill.
4. Returns to clinic for assistance with problems or change of method.

NURSING INTERVENTIONS

1. Determine level of understanding before orientation to methods. Relate contraindications that may be apparent in her life-style.
2. Review side effects, risks, and rates of pregnancy. Provide literature to reinforce instruction. Support Lucille's informed decision to use IUD.
3. Prepare her for fitting and pelvic examination. Review adverse effects and how to contact clinic for help. Encourage adherence to follow-up schedule.

EVALUATION

1. Does she state satisfaction with method?
2. Can she accurately describe expected side effects, method of checking for strings, what to do if IUD appears to have come out?
3. Can she state when to notify health care provider of problems?
4. Did she return for first follow-up visit as arranged?

KEY POINTS

- Methods based on natural body rhythms are gaining wide acceptance because of low cost and increased effectiveness.
- The HIV epidemic has altered the emphasis to methods that focus on an effective barrier, such as the correct use of the condom.
- Over-the-counter methods are popular but expensive for consistent use. Thus user "forgetfulness" plays a major role in lowered success ratings.
- Toxic shock syndrome has occurred with the diaphragm, the cap, and the sponge when these devices are left in place longer than recommended.
- Exposure to STDs must be taken into account in the choice of a method.
- The effectiveness of the intrauterine device (IUD) depends on the woman's reaction to bleeding, inflammation, and cramping. Those who can tolerate these early effects will find this coitus-independent method quite satisfactory.
- Hormonal control of fertility seeks to mimic body responses to pregnancy—inhibition of hypothalamus and pituitary and ovarian hormones.
- Side effects of the pill mimic early pregnancy. Low-dose preparations today are prescribed according to a woman's body type.
- Low-dose progesterone is an increasingly popular method with few side effects.
- Sterilization is a widely used method because its effects persist. Minisurgery has increased the popularity for both men and women.

STUDY QUESTIONS

5-1 Select key terms that described the following statements.
   a. Hormonal methods and sterilization are unrelated to the intercourse event and thus are _____ .
   b. The latex version of the _____ is protection against HIV infection if used correctly.
   c. The rate of effectiveness that includes reality factors is called _____ .
   d. A chemical that slows motility of sperm is _____ .
   e. Inflammation ascending into the fallopian tube results in _____ .

5-2 Rates of effectiveness are described as:
   a. Acceptability by the user and partner.
   b. Accounting for user forgetfulness.
   c. Degree to which pregnancy is prevented.
   d. Predictability about results.

5-3 Decide whether each of the following statements is *true or false*.
   a. The most effective contraceptive today is Norplant.
   b. Lowered fertility for 6 to 12 months results after stopping the combined contraceptive pill.
   c. The LAM method works only if a woman is amenorrheal during lactation.
   d. Toxic shock syndrome is a risk only with use of the vaginal sponge.
   e. Coitus interruptus is a prevention against HIV infection if used correctly.

5-4 The markers of the end of the "unsafe" period in the rhythm method include:
   a. Three full days of elevated BBT plus sticky cervical mucus.
   b. A return to preovulatory BBT and absence of any discomforts.
   c. Breast tenderness and one full day after mittelschmerz.
   d. A rise of BBT 0.8° to 1.0° F above the lowest temperature of the cycle.

5-5 Which of the following is the main advantage of Norplant?
   a. Women cannot discontinue the method on their own.
   b. Low dosage means effectiveness with few side effects.
   c. Cost over 5 years is low.
   d. Its effectiveness rate is higher than the mini-pill.

Answer Key

5-1 a. Coitus independent, b. Condom, c. Typical use, d. Spermistatic, e. Pelvic inflammatory disease 5-2 c 5-3 a. False, b. True, c. True, d. False, e. False 5-4 a 5-5 b

REFERENCES

Beral Z et al: Oral contraceptive use and malignancy of the genital tract *Lancet* 2:1331, 1988.

Board of Trustees, American Medical Association: Requirements or incentives by government for use of long-acting contraceptives, *JAMA* 267(13):1818, 1992.

Bowman M: Hormone replacement therapy: a new look at the combination regimen, *Female Patient* 15:63, 1990.

Brown RT et al: Adolescent sexuality and issues in contraception, *Obstet Gynecol Clin North Am* 19(1):177, 1992.

Charo, RA: Mandatory contraception, *Lancet* 339:1104, 1992.

Contraceptive use in older women—the rationale underlying new labeling, *Contraceptive Report* 1(2):4, 1990.

Diczfalusy E: Contraceptive prevalence, reproductive health, and our common future, *Contraception* 43(3):201, 1991.

Diczfalusy E: Contraceptive prevalence, reproductive health and international morality, *Am J Obstet Gynecol* 166(4):1037, 1992.

Fehring RD: New technology in natural family planning, *JOGNN* 20(3):199, 1991.

Franklin M: Reassessment of the metabolic effects of oral contraceptives, *J Nurse Midwife* 35(6):358, 1990.

Franklin M: Recently approved and experimental methods of contraception, *J Nurse Midwife* 35(6):365, 1990.

Gladwell M: Rating contraceptives, *Washington Post* (national weekly edition), p. 37, Jan 4-10, 1993.

Hatcher RA et al: *Contraceptive technology: 1990-1992*, ed 15, New York, 1990, Irvington Publishers.

Helbig D: Components of effective fertilization regulation, Report # R 01-HD-16504, Washington DC, 1987, National Institute of Child Health Development.

Hoffman, J: The morning-after pill, *New York Times* (magazine section), p. 12, Jan 10, 1993.

Hormonal contraception: new long-acting methods, *Popul Rep* [K] (3):1557, March-April, 1987.

IUDs—a new look, *Popul Rep* [B] 16 (1):1, No 5, March 1988.

Jones EF, Forrest JD: Contraceptive failure in the United States: revised estimates from the 1982 national survey of family growth, *Fam Plann Perspect* 21:103, 1989.

Kennedy KI et al: Contraceptive efficacy of lactational amenorrhea, *Lancet* 339 (8787):227, 1992.

Kestelman P, Trussell J: Efficacy of the simultaneous use of condoms and spermicides, *Fam Plann Perspect* 23(5):226, 1991.

Kost K et al: Comparing health risks and benefits of contraceptive choices, *Fam Plann Perspect* 23(2):54, 1991.

Lethbridge DJ: Choosing and using contraception: toward a theory of women's contraceptive self care, *Nurs Res* 40(5):276, 1991.

Lethbridge DJ: Coitus interruptus: considerations as a method of birth control, *J Obstet Gynecol Neonatal Nurs* 20(1):88, 1991.

Letterie GS, Chow GE: Effect of "missed" pills on oral contraceptive effectiveness, *Obstet Gynecol* 79(6):979, 1992.

Lynn MM, Holdcroft C: New concepts in contraception: Norplant subdermal implant, *Nurse Pract* 17(3):85, 1992.

Mishell DR: Norplant: subdermal implant system for long term contraception, *Am J Obstet Gynecol* 160:1286, 1989.

Moore SN and Rosenthal D: Condoms and coitus: adolescent attitudes to AIDS and safe sex behavior, *J Adolesc* 14:211, 1991.

Mosher WD: Contraceptive practice in the United States, 1982-1988, *Fam Plann Perspect* 22(5):198, 1990.

Petitti DB, Porterfield D: Worldwide variations in the lifetime probability of reproductive cancer in women: implications of best-case, worst-case, and likely-case assumptions about the effects of oral contraceptive use, *Contraception* 45(2):93, 1992.

Queenan JT, Moghissi KS: Natural family planning: looking ahead, *Am J Obstet Gynecol* 165(6 Pt 2):1979, 1991.

Rosenberg MJ et al: Barrier contraceptives and sexually transmitted diseases in women: a comparison of female-dependent methods and condoms, *Am J Public Health* 82(5):669, 1992.

Sharts-Engel NC: Levonorgestrel subdermal implants (Norplant) for long-term contraception, *MCN* 16:232, 1991.

Shoupe D and Mishell DR: Norplant subdermal implant system for long term contraception, *Am J Obstet Gynecol* 5(160):1286, 1989.

Silvestre L et al: Postcoital contraception: myth or reality? *Lancet* 338:39, 1991.

Soskkolne V et al: Condom use with regular and casual partners among women attending family planning clinics, *Fam Plan Perspect* 23(5):222, 1991.

Speroff L et al: *Clinical gynecology, endocrinology and infertility*, ed 4, Baltimore, 1989, Williams & Wilkins.

Tanis JL: Recognizing the reasons for contraceptive use, non-use and abuse, *Am J Maternal Child Nurs*, 2(3):364, 1977.

Winter L and Breckenmaker LC: Tailoring family planning services to the special needs of adolescents, *Family Planning Perspectives* 23(1):24, 1991.

📚 STUDENT RESOURCE SHELF

Fehring, R: New technology in natural family planning, *J Obstet, Gynecol Neonatal Nurs* 20(3): 199, 1991. Illustrates the new devices for monitoring the menstrual cycle.

Labbock MH, Howie PW: Overview and summary: the interface of breastfeeding, natural family planning and lactational amenorrhea method, *Am J Obstet Gynecol* 165(6 Pt 2):2013, 1991.

May K: Home tests to monitor fertility, *Am J Obstet Gynecol* 165(6 Pt 2):2000, 1991. This issue has a number of update articles on family planning.

Moore SM, Rosenthal D: Condoms and coitus: adolescent attitudes to AIDS and safe sex behavior, *J Adolesc* 14:211, 1991. The AIDS crisis is rapidly invading the adolescent world. Education is only part of the answer

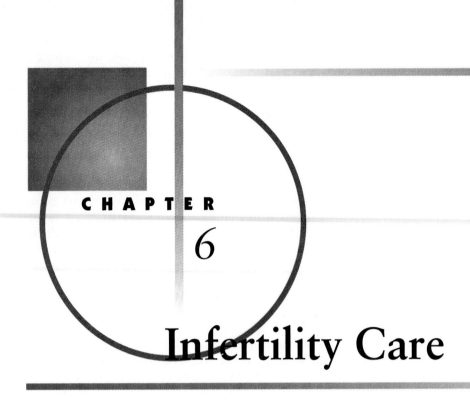

Infertility Care

LEARNING OBJECTIVES

1. *Name the major causes of male or female infertility.*
2. *Identify nursing responsibilities for the infertile couple while in therapy.*
3. *Relate health management principles for each preventable cause of infertility.*
4. *Describe nonjudgmental support measures for the infertile couple.*
5. *Compare the choices facing a couple for whom treatment is unsuccessful.*

Analysis of Infertility

The desire to give birth, to nurture an infant, and to experience parenthood is a basic human desire. Therefore impaired fertility affects a couple's self-esteem on many levels. In addition, a couple may not realize the extent and cost of the process of diagnosis and treatment when they seek assistance for their inability to conceive. Recommended treatments and supportive care needed for impaired fertility are now a subspecialty of health care. Nurses in this field need a special sensitivity to the crisis that infertility produces.

Infertility is the inability to achieve conception after 1 year of unprotected intercourse. **Primary infertility** occurs when a couple has never had a child; either the woman has never conceived, or the man has never

fathered a child. **Secondary infertility** occurs when a couple has been able to conceive one or more times (regardless of outcome) but has not been able to sustain pregnancy. In unexplained or **idiopathic infertility,** no definite cause for the infertility can be found.

Approximately 15% of couples of childbearing age in the United States are infertile. Factors that cause infertility are almost equally divided between male and female. Unexplained infertility may be the cause of 10% to 20% of the problems (Mosher et al, 1991).

Nursing care for the infertile couple is unique in one aspect: the *couple* is the client. In other areas of nursing care, you care for the couple during pregnancy, childbirth, and child rearing, but with infertility, care is intensely aimed at the partnership. With this in mind, be aware that every intervention has an impact on two people. Even if one partner is diagnosed as infertile, the partnership and relationship as a whole are affected. You must be sensitive and supportive in the care of this couple.

The success or failure of conception depends on many factors, all of which rely on appropriate physiologic function of the reproductive organs. Elements favoring conception are listed in Table 6-1.

CAUSES OF INFERTILITY

Early investigation into the causes of infertility involves a detailed history and physical examination of each partner so the obvious causes of infertility can be ruled out before the couple undergoes further costs in time, money, and emotional and physical stress. For example, timing, frequency of intercourse, chronic disease, nutritional deficiencies, alcohol or drug dependencies, psychologic problems, or treatable infections may be found to be the cause for infertility at the beginning of the work-up.

Certain occupations or life-styles pose an increased risk for men and women (for example, firefighters and workers exposed to hazardous wastes or radiation). In addition, women who have had multiple elective abortions with cervical scarring, multiple sexual partners, dramatic alterations in weight, or untreated pelvic infections are at a higher risk for infertility. Factors that contribute to infertility are outlined in Table 6-2.

Endometriosis

Nearly one third of infertile women have endometriosis. In this condition, endometrial tissue normally found inside the uterus is located outside the uterus. The cause is unknown. Recent research indicates that it may be an autoimmune response involving many organs, including the reproductive organs (Devore and Baldwin, 1986). Cyclic bleeding occurs in response to hormonal stimulation, but this tissue cannot be eliminated from the body as menstrual flow. Retention leads to reabsorption and causes scarring and adhesions within the tubes and in the peritoneal cavity. Some investigators theorize that endometriosis induces changes in the peritoneal fluid, which may create a hostile environment for optimum sperm-oocyte interaction or sperm motility (Moghissi and Wallach, 1983). The endometrial tissues that adhere to surrounding organs are known as "implants." These implants within or around the tubes also prevent clear passage of the ovum and sperm.

Symptoms (irregular menses, heavy bleeding, and severe dysmenorrhea) are often severe enough for the woman to seek help; however, many women have no symptoms until they try unsuccessfully to become pregnant. Surgical treatment or drug therapy is possible in all but the most severe cases.

TABLE 6-1   Factors Favoring Fertility

MEN	WOMEN
REPRODUCTIVE FACTORS	
Genital tract	Tubal factors
Unobstructed urethra	Unobstructed tubes
Functioning epididymis, vas deferens, and prostate	Tubal fluids and cilia fostering proper movement of ovum and sperm in tube
Descended testes	Uterine structure and function
No congenital anomalies	Endometrium adequately prepared to receive fertilized ovum
Normal secretions of genital tract	Cervical mucus receptive to sperm
Ability to penetrate vagina	Cervix competent
Ejaculate deposited at cervix (that is, no retrograde ejaculation or hypospadias)	No congenital anomalies impairing free passage between cervix and tubes
SEX CELL REPRODUCTION	
Normal spermatogenesis producing mature spermatozoa	Normal maturation of graafian follicle and release of ovum
Spermatozoa with adequate numbers and motility	Normal oogenesis producing mature ova
HORMONAL FACTORS	
Hypothalamus-pituitary-gonadal functioning intact	Hypothalamus-pituitary-gonadal functioning intact
Adequate testosterone production	Adequate ovarian hormone production

TABLE 6-2 Factors Contributing to Infertility

MEN	WOMEN	MEN	WOMEN
GENETIC OR DEVELOPMENTAL FACTORS		**CHEMICAL OR ENVIRONMENTAL FACTORS**	
Production of deformed sperm	Chromosomal abnormalities: trisomy or deletions of chromosomes, Turner's syndrome (45 X0), mosaicism of sex chromosomes	Drug abuse	Drug abuse: tranquilizers, alcohol, or nicotine
Abnormalities of testicles		Alcoholism causing reduced testosterone levels	Strenuous exercise over prolonged period
Absence or diminished number of sperm		Nicotine reducing number and motility of sperm	Use of phenothiazines and reserpine
Abnormal genitalia	Abnormal genitalia	Tight underwear	Exposure to toxic chemicals, pesticides, radiation, or heavy metals
Epispadias or hypospadias	Vaginal, uterine, ovarian abnormalities, cervical stenosis	Excessive hot tub use	
Undescended testes (both usually surgically repaired during childhood)		Exposure to toxic chemicals, radiation, pesticides, or heavy metals	Obesity or extreme underweight
Varicocele		Agent Orange exposure (in veterans)	
Chromosomal trisomy (XXY)		Strenuous exercise	
HORMONAL FACTORS		**INFLAMMATORY PROCESS AND IMMUNOLOGIC FACTORS**	
Hyposecretion of pituitary, thyroid, adrenal, or gonadal hormones	Hypersecretion of hormones released by pituitary-gonadal activity	Mycoplasma infection	Gonorrhea
	Luteal phase defects	Prostatitis	Endometriosis
	Excessive production of androgens	Mumps orchitis	Postabortion sepsis
	Polycystic ovarian disease (PCOD)	Epididymitis	Sperm antibodies in vaginal mucus
	Hyposecretion of hormones	Other infections with high fevers	
	Amenorrhea	Sperm antibodies—autoimmunity	
	Anovulation	**PSYCHOGENIC FACTORS**	
	Premenopause or postmenopause	Physical or mental stress resulting in impotence, retrograde ejaculation, or oligospermia	Anorexia nervosa
MECHANICAL OBSTRUCTION			Excessive weight loss
Retrograde ejaculation	Adhesions from previous surgery		Amenorrhea
Repair of vasectomy	Endometriosis	Poor information regarding sexual techniques	
Spinal cord injury or disease	Salpingitis	**CHRONIC ILLNESSES OR DEFICIENCIES**	
Urethral trauma causing scarring	PID	Rare pituitary or adrenal tumor	Rare pituitary or adrenal tumor
	Repair of ectopic pregnancy	Cancer of reproductive organs	Cancer of reproductive organs
	Uterine polyps	Severe diabetes	Severe diabetes
	Previous rupture of appendix with peritonitis and scar formation on fallopian tubes	Thyroid disease	Thyroid disease
		Renal disease	Renal disease
		Cardiac disease	Cardiac disease
		Severe nutritional deficiencies	Severe nutritional deficiencies
		Anemia	Anemia

PID, Pelvic inflammatory disease.

Tubal Blockage

Blockage of the fallopian tubes is often caused by pelvic inflammatory disease (PID), which leaves scar tissue and adhesions as a result of inflammation. Sometimes the tubes become kinked or twisted. Growths inside the uterus called *fibroids* may block the free passage of the sperm or ovum. Previous pelvic surgery such as an appendectomy, ovarian wedge resection, or repair of a tube after an ectopic pregnancy may result in adhesions or scarring. Use of an intrauterine contraceptive device

(IUD) or the progesterone-only oral contraceptive increases the risks of ectopic pregnancy. Tuboplasty or surgical repair of the tubes may be possible by microsurgical techniques; however, fertility rates after surgical repair of the tubes are not encouraging.

Ovulation Anomalies

The most common cause of **anovulation**—failure of the ovaries to produce, mature, or release eggs—is an imbalance of hormones that can occur at any point in hypothalamic-pituitary-ovarian interaction. Extensive testing is required to determine the source of the imbalance. In many cases ovulation is induced by the use of fertility drugs. Treatment can be extremely costly, but the resulting pregnancy rate ranges from 30% to 60%.

Cervical Mucus Problems

Cervical mucus problems may arise from vaginal infections or hormonal deficiencies that maintain the thick, acidic property of cervical mucus so it is hostile to sperm. In the case of infection, appropriate antibiotic therapy may alleviate the problem. Other cervical mucus problems may be caused by inadequate ovarian function, as in luteal phase defects (LPDs), insufficient estrogen or progesterone production, excessive androgen production, and elevated or depressed follicle-stimulating hormone (FSH) or luteinizing hormone (LH) levels. Once the problem is found, however, hormone replacement therapy may result in conception.

Varicocele

A **varicocele** is a varicose or swollen vein in the testicle. The swelling elevates the temperature within the testis and thus retards or destroys the process of spermatogenesis. The incidence of varicocele is as high as 35% in the infertile population. However, when surgical intervention alleviates the varicosity, conception results in 30% to 70% of cases.

Immunologic Factors

When a couple is infertile despite normal sperm and hormone levels, assessment of immunologic causes is the next step. Many antigens are present in semen and in the acrosome (head), midpiece, and tail of a sperm. In some cases both men and women produce antibodies against these antigens.

Sperm antibodies exist in the serum of about 12% of infertile women; research has also shown that sperm antibodies are present in the cervical mucus of about 19% of infertile women. These antibodies may be responsible for many cases of idiopathic infertility because the sperm may be unable to move freely into the uterus. In addition, nonvaginal coitus may increase this **immune response** because the mouth and anus are highly vascular areas that allow for quick entry of the

antigen into the body, triggering a large antibody response (Moghissi and Wallach, 1983).

Men who have undergone vasectomies still produce sperm; however, these sperm are absorbed into the body, not ejaculated into semen. This reabsorption sometimes promotes antibody production. This *autoimmune response* is often the cause of infertility in a man who has had vasectomy reversal.

TESTING FOR INFERTILITY

Infertility testing may be extensive before the cause of the problem can be determined (Table 6-2 and Figure 6-1). Often these tests investigate the function of each partner's reproductive organs. In women tests assess ovulatory function, presence of sexually transmitted diseases (STDs), tubal patency, and hormonal function. Testing for men centers around the presence of STDs, patency of the male ductal system, and adequacy of sperm function.

A physical examination is performed on both partners to rule out obvious signs of infertility such as abnormalities of the pelvic organs, congenital absence of organs, undescended testes, and varicocele. Thereafter tests involve internal analyses of reproductive ability.

Test Yourself
- List potential environmental causes of infertility.
- Which causes could be eliminated by general education about infertility?

Ovulatory Analysis

Poor ovulatory function may be responsible for 15% to 20% of infertility cases in women. Tests are performed to assess adequate function, as indicated in the following descriptions.

Detection of ovulation. Daily basal body temperatures (BBTs) are used routinely as a means of determining the approximate time of ovulation. Many clinics rely on the use of BBT, although it has been found to be tedious and frequently is interpreted incorrectly. A more favored means of ovulation detection is the use of an ovulation detection test (available in most pharmacies). The urine is tested for the surge in the LH levels that indicates follicular development and ovulation. Computerized fertility testing may become less expensive and more readily available in the future.

Cervical mucus testing. The appearance of *spinnbarkeit* or evidence of *ferning* indicates estrogenic influences to make mucus receptive to sperm. Spinn-

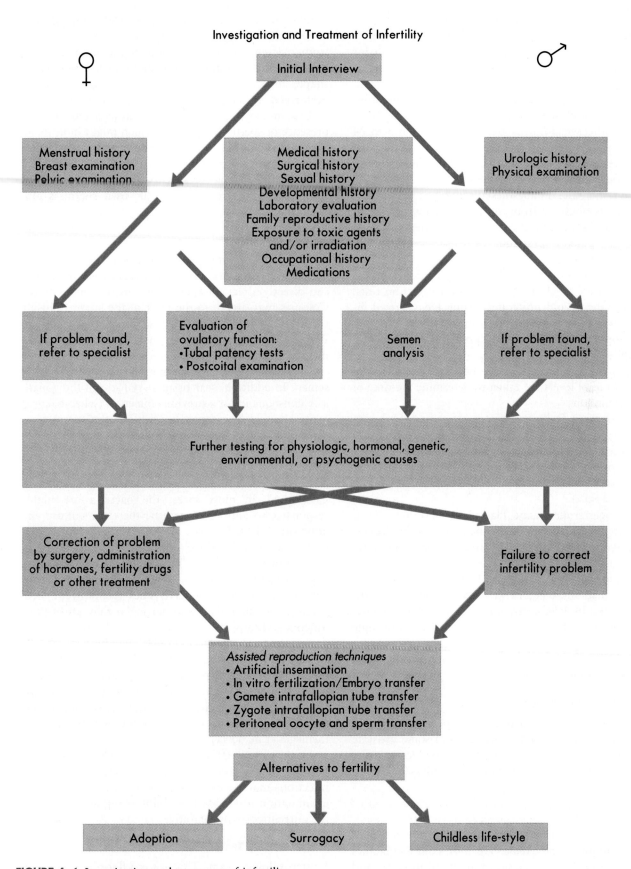

FIGURE 6-1 Investigation and treatment of infertility.

barkeit is the clear, slippery, elastic consistency of cervical mucus during ovulation, and ferning is the fernlike pattern of cervical mucus when dried on a glass slide for testing (see Figure 5-2).

Postcoital testing. Postcoital testing is performed after intercourse, as close to the time of ovulation as possible. Semen and cervical mucus are retrieved within 3 to 24 hours of intercourse to determine the adequacy of penile penetration, quality of cervical mucus, and ability of the sperm to penetrate the mucus.

The test is safe; no anesthesia is involved because the specimen is obtained from the vagina. However, many couples find that having intercourse "on demand" and then being tested is stressful.

Hormonal function tests. Hormonal function tests assess ovulatory function after ovulation detection tests, cervical mucus, and postcoital testing have proved inconclusive; these tests are performed with an endometrial biopsy for data regarding progesterone influence. The following tests are usually performed:

1. *Estrogen assay.* Midcycle measurement of serum estradiol levels are taken to determine the time of ovulation.
2. *LH assay.* Daily assessments of serum LH during the middle of the cycle are used to detect the LH surge that should occur immediately before ovulation. (LH levels are also tested in men because testicular function is controlled by pituitary gonadotropins.)
3. *Progesterone assay.* Plasma progesterone levels are measured late in the menstrual cycle. Progesterone usually rises with the LH surge and stays elevated for 8 to 10 days.
4. *Other hormone analyses.* FSH levels are tested in women and men; 17-ketosteroid and hydrocorticosteroid levels, thyroid function, and glucose tolerance tests may be necessary to determine adequate endocrine function. LTH or prolactin levels may be calculated to determine the presence of a pituitary tumor.

Ultrasound Examination

Ultrasonography is used to identify pelvic abnormalities, cysts, ovarian disease, masses, and some prostate and testes problems. Ultrasonography involves no anesthesia and is primarily noninvasive (unless a vaginal transducer is used).

Sperm Analysis

Male infertility is usually suspected when no abnormalities are found in the female. The most common factors in male infertility are sperm production, motility, and basic structure. Adequate numbers of sperm are essential for fertilization. Impairment in the shape or motility (e.g., infection, antibody production, genetic abnormalities, or environmental causes) prevents sperm from reaching their destination in the fallopian tube (Table 6-3). In addition to evaluation of the numbers, shape, and motility of the sperm, other tests are performed to aid in the diagnosis, including urinalysis and sperm antibody analysis. Urinalysis determines the presence of sperm in the urine, which might indicate an anomaly in the ducts or urethra. Urinalysis may also reveal *pyuria,* a sign of infection in either the urethra or the prostate. Testing for sperm antibodies that may be produced by the man against his own sperm is also performed.

Testing for STDs

Chlamydia trachomatis, gonorrhea, syphilis, and *Mycoplasma* infections have serious effects on fertility. They can directly affect the quality of semen in many ways. Colonies may attach to the neck of the sperm, causing them to swim in tight circles rather than straight. Bacteria may ingest substances vital for sperm nourishment or may stimulate production of antibodies. Bacteria may cause an inflammation in the glands that secrete semen. In addition, scar tissue may form in the gonads as a consequence of a previous infection (when bacteria can no longer be cultured) and block the sperm from exiting. Bacteria in seminal fluid can play a role in development of PID with subsequent salpingitis in the female.

The infections must be diagnosed to be treated (see Chapter 4). In most cases, the bacteria are highly responsive to antibiotic therapy; therefore culture and antibiotic sensitivity tests are essential. Certain antibiotics may have adverse effects on spermatogenesis, sperm function, or both. The categories of nitrofurans (e.g., Furacin), macrolides (lincomycin, chloramphenicol), tetracyclines, aminoglycosides (gentamycin, neomycin), and sulfasalazine in particular may affect these functions. Many of these drugs may impair fertility during the treatment period only. The physician usually weighs the benefits against the risks of each antibiotic therapy. Often both partners are treated, even if only one is diagnosed with the infection. After the infection has been treated with the appropriate antibiotic (see Appendix 5), conception may occur in many couples (Schlegel et al, 1991).

In the future it is hoped that cervical smears for *Chlamydia trachomatis,* gonorrhea, and *Mycoplasma* infections may become a routine part of a gynecologic examination for women of childbearing age. However, the current cost is prohibitive.

Tubal Patency Tests

Hysterosalpingogram. This test is a fluoroscopic examination that assesses tubal patency. It is performed immediately after menstruation in the absence of any

TABLE 6-3   Normal Values in Semen Analyses

CHARACTERISTICS	DESCRIPTION	COMMENTS
Color	Opaque	
pH	7.2-7.8	Sperm movement inhibited by lower pH levels.
Consistency	Fluid; quickly gels and then liquefies before 20 minutes	
Volume	3-6 ml; mean volume: 3.2 ml	Over 6 ml causes low concentration of sperm at cervical os.
Count	≥20 million to 100 million ml	Count may depend on frequency of ejaculation.
	>30 million more frequent	Allow 48-72 hours of abstinence before specimen is obtained.
Motility	≥50%-60% with good forward progression; evaluated at grade 2+ to 4 is normal	Graded on a scale of 0-4 measured 2 hours after ejaculation.
Morphology (structure)	≥60% normal, oviform	Higher percentage of tapering forms and spermatids is associated with varicocele.
Viability (eosin)	≥50%	
Cells (WBC and others)	None to occasional	Increased WBC count indicates infection.
Agglutination	None	If persistent, *Escherichia coli* infection or sperm antibodies are present.

Data compiled from Speroff L, Glan RH, Kase NG: *Clinical gynecology and endocrinology,* ed 2, Baltimore, 1979, Williams & Wilkins; and from Insler V, Lunenfield B: *Infertility: male and female,* New York, 1986, Churchill Livingstone.

infection. The absence of infection is essential because injection of the dye into the area may cause further spread of any existing infection.

Laparoscopy. This surgical procedure requires use of anesthesia for the client in most cases. After a small incision is made in the area of the umbilicus, the clinician can view the pelvic area with a laparoscope, an illuminated tube with an optical system. Minor surgical repairs such as removal of adhesions of the tubes or lesions from endometriosis may be performed. Because carbon dioxide is used to lift the abdominal wall for a clear view of the pelvic organs, referred shoulder pain may occur after the procedure.

Analysis of Male Tubes and Ducts

X-ray examination using contrast medium visualizes the vas deferens and epididymis to determine whether there are any obstructions or abnormalities. Transrectal ultrasound (TRUS) has become a more widespread and less invasive means to evaluate both the prostate and the seminal vesicles. It may also help to diagnose ejaculatory duct obstruction or stenosis. Biopsy of the testicle can also be performed if there is an obstruction.

TREATMENT FOR INFERTILITY

The approach for treatment of the infertile couple is based on the particular diagnosis. Cases of idiopathic infertility may occur in as many as 15% of infertile couples (Moghissi and Wallach, 1983). Because the field of infertility is still relatively new, there is ongoing research into causes, prevention, and cures.

Hormonal Therapy

Replacement therapy often cures infertility problems involving hormone deficiency. For instance, in cases of infertility caused by poor ovulatory function, medications to induce ovulation are available (Table 6-4).

Depending on the cause of amenorrhea or anovulation and the length of treatment, the incidence of multiple ovulation with conception of two or more ova may be as high as 30%. With the latest methods of cryopreservation, however, couples undergoing assisted reproductive techniques may elect to preserve or "freeze" their extra embryos for future use. It is thought that combining an ovulation-inducing drug with a gonadotropin-releasing hormone agonist (GnRHa) helps prevent the premature surge of LH, which in the past had led to faulty or multiple ovulation. Careful monitoring of ovulation through the use of ultrasound techniques helps reduce the risks.

Surgical Intervention

Surgical intervention can provide promising results for couples eligible for it. The couple should be given the most recent information on the probable outcomes so their ability to make decisions is not clouded. Every client undergoing reproductive surgery—and the partner—must be prepared for the possibility that

TABLE 6-4 Drug Therapy for Infertility

CATEGORY	DOSAGE	USES	PRECAUTIONS
OVULATION-INDUCING DRUGS			
Clomiphene citrate (Clomid)	Start with 50 mg every day for 5 days beginning on the third to fifth day after the LMP for three cycles. Use of high doses of Clomid (> 150 mg/day) only for women weighing > 180 lb.	Nonsteroid estrogen antagonist modifies hypothalamic activity, resulting in release of GnRH, which causes increase of FSH and LH and development of the graafian follicle. Ovulatory surge should begin 5-10 days after last pill is taken. Advise coitus every other day for one week beginning 5 days after clomiphene tablets are stopped.	Evaluate ovulation and plasma progesterone and estrogen levels. Endometrial biopsy may be done in third week. *Side effects:* Flushing, abdominal distension, bloating, breast tenderness, nausea, vomiting, visual disturbances, dryness of hair, hair loss. Symptoms cease at the end of treatment. *Adverse effects:* Ovarian enlargement. Medication not reused if visual disturbances occur. Used alone, multiple pregnancy risk is 6% to 18%. High doses may lead to significant antiestrogenic effects and abnormal folliculogenesis.
Human chorionic gonadotropin (hCG)	10,000 IU IM 7-10 days after clomiphene citrate.	hCG is added to clomiphene regimen if there is no effect or a short luteal phase. Used to trigger ovulation from a ripe follicle.	Ultrasonography is used to measure follicle development before administration. Intercourse is planned for evening of first day after injection and for next 2 days. *Side effects:* Contributes to hyperstimulation syndrome if given with hMG. *Adverse effects:* Multiple pregnancy risk at 20%–40%.
Human menopausal gonadotropin (hMG, Metrodin, Pergonal, menotropin)	Purified gonadotropins contain 75 IU of FSH and 75 IU of LH given IM, 1 ampule every day. If no response after 5 days, increase dosage.	Given for 9–12 days only to affect maturation of follicle. Must be followed by 10,000 IU hCG for rupture of follicles when appropriate size and when estrogens and cervical mucus are ready. Used for women who do not ovulate with clomiphene treatment.	Maturation of follicle followed closely to avoid overstimulation. *Side effects:* Not given if FSH or LH is already elevated, or if thyroid or adrenal problems or ovarian cyst present. Client may have febrile reaction related to possible allergy to drug. *Adverse effects:* After treatment is finished abdominal distension may indicate ovarian overstimulation. Mild to severe pain may occur.

TABLE 6-4 **Drug Therapy for Infertility—cont'd**

CATEGORY	DOSAGE	USES	PRECAUTIONS
OVULATION INDUCING DRUGS—cont'd			
Bromocriptine	1.25 mg/day for 1 week. If tolerated, dosage increased to 1–2 tablets daily (2.5–5 mg/day).	In people with persistent hyperprolactinemia. Dopamine agonist to reduce serum prolactin levels. Helps restore normal menstrual cycles and inhibits lactation.	*Side effects:* lowered BP, nausea, headache, fatigue, nasal congestion.
TESTOSTERONE PRODUCTION			
Human chorionic gonadotropin for men	5000 IU IM 3 times a week may be necessary for 4-6 months.	For primary or secondary hypo-gonadotropic gonadotropism (lack of secondary sex characteristics). Stimulates testosterone production. hMG with hCG may stimulate spermatogenesis, induce development of secondary sex characteristics, or produce more active and more numerous sperm.	*Side effects:* Possible gynecomastia. Treatment is expensive and time consuming.
GONADOTROPIN-RELEASING HORMONE THERAPY (GnRH)			
Factrel Lutre pulse	Injection administers automatic pulse dose between 1-20 mg/pulse. A belt is worn around the waist for administration of this drug.	For induction of ovulation in patients with amenorrhea with intact pituitary function who fail to respond to clomiphene treatment. Stimulates release of FSH and LH; leads to folliculogenesis. 1000-2000 IU hCG given at 3-to 4-day intervals to maintain corpus luteum function.	*Adverse effects:* Rare localized phlebitis from pulse injector.
SUPPRESSION OF PITUITARY FUNCTION			
Gonadotropin-Releasing Hormone Agonist (GnRHa) Lupron (leuprolide), synarel (inhalant), Zoladex ("Depo") Buserelin acetate	Begins on day 3 of menses. 1 mg SC daily. Lower dose after estrogen levels checked. hMG may be started.	Alleviates a major problem of LH surges associated with sole use of hMG to stimulate ovulation. Down-regulates pituitary (depletes LH stores for 2 weeks, followed by hMG) or GnRHa and hMG given concurrently. Close monitoring of estrogens and follicles required.	*Side effects:* Hot flashes, memory and sleep disturbances, irritability.

Continued.

TABLE 6-4   Drug Therapy for Infertility—cont'd

CATEGORY	DOSAGE	USES	PRECAUTIONS
ENDOMETRIOSIS SUPPRESSION			
Danazol (danocrine)	600-800 mg in 3 or 4 divided doses daily for 4-6 months, starting on day 5 of menses.	Synthetic weak androgen prevents midcycle LH surge, so endometriosis is inhibited and tissue regresses and atrophies. Stimulates menopausal effect on endometrial tissue suppressing ectopic implants. It is sometimes used in fibrocystic breast disease to relieve pain and tender nodules.	*Side effects:* Related to reduced gonadotropins: amenorrhea, weight gain, acne, increased skin oils, vasomotor flushing, vasomotor instability, voice changes, fluid retention. Return of ovulation occurs in 60-90 days. Care needed to monitor ovulation (either with the kit or with BBT charts) because drug should not be used during pregnancy (may cause clitoral hypertrophy and labial fusion in female infants).
Provera (medroxy-progesterone acetate)	10-30 mg/day orally or 200 mg IM ("Depo") once a month for 6 months.	Sustained progestational effect causes atrophic changes in the endometrial implants.	*Side effects:* Abdominal bloating. *Adverse effects:* Prolonged anovulation after discontinuing treatment. Not usually recommended for women with primary infertility.

pregnancy may still not be achieved afterward. Among surgical interventions that may be considered are repairs of congenital anomalies, tubal adhesions, vasectomies, varicoceles, ductal obstructions, and removal of tumors affecting reproductive ability. Certain chronic infections of the vaginal tract may respond to a procedure called conization, which is removal of a cone-shaped portion of the endocervix.

Treatment for Immunologic Infertility

Several options are available for the treatment of immunologic infertility. The most promising pregnancy rates occur in couples who elect to undergo assisted reproductive techniques—such as in vitro fertilization (IVF), gamete intrafallopian tube transfer (GIFT), and zygote intrafallopian tube transfer (ZIFT)—because these processes all involve sperm "washing" (Hammond and Talbert, 1992). Other methods used with less success are separation of sperm from the cervical mucus by condoms for 6 to 12 months until the serum antibody titer is lowered in the woman; then condoms are used at all times except at ovulation. The couple should avoid anal and oral intercourse, which could increase the antibody titer in the body. "Washed" spermatozoa from the partner may be inserted into the cervical canal for insemination. Antibiotic therapy eliminates bacteria that may have contributed to antibody formation in the man or the woman.

Alternate Methods to Promote Fertility
ARTIFICIAL INSEMINATION

Artificial insemination can be performed using the husband's sperm (homologous insemination [AIH]), a donor's sperm (heterologous insemination [AID]), or a combination of both. The sperm may be fresh or frozen. The success rate is as high as 70% to 90%. Artificial insemination is carefully timed to coincide with ovulation. This method is usually used when the male partner is infertile or if there is an immune problem.

The ejaculate is deposited into the cervical canal or vaginal vault and kept in place with a diaphragm or cervical cap for 8 hours. Two or three inseminations may be required within one monthly cycle; the process may continue for 6 to 12 months until pregnancy occurs.

Ethical, legal, and moral questions occur with donor inseminations. However, many legal safeguards have been established, including the anonymity of the donor and recipient, use of only one donor for each attempt, and screening the donor for genetic defects, infectious processes, drug abuse, and blood type. Screening for the HIV virus is a routine part of the donor process. The couple requesting artificial insemination must sign an informed consent and a contract accepting the resultant offspring as their legal heir.

IN VITRO FERTILIZATION/EMBRYO TRANSFER (IVF/ET)

The first successful *in vitro fertilization (IVF)* (test tube conception) was performed in Great Britain in 1978. The most likely candidates for this approach are women whose oviducts have been irreparably damaged.

The success rate of IVF/ET is only 15% to 20%. Because most fertility clinics calculate their success rates according to the number of pregnancies per IVF/ET, it can be a misleading statistic for couples. The delivery rate is substantially lower as a result of spontaneous abortions, preterm deliveries, and stillbirths. However, because it is usually a last resort, almost every couple expects success. Thus the process is very stressful. In addition, the cost is high, between $2000 and $5000 per attempt, which may or may not be covered by the couple's health insurance.

Seven steps are involved in the process of IVF/ET: (1) patient selection, (2) induction of ovulation to ensure the release of ova and their subsequent retrieval, (3) oocyte retrieval, (4) semen collection, (5) fertilization and cleavage in the laboratory with "washed" sperm, (6) transfer of the embryo to the woman's uterus, and (7) establishment of pregnancy (Good and Hahn, 1993). Many infertility centers use transvaginal ultrasonography to retrieve the ova; this procedure can be performed without general anesthesia on an outpatient basis. The goal for many centers is to perform the entire IVF/ET process on an outpatient basis, thus lowering costs in terms of time and fees as well as lowering the incidence of physical complications of surgery.

A new method that may become more widespread is intravaginal fertilization after oocyte retrieval (Taymor, 1992). With this process the oocytes are retrieved by use of ultrasound guidance; they are then mixed with sperm in the laboratory, positioned in a sealed "envelope" in the vagina (to incubate the ova and sperm under more optimal conditions), and removed 48 hours later to determine whether fertilization occurred. The embryo is then transferred to the uterus. Because this method is still under investigation, its use is not yet routine.

GAMETE INTRAFALLOPIAN TUBE TRANSFER (GIFT)

Gamete intrafallopian tube transfer (GIFT) is a process that closely approximates the process of IVF/ET except that the embryo is placed in the fallopian tube. Many problems can be overcome with this method, including cervical mucus abnormalities, low sperm count or motility, and some cases of idiopathic infertility. The couple is followed closely as with IVF and given hormonal therapy to stimulate ovulation. Daily ultrasound evaluations determine follicular maturation. After confirmation of mature follicles, the ova are retrieved and placed with the partner's sperm. The combined ova and sperm are then immediately returned to the woman's fallopian tubes. There is no waiting period in the laboratory for confirmation of fertilization. Progesterone therapy to support implantation is used when necessary. GIFT is a technique that can sometimes be used without religious objection because fertilization actually occurs in the fallopian tubes.

This program involves intense couple participation on a daily basis. The potential for stress is high. There is also a risk of ectopic pregnancy, multiple births, and surgical complications (placement of the embryo in the fallopian tubes must be done surgically with the woman under anesthesia).

ZYGOTE INTRAFALLOPIAN TUBE TRANSFER (ZIFT)

Zygote intrafallopian tube transfer (ZIFT) is the same process as GIFT except that the ova and sperm are returned to the fallopian tubes after fertilization occurs in the laboratory.

GIFT and ZIFT are options used only in women who have at least one functioning fallopian tube. Some researchers believe that success rates are higher because the ova and sperm are placed in the tubal area where fertilization ordinarily occurs, thus providing the fertilized ovum a chance to become acclimated and move through the tube to the uterus, not arriving there prematurely as in some IVF procedures (Guirgis et al, 1992).

Although the tubal transfer procedures may be more beneficial to pregnancy outcome than uterine transfer, tubal transfer procedures have several disadvantages because of the need for general anesthesia, laparoscopy, and hospitalization.

PERITONEAL OOCYTE AND SPERM TRANSFER (POST)

Peritoneal oocyte and sperm transfer is a procedure that uses ultrasound guidance for retrieval of oocytes to which sperm are added. The mixture is then placed in the peritoneal cavity near the fimbriae of the tubes. Luteal support may be necessary in the form of hCG therapy. This procedure has been used successfully for the treatment of unexplained infertility and failed donor insemination. As with GIFT, POST allows accurate control of the number of oocytes transferred; any excess oocytes may be inseminated and frozen for future use. Currently scientists are unable to successfully cryopreserve oocytes alone. POST is done with local anesthesia for the woman; no abdominal surgery is necessary and the procedure can thus be performed on an outpatient basis (Bongers, 1991; Sharma et al, 1991; Tan, 1992).

INTRAUTERINE INSEMINATION (IUI)

Intrauterine insemination (IUI) is used in cases in which cervical mucus properties (possibly altered by infection or antibody formation) cause infertility. IUI involves hormonal stimulation of the ovaries with artificial insemination inside the uterus, thus bypassing the cervix. IUI can be performed on an outpatient basis and requires little or no anesthesia for the woman.

MICROMANIPULATION

Zona drilling is a new approach that is used when semen is repeatedly unable to fertilize the ova in the laboratory (in vitro). The zona pellucida is the protective layer of cells surrounding the ovum. For fertilization to occur (in vivo or in vitro), the cell membrane must be penetrable by the sperm. The following methods aid in that process: (1) *partial zona dissection*

involves making a small slit in the zona pellucida, which allows the sperm direct access to the oocyte, and (2) *subzonal insertion* involves puncturing the zona with a fine pipette through which a small number of spermatozoa are injected (Figure 6-2).

Alternatives to Fertility
SURROGACY/HOST MOTHERHOOD

In surrogacy, a surrogate or substitute mother accepts an embryo and agrees to carry the pregnancy to term for the infertile couple. The ova and sperm may be donated from the infertile couple or donor ova and sperm may be used. There are cases of the infertile woman's own mother accepting her daughter's fertilized ovum and carrying her own grandchild to term. Hormonal replacement therapy enables even the menopausal woman to support the pregnancy. When the infertile woman produces no ova, donor embryos may be used from cryopreservation units.

Many states lack legislation to protect the rights of all parties involved in a surrogate program. As a result the risk of exploitation on both sides is high. Many safeguards must be provided for the infertile couple as well as the surrogate mother. These safeguards include written agreements of assumption of responsibility for the infant, counseling, psychologic screening, screening for genetic diseases or STDs, legal counsel, and tissue typing to determine paternity.

The potential for surrogate attachment to the infant is significant. Some grief or mourning over giving up the

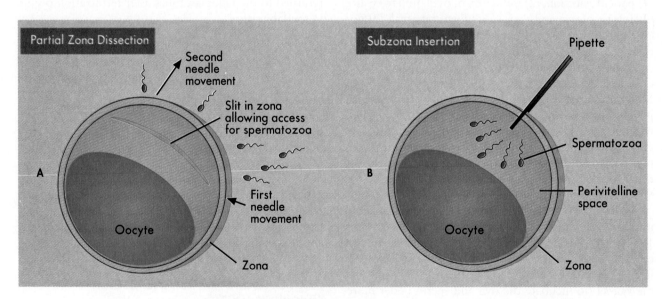

FIGURE 6-2 Micromanipulation is a new technique for assisting fertilization when sperm quality is poor. **A,** A slit is made in the zona, allowing sperm to enter. **B,** Sperm are inserted through the zona by means of a pipette. (Redrawn from Waterstone J: Investigations in subfertility, *Practitioner* 236:144, 1992.)

infant can be expected. Counseling the surrogate by providing all information may help her overcome feelings of loss. The surrogate may also benefit from the nurse's availability for counseling for a period of time after the birth.

ADOPTION

When the infertile couple consider adoption, the solution to their infertility problem may or may not be resolved. They may have undergone years of testing, probing, and questioning about their private lives and habits but are still faced with the inability to conceive. In such cases the couple may need to isolate their desire to reproduce themselves from their desire to parent a child. Only the latter need can be met by adoption (Valentine, 1986) (see Chapter 20).

CHILDLESS LIFE-STYLE

For most people childbearing and parenthood are major life events involving goals and plans for the future. When childbearing does not take place, a deep sense of loss is perceived. Couples who have already undergone the process of infertility testing and treatment are frequently faced with intense stress, anger, and rage. If the couple chooses to remain childless, they may need to grieve and mourn for their lost role as parents. Although males and females may differ in their particular adjustment, a sense of shared values, goals, and interests helps the couple adjust to a childless life-style. The couple may need much support during this time of transition. Helping them to refocus their goals for their marriage, review career options, and establish hobbies or outside interests may foster the adjustment to childlessness. Acceptance of a childless life-style may be associated with greater marital adjustment over time (Ulbrich et al, 1990).

ISSUES TO CONSIDER

Children born as a result of assisted reproductive technologies require extensive follow-up care. Many women deliver their infants in centers that are not associated with their infertility clinic, and they may not receive thorough follow-up. Infants should be evaluated for physiologic problems (i.e., congenital anomalies such as spina bifida, transposition of the great vessels, hypospadias, adolescent cancers in reproductive organs) as well as behavioral and psychologic sequelae (attention deficit problems, "miracle or precious child" problems resulting from overattention).

As the technology increases in sophistication, ethical, moral, and social issues surrounding assisted reproduction are being debated. Some concerns involve whether embryos should be frozen or used in experiments for research purposes. Other concerns revolve around the risks to mother, father, and offspring.

The increasing reliance on expensive technology and the use of money, resources, medical education and expertise for assisted reproduction for a few clients as compared to more urgent community health needs should be discussed so that legislation for funding can become more equitable.

Nursing Responsibilities
▶ NURSING DIAGNOSES

Nursing diagnoses for infertility are related to the physical and emotional impact on the couple, invasive procedures, and teaching involved. Examples are:

1. Altered health maintenance. One or both partners may use ineffective methods of coping.

2. Self-esteem disturbance. The loss of reproductive abilities may change image of self.

3. Altered family or individual coping.

4. Health-seeking behavior concerning menstrual cycle, sexual reproductive physiology, and medical interventions. These behaviors may be impaired by the fear of the unknown.

5. Altered patterns of sexuality related to invasion of privacy, loss of spontaneity in the sexual relationship, or extensive diagnostic testing.

6. Decisional conflict during the process of treatment or in choosing alternatives to fertility.

▶ EXPECTED OUTCOMES

An essential aspect of care for the infertile couple is helping them maintain a sense of control. Fostering a sense of active participation in the management and treatment of the problem is an integral part of the goal. The couple should be able to:

1. Accurately describe the physiologic and psychologic factors influencing their fertility.

2. Compare the costs, purposes, and progression of fertility testing before decision making.

3. Attend counseling and treatment sessions to foster progress through the infertility work-up.

4. Comply with the regimen by maintaining accurate ovulation/intercourse/menstrual charts. The couple will

  Self-Discovery

How do you feel about a couple's options for use of AID, AIH, adoption, or surrogate motherhood?

BOX 6-1 Fertility Promotion for Couples

- It takes the average couple 6 to 9 months of unprotected intercourse to achieve pregnancy.
- Women who ovulate regularly do so 14 days ±2 before the *next* menstrual period. Distinctive changes in cervical mucus indicate that ovulation has probably occurred.
- Use of ovulation predictor tests is very helpful.
- The woman may be asked to keep a record of distinctive changes in cervical mucus. This clear, abundant mucus precedes the day of ovulation and provides a transport medium for the sperm. If these changes do not occur, the physician will evaluate hormonal levels.
- The normal fertile man needs 30 to 40 hours to return to his usual sperm production levels after an ejaculation. A man with low sperm count may need as long as 48 hours.
- With a typical menstrual cycle of 28 days (there are many variations in cycle length), intercourse should occur in the following pattern when a woman is trying to conceive:
    Nights 9 and 12
    Morning 14
    Night 15
    No times in between
  This schedule allows the pituitary gland to stimulate sperm production and provides time for sperm production to return to peak levels. It also maintains active sperm in the female reproductive tract.
- Intercourse should occur three to four times per week during the month to stimulate sperm production.

- Positions are important. The superior (man above) position is best for intercourse aimed at fertility. The woman's hips should be elevated on a small pillow to facilitate sperm collection in the seminal pool near the opening of the cervix.
- The deepest penetration is advised. The woman may fold her knees on her chest and spread them as far apart as possible.
- At ejaculation, the man should penetrate as deeply as possible and stop thrusting so ejaculation occurs as near the cervix as possible. Withdrawal should occur just after ejaculation.
- When female orgasm occurs during or after ejaculation, the cervix is allowed to dip into the seminal pool.
- The woman should remain in bed for 1 hour after ejaculation to hold the seminal pool near the cervix.
- No artificial lubricants should be used. However, saliva, egg white, or olive oil are physiologic and will not hinder sperm mobility.
- No douching should be used before or after intercourse.
- Because intercourse "on demand" or on a "medical schedule" may seem artificial, care should be taken that technique and timing do not destroy an atmosphere of making love. Some men experience temporary impotence. Talking this over with the fertility nurse or physician may lessen tension and promote appropriate function.

From Dickason EJ, McKenzie CA: The infertile family. In Howe J et al, eds: *The handbook of nursing,* New York, 1984, John Wiley & Sons.

---

adhere to the schedule of sexual intercourse and the medication regimen.

5. Express a sense of self-worth and adequacy or be able to verbalize the need for help.

▶ NURSING INTERVENTIONS

Nursing care for the infertile couple requires a great deal of sensitivity, maturity, and empathy. Couples may need an honest listener who is neither authoritarian nor emotionally involved with their complex problems. As the nurse you will not be able to provide the "right answers" to "fix" their problems. You may need to help the couple grieve for the loss of the "perfect" body and help them find a means of coping with their new physical and sexual identities (Hammond and Talbert, 1992). Nursing care also involves a documentation of the records. A nursing care plan will include*:

1. Providing privacy.

2. Encouraging discussion to lay the groundwork for a trusting nurse-couple relationship.

3. Identifying areas of lack of knowledge and teaching self-help techniques (see Box 6-1).

4. Determining the couple's readiness to learn and absorb information along with the physician or other members of the health team.

5. Assisting the couple in identifying long-range plans, including setting a time limit on the treatments and choosing artificial insemination, adoption, or remaining childless if infertility cannot be overcome.

6. Helping the couple identify and use outside support systems, other family members, or religious or support groups.

7. Helping the couple nurture the marriage through this stressful time.

8. Respecting and preserving the couple's choice and manner of reproduction.

*From the Statement of Standards' Committee of the American Fertility Society Nurses' Special Interest Group (Hammond and Talbert, 1992).

▶ EVALUATION

Evaluation of care requires follow-up for the infertile couple. Many couples become frustrated and discouraged from the time-consuming and painstaking nature of the process. A man may experience temporary impotence from intercourse on demand. Time out from the regimen to restore the romance in making love may be necessary. If pregnancy results, however, follow-up care is still necessary because of the drastic change in the couple's life-style, self-image, and future plans. Previously infertile women may have more difficulty adapting to the role of mother. The infertile couple is confronted with many experiences of failure and may insulate themselves psychologically from yet another failure. The couple may delay preparing for the arrival of the baby and exhibit less self-confidence once parenthood occurs (Dunnington et al, 1991).

If the couple does not conceive, long-range follow-up depends on the decisions they make about alternative options. Evaluation of outcomes shows that:

1. Communication remained open between the couple and the health care team.
2. Couple expressed positive self-esteem.
3. Couple used support resources as needed and contemplated alternatives.
4. Each partner was able to follow directions for testing and treatment.

(KEY) POINTS

Infertility may be found in as many as 15% to 20% of the childbearing population.

- A couple is considered infertile after 1 year of unprotected intercourse without conceiving.
- To determine the cause of infertility, the couple is evaluated for reproductive organ function, and sperm and ova adequacy.
- Causes of infertility are almost equally divided between male and female. Approximately 10% to 20% of all cases of infertility are related to unexplained or idiopathic causes.

- Treatment may be multifaceted and may involve administration of hormones and antibiotics, surgical repair of structural abnormalities, or removal of adhesions or tumors.
- Advanced technologies to assist reproduction include IVF/ET, GIFT, and ZIFT. Other microtechnologies are being developed.
- Nursing care for the infertile couple focuses on support and assessment. Active listening, teaching, counseling, information about referral systems and support groups, and documentation of events are essential aspects.

STUDY QUESTIONS

6-1 Apply Key Terms to the following descriptions:
  a. The introduction of semen directly into the uterine cavity _____
  b. Artificial insemination with the husband's sperm _____
  c. A male forms antibodies against his own sperm _____
  d. A female forms antibodies against her partner's sperm _____
  e. A swollen, twisted vein in the testicle _____

6-2 Select the true statements about infertility in the list below.
  a. Highest rate in men working in hot environments
  b. Usually caused by unexplained factors
  c. Antibiotic therapy may have adverse effects on spermatogenesis
  d. Approximately evenly divided between male and female
  e. Can usually be altered by improved coital techniques

6-3 The Smiths had one child 5 years ago. They have tried to conceive with no success. They will be assessed at the clinic for:
  a. Idiopathic infertility
  b. Primary infertility
  c. Secondary infertility

6-4 Which of the following statements about endometriosis are usually true?
  a. Results in permanent infertility
  b. Involves all the reproductive organs
  c. Increases discomfort during menses
  d. May scar the fallopian tubes

6-5 Match the conditions below with the most likely causes or etiologic factors.

1. Anovulation	a. Autoimmune response
2. Endometriosis	b. Infection
3. Postvasectomy repair infertility	c. Inadequate ovarian function
4. Low sperm production	d. Chemical/environmental factors

Answer Key

REFERENCES

Abbey A et al: Psychosocial, treatment and demographic predictors of the stress associated with infertility, *Fertil Steril* 57(10):122, 1992.

Bongers MY et al: Peritoneal oocyte and sperm transfer; a prospective pilot study, *Fertil Steril* 56(1): 147, 1991.

Chang SY et al: A clinical pregnancy after a simple method of zona cutting, cryopreservation and zygote intrafallopian tube transfer, *Fertil Steril* 55(2): 420, 1991.

Davis DC, Dearman CN: Coping strategies of infertile women, *J Obstet Gynecol Neonatal Nurs* 20(3): 221, 1993.

Devore N and Baldwin K: Ectopic pregnancy on the rise, *Am J Nurs* 86(6): 674, 1986.

Dunnington RM et al: Potential psychological attachments formed by donors involved in infertility technology—another side to infertility, *Nurse Pract* 16(11): 41, 1991.

Dunnington RM et al: Maternal identity and early mothering behavior in previously infertile women, *J Obstet Gynecol Neonatal Nurs* 20(4): 309, 1991.

Fischel S et al: Evaluation of 225 patients undergoing subzonal insemination for the procurement of fertilization in vitro, *Fertil Steril* 57(4): 840, 1992.

Fischel S et al: Subzonal insemination for alleviation of infertility, *Fertil Steril* 54:(5): 828, 1990.

Gant NF: Infertility and endometriosis: comparison of pregnancy outcomes with laparotomy versus laparoscopic techniques, *Am J Obstet Gynecol* 166(4):1072, 1992.

Guirgis RR et al: GIFT in women who had ectopic pregnancy previously, *Obstet Gynecol* 79(4):586, 1992.

Hammond MG, Talbert LM, eds: *Infertility: a practical guide for the physician,* ed 3, Boston, 1992, Blackwell Scientific.

Harris BG et al: Infertility . . . a new interpretation of pregnancy loss, *MCN Am J Matern Child Nurs* 16(4):217, 1991.

Hirsch AM, Hirsch SM: The effect of infertility on marriage and self-concept, *JOGNN* 18(1) 13, 1988.

Keleher KC: Occupational health: How work environments can affect reproductive capacity and outcome, *Nurse Pract,* 16(1):23, 1991.

McClusky S et al: Infertility and eating disorders [letter], *Am J Obstet Gynecol* 165:1576, 1991.

Millard S: Emotional responses to infertility: understanding patients' needs, *AORN J* 54(2):301, 1991.

Moghissi KS and Wallach EE: Unexplained infertility, *Fertil Steril* 39(1):5, 1985.

Mosher WD et al: Fecundity and infertility in the US: incidence and trends, *Fertil Steril* 56(2):192, 1991.

Nachtigall RD et al: The effects of gender-specific diagnoses on the male and female response to infertility, *Fertil Steril* 57(1): 113, 1992.

Sandelowski M: The color gray: ambiguity and infertility, *Image* 19(2): 70, 1987.

Sandelowski M: Women's experiences of infertility, *Image* 18(4): 140, 1986.

Schlegel PN et al: Antibiotics: potential hazard to male fertility, *Fertil Steril* 56(2):1235, 1991.

Sharma R et al: Establishment of pregnancy after removal of sperm antibodies in vitro, *Br Med J,* 304:640, 1992.

Sharma R et al: Experience with peritoneal oocyte and sperm transfer as an outpatient based treatment for infertility, *Fertil Steril* 55 (3): 579, 1991.

Speroff L, Glass RH, Kase NG: *Clinical gynecology endocrinology and infertility,* ed 4, Baltimore, 1989, Williams & Wilkins.

Stewart S, Glazer G: Expectations and coping of women undergoing in vitro fertilization, *MCN Am J Matern Child Nurse* 15(2): 103, 1986.

Tan SL: Transvaginal peritoneal oocyte and sperm transfer for the treatment of nontubal infertility, *Fertil Steril* 57(4): 850, 1992.

Ulbrich PM et al: Involuntary childlessness and marital adjustment: his and hers, *J Sex Marital Ther* 16(3): 147, 1990.

Valentine D: Psychological impact of infertility: identifying issues and needs, *Soc Work Health Care* 11(4): 61, 1986.

Wright J et al: Psychological distress and infertility: males and females respond differently, *Fertil Steril* 55(1):100, 1991.

Wessels PH et al: Cost effectiveness of gamete intrafallopian tube transfer in comparison with induction of ovulation with gonadotropins in the treatment of female infertility: a clinical trial, *Fertil Steril* 57(1): 163, 1992.

STUDENT RESOURCE SHELF

Good CJ, Hahn SJ: Oocyte donation and in vitro fertilization: The nurse's role with ethical and legal issues. *J Obstet, Gynecol Neonatal Nurs* 22(2)-106, 1993.

Harris. BA, Sandelowski M, Holditich-Davis D: Infertility and new interpretations of pregnancy loss, *Am J Maternal/Child Nurs* 16(4): 217, 1991.

Nursing interventions for couples losing a pregnancy after infertility work-up.

Sandelowski M et al: Pregnant moments: the process of conception in infertile couples, *Res Nurs Health* 13(5) 273, 1990.

A complex problem continues to be a subject for nursing research.

BOOKS FOR COUPLES

Bellina JH, Wilson J: *You can have a baby: everything you need to know about fertility,* New York, 1985, Crown Publishers.

Carter JW, Carter M: *Sweet grapes: how to stop being infertile and start living again,* Indianapolis, 1989, Perspectives Press.

Harkness C.: *The infertility book: a comprehensive medical and emotional guide,* San Francisco, 1987, Volcano Press.

Lasker JN, Borg S: *In search of parenthood: coping with infertility and high-tech conception,* Boston, 1987, Beacon Press.

Mason MM: *The miracle seekers: an anthology of infertility,* Chicago, 1987, Perspectives Press.

Menning BE: *Infertility: a guide for the childless couple,* ed 2, New York, 1988, Prentice Hall.

Perloe M, Christie LG: *Miracle babies and happy endings for couples with fertility problems,* New York, 1986, Penguin Books.

Stephenson LR: *Give us a child: the personal crisis of infertility,* New York, 1987, Harper & Row.

VanRegenmorter J, VanRegenmorter S, McIlhaney JS: *Dear God, why can't we have a baby? A guide for the infertile couple,* Grand Rapids, Mich, 1986, Baker Book House.

Winston R: *What we know about infertility: diagnosis and treatment alternatives,* New York, 1987, Free Press.

RESOURCES FOR COUPLES

Organizations

American College of Obstetricians and Gynecologists (ACOG)
  ACOG Distribution Center
  PO Box 91180
  Washington, DC 20090-1180

American Fertility Society
  2140 Eleventh Avenue South
  Suite 200
  Birmingham, AL 35205-2800

National Infertility Network
  Networth Exchange
  PO Box 204
  East Meadow, NY 11554

RESOLVE Inc.
  5 Water Street
  Arlington, MA 02174

Serono Symposia USA
  100 Longwater Circle
  Norwell, MA 02061

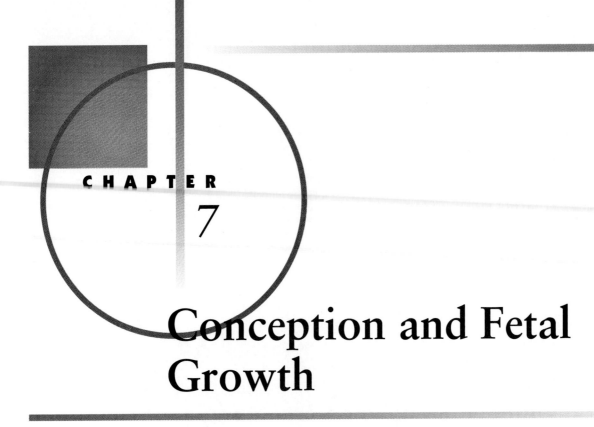

Conception and Fetal Growth

KEY TERMS

Amnion
Anencephaly
Autosomal
Blastocyst
Brown fat
Chorion
Dermatoglyphics
Ductus Arteriosus
Ductus Venosus
Embryo
Fertilization Age
Fetal Germ Layers
Fetal Viability
Foramen Ovale
Germinal Matrix
Gestational Age
Hematopoiesis
Meconium

Meiosis
Mitosis
Morula
Myelin
Organogenesis
Passive Immunity
Surfactant
Syngamy
Trophoblast

Teratogen
Testes Determining
  Factor
Umbilical Artery
Umbilical Vein
Vernix Caseosa
Viable
Wharton's Jelly
Zygote

LEARNING OBJECTIVES

1. *Distinguish between growth and development.*
2. *Compare meiosis and mitosis.*
3. *Describe the process of fertilization.*
4. *Distinguish between the embryonic and fetal periods.*
5. *Explain the sequence of development of the placenta, umbilical cord, and fetal circulation.*
6. *Relate fetal structures to prenatal and postnatal function.*
7. *Identify important milestones in embryonic and fetal growth and development.*

Between conception and birth, health care begins for the prospective mother and the growing fetus. Many factors are involved in the growth and development of the infant as a separate and unique individual, including the configuration of genes from both parents, intrauterine environment, and external environmental influences.

It is important to distinguish between growth and development. *Growth* is an increase in the size and number of cells that causes an organism to gain weight

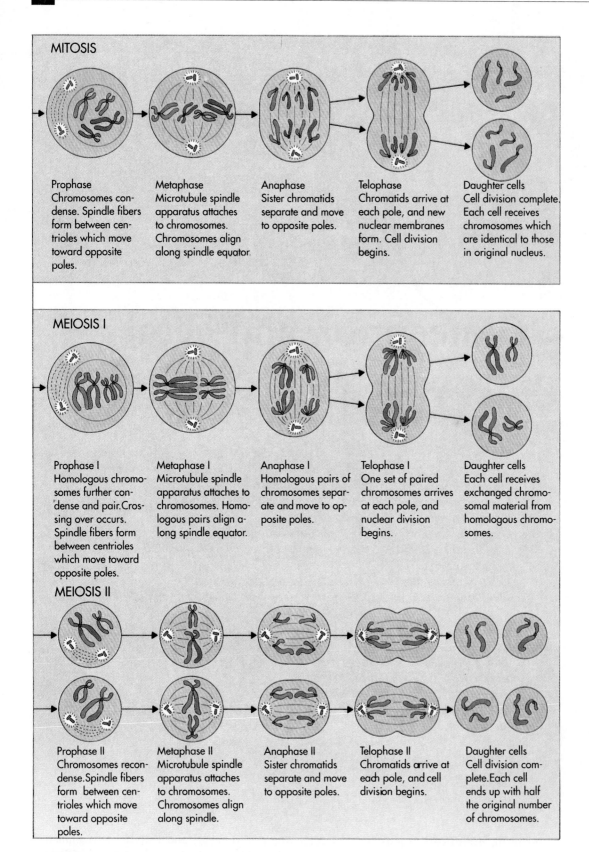

MITOSIS

Prophase
Chromosomes condense. Spindle fibers form between centrioles which move toward opposite poles.

Metaphase
Microtubule spindle apparatus attaches to chromosomes. Chromosomes align along spindle equator.

Anaphase
Sister chromatids separate and move to opposite poles.

Telophase
Chromatids arrive at each pole, and new nuclear membranes form. Cell division begins.

Daughter cells
Cell division complete. Each cell receives chromosomes which are identical to those in original nucleus.

MEIOSIS I

Prophase I
Homologous chromosomes further condense and pair. Crossing over occurs. Spindle fibers form between centrioles which move toward opposite poles.

Metaphase I
Microtubule spindle apparatus attaches to chromosomes. Homologous pairs align along spindle equator.

Anaphase I
Homologous pairs of chromosomes separate and move to opposite poles.

Telophase I
One set of paired chromosomes arrives at each pole, and nuclear division begins.

Daughter cells
Each cell receives exchanged chromosomal material from homologous chromosomes.

MEIOSIS II

Prophase II
Chromosomes recondense. Spindle fibers form between centrioles which move toward opposite poles.

Metaphase II
Microtubule spindle apparatus attaches to chromosomes. Chromosomes align along spindle.

Anaphase II
Sister chromatids separate and move to opposite poles.

Telophase II
Chromatids arrive at each pole, and cell division begins.

Daughter cells
Cell division complete. Each cell ends up with half the original number of chromosomes.

FIGURE 7-1 A comparison of mitosis with meiosis. During mitosis, chromosomes are duplicated and the cell divides, producing two new cells identical to the first. During meiosis, chromosomes are duplicated only once, but there are two consecutive cellular divisions. This yields four daughter cells, each with half the maternal number of chromosomes. (Courtesy Raychel Ciemma.)

and length. *Development* refers to the changes that occur in primitive cells as they differentiate into tissues that will perform specific functions. In this chapter you will learn how these processes interact during gestation.

When prospective parents inquire about the formation, growth, and development of their infant, you will be in an ideal position to encourage their interest and help them to understand factors that can affect the health of the fetus.

Cellular Reproduction

In all body tissue, cells multiply by a process called **mitosis**. To divide, the parent cell duplicates each chromosome so each new cell is an exact replica (copy) of it. First, there is separation to the opposite sides of the cell before division; an indentation develops in the center so two identical cells result.

In contrast, a special type of cell division, **meiosis** (Figure 7-1), must take place in the ovum and sperm to assure that there will be exactly 23 pairs or 46 chromosomes in the new embryo's cells. Meiosis causes each oocyte and spermatocyte to contain one member of each pair of chromosomes. This reduction in chromosomes is made possible by a two-step process. The first meiotic division begins much earlier than fertilization. During this step, the primary oocyte and primary spermatocyte duplicate their deoxyribonucleic acid (DNA) and double their chromosomes, producing double strands or chromatids.

At the same time, the two members of a chromosome pair often exchange segments of genetic material (Figure 7-2). During this "crossing over" between homologous chromosomes, paternal and maternal genetic material is randomly recombined so that the genes passed to the infant may be quite different from those in either parent. This is one of the reasons a child may not look or act like either parent. After the exchange, the chromosomes line up near the middle of the cell, and the cell and chromosomes divide into two new cells. Thus two nonidentical daughter cells result from this division.

Double strands of genetic material are still in these cells, however. In the second meiotic division, the double-structured chromosomes divide, and the reduction is completed. The resulting cells are ready for fertilization. Each of the four cells that result from the two oocyte maturational divisions contain 22 autosomes (body cell chromosomes) and one X (sex) chromosome. Only one of these cells develops into a mature oocyte. The other three become polar bodies, which receive chromosomes that eventually degenerate and dissolve. In contrast, a spermatocyte divides into four types of cells, two containing 22 autosomes and one X chromosome and two containing 22 autosomes and one Y chromosome. All these cells become active sperm (Figure 7-3).

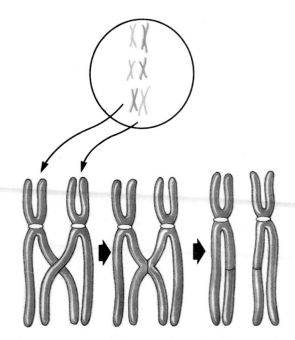

FIGURE 7-2 Crossing over. Genes (or linked groups of genes) from one chromosome are exchanged with matching genes in the other chromosome of a pair during meiosis. (Courtesy David J. Mascaro & Associates.)

OOGENESIS

During embryonic life, the primary oocytes undergo only a part of the first meiotic division. Then these same primary oocytes enter a resting phase until puberty. (This resting phase may vary from 12 to 50 years, providing ample opportunity for damage to the oocytes' genetic material.) When puberty begins, these primary oocytes complete the first meiotic division so ovulation can occur in monthly patterns. Each month, usually a single primary oocyte begins to increase in size and thickness and develops a protective membrane, the *zona pellucida*. The graafian follicle enlarges, and follicle cells form a thick, fluid-filled layer around the oocyte (see Figure 7-6). As soon as the graafian follicle matures, the oocyte resumes a meiotic division to produce two cells of unequal size: the secondary oocyte and the first polar body. The secondary oocyte receives all the cytoplasm and enters into the second meiotic division. This second division is completed only if the ovum is fertilized. Otherwise the ovum degenerates and is passed out of the body.

SPERMATOGENESIS

Spermatogenesis starts as puberty begins and can continue well into the eighth decade of life. Once it begins, it is a continuous process, not cyclical. It takes about 72 hours for a primary spermatocyte to develop into a mature sperm (see Chapter 3). Primary spermatocytes begin

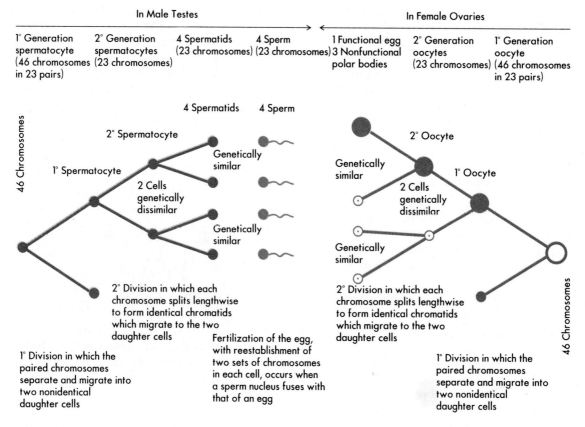

In Male Testes				In Female Ovaries		
1° Generation spermatocyte (46 chromosomes in 23 pairs)	2° Generation spermatocytes (23 chromosomes)	4 Spermatids (23 chromosomes)	4 Sperm (23 chromosomes)	1 Functional egg 3 Nonfunctional polar bodies	2° Generation oocytes (23 chromosomes)	1° Generation oocyte (46 chromosomes in 23 pairs)

FIGURE 7-3 Ovum and sperm maturation. Spermatogenesis results in four spermatids, but oogenesis results in only one functional ovum and three polar bodies.

the first meiotic division, which results in two secondary spermatocytes. Immediately, the secondary spermatocytes undergo the second meiotic division to result in four spermatids. These spermatids contain half the number of chromosomes of the primary spermatocyte, as shown in Figure 7-3. (Figure 3-3, *A*, illustrates the anatomic location of the spermatocytes in the seminiferous tubules.) Several stages of the process may occur simultaneously in different parts of the seminiferous tubules.

Mature sperm have virtually no source of nutrition when separated from the semen. Therefore after ejaculation, only some will survive as long as 72 hours.

Fertilization

Many factors are necessary for effective fertilization of the ovum. Coitus causes an average of 200 to 300 million sperm to be deposited in the vaginal canal close to the cervical os. After ejaculation, the life span of sperm is relatively short, and they must quickly move toward the *outer* distal portion of the fallopian tube where fertilization normally occurs. Many factors may impede the journey, a distance of about 21 cm. These factors include incompatible vaginal or cervical fluids, an extremely acidic environment, or possible narrowing

of the cervix, uterus, or tubes (see Chapter 3). Yet, the estrogenic influences that help to change cervical mucus properties to allow for easier sperm penetration are at a peak at ovulation. At the same time, the peristaltic actions of the uterine and tubal muscles foster the movement of sperm toward the tube and move the ovum toward the sperm. Prostaglandins found in semen might aid in the rapid transport of sperm toward the tube by affecting the smooth muscle contractions of the uterus. Approximately 2000 sperm reach the fallopian tubes.

Normally, only one of the many sperm reaching the ovum will enter it. The others secrete hyaluronidase, an enzyme found in the acrosome or outer covering of the head of each sperm that helps to penetrate the zona pellucida. As fertilization occurs, a process called **syngamy** acts to protect the fertilized ovum. During syngamy, the ovum completes its second maturational division and extrudes a polar body (Figure 7-4). A reaction that causes the membrane to form a barrier preventing other sperm from entering the cell occurs in the oocyte cytoplasm just below the cell membrane. The tail of the sperm disappears, and the nucleus becomes larger, revealing its chromosomal content. At this point, the structure becomes known as the *male*

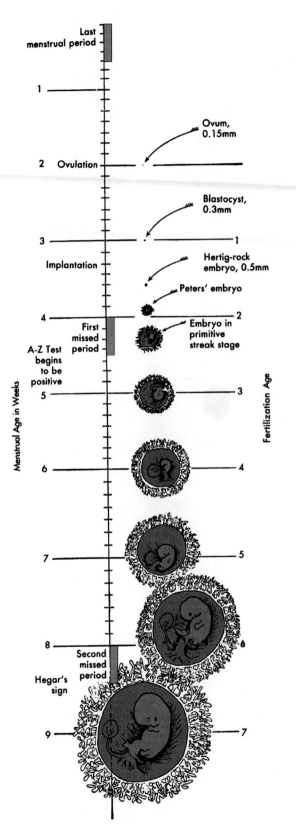

Last menstrual period

1

Ovum, 0.15mm

2 Ovulation

Blastocyst, 0.3mm

3 ————————— 1

Implantation

Hertig-rock embryo, 0.5mm

Peters' embryo

4

First missed period

Embryo in primitive streak stage ———— 2

A-Z Test begins to be positive

Menstrual Age in Weeks

Fertilization Age

5 ————————— 3

6 ————————— 4

7 ————————— 5

8

Second missed period

Hegar's sign

6

9 ————————— 7

FIGURE 7-4 Actual size of embryos in relation to mother's menstrual history. *Left,* Gestational age; and *right,* fertilization age of embryo. Based on a 28-day cycle. (From Corliss CE: *Patten's human embryology,* ed 4, New York, 1976, McGraw-Hill.)

pronucleus, the sperm nucleus before it fuses with the nucleus of the ovum. The *female pronucleus,* the nucleus of the ovum before it fuses with the nucleus of the sperm, swells. The pronuclei gravitate toward one another and fuse, thus completing fertilization by restoring the full diploid number of chromosomes to the fertilized ovum, which is now the **zygote.** At this point, the genetic foundation is laid for the growth and development of the infant.

Test Yourself

- After completion of meiosis, each oocyte or spermatozoan will contain only _____ autosomal and _____ sex chromosomes.
- Exchange of genetic material occurs during _____ of chromatids.
- Why is the genetic material contained in oocytes at higher risk for damage than that contained in spermatocytes?
- After the male and female pronuclei fuse, the fertilized ovum is called a _____.

DETERMINATION OF SEX

The twenty-third pair of chromosomes are the sex chromosomes (either XX or XY). Females have two X chromosomes; males have an X and a Y chromosome.

The sex of an individual is determined by the presence or absence of the Y chromosome. Not until 1959 did scientists discover that embryos carrying the Y chromosome developed as males; embryos lacking a Y chromosome developed as females.

A **testes determining factor** is thought to be a single gene on the Y chromosome. Before 6 weeks, the male and female genitalia are undifferentiated or in the *indifferent stage.* Then it is thought that the gene triggers signals that lead to development of the Leydig's cells that produce testosterone to induce masculinization of the external genitalia. In the absence of the gene (regardless of whether there is a Y chromosome), the embryo becomes a female. Similarly, there may be a single gene on the X chromosome to control a chain of events that triggers feminization of external genitalia.

GESTATIONAL VS FERTILIZATION AGE

When clinicians calculate the embryo's age from the first day of its mother's last menstrual period (LMP), they are calculating its **gestational age,** or menstrual age. Calculating the gestational age is easy because most women are able to remember when their LMP began. However, calculating the time of ovulation, the **fertili-**

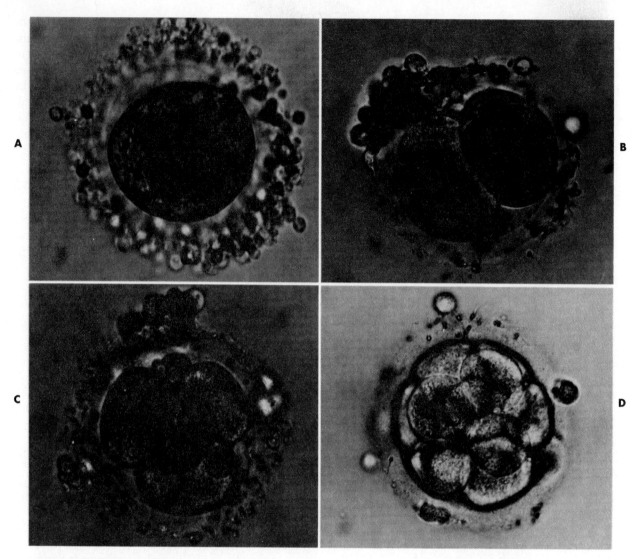

FIGURE 7-5 Early stages of human development. **A,** Fertilized ovum, or zygote. **B** to **D,** Early cell divisions produce more and more cells. The solid mass of cells shown in **D** forms the morulan early stage in embryonic development. (Courtesy Lucinda L. Veeck, Jones Institute for Reproductive Medicine, Norfolk, Va.)

zation age, is difficult because the duration of the *follicular phase* of the menstrual cycle varies from month to month and woman to woman. Figure 7-4 compares gestational age with the fertilization age.

In this chapter, discussion of fetal growth and the age in weeks refers to the time since fertilization rather than the time since the **LMP.** Calculations for determining the expected date of birth are given in Chapter 9.

Embryonic Period
CLEAVAGE

About 24 to 48 hours after fertilization, the zygote divides; the daughter cells resulting from this mitosis are half the size of the fertilized ovum. Continued division results in progressively smaller cells because during this phase the zona pellucida remains intact, keeping the mass of dividing cells at about the same size as the fertilized ovum (Figure 7-5). As cleavage occurs, the zygote travels down the fallopian tube toward the uterus. After 3 or 4 days, it begins to look like a solid ball of cells, the **morula,** which resembles a mulberry.

IMPLANTATION

Approximately 3 to 4 days after fertilization, the morula enters the uterus. Cells can be distinguished according to function. Fluid enters the morula and divides the cells into inner and outer cell masses. A

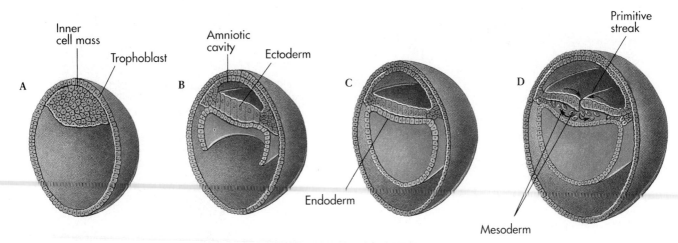

FIGURE 7-6 Formation of the three primary germ layers. **A,** 3 to 4 days. The amniotic cavity forms within the inner cell mass. **B** and **C,** Second week. Two germ layers are seen—ectoderm and endoderm. The yolk sac is surrounded by endoderm. **D,** During the third week cells that will become the mesoderm (third germ layer) are sent throughout the embryo by means of the primitive streak. (Courtesy Kevin Sommerville after Bill Ober.)

cavity (blastocyst cavity) forms and the zona pellucida gradually disappears. The embryo is now called a **blastocyst.** Over the next $2\frac{1}{2}$ weeks the inner cell mass differentiates into three layers: ectoderm, endoderm, and mesoderm (Figure 7-6). These primary germ layers are the tissues from which all body systems are formed (Box 7-1).

Approximately 7 days after ovulation, the trophoblast begins to burrow into the lining of the uterus; this burrowing is called *implantation* or *nidation.* Trophoblastic cells secrete enzymes that digest or liquefy endometrial tissue. The blastocyst sinks deep into the endometrium, which becomes the decidua basalis. Fingerlike projections, villi, of the trophoblast "dig into" and break down tissue and firmly anchor the blastocyst

in the decidua basalis, an area with a rich source of nourishment and oxygen. This may be confused with a menstrual period. Some women may experience slight vaginal bleeding at this time. However, by the ninth or tenth day, the epithelium, now called the *decidua capsularis,* has begun to heal over the area in which the blastocyst became embedded (Figure 7-7).

By day 13, the trophoblast has become the chorion, and the villi have become the chorionic villi. By the end of the third month when the growth of the embryo causes the decidua capsularis and decidua parietalis (uterine lining farthest from the implantation site) to compress one another, the chorionic villi (also called the *chorion frondosum*) remain only in the decidua basalis. These chorionic villi make up the fetal portion of the placenta.

BOX 7-1   Organs and Tissues Derived from Germ Layers

Ectoderm
- Central nervous system
- Peripheral nervous system
- Sensory epithelium of sense organs
- Epidermis of hair, nails, subcutaneous glands
- Hair follicles
- Lens of eye
- Enamel of teeth
- Hypophysis
- Mammary glands

Mesoderm
- Heart
- All connective tissue layers
- Bone
- Muscles
- Cartilage
- Blood
- Kidneys
- Urinary tract
- Lymphatic system
- Gonadal system
- Spleen

Endoderm
- Gastrointestinal tract
- Epithelium of respiratory tract, pharynx, tongue, thyroid, parathyroids
- Liver
- Pancreas
- Epithelial lining of bladder and urethra

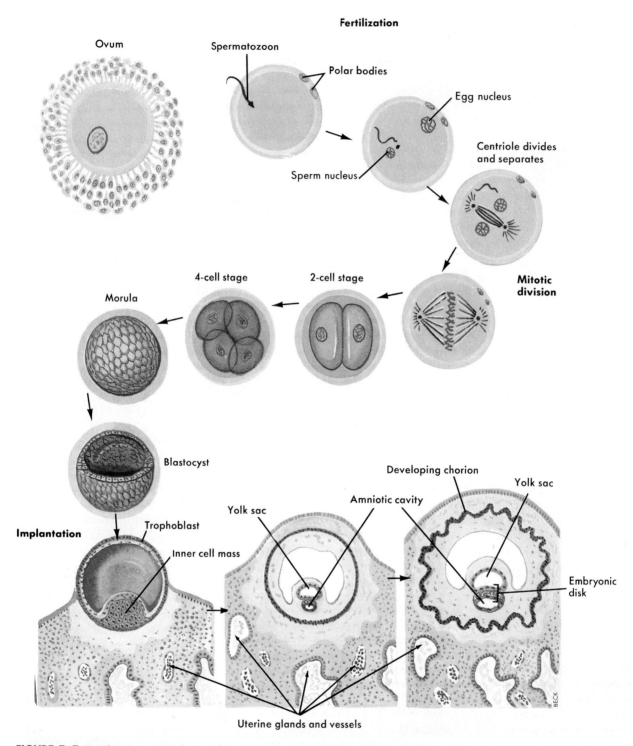

FIGURE 7-7 Fertilization to implantation and development of the yolk sac. Rapid growth of uterine glands and vessels covers the developing blastocyst at the time of implantation. (Courtesy Ernest W. Beck.)

Chorion

The **chorion** develops from the trophoblast and is the outermost membrane and closest to the uterine lining (Figure 7-8). The trophoblast infiltrates maternal tissues with chorionic villi, which are embedded in the decidua basalis. These villi form the fetal side of the placenta. Thus the villi become bathed with maternal blood rich in oxygen and nutrients.

Exchange of fetal and maternal material takes place through osmosis, diffusion, active transport, and pi-

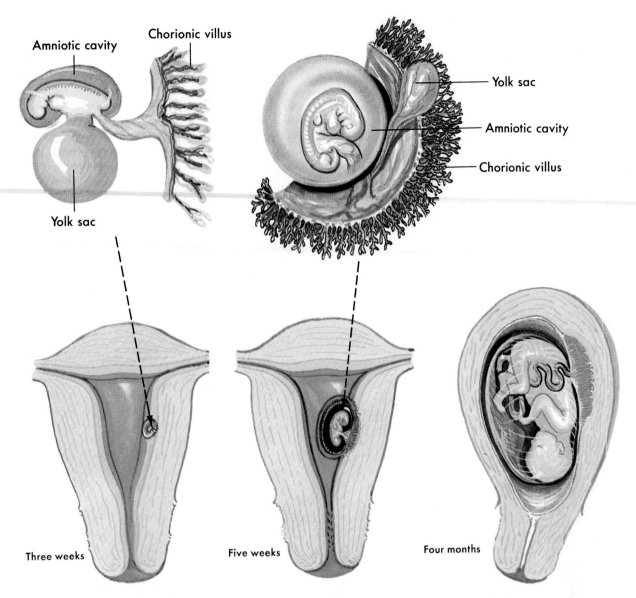

FIGURE 7-8 Development of the chorion and amnion. Development of the chorion and amniotic cavity to 4 months of gestation. (Courtesy Ernest W. Beck.)

nocytosis (ameboidlike action). There are also other complex transfer mechanisms. There is no direct mingling of fetal and maternal blood. However, there may be very isolated exchanges of fetal and maternal blood cells when small leaks occur in the trophoblast or during threatened abortion or diagnostic tests such as *chorionic villus sampling* (CVS) and *amniocentesis* (see Chapter 11).

The chorionic villi enlarge by the end of the fourth and fifth months to form 15 to 20 visible placental partitions (cotyledons or little trees).

In addition, part of the chorion produces hCG, which helps to sustain pregnancy by preventing the involution of the corpus luteum.

Amnion

The **amnion** appears very early in embryonic life, even before the embryo has taken form. At first, the amnion is small, but as it fills with fluid and the embryo grows, it becomes much larger and eventually surrounds the embryo and umbilical cord. Later in pregnancy, the amnion expands to fill the entire space and adheres to the other membrane, the chorion. Together, the amnion and chorion are known as the fetal membranes (Figure 7-11).

At term, the amniotic sac contains almost a liter of amniotic fluid, which forms from amniotic cells, urine, and secretions from the lungs and skin of the fetus. This fluid contains albumin, urea, creatinine, lecithin, sphingomyelin, bilirubin, fat, fructose, lanugo hairs, uric acid, and inorganic salts and is slightly alkaline. It cushions the fetus against injury, prevents adhesions of the sticky skin and umbilical cord compression, equalizes pressure, and provides thermal regulation, a medium for fetal movement, and fluid for the fetus to swallow. The fluid is replaced approximately every 3 hours. This secretion and reabsorption is regulated by the amnion cells and fetal swallowing and urinating.

At term, this fluid provides a "wedge" to help to soften and dilate the cervix during labor. Amniotic fluid can also provide the physician with valuable diagnostic information when its components are analyzed in high-risk pregnancies. Volumes of amniotic fluid greater (hydramnios) or less (oligohydramnios) than average are significant because these variations may be associated with fetal abnormalities (see Chapter 21).

Placenta

The development and circulation of the placenta (Figure 7-9) occurs during the third week. It is formed at the site of attachment of the chorion to the uterine wall. The placenta and membranes are completely functional by the twelfth week. The placenta expands until it covers about half of the internal surface area of the uterus by the twentieth week.

The placenta secretes hormones essential for maintaining pregnancy. By the third month, it takes over production of progesterone from the corpus luteum. It also secretes estriol, an estrogen.

Human placental lactogen (hPL), a hormone similar to prolactin, is also produced by the placenta. hPL stimulates changes in the mother's metabolic process to ensure that the mother's body is prepared for lactation.

The placenta grows until late in the eighth month. Toward the end of pregnancy, it begins to age, secreting hormones in decreasing amounts and becoming gradually less able to effectively exchange nutrients, oxygen, and wastes. Placental aging may be assessed during ultrasound examination (see Chapter 11).

The placental barrier is composed of layers of fetal tissue (trophoblast, connective tissue, basement membrane, and fetal capillary endothelium). It provides some protection to the fetus, but as pregnancy progresses the membrane becomes thinner. The preg-

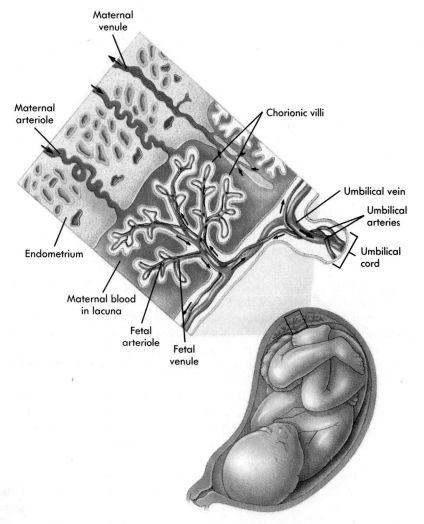

FIGURE 7-9 Mature placenta. Embryonic blood vessels and maternal blood vessels are in close contact, but there is no mixing of fetal and maternal blood. (Courtesy Christine Oleksyk.)

Maternal venule

Maternal arteriole

Chorionic villi

Umbilical vein

Umbilical arteries

Umbilical cord

Endometrium

Maternal blood in lacuna

Fetal arteriole

Fetal venule

nant woman must understand that virtually *everything she puts into her body may cross the placenta.* The placenta acts as the lungs, kidneys, endocrine and digestive system, liver, and immune system until fetal systems are mature enough to function.

Placental exchange is by *simple diffusion* for oxygen, carbon dioxide, fat-soluble vitamins, lipids (including narcotics, anesthetics, and barbiturates that are fat soluble). *Facilitated diffusion* and active transport govern glucose, amino acids, calcium, iron, and water-soluble vitamins. *Pinocytosis* controls larger molecules such as globulins, viruses, and antibodies. Other substances pass by additional means. Some large molecules such as IgM, heparin, insulin, or complex cells such as blood cells do not cross the placenta unless there is damage to the placental membrane (Blackburn and Loper, 1992).

Umbilical Cord

While the placenta develops, the **umbilical cord** is also forming. Blood vessels establish a connection between the developing embryo and the placenta via the body stalk. Together the body stalk and remnants of the yolk sac form the primitive umbilical cord.

Originally there are four cord vessels. Early in gestation, one vein atrophies, leaving one larger vein to carry blood from the placenta to the fetus and two small arteries to return deoxygenated blood to the placenta. Approximately 400 ml/min flows through the cord; this flow helps to stabilize the soft cord. The cord vessels also are supported by a substance, **Wharton's jelly,** made up of connective tissue, mucopolysaccharides, and covered by amnion that extends up from the fetal side of the placenta and ends at the skin of the abdomen of the fetus. The amount of Wharton's jelly varies widely; it is especially influenced by fetal nutrition, activity, and gestational age. Cord vessels may be constricted in response to stimuli or drugs. The surface of the cord contains no pain receptors; thus cutting the cord is painless.

Test Yourself

- The segment of the Y chromosome thought to direct male sexual development is the _____.
- The embryonic tissue that will become the chorion and placenta is called the _____.
- Name three functions of amniotic fluid._____

DEVELOPMENT OF THE EMBRYO

The time between fertilization and the first 14 days of development is the preembryonic period. It is a time of rapid cell division, with differentiation of tissues and the development of the primary germ layers, the ecto-

derm, endoderm, and mesoderm. These three germ layers are the tissues from which all body structures are formed (see Box 7-1).

At the third week, the mass of growing cells becomes an **embryo.** The embryonic period is marked by rapid growth and further tissue differentiation, including **organogenesis,** the differentiation and formation of organs. Many organs are developed before the mother realizes she is pregnant. This period is also characterized by extreme susceptibility to adverse environmental influences such as radiation, infection, drugs, or smoking. The shape of the embryo changes dramatically (Figures 7-10 and 7-11).

By the end of the third week, germ layers have begun to form distinct tissues. The ectodermal layer develops into the organs and structures such as the central nervous system and brain that maintain interaction with the outside world. The mesodermal layer develops into the supporting tissues of the body (muscle and bone) and the vascular and urinary tract systems so the body can maintain movement and internal function. Finally, the endodermal layer provides for the epithelial linings of most of the systems of the body.

Fetal Period

By the ninth week of gestation, the embryo has developed sufficiently to be called a fetus. The fetal period continues until birth and is a time of rapid growth (Box 7-2). Some tissue differentiation still occurs in the genitourinary tract, eyes, and lungs.

By the end of the *first trimester,* the fetus appears to be a miniature human being. All organ systems have formed and continue to develop the ability to function. However, the fetus is not yet viable outside the uterus because its systems are unable to function independently.

Neurons within the CNS, especially those in the brain, continue to differentiate, proliferate, and grow throughout gestation. Adequate nutrition and avoidance of **teratogens** (substances that can harm the growing fetus) are vital if development is to proceed normally. Teratogens are discussed fully in Chapter 27.

The *second trimester* lasts from week 13 to the end of week 26 (Box 7-2). It is characterized by rapid fetal growth, especially in length, and continued cellular differentiation. By the end of the second trimester, the infant is viable.

The *third trimester* begins in week 27 and lasts until term (38 weeks). During this period subcutaneous fat is deposited and the refinement of organ development continues. As you read the following system-by-system descriptions, keep in mind that these amazing processes occur simultaneously, and that they are interdependent. Therefore the health of one system often influences the health of others.

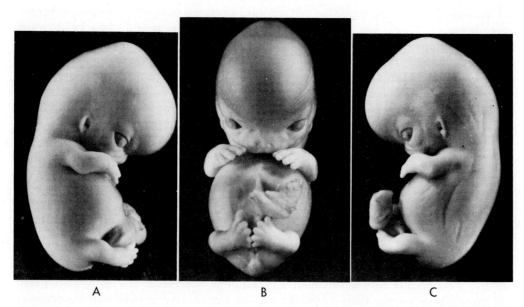

A   B   C

FIGURE 7-10 Human fetus at 54 days (22.5 mm or ⅞ inch). **A,** Right side. **B,** Front. **C,** Left side. (Photo by E. Ludwig. From Rugh R and Shettles LB: *From conception to birth: the drama of life's begining.* Copyright by R Rugh and LB Shettles. Reprinted by permission of HarperCollins.)

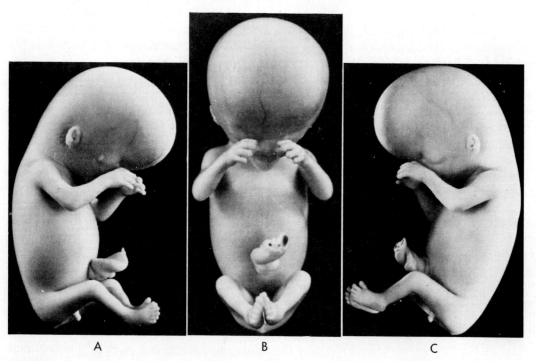

A   B   C

FIGURE 7-11 Human (male) fetus at 68 days (47 mm). **A,** Right. **B,** Front. **C,** Left. (Photo by E. Ludwig. From Rugh R and Shettles LB: *From conception to birth: the drama of life's begining.* Copyright by R Rugh and LB Shettles. Reprinted by permission of HarperCollins.)

BOX 7-2 Embryonic, Fetal, and Placental Milestones at Fertilization Age*
Development of Embryo and Fetus

Preembryonic period
3 minutes-48 hours

Fertilization, syngamy occur

24-48 hours

First cleavage of zygote occurs

3-4 days

Morula enters uterus

4-5 days

Blastocyst reaches uterus

6 days

Zona pellucida lost
Trophoblast invades decidua basalis, becomes chorion

7-8 days

Implantation occurs
Ectoderm, endoderm appear

8-10 days

Clefts in ectoderm form amniotic cavity
Amnion, yolk sac begin to form
Amniotic cells secrete amniotic fluid to protect embryo

13 days

Trophoblast becomes chorion
hCG appears in urine, serum 10 to 21 days after
    fertilization
Primary chorionic villi form

Embryonic period
15 days

Implantation complete
Blood vessels form from yolk sac, body stalk, chorion
Primitive streak, mesoderm form
Germ layers begin cell specialization or differentiation
Chorionic villi have circulatory core

18-21 days

Primitive nervous system folding occurs
Heart begins to twitch
Primitive eyes, ears exist
Primitive red blood cells differentiate
Placenta covers approximately one fifteenth of uterus,
    begins to function

4 weeks (1 month)

Heart folds, begins asynchronous pulsations; blood
    pumped

*Length of pregnancy is 266 + 8 days, 38 weeks, or $9\frac{1}{2}$ months, from fertilization.
†C-R (crown-rump) length is the measurement used to determine the fertilization age; it is usually determined by ultrasonography.

Yolk sac produces blood cells
Brain differentiates into forebrain, midbrain, hindbrain
    Head large in proportion to body
Outlines of eyes seen above primitive mouth cavity
    Lung buds appear
Gastrointestinal tract, liver, thyroid gland, pancreas,
    gallbladder can be identified
Somites (future vertebrae) appear on sides of midline
Crown-rump (C-R) length† is 4-5 mm

5 weeks

Limb buds appear
Rapid brain growth occurs
Cranial, spinal nerves develop
Primitive nose, ears, jaws, eyes form
Germ cells migrate toward gonads
Umbilical cord forms from body stalk
Heart forms septa
C-R length is 6-8 mm

6 weeks

Trachea, bronchi, lung buds, lips form
Liver produces red blood cells
Central, autonomic nervous systems form
Rudimentary kidney, penis exist
Eyes move to front of face; sensory retinal ends form;
    pigmentation occurs
Cartilage forms; rudimentary bone present
Differentiation of muscles occurs; muscle mass forms
    over primitive skeletal shape
C-R length is 10-14 mm

7 weeks

Eyelids form
Gallbladder forms
Liver forms blood cells
Yolk sac declines
Palate, tongue form
Bone cells begin to replace cartilage
Arms, legs move
C-R length is 22-28 mm

8 weeks (2 months)

Hands, feet well formed
Eyes move to front of face; eyelids fuse
Heart has four chambers, beats 40-80 times per minute
Major blood vessels form; circulation through umbilical
    cord occurs
Thyroid, adrenal glands, taste buds well formed
External genitalia can be distinguished as male or
    female
Placenta covers one third of uterine lining
C-R length is 3 cm; weight is 2 g

BOX 7-2   Embryonic, Fetal, and Placental Milestones at Fertilization Age*
Development of Embryo and Fetus—cont'd

Fetal period
9 weeks

Fingernails, toenails form
Heartbeat can be heard faintly by ultrasound instruments
Genitalia well developed

10 weeks

Head growth slows; body begins to develop in proportion
   to it
Limbs reach relative lengths
Bone marrow forms, produces red blood cells
Bladder sac forms; kidneys make urine

11 weeks

Tooth buds appear for temporary teeth
Salivary glands form. Peristalsis begins
Thyroid gland secretes hormones
Insulin forms in pancreas. Liver secretes bile
Urinary tract passages function

12 weeks (3 months)

Lungs take shape; respiratory motion seen
Thumb, forefinger oppose
Vocal cords form. Palate fuses
Swallowing reflex present
Liver begins production of red blood cells
C-R length is 9 cm; weight is 45 g

Second trimester
16 weeks (4 months)   (18 wks gestational age)

Fingerprints develop
Arms, legs move frequently
Lips form; facial contours fill out
Skin still loose, wrinkled, pink
Brain forms ridges, cerebrum grows rapidly
Bladder fully formed
Oocytes form in fetal ovaries
Fetus sensitive to light
Meconium (dead cells, mucus, gland secretions) forms,
   will make up newborn's first stool   4oz
C-R length is 14 cm; weight is 180-200 g
200 ml of amniotic fluid present
Amniocentesis possible by weeks 14-16.

20 weeks (5 months)

Anabolic-catabolic exchange begins
Eyelashes, eyebrows, hair on head more abundant
Vernix caseosa (grayish-white, cheeselike substance),
   lanugo (soft hair) cover, protect fetus
Fetus sucks, swallows, hears sounds
Brown fat deposits form
Circadian rhythm begins
Respiratory movements occur, become more regular
Myelinization of spinal cord begins
C-R length is 19 cm; weight is 430-480 g

Placenta covers half of uterine lining, weighs 120 g
400 ml amniotic fluid present

24 weeks (6 months)

Eyes complete; eyelids open, close
Alveolar ducts, sacs present; alveolar cells produce
   pulmonary surfactants (phospholipids that minimize
   surface tension of respiratory fluids)
Bone ossification begins
Thick vernix covers fetus; head hair very long
Skin layers on hands, feet thicken
Many reflexes appear   1# 11z
C-R length is 23-24 cm; weight is 700-800 g

Third trimester
28 weeks (7 months)

Respiratory, circulatory systems function
Respiratory movements in utero seen by ultrasound
Testes begin to descend
Skin very thin, red, wrinkled, with prominent capillaries
   underneath
Eyebrows, eyelashes prominent; nails appear. Lanugo
   begins to disappear
C-R length is 28 cm; weight is 1000-1200 g

32 weeks (8 months)

Subcutaneous fat deposits form to insulate fetus from
   temperature changes at birth
Skin becomes less wrinkled, red
Fingernails, toenails complete
Alveoli fill; ratio of lecithin, sphingomyelin (L/S) (sur-
   factants) is 1.2:2
More reflexes present
C-R length is 29-32 cm; weight is 1300-2100 g

36 weeks

Brain myelination begins, continues through birth
L/S ratio is 2:1
Sleep-wake cycle more definite
Maternal antibodies transfer to fetus and last for ap-
   proximately 6 months
C-R length is 32-35 cm; weight is 2500-2800 g
Approximately 1000 ml of amniotic fluid present

38 weeks (term)

Fetus less active due to limited space
Meconium accumulates in intestines
Nails have grown to tips of toes, fingers; creases promi-
   nent on soles of feet
Fetus may be able to lift head
Fetal circulation developed (see Chapter 16)
C-R length is 35-37 cm; crown-heel (C-H) length is
   46-52 cm. Weight is 3000-3600 g
800 ml of amniotic fluid present

RESPIRATORY SYSTEM: DEVELOPMENT AND FUNCTION

In utero the placenta is a substitute for the nonfunctioning fetal lungs. Oxygenated blood comes to the fetus from the placenta via the umbilical vein. Although lungs are not being used for ventilation and oxygenation, the normal fetus makes respiratory movements in utero. These movements have been demonstrated by real-time ultrasound and are one of the parameters of the biophysical profile (see Chapter 11). These "practice" respiratory movements normally do not draw amniotic fluid into the fetal lungs; they are merely small movements of the chest wall. The respiratory system develops from the endoderm (the same tissue that will give rise to the gastrointestinal system) during day 24 of embryonic life. Bronchi are formed by the sixteenth week of fetal development, and there are primitive lungs by 23 weeks. However, these can function only with great difficulty, since there are not enough alveoli for the necessary exchange of gases. Blood flow to the lungs is also inadequate at this time. Figure 7-12 illustrates the anatomic development of the respiratory system.

Two distinct types of cells are found in the lungs: type I cells, which allow for exchange of gases, and type II cells, which produce **surfactant** at 20 to 24 weeks of gestational age. Surfactant is composed of surface-active compounds that stabilize the alveoli and prevent their collapse with each exhalation. There are two pathways

of surfactant production. The first pathway functions from 20 to 24 weeks and continues until birth. However, it is an unstable pathway—easily inhibited after birth by hypoxia, hypothermia, and acidosis. The second pathway is much more resistant to these stressors but does not fully mature until 35 to 37 weeks of fetal life. Interestingly, stresses on the health of the mother, such as hypertension, preeclampsia, or heroin use, can stimulate the production of surfactant. It is thought that increased amounts of steroids are produced by a mother who is stressed. Pulmonary maturity can be accelerated by giving steroids to a mother before term if enough time is available before delivery of the infant (see Chapter 21).

Respiration is regulated by the respiratory center in the brainstem. Maturation of the central nervous system progresses as pregnancy continues, with coordination of feeding and respiration occurring at about 34 weeks of gestation. All of these developmental milestones are vital to the discussion of **fetal viability**. The fetus is considered to have reached the age of viability at 20 weeks gestation, although extrauterine survival at this stage of development is currently almost impossible. When an infant of 20 weeks seems to be surviving, it is often because there is a discrepancy between the expected date of birth and the real gestational age. The lungs become capable of *borderline* support of extrauterine respiration sometime after 23 weeks of gesta-

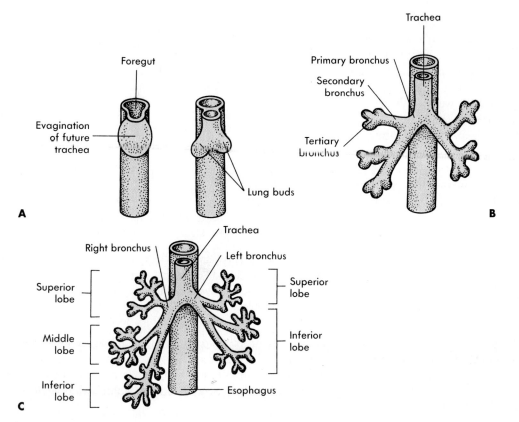

FIGURE 7-12

Development of the lung. **A,** 28 days—a single lung bud forms and divides into two buds, forming primary bronchi. **B,** 35 days—tertiary bronchi branch to form lobules. **C,** 50 days—continued branching. (Courtesy David J. Mascaro & Associates.)

tion. Adequate respiratory function also depends on maturation of surfactant production and neurologic control of respiration. There is great variation between humans; therefore there is no "magic week of gestation" during which pulmonary maturity is certain.

Test Yourself

- Which germ layer will form the body's support structures?
- The second trimester extends from week _____ to week _____; the third trimester extends from week _____ to week _____.
- If primitive lungs are present by the twenty-third week of gestation, why do you think respiration is so difficult for the infant delivered prematurely?

CARDIOVASCULAR SYSTEM: DEVELOPMENT AND FUNCTION

With blood circulating by the end of the third week of gestation, the cardiovascular system is the first system to function in the embryo (Figure 7-13). This is necessary because the rapidly growing embryo requires a large quantity of nutrients and produces an equally large amount of waste products. Humans, unlike other animals, have a small yolk sac for nutritional support during early gestation.

The first indication of cardiac development is seen on day 18 to 19 in the cardiogenic area where cells cluster to form the cardiogenic cords. These are two tubes, which fuse and then develop strictures and outpouchings that form the primitive heart chambers and vessels. By the end of the fifth week, cells around the heart tubes differentiate into myocardial and pericardial cells. The primitive heart begins beating by day 22, even before the four chambers are well defined. Cardiac muscle develops from mesenchyme, which is around the embryonic cardiac tubes. Some of these cells will later form Purkinje's cells, which are the conducting system.

Fetal Circulation

The three purposes for fetal circulation are accomplished through the following specialized fetal structures and their functions:
1. To decrease blood flow to the fetal lungs.
2. To increase blood flow to the head and the heart.
3. To direct blood to the placenta.

Fetal circulation differs from adult circulation in several ways. Blood pressure in the adult is lower in the lungs (pulmonary blood pressure) than it is in the rest of the

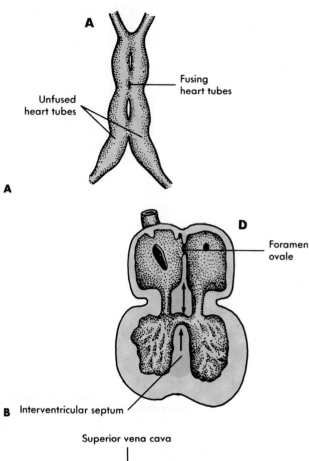

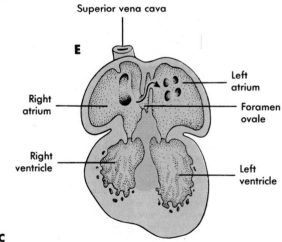

FIGURE 7-13
Development of the heart. **A,** At 20 days after fertilization—two-tubed heart. **B,** At 31 days; note the foramen ovale. The interventricular septum is nearly complete. **C,** The flap of the foramen ovale is a one-way door allowing blood to shunt from the right side of the heart to the left. After birth, the increased blood flow from the newly expanded lungs into the left atrium will force the flap shut, ending the shunt. (Courtesy David J. Mascaro & Associates.)

body (systemic blood pressure). In fetal life, this condition is *reversed*. Fetal pulmonary blood pressure is higher because fetal pulmonary blood vessels are constricted to divert blood flow away from the nonfunctioning fetal lungs. Fetal systemic blood pressure, however, is lower because flow leads to the placenta through blood vessels that are not constricted. Follow Figure 7-14 as you read the following description of fetal circulation:

1. Highly oxygenated blood comes to the fetus from the placenta *via*
2. The **umbilical vein.**
3. This is shunted past the liver *via* the **ductus venosus** *and*

4. Continues through the inferior vena cava to the right atrium.
5. Poorly oxygenated blood from the lower body flows from the inferior vena cava through the liver and also continues through the inferior vena cava to the right atrium.
6. Most of the highly oxygenated blood from the inferior vena cava is diverted to the left atrium through the **foramen ovale,** a flap that allows blood

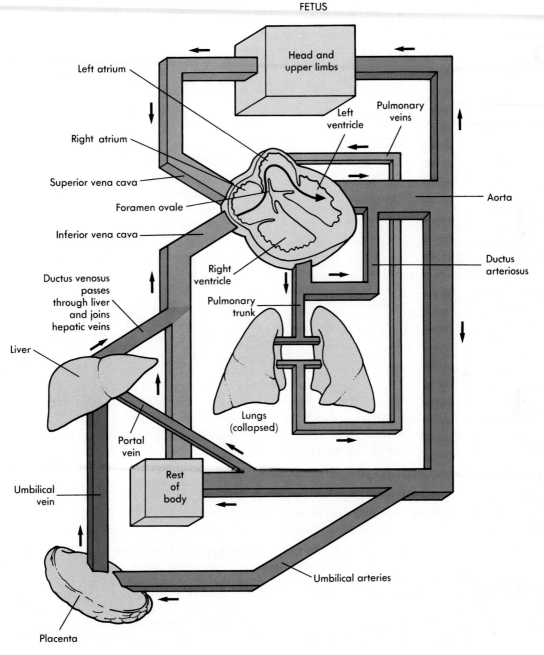

FIGURE 7-14 The architecture of the fetal circulatory system, showing levels of oxygen saturation in different parts of the system. Blood with the highest oxygen levels is indicated by scarlet color; intermediate values are shown in darker red and purple and the lowest values in blue. (Courtesy G. David Brown.)

to flow only from the right to left sides of the heart ("right-to-left shunt").

7. Poorly oxygenated blood from the upper body flows through the tricuspid valve into the right ventricle and *through*

8. The pulmonary artery to the fetal lungs, but

9. Increased pressure caused by fetal pulmonary constriction directs most of this blood away from the pulmonary vessels and to the aorta through the **ductus arteriosus**; this is another "right-to-left shunt."

10. Simultaneously, highly oxygenated blood in the left atrium, mixed with a small amount of blood from the nonfunctioning fetal lungs, flows through the mitral valve into the aorta. This allows highly oxygenated blood to be directed to the myocardium and the brain, a major benefit.

11. Blood from the ductus arteriosus and the aorta mixes and supplies the rest of the body.

12. The two umbilical arteries (branches of the internal iliac arteries) carry mixed blood back to the placenta for reoxygenation.

Test Yourself

- Name three purposes of fetal circulation.
- Which fetal structure diverts blood from the right atrium to the left atrium?
- Which fetal structure diverts blood from the pulmonary artery to the aorta?

METABOLIC CONTROL

Thermal Control

The fetus produces heat in utero, which is dissipated through the placenta to the mother if the mother's temperature is less than that of the fetus (the maternal-fetal thermal gradient). The temperature of the fetus is about 0.5° C (0.9° F) above maternal core temperature, which ranges from 37.6° C to 37.8° C (99.8° F to 100.0° F). If the mother becomes febrile, this mechanism can fail, allowing fetal core temperature to rise. Maternal hyperthermia may not be related to illness. Strenuous exercise or increased environmental temperatures such as those found in hot tubs, saunas, and steam baths can lead to fetal hyperthermia. It has been suggested that early fetal/maternal hyperthermia may cause central nervous system defects such as **anencephaly** (Pleet et al, 1980).

Newborns produce most of their body heat by metabolizing a specialized tissue called **brown fat,** which develops progressively during the last trimester of pregnancy. Sites for brown fat storage in the term infant: the nape of the neck, between the scapulae, in the mediastinum, and surrounding the kidneys.

The control center for heat regulation is located in the hypothalamus and is fully functional in the healthy newborn. It is therefore the lack of brown fat and not the lack of temperature control that places healthy but premature and growth-retarded infants at risk for hypothermia. An insulating layer of fat (white fat) is also deposited during the third trimester. With maturation of the hypothalamus, central control of temperature is further developed. However, the neonate does not adapt well to extremes of temperature; mechanisms for maintaining temperature are still immature at birth.

Test Yourself

- How is fetal temperature controlled in utero?
- Why is maternal hyperthermia so serious?

Glucose and Calcium

Fetal energy requirements are supplied by maternal metabolism in the form of glucose, lactate, free fatty acids, and amino acids; fetal gluconeogenesis also contributes to energy supplies. This energy is used for both fetal growth and storage of energy for future needs. The rate of energy storage increases toward term as glycogen is stored in the fetal liver and cardiac muscle.

Calcium is supplied to the fetus via active transport mechanisms in the placenta that facilitate transfer from the maternal circulation. Fetal calcium levels are maintained 1 mg/100 ml of blood higher than maternal levels. Maternal calcium levels drop slightly toward term because of fetal needs. Because the growing fetus needs calcium for development of the bony skeleton, during the last trimester of pregnancy, fetal calcium content increases fourfold as bone density progresses. Thus the infant who is delivered prematurely will have decreased calcium stores. If nutritional intake of calcium is inadequate, fetal calcium needs will be taken from maternal stores. Chapter 10 discusses maternal nutritional needs.

INTEGUMENTARY SYSTEM: DEVELOPMENT AND FUNCTION

Although the **skin** is considered a single organ, it arises from two separate embryologic germ layers. The epidermis, or outermost layer, develops from the surface ectoderm. The dermis is derived from mesenchyme. The skin and its products (mainly vernix caseosa) function mainly in fetal life as protection for underlying structures. Tactile sense is present in utero—a fetus accidentally touched by the needle during amniocentesis will move away from it.

During gestation, cells from the epidermis proliferate, are shed, and replaced. These cells form part of the **vernix caseosa,** a white cheesy substance that protects the skin in utero. The amount of vernix decreases as gestation proceeds, until at term only a small amount is seen in the thigh and axillary creases. Therefore you will observe the extent and location of any vernix when you assess the infant's gestational age.

During the eleventh week of gestation, cells proliferate downward and form epidermal ridges in a pattern of grooves and ridges on the soles, fingers, and palms. A unique, genetically determined, permanent design forms by 17 weeks of gestation. **Dermatoglyphics,** or the study of epidermal ridges and lines, is part of the examination of infants with possible genetic disease, because distinct patterns are sometimes associated with specific syndromes.

Skin color begins to develop prenatally as some cells differentiate into melanoblasts and then melanocytes. The amount of melanin produced in utero varies with race. Infants of black parents may vary in skin color from very light to very dark, with darker skin found nearest the nail beds and on the scrotum.

The hair that becomes visible during the twentieth week of fetal life has a fine downy quality and is called **lanugo.** Lanugo is found over the entire fetal body and then recedes with increasing gestational age (see Figure 7-22). By 36 weeks it can be found only on the fetal shoulders and forehead. By term most is gone.

Sebaceous glands develop along with the hair follicles. Sweat glands develop as growths from the epidermis downward into the dermis.

Nails begins to appear at the tips of digits during the tenth week of gestation, with fingernails appearing before toenails (Figure 7-15). (Arm development precedes leg development as well.) Nail growth is used to assess gestational age; at 32 weeks the fingernails are at the fingertips; by 36 weeks the toenails have reached the ends of the toes.

The *teeth* arise from two embryologic layers. The enamel is derived from ectoderm; all other tissues have the mesenchyme as their source. Teeth begin to appear in the primitive jaws during the sixth week of gestation.

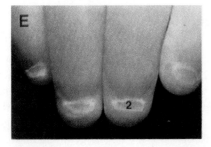

FIGURE 7-15 Fingernails on a fetus of 15 weeks gestation. (From England MA: *A color atlas of life before birth: normal fetal development,* St Louis, 1990, Mosby.)

Early proliferations of cells, or tooth buds, will later become the primary or deciduous teeth, which are shed during childhood. Each jaw contains 10 tooth buds that start developing from the anterior region of the jaw with progression posteriorly. Some precursors to the permanent teeth appear later in gestation, at 10 weeks, while others appear even later in the pregnancy. Tooth buds for second and third permanent molars, however, do not appear until after birth, during the fourth month and fifth year.

Mammary glands develop along the mammary ridges, commonly called the milk lines, during the sixth week of gestation. Normally, only those breast buds located in the pectoral region persist. The mammary buds that remain divide and develop the main lactiferous ducts. Further development of lactiferous ducts in the female is postponed until the onset of puberty and continues during pregnancy under the influence of estrogen and progesterone.

GASTROINTESTINAL SYSTEM: DEVELOPMENT AND FUNCTION

The gastrointestinal tract, or gut, appears during the fourth week of gestation as the embryo folds on itself and incorporates part of its yolk sac. Epithelium, glands, muscles, and fibrous tissues are derived from separate fetal germ layers. Because of the separate arterial supply of each, the gastrointestinal tract is divided into three anatomic areas: foregut, midgut, and hindgut.

The mouth first appears as a slight depression on the embryo's surface. The lips and palate arise from separate tissue masses of the head and face that grow inward and merge in the midline of the fetus. Clefts in lips or palate occur when either of these masses fails to merge completely. The esophagus grows from the foregut and a partition, the tracheoesophageal groove, divides it from the beginning trachea. The stomach begins as a dilated area in the foregut as it nears its caudal end. The duodenum forms just past this joint, at the junction between the foregut and midgut. The liver, pancreas, and spleen develop from specialized layers of foregut and midgut. All structures from the common bile duct to the proximal part of the transverse colon are midgut derivatives. The hindgut gives rise to the distal colon, rectum, part of the anal canal, and the urogenital system.

The anus and rectum develop from the *cloaca* (end of the hindgut) as it is divided by the urorectal membrane into the rectum posteriorly and urogenital sinus. The cloaca is covered externally by the cloacal membrane, which must rupture to establish a route for excretion. See Chapter 27 for anomalies of this system.

Development of digestive enzymes continues throughout gestation. Intestinal *disaccharidase* function develops earliest, with mature levels of *maltase* and *sucrase* observed at 6 to 8 months of gestation and mature levels of *lactase* only at term. However, if an infant is born prematurely, lactase levels will reach normal levels soon after delivery. Production of some enzymes responsible for protein metabolism does not reach mature levels until term, making an external source of some amino acids vital.

The fetus will "rehearse" later feeding behavior by swallowing amniotic fluid. This does not provide any nutrition to the fetus, but the cellular components of amniotic fluid contribute to the production of meconium. Coordination of suck and swallow reflexes does not occur until about 34 weeks of gestation, but this does not stop the fetus from swallowing amniotic fluid. A fetus will also turn toward his or her fingers if they brush the face (the rooting reflex) and begin to suck on them. Another reflex important for successful feeding without aspiration is the gag reflex. This does not fully mature until the eighth month of gestation.

Meconium, a tarry black substance, begins to form in the fetal intestine during weeks 13 to 16 of gestation. It consists of secretions from the gastrointestinal tract, including bile pigments, fetal cells and hair contained in swallowed amniotic fluid, and cells sloughed from the intestinal walls.

Although meconium is formed early in fetal life, there should be no passage of it in utero. During a breech position delivery, meconium may be passed as the infant's abdomen is compressed by maternal tissues and perhaps other fetal parts. During times of stress, especially hypoxic stress, the fetal anal sphincter may relax and meconium may be passed, causing the amniotic fluid to become "meconium stained" (see Chapter 14).

Test Yourself

- What are the components of meconium?

GENITOURINARY SYSTEM

Renal Development and Function

Developmental problems of the renal and reproductive systems are relatively common because they develop in close proximity to each other and derive from several common sources of tissues; therefore, malformations of either system may occur together.

Kidneys. The kidneys develop low in the pelvis and seem to move up as they develop, but their location only seems to move because of the growth of the lower part of the body. At about 12 weeks of gestation the fetal kidneys start to produce hypotonic urine, which contributes to amniotic fluid volume. Absent or malformed kidneys lead to a decrease in amniotic fluid volume, or oligohydramnios. This is an important observation during the antepartal period. Although urine production has begun in utero, the placental and maternal kidney functions eliminate fetal waste products.

At birth, the term newborn has all the nephrons that will be produced during his or her lifetime. Further growth of the kidney is by hypertrophy, not hyperplasia.

Bladder and urethra. The cloaca is a dilation at the caudal end of the hindgut, divided into the rectal/anal canal and the urogenital sinus by the urorectal septum. The bladder and urethra develop from the urogenital sinus, with additional contributions from surrounding tissues. In the male, production of androgens is vital to the closure of tissues around the urethral tube. If this tube closes abnormally, the urethral meatus will be located on the dorsal (hypospadias) or ventral (epispadias) surface of the penis, rather than at the tip. In very rare instances, the abdominal wall fails to close around the bladder, causing extrophy of the bladder.

Adrenal Development and Function

The adrenal glands, although in direct contact with the kidneys, have different embryologic origins. Even the cortex and medulla are derived from separate germ layers. The adrenal cortex, which secretes corticosteroids and some androgenic hormones, arises from the mesoderm, while the adrenal medulla, which secretes neurohormones (epinephrine and norepinephrine), has the neuroectoderm as its source. The adrenal glands also secrete androgens. Adrenal hyperplasia during gestation can cause masculinization of the female fetus because of the increased amounts of androgens secreted.

During the first half of pregnancy the fetal adrenal glands are large but they decrease in size as term approaches. Fetal adrenal function may be vital to maintenance of the pregnancy through the active production of steroids. Fetal lung maturity is accelerated by increased fetal steroid production, which occurs during pregnancies complicated by hypertension or preeclampsia and also during labor. Development of the fetal adrenals depends on a functioning hypothalamic-pituitary axis. A fetus with major defects in cerebral development, such as anencephaly, also has adrenal hypoplasia.

Reproductive Development and Function

The reproductive system develops along with the urinary system. Testes develop in the fetal abdomen and can be recognized after 7 weeks of gestation. By week 30 of gestation, testes begin to descend through the inguinal canal into the scrotum. Ovaries develop in the abdomen and remain in the pelvic cavity. Figure 7-16 shows development of external genitalia in the male and female fetuses (see Chapter 27).

Sexual development continues throughout gestation as the external genitalia change in appearance. These

Cryptorchidism – undescended testicles

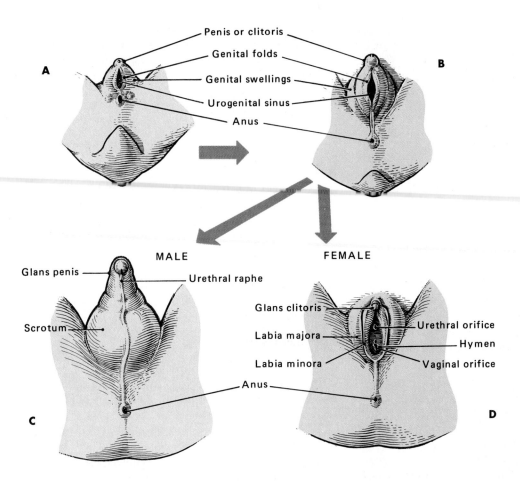

FIGURE 7-16 Embryonic development of external genitalia. **A** and **B**, Early undifferentiated stages. **C** and **D**, Differentiation into male and female genitalia. (From Langley LL, Telford IR, Christensen JB: *Dynamic anatomy and physiology*, New York, 1980, McGraw-Hill. © by Mosby.)

changes are an important part of gestational age assessment. Sexual maturity continues with identification of the infant's somatic sex by both infant and parents, and then with the onset of sexual maturity during puberty.

MUSCULOSKELETAL SYSTEM: DEVELOPMENT AND FUNCTION

The musculoskeletal system develops from embryonic mesoderm. Cells from the mesoderm give rise to the embryonic connective tissue, called mesenchyme. Some mesenchymal cells differentiate into myoblasts, the precursors of muscle tissue. Others form fibroblasts (connective tissue), chondroblasts (cartilage), or osteoblasts (bone).

The limbs begin as limb buds that appear on the ventrolateral aspect of the embryo's body near the end of the fourth week. Development proceeds in a proximal-distal manner and is completed by the end of the eighth week of gestation, with completion of the arms preceding the legs by a few days. Limb development is illustrated in Figures 7-17 and 7-18. Bones of the upper and lower extremities that are homologous are the radius, tibia, ulna, and fibula; the thumb and big toe are homologous digits. The growth of the infant's entire skeleton is determined both by genetic endowment and perinatal environment (see Chapter 27).

Cartilage is seen in the embryo at about five weeks of gestation. Bone may develop directly from mesenchymal cells or from cells that first become cartilage and then ossify. Ossification begins in the *diaphysis,* or shaft of long bones, and proceeds in all directions (Figure 7-19). At term, ossification is mostly completed at the diaphyses but has only begun to appear at the *epiphyses,* or ends of the bones. You can notice the soft pliability of the skull bones at birth. Development of the fetal skeleton depends on maternal supplies of calcium and phosphorus, especially from the end of the embryonic period (8 weeks of gestation) until term, since this is the period of ossification; thus maternal nutrition is important.

Smooth muscles arise from mesenchymal cells located near their associated organs (the digestive tract and elsewhere). *Skeletal muscle* is derived from myoblasts and begins to show its characteristic striations and involuntary movements by the end of the third fetal month. Each skeletal muscle develops near the bone that will be moved by the muscle. It then becomes associated with motor nerves. Adequate development of skeletal muscle depends on adequate amniotic fluid volume. Therefore the fetus crowded into the intrauterine environment because of oligohydramnios will be born with contractures because of lack of movement.

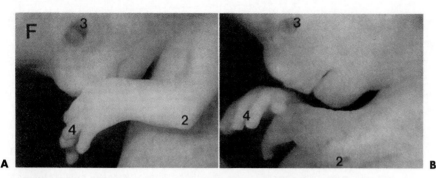

FIGURE 7-17 Arm development from day 44 to 46. **A,** The arm has bent at the elbow, which points caudally. The arms move in utero from week 7 to 8. **B,** The hands meet and cross in the midline over the thorax. (From England MA: *A color atlas of life before birth: normal fetal development,* St Louis, 1990, Mosby.)

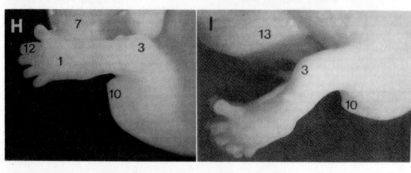

FIGURE 7-18 Leg development from day 44 to 46. **A,** The soles of the feet face each other. **B,** The knee points cranially. (From England MA: *A color atlas of life before birth: normal fetal development,* St Louis, 1990, Mosby.)

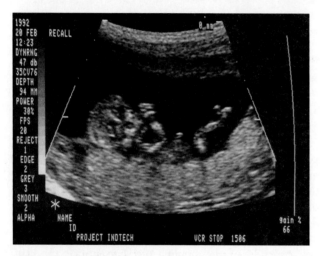

FIGURE 7-19 Ultrasound print of infant's arms and legs (12 weeks). (Courtesy Advanced Technology Laboratories, Bothell, Wash.)

The normal fetus can perform a wide variety of voluntary and involuntary movements. Both muscle tone and movements change with increasing gestational age. This is known via ultrasonic examination and maternal reports of fetal activity, as well as direct observations of premature infants. Table 7-1 summarizes characteristics of movement and tone in the development of the infant.

NEUROLOGIC SYSTEM: DEVELOPMENT AND FUNCTION

Human development both prenatally and postnatally proceeds in a cephalocaudal, mass-to-specific, gross-to-

fine direction. The nervous system develops from a specialized area of ectoderm called the neural plate about 18 days after conception. The neural plate differentiates into the neural crest and the neural tube. The neural crest becomes the peripheral nervous system, and the neural tube becomes the central nervous system (brain and spinal cord) (Figure 7-20). The tube is open at the cranial and caudal ends (anterior and posterior neuropores). From day 22 to day 26 after conception these ends will close by "zipping up" from the thoracic area and proceeding toward the top of the head and "zipping down" from the same area to the base of the spine. Severe developmental defects result from failure of closure in the early days. If the anterior neuropore does not close, the fetus will be *anencephalic.* If the posterior neuropore does not close, the fetus will have some form of *spina bifida.* Fortunately, prenatal diagnosis is available for many of these major defects (see Chapter 11).

Neural tube growth is greater at the cranial end of the fetus, which will accommodate the brain. The size of the fetal head is related to brain growth and amount of cerebral spinal fluid.

Development of the brain influences the infant's neurohormonal function, as well as intellectual capacity. The pituitary gland or hypophysis is referred to as the "master gland" because of its powerful influence on human function. The two lobes of the pituitary are derived from separate tissues, which explains their separate functions. The anterior pituitary develops from oral ectodermal tissue and is the glandular portion that secretes trophic and growth stimulating hormones. The posterior pituitary develops from neuroectoderm and secretes antidiuretic hormone and oxytocin. The pitu-

TABLE 7-1   Development of Movement and Tone

GESTATIONAL AGE	TONUS	MOVEMENTS
28 weeks	Absent. Infant lies in extension.	Spontaneous movement when awake. Slow and twisting or rapid movements of entire limb.
32 weeks	Flexor tone begins in lower extremities. Upper still extended.	Flexor movements in lower extremities occur in unison. Onset of head turning.
36 weeks	Flexor tone increases in lower extremities. Begins to flex upper extremities.	Vigorous flexion movements of lower extremities now alternate. Flexion movements of upper extremities begin. Onset of neck extension.
Term	Flexor tone in all extremities.	Alternating movements of all limbs. Neck extension continues to improve. Neck flexion begins.

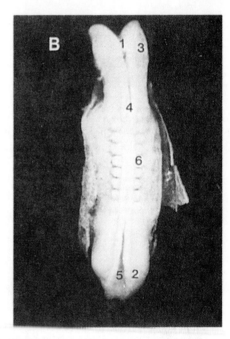

FIGURE 7-20 The neural tube is fusing, but the anterior and posterior neuropores are still open (day 22 to 23). (From England MA: *A color atlas of life before birth: normal fetal development,* St Louis, 1990, Mosby.)

itary gland forms in a specialized area called Rathke's pouch, located in the roof of the fetal mouth. The gland migrates into the base of the brain as development proceeds, but the original site of Rathke's pouch can be felt as a small indentation on the hard palate.

Protection of the brain is a priority of prenatal development. Premature birth threatens neonatal neurologic function in several ways. Because the third trimester is the period of increased brain growth, delivery before term forces completion of brain growth in the less than ideal extrauterine environment. The germinal matrix is an area of the brain especially vulnerable to damage before 32 weeks of gestation. It is richly supplied with blood vessels that can be easily ruptured, leading to intraventricular hemorrhage (see Chapter 28).

Myelination

Impulses created by neurons must be transmitted throughout the body. **Myelin** forms an insulating sheath around axons and allows the conduction of impulses in an organized manner. Myelination begins during the middle of gestation and continues through adolescence. Maturation of sensory and motor functions follows the sequence of myelinization, with mastery of gross motor movements preceding mastery of fine movements.

Fetal responses to external stimuli can be voluntary or involuntary. Motor activity begins early in development with reflex movements occurring at about 7 weeks gestation. Spontaneous movements follow at about 8 weeks gestation, with swallowing, breathing, and grasping movements (all necessary for postnatal survival) appearing early. By about 16 to 20 weeks of gestation, fetal movements are strong enough to be felt by the mother.

Motor Activity   *Fetal movements noted @ 7wks.*

Increased fetal movements and changes in fetal heart rates have been noted when mothers are exposed to a loud noise or if a strong light is directed toward the maternal abdomen. Maternal hunger and anxiety also cause changes in fetal status; it becomes tachycardic in response to maternal catecholamine secretion during maternal anxiety. The normal fetus alternates periods of rolling and stretching movement with periods of sleep. Each part of the cycle lasts about 20 minutes. Heart rate variability decreases during fetal sleep and increases during periods of fetal activity. Reactivity of the cardiac

Fetal movement felt by mother @ 16-20 wks

control center to fetal movement is an index of an intact central nervous system examined by the nonstress test (NST) (Chapter 11).

SPECIAL SENSES: DEVELOPMENT AND FUNCTION

The sensory systems develop chronologically—touch, smell, vestibular, taste, hearing, vision (Haith, 1986). The fetus responds to *touch* through the maternal abdominal wall; mothers feel this response. Movement in the uterus provides development of *vestibular function*. Preterm infants born by 26 to 30 weeks respond to odors. Finally, it is known that newborns discriminate between varying tastes (see Chapter 20).

Vision

Development of vision begins in the fourth week of life. The eyes appear as optic grooves at about 22 days. Very complex in construction, all three layers of embryonic tissue are involved (Figure 7-21). A fetus of about 16 weeks is able to react to light, as evidenced by its startle reflex when a strong beam of light is shone on the mother's abdomen. Later in gestation, at 29 weeks, the same fetus turns toward the light. There is some indication that eye and respiratory movements together can be used to assess prenatal central nervous system function (Figure 7-22).

Hearing

The ears develop from several separate structures. The internal ear develops first, beginning with the *otic pit*. Ear structures mature at about 24 to 28 weeks, enough to demonstrate a response to sound. Auditory acoustic stimulation is used during prenatal testing to stimulate a fetus. (There is debate about the level of decibels to use; only sounds of low frequency seem audible. As gestation progresses, the fetus is able to hear sounds of higher frequency. The fetus is in a "noisy" environment where maternal heartbeat, breathing, and placental and intestinal sounds are heard. Mothers have long reported increased fetal movement in response to loud music, and fetal soothing with more placid music.

HEMATOLOGIC SYSTEM: DEVELOPMENT AND FUNCTION

Formation of blood, or **hematopoiesis**, parallels cardiovascular development. At about 13 to 15 days of gestation, **angioblasts** organize as "blood islands" in the mesoderm of the yolk sac. Spaces develop within these islands and become lined with the angioblasts, forming the primitive blood vessels and endothelium. Cells of the endothelium give rise to primitive blood cells. This all occurs outside the embryo, *in the yolk sac.* Blood is not formed within the embryo until the fifth week of

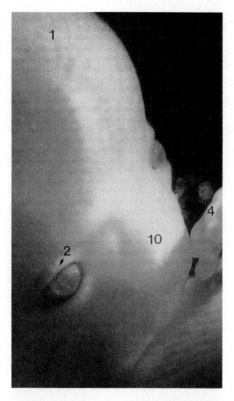

FIGURE 7-21 At 44 to 46 days of gestation the eyelids have not yet formed. (From England MA: *A color atlas of life before birth: normal fetal development*, St Louis, 1990, Mosby.)

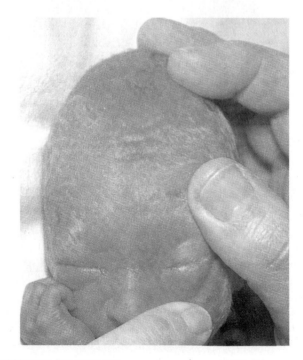

FIGURE 7-22 Tiny preterm infant whose eyelids do not open (24.6 weeks). (Reprinted with permission of Harcourt Brace Jovanovich Group [Australia]. From Beischer MA and MacKay EV: *Obstetrics and the newborn*, ed 3, Philadelphia, 1993, WB Saunders.)

blood is formed by 5 wks

gestation. The primary site for *hematopoiesis* in the embryo is the liver, which grows larger as this process continues. The liver increases in size until, by the ninth week of gestation, it is responsible for about 10% of total fetal weight. Hematopoiesis also gives the liver its red color.

Later in gestation the **reticuloendothelial system,** comprised of the liver, spleen, bone marrow, and lymph nodes, becomes the primary site of hematopoiesis. By term, the bone marrow is the main site for production of all red cells and most other cellular blood components. However, the liver, spleen, and lymph nodes can be stimulated to produce blood cells during periods of extreme and continued demand.

The **reticulum cell,** the germinal cell for all blood cell production, is found within the reticuloendothelial system. In the lymph nodes, reticulum cells develop into lymphocytes and monocytes. Elsewhere reticulum cells will yield plasma cells, which provide immune factors. In the bone marrow, the reticulum cell will differentiate into either a hemoblast or myeloblast. Hemoblasts undergo several other stages of transformation before emerging as erythrocytes, while myeloblasts differentiate into granulocytic leukocytes or megakaryocytes (platelet precursors).

There are many differences in the anatomy and function of fetal blood cells. Fetal erythrocytes are larger in size than adult erythrocytes; however, they also have a shorter life span (80 to 100 days vs 120 days for adult cells). Fetal leukocyte function is not always adequate for defense against infection. Implications for these differences are discussed later in Chapter 28.

Hemoglobin

Fetal hemoglobin, or Hgb F, is a specialized form of hemoglobin found only during gestation and in early infancy. Hgb F accounts for 70% to 90% of the hemoglobin found in the perinatal period. It has a high affinity or attraction for oxygen. This ensures an adequate supply for the rapidly dividing fetal cells.

Blood Type

Blood type is determined at conception. As with other genetically transferred traits, different blood factors may be dominant or recessive. Incompatibility between maternal and fetal blood may cause fetal and neonatal hemolysis and neonatal jaundice (see Chapter 9).

Coagulation

The ability of the fetus to synthesize clotting factors is genetically determined. A fetus with inherited defects in production of clotting factors usually does not show symptoms in utero, even though clotting factors cannot pass from mother to fetus through the placental circulation. In fact, the infant may appear normal for the first few weeks of life.

In the genetically normal fetus and newborn, production of adequate amounts of clotting factors depends on maturation of the liver and the presence of vitamin K. This vitamin is produced in the gastrointestinal tract through the interaction of bacteria, food, and time. Synthesis of prothrombin and factor VII cannot occur without it (see Chapter 19).

> **Test Yourself**
> • How does fetal hemoglobin differ from adult hemoglobin?

IMMUNOLOGIC SYSTEM: DEVELOPMENT AND FUNCTION

The development of immune capability begins in the human fetus between the eighth and fifteenth weeks of gestation. The fetus normally lives in a sterile environment, and the immune system is therefore functioning only in a rudimentary manner. Passive immunity, acquired from the mother across the placenta late in pregnancy, offers protection from several pathogens in the early infancy period. *Only IgG antibody cross*

As described in the hematologic system, the cells of the immune system arise from stem cells, which then become **lymphopoietic** cells (precursors to tissues of the immune system). One type of lymphopoietic cell, called the T cell, is produced first in the thymus and then throughout the body's lymphoid tissues. Another type, the B cell, is produced in an unknown site within the human body. T cells destroy pathogens by phagocytosis; B cells produce antibodies to these pathogens. T-cell function is referred to as **cellular immunity;** B-cell function is called **humoral immunity.** (For more on immunity, see Chapter 25.)

Antibody Production

There are five different classes of antibodies produced by humans: immunoglobulin (Ig) G, M, A, D, and E, each with its own unique chemical structure. IgG, IgA, and IgE are produced by the fetus before the twentieth week of gestation. The **IgG** group is the largest and also provides the most immunity. Only small amounts of IgG are produced by the human fetus, but maternal IgG is actively transported across the placenta. Maternal IgG provides passively acquired immunity against many infectious diseases. Blood group antibodies are also in the IgG class, and therefore can freely cross the placenta to cause hemolytic disease of the newborn (see Chapter 9).

IgA is the second largest group of immunoglobulins and is produced by lymphoid tissues within the gastrointestinal, urinary, and respiratory tracts. This immunoglobulin protects against local infections, such as those of the respiratory and gastrointestinal tracts. Its presence in human breast milk lowers the incidence of enteric infections in breast-fed infants. IgA can be found in the saliva of neonates after several days of life.

The **IgM** molecule is the largest of all the immunoglobulins and *cannot cross the placenta*. It also is the immunoglobulin that is formed early in the immune response. Therefore any IgM found in the fetus or neonate must be of fetal origin; examination of cord blood for IgM levels can reveal the existence of congenital infection (see Chapter 28).

The exact role of IgD immunoglobulin is not known. IgE is found in elevated amounts in persons with atopic allergic disorders. IgE and IgA are produced by the same tissues and are found in external secretions.

Test Yourself

• Name the primary differences between fetal and adult red blood cells.
• How does the fetus acquire passive immunity?

KEY POINTS

• Growth and development are distinct but related concepts.
• Fetal growth and development depend on genetic quality and intrauterine and extrauterine environments.
• Mitosis produces cells with the same chromosomal number as the parent cells, whereas meiosis yields cells with one member of each chromosome pair.
• Meiosis allows for variations in genetic makeup.
• Support structures and circulation arise early in development so as to supply nutrition for rapid growth.

• Both anatomic (structural) and biochemical (functional) development occur during embryonic and fetal life.
• Although substantial organ system development occurs during the first trimester, the fetus is vulnerable to the effects of teratogens throughout gestation.
• Normal growth and development yield a newborn well equipped to adapt to a supportive extrauterine environment.

STUDY QUESTIONS

7-1 Match key terms with the definitions below.
   a. Layer of the embryo from which skin, hair, and nails are created *Ectoderm*
   b. Body cell chromosomes *autosomes*
   c. Double strands of genetic material *DNA*.
   d. Increase in the size or number of cells *growth*.
   e. Process by which primitive cells mature *development*
   f. Process by which the chromosome number is halved *meiosis*
   g. Structure consisting of two arteries, one vein, Wharton's jelly, and amnion *umbilical cord*
   h. Process by which the embryo attaches to the uterine wall *implantation*
7-2 The three germ layers are formed and begin differentiation by the end of the second week. The endoderm layer will become:
   a. Linings of the body organs
   b. Muscle, bone, and cartilage
   c. The brain and central nervous system
7-3 Which of the following statements would best describe the 12-week fetus?

   a. It is capable of extrauterine life.
   b. All organs and body systems are completely differentiated.
   c. Although much development has occurred, the fetus is still vulnerable to the action of teratogens.
   d. The placenta forms a complete barrier from the external world.
7-4 What milestone in development occurs around 23 weeks?
   a. The fetal lungs are capable of respiration.
   b. The fetal cardiovascular system is fully formed.
   c. The fetal fingernails have reached the ends of the fingertips.
   d. The fetal brain is completely differentiated.
7-5 Select the correct answer from these true-false choices:
   a. Suck and swallow are coordinated by 32 weeks of gestation.
   b. Amniotic fluid cellular components become part of meconium.
   c. The fetus swallows and voids into the amniotic fluid.

d. There is a time in development when sex appears "neutral."

7-6 The reticulum cell is amazing because it develops in different locations into different cells. Match location with cell type below:

Cell Type

1. Lymphocyte *B*
2. Hemoblast *a*

3. Myeloblast *A*
4. Monocytes *B*

Location

a. Bone marrow
b. Lymph node
c. Other reticuloendothelial tissues

REFERENCES

Bernhardt J: Sensory capabilities of the fetus, *MCN Am J Matern Child Nurs* 12:44, 1987.

Blackburn ST, Loper DL: *Maternal, fetal and neonatal physiology*, Philadelphia, 1992, WB Saunders.

Carlson BM: *Patton's foundations of embryology*, New York, 1981, McGraw-Hill.

Haith MM: Sensory and perceptual processes in early infancy, *J Pediatr* 109:158, 1986.

Page DC: The sex-determining region of the human Y chromosome encodes a finger protein, *Cell* 51:1091, 1987.

Pleet HB et al: Patterns of malformations resulting from teratogenic effects of first trimester hyperthermia, *Pediatr Res* 14:587, 1980.

 STUDENT RESOURCE SHELF

England MA: *Color atlas of life before birth: normal fetal development*, Chicago, 1990, Mosby.

A fascinating look at the process of fetal development through pictures of fetuses at various stages of gestation. Anatomy, function, and relation of these to newborn life are emphasized.

Moore KL: *The developing human: clinically oriented embryology*, ed 4, Philadelphia, 1988, WB Saunders.

The classic textbook of human fetal development. Moore extensively illustrates the descriptions, relates influences of parental health and effects of abnormal development on the newborn.

Sadler TW: *Langman's medical embryology*, ed 5, Baltimore, 1985, Williams & Wilkins.

Smaller in size than the Moore text, but similar in scope. Descriptions of developmental processes are more succinct than in Moore.

UNIT
Two

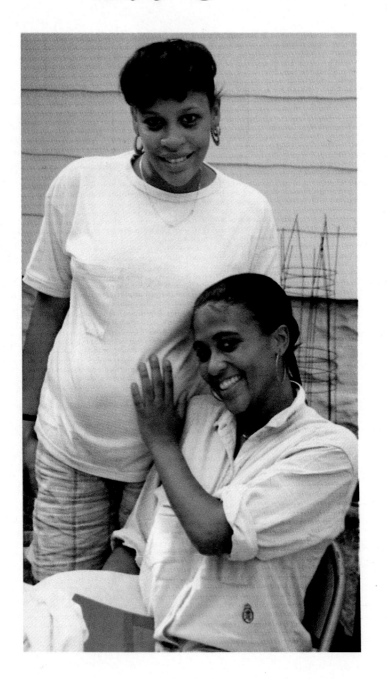

PREGNANCY

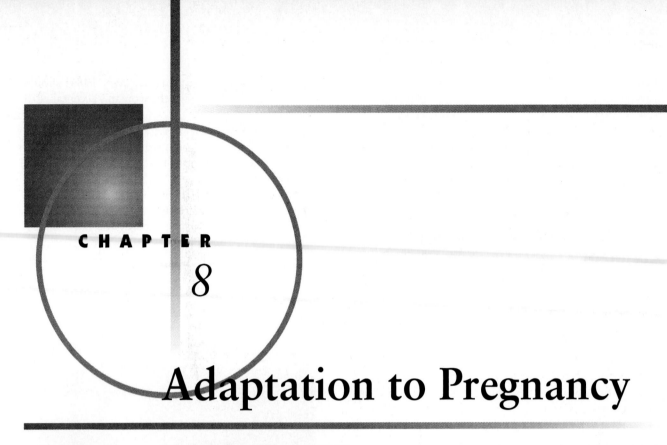

Adaptation to Pregnancy

KEY TERMS

Acquaintance
Ambivalence
Attachment
Avoidance
Bonding
Couvade
Developmental Tasks
Differentiation
Imagery
Incorporation
Tentative Pregnancy
Visualization

LEARNING OBJECTIVES

1. *Identify the prospective mother's major developmental tasks of pregnancy. Separate them into first-, second-, and third-trimester tasks.*
2. *Discuss psychosocial factors that have an effect on these developmental tasks.*
3. *Relate how the biologic age and developmental phase of expectant parents influence the tasks of pregnancy.*
4. *Compare developmental tasks of the expectant mother and father.*
5. *Recognize the initial steps in the bonding process.*
6. *Describe how acquaintance and bonding may be interrupted.*

People learn how to be mothers or fathers from their own parents. Memories of their parents' behavior and attitudes lead them to develop ideas about what a parent is or should be. Once formed, these ideas are extremely difficult to change. If parent-child relationships were loving, individuals are likely to become loving parents. If relationships were full of distrust and abuse, these patterns are also likely to be repeated in the next generation.

Because parents are role models, children at play often mimic parents' acts. As children mature, play is replaced by a more inward rehearsal. The adolescent dreams of future roles and rehearses them in the mind. In adulthood, this process occurs through a series of images. During times of change, particularly when a major change in life-style is anticipated, a person imagines himself or herself in the situation. For example, an expectant mother imagines herself rocking her baby, or an expectant father pictures himself comforting a crying child.

Motivations for pregnancy vary widely. The couple may want to prove their ability to reproduce or to achieve adult status. They may be fulfilling the cultural expectation that "everyone" wants children or may wish to fulfill their parents' wish for a grandchild. A woman may desire to again experience the closeness of the mother-child relationship or to strengthen ties with her partner. More positively, having a child may be

161

viewed as a new beginning, an enriching life experience leading to feelings of creativity and competence. The woman may be reaching the age when she feels that "it's now or never," that she must soon decide to have a baby or risk the inability to conceive or carry the baby to term. However, when the time comes, transition to first-time parenthood is abrupt; the new parents often feel unprepared for the reality of the responsibility.

Developmental Tasks During Pregnancy

Many **developmental tasks** occur during the psychologic transition from nonparent to parent. This transition parallels and is stimulated by the development of the child within the womb.

During the early weeks, the expectant mother tests the reality of the pregnancy. Even after she has confirmation through tests, she looks for affirmation in other signs and symptoms. These symptoms reassure her that the pregnancy is real.

FIRST TRIMESTER

First-trimester needs vary, depending on whether the pregnancy is the woman's first. A first pregnancy is like any other first experience. The expectant mother feels curiosity and concern about the changes ahead. Even the most carefully planned educational program does not fully relieve the anxiety.

Although the woman may have chosen to become pregnant, there is always an ambivalence until the idea of being pregnant becomes a reality and an acceptance of the growing fetus, *integration* or **incorporation,** takes place (Tanner, 1969; Rubin, 1984).

Acceptance

The expectant parents' conscious or unconscious motivation and eagerness for pregnancy change the normal degree of **ambivalence** about anticipated life changes pregnancy causes. For the first-time mother, the infant is a final step away from the girl she once was. She must give up her image of herself as a childless person before she can accept her pregnant self. Some women experience considerable nostalgia for the person they once were, feeling unready for the "mother person" they will become. This is often expressed in dreams and images of younger days.

Occasionally, unresolved ambivalence can interfere with acceptance of pregnancy. Inconvenient social circumstances such as being young and single may cause the expectant mother to deny the existence of the pregnancy. A disintegrating relationship with the expectant father can cause anger, which may lead to maternal rejection of the fetus.

The following dimensions (Lederman, 1984) should be considered when assessing the woman's acceptance of the pregnancy:

1. *The desire for the pregnancy and/or infant.* In Lederman's study, some women wanted an infant but disliked being pregnant. In less healthy cases, some loved the warm feelings related to being pregnant but could not look ahead to actually nurturing an infant. However, resolution of negative feelings usually occurred by the third trimester (Lederman, 1984).

hopefully by 1st trimester

 Self-Discovery

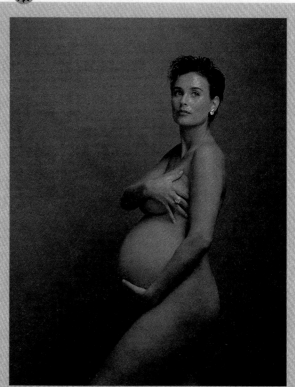

Copyright Annie Leibovitz/Contact Press Images.

- *How do you respond to this photograph?*
- *How do the media influence the way women feel about their bodies?*
- *Has this photograph helped women feel that the pregnant body is beautiful? Normal? Natural?*
- *What were women's attitudes about their bodies during pregnancy in your mother's generation? Your grandmothers'? Have they changed?*
- *How would you encourage a woman who feels ugly during pregnancy?*

2. *Amount of happiness or unhappiness.* For some women in the study, emotional gratification came from feelings of biologic fulfillment and from their conscious desire for a child despite mood swings and emotional lability. In women with a history of depression, however, the pregnancy tended to trigger recurrence. Low self-esteem greatly increased fears related to labor and/or the ability to mother the newborn.

3. *Discomfort during pregnancy.* The amount of discomfort experienced during pregnancy varies considerably from woman to woman. When discomfort seems intensified and markedly prolonged, it may indicate a problem with acceptance of the pregnant state.

4. *Acceptance of body changes.* In our society, the media have promoted the idea that the skinny body is the model for beauty. Many women fear being viewed as "fat" and feel relieved when they look obviously pregnant. Such women look forward to wearing maternity clothing and may choose to wear it early in the pregnancy. New views expressed in the media may change perceptions.

5. *Amount of unresolved ambivalence.* Most women accept pregnancy by the beginning of the third trimester. To assess how well the woman has accomplished this task, discuss her feelings about the infant and help her to express how she sees herself as a new mother. Some mothers accept pregnancy but are still unable to imagine themselves as mothers. Women who receive little or no psychologic support may have particular difficulty.

As a nurse, you will need to assess the degree of interference with the woman's acceptance process. For example, ambivalence is natural if a woman must give up a rewarding career or if financial considerations mean that the timing of the pregnancy is poor. These feelings do not mean that the woman has rejected pregnancy; her attitude of happiness or unhappiness is a far more accurate indication of her state of mind. She is in the period of *pregnancy validation,* a necessary developmental phase of pregnancy.

Concerns

Most pregnant women are concerned during the first trimester with the changes in their own bodies and how these changes will affect their lives. Some of their expressed concerns have to do with the following:

1. Normal symptoms of pregnancy ("Should I worry? Am I normal? What shall I do?")
2. Changes in life-style that will result from the pregnancy ("I wonder how pregnancy will make me different.")
3. Changes in relationship with the partner ("How will he accept this pregnancy? How will it change our sexual responses?")

4. Medical care—the sequences and reasons for visits ("How can I get help between visits?")

The woman may appear to be very self-concerned. Because she probably will not be able to focus on instructions concerning future events such as labor, delivery, child care, or contraception, such topics are best discussed in later visits.

Practical concerns may center around finances, especially if the new infant's arrival will mean curtailment of the woman's income, or about the expenses of having and raising a child. Women may worry about loss of freedom, increased dependency, or other changes in relationships. Although these concerns are most evident in the first pregnancy, relationships also shift and change with later children.

Signs of Difficulty

Signs of difficulty in first-trimester tasks may be demonstrated as exaggerated discomforts such as severe nausea, sleeplessness, and fatigue. In addition, she may have unresolved anger, feel depressed, and be hostile toward her partner. Interventions may assist her to resolve these conflicts.

SECOND TRIMESTER

By the end of the first trimester, discomforts from physiologic changes have usually disappeared. The expectant mother settles down and her concerns begin to shift from her own bodily changes to the growing infant. During this trimester the infant takes on its own identity as a separate being. The psychologic task of perceiving the fetus as a growing infant, separate from herself, or fetal **differentiation,** is normally completed by the end of the trimester.

Infant as Non-Self

Beginning with quickening, the parents' thoughts turn inward to the separateness of the child. The infant is part of them but is distinct and familiar; however, they can't guess how he or she will look. Physical sensations, which at first are described as light, fluttering, and exciting, may later seem disruptive. Women complain, "He never leaves me alone! Always giving me a thump when I want to sleep" (Lederman, 1984). This period has been called *fetal embodiment,* a developmental task of the second trimester (Starn & Niederhauser, 1990).

Visualization. Through **visualization** the woman imagines what her child is like and becomes acquainted with it as she notices what disturbs and what soothes it. For instance, most fetuses react to loud music such as rock music with strong movement, yet quiet down and are soothed by smooth, lilting melodies. An expectant mother may experiment with and note reactions to rhythmic sensations such as when she leans against the spinning dryer or when she rubs firmly in a particular spot. Many "play" with the fetus by pushing against a protruding spot and waiting to be kicked in return.

When the expectant mother has a sonogram early in pregnancy, she can actually see her child moving about within her. Women frequently report that this was the first time they experienced the feeling that another person was really there. Encourage the mother to ask for an ultrasound "photo" of her infant to help her picture the child and develop feelings for it.

Dreams. Fears often arise as an expectant mother begins to accept this separateness. Low self-esteem intensifies the woman's fear that her child will not be perfect. This fear does not diminish with later pregnancies, even when the first infant was healthy. This woman may believe that she could not possibly be lucky again after her first infant was "perfect."

These are often fears expressed in dreams. A theme common in dreams is the monster-child, devouring from within, or the wolf-child suckling at the breast. These themes may indicate that the woman feels ambivalence and fear toward the unknown "other" or that she will be so consumed by the coming infant that she will never again regain her sense of self.

Emotional separateness. Emotional separation between self and the infant is important. In image-making, some women report feeling that the infant is a total stranger and are surprised that the infant may have reactions different from their own. For example, the expectant mother may be fond of rock music and be amazed to find that her unborn child is clearly restless when it is played. For women who have not completed the process of *individuation* (adolescents, for example), this realization is especially difficult.

Maternal role attainment. The newly pregnant woman begins to "put on" her new role in the first trimester. She looks for role models who have had this experience. Rubin (1984) calls this activity *replication*, copying behaviors in other pregnant women or successful mothers. The pregnant woman then plays these roles and tries the various ways of interaction. During the second trimester, the process moves a step further to *internalization*, when the woman lingers over images of herself in various situations. Using **imagery**, she begins adapting to the future.

In the third trimester, as the woman's focus shifts to look forward to the end of pregnancy discomforts, the fetus may be a threat and cause anxiety. Role assumption behaviors, according to Rubin, now focus on evaluation and criticism of others, including her own mother. She is *differentiating* herself from others to become the kind of mother she imagines.

Relationship with Her Own Mother

The need of expectant mothers to get reacquainted with their own parents is universal. Expectant parents relive past and present relationships with their parents in their minds and try to come to terms with them.

If her own mother is available, the expectant mother may attempt to get closer to her. If there are still unresolved issues of separation and power between them, she may exclude her mother from participation. Rivalry between the expectant mother and her mother may cause friction in everything from naming the infant to whether or not the new grandmother will be invited to come to help out when the baby comes home.

If her own mother is unavailable, the woman may try to befriend another motherly person to serve as her alternate maternal role model. This person may be a friend with children whom the expectant mother admires and wishes to emulate.

Concerns

In general, in the second trimester, the mother is interested in protecting the health of the infant, and her concerns will reflect her awareness of its needs. The general concerns are as follows:

1. Nutritional intake (Am I gaining too much? Too little?)
2. Amount of exercise, travel (What restrictions are necessary?)
3. Progression of fetal growth (How big is the baby this month?)
4. Warning signs of problems
5. Changing body image (how reflected in clothes, hygiene, hair, skin)
6. Changes in sexual desires (concern about restrictions and misconceptions)

Signs of Difficulty

Signs of difficulty with second-trimester tasks may include continuing anger and depression because of lack of acceptance. Physical complaints and a focus on her own concerns rather than thoughts of the fetus may indicate problems. Clues to difficulty in parenting may become evident in self-involvement or in regression to more childish behavior.

THIRD TRIMESTER

Separation and Birth

In the final weeks the mother's task is to prepare for the end of the pregnancy and for the birth itself. As the mother looks forward to the birth, she may again feel considerable ambivalence. She must prepare for *letting go* of the pregnancy and all its warm feelings of fusion and creativity, or *fetal separation*. Conscious or unconscious fears of mutilation, death, or abandonment often surface at this time. Anticipatory anxiety is considered in this phase to be normal and healthy. As the birth nears, the overriding concern is how to cope with the stresses of labor and delivery and whether there will be a safe passage. As they work on structuring a mental image of what labor and birth will be like, many couples seek out other new parents for advice and questioning and listen to their stories of how they dealt with their birth experiences.

Increasing Dependency Needs

During pregnancy, dependency needs increase and reach a peak in the third trimester, labor, and the early nurturing period after birth. The expectant mother needs to be nurtured to store up reserves for the time when she is nurturing the infant. This is not limited to the first pregnancy, only to expectant women. Men, also, feel a heightened need to have someone dependable to care for them, particularly because the expectant mother becomes more introspective with advancing pregnancy and perhaps withdraws some of the "mothering" attention he usually gets from her.

By becoming a parent, a person is no longer the child in the relationship with parents. As a parent, a person becomes the provider rather than the recipient. In this sense, becoming a parent for the first time means that the new parents can never return to childhood.

Childbirth Education

Many couples seek childbirth classes to make them feel prepared. In these classes, expectant parents learn the facts and techniques of childbirth but also receive support (see Chapter 12).

The woman is eager to learn any methods and techniques to relieve discomforts and to assist her during the later part of pregnancy and labor. She will use exercises and practice breathing in these weeks. Counseling continues on an individual basis and may now include preparation for infant's arrival and care. In the third trimester, information for recovery, self-care, and infant care should be presented because early discharge does not allow adequate time to teach these things.

Concerns

Expectant mothers' needs in the third trimester are expressed in approximately the same ways despite differences in background, educational level, and experience. A woman focuses on the infant, the process of labor, and her own changing physical condition and emotions. Even multiparas have questions about the differences in labor and delivery with each infant. Concerns expressed in this trimester tend to pertain to the following:

1. The infant's well-being (questions on birth defects, signs of fetal well-being, how birth affects the infant, effects of medication and anesthesia)
2. The costs of having an infant (fees, having to stop work, expenses for equipment)
3. The process of labor and delivery (pain, fears, misconceptions, when to go to the hospital)
4. Family (how other children will accept the infant, how to plan for them during hospitalization, how her partner will respond to the infant)

The changing contours of the woman's body become more prominent; backaches, leg aches, lower abdominal pressure, ligament pain, fatigue, extra weight, cause her to be impatient for labor to begin (Table 8-1).

"Nesting." Some women are superstitious about buying anything for the infant before its birth; to do so might risk death or injury to the child, they have been told. You may acknowledge that some hold this belief but should turn the conversation to the equipment that will be needed by the new infant, even though purchasing will begin later. The father or grandparents may have this task during her hospitalization, but the mother will want to know how to plan. The only important fact to emphasize is that planning should be done before taking the infant home. Mothers who have limited apartment space or income will usually welcome suggestions on how to economize. All women feel the "nesting" impulse, an urge to prepare for the infant.

Signs of Difficulty

Signs of difficulty in the third trimester include a continuing high level of anxiety about herself, labor, or the discomforts of pregnancy. If the woman neglects health practices or cannot prepare for or focus on the needs of the coming infant, she may be indicating that she cannot adjust to what is happening in her body.

EXPECTANT FATHER'S TASKS

Like his mate, the expectant father must make the psychologic shift from his idea of himself as a man or boy without children to that of a *man with a child,* a father. The ease with which he is able to do this is related to his readiness for the pregnancy and the amount of ambivalence he has experienced. Antle-May (1982) states that readiness is related to the man's sense of financial security, of stability in the couple relationship, and of readiness to end the childless state within the couple's relationship. Although his experience lacks the immediacy of the expectant mother's role shift, it follows a similar pattern.

In the beginning tests confirm the pregnancy, and couples tell their significant family and friends. This early phase is called the **announcement** phase and does not last long. After this period, many men pull away psychologically and may distance themselves and avoid discussion of the coming infant, postponing emotional investment. The father's acceptance frequently lags be-

TABLE 8-1   Maternal Tasks, Concerns, and Problems

TASKS	CONCERNS	PROBLEMS
FIRST TRIMESTER		
To acknowledge pregnancy To begin to work through conflicts with own mother to begin to develop own mothering role Pregnancy validation and acceptance	Normality of symptoms, future changes in life-style Changes in relationship with partner Cost of care, how to manage Normality of ambivalence	Exaggerated discomforts such as nausea, sleeplessness Excessive need for reassurance that she is pregnant Anger, rejection of idea of pregnancy Depression, crying, extreme mood swings Distance from sexual partner
SECOND TRIMESTER		
To regard fetus as a reality, fetal embodiment To manage shifts in dependency from the role of daughter to the role of mother To continue working through conflicts with own parents To use mimicry, role playing, imagery to help herself to assume the role of mother	Nutritional intake Changing body image Changing life-style, sexual needs Progression of fetal growth Warning signs of problems	Lack of acceptance of pregnancy Depression, anger, anxiety continue Numerous physical complaints, focus on own concerns Indications of no family support Indication of inability to plan ahead
THIRD TRIMESTER		
To view fetus as a separate individual to be "let go" through birth To accept physical, psychologic changes To prepare for parenting To prepare for labor, birth, and accept the risk of "safe passage"	Infant's well-being, factors affecting labor and birth Anxiety over possibility of deformed baby Expenses Process of labor, delivery Acceptance of infant by other children Present discomforts	High level of anxiety about self, labor Continued nonacceptance of pregnancy Behavior that neglects health practices Lack of support from family or spouse Lack of preparation for or focus on needs of new infant

hind the mother's. Until he is able to imagine that he will actually be a father and have a real child to raise, the whole process may not have an impact. He may involve himself in other pursuits for long periods of time, "forgetting" about the pregnancy. This is the **avoidance** phase of acceptance.

Test Yourself

Name three developmental tasks of an expectant mother during pregnancy.

As the expectant father adjusts to the reality of the situation, his partner experiences her own increased need for support and reassurance. Sensing his withdrawal, she may attempt to involve him more closely. Frequently he withdraws even more (Antle-May, 1982). Disagreements between marital partners are common, and the expectant mother feels that his lack of enthusiasm is a lack of caring. The expectant father feels pressured to organize himself and his priorities around the pregnancy. He may desire a moratorium on pregnancy talk, having trouble with its reality.

In the third phase described by Antle-May, the man focuses on the pregnancy. In research findings, the transition from the avoidance phase takes place near the start of the third trimester and in many cases is quite abrupt. For some men, emotional investment is triggered by the physical reality of the infant, of noticing the obvious changes in his partner's body, feeling fetal movements, or by actually becoming involved in preparations. He suddenly realizes that he will be the father of the child, and he begins to define himself as a father through image-making. Like his partner, he begins to imagine himself as a father, remembering how he was fathered and accepting or rejecting that role. Other relationships are examined (for example, his parents as grandparents). He seeks friendship with others who have children and tends to drift away from those who do not. Jordan (1990) calls this "laboring for relevance" as the father works through phases to become ready for parenting.

He and his partner must also work out the degree of involvement he will have in childbirth and later in parenting the child. This decision is highly individual; yet, the decision needs to be made by both partners. If a couple's expectations differ, they need to reach a compromise before the birth, or unmet expectations may lead to conflict or rejection.

Somatic Symptoms: Couvade

The father's adjustment may include a migrating series of health symptoms and complaints, termed **couvade**. It is thought that this demonstrates a positive level of identification with the pregnant partner. Longobucco and Preston (1989) found that men who experienced symptoms scored higher on scales measuring paternal-role preparation than men who reported no symptoms. Because paternal bonding begins during the pregnancy, this finding seems logical. One father's experience is recorded below:

One father left the scene of the birth of his first child, to cry alone. He shared with me his deep sadness that he could not also bear a child. He has continued to be a very nurturing father.

A recent study identified 39 symptoms reported by the men in the survey. These symptoms included intestinal gas pains, nausea, hunger and weight gain, restlessness, sleeping difficulties, and bad dreams. These symptoms may persist into the early postbirth period. In Clinton's study (1986), men reported 12.5 couvade symptoms per month in the second and third trimesters.

Test Yourself

- According to the studies by Antle-May, the expectant father's readiness for pregnancy is related to _____ .

- When a man is working through his own feelings, it could be called a form of labor. List some steps in the process.

COPING DURING PREGNANCY

Most women do well with support. Others find pregnancy an additional stress that puts them off balance. With an understanding of the normality of body changes, the woman may enjoy her progress. If she is uninformed, she may resent or be fearful of what is happening. If she looks forward to and recognizes the steps of pregnancy, she will feel pride and enjoyment. If she is stressed, her changing body responses may cause anger and frustration.

Any inhibition of the mother's progress through the developmental steps may result in anxiety or conflict that further hinders her ability to form an image of her maternal self. Such impediments can arise from low self-esteem, lack of a maternal role model, or conflicts between the mother-self and career-self roles. If the woman is very young or is older, or when medical or social problems occur, maternal role attainment may be more troublesome.

Low self-esteem makes it difficult for the expectant mother to visualize herself in labor or as a competent mother. Her poor self-image projects itself onto her idea of what kind of parent she will be. She will need strong support and reinforcement for her abilities.

Nursing Responsibilities
▶ ASSESSMENT

You may use the questions in Table 8-2 to elicit information regarding family and individual situations that may precipitate stress during pregnancy. Often when questions focus on what the woman really needs or is concerned about, the presenting need is far from what the nurse assumes it to be. Always *listen* first, before giving instructions or advice. See Chapter 26 for the model that has been developed for care of high-risk teens and women with psychosocial problems or problems that place mother and infant at risk.

You can determine whether the woman has positive role models by asking her who she will talk with about her pregnancy. Find out if the woman is socially isolated (even within a marriage) by asking her how she spends time with friends or family.

▶ NURSING DIAGNOSIS

Whenever a nurse works with expectant parents the following should be considered.

- Altered role performance related to adaptations to the pregnancy.
- Family coping: potential for growth related to anticipation of parenting.
- Ineffective coping compromised by inadequate family support or disengagement.
- Situational low self-esteem related to prior life experiences or level of support during pregnancy.

TABLE 8-2   Initial Questions to Elicit Status Regarding Pregnancy

QUESTIONS	FACTORS INFLUENCING PLANNING
SUPPORT AVAILABLE	
Length of time living in this location?	An isolated couple will need encouragement to seek support.
Support system in this locality?	Referrals must be considered. Exploration with family about resources is important.
Who is available to help with siblings or during the early postpartum period?	
What emotional supports are available for each partner?	A major component of parenting classes is to foster sharing about these issues.
Financial plans to cover costs of pregnancy?	Location and type of medical service influence available referrals.
What are their needs for assistance?	Working may be beneficial or harmful, depending on risk status.
Are there needs that will keep the woman working throughout pregnancy?	
RESPONSE TO PREGNANCY	
What are the most direct concerns about the idea of being pregnant at this time?	Ambivalence about pregnancy is usual in first months but may be a clue to difficulty if still present toward the end of pregnancy.
What interruptions in life goals?	Partner's responses need to be elicited. His attendance at one prenatal visit and at parenting classes is highly recommended.
What sense of "this is the right time"?	
What are the reactions of other family members to the pregnancy?	Single mothers need extra support, as do those in hostile environments.
Are there strong desires to bear only a son or daughter?	Fixation on sex of infant may hinder bonding after delivery; some opportunity to talk about this aspect is important.
Has there been exploration about acceptance of either sex in the infant?	
PROCESS	
What needs for information do the future parents have?	Information giving must be preceded by a determination of what the person already knows.
Fetal growth and development?	
Sexuality during pregnancy?	
Care of woman to promote health?	
Other questions?	
What plans for or fears of delivery are present?	Fears are not easily elicited. Sharing common misconceptions that other mothers have had may prompt a person to recognize her own fears.
Which questions need to be asked of physician (anesthesia, type of delivery)?	
What fears can be identified?	Fearful women need special assistance and perhaps some group discussions before they can openly admit fears.
How do they feel information can help?	Encourage attendance when possible if classes are supportive.
What interest in parenting classes is expressed?	Provide several options for differing approaches and needs.

REMEMBER: "Parents who are secure, supported, valued, and in control of their lives are more effective parents than those who feel unsure and who are not in control" (Keniston, 1977).

▶ EXPECTED OUTCOMES

Consider these examples of outcomes to direct patient care.

- Seeks assistance from appropriate resources and referrals.
- Verbalizes changes that are taking place.
- Seeks involvement of the partner in the care process.
- Father participates in care and preparation for birth.
- Increases understanding of self as a future parent.
- Works on problem resolution.

▶ NURSING INTERVENTIONS

You must be perceptive to identify some of the subtle indications of problems and need to recognize the importance of psychosocial adaptation in planning care during pregnancy and recovery. The following examples of questions that may elicit the woman's perception of her life events are adapted from suggestions by Kleinman, Eisenberg, and Good (1979):

1. What do you think caused your problem?
2. Why do you think it started when it did?
3. What do you think the problem does to you? To your infant?
4. How do you think you can resolve this problem?
5. Can you express the anxiety that comes from this problem?

The woman will often articulate a different emphasis than the health care professional would have expected. The cultural differences play a significant part in the emphasis placed on the meaning of the problem. If you note a depressed affect or lack of grooming, further assess for more severe problems and make appropriate referrals.

Plans to help the mother become more active in her own self-care can be as simple as reinforcing her ability to make appropriate choices. To do this, you will have to allow her to make choices about her care and to give her the responsibility of carrying them out. Self-care means that you must treat the expectant parents as adults, even when they are adolescents.

In addition, refer to social service any woman with stressed life circumstances or economic problems that interfere with adequate nutrition, housing, or future care of the infant and herself.

▶ EVALUATION

Sample questions to evaluate if the mother reached outcomes are listed below.

- Did the partners seek to learn about pregnancy and parenting?
- How was her partner planning to be involved?
- Were clinic appointments kept and outside resources used?
- Did she indicate adequate social support?
- Has she received and followed through on referrals for unresolved problems?

SEXUAL RESPONSES DURING PREGNANCY

Woman's Responses

In the course of prenatal counseling, a woman may express anxiety about sexuality during pregnancy. She may allude to particular problems. Even if she does not, you should approach the subject in a nonthreatening way, either individually or in prenatal classes. A number of women react positively to their changing body image, feeling less restricted in their sexual expression. Some experience a sense of fulfillment when pregnant or feel more attractive than before. For these women, there may be heightened interest in sexual activity. Other women feel less desirable and awkward and because of discomforts express less interest in sexual activity.

For many couples, sexual responses may differ between the woman and her partner. (see Chapter 3). She may be more interested, he less. Interest levels also change as the pregnancy progresses. Research studies have shown that each trimester may have a different set of responses. Regardless of which responses are expressed, most women indicate an increased need to be nurtured and held closely (Reamy et al, 1982).

Partner's Responses

Although many men have no change in sexual desires because of pregnancy, some feel an increased closeness, intimacy, and eroticism. Certain men express a fear of harming the woman or fetus or have questions about whether intercourse is "right" when the woman is pregnant. They may have fantasies about the fetus or about being inadequate to satisfy the woman's increased desires. Other men may withdraw or seek a sexual outlet outside the partnership.

Changes During Phases of the Sexual Response Cycle

When pregnancy responses are placed within each phase of the sexual cycle, the differences may be seen more clearly (Mueller, 1985).

Desire. Changes in body image may increase or decrease sexual interest. A woman may be more tense or relaxed. If she enjoys her body changes, there will be increased interest in more frequent intercourse. Any pregnancy discomforts reduce desire.

Excitement. The phase of physiologic excitement includes vasocongestion of vaginal and labial tissues and clitoral enlargement. Pregnancy increases lubrication and vasocongestion, and excitement may come more quickly. Breasts, too, are already enlarged and may be tender or even sore. Sexual excitement makes nipples erect and may bring discomfort for some; breasts may be a new focus in sex play because all women have enlargement. In some cases the woman may be increasingly uncomfortable with the enlargement, whereas her partner finds it stimulating.

Plateau and orgasm. The vaginal tract becomes engorged during pregnancy. Because muscle tension and venous engorgement increase, many women experience orgasm quickly and may have several during sexual activity. Some women describe orgasm as "fulminating" (Reamy and White, 1985). Mild uterine contractions during orgasm do not appear to harm the fetus.

Resolution. The period of decrease in tissue engorgement and relaxation is often changed. Vasocongestion does not diminish quickly. Some women have continuing discomfort and take longer to relax.

Nursing Responsibilities

 ASSESSMENT

If you are working with different ethnic groups, you should seek information about any cultural sexual taboos during pregnancy and recovery. By seeking this information from each client, you can avoid stereotyping and plan care based on individual needs.

NURSING DIAGNOSIS

There are only a few possible diagnoses to use for this concern, depending on whether the problems expressed are related to the partner or to the woman, or stem from a medical complication during pregnancy.

- Altered sexuality patterns related to differing responses to pregnancy.
- Individual coping stressed by changes demanded by complications of pregnancy.
- High risk for sexually transmitted infection depending on partner's status.

EXPECTED OUTCOMES

- Expresses feelings regarding sexual responses during pregnancy.
- Incorporates anticipatory guidance.
- Protects herself from sexually transmitted diseases (STDs).

NURSING INTERVENTIONS

The most effective intervention for sexual problems expressed by the client during pregnancy is *anticipatory guidance.* On the basis of current understanding of the physiologic changes of pregnancy, the following may be taught regarding sexual activity during pregnancy:

1. There is little potential for injury.
   a. The fetus is not injured by normal coitus because it is cushioned by amniotic fluid and protected by the cervix and uterus.
   b. In the last few weeks, after the fetal head has descended into the pelvic canal, a woman may find deep thrusting uncomfortable.
2. There is little potential for harm by stimulating uterine contractions.
   a. Miscarriage in the first 3 months is rarely caused by coitus. Almost all reasons for spontaneous abortion are intrinsic, related to genetic causes or poor development of the embryo.
   b. If there is threatened abortion, abstinence is suggested until it is clear that the pregnancy will continue.
   c. Prostaglandins in semen may stimulate mild uterine contractions, especially a few days before labor begins. For this reason, women who

have threatened premature labor onset or third trimester bleeding should abstain for a number of weeks (determined by their condition) before their due date. Conversely, if the infant is overdue, some encourage the couple to have intercourse in hopes of stimulating labor. Most research, however, has shown no association between maternal orgasm and premature labor (Reamy and White, 1985). One study recommends that condoms should be used with coitus occurring during the last month to prevent potential infection or stimulation of labor.

3. STDs and infection have adverse effects on the fetus.
   a. STDs should be taken very seriously. Both partners should be treated if an infection is diagnosed (see Chapter 25). Inform the woman how to seek personal protection.
   b. Women with new partners or multiple partners must insist that partners use a condom for protection. Women whose partners are at risk should always insist on condom use, but may not be able to do so (see Chapter 25).
4. Air must never be blown into the vagina during sexplay because there is a rare chance of death due to air embolism (Reamy and White, 1985). Because of partial dilation of the cervix, air forcibly blown may enter the uterus and through the placenta find a way into maternal circulation.
5. Variations in sexual interest are normal and reflect physiologic changes.
   a. First trimester: Because of increased blood supply to vaginal tissue and the enlarging uterus, some women have a more total orgasmic response. Nulliparas may have a decreased response, often because of discomforts and fatigue. Multiparas often find relief in not needing contraception.
   b. Second trimester: There is an increase in eroticism and orgasmic response noted by all women. Most women indicate increased interest. The enlarging uterus begins to require changes in position for coitus, including side to side, rear entry, and woman-superior, for instance.
   c. Third trimester: As the due date approaches, the frequency of intercourse is reduced for all women. Fatigue and discomfort play a part, but women may also be worried about arbitrary instructions by health professionals. It is common to hear "6 weeks before and 6 weeks after" as the period of abstinence. Such instruction should no longer be provided.

EVALUATION

Evaluation questions that may be asked to determine progress toward the outcomes include the following.

- Did the couple/woman ask appropriate questions and indicate understanding of the effects of pregnancy on sexuality?
- Did she state that she used precautions to protect against STDs?
- Did a medical condition during pregnancy cause stress between partners? Were they able to resolve these problems?

Increased Psychosocial Risk

When the parent-child relationship is healthy, the child learns to socialize with others from parents and becomes an adult who can complete the developmental and pregnancy-related tasks in preparation for becoming a parent who can form bonds to her or his own children.

People in urban societies move away from the family of origin; extended kinship groups may not exist. Parents often raise their children without the support of a group. Without an extended family on which to depend, the *parent-child relationship is absolutely crucial to the child's psychologic growth*. Today's new mother may have only her own family as a role model or may come from a single-parent family; as a result, her problem is compounded.

Women at either extreme of reproductive age—the older, **mature gravida** and the **adolescent gravida**—are at increased psychosocial risk. These risks vary with and correspond to developmental stages.

MATURE GRAVIDAS

The pregnant woman over 35 faces unique problems. The primigravida in this age category has generally decided to postpone childbearing until her career is well established. Although the child may be wanted and anticipated, she will often have much ambivalence and concern about how motherhood will affect her life-style and how it will affect her relationship with the father of the baby. She might be a single woman deciding to have a child on her own, perhaps even by artificial insemination. She may have conceived after treatment of infertility or in vitro fertilization. She might be having a child later in her childbearing years because of remarriage or by "accident." This child may be much desired

Cultural Aspects of Care

Many Haitian women and some Israeli women believe that sexual intercourse should be continued throughout pregnancy to lubricate the birth canal. Many Hispanic men believe that vaginal intercourse during late pregnancy will hurt the fetus.

or unwelcome. You need to ascertain this information because the woman's and her family's responses are closely tied to their feelings.

Developmental Stage

Women over 35 are generally in the developmental stage of *intimacy vs isolation*, which is described by Erikson (1963) as the time in which

The young adult, emerging from the search for and the insistence on identity, is eager and willing to fuse his identity with that of others. He is ready for intimacy, that is the capacity to commit himself to concrete affiliations and partnerships and to develop the ethical strength to abide by such commitments even though they may call for significant sacrifices and compromises.

The woman over 40 may have entered the life stage of *generativity vs stagnation* defined by Erikson (1963) as "primarily the concern in establishing and guiding the next generation."

Concern is accentuated in women who realize that the time in which to have a baby is running out, often referred to as hearing the "biological clock" ticking louder. Even women who have other children may feel the desire to have another before it is too late.

It may seem that these women are the best prepared psychologically for the demands of pregnancy and parenthood because their lives are stable. This readiness intensifies their need for nursing care. They are heavily invested in these pregnancies because of the need to have the first, the only, or the last child or because they have decided to carry and deliver an unplanned pregnancy because it may be their last chance. When something goes wrong or threatens to go wrong, there may be guilt and sorrow.

Genetic Concerns

Genetic concerns complicate the psychosocial needs of these women and their families. The decision to undergo genetic testing is not always easy. Some women are certain that they would abort a genetically defective fetus; others are equally resolute that they would not. Others agonize over what they would do. These additional concerns are superimposed on normal worries. This phenomenon, called the **tentative pregnancy**, occurs when women are unsure whether they are mothers or "carriers of a defective fetus" (Katz-Rothman, 1986). They are concerned because there is a higher ratio of Down syndrome and other autosomal trisomies (see Chapter 27).

Chorionic villus sampling shortens the waiting period for genetic diagnosis. Even so, a considerable amount of anxiety is generated. Genetic counselors can furnish the client with statistics that can put risks into perspective and aid in the decision to undergo or to forego genetic testing (see Chapter 4).

Issues of Control

Issues particularly important are control and past coping behaviors. Many women have been successful in their careers by manipulating situations to their advantage. When faced with a situation in which they are not in control and must trust others, severe anxiety develops. Their past coping behaviors will not be effective, and this will intensify their anxiety. They feel unable to take care of themselves and often have little experience in relying on others during times of need. The educational level of the client must be considered when recommending literature.

An important part of *anticipatory guidance* is letting the client know that her old ways of dealing with situations need to change during the pregnancy. A newborn disrupts its parents' life-style tremendously, and the client needs to begin to consider this during pregnancy.

Reassurance

In the past, many studies grouped genetic defects with all other problems for the older woman. In fact, some research shows a better outcome when the mother is older. There is a reduced risk of preterm birth, infant mortality, and sudden infant death syndrome (Harker and Thorpe, 1992). It is important to distinguish between women delaying childbirth to have the first child and women who have had several children before age 35. For the latter group of women, there is an increased rate of twins and triplets.

For women having a first pregnancy later in life, fear about the infant's health and survival often becomes the dominant feeling. This may be the "last egg in the basket" and thus very much valued (Harker and Thorpe, 1992). As a result, cesarean birth is chosen more often by obstetricians, and indicates an overcautious approach to birth problems. Nonetheless, the woman approaching a first birth in her later reproductive years may be encouraged by the positive findings of greater satisfaction with motherhood and greater commitment to parenting.

ADOLESCENT GRAVIDA

The adolescent mother and her family create a particularly difficult problem. The needs can be so extensive that care will be fragmented and ineffective unless an interdisciplinary team approach coordinates the school, social, and health care services.

Incidence of Adolescent Pregnancy

The scope of adolescent pregnancy is enormous. The mean age of menarche in the United States is 12.3 years. In contrast to other developed countries, the pregnancy rate among U.S. teenagers is quite high; approximately 1 million teenagers become pregnant each year (National Research Council, 1987). Forty-two percent of girls and 64% of young boys are sexually active by age 18 (see Chapter 2).

A family's reaction to teenage pregnancy varies considerably (Figure 8-1). In certain ethnic and cultural groups, teenage parenting is common. Indeed, the girl's mother may have been a teenage parent herself. *In these cases, the situation is not a crisis.* In other families, major problems result.

Developmental Stage

The developmental stage of adolescence is described as *identity vs role confusion.* Erikson speaks about the essence of the crisis of adolescence, including the dramatic body changes and drives, and the need to be accepted to conform and to be someone. Teenagers' role models are their peers and television and movie personalities, not their parents, older siblings, or teachers.

Need for Sex Education

Adolescents lack knowledge about their bodies and bodily changes. Many parents find it difficult to talk

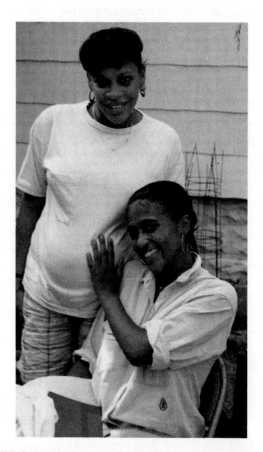

FIGURE 8-1 When pregnancy is supported in the family, self-esteem grows. (Courtesy Camille Bodden.)

with their children about maturation, sex, birth control, and parenting. Parents may not understand that this information is vital and that it must be given early. Furstenberg (1980) found that, although 59% of mothers frequently talked to their daughters about sex and 92% occasionally talked to their daughters about sex, most of the messages were "not to get mixed up with boys" and "not to do anything she would be sorry for later." This is hardly the information teenagers require. On the other hand, 50% of the young girls whose mothers discussed methods of birth control used contraception at least occasionally.

Need for Family Planning

Hatcher et al (1990) state that the pregnancy rate among teenagers is so high because only *one in three* sexually active teens always uses contraceptives. Only about half of these use the most effective methods. The most common reasons given by teenagers for not using contraception are (1) they do not feel they will get pregnant and (2) they did not anticipate having intercourse. In Piaget's cognitive framework, adolescents are in the transition from the phase of concrete operations to the phase of formal operations, which is usually not reached until adulthood. In formal operations, the individual can think abstractly, consider alternatives, and recognize the consequences of behavior. Until the adolescent reaches this stage, she will be likely to take risks without considering consequences.

On the average, teenagers wait almost one year to attend a family planning clinic after initiating intercourse. Half of all teenage pregnancies occur in the first 6 months after initiation of intercourse and 20% in the first month alone (Zabin, Kantner, and Zelnick, 1979).

Experience in other countries where teenage sexual activity is just as prevalent as in the United States shows that the rate of pregnancy can be reduced by making effective contraception readily available. High-quality sex education programs have been found to be useful only if accompanied by provision of supplies (Hatcher et al, 1990). Programs designed to reach out to sexually inexperienced teenagers to inform them about contraceptive methods and where to obtain them are most effective (Chilman, 1983).

While the national debate continues over where and by whom sex education programs should be taught, research is clear: we must begin early and be specific. Teenagers are at risk not only for pregnancy but also for STDs, including HIV infection. It is unlikely that the United States will soon develop policies to encourage early sex education programs even though the urgency of the rates of HIV infection and of teenage pregnancy demand it. The media has begun to modify its approach to sexuality because of the risk of HIV infection, but there is still much to be done. The emphasis needs to be on responsible sexuality, including abstinence, as well as on contraception.

As a nurse, your role is twofold: you must care for adolescent parents and support their parents and teachers in efforts to communicate about responsible sexual behavior before pregnancy occurs and after its termination, either by abortion or delivery. Parents and teachers need education also. The fears that talking about sex encourages earlier sexual activity are unfounded. In communities where human sexuality is discussed, the number of teenage pregnancies is reduced and healthy attitudes toward childbearing and child-rearing are acquired (Furstenberg, 1980).

Influences. Some teenagers, either consciously or subconsciously, want to have babies because their friends have them, or because they want something they can succeed in doing, something to love, or something to make them feel important or special (Figure 8-2). Some teenagers want to keep their boyfriends and fear that refusing to have sex will drive them away. Some want to gain attention from their parents. These are all adoles-

Self-Discovery

* *Think about when you first learned about sex and birth control. Who gave the information to you? Was the information correct? How did you respond at that time? How would you do it differently for your own child?*

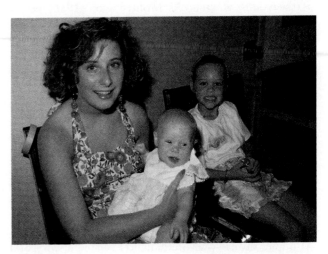

FIGURE 8-2 The teenage mother may think of her baby as a doll. (Marjorie Pyle, RNC, *Lifecircle.*)

cent ways of expressing basic needs for belonging, love, and self-esteem.

Denial of pregnancy. Many adolescents do not expect to become pregnant. They may deny it until the signs are so obvious they can no longer be ignored by family members. It is common for teenagers to diet and wear constricting clothes to hide their condition and to succeed in hiding the pregnancy until it is quite advanced, sometimes until delivery. The levels of denial in some teenagers and their families can be quite high. You must be especially concerned about a teenager who arrives in labor and delivery claiming she did not know that she was pregnant. She may have been brought in by her family, with whom she was living, who also claim they were unaware of it. This may truly be denial or a way for her family to hide their embarrassment about the pregnancy or the delay in care. Nevertheless, the ability of the family to care for the infant in these cases requires further assessment by the interdisciplinary team members.

ADOLESCENT FATHERS

The adolescent father is often neglected in these situations. Some families are angry and upset and will ostracize him. At other times, both families pool their financial, physical, and emotional resources to support the young parents as they care for their infant. Some young men are not involved by their own choice, but others may distance themselves because they assume that they do not have a role to play or they are not needed by their partner for support. They may fear that they will be forced to marry and provide financial support before they are capable of doing so or be "saddled" with 20 years of child support payments. These young men are in the same developmental stage as the young women. As Montemayor (1986) points out, "Teenage fathers have many problems. They are young; are capable of sexual reproduction, but not considered adults; are cognitively and psychologically immature; possess few legal rights and are out of life cycle synchrony with their peers."

Adolescent fathers are less likely to receive a high school diploma or general education diploma by age 20. Fathering a child as an adolescent is associated with reduced levels of education in general. Lower educational levels limit career choices and earning potential. Adequate wages for male employment have been found to be important in determining the success of early marriage (Chilman, 1983).

At dinner my 16-year old daughter related a story of a girl in her class who had announced she was pregnant. My 14-year-old son was not interested in this "girl talk." Kelly and her friends had asked Nancy why she wanted a baby and got the classic answer: "I wanted a baby so I'll have someone who will always love me." The girls then asked Nancy if she and her boyfriend were going to get married, and Nancy said, "No. He didn't even want a baby, so I told him I was on the pill." Then Kelly's friends asked how she was going to support herself and the baby, and Nancy responded that she was going to sue her boyfriend for child support. Suddenly intensely interested, Bill exclaimed, "But she can't do that! She lied!" I assured Bill that she could indeed, and the "girl talk" became a discussion of shared responsibilities, consequences, and maturity.

Problems with Economic Support

Adolescent parents are rarely able to support themselves and their children. Optimally, the family should be involved early. Detailed arrangements must be worked out, and allowing enough time before delivery makes the crisis less overwhelming. Building on and supplementing family resources and only substituting for families when absolutely necessary is believed to be the most effective way to help adolescents and their infants (Ooms, 1984).

Women who become parents as teenagers are *less likely to complete their education or to be employed*, especially if they are younger than 17. Availability of child care, especially by family members, is a crucial factor in the mothers returning to school (Chilman, 1983; National Research Council, 1987).

Women who become parents as teenagers are *more likely to be welfare dependent*, especially those who are very young at the birth of their first child (Chilman, 1983). They are *more likely to have large families*, especially if they get married. They are also *less likely to be happily married* (National Research Council, 1987).

After the first child, 80% of teenage mothers state that they plan to wait at least 2 years before having another child. In Furstenberg's study, less than half did. He found some had already reached or exceeded the number of children they ever wanted within 5 years. Those who returned to school had a lower rate of recurrent, early pregnancy (Furstenberg, 1980). Salguero (1984) found that the average length of time between pregnancies was 7 to 9 months when young parents did not return to school.

Parenting Success

Adolescents generally have unrealistic expectations of the abilities and needs of an infant (Figure 8-3). Responsibilities of parenting may be difficult. Sacrificing personal pleasure for the needs of another is a developmental growth task not usually completed by this age. There is evidence that the majority of teenage parents

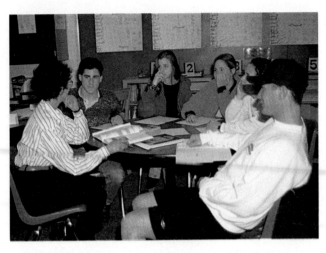

FIGURE 8-3 Adolescent learning groups where free discussion about parenting may be held. (Marjorie Pyle, RNC, *Lifecircle*.)

do well with proper intervention. Teenage mothers have been observed to have adequate maternal warmth and physical interaction. Many, however, do not talk much to their infants (Chilman, 1983).

These findings indicate a need for more parenting education as well as assessment for potential problems. Child abuse is not more common, as some have thought. The presence of a supportive extended family is an essential factor in development of good parenting skills.

Choices

Today, a pregnant woman has three choices: to abort, to have the child and place it for foster care or adoption, or to have the child and raise it. Adolescent parents have the same choices, but may need to be guided through the decision-making process. In some areas legal requirements for a waiting period before elective abortion and parental notification affect these choices. Some teenagers have sought confirmation of pregnancy and then chosen abortion without involving family members. They tend to be older and more goal directed. Others tell their parents or a relative and enlist their support. The way in which the situation is handled depends on the teenager's relationship with the father of the child and his family, and their cultural and ethnic backgrounds and beliefs. These and other variables may interact in a variety of ways. More teenagers are intending to raise their children with the help of grandmothers or aunts than in previous decades.

Nursing Responsibilities
▶ NURSING DIAGNOSES

These diagnoses may be selected to be included in a complete nursing care plan for the pregnant adolescent or the more mature gravida.

- Ineffective individual coping related to developmental level, situation in which pregnancy occurs.
- Coping, family: potential for growth related to responses to adolescent or mature pregnant woman.

▶ EXPECTED OUTCOMES

- Recognizes potential for growth in the situation.
- Chooses to obtain prenatal care.
- Follows through on referrals.
- Seeks support for expressed needs.
- Recognizes fetal needs for a healthy start.

▶ NURSING INTERVENTIONS

You must first gain an understanding of the teenager's situation when she comes in for the visit. She has chosen to come in, which reflects a big decision for her. She may be afraid to tell her parents and may need assistance. Or, she may have been brought in by her mother, and the dynamics between them will reveal much about the situation. She and her family may need a variety of assistance programs such as WIC, public assistance, or general social service. Unless you learn this at the *first encounter,* the young woman may be lost to follow-up. Do not wait for her to volunteer information. It is important to engage her trust, a difficult task because an adolescent may not trust easily and may have difficulty relating to authority figures. The adolescent fears *breach of confidentiality.* A climate of *strict confidentiality* is vital in all nursing situations, but is crucial for adolescents. For these reasons, care is best given in a setting that has providers who specialize in adolescent health care (Figure 8-4).

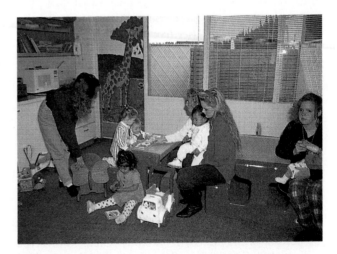

FIGURE 8-4 Teenage mothers in a day-care facility learn child care. (Marjorie Pyle, RNC, *Lifecircle*.)

Respond to the adolescent's needs rather than to her behavior. For example, when asked how her mother feels about the pregnancy, a teenager may state, "Fine." When probed further, she may get angry and respond, "Why do you care?" Perhaps she is afraid to tell you that she has not told her mother or that her mother is insisting that she have an abortion. Respond to the need; do not react. For example, state, "Lots of pregnant girls your age have real problems when they tell their parents or are even afraid to tell them. Let's talk about that." In this way, she is given the opportunity to talk to a provider who shows caring and understanding.

Because she may not want her parents to know where she is going and is concerned that you will call them, a teenager may not give correct information. She may not be able to secure the insurance information on her own. Ability to pay or provide insurance information should also never become a barrier to provision of care of adolescents.

Identify the girl's readiness to use referrals. Ask her to write down the sequence of what has been planned together, because tension will prevent her remembering what to do. Follow through with telephone contact if she skips appointments—if her family is aware of her condition. If she still does not tell them early in the pregnancy, ask her for a way to establish contact. Keep gently urging full disclosure to the family, because it will become evident in a very short time that she is pregnant. Help her identify other sources of support in her extended family circle.

The key is to keep the teen parent in the health care system and to keep her in school. Since there appear to be no adverse effects on the mothers and infants if quality care is provided, such care becomes of prime importance. In the most effective settings, the supportive primary nurse adds the new client to her case load and follows through the pregnancy with her. The impersonal nature of large clinics is counterproductive for the adolescent mother (see Chapter 26 for a model of care).

Peer support groups in schools for pregnant adolescents or in clinics are helpful in preparing teens to cope with the demands and sacrifices of parenting (Figure 8-5). Educational programs and literature should be geared to teens. Providers must like working with teens and understand their unique problems and responses. The teen father needs to be involved as much as possible. He should be invited to clinic visits and parenting classes and assisted to see his role in providing physical and emotional support for his partner and his child. Furstenberg (1980) found that with support, 63 percent of the fathers in his study remained involved with their children, regardless of whether they married the child's mother.

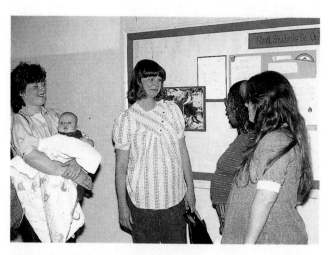

FIGURE 8-5 Sharing experiences in prenatal clinic may help anxiety for teenage mothers. (Marjorie Pyle, RNC, *Lifecircle.*)

The nurse, by her own attitude, will influence how well the teen follows through on care (See Nursing Care Plan).

▶ EVALUATION

The results of comprehensive care for a teenage mother would show some of the following:

- Stated she learned a great deal about herself and problem solving.
- Followed through on referrals and obtaining assistance.
- Involved father of child in planning and in care of infant.
- Followed guidelines for nutrition and self-care during the pregnancy.
- Attended school and parenting classes.

 Self-Discovery

What is your opinion about:
- *Involving parents and teachers in early, comprehensive programs about sexuality?*
- *Limiting availability of contraceptives to decrease incentives for teenagers to become sexually active?*
- *Educating teenagers in the consequences of early parenting on the success of marriages and careers?*
- *Leaving sex and parenting education to parents because it is their responsibility?*

NURSING CARE PLAN • Adolescent Pregnancy

CASE: Sixteen-year-old Cathy was brought to the emergency department by her anxious father. She had vaginal bleeding. On admission, she was found to be in preterm labor. A 32-week-old infant was born in good health. Cathy was upset, more by her parents' angry, blaming response because she had hidden the pregnancy from them. No one could focus on the baby or make plans for her. The baby was to remain in the neonatal intensive care unit (NICU) for 3 to 4 weeks. Cathy would not name the father of the baby.

ASSESSMENT DATA

1. Unprepared for pregnancy, no prior experience or support during pregnancy.
2. Evidence of low self-esteem and difficulty with parental communication.
3. May be in conflict with mother and father, no siblings.
4. Physical condition seems healthy, no signs of high blood pressure, anemia, excessive weight gain.
5. Unwilling to name father of child, potential for relative incest.
6. Factors precipitating preterm labor need investigation.
7. Baby is preterm, in NICU for three to four weeks. Condition stable.

NURSING DIAGNOSIS

1. Denial of pregnancy.
2. Altered role performance related to keeping secret/lack of affirmation.
3. Lowered self-esteem related to teen pregnancy and potential victimization.
4. High risk for altered parenting related to prematurity of infant and adolescent, unsupported pregnancy.

EXPECTED OUTCOMES

1. Expresses concerns to health care team member.
2. Seeks information about pregnancy and self-care during recovery.
3. Shows evidence of self-esteem by following through on recommended self-care activities and referrals.
4. Attempts communication with parents.
5. Shows evidence of beginning attachment to infant.
6. Discusses potential of infant's future with NICU nurses.

NURSING INTERVENTIONS

1. Assign one primary nurse for the whole stay. Assess level of acceptance of infant. Affirm Cathy's need to talk about experience.
2. Assess mood and reactions to birth.
3. Encourage problem solving and provide information about resources.
4. Educate regarding self-care during recovery; include family planning.
5. Involve significant other person, if parental anger continues.
6. Collaborate with social service to build a support network involving extended family.
7. Refer to social service counseling because of unwillingness to involve infant's father, financial needs, outcome for infant.
8. Communicate with NICU regarding outcome for infant; homegoing, foster care, or adoption.

EVALUATION

1. Did Cathy understand and agree to follow through on self-care activities?
2. Did she seek information to prepare herself for new infant?
3. Has communication with family members improved?
4. Has beginning attachment started?
5. Were resources found in support network or through referrals?

Attachment and Bonding
BACKGROUND OF BONDING THEORY

As early as 1952, scientists wrote about imprinting behavior in birds and other animals and described a critical period during which attachments between the mother and her young must be formed. Separation during this critical time resulted in rejection of the young. Researchers observed that human mothers separated for long periods of time from premature or sick infants often had difficulty in accepting them when the emergency was over; this observation led researchers to wonder whether there was a time for attachment in humans.

Klaus and Kennell (1976) demonstrated that this period exists in the first few hours after birth. They noted that close physical contact between an infant and its mother set in motion an intricate set of reciprocal actions whereby each stimulated and rewarded the other (Figure 8-6). Based on their research on animals and humans, they hypothesized that around the time of delivery, hormonal stimulation prepared the mother to receive and respond to her newborn. If this opportunity were missed, the mother-infant pair never bonded.

Humans give birth throughout the year and bear young that are wholly dependent for an extended period, requiring a relationship that is specific, stable, and enduring. Strong feelings of protectiveness and caring are evoked in human mothers even after their children have reached adulthood and may have been separated from them for years. Furthermore, unlike maternal behavior in animals, maternal behavior in humans must be flexible, adapting to the circumstances and the developmental level of the child.

Klaus and Kennell also studied the effects of early skin-to-skin contact on later mothering behavior. In their study, a group of poor, inner city mothers who had 1 hour of contact immediately with their newborns and 5 hours of contact each day in the hospital were compared with a control group who received traditional, more isolated contact, only during four hourly feeding periods. These early-contact mothers showed differences in maternal behavior, including holding their infants more affectionately and showing more concern for them three months and one year later.

Early and unlimited access to the infant is desirable because it enhances the mother's feeling of competence and self-esteem (Figure 8-7), but the early studies are flawed. Although the study group of early-contact mothers showed positive changes in expected behavior patterns, the effects of the extra attention by nurses and others given to this group were not taken into account. Moreover, existing differences in temperament of mothers and infants were not considered. Later studies failed to demonstrate any lasting differences.

Changes in maternity care now allow extended contact between parents and infants. If a baby is high-risk or ill and separated from its parents in the ICU, the parents may be anxious about "Nursing" bonding. The nurse can be very helpful by assuring them that although the early recovery period is the ideal time for attachment to take place, it is not the only time. The mother who began attachment with visualization early in pregnancy is unlikely to be seriously hindered if initial interaction with her newborn must be deferred. Hormonal stimulation may contribute to the attachment, but social and cultural components play a far more influential role.

ENCOURAGING ATTACHMENT AND BONDING DURING PREGNANCY

Around the fourth month of pregnancy the expectant mother becomes increasingly aware of her fetus as a

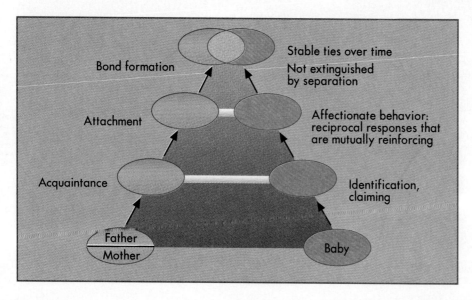

FIGURE 8-6 Model of the bonding process.

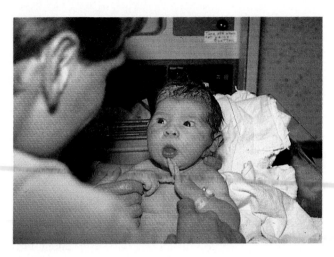

FIGURE 8-7 Fingertip exploration and eye-to-eye contact. (Courtesy Ross Laboratories, Columbus, Ohio.)

separate individual through movement (see the section on developmental tasks during pregnancy) and begins to develop feelings for it. Before this time, her feelings for it were for an abstract notion of what "a baby" is like. From the time of quickening onward, she becomes acquainted with her infant by identifying fetal parts, and by noting its response to changes in its environment such as when she is anxious or taking a warm shower or is listening to loud or soothing music. The more she becomes familiar with her infant's responses to her actions, the more she feels she "knows" the infant before birth. The fact that mothers form an attachment to their unborn fetuses is indicated by their grief when their infants are stillborn.

You can encourage prenatal attachment as you perform your usual care-giving tasks. Ask the woman what she calls her infant; it can be the name that will be put on the birth certificate or an affectionate nickname such as "the lump" or "Thumper." This name helps her to personalize the infant within. Help her to examine behaviors to identify "who the infant is like" in her or her partner's family. When the woman complains "This baby is always moving," ask, "Who in your family is like that?" Encourage her to pay attention to fetal activity and to note what behavior on her part seems to influence the infant to move or kick.

An ability to identify fetal parts can be encouraged by guiding the pregnant mother's hands to identify the hard, round head; the long, curved back; the softness of the rump; the fleeting movements; and a surprisingly large number of prods from heels, toes, knees, shoulders, elbows, and hands. She can be urged to soothe and quiet her baby by massaging, stroking, or rocking.

You can also use a Doppler that amplifies fetal heart tones during prenatal visits to help parents identify its various sounds: the hoofbeat rhythm of the fetal heart tones; the slower, more measured rate of the mother's heartbeat; the swooshing sound as the blood rushes through the umbilical cord; and the gurgling of the mother's intestines. Time spent in this way gives the parents a feeling of increased knowledge and reduced uncertainty.

When a sonogram has been done, this can also be used as an aid for discussion on attachment. Some women report that they felt that the infant was real for the first time when they saw its features in the sonogram. The literature has shown that women who are concerned for the infant's survival often fear attachment. However, women who have experienced threatened miscarriage or similar problems often express positive feelings for their infants after viewing the sonogram. Encourage parents to request a copy of their infant's "picture."

By the end of the third trimester a strong attachment should have formed for the infant (Rubin, 1984). If the mother demonstrates obvious negative behaviors during later pregnancy, closely observe postdelivery interactions. Phases of bonding occur throughout pregnancy and parenting. The process goes through phases of **acquaintance,** with cues of acceptance being exchanged, to **attachment,** with affectional exchanges when parents and the infant are in close contact. These exchanges are more positive than negative. You can observe these initial acquaintance and attachment behaviors by using tools such as the FIMI tool seen in Table 20-3. Nursing interventions during prenatal care can be very supportive of the young family. Bonding after the birth of the baby is discussed in Chapter 20. Remember, in most family-infant groupings bonding will occur—a positive, loving relationship that will be able to endure over time and distance.

KEY POINTS

- Major developmental tasks of pregnancy follow a step-by-step progression. Any lag will delay the next phase.
- Adjustment proceeds through phases that may be described by fetal incorporation, fetal differentiation, and fetal separation with safe passage into newborn life.

- Women seek maternal role models, and men paternal role models to help imagine how they will respond as parents. This task is more difficult when there are dysfunctional families or life circumstances.
- Parental adjustments in role responsibility and in self-concept take emotional energy. Future parents

need support while the psychologic tasks of pregnancy are being achieved. Single mothers often may feel isolated.

• Family networks provide most women with support, but young, single, or older women may need additional support.

• Pregnancy modifies sexual responses. Anticipatory guidance may help the woman to understand and explain these changes to her partner.

• Young gravidas are coping with role confusion and with gaining a sense of identity and positive self-esteem.

• Knowledge and use of family planning must be a focus for teaching the sexually active teenager.

• With support and continued schooling, the outlook is positive for teenage parents.

• Bonding occurs throughout pregnancy and parenting. The process goes through phases and is reinforced by nurses who understand the importance of the parent-infant bond.

STUDY QUESTIONS

8-1 Which Key Terms fit the following descriptions?
  a. Including the idea of being pregnant into ones life-style and plans _Acceptance_
  b. Thinking about the fantasy-child's characteristics and how it will feel to be a parent _____ . _Visualization_
  c. A positive emotional connection that persists over time and distance ___ _Bonding_
  d. The woman recognizes that the fetus is separate from herself ___ _Individualization_
  e. Father has more physical discomforts during his partner's pregnancy _Couvade_

8-2 Pregnancy in the later reproductive years is becoming more commonplace. The older woman's chances of carrying the pregnancy to term and giving birth to a healthy baby are:
  a. About the same as reported in early studies because the incidence of age-related diseases such as hypertension and diabetes remains unchanged
  b. Decreased because the risk of Down syndrome increases to about 1% by the time a woman is 36

  c. Not significantly different from that of younger women in the same health category

8-3 The best time to teach expectant mothers about parenting is:
  a. During the first trimester because there is enough time to explore all the issues
  b. During the second trimester because the mother is beginning to realize that the infant is a separate individual
  c. During the third trimester because the imminent birth gives a feeling of immediacy and a need to get organized

8-4 The expectant mother's attachment to her infant occurs by:
  a. Visualizing herself as a mother
  b. Getting to know the infant by identifying its behaviors
  c. Learning all she can about fetal development
  d. Trial and error

Answer Key   8-1 a. Acceptance b. Visualization c. Bonding d. Individuation e. Couvade 8-2 c 8-3 c 8-4 a,b

REFERENCES

Antle-May K: Three phases of father involvement in pregnancy, *Nurs Res* 31:337, 1982.

Berkowitz GS et al: Delayed childbearing and the outcome of pregnancy, *N Engl J Med* 322:659, 1990.

Chilman C: *Adolescent sexuality in a changing American society,* New York, 1983, John Wiley & Sons.

Clinton R: Expectant fathers at risk of couvade, *Nurs Res* 35:290, 1986.

Elster A, Lamb M, eds: *Adolescent fatherhood,* NJ, 1986, Lawrence Erlbaum Associates.

Erikson, E: *Childhood and society,* New York, 1963, WW Norton.

Furstenberg F: The social consequences of teenage parenthood. In *Adolescent pregnancy and childbearing: findings from research,* Pub No 81-2077, Washington, DC, 1980, National Institutes of Health, Department of Health and Human Services.

Gaffney KF: Maternal-fetal attachment in relation to self-concept and anxiety, *Matern Child Nurs J* 15:91, 1986.

Grimes DA, Gross GK: Pregnancy outcomes in black women aged 35 and older, *Obstet Gynecol* 52:7, 1981.

Hall LA: Prevalence and correlates of depressive symptoms in mothers of young children, *Pub Health Nurs* 7:71, 1990.

Harker L, Thorpe K: "The last egg in the basket?": elderly primiparity—a review of the findings, *Birth* 19:23, 1992.

Hatcher R et al: *Contraceptive technology 1990-1992,* New York, 1990, Irvington.

Horowitz SM et al: School-age mothers—predictors of long-term educational and economic outcomes, *Pediatrics* 87:862, 1991.

Jordan, PL: Laboring for relevance: expectant and new fatherhood, *Nurs Res* 39:11, 1990.

Katz-Rothman B: *The tentative pregnancy,* New York, 1986, Viking Penguin.

Keniston K and the Carnegie Council on Children: *All our children: the American family under pressure,* New York, 1977, Harcourt Brace Jovanovich.

Kirz DS, Dorchester W, Freeman RK: Advanced maternal age: the mature gravida, *Am J Obset Gynecol* 152:7, 1985.

Klaus MH, Kennell JH: *Maternal-infant bonding,* St Louis, 1976, Mosby.

Kleinman A, Eisenberg L, Good B: Culture, illness and care: clinical lessons from anthropological and cross-cultural research, *Ann Intern Med* 88:251, 1979.

Lederman RP: *Psychosocial adaptation in pregnancy,* Englewood Cliffs, NJ, 1984, Prentice Hall.

Light HK, Fenster C: Maternal concerns during pregnancy, *Am J Obstet Gynecol* 118:47, 1974.

Longbucco DC, Preston MS: Relation of somatic symptoms to degree of paternal role preparation, *JOGNN* 18(6):482, 1989.

Mansfield PK, Cohn MD: Stress and later-life childbearing: important implications for nursing, *MCN Am J Matern Child Nurs* 15:139, 1986.

Montemayor R: Boys as fathers: coping with the dilemmas of adolescence.

Mueller LS: Pregnancy and sexuality, *J Obstet Gynecol Neonatal Nurs* 6:298, 1985.

National Research Council: *Risking the future: adolescent sexuality and childbearing,* Washington, DC, 1987, National Academy Press.

Ooms T: The family context of adolescent parents. In Sugar M, ed: *Adolescent parenthood,* New York, 1984, SP Medical Scientific Books.

Piaget J: *The language and thought of the child,* New York, 1926, Harcourt Brace.

Reamy KE et al: Sexuality and pregnancy, *J Reprod Med* 6:321, 1982.

Reamy KE, White SE: Sexuality in pregnancy and the puerperium: a review, *Obstet Gynecol Surv* 40:1, 1985.

Rubin R: Maternal identity and the maternal experience, New York, 1984, Springer.

Salguero C: The role of ethnic factors in adolescent pregnancy and motherhood. In Sugar M, ed: *Adolescent pregnancy,* New York, 1984, SP Medical and Scientific Books.

Sosa R et al: The effect of a supportive companion on perinatal problems, length of labor, and mother-infant attachment, *N Engl J Med* 303:597, 1980.

Starn J, Niederhauser V: A MCN model for nursing diagnosis to focus nursing intervention 15(3): 180, 1990.

Tanner LM: Developmental tasks of pregnancy. In Bergeson BS, ed: *Current concepts of clinical nursing,* St Louis, 1969, Mosby.

Tunis SL, Globus MS: Assessing mood states in pregnancy: survey of the literature, *Obstet Gynecol Surv* 46:340, 1991.

Weinberg JS: Body image disturbance as a factor in the crisis situation of pregnancy, *J Obstet Gynecol Neonatal Nurs* 7:817, 1978.

Weiser MA, Castiglia PT: Assessing early father-infant attachment, *MCN Am J Mother Child Nurs* 9:104, 1984.

Zabin, L, Kantner J, Zelnick M: The risk of adolescent pregnancy in the first months of intercourse, *Fam Plann Perspect* 11:215, 1979.

STUDENT REFERENCE SHELF

Gaffney KF: State of the science: prenatal maternal attachment, *Image* 20:106, 1990.
   Overview of maternal steps in bonding.

Hall LA et al: Psychosocial predictors of maternal depressive symptoms, parenting attitudes and child behaviors in single-parent families, *Nurs Res* 40:214, 1991.
   Depressed mothers affect their children. Stressors are identified for single-parent families.

Norbeck JS, Anderson NJ: Psychosocial predictors of pregnancy outcomes in low income black, Hispanic, and white women, *Nurs Res* 38:204, 1989.
   Nursing research clarifies vague psychosocial issues. This study identifies stress responses in three groups of women.

Symanski ME: Maternal infant bonding: practice issues for the 1990s, *J Nurs Midwifery* 37:67S, 1992.
   A review of bonding issues with an extensive bibliography.

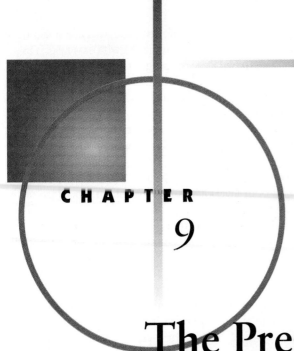

CHAPTER

9

The Pregnancy Process and Nursing Care

KEY TERMS

Anticipatory Guidance
Asymptomatic Bacteriuria
Carpal Tunnel Syndrome
Changes of Accommodation
Colostrum
Diabetogenic Response
Due Date (DD)
Erythema
Expected Date of Birth (EDB)
Expected Date of Childbirth (EDC)
Gravidity
Heartburn
Isoimmunization
Kegel Exercises
Last Menstrual Period (LMP)
Leopold's Maneuvers

Leukorrhea
Lightening
Linea Nigra
Lordosis
Mean Arterial Pressure (MAP)
Melasma
Mucous Plug
Nocturia
Orthostatic Hypotension

Parity
Pruritus
Relaxin
Spider Angioma
Striae Gravidarum
Supine Hypotension Syndrome (SHS)
Syncope
Vena Caval Syndrome (VCS)

LEARNING OBJECTIVES

1. Explain the relationship of maternal physiologic adaptations to pregnancy and common, minor discomforts of antepartum.
2. Identify significant prenatal health and history information required to formulate a plan of care.
3. Correlate appropriate anticipatory guidance by trimesters.
4. Describe major hazards to be avoided during pregnancy.
5. Recognize rationale for changes in exercise and activity levels during pregnancy.
6. Describe screening and monitoring steps in prenatal care.
7. Individualize a nursing care plan for prenatal care, including cultural adaptations.
8. Identify referral needs according to a pregnant woman's physical and emotional adjustment.

Changes during the Pregnancy Process

Pregnancy triggers a complex chain of events. Energy is required to fuel the rapidly dividing cells on the journey toward implantation and development. At the same time hormones begin sending messages throughout the body, preparing the organ systems for the **changes of accommodation** during pregnancy.

CARDIOVASCULAR SYSTEM

Blood volume expansion is one of the earliest and most basic of changes in pregnancy (Table 9-1). It occurs to provide circulation to all the developing organs and body parts. To accommodate the expansion, progesterone causes relaxation of smooth vascular tissue. The intravascular space is expanded, allowing greater blood volume to meet the increased needs of the mother and fetus. The average increase of 45% may occur as early as 6 weeks, although it generally rises slowly in the first trimester, reaching a peak around 30 to 34 weeks. Most of the increased volume (1200-1500 ml) is plasma, with about 300 to 450 ml composed of red blood cells (RBCs). Because of this imbalance the ratio of RBCs to plasma (the hematocrit) will decrease. This is called **hemodilution** of pregnancy. What appears to resemble anemia is a normal event. The RBC count may fall from a prepregnancy count of 4.0 to 5.5 million/mm^3 to 3.75 to 4.5 million/mm^3 (written on laboratory reports as 3.75^6, meaning six places to the right of the decimal point, which takes its place with a comma—3,750,000). The hematocrit decreases from a ratio of 37% to 45%, falling to 34% to 40% (Figure 9-1). Hemoglobin levels also may drop slightly because of the demand for extra iron.

During pregnancy there is an increase in platelets, fibrin, fibrinogen, and coagulation factors, especially factors VII, VIII, IX, and X. These changes are necessary to protect the mother from bleeding at the time of delivery. However, this hypercoagulability makes her more susceptible to thrombus development during pregnancy and the *puerperium,* the postbirth period.

The normal white blood cell count in the nonpregnant state is between 5000 and 10,000/mm^3. The count begins to rise during the second month to about 10,000 mm^3 and by late pregnancy and labor can reach levels of 18,000 or more. This count is within normal limits for pregnancy and recovery. An increase in the granulocytes, particularly neutrophils (which are polymorphonuclear [PMN] cells), causes this increase. Neutrophils, which normally constitute more than half of the white blood cell profile, increase in the body in response to inflammation, pain, anxiety, stress, and labor and delivery; protect against invading organisms, engulfing them through phagocytosis; and débride the decidual tissues of dead cells during the healing process.

TABLE 9-1   Laboratory Values during Pregnancy

DETERMINATION	VALUE
CARDIOVASCULAR SYSTEM	
Blood volume	+30%-50% (+1500-2000 ml)
RBC mass	+ 30% (250 to 450 +), 3.75^6 - 4.5^6/mm^3
Hematocrit (Hct)	34%-40%
Hemoglobin (Hb)	11.5-14 g/dl
White blood cells	5000-15,000/mm^3
Heart rate (HR)	+15-20 beats/min
Cardiac output (CO)	+ 30%-50% (to 6 L/min)
First-stage labor	+60%
Second-stage labor	+80%
Blood pressure (BP)—second trimester	90/60-128/79 mm Hg
Mean arterial pressure (MAP)—second trimester	
Adult	< 100 mm Hg
Adolescent	< 85 mm Hg
RESPIRATORY SYSTEM	
P$_{AO_2}$	104-108 mm Hg
P$_{ACO_2}$	27-32
pH	7.40-7.45
Sodium bicarbonate (NaHCO$_3$)	18-22 mEq/L

Values higher for multiple pregnancy.

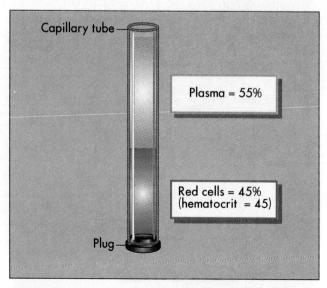

FIGURE 9-1 After centrifuge, the hematocrit is the volume of red cells per 100 ml whole blood, expressed as a percent.

Pulse and Blood Pressure

The heart makes several adaptations to accommodate these changes. Viewed during x-ray examination, it is more prominent because of its increased work load. The *heart rate* (HR) increases by 15 to 20 beats/min; the *cardiac output* (CO), the amount of blood pumped from the heart in 1 minute, increases by 30% to 50% very early in the pregnancy. Cardiac output is determined by multiplying the stroke volume times the heart rate in 1 minute:

$$CO = \text{Stroke volume} \times \text{Heart rate per minute}$$

The stroke volume does not usually increase, but the heart rate increases, resulting in the increased cardiac output. (See Chapter 22 for cardiovascular alterations that result in problems during pregnancy.)

Blood pressure (BP) in the first 24 weeks usually decreases 5 to 10 mm Hg systolic and 10 to 15 mm Hg diastolic, producing a widening of the *pulse pressure*. These changes are caused by (1) relaxation of the vascular smooth muscle layer and (2) formation of new peripheral vascular beds in the breasts, uterus, and placenta. BP levels usually rise to stabilize at nonpregnancy levels by the time labor begins.

Mean Arterial Pressure

The **mean arterial pressure (MAP)** is computed by the following formula, which uses the systolic (S) and diastolic (D) readings:

$$MAP = D + \frac{(S - D)}{3} \text{ (pulse pressure)}$$

In the second trimester a mean arterial pressure (MAP-2) of more than 100 mm Hg after 20 weeks can be interpreted as hypertension. Adolescents with lower baseline pressures may have hypertension with an MAP after 20 weeks of >85. These figures are general guidelines; remember that BP readings must be measured against a woman's baseline. Accuracy of readings can be ensured by consistent measurement on the same arm (and during labor, between contractions). Readings also are influenced by maternal factors such as anxiety, pain, and drug use.

Figure 9-2 shows the Finipres cuff attached to the BP monitor with an MAP readout.

Test Yourself

- In the prenatal clinic, what additional information should you first obtain if a woman's laboratory report at 18 weeks shows the following values: red blood cell count $3.9^6/mm^3$, Hb 11.5 g/dl, and Hct 30%?

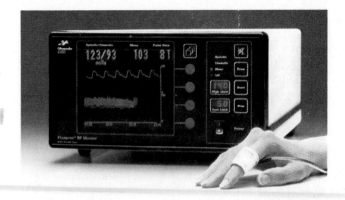

FIGURE 9-2 New techniques of blood pressure monitoring save time for the nurse. Note that the MAP is obtained with each reading on the Finipres monitor. (Courtesy Ohmeda Corp., Englewood , Colo.)

Vena Caval Compression

Maternal position can cause the enlarging uterus to compress the inferior vena cava, impeding venous return, thus decreasing the CO and lowering BP. This problem occurs more often in the later stages of pregnancy, particularly when the woman is lying in the supine position (Fig. 9-3). This resultant **supine hypotension** occurs in up to 10% of women, who experience dizziness, light-headedness, nausea, pallor, clamminess of skin, and even syncope, or fainting. Treatment consists of changing the maternal position from supine to left side-lying and explaining to the woman the cause of the symptoms. This problem also is referred to as the **vena caval syndrome (VCS)** or **supine hypotension syndrome (SHS)** and must be avoided during pregnancy.

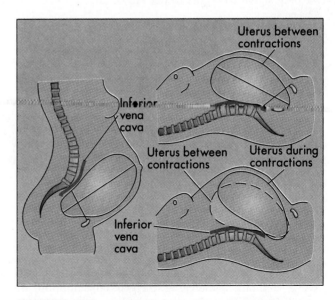

FIGURE 9-3 Vena caval syndrome. Large uterus presses on vena cava as it lies beside the spine. Side-lying position relieves pressure, and blood pressure returns to normal.

Femoral Venous Pressure

An increase in femoral venous pressure is related to the weight of the uterus. Venous return from the femoral veins is affected by the enlarged organ and by increased blood volume. Femoral venous pressure rises in the legs up to 18 mm Hg from a normal of below 10 mm Hg. This contributes to a feeling of fullness in the legs and to *dependent edema,* which is more noticeable in the evening or after standing or sitting for a long time. Varicose veins may appear early in the second trimester and worsen as pregnancy progresses (see Chapter 22).

Varicose veins of the saphenous system and of the vulva and rectum (hemorrhoids) are affected primarily by the rising venous pressure in the lower extremities. Varicosities usually are more common and pronounced in the multigravida but may occur for the first time in a young primigravida with a family history of varicose veins. In addition to being unsightly, these enlarged superficial veins may be painful and throbbing, especially those in the vulva and rectal/anal area.

Walking and positional change to facilitate venous return is helpful. A woman with a tendency toward varicosities should wear support hose during pregnancy to give support and counterpressure to the walls of the distended veins.

Dependent edema of the lower extremities also is related to venous return. Standing or sitting for long periods of time and pressure of the uterus on large veins returning from the legs tend to hinder the venous return (against gravity). Positional change to facilitate venous return helps reduce this *gravity-based edema.* The side-lying position during sleep and rest provides maximal kidney blood flow and function. Edema that persists is a warning signal to report to the physician.

Orthostatic Hypotension

A decrease in the CO caused by the interference of venous return can result from the effects of **orthostatic hypotension,** which occurs when a woman moves from a recumbent to a standing position. Normal, uncomplicated pregnancies usually can withstand this stress without harm to the fetus. However, it might cause problems in pregnancies with preexisting uteroplacental insufficiency. For such women, bed rest is recommended.

β RESPIRATORY SYSTEM

Oxygen Demands

Changes in the respiratory system are caused by the increased need for oxygen intake and carbon dioxide (CO_2) discharge. Increased oxygen consumption of 20% to 30% during pregnancy is the result of cardiac work, renal performance, respiratory performance, and breast, uterine, and placental demands.

Progesterone lowers the CO_2 threshold in the respiratory center, thus increasing sensitivity to CO_2. This hormone decreases pulmonary resistance, thereby promoting an environment for increased alveolar function, allowing the thoracic cage to expand and the diaphragm to become more mobile. The result is a 30% to 40% increase in tidal volume; thus the lungs have a greater capacity to exchange gases. Although these events increase the depth of respiration, the rate remains stable.

Blood Gases

To facilitate CO_2 transfer from the fetus, the pregnant woman is in a state of compensated respiratory alkalosis with a lowered carbon dioxide pressure (Pco_2) and an elevated oxygen pressure (Po_2) (Blackburn and Loper, 1992). Maternal Po_2 increases to 100 to 108 mm Hg during pregnancy. At that level, 100% of maternal hemoglobin is oxygen-saturated, thereby readily allowing maternal red cells to give up oxygen to the fetus. Fetal oxygen levels are much lower, 25 to 35 mm Hg. Fetal hemoglobin (HbF), however, has an extremely high affinity for oxygen, and the *maternal-fetal oxygen gradient* promotes fetal uptake (see Chapter 7).

Maternal $Paco_2$ values are decreased from 35 to 45 mm Hg to about 27 to 32 mm Hg during pregnancy, which promotes elimination of fetal waste CO_2. To maintain a mild alkalosis, the concentrations of sodium bicarbonate ($NaHCO_3$) become lower in pregnancy, averaging 18 to 22 mEq/L. The maternal pH remains stable at about 7.4 to 7.42 because bicarbonate is efficiently eliminated from the kidneys (see Table 9-1).

Dyspnea

About 60% to 70% of women suffer dyspnea, probably related to hyperventilation during pregnancy. Changes in the CO_2 level cause some women to become more aware of the desire to breathe. The onset of this condition usually is early and becomes more marked as the pregnancy progresses, provoking anxiety. In addition, by the eighth or ninth month, the enlarged uterus crowds the diaphragm sometimes by as much as 4 cm. The discomfort may be temporarily alleviated by a change in position, which allows freer excursion of the diaphragm. Later, discomfort is relieved by **lightening,** or the descent of the presenting part as the body prepares for delivery (see Figure 9-10).

Hyperemia

Nasopharyngeal congestion occurs as more blood enters the system. Secretions increase and sometimes cause discomfort because of edema, tissue fragility, and even nosebleeds. Because of increased edema in the upper airway, care must be taken to prevent damage or bleeding if any manipulation of the passage is necessary, such as with intubation or suctioning at the time of delivery. A few women complain of chronic nasal stuffiness and may have a hoarse voice. The pitch of the voice may change. These women feel as if they always have a cold. A humidifier may help this discomfort. The symptoms recede without treatment in the postbirth period.

RENAL SYSTEM

The kidneys increase in size and weight to enable greater filtration volume and reabsorption. No real increase in output occurs in spite of the 50% increase in flow. Changes occur because of increased CO, decreased renal vascular resistance, plasma volume expansion, decreased viscosity of the blood, and other endocrine changes. The pelves, calyces, and ureters are dilated because of hormonal stimuli and the physical presence of a more filtered load.

Hemodynamic Changes

Hemodynamic changes include increases in the *glomerular filtration rate (GFR)*, *renal plasma flow (RPF)*, excretion of amino acids, and elimination of water-soluble vitamins. Early in pregnancy, creatinine excretion levels also increase, and there is increased reabsorption of sodium, chloride, and water. A trace of *glycosuria* and *proteinuria* may develop; any greater amounts should be investigated because they could signal other disorders.

Positional changes affect kidney function. In the supine position the uterus presses on renal veins and arteries, reducing effective flow. Best function is produced during rest in a side-lying position (see Figure 24-5).

Frequency of Urination

Some common urinary complaints during pregnancy arise from physiologic adaptations. Urinary *frequency* usually occurs in the first and third trimesters. In the first trimester the enlarging uterus presses or impinges on the bladder, stimulating the sensation of needing to void even though the bladder is not full. During the second trimester the uterus rises out of the pelvic cavity and into the abdominal cavity, reducing pressure on the bladder. Later, during the third trimester when *lightening,* or descent of the presenting part, occurs, the enlarged uterus will again compress the bladder.

Nocturia

The horizontal position for sleep promotes renal flow, with the result that more urine is produced during rest and sleep. This may be a positive benefit in reducing lower extremity edema, or it may be a problem because sleep is interrupted several times during the night. The woman can plan to avoid fluid intake after the evening meal to help reduce the number of times she must void during the night.

Urinary Tract Infections

Although only a small number of women are affected by urinary tract infection with symptoms, many more women may have **asymptomatic bacteriuria,** that is, bacteria in the urine. The changes of pregnancy promote growth of bacteria because of (1) obstruction of free flow of urine by the pressure of the uterus on the ureters and (2) the relaxing effect of progesterone on smooth muscle. The bladder may contain residual urine, and the ureters loop and dilate. Stasis of urine provides a medium for bacterial growth. (See Chapter 24 for interventions for more severe urinary tract infections.) Nursing interventions include teaching the woman to take adequate amounts of fluid each day and to report signs and symptoms of urinary tract infections: dysuria, pain, blood in urine, and urgency. Because there may be a strong link with preterm labor, some physicians treat bacteriuria with antibiotics.

Test Yourself

Which of the following changes in the renal system may lead to significant health problems and why?

- A trace of glucose in the urine
- Smooth muscle relaxation of the urinary tract
- Nocturia that leads to voiding at least three times during the night

---

GASTROINTESTINAL SYSTEM

Pregnancy causes profound changes in the gastrointestinal (GI) system; many of these changes result in the common discomforts women report. Progesterone causes the GI system to relax, and the growing fetus causes crowding of the surrounding organs.

Several changes occur in the *mouth.* The gums become more vascular and are more likely to bleed when the woman brushes her teeth or even eats crunchy foods. Dental care is important for the treatment of gingivitis, which is common. There is no evidence to support the myth that dental caries is more common at this time. The production of saliva and its pH usually are unchanged during pregnancy. However, some women experience *ptyalism,* an increased secretion of saliva. These women usually experience extreme discomfort from nausea, and the amount of saliva is increased. Women wipe their mouths frequently and complain of an enlarged, reddened tongue (Van Dinter, 1991). This discomfort is related to increased circulation to peripheral tissues and cannot be reversed.

Changes within the *stomach* are the result of smooth muscle relaxation, which decreases motility and cardiac sphincter control. Gastric emptying time is diminished, and acid reflux into the esophagus may cause heartburn. The normal amount of gastric secretions is somewhat lower in the first and second trimesters but increases dramatically in the third. Throughout gestation, however, mucus production increases, which produces a soothing, protective effect on the gastric lining. The mucosa needs this effect because delayed emptying time means that irritating gastric juices remain in the stomach longer. Acid indigestion, or *pyrosis* (heartburn), may include burping and an acidic taste in the mouth (see Chapter 10 for interventions).

Motility is reduced in the *small bowel*. Absorption of nutrients generally is unchanged; the absorption of iron, however, is increased.

The size of the *liver* and blood flow to it are unchanged during pregnancy. Normal function is altered, mostly from the influence of progesterone. Serum albumin levels fall gradually; serum alkaline phosphatase and serum cholesterol levels rise by the end of pregnancy. Serum concentrations of many proteins also are elevated. *↑absorption is ↑*

Nausea and Vomiting

Nausea and vomiting in about 50% of all pregnancies generally are attributed to changes within the GI tract and higher systemic hormone levels. The problem usually surfaces early in the first trimester, around 4 to 6 weeks, and persists until the early part of the second trimester. The incidence of nausea parallels the curve of human chorionic gonadotropin (hCG) and the increase in steroidal hormones (Figure 9-4). By 100 days most nausea has subsided. A study using ultrasonography determined that the corpus luteum was on the right ovary in most women who complained of nausea. It is possible that ovarian steroid hormone concentration increased because of the more direct blood flow from the right ovary through the portal vein to the liver; in contrast, blood flow from the left ovary carries steroids through the circulatory system before they reach the liver. Samisoe (1987) found that women who have been pregnant more than once are more prone to morning nausea and noted that the same women may feel nausea in one pregnancy but not in another.

expec in multigravida, due to ↑hCG levels

Constipation

Women may find constipation a major discomfort. During pregnancy some relaxation of the intestinal smooth muscle results in slowing of motility with removal of more water from the *lower bowel*. In later pregnancy, displacement of the bowel by the enlarging uterus may intensify the problem. If the woman is taking prescribed iron supplements, constipation may

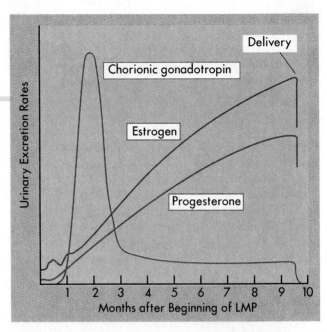

FIGURE 9-4 Urinary excretion of estrogen, progesterone, and hCG during pregnancy. (From Vander AJ, Sherman JH, Luciano D: *Human physiology,* New York, 1970, McGraw-Hill.)

be further aggravated unless medication contains a stool softener, such as ferrous fumarate plus docusate sodium (Ferro-Sequels). Increasing fluid intake to 8 glasses a day, as well as increasing the exercise level and intake of fiber, may help alleviate constipation (see Chapter 10). *↑walking, ↑venous return*

Diarrhea

Diarrhea during pregnancy may precipitate hemorrhoids. It usually does not last long and is usually related to a food source or a viral infection. If it does not subside within 24 hours, medical attention should be sought. Over-the-counter (OTC) medications should not be taken without medical advice.

Diarrhea may occur normally as labor begins and uterine activity increases. Uterine contractions stimulate bowel activity, causing frequent bowel movements. For this reason the routine enema in early labor has largely been abandoned, except for constipated women. (For a complete discussion of other GI minor discomforts, see Chapter 10.)

Hemorrhoids

Hemorrhoids are painful outpouchings of varicose veins in the lower rectal and anal area. Because of increased femoral and portal venous pressure and increased blood volume, hemorrhoids may worsen toward the end of pregnancy. The following interventions should be encouraged to prevent or minimize hemorrhoids and varicose veins in the pelvic area.

1. Elevate legs and the lower pelvis to facilitate venous return.
2. Use support hose, take more frequent rest intervals, decrease standing, and increase walking.
3. Use sitz baths or sit in a bathtub in 2 to 3 inches of warm water as needed.
4. Insert a glycerin suppository before stooling.
5. Apply witch hazel wipes to anal area.
6. Perform frequent perineal hygiene.
7. With lubricated glove, replace external hemorrhoids after each bowel movement.

If additional medication is needed, it is prescribed for constipation and as a local anesthetic in ointment or suppository form (for example, Anusol) may ease evacuation.

INTEGUMENTARY SYSTEM

Vascular Changes

As a result of higher estrogen levels, superficial vascular changes related to increased blood flow can occur. Spider angioma, commonly seen in light-skinned women, consists of tiny vessel networks that appear mainly on the face, chest, and arms. Many women notice erythema or redness of the palms and soles of the feet. Nosebleeds, nasal congestion, and increased bleeding of the gums also can occur. In addition, many women who are usually intolerant of cold weather are more comfortable during pregnancy because of increased peripheral circulation.

Striae gravidarum, commonly called *stretch marks*, appear as pink or purple lines on the breasts, lower abdomen, or thighs. In time, they become brown or silvery but never completely disappear. There is no preventive treatment; striae occur in women who are genetically predisposed to these changes, regardless of the amount of weight gained.

Glandular Changes

Sweating and the excretion of sebum increase during pregnancy, necessitating more frequent cleansing for comfort. Oily skin and sometimes acne may recur in women with a history of this problem. In contrast, some women complain of pruritus (itching) caused by dry skin. If it persists, the women should be evaluated for liver function.

PUPPP

Pruritic urticarial papules and plaques of pregnancy (PUPPP) is a dermatologic condition that may affect a primigravida in her third trimester. The condition is thought to occur in 1 in 200 pregnancies. The rash usually starts as eruptions in the stretch marks (striae) and spreads across the abdomen and buttocks to the arms and legs. The rash resembles poison ivy rash,

according to one affected mother. Women affected by this pruritic rash tend to have excessive weight gain.

Treatment consists of oatmeal baths, topical ointment, and antihistamines, usually diphenhydramine (Benadryl). According to Rook et al (1979), the eruptions usually clear within a few days of delivery. Blackburn and Loper (1992) report spontaneous clearing within 3 weeks after birth.

Hormonal Changes

The actions of hormones during pregnancy spur increased pigmentation, especially on the nipples and areolae, umbilicus, axillae, and perineum. On the lower portion of the abdomen, the line between the symphysis and the umbilicus, the *linea alba*, will darken, to become the linea nigra. Melasma, a blotchy, irregular hyperpigmentation of the forehead, cheeks, nose, and upper lip, commonly referred to as the "mask of pregnancy," occurs more frequently in women with dark complexions (see Figure 22-7). This condition, which formerly was called *chloasma*, fades after delivery, but in some women it never disappears completely. Pigmented nevi are stimulated and become darker and larger; new moles may even appear but usually regress after delivery.

Growth of hair and nails is accelerated during pregnancy. Hair growth quickens, and more follicles become active. After delivery, this rate slows, the follicles cease activity, and hair loss increases. Some women are frightened by this and must be reassured that their prepregnancy hair-growth pattern will return.

MUSCULOSKELETAL SYSTEM

As pregnancy progresses, the skeleton makes several adjustments to accommodate the growing uterus and to prepare for delivery. Progressive *lordosis* (abnormal increased degree of forward curvature) of the spine develops to keep the center of gravity over the woman's legs. Although this measure allows her to maintain her upright posture, the abnormal curvature causes backache. Posture is affected by the hormonal changes and the weight of the uterus. The hormone relaxin loosens the cartilage and connective tissues of the symphysis pubis and sacroiliac joints to facilitate vaginal delivery. This relaxation, however, can lead to pelvic discomfort, particularly in late pregnancy.

As a result of these adjustments, the pregnant woman acquires a characteristic carriage and *gait*. The compensatory changes, although helpful, do not allow her to maintain full control of balance and mobility, a situation distressing to many women who want to be active throughout pregnancy.

Calcium Metabolism

Although maternal calcium levels fall during pregnancy, the serum ionized calcium concentration remains at nonpregnancy levels, probably a result of the increased action of maternal parathyroid hormone (PTH). PTH acts on the intestines to increase absorption of calcium and on the kidneys to decrease filtration. As a result, more calcium is recovered from dietary sources, thereby ensuring a supply for maternal and fetal needs. There is no loss of bone density from pregnancy.

Leg Cramping

Muscle cramping is a common complaint. It occurs later in pregnancy and often at night. The cause may be related to a change in electrolyte, calcium, and phosphorus levels. Usually medical intervention is not indicated. The woman may stretch the muscle by sitting up and pulling hard on her toes or by standing at the bedside and, with her foot flat, flexing the foot to stretch the calf muscle. Gentle massage of the muscle also seems to help. Some women occasionally are treated with calcium lactate or vitamin B complex, but no standard intervention exists.

Backache and Neuralgia

Strain on weak abdominal muscles and lower back muscles and increased weight of the uterus may cause backache. A few women have a serious problem with backaches or with pain radiating along the nerve to the leg. Sacroiliac joint strain is common, with tenderness over the posterior aspect of the joint (Beischer and MacKay, 1993). Separation of the symphysis pubis is uncommon but very distressing. The woman has pain while walking, and the pubic joint is tender to touch. This problem may appear at the time of childbirth, and a client who reports severe pain during ambulation should be examined for symphysis separation.

Exercise to strengthen the lower back is basic to improved status. Some women need to wear a supportive girdle. Warmth to the affected area and physical therapy may be advised. Remember, pain during pregnancy is a sign of a problem. The woman should be referred for evaluation.

Sacroiliac joint strain, which is affected by relaxin, also is common in pregnancy. Very few women have *sciatic nerve pressure* with significant pain.

Bed rest is required in these cases. Others have **carpal tunnel syndrome:** the radial side of the hand may be numb or painful. The median nerve is compressed in the fibrous tunnel through which it passes. Treatment to moderate the condition is not given until after childbirth, when it may disappear. The lateral cutaneous nerve of the thigh also runs in a restricted space under the inguinal ligament and may be compressed during later pregnancy, resulting in sensory changes.

Strain on weak abdominal and lower back muscles because of the weight of the uterus may lead to *lordosis* and backache. Women should be instructed to recognize

postural changes, to use low-heel, comfortable shoes, and to strengthen lower back muscles with exercise. She should be taught proper body alignment for standing, stooping, and lifting (Figure 9-5). Squatting instead of stooping is beneficial; yet women who are unaccustomed to squatting fall when they attempt that posture. Women in other countries find squatting very comfortable, and a number of these women give birth in this position. Walking upstairs also is a function that demands good posture (Figure 9-6).

To balance and compensate for the weight at the front of the body, the woman should learn appropriate ways to get out of a chair or out of bed. In this technique, she moves to the edge of the chair and leans forward until the weight of her body is over the feet. To arise from a bed, she should move to the edge of the bed while lying on her side. She pushes up with her depen-

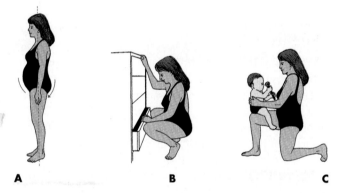

A   **B**   **C**

FIGURE 9-5 Correct posture during pregnancy. **A,** Standing. **B,** Stooping. **C,** Lifting.

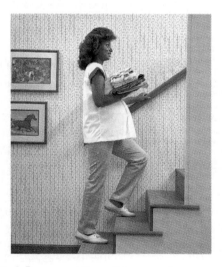

FIGURE 9-6 Posture while walking upstairs or carrying loads is important to discuss during prenatal teaching. (Courtesy Ross Laboratories, Columbus, Ohio.)

dent elbow and opposite hand to a sitting position and waits for dizziness to pass before standing upright.

Posture

Proper posture, good body mechanics, and exercise cannot be ignored by the expectant mother. Women need to recognize the value of good body condition. Although many participate in exercise programs, others are not active and become less so during pregnancy.

Exercise

In our health-conscious society, there has been a surge of interest in physical fitness and exercise programs. Aware of the difficulties produced by the changing body, frustrated in their attempts to lead an active life-style, and motivated to be physically fit for vaginal delivery, women have extended this pursuit to pregnancy. In most communities exercise classes are readily available through fitness centers and childbirth educators. Swimming is a recommended activity during pregnancy (Figure 9-7).

Physiologic responses. Exercise physiology is a new field that explores the effects of exercise on pregnancy and the fetus. Current guidelines are based on extensive studies and anecdotal observations of women who choose to engage in work and fitness programs. Precautions surround the increased oxygen consumption and cardiac workload needed for exertion before and during pregnancy; there is also concern about the effect on the fetus of the temperature increase produced during a workout.

During exercise, vasodilation to the heart, muscles, and brain occurs, thus decreasing the blood supply, particularly to the viscera. Stress is placed on joints already weakened by hormonal influence. Oxygen uptake is increased to meet the demands of the heart and muscles. The respiratory rate, tidal volume, heart rate, cardiac output, body temperature, and metabolic rate rise. If exercise is

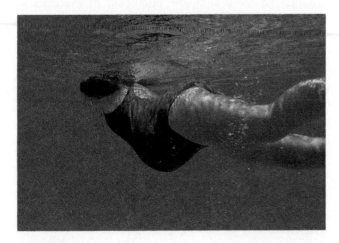

FIGURE 9-7 Swimming is a recommended exercise during pregnancy. (Courtesy Ross Laboratories, Columbus, Ohio.)

prolonged and strenuous, the oxygen supply may be exceeded, leading from an aerobic (with oxygen) to an anaerobic (without oxygen) state. If the latter occurs, metabolic acidosis arises, which may compromise the fetus.

Fetal responses. Fetal responses to maternal exercise can be transitory or long-term. Fetal heart rate and breathing movements increase with moderate exercise. The greatest concern is that regular strenuous exercise, particularly in the first trimester, could raise the body temperature core sufficiently to manifest the teratogenic effects of heat on the growing embryo. For this reason, moderation is advised during this period (De Grez, 1988).

Another concern for the fetus is the adequacy of uteroplacental blood flow. Studies of working mothers and those who have engaged in active fitness programs have shown that birth weights are consistently somewhat lower. Because of design limitations, these studies cannot be judged as definitive; however, most physicians advise limiting activity for women with known uteroplacental deficiency problems such as hypertension and intrauterine growth retardation. In addition, women who engage in strenuous activity should be monitored for signs of compromise before continuing regular exercise.

Basic Exercises

Basic exercises to strengthen the abdominal muscles and lower back are curl-ups or partial sit-ups and the pelvic tilt. The nurse should inform the woman of the guidelines of exercise and inquire about her exercise, posture, and fatigue at each clinic visit. In addition, conditioning exercises for childbirth preparation should be encouraged (see Chapter 12). The woman should be taught Kegel exercises in preparation for birth and recovery. To perform Kegel exercises, the woman should sit or lie supine and alternately tighten and then relax the muscles of the pelvic diaphragm and perineum for 6 seconds at a time. Samples et al (1988) and Dougherty et al (1989) suggest that women increase the tightening time to 12 seconds per exercise and work up to at least 12 minutes of exercise a day.

Wallace (1986) compared exercising with nonexercising women and found that women who exercised had significantly higher self-esteem and lower rating for physical discomforts than did the nonexercising group. This study's findings point to the importance of exercise during pregnancy.

Guidelines. The American College of Obstetrics and Gynecology (ACOG, 1985) has proposed guidelines for exercise during pregnancy and suggests that strenous exercise be limited to 15 minutes (Box 9-1). Before a pregnant woman begins a new exercise program or considers a strenuous new activity, risks and benefits must be

BOX 9-1 American College of Obstetricians and Gynecologists Guidelines for Exercise during Pregnancy and Postpartum

Pregnancy and postpartum

1. Regular exercise (at least three times per week) is preferable to intermittent activity. Competitive activities should be discouraged.
2. Vigorous exercise should not be performed in hot, humid weather or during a period of febrile illness.
3. Ballistic movements (jerky, bouncy motions) should be avoided. Exercise should be done on a wooden floor or a tightly carpeted surface to reduce shock and provide sure footing.
4. Deep flexion or extension of joints should be avoided because of connective tissue laxity. Activities that require jumping, jarring motions, or rapid changes in direction should be avoided because of joint instability.
5. Vigorous exercise should be preceded by a 5-minute period of muscle warm-up. This can be accomplished by slow walking or stationary cycling with low resistance.
6. Vigorous exercise should be followed by a period of gradually declining activity that includes gentle stationary stretching. Because connective tissue laxity increases the risk of joint injury, stretches should not be taken to the point of maximum resistance.
7. Heart rate should be measured at times of peak activity. Target heart rates established in consultation with the physician should not be exceeded.
8. Care should be taken to gradually rise from the floor to avoid orthostatic hypotension. Some form of activity involving the legs should be continued for a brief period.
9. Liquids should be taken liberally before and after exercise to prevent dehydration. If necessary, activity should be interrupted to replenish fluids.
10. Women who have led sedentary life-styles should begin with physical activity of very low intensity and advance activity levels very gradually.
11. Activity should be stopped and the physician consulted if any unusual symptoms appear.

Pregnancy only

1. Maternal heart rate should not exceed 140 beats/min.
2. Strenuous activities should not exceed 15 minutes in duration.
3. No exercise should be performed in the supine position after the fourth month of gestation is completed.
4. Exercises that employ the Valsalva maneuver should be avoided.
5. Caloric intake should be adequate to meet not only the extra needs of pregnancy but also of the exercise performed.
6. Maternal core temperature should not exceed 38° C (100.4° F).

From American College of Obstetricians and Gynecologists: *Exercise during pregnancy and the postnatal period. Home exercise programs,* Washington, D.C., 1985, The College, p. 4.

Clinical Decision

Jane is accustomed to doing an aerobic workout three times a week. She asks about precautions during the second trimester. What would you tell her? Give rationale.

presented to her as well as precautions. For example, activities that require the supine position and could lead to supine hypotensive syndrome should be avoided. High-impact aerobics and aggressive contact sports also should be questioned because low-impact aerobics are safer for the pregnant woman and provide equal benefit. Skydiving, scuba diving, and similar activities in which atmospheric and oxygen pressure changes occur should be avoided during pregnant.

Exercise in moderation benefits both the mother and fetus. Pregnant women should be encouraged to en-gage in some form of exercise or activity program to promote physical and psychologic well-being. (See Chapter 12 for a complete discussion of exercises in preparation for childbirth.)

ENDOCRINE SYSTEM AND METABOLISM

Thyroid Function

In the first trimester the thyroid gland increases in size and is readily palpable. This results in a normal increase in thyroid hormone (triiodothyronine [T_3] and thyroxine [T_4]) synthesis to support gestational growth. In spite of this increase the hypothalamic-pituitary-thyroidal relationship remains stable.

Normal pregnancy mimics a mild *hyperthyroid* state; the basal metabolic rate (BMR), CO, heat intolerance, and emotional lability increase, and menses stop. The BMR rises gradually during pregnancy to a 25% increase. The thyroid hormones function to increase the production of intracellular proteins and energy, which increases the rate of consumption of carbohydrates, fats, and oxygen, resulting in increased heat production. Because of increased heat production and expanded vascular supply, many women complain of being warm and flushed. This change is normal and subsides after childbirth.

Adrenals

The adrenal glands produce glucocorticoids during pregnancy. Free plasma cortisol levels rise to 2.5 times higher at full term than they were before pregnancy. Cortisol regulates carbohydrate metabolism and influences insulin production.

Pancreas

The insulin-producing cells of the pancreas increase in size and number during pregnancy. Thus an accelerated starvation effect is produced by maternal fasting. During fasting, the woman's blood glucose levels will drop 15 to 20 mg/dl below nonpregnancy levels as a result of fetal drain on the maternal supply. The fasting levels of insulin also are lower, resulting in the potential for ketosis. Ketosis must be avoided because ketone bodies have been implicated in fetal brain damage.

Maternal eating, on the other hand, produces an extreme opposite response. Blood sugar levels rise sharply, as do insulin and triglycerides, and there is decreased tissue sensitivity to the action of insulin. This diabetogenic response, or insulin antagonism, is heightened by the action of human placental lactogen (hPL) and, to a lesser extent, is related to the higher levels of estrogen, progesterone, and free cortisols. This is the reason for encouraging six small meals a day in place of three large meals.

Pregnancy impairs insulin action, and the decreased responsiveness of tissue to the effect of insulin results in elevated glucose levels. Although maternal insulin does not cross the placenta, the fetus relies on facilitated diffusion of maternal glucose for energy needs. If maternal hyperglycemia is present, fetal levels are elevated. (See Chapter 24 for detrimental effects of hyperglycemia on the fetus.)

Parathyroid

Activity of the parathyroid glands increases during pregnancy. With more parathyroid hormone (PTH) released, the body is able to absorb more calcium from the GI tract, ensuring sufficient calcium for maternal and fetal needs.

Pituitary

Because the menstrual cycle has been interrupted, the anterior pituitary gland ceases its release of follicle-stimulating hormone (FSH) and luteinizing hormone (LH). After birth, prolactin or luteotropic hormone (LTH) is secreted in response to nipple stimulation and breast-feeding. The posterior pituitary secretes small amounts of oxytocin late in pregnancy, which stimulates uterine contractions of labor. After delivery, nipple stimulation with breast-feeding triggers release of oxytocin (1) to contract uterine muscle and thus prevent bleeding, (2) to release prolactin, and to (3) contract the ducts, which causes the let-down reflex whereby milk is ejected as the baby sucks on the nipple.

REPRODUCTIVE SYSTEM

Hormones

Estrogen. Estrogen is secreted by the ovary at the beginning of pregnancy and then by the placental cells. Estrogenic effects on most of the body systems have been indicated earlier (see Chapter 3). Acting alone or in conjunction with other hormones, it stimulates the following groups of actions:

- Alteration in vaginal pH and glucose levels
- Increase in uterine size and weight
- Breast and mammary duct development and changes in nipple consistency and color
- Various skin changes, including darker coloration of melana-influenced cells
- Nasopharyngeal edema
- Diabetogenic response, partially as the result of estrogen levels
- Increased blood flow to tissues, stimulated by estrogen

Progesterone. The hormone that maintains the pregnancy is named for its action—progestation. Progesterone inhibits uterine motility, increasing potential for implantation, allowing the uterus to contain the fetus. Progesterone is first secreted by the corpus luteum in the ovary, but by the twelfth week it is secreted primarily by the placental tissue. It maintains the decidual lining, relaxes smooth muscle throughout the body, and contributes to the vascular changes. The following categories of effects are seen:

- Cardiovascular system: relaxed vessels allow for blood expansion
- Respiratory system: decreasing pulmonary resistance
- Renal system: relaxing its structures to allow for higher volume
- Breasts: development of lobes and alveoli in preparation for breast-feeding
- Liver: decreasing levels of serum albumin and increasing levels of serum phosphatase and cholesterol
- Pancreas: contributes to diabetogenic effects
- Gastrointestinal system: reducing motility

Human chorionic gonadotropin. Human chorionic gonadotropin (hCG) is secreted by the trophoblastic layer of the blastocyst. This hormone maintains the corpus luteum until the placental tissue can produce adequate amounts of pregnancy hormones. This hormone has been implicated in the cause of morning sickness; nausea of pregnancy follows closely the curve of hCG in the first trimester (see Figure 9-4). hCG levels in urine or serum provide the basis for pregnancy tests. The hormone also may be referred to as *urinary chorionic gonadotropin* (UCG).

Relaxin. Relaxin is secreted during pregnancy, first by the corpus luteum and then by the placenta. Its actions are not precisely known, but it appears to work in conjunction with progesterone, quieting uterine muscular activity and preventing loss of the conceptus. It may contribute to the fatigue and tiredness experienced early in pregnancy. Later in pregnancy it may relax the connective tissue, especially in the sacroiliac and symphysis pubis in preparation for labor. Softening of the cervix also is partially attributed to relaxin.

Human placental lactogen. When human placental lactogen (hPL) was first isolated from the placenta, its similarity to both human growth hormone (hGH) and prolactin was noted. Because its effect on the mammary gland is greater than its effect on growth, it is called *hPL*. Later, because it possessed somatropic and lactogenic properties, the name *human chorionic somatomammotropin* (hCS) was proposed. Both names are still used.

hPL prepares the body for lactation by stimulating the development of the breast and milk production. Other possible effects are attributed to this hormone; it may assist hCG in prolonging the life and activity of the corpus luteum. Blackburn and Loper (1992) suggest other influences of hPL, including enhancement of carbohydrate metabolism, promotion of fat storage, increase of free circulating fatty acids, and stimulation of erythropoiesis (erythrocyte production) and aldosterone secretion.

Prolactin Prolactin (PRL, PL) is secreted by the chorionic layer of the placenta and the pituitary gland. Its major influence is indicated by its name, *pro-lactin* (for lactation), although the hormone also is known as galactopoietic hormone, lactogenic hormone, luteotropic hormone (LTH), and mammotropin.

Prolactin has 82 groups of actions, including breast growth, osmoregulation, reproductive activity, integumentary action, synergism with steroids, and lactogenesis. Medications, exercise, and anesthesia can influence its release.

Serum levels rise from 30 ng/ml in the first trimester to a high of 200 ng/ml at term. Amniotic fluid contains 5 to 10 times more prolactin than does maternal serum. After delivery, prolactin levels diminish in 1 week if bottle feeding is chosen. If the mother chooses breast-feeding, levels remain high during the first week and rise even higher after a feeding. After lactation is established, however, the base level is lower, with continued peaks of release within 30 minutes of suckling by the infant. There is indication that prolactin plays some part in inhibiting ovulation during the period of breast-feeding by inhibiting release of LH by the anterior pituitary. Continued release of prolactin occurs in response to infant sucking, but levels eventually decrease and menses resumes. Thus frequent nursing and vigorous sucking of the infant seem to be the key to preventing the return of ovulation for at least 3 to 6 months after birth.

Uterus

To accommodate the growing fetus the smooth muscles of the uterus enlarge, stretching to at least eight times the prepregnant size. As already noted, the nonpregnant uterus weighs approximately 60 g (2 oz). The once pear-shaped organ enlarges first to a globular shape and then to an ovoid or egg shape weighing more than 1000 g. The increase in size depends on fetal size, the shape of the placenta, and the volume of amniotic fluid. Most of the increase is in the fundal portion and is due not to an increase in the number of cells but rather to cell size. This hypertrophy contributes to the remarkable changes just after the birth.

Uterine growth follows a pattern, and measurement of the height of the uterine fundus gives clues to deviations that may indicate a problem with pregnancy. By week 12 the uterus is palpable at the symphysis pubis; by week 20 the fundus should reach the umbilicus, and by week 36 it should be at the xyphoid process (Figure 9-8). Within 2 weeks of birth, as the fetus settles into position for birth, the uterus shifts position

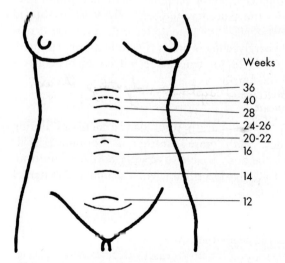

	Weeks
	36
	40
	28
	24-26
	20-22
	16
	14
	12

FIGURE 9-8 Expected changes in height of uterine fundus in relation to weeks of gestation.

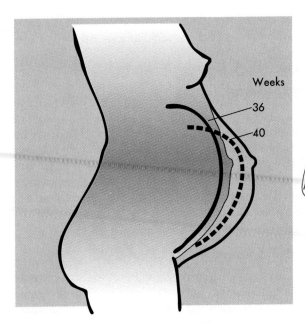

FIGURE 9-9 Changes in uterine position as lightening occurs. Lordosis may become discomfort of pregnancy.

and moves away into a more forward angle, relieving pressure on the diaphragm. This final shift in position is known as *lightening* for the sense of relief that is experienced. Figure 9-9 illustrates the positions of the uterus during pregnancy.

The myometrium is thick and firm and becomes progressively stretched and thinner in the second half of gestation. Toward the end of pregnancy, it is thin enough to allow the fetal head and extremities to be palpated easily.

The isthmus or juncture between the body of the uterus and the cervix is softened by hormonal influence. By bimanual examination, the isthmus can be compressed to almost paper thinness, a condition called *Hegar's sign* (Figure 9-10). Another early sign of pregnancy is *Ladin's sign,* a softening of a spot on the anterior portion just above the uterocervical juncture.

(pg 199 Leopold's maneuver.)

Cervix

The nonpregnant cervix has the firmness and feel of the tip of a nose. Because of expanded blood circulation and hormonal activity, it becomes increasingly soft. The softening is known as *Goodell's sign,* one of the early indications of pregnancy. The cervical os is lined with mucus-secreting glands that enlarge to secrete a thick, tenacious mucus that effectively closes the os for the duration of pregnancy. This seal, or **mucous plug,** prevents ascending infection from contaminating the fetus. In the few weeks before birth, the cervix becomes gradually softened, or it ripens. Toward the beginning of labor, it gradually shortens (*effaces*) and begins to open (*dilates*). As the uterus begins the work of labor to open and thin the cervix, the mucous plug (called "show") is expelled from the cervical canal. The show is one of the first indications that effective labor has begun. Because small capillaries in the cervix may be broken, blood mixes with the mucus and hence the term *bloody show.*

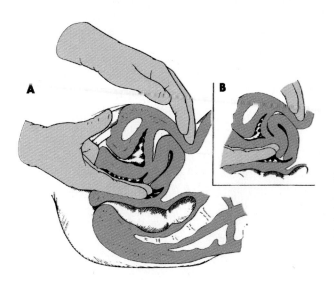

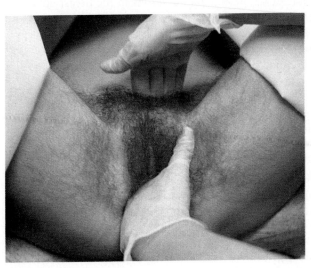

FIGURE 9-10 Bimanual examination. **A,** Palpation of cervix to determine size, shape, consistency, and its relation to axis of vagina. **B,** Palpation of uterus for size, shape, consistency, mobility, and tenderness; its anterior position is best determined when corpus can be "grasped" between fingers of two hands. **C,** Position of gloved hands for vaginal examination. (**C** from Seidel HM et al, eds: *Mosby's guide to physical examination,* ed 2, St Louis, 1991, Mosby.)

Vagina

During pregnancy the vaginal rugae enlarge and become more elastic in preparation for the passage of the fetus and placenta. Because of hormones, especially estrogen, there is increased sloughing of cells from the cervical and vaginal walls, causing increased amounts of vaginal mucus or **leukorrhea**. Leukorrhea may be thin and milky or thick and sticky but should not cause itching or irritation to tissues unless infection such as *Trichomonas vaginalis* or *Candida albicans* is present. The vaginal pH changes from a low of 4 to 5 to a less acidic 5 to 6. This change, with increased glycogen content in cells, may foster growth of organisms in the vagina (see Chapter 4). Circulation to the vaginal and cervical tissues increases, and the vaginal mucosa and cervix take on a bluish-purple hue; this change is *Chadwick's sign* and can be seen by the eighth week of pregnancy. Vaginal birth weakens the circumvaginal muscles (CVM), and *Kegel exercises* can help to strengthen the CVM (Dougherty, 1989).

Breast Changes

For many women, one of the first signs of pregnancy is a fullness or tingling of the breasts very similar to the fullness and tingling experienced during the premenstrual period. During pregnancy, however, the fullness can cause discomfort. The tenderness continues for some time because the hormones of pregnancy, particularly estrogen and progesterone, prepare the body for breast-feeding; most changes are influenced by both hormones. Estrogen influences the development of the ducts, whereas progesterone influences alveolar and lobule development. Blood vessels in the breast enlarge and become prominent, showing visible, blue, twisting patterns. The enlargement and mobility of the nipple and darkening and enlargement of the tubercles of Montgomery are attributed in part to the action of estrogens (see Figure 3-8).

Additional hormones are necessary for breast development; these include pituitary hormones (prolactin, adrenocorticotropic hormone [ACTH], hGH, FSH, LH, thyroid stimulating hormone [TSH], and hCS).

Colostrum, a fluid full of nutrients and antibodies, is secreted in small amounts as early as the second trimester. Some authors recommend no breast preparation or expression of colostrum during pregnancy. Storr (1987), however, recommends that nipple preparation and prenatal breast massage be begun in the third trimester to more quickly establish lactation.

Breast stimulation during later pregnancy has been out of favor because nipple stimulation triggers the release of oxytocin from the posterior pituitary. Oxytocin is a factor in the initiation of labor. If there is doubt about stimulation or if the woman is threatened with early labor, such a practice is not recommended in the last few weeks of pregnancy. (See Chapter 17 for complete discussion of breast-feeding.)

Signs and Symptoms of Pregnancy

Several weeks or 2 months may pass before a woman suspects she is pregnant because early symptoms may be confusing. Although fatigue and breast changes often are the earliest symptoms, amenorrhea or scanty, brief menstrual flow usually signals possible pregnancy. Other women report nausea or taste and olfactory disturbances as early clues.

POSSIBLE SIGNS AND SYMPTOMS

Signs that indicate a growing embryo might also occur with another condition. In the past the term *presumptive* referred to signs most likely to indicate pregnancy; this distinction no longer is necessary. If pregnancy is suspected, it may be verified by a urine test for the presence of hCG or by ultrasound examination. Table 9-2 summarizes signs and symptoms of pregnancy by trimester.

Subjective Signs

Tender breasts occur because of increased blood supply. Nipples and areolae darken and become more prominent. By 14 weeks, colostrum, the precursor of breast milk, is being produced. Many women experience breast tenderness or tingling as one of the first symptoms (Box 9-2).

Nausea is experienced by approximately 50% of pregnant women. It is easy to identify and often occurs on awakening. With onset about the fourth week nausea usually lasts until the thirteenth week.

Frequency of urination occurs during the first trimester because of the enlarging uterus. With no other signs of infection, frequency usually indicates pregnancy.

Abdominal enlargement does not become evident until the second trimester. By the sixteenth week a woman will find it difficult to wear her normal waistband size. The rise of the uterus into the abdominal cavity is gradual and reaches the symphysis pubis by the twelfth week. From that time the height of the fundus becomes a guide to the progress of fetal growth. Measurements are changed by obesity, multiple pregnancy, and a smaller or larger than average amount of amniotic fluid.

There are a few cases of *pseudocyesis,* or pseudopregnancy, when a woman, believing strongly that she is pregnant, appears to have all the early signs. The physiologic basis for such a condition was documented by Brown and Barglow (1971) and showed that the corpus luteum can remain active under the influence of stress-induced hormones, although conception has

TABLE 9-2   Subjective and Objective Signs during Pregnancy

SUBJECTIVE	OBJECTIVE
FIRST TRIMESTER	
Weeks 1-4	
Fatigue, thought to be due to relaxin	Amenorrhea, but possible spotting at time of expected period
Nausea, peaking 60 to 100 days after conception	Elevated hCG levels
Soreness, tingling of breasts	Elevated BBT because of progesterone secretion
Weeks 5-8	
Enlarging uterus causing pressure on bladder and frequency of urination	Breast enlargement, darkening of areolas, enlarged Montgomery's tubercles
Possible decrease in desire for sexual relations	Signs (weeks 5-7):
	Ladin's
	Goodell's
	Hegar's
	Positive pregnancy test for hCG using isoimmunologic methods
	Chadwick's
Weeks 9-13	
Nausea subsiding by 13 weeks	Weight gain of 0-3 lb but also possible weight loss
Frequency of urination subsiding by 12 weeks	Height of fundus at the symphysis pubis, rising about 1 cm/wk thereafter
Gingivitis and hypertrophy of gums	9-12 weeks—detection of fetal pulse by ultrasonic techniques
SECOND TRIMESTER	
Weeks 14-20	
Breast fullness	Colostrum present
Headaches	Mucous plug formation in cervical canal
	Leukorrhea; report if pruritus or foul odor develops: *Candida albicans*, trichomonal infections
	Abdominal appearance of pregnancy
	Height of fundus between symphysis and umbilicus
	Increase in total blood volume contributing to lightheadedness or fainting; occurs by 10-14 weeks; peaks at 8½ months (34-36 weeks)
Weeks 20-24	
Quickening	Hemodilution of pregnancy resulting from increased plasma (40%) and small red blood cell increase; Hb of 11-12 g and possible Hct of 33%-35%
Often increased sexual desire	
	Fundus at umbilicus (20 weeks)
	Pelvic joints relaxing because of hormone relaxin
	Possible pigment changes in skin: melasma, linea nigra, striae gravidarum
	Increased perspiration, oily secretions
	Dilation of right ureter as a result of pressure from dextrorotated uterus
Weeks 25-28	
Leg cramps caused by decreased calcium when phosphorus level is increased	Constipation and hemorrhoids because of slowed peristalsis and pressure of uterus on lower colon and rectum
Fatigue	

BBT, Basal body temperature.

Continued.

TABLE 9-2   Subjective and Objective Signs during Pregnancy—cont'd

SUBJECTIVE	OBJECTIVE
THIRD TRIMESTER *Weeks 29-33*	
Fatigue	Heartburn caused by pressure of uterus on stomach, causing mild hiatus hernia and regurgitation of stomach acid into esophagus
Anxiety about future	BP returning to prepregnancy level after slight drop as a result of vasodilation
Bad, fearful dreams	Pulse rate at 15 beats/min over normal from increase in cardiac work
Possible faintness in supine position from pressure on inferior vena cava	Braxton Hicks contractions (painless, intermittent contractions)
Decrease in sexual desire because of physical discomfort	Fundus midway between umbilicus and xiphoid
Weeks 34-38	
Backache, change in gait	Increase in shortness of breath and other pressure symptoms (heartburn, feeling of fullness after eating, constipation, varicose veins, dependent edema, hemorrhoids)
Impatience for end of pregnancy	
Mood swings because of ambivalence about future	
Just before labor	
Lightening	Fundus just below diaphragm until lightening, then appears to tip forward
Aching in lower abdomen	

BOX 9-2   Signs and Symptoms of Pregnancy

Possible signs and symptoms
Subjective
- Breast tingling
- Nausea
- Frequency of urination
- Fatigue
- Increased abdominal girth
- Quickening

Objective
- Breast enlargement
- Amenorrhea
- Changes in uterus and cervix
- Vaginal hyperemia
- Positive pregnancy tests
- Ballottement

Positive signs
- Ultrasonic visualization of moving embryo or fetus and fetal heart movements
- Auscultation of fetal heartbeat
- Fetal parts or movement palpated by examiner

not occurred. Of course ultrasound examination would confirm the absence or presence of an embryo.

Quickening occurs by the sixteenth to eighteenth week and certainly by the midpoint of pregnancy. A woman will feel the baby move—"feeling life." It is a significant point in pregnancy for many women. Even the woman who is anxiously waiting for the signs may mistake it for flatulence because fetal movement is so slight at the beginning.

Objective Signs

Breast enlargment, under the influence of hormones and with increased vascular supply, begins soon after the woman becomes pregnant. By term the breast may have doubled in size. Superficial veins become more prominent.

Amenorrhea is a sign that may be caused by other factors such as stress, anemia, illness, and approaching premenopause. Also, some women may have spotting during the early weeks of pregnancy, particularly at the time of implantation or expected menstrual period.

Uterine and cervical changes occur as a result of hormonal activity and increased blood supply to these tissues. The isthmus or juncture between the body of the uterus and cervix is softened under hormonal influence. On bimanual examination the isthmus may be compressed to almost paper thinness, a condition called *Hegar's sign*. Because of expanded blood circulation and hormonal activity, the cervix becomes increasingly soft, known as *Goodell's sign*. Today, with the use of ultrasound, these tests are used less frequently for determining pregnancy status.

Vaginal hyperemia results from increased circulation in the pelvic area that causes the tissues to take on a bluish-purple hue. The color change of vaginal mucosa and cervix is called *Chadwick's*.

Pregnancy tests based on isoimmunologic reactions are in common use. Kits available OTC provide a 70% to 85% accuracy rate (Doshi, 1986). A fresh urine sample is tested together with hCG-coated particles and antiserum. As early as 15 to 20 days after conception, if enough hCG is present in the urine, the particles will not agglutinate. The later the test is performed, the more accurate it will be, with positive results reflecting higher levels of hCG. Monoclonal antibody tests are more accurate but more costly.

Positive Signs and Symptoms

Visualization of the fetus by ultrasonic examination will demonstrate the amniotic sac, fetal parts, and heart rate movements. It also is used at 16 to 18 weeks to confirm the expected date of childbirth.

Auscultation of a faint fetal heartbeat may be noted at 9 weeks with a Doppler scan or fetal monitor. Auscultation with a stethoscope must wait until 18 or 20 weeks.

Palpation of the fetal outline by the use of *Leopold's maneuvers* (Figure 9-11) allows the examiner to feel for parts of the fetus, including the head, knees, and back. By week 20 an observer also may see fetal movements by watching the surface of the abdomen when the fetus is active.

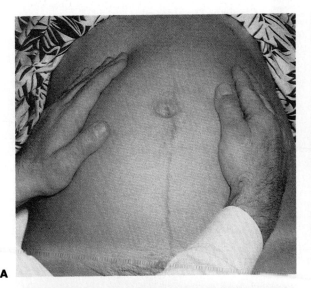

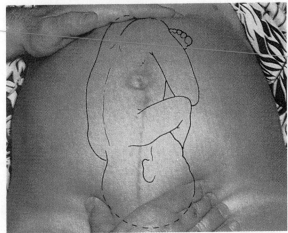

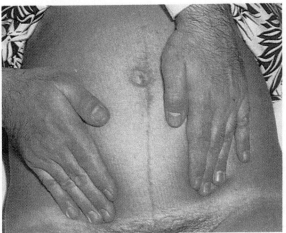

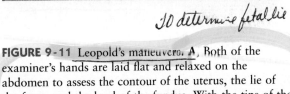

to determine fetal lie

FIGURE 9-11 Leopold's maneuvers. **A,** Both of the examiner's hands are laid flat and relaxed on the abdomen to assess the contour of the uterus, the lie of the fetus, and the level of the fundus. With the tips of the fingers, the examiner then assesses which part of the fetus occupies the uterine fundus. **B,** The fetal part above the symphysis pubis is grasped gently but firmly with the thumb and fingers of the right hand. The contour and consistency of the fetal part can then be examined and compared with the opposite part in the fundus. **C,** If the presentation is cephalic, the examiner faces the mother's feet and presses with the first three fingers of each hand on the sides of the fetal head, in the direction of the pelvic inlet. (From Al-Azzawi F: *Color atlas of childbirth and obstetric techniques*, St Louis, 1990, Mosby.)

ref to pg 316 for toco placement to assess FHT

Fetal Maturity

GESTATIONAL AGE

The preterm or premature infant is born after week 20 and before the end of week 37. The term or mature infant has developed for 266 to 287 days, or 38 to 41 weeks. The postterm or postmature infant's gestational age is 42 weeks or longer.

The *previable* period extends to week 20; if the pregnancy ends, the fetal product is an abortion, even if it occurs spontaneously (see Chapter 21). To be considered *viable* or able to live, the fetus must weigh more than 499 g. After 20 to 24 weeks a fetus is considered potentially viable. Therefore any fetus who dies in utero after 20 weeks of gestation is considered a *stillbirth* that must be recorded in the statistics of fetal mortality. Very few premature infants survive intact (that is, without residual problems) between weeks 20 and 28. By week 28 the fetus's chances have improved (Figure 9-12).

These facts reinforce the importance of determining the gestational age of the pregnancy. Because the first phase of the menstrual cycle may be longer or shorter than 14 days, women often do not give birth on their predicted days.

ESTIMATING DURATION OF PREGNANCY

Because the exact day of fertilization rarely is known, calculation is based on the first day of the **last menstrual period (LMP)**. Thus approximately 14 extra days are added to the conception age; as a result the gestational age is based on 280 days from the LMP. All calculations are based on a 28-day cycle in which ovulation occurs 14 ± 2 days after the menstrual period begins, even though 50% of all women have a shorter or longer interval between menses.

The full-term date is indicated by many terms, most commonly **estimated date of childbirth (EDC)**, **estimated date of birth (EDB)**, and **due date (DD)**.

Several methods are used to calculate the EDB. Using *Nägele's rule*, for example (first formulated in 1812), the EDB is calculated by adding 7 days to the first day of LMP and then subtracting 3 months from the months of LMP. Using the LMP date of July 5 the following calculation is made:

	Day	Month (July)
LMP	5	7
	+7	−3
	12	4

EDB = April 12

Clinical Decision

During the physical examination at 14 weeks, the midwife determines that the uterine fundus is 2 cm above the symphysis pubis. Which other physical findings should accompany a normal pregnancy at this stage?

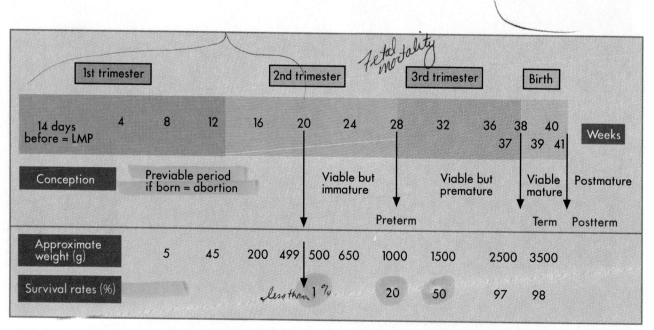

FIGURE 9-12 Fetal maturity and relative risk.

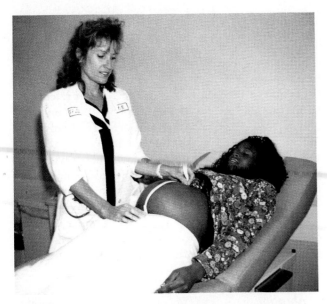

FIGURE 9-13 Measuring the height of the fundus. A tape measure is used to measure the distance between the symphysis pubis and the level of the uterine fundus. After 20 weeks' gestation the measurement in centimeters approximately corresponds to the duration of pregnancy in weeks. (Courtesy Marjorie Pyle, RNC, *Lifecircle*.)

Remember to account for the number of days in a month. For instance if a calculation resulted in the figure July 32, move forward to August 1. A newer method uses +9 days +9 months from LMP. This measure is the *method of nines.*

> **Test Yourself**
>
> • Using the LMP of May 27, calculate Amy's EDB by Nägele's rule and by the new method of nines. How much variation do you find?

A simple guide to the progress of pregnancy is to measure from the symphysis pubis to the top of the fundus (Figure 9-13) and to add 12 weeks to the centimeter reading on the tape (Engstrom, 1988). The fundus rises about 1 cm per week after the twelfth week. When it reaches the umbilicus, 20 weeks should have elapsed; when it reaches the xiphoid process, 36 weeks should have elapsed. Another quick and simple means to determine DD is by using the birthing wheel (Figure 9-14).

A more precise estimation is possible by *ultrasound evaluation* of the biparietal diameter of the fetal head or

FIGURE 9-14 Gestational age wheel makes calculation easy. (Courtesy Tokos Medical Corp., Los Angeles, Calif.)

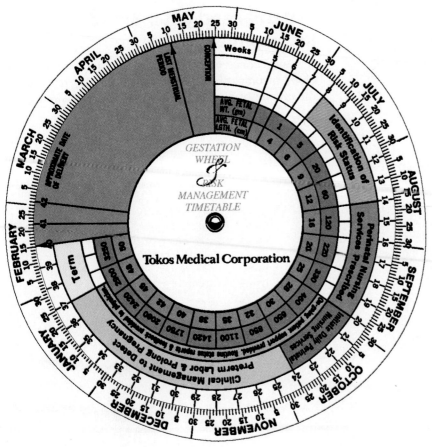

BOX 9-3   Definitions

- *Gravidity (gravida):* The number of times a woman has ever been pregnant.
- *Primigravida:* A woman pregnant for the first time
- *Multigravida:* A woman who has been pregnant more than once
- *Parity (para):* Pregnancies carried 20 weeks or longer. The infant is considered viable (whether alive or stillborn)
- *Nullipara:* A woman pregnant for the first time but undelivered
- *Primipara:* A woman who has had one delivery of a viable infant
- *Multipara:* A woman who has had two or more deliveries of viable infants

of the length of the femur (see Chapter 11). Commonly performed at 16 weeks by use of a table of expected measurements, ultrasound evaluation is accurate to ±6 days. In any case the woman should know that the EDB is approximate so she will not worry unnecessarily.

Crown to rump measure.

Test Yourself

- Amy Jones wants to know when she will have her baby. The ultrasound examination shows a biparietal diameter consistent for 16 weeks of development. What can you explain about the DD?

TERMINOLOGY OF PREGNANCY

Terms are used in obstetrics to refer to a woman's obstetric history (Box 9-3). **Gravidity** means that a woman has conceived a baby or has been pregnant, regardless of the length of time she is or was pregnant; it refers only to the number of conceptions, not to the number of babies born. **Parity** refers to the delivery of any fetus older than 20 to 24 weeks. If a woman miscarried before week 20 of gestation, it is recorded with her gravidity but not in her parity. Parity does not refer to the number of babies, just the number of times a woman has delivered. Thus multiple births still count as one parity.

In an effort to clarify and provide more detail in describing obstetric history, a second system was developed. In this system, parity is listed in four categories:

Full-term (F/T) delivery: 38+ weeks
Preterm (P) delivery: 20 to 37 completed weeks
Abortion (A): loss of pregnancy before viability (spontaneous or elective)
Living offspring (L): number of children, whether or not living with the family (covers multiple gestations).

If a child has died, however, the notation will seem inaccurate, and additional comments must be made to explain the (L) column. Occasionally a fifth column is added to detail the outcome of multiple pregnancies. Try transferring between systems for the examples in Box 9-4.

Maternal and Fetal Blood Incompatibility

A major concern during pregnancy is maternal-fetal blood incompatibility. An antigen-antibody reaction to the mixing of fetal blood into the maternal circulation

BOX 9-4   Comparison of Gravidity and Parity

Case A: A woman is pregnant; she has had one delivery at term, and this child is living.
Case B: A woman is not pregnant; she has had one delivery at term, one abortion (spontaneous or induced), and has one living child.
Case C: A woman is pregnant; she has had three deliveries at term, one preterm delivery, and two abortions. She has four living children.
Case D: A woman is not pregnant; she has had one preterm delivery (at 33 weeks) and has two living children.

	SYSTEM 1		SYSTEM 2 (PARITY ONLY)			
Case	Gravidity	Parity	Term	Preterm	Abortion	Living
A	II	I	1	0	0	1
B	II	I	1	0	1	1
C	VII	IV	3	1	2	4
D	I	I	0	1	0	2 (twins)

may occur in the same way that a reaction to a poorly typed blood transfusion may occur. The mechanism of becoming sensitized or forming antibodies against antigens from the same species is *isoimmunization,* or alloimmunization. When two parents have different blood types, their infant may inherit from the father an RBC group that differs from the mother's. As a result, specific antibodies may be produced in the mother's serum if the fetal erythrocytes enter her system, and these antibodies can cross the placenta to destroy fetal erythrocytes.

RH FACTOR INCOMPATIBILITY

The Rh factor is a group made up of the C, D, and E factors of the red cell (there are more than 50 blood factors). In the United States the Rh group is referred to with CDE typing; other countries may refer to the Rh-Hr system (Table 9-3). The D factor (positive or dominant) is the major stimulus, although in rare instances the infant may be affected by C or E alone. (Refer to Chapter 27 to review the way parents' genes affect the infant.)

Because the Rh-negative cell group is inherited as a recessive trait, a child must inherit the same gene from both parents to show Rh negativity. This is why only approximately 15% of the white population in the United States has the Rh-negative factor. Incidence is lower in the African-American population (5%) and the Asian-American population (1%).

Mechanism

The placenta is usually an effective barrier to the transfer of fetal red blood cells. Minute breaks in the placental interface may occur in cases of infection of the placenta; trauma during abortion, ectopic pregnancy, or birth; or small tears occurring as the placenta separates from the wall of the uterus. Intermingling of maternal and fetal blood also may occur during or after amniocentesis. In another way an Rh-negative woman may build up

anti-Rh antibodies after receiving even a brief transfusion of Rh-positive blood. The antibody build-up is detrimental to an Rh-positive infant (Figure 9-15).

Prevention

The best solution is prevention of the initial reaction. Today, few cases of Rh incompatibility are seen in women who receive adequate medical care during their reproductive lives. Women, particularly those who have immigrated from other countries or have received little or no prenatal care during a prior pregnancy, need to be screened early in pregnancy.

Coombs' test. The Coombs' test detects the presence of antibodies in maternal serum (indirect Coombs') or detects if antibodies are attached to the infant's red blood cells (direct Coombs'). A woman with Rh-negativity is tested early in pregnancy and is retested several times during the pregnancy. If she is sensitized already (has Rh D antibodies), her antibody titer is checked frequently. An increase in the titer indicates that the process is continuing and the fetus will be in jeopardy unless intervention occurs.

Passive immunization. Passive immunization is performed to prevent isoimmunization of the Rh-negative woman who bears an Rh-positive fetus. A serum concentrate containing pooled anti-Rh D antibodies (immune globulin) is administered after a potential "insult" or infusion of fetal blood into the maternal system. These extrinsic antibodies (not the mother's) will "recognize" the antigen (RhD) and begin the destruction of the foreign fetal cells. The maternal system then is protected from receiving an imprint, a code to make such antibodies again. The woman must be reimmunized each time a fetal or maternal transfusion occurs, after an abortion of any kind, after amniocentesis, and within 48 to 72 hours of a live birth or stillbirth (especially after a cesarean birth). Currently, each woman also receives Rho(D) immune globulin at 28 weeks. It may also be given at 34 weeks of gestation to protect the mother and fetus (Thornton et al, 1989).

Dosages of immune globulin may vary according to the estimate of fetal transfusion. This may be confirmed by maternal blood testing by use of the Fetaldex or Kleihauer-Betke test to determine the presence and amount of fetal red blood cells. The woman's blood is crossmatched with the dose, and the immune globulin is given by deep intramuscular injection using the Z-track method. There should be no side effects. The woman is given complete information about her condition and the injection and takes home a card with the date of immunization. Administration of Rho(D) immune globulin is a standard of care, and omission by neglect or error constitutes malpractice (see Chapter 30 and Drug Profile 9-1).

TABLE 9-3 **Typing of Rh Groups**

GROUP	CDE TYPING
POSITIVE	
Rh 1	D
Rh 2	C
Rh 3	E
NEGATIVE	
Rh 4	c
Rh 5	e

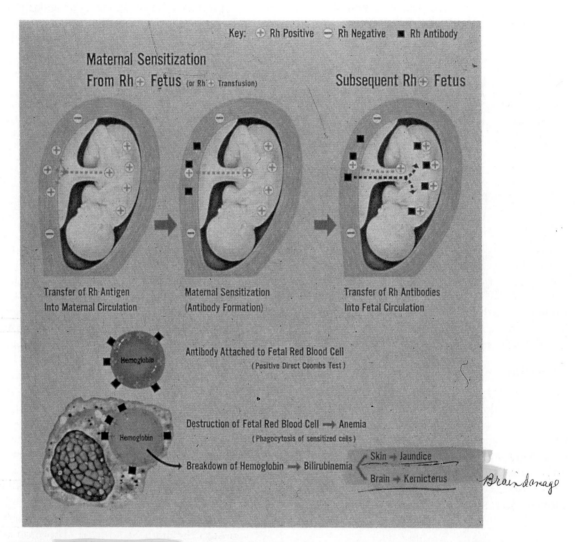

FIGURE 9-15 Rh incompatibility. (Used with permission of Ross Laboratories, Columbus, Ohio. From Clinical Education Aid No. 9, © Ross Laboratories.)

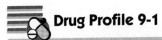

Drug Profile 9-1

Rh (D) immune globulin (RhIG)

(RhoGAM, Gamulin Rh, HypRho-D, WinRho)

Action: Suppresses reaction of Rh-negative woman exposed to Rh-positive blood cells in transfusion or across placenta from an Rh-positive fetus. Prevents isoimmunization after spontaneous or elective abortion, ectopic pregnancy, amniocentesis; routinely given at 28 weeks of pregnancy if father is Rh-positive. Must be given to women with Rh and Coombs' negativity as soon as possible after childbirth, usually within 24 to 48 hours, but always before 72 hours. Blood type is cross-matched, and blood bank reports eligibility status.

Dose/route: Deep intramuscular injection by Z track
Prophylaxis: At 28 weeks' pregnancy—one vial (300 μg); may also be given at 34 weeks.
After abortion, miscarriage <13 weeks: one MICRhoGAM (50 μg) dose
After ectopic pregnancy or amniocentesis, abortion >13 weeks: one vial (300 μg)
After birth: As early as possible, before 72 hours with negative Coombs' reaction and and Rh-positive infant: one vial (300 μg)
Betke-Kleihauer stain will assess amount of fetal RBC in maternal circulation, and dosage may be adjusted accordingly.

Side effects/adverse effects: Only local warmth, aching; very rare allergic reaction

Precautions: Inform woman of dosage, and give ID card. Drug is needed during and after each pregnancy if baby shows Rh positivity.

? dose ? for C-sections

If a woman has a positive Coombs' titer, it is *too late* to prevent isoimmunization. A positive indirect Coombs' result means that her body is already producing antibodies against the fetal Rh factor.

ABO INCOMPATIBILITY

So far no procedure exists for preventing ABO incompatibility. There are no blood or amniotic fluid tests to distinguish between naturally present a or b agglutinins (antibodies) in an O mother's serum and an increased titer resulting from introduction of fetal red blood cells with A or B antigens. Fortunately ABO incompatibility usually is less severe because maternal natural antibodies are weaker in hemolytic effect than are Rh antibodies. No special testing is performed before birth.

Genetic inheritance of one factor from each parent leads to six possible genotypes in the ABO blood groups:

TABLE 9-4   ABO Antigen Placement

TYPE	ANTIGEN IN RED CELL	ANTIBODIES IN PLASMA *maternal*
O	None	Anti-A, anti-B
A	A	Anti-B
B	B	Anti-A
AB	A and B	None

Homozygous	Heterozygous
OO	AO
AA	BO
BB	AB

The antibody in the serum depends on the antigen in the red cell. For example, if a person has type B antigen, anti-A antibodies are in the serum (Table 9-4).

This problem is more frequent in the type O mother because she already possesses a and b agglutinins (that is, anti-A and anti-B antibodies), which may cross the placental barrier and interact with the A or B factors in the erythrocytes of the fetus. Interestingly, when Rh and ABO incompatibility exists, anti-A or anti-B antibodies in the maternal serum usually suppress her production of Rh antibodies.

ABO may account for about two thirds of the maternal isoimmunization that leads to neonatal problems, but the effects are less severe. Three combinations are possible:

Mother	Infant
O	A, B, or AB
A	B
B	A

most common

Problems occur most frequently with an O mother and an A infant, less commonly with the O mother and B infant, and very rarely in the other combinations.

Newborns who are affected by either Rh or ABO incompatibility will show evidence of problems by a positive direct Coombs' test result and will have jaundice in the first 3 days of life. (See Chapter 18 and 28 for assessment and care of these infants.)

In every case of an Rh-negative woman's care during pregnancy, birth, and recovery the following measures must be ensured.

1. Check mother's blood type and Rh factor on clinic laboratory reports.
2. With Rh-negative status, alert midwife or physician; flag chart to note Coombs' test administration and results.
3. If invasive procedure is performed during pregnancy (amniocentesis, chorionic villus sampling), ensure that immune globulin is given on schedule.

(Caution for jaundice)

4. After abortion at any week, ensure that immune globulin is given on schedule.
5. Alert labor and postpartal nursing staff to woman's Rh and Coombs' titer status.

Nursing Responsibilities in Prenatal Care

Each pregnancy is special and unique for the woman and her partner. They bring to the pregnancy their own concepts, feelings, and, with second or third pregnancies, previous positive or negative experiences. The prenatal period is a time for the couple to correct misconceptions regarding pregnancy and childbirth. Anticipatory guidance—assessment of maternal and fetal status—makes a significant difference in a healthy outcome. Assessment should include psychosocial factors that may place stress on the family (discussed in Chapter 8), as well as the couple's response to the pregnancy. The physiologic adjustments are only part of the assessment.

Providing an atmosphere for open communication allows the woman to explore feelings and gain knowledge about self-care and new role demands. The nurse works in partnership, engaging the woman in self-monitoring, including reporting minor discomforts or warning signals. Such an increase in knowledge also will benefit her future health care because she understands the importance of nutrition, exercise, weight gain, and protection from hazards. For many women, prenatal care is their first entry since childhood into such an assessment and opportunity for health education.

Assessment of cultural differences is a factor—whether the woman's practices are neutral, functional, or dysfunctional (see Chapter 2). It is especially important to ascertain if the woman would be most comfortable seeing a woman health care practitioner and if the partner wants to participate in the pregnancy and birth. If the woman can see the same health care professional at each visit, she has the opportunity of developing rapport and may discuss problems, questions, and needs more openly.

Preventive care obtained though regular visits is the key to improved outcomes. Assessment can be accomplished and early problems identified. In particular, women at risk of premature labor may be identified and counseled. As couples become partners in care, they may enjoy the rhythm of life and anticipate the changes in roles.

▶ **ASSESSMENT**

Interview

The nurse interviews the client during her first visit to the clinic or office. If her reading level is adequate, she can respond to a questionnaire, which will save time. Because of the wide variation in ethnic groups, the nurse needs to develop considerable knowledge and cultural sensitivity to obtain useful data. Reluctance to answer some questions will be evident if the woman perceives that the information seems unnecessary to health care. Therefore the nurse may be able to gain her cooperation by fully explaining the purpose and use of the information.

All data gathered in the interview help to assist in determining the direction of the client's care. To individualize care the physician, midwife, and nurse need to know the woman's idiosyncrasies. Each woman requires counseling and teaching according to her particular life circumstances without generalizing or making assumptions.

Family history. *Family history* includes ethnic and cultural factors and family problems that may have a genetic or social impact on the woman and her pregnancy. The nurse asks about the current status of the family's health and immunizations, especially if there are children in the home, and whether any family members have chronic illnesses that the woman might develop during her pregnancy, for example, diabetes, hypertension, and certain anemias.

Health history. A woman's *health history* includes allergies, medications regularly used, and her immunizations and childhood diseases because infection and medications may be detrimental to the fetus. The physician will want to know if there has been any injury or surgery in the pelvic or abdominal area. Finally, knowledge of prior health problems in any body system provides aid in screening for current health and well-being.

Reproductive history. The *reproductive history* begins with menstrual history, including onset, duration each month, and interval. If a woman has discomfort with menses or if it began later than normal, the presence of hormonal imbalances should be considered. The nurse asks about prior pregnancies and any complications that developed during those pregnancies (GP/TPAL). The ages of any children should be recorded, as well as her contraceptive practices and whether or not this is a planned pregnancy. Specific details are important in eliciting history of exposure to sexually transmitted diseases.

Stress impact of STD during pregnancy

Current status. A woman's *current status* includes reasons for seeking care. What symptoms does she describe? In this section of the interview her birthplace, education, occupation, marital status, and support system are recorded. How does she perceive this pregnancy? What are her expectations of health care?

Social history. Her *social history* includes habits such as customary amount of drinking or smoking and use of drugs. Often this information is sought at the second visit rather than at the first, or it is asked again because the woman may have been tense and unsure about what the interviewer needed to know during the first visit. Information may be elicited about social and family factors that may complicate adjustment during pregnancy.

Physical Examination

For many healthy women, this may be the first physical examination as adults. Therefore explanations of each step will ease anxiety. The physical examination is performed by the physician or midwife during the first or second visit. If a confirming pregnancy test is needed, it is performed at the first visit, and the result is made available before the woman leaves.

Overall appearance. During the general examination, an overview of the whole person should be obtained. Does the woman look happy, sad, or depressed? Is she clean or dirty? Is she overweight or underweight? Is there a sense of alertness or does she seem less alert? Does she seem tired, harassed, or upset? The physical examination begins with the head and proceeds caudally; the vaginal examination is performed last.

Skin and hair. Skin and hair are assessed during the examination. Their condition gives clues to overall health. A skilled examiner can gain a general impression of adequate diet and self-care by observing color, turgor, and condition of the skin and quality of the hair.

Head, ears, eyes, nose, and throat. During a head, ears, eyes, nose, throat (HEENT) examination, funduscopy—examination of the fundus of the eye—may give clues to chronic diseases. Hypertensive or diabetic changes may be observed in the blood vessels in the fundus of the eye. Indications of anemia or infection may be seen in mucous membranes of the eyes, nose, and throat. Dental caries or gum problems may be observed in the mouth.

Neck and chest. Neck and chest examination yields information about the thyroid gland, lymph nodes of the axillary area, and neck. The breasts are examined for asymmetry, dimpling, and retraction of the nipple or skin surface. With the client supine, the breasts are palpated for masses. Every woman should be taught about breast self-examination. Later in pregnancy when breasts are enlarged, examination may not be valid, but teaching should take place.

Heart and lungs. The heart and lungs should be auscultated for irregularities in function. These findings and a medical history may permit diagnosis of a borderline cardiac condition.

Extremities. Extremities are examined for varicose veins and edema, signs of infection or restriction of movement are noted, and pulses and color in the extremities are checked.

Abdomen. Abdominal examination is performed to find any tenderness or masses. The size and shape of the uterus and the fundus usually are measured during each visit to permit recording of the rate of fetal growth (see Figure 4-4). Clients often are very tense about abdominal palpation and need help in relaxing.

Pelvic examination. A pelvic examination is performed with the woman placed in lithotomy position. The external genitalia are examined for lesions, scars, or infection. A vaginal speculum is inserted to provide a clear view of the cervix (see Figure 4-4). The color and condition of cervix and amount of *leukorrhea* are observed. At this time a Pap smear is obtained to screen for cervical cancer cells. A specimen of cervical mucus for detection of infections such as gonorrhea also is taken. The speculum is removed, and a bimanual examination is performed to determine pelvic and uterine size.

Pelvic measurements. *Pelvic measurements* are obtained, including the *biischial diameter,* the distance between the ischial tuberosities (normally 8 cm or more), and the *diagonal conjugata,* the distance between the lower margin of the pubic bone to the promontory of the sacrum (normally 11.5 cm or more). Measurements of the birth canal are discussed in detail in Chapter 13.

After completion of the examination, the health care provider will discuss the findings with the woman and make recommendations for self-care. Screening tests will be arranged and referrals made for anticipatory instruction, nutritional care, or social service involvement. It is important to encourage the woman to voice her concerns.

Vital Signs

The nurse records vital signs during every visit. BP is the most important indication of a potential problem. An

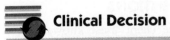

Clinical Decision

Marie Rodriguez comes to the clinic with a friend for her first prenatal visit. She is given a questionnaire to complete but stares at it for a long time without writing. You come back to collect the form and find it empty. What would you do next?

early baseline reading is essential for comparison with later changes. A slight drop in pressure is expected in the first half of pregnancy, with a return to normal or slightly above baseline in the last trimester. An elevation above baseline of 30 points systolic and 15 points diastolic or an elevated MAP reading may indicate hypertension or preeclampsia. If BP is elevated, the nurse checks for signs of headache, dizziness, epistaxis, and increased edema in the extremities (see Chapter 22).

Screening Tests

Problems will be detected by screening tests performed during prenatal visits. Table 9-5 lists the most frequently performed tests.

Blood tests. Blood tests include a complete blood count. Hct is repeated at 32 to 36 weeks. If the reading is 32% or less, a complete work-up is performed for anemia and intestinal ova and parasites. Folic acid, 1 mg, and ferrous gluconate are prescribed.

Blood is tested for AB or O categories and the Rh factor. The partner's type should be ascertained if possible because of the potential for incompatibility of type between mother and fetus. If the client is Rh negative, the Coombs' test is done. If antibody titer is negative at 28 weeks, RhD immune globulin is given and repeated at 34 weeks.

Genetic screening. Screening for genetically carried diseases is performed routinely for sickle cell trait and for determination of other problems such as *thalassemia* and *glucose-6-phosphate dehydrogenase* (G-6-PD) *deficiency* (see Chapters 22 and 23).

Screening for *glucose* is done in several ways. If there is a history of diabetes or if any risk factors are present, the woman is tested for hemoglobin A_{1c}, which would indicate a history of hyperglycemia. If the test result is positive, the woman will be tested for the onset of diabetes. All women are tested at 28 weeks with a 1-hour glucose load test to determine if gestational diabetes is developing (see Chapter 24).

Urine tests. For urine tests a fresh urine specimen is obtained and a urine test strip is used during each visit (and may be performed by the woman herself as part of her participation in care). Screening for glucose and protein provides approximate results but indicates if further testing is required. Urinalysis determines cells, casts, and specific gravity. If there are any signs of infection, a careful midstream, clean-catch voided specimen for testing is preferable to a catheterized specimen.

Infection screening. There are various screens for infections (see Chapter 25). The rubella titer determines if the woman is susceptible to rubella. If, for example, her titer is below 1:10, she must be immunized after the pregnancy is over. Recently the number of tuberculosis cases has risen. It is especially important that women in susceptible populations be screened by skin test and a chest x-ray obtained if the test result is positive. Finally, the presence of any STD must be discovered. Syphilis, gonorrhea, and *Chlamydia* tests are done routinely. Human immunodeficiency virus (HIV) tests also may be performed, with consent, especially for high-risk populations. Routine toxoplasmosis screening during pregnancy is not currently recommended unless definite exposure has occurred (see Chapter 25). *Can cause birth defects*

▶ NURSING DIAGNOSES

Nursing diagnoses relating to the pregnancy process include the following:
1. Health-seeking behaviors regarding self-care during pregnancy and fetal health
2. Knowledge deficit related to pregnancy process and labor expectations
3. Sleep-pattern disturbance related to discomforts of pregnancy
4. High risk for injury related to environmental toxins, pharmaceuticals, Rh incompatibility, or adverse responses to exercise

▶ EXPECTED OUTCOMES

The following examples of expected outcomes of prenatal care are discussed in this chapter:
1. Participates in prenatal care and follows through on referrals
2. Describes alterations in health maintenance
3. Follows health practices that demonstrate new knowledge
4. Recognizes and reports occurrence of warning signs
5. Describes ways of avoiding potential hazards during pregnancy; reports the faithful use of seat belts
6. Evidences preparation for birth and infant care; involves partner

▶ NURSING INTERVENTIONS

To perform self-care, the client must know what is important for health. A woman in her first pregnancy usually is unaware of health maintenance unless she has read literature or is a member of an extended family and has observed other pregnant women. She needs **anticipatory guidance** about the events of each trimester and the growth patterns of the baby (Figure 9-16). People learn in different ways and learning may be

TABLE 9-5   Screening Tests during Pregnancy

TEST	RESULTS AND COMMENTS
COMPLETE BLOOD CELL COUNT	
Hemoglobin	Measured as g/dl. May drop to 11.5 g/dl later in pregnancy because of increase of plasma in ratio to RBCs.
Hematocrit	Volume of RBCs in 100 ml blood, measured in a percentage; 33% is lowest acceptable level.
Mean corpuscular volume	Average volume of individual RBC; below average indicates some types of anemia.
RBC count	Number of RBCs in each microliter of blood. In pregnancy, hemodilution level may drop to 3.75 million/mm^3
WBC count	Neutrophils (50%), lymphocytes (21%-35%), monocytes (4%), basophils (0.3%), eosinophils (2.7%). Total count is 7000-10,000/mm^3. Rises to 18,000 by late pregnancy in preparation for the healing process after birth.
Hemoglobin electrophoresis	Determines sickle cell trait.
GLUCOSE	
Hemoglobin A$_{1c}$	Less than 3.5% is normal; if over, indicates hyperglycemia within 6 weeks. Used to identify diabetic problems.
1-hr 50-g glucose load test	Load at 28 weeks; if 1-hr level is under 135, it is normal. If over, then glucose tolerance testing is done.
BLOOD TYPE (ABO)	Check partner's blood type and potential for incompatibility.
Rh factor	Indirect Coombs' should remain negative.
Coombs' test	Retested at 28 weeks in Rh-negative woman.
INFECTION*	
Rubella titer	Less than 1:8—immunize after birth. If titer more than 1:128 in early pregnancy, repeat test.
STD: serum	
Venereal Disease Research Laboratory (VDRL) or fluorescent treponemal antibody absorption (FTA-ABS) test	False positive results may occur with VDRL. FTA-ABS specific for antitreponemal antibodies. Repeat VDRL at 32 weeks.
STD: vaginal and cervical smear	Gram stain or enzyme-linked immunosorbent assay
Gonorrhea	(ELISA) test; repeat at 28 weeks.
Chlamydia	Direct examination of smear on slide.
Gram-positive Streptococcus	Direct slide examination.
Hepatitis B surface antigen	Hepatitis B virus–infected infant can be treated if mother is diagnosed early.
Tuberculosis	Screen for tuberculosis.
Skin tests: Tine, Mantoux	X-ray examination performed after positive finding.
URINE	
Glucose, ketones	Urinalysis performed during each visit. Catch clean, mid-stream specimen for culture if cells present.
Albumin	
Cells: leukocyte, red blood cells, bacteria casts	
Specific gravity	

*Some physicians also check all women for toxoplasmosis. See Chapter 25 for complete discussion of infection.
RBC, Red blood cell; *WBC,* white blood cell.

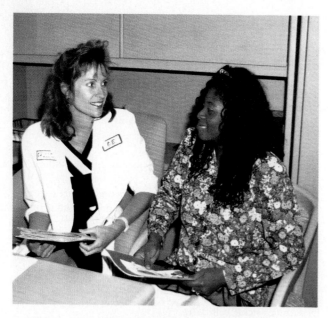

FIGURE 9-16 Expectant mother and nurse discuss prenatal care concerns. (Courtesy Marjorie Pyle, RNC, *Lifecircle*.)

inhibited for a number of reasons. The skill to work with women of various backgrounds or with those who speak English as a second language is a requirement.

Women are asked to monitor themselves, and the nurse emphasizes these self-monitoring activities, including regular weighing and noting and reporting any difficulties. They are taught requirements for food and fluid intake and encouraged to report difficulties. Questions about labor onset or fetal condition are addressed in the last trimester, and the woman is taught to self-monitor contractions and fetal movements. An important part of helping the woman to self-monitor progress is a clear description of the warning signals of potential complications.

Warning Signs

Warning signals of problems other than normal minor discomforts should be taught early. If the warning signs are not taught, a woman may not report a pathologic change in her condition under the assumption that it is supposed to happen. Every pregnant woman should be taught to report the following *signs of premature labor* immediately:

1. *Bleeding.* Bleeding during pregnancy is abnormal. It may warn of impending abortion, a poorly implanted placenta, or a sudden separation of the placenta. A few women have vaginal bleeding from cervical erosion caused by chronic infection.
2. *Infection.* Signs of infection in any part of the body are warning signals, but during pregnancy, conditions that might affect fetal condition are especially serious. Fever, chills, and signs of kidney, bladder, or vaginal infection should be reported.
3. *Pain.* Pain is usually abnormal. Exceptions are the abdominal aching and perineal pressure of prelabor or a brief pain in the side caused by a pulling sensation of the round ligament. Occasionally, pain radiates through the groin or down the line of the sciatic nerve as a result of pressure on the nerves in the pelvic region.
4. *Preeclampsia.* Signs and symptoms related to developing preeclampsia are severe continuous headache; edema in the face, hands, or legs on arising in the morning; scanty, concentrated urine; visual disturbances, and epigastric pain. Any of these symptoms must be reported at once because hypertension can develop very rapidly.
5. *Severe nausea and vomiting.* Severe nausea and vomiting may escalate to cause ketosis, dehydration, and treatment for *hyperemesis*.

The pregnant woman should be taught the early signals of problems during the first trimester. These include bleeding or spotting, pain in the pelvic region, or cramping, which may indicate abortion or ectopic pregnancy, and should be reported immediately. Other areas of teaching include signs and symptoms of vaginal and urinary tract infection (see Chapter 4 for vaginal infections and Chapter 25 for urinary infections). The woman needs to know the difference between frequency caused by the changes of pregnancy and those of urinary infections, which are accompanied by fever, burning on urination, cloudy urine, dysuria, and occasionally blood-tinged urine (Box 9-5).

Women do best in self-care activities when they are asked to take responsibility. Effective compliance with clinic visits has been demonstrated by those women who have been given copies of their medical screening records (Diamond, 1990) (Figure 9-17). The results of each visit's activities—such as vital signs, urine tests, weight changes, and fetal assessment—are recorded. The woman receives the record at the first visit and is asked to bring it to each visit, including any emergency visit.

Sleep Patterns

Causes of sleep disturbance vary according to the trimester. Early in pregnancy, fatigue related to relaxin and other hormonal effects may lead the woman to take naps and then to be wakeful at night.

Later, discomforts of pregnancy interrupt rest. Nasal congestion is a major problem for some because of increased peripheral circulation to nasal tissues. Because use of antihistamines usually is not advised, humidified air may relieve breathing. When positional dyspnea occurs, the woman may use semi-Fowler's position for sleep. Use of extra pillows helps her to maintain a side-lying position. During later pregnancy the supine position must be avoided to prevent the supine hypotension syndrome (see Figure 9-3).

BOX 9-5 Prenatal Teaching Plan

First trimester
Describe pregnancy changes and minor discomforts

- Nausea, vomiting, ptyalism
- Breast tenderness and care
- Fatigue, rest and activity, frequency

Explain safety concerns

- Hazards in home and workplace
- Smoking, drugs, and alcohol cessation
- OTC drugs and vitamin precautions
- Hot tubs and dangers of hyperthermia

Discuss schedule of clinic visits and clinic resources

- Calculate EDC; discuss weight, nutrition
- Screening tests: tuberculosis, blood, urine

Interpret psychosocial adjustment and concerns
Identify warning signals

- Spotting, bleeding, cramping, pain
- Infection signs and symptoms

Second trimester
Describe pregnancy changes and minor discomforts

- Backache, constipation, hemorrhoids, varicose veins
- Hygiene, leukorrhea
- Breast changes and care

Discuss fetal growth and development
Discuss nutrition and weight management
Explain safety concerns

- Seat belts and travel
- Employment
- Exercise and activity

Identify reasons for screening tests

- MASFP, ultrasound, glucose load test

Interpret psychosocial concerns

- Sexuality and partner's concerns

Identify warning signals

- Bleeding, pain, leaking membranes
- Preterm labor signs and symptoms
- Hypertension

Third trimester
Describe pregnancy changes and minor discomforts

- Pressure symptoms: dependent edema, leg aches, leg cramps, round ligament pain
- Dyspnea, frequency, pyrosis

Identify screening tests: nonstress test (NST), biophysical profile
Discuss preparation for childbirth

- Planning for siblings, sibling classes
- Exercises, breathing, relaxation
- Birth plans
- Emergency arrangements for transport, child care

Explain safety concerns

- Review signs and symptoms of preterm labor/term labor
- Body mechanics/posture/positions in bed
- Exercise and activity, travel

Interpret psychosocial concerns

- Sexuality
- Support system for homecoming and care

If fatigue is related to anemia, the cause should be corrected, if possible. If fatigue is related to night wakefulness, the woman should be asked about feelings of anxiety, dreams, environmental noise, overfatigue during the day, muscle cramping, and nocturia.

A woman may have a life situation, such as work or several small children, that prevents a rest period during the day. She should be encouraged to analyze her situation to determine how to obtain additional rest. In this way she learns coping skills and may be able to solve the problem herself.

Hygiene

Hygiene during pregnancy may be a problem for some women because of increased oil and perspiration. Safety during bathing should be emphasized. The most important point to discuss is maintaining balance. Tub and shower baths may be taken up to the time of birth, but a woman may find it awkward to move in and out of a tub because of the altered center of gravity.

Reinforcing good dental hygiene is important. Dental plaque should be removed by floss once a day and teeth brushed with a soft tooth brush to prevent injury to tender or bleeding gums.

Preventing Hazards

Every pregnant woman should be informed regarding the dangers of self-medication (see Chapter 16) and cautioned that home remedies may contain substances that can affect the infant. She should be asked to list any OTC and prescription medications she takes.

OTC drugs. Drugs for pain relief are available OTC. *Acetaminophen* is the only analgesic medication recommended during pregnancy and lactation (and for children). It works as an antiprostaglandin but has less antiinflammatory effect than aspirin or ibuprofen. It is also an antipyretic, producing peripheral vasodilation through action on the heat-regulating center. Listed in risk category B (see Table 27-6), the drug should not be taken often because it is metabolized in the liver, crosses the placenta, and is metabolized by the fetal liver as well. Drug interactions must be observed. With caffeine combinations, central nervous system stimulation is increased. Laboratory test readings for glucose may be reduced, and prothrombin time and bilirubin concentrations may be increased.

Acetylsalicylic acid (ASA) may be found in many OTC combinations (more than 400). This drug is not recommended during pregnancy and is classified as risk category C (see Table 27-6) because of potential harm to the developing fetus. When the drug crosses the placenta, its anticoagulant action results in a reduction in clotting time and in fetal bleeding. The antiprostaglandin action may promote closure of the ductus arteriosus before birth and may prolong gestation and labor. In addition, the mother may have bleeding after delivery.

Nonsteroidal prostaglandin inhibitors (*ibuprofen*) are the newest analgesics. They inhibit prostaglandin synthesis and decrease inflammation by inhibiting local inflammatory responses. Women have discovered the effectiveness of these drugs for menstrual cramping and may be inclined to continue to use them during pregnancy. These drugs are not recommended because they prolong gestation and labor and may prematurely close the ductus arteriosus, acting somewhat like ASA.

Women should be encouraged to read the labels on all drugs and taught self-care and avoidance of drug-related hazards. OTC medications should be cleared with the physician before use. A woman will be more sensitive to drug effects during pregnancy because of changes in her metabolic rate. Therefore she should

BRIGHAM AND WOMEN'S HOSPITAL
A Teaching Affiliate of Harvard Medical School
75 Francis Street, Boston, Massachusetts 02115

Ambulatory Services
Monday – Friday 8:00 am to 4:30 pm

Phone: ____________________

After 4:30 pm and on weekends call
732-6987, ask for

OB ____________________ on call.

Site: Health Care Provider:

LMP: EDC DATES: EDC U/S: EDC CORRECTED:

Test	Date	Result	Test	Date	Result	Test	Date	Result
Bld. tpe. & Rh			HCT			3rd Δ HCT		
Anti-bodies			HBsAg					
Serology			Urine C & S					
Rubella			Sickle Prep					
G/C			GLT					
Pap			GTT					
PPD								
AFP								
U/S Dates								
Presentation								
Placenta								
Fluid volume								
G.A.								
Wt.								
BPP								
Other								

A

FIGURE 9-17 **A,** The front of the prenatal medical record precis.

CONTACT THE HOSPITAL AT ONCE IF YOU HAVE —

1. Any vaginal bleeding.
2. Persistent severe headaches.
3. Swelling of ankles, legs or face.
4. Nausea or vomting.
5. When your labor pains come every ten minutes.
6. If your water breaks even though you are not yet in labor.
7. If in doubt, phone doctor at hospital.

PONGASE EN CONTACTO CON EL HOSPITAL SI USED TIENE —

1. Derrame Vaginal.
2. Dolores de cabeza fuertes.
3. Hinchazon de los tobillos, piernas, o de la cara.
4. Nauseas o Vomito.
5. Cuando le den los dolores de parto cada diez minutos.
6. Si se rompe la bolsa de agua sin tener dolores de parto.
7. Si Tiene Alguna Duda Llame El Medico En El Hospital.

OB HISTORY

# Pregnancies	Illnesses
	Past
	Present

OB Problems	Current Meds
Past	
Present	Allergies

Other Delivery Needs

☐ MMR Post Partum   ☐ Booked C/S   ☐ Desires VBAC
☐ PPS Signed   ☐ PPS Post Partum   ☐ Rhogam
☐ Social Service _____

B

FIGURE 9-17, cont'd B, The back of the prenatal medical record precis. C, The inside of the prenatal medical record precis. (This is a duplication of the prenatal flow sheet.) (Courtesy Frieda B. Diamond and Antenatal Diagnostic Center, Brigham and Women's Hospital, Boston, Mass.)

Name: _____   G   P   AGE: LMP: CORRECTED EDC:

DATE	GEST AGE	WGT.	BP	PROT/ GLU	FHR/ Pres.	FUNDAL HEIGHT	EDEMA	FETAL ACTIV.	TREATMENT/REMARKS	SIG.

C

check dosages with the physician. This is especially true for a woman who must take insulin or other medications for chronic diseases.

Women have read about teratogenic substances and may ask about drug safety. In addition, substances and chemicals in the work and home environment are a source of concern. (See Chapter 10 for discussion of cigarettes, alcohol, coffee, and saccharine and Chapter 27 for hazards of drug abuse.)

Work precautions. Despite the fact that 60% to 65% of women between the ages of 18 and 64 have jobs, there is still no uniform policy on pregnancy and recovery leave in the United States. Therefore work during pregnancy is a major issue. Working conditions for women vary throughout the country, and each job causes potential difficulties. Women who work on assembly lines and farms, for example, may have to perform heavy lifting, whereas teachers, nurses, and other health-related workers spend most of their day on their feet. These women also may be exposed to chemical and environmental hazards. Even a "safe" position as secretary or office worker may cause problems because of long periods of sitting, standing, or working at computer terminals. Neck, back, and eye strain are major complaints, and there is growing concern about possible effects on the fetus of low-level magnetic field emissions emanating from elements that coat video display terminals (Blackwell and Chang, 1988). See Chapter 27 for reproductive hazards in the workplace.

The Occupational Safety and Health Administration (OSHA) has published guidelines for hazards in the workplace. Women who are concerned are encouraged to check that the employer has received and is following these guidelines (Bernhardt, 1990).

It is now acceptable and expected that a woman continue to work while pregnant. This may be a satisfying or an exhausting experience for the woman, depending on physical fitness, discomforts, and stress of the job. Many women worry about endangering or even losing their positions when they need to take extra time off for complications or even normal maternity leave. Often it is only when this extra time is needed that the woman finds that her job does not provide enough sick leave. This may be especially true for women with prior health problems or low-income work situations that traditionally offer few or no health care benefits. For the woman whose financial situation demands work, stress and fear of losing her job may prevent compliance with prescribed regimens of rest and treatment (Figure 9-18).

The woman should be asked about her job, including its responsibilities, environment, and sick and maternity leave policies. She should be encouraged to plan realistically to maintain her financial security while caring for herself and her child. If there is or may be a serious problem, referral to social services for assistance and guidance is appropriate.

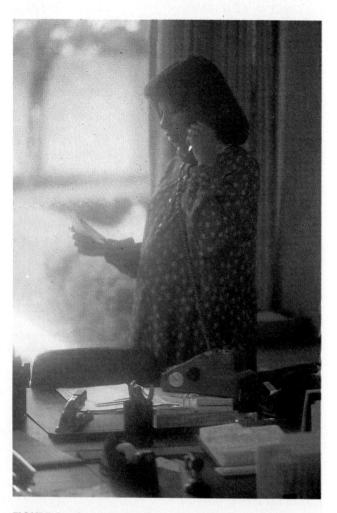

FIGURE 9-18 Many women work throughout the entire pregnancy. Rest periods are important and provide a chance to elevate the legs for several periods during the day. (Courtesy Ross Laboratories, Columbus, Ohio.)

Rest periods with legs elevated whenever possible should be encouraged, and support hose should be worn when the woman must stand for long periods. If she sits for most of the day, she should change position frequently, walk, or elevate her legs on a stool.

Hyperthermia. Heat may be a hazard to the developing embryo in the first trimester because it cannot be dissipated if the mother has hyperthermia. The fetus already is 0.5° to 1° F warmer than the mother; thus a fever could cause adverse fetal effects. Offspring of laboratory test animals that had suffered hyperthermia developed smaller brains and learning dysfunction (Smith, Edwards, and Upfold, 1986). Thus it is indicated that a woman should not allow a temperature elevation above 103° F (38.9° C) during the critical time of organogenesis, the first 12 weeks of pregnancy (Smith, Edwards, Upfold, 1986).

Hyperthermia may result from excessive aerobic exercise, use of a sauna or hot tub, and fever. As a result of vasodilation, most pregnant women report that they feel warmer and usually do not choose to voluntarily become warmer. In climates that are humid and warm, however, special efforts should be taken to maintain a lower temperature. Antipyretics such as acetaminophen and cooling sponge baths are used to reduce body temperature during illness.

Infection. Women must understand that infection may adversely affect the fetus. Information should be provided from the beginning regarding STDs, other vaginal infections, and urinary infections. Primary prevention avoids exposure (see Chapter 25).

Immunizations should be checked. If a woman is unprotected against rubella, she should be scheduled for inoculation after childbirth and should avoid exposure during pregnancy, particularly in the first trimester. Exposure is more common than would be expected because so many children are not immunized adequately. She will not be immunized with vaccinations that contain live attenuated preparations.

Because of vaginal changes during pregnancy, the presence of *Lactobacillus* species increases and anaerobic bacteria decrease. Increased vaginal secretions may become a problem. The woman may have to wear a pant liner because of leukorrhea. If leukorrhea is odorous, discolored, or causes itching or pain, the physician should be notified and treatment prescribed. Douching should not be done without the physician's recommendation, and tampons, feminine deodorants, and suppositories are prohibited. Perineal care should relieve any discomfort.

During each visit the woman should be queried about the status of vaginal or urinary infections because recurrence is common. The common vaginal infections, *Trichomonas* and *Candida*, are most troublesome during pregnancy (see Chapter 4). A recent study reported that monilial spores are not destroyed by normal laundry temperatures and thus may remain on underwear to reinfect the woman. These findings lead to recommendations for microwaving wet cotton underwear (for 5 minutes on a high setting) or using a hot iron before wearing them when a monilial infection is being treated (Friedrick and Phillips, 1988).

Travel and Accidents

After midpregnancy, trips of more than 2 to 3 hours by car, train, or plane are unwise because of prolonged sitting. If a trip must be made, the woman should change positions frequently and, when possible, walk to promote circulation. Prolonged sitting or standing is related to a marked increase in sodium retention, a change initiated by the postural effect on renal blood flow. Sodium retention leads to water retention and edema. Compression of the veins leading from the legs also occurs, with elevated femoral venous pressure and edema.

Automobile accidents are the leading reason for maternal mortality unrelated to pregnancy. The woman restrained by a seat belt comes to a stop with the car, rather than leaving the seat and flying through the windshield or door. This force is dissipated more evenly when a seat belt is used correctly (see Trauma, Chapter 23).

Seat belts. It is possible to sustain injury in an accident from the improper use of belts. Lap belts or shoulder belts should not be used alone. Lap belts used alone or not fastened below the abdominal bulge may cause injury from the pressure of the buckle; sudden flexion may cause injury to the intestines, spleen, kidneys, pancreas, stomach, bladder, and uterus. Shoulder belts used alone may injure the ribs, spine, neck, or sternum.

In contrast, injuries tend to be minor with the three-point belt. These injuries include lacerations on the shoulder area, thighs, or chest. The three-point belt is by far the safest restraint system. In addition to use of this belt, the headrest should be adjusted correctly to avoid whiplash (Schoenfeld et al, 1987).

Every pregnant woman should be told about the correct method of applying a seat belt. The restraint should be a lap belt worn as low as possible over the pelvic bones and below the abdominal bulge. The strap across the shoulder, chest, and upper abdomen should be firm but comfortable. A pad may be attached to the shoulder strap if the belt touches the side of her neck (Figure 9-19). The woman should be questioned about consistent seat belt use and introduced to guidelines for infant car seats (see Chapter 20).

Clinical Decision

During the prenatal visit at 24 weeks, Hannah asks whether she should continue working as a secretary. Give the rationale for and debate the pros and cons of the following statements:

a. *Sitting without moving or walking at intervals adversely affects venous circulation in the lower extremities.*

b. *If a woman is able, she needs time at home to adapt to the developmental tasks of pregnancy.*

c. *Women today are in better condition than ever, and working is not a health hazard as long as the woman gets enough rest.*

d. *Pregnant women are self-involved in the last part of pregnancy and do not concentrate well for long periods.*

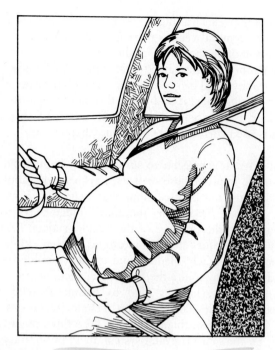

FIGURE 9-19 Proper use of seat belt and headrest. (From Bobak IM, Jensen MD: *Maternity and gynecologic care: the nurse and the family,* ed 5, St Louis, 1993, Mosby.)

Referrals

Before the end of their first or second visit, women receive referrals to the dentist to provide dental screening for those whose teeth may be neglected, to prevent decay if sufficient calcium is not ingested, and to obtain an assessment of dental health from the beginning of pregnancy. Dental health contributes toward her total health status.

In clinic care, referrals are made to the social worker for assistance with family or economic concerns. The nutritionist also is available for women who are overweight or underweight and for those with chronic diabetes, hypotension, hypertension, or anemia (see Chapter 10).

Revisits

The interval for subsequent visits may vary. The usual pattern is one visit per month until week 32, after which visits are scheduled according to the woman's progress. Most physicians schedule weekly visits during the last few weeks. (For psychosocial care see Chapter 8 and for nutritional care see Chapter 10.)

Summary of Nursing Interventions during Prenatal Care

- Introduce yourself to the client and partner, and welcome them to the beginning of prenatal care. Help them feel that care will be individualized.
- During the interview, listen to the woman's responses to identify unspoken concerns. Foster communication between staff members and couple.

- Ask personal and potentially awkward questions (about family matters, use of adverse substances) in a nonthreatening, nonjudgmental manner.
- Explain sequences of the visit and all procedures. Begin Care Plan.
- Stay with the woman during the vaginal examination if the physician is male. Find a female care giver if the woman indicates that care by a male is unacceptable. Protect her privacy, and identify cultural roots of any problems she expresses concerning the examinations.
- Be aware of cultural differences that may affect care in pregnancy and labor. Discuss these with client, making sure she understands instructions that do not counteract her cultural patterns. If practices conflict with her customs or practices, work with her to find neutral practices to substitute for routine instructions on nutrition, activities, and hygiene.
- Describe self-care activities such as urine testing and weighing. Include rationale for monitoring during pregnancy. Begin prenatal record for client to keep.
- Explain warning signals. Provide the client with the clinic telephone number and 24-hour telephone number.
- Discuss minor changes of accommodation and discomforts. Discuss nonpharmacologic interventions she may use.
- See partners together some time during each visit to answer questions and observe responses. Elicit from partner his feelings about participation in labor and birth support.
- Make referrals to other health professionals, dentist, nutritionist, social worker. Set up appointments while the client is in clinic.
- Refer the client and partner to childbirth education classes, or provide them in your setting. Give literature in client's own language.
- Discuss labor plans with couple. Ascertain if there are birth plans they feel are important to them.
- Introduce the need to make decisions about breast-feeding and infant circumcision. Provide literature.
- Keep the client informed of progress and results of testing.

▶ EVALUATION

A number of questions can be asked to evaluate the outcomes of the course of prenatal care.

- Were guidelines for health maintenance followed?
- Were deviations from normal promptly reported?
- Did dietary intake and exercise result in adequate weight gain and nutritional status, as well as soft stools?
- Did the client state that hazards were avoided and seat belts used at all times?
- Were plans discussed for labor and birth and recovery support?

NURSING CARE PLAN • Prenatal Care

CASE: Mary, age 18, and Leonard, age 20; first pregnancy. LMP Sept. 1; vital signs: temperature, pulse, respiration—98.8/80/24; BP 106/74; ht. 5 ft 6 in, wt. 106 lb; complains of "nauseated for a few weeks; wants to sleep all the time; takes naps after work and finds it hard to sleep at night between running to the bathroom and restlessness." Works at local fertilizer plant. Eats out often at fast food restaurants (mainly french fries and hamburgers). Has lost 2 lb in the last month. Smokes two packs/day. Drinks beer with coworkers after work.

ASSESSMENT DATA

1. History
   - Patient's age, parity
   - Knowledge of pregnancy—Signs and symptoms of pregnancy: possible and positive
     — Determine EDB
     — Assessing self-care activities regarding pregnancy
   - Role expectations
   - Support systems
2. Knowledge of minor discomforts in pregnancy
3. Knowledge of nutrition, diet habits
4. Knowledge of safety habits
   - Employment setting
   - Smoking
   - Alcohol

NURSING DIAGNOSES

1. Knowledge deficit regarding self-care in pregnancy related to inexperience
2. Sleep-pattern disturbance related to frequent daytime naps and nocturia
3. Altered nutrition: less than body requirements related to inadequate food intake as a result of nausea and poor eating habits
4. Injury, high risk for, related to nicotine, alcohol, and possible chemical inhalation in workplace

EXPECTED OUTCOMES

1. Actively participates in pregnancy-related care. Pregnancy monitoring progress and reporting warning signs promptly
2. Adjusts activities of daily living (ADL) to gain sufficient rest and sleep
3. Reports intake of adequate nutrients for sufficient weight gain
4. Reports reduction or cessation of smoking and drinking; negotiates work responsibilities and schedule to minimize hazards

NURSING RESPONSIBILITIES

1. Education
   - Discuss signs and symptoms of pregnancy and changes during pregnancy that precipitate minor discomforts.
   - Discuss nonpharmacologic remedies during pregnancy.
   - Discuss warning signals of pregnancy. Encourage prompt reporting.
   - Discuss support systems available.
   - Make referrals to appropriate departments.
2. Assist client to evaluate and to modify ADL—including nap times, limiting fluid intake in the evening, and work schedule—to ensure adequate rest
3. Nutrition
   - Obtain complete nutritional and diet history.
   - Discuss nutritional requirements of pregnancy and how to meet them.
   - Collaborate to develop a diet plan that will encourage adequate intake.
   - Refer to nutritionist if necessary.
4. Preventing hazards
   - Explain dangers of smoking and alcohol and possible workplace hazards to self and fetus.
   - Encourage reduction or elimination of hazards.
   - Encourage client to seek assistance if needed for these problems (such as Alcoholics Anonymous [AA]), and make referrals to appropriate agencies as needed.

Continued.

EVALUATION OF OUTCOMES

1. Did she monitor self-care and report problems promptly?
2. Did she report that she got adequate rest?
3. Does dietary diary indicate a nutritionally adequate diet as evidenced by appropriate weight gain and discussion of her dietary intake?
4. Does she report reduction in or elimination of her smoking and drinking behaviors?
5. Does she report employer cooperation regarding work environment and schedule?

KEY POINTS

- Changes in pregnancy are accomplished by the delicate balancing of bodily functions, that is, the changes of accommodation.
- Every body system is affected by the pregnancy and is under the influence of hormones of pregnancy.
- Minor discomforts occur as a result of the changes of accommodation, and women benefit from instruction that teaches them how their bodies work.
- Each woman should be taught self-monitoring techniques and given information that includes warning signs and record keeping.

- Increasing women's participation in self-care increases compliance with health maintenance behaviors and prenatal clinic visits.
- Safety from hazards related to employment, travel, home environment, and drug use is an important part of prenatal teaching.
- Warning regarding self-medication with OTC drugs should be given early in pregnancy.
- Individual instruction on activity and exercise is an important part of prenatal care.

STUDY QUESTIONS

9-1 Match key terms with the following statements:
   a. Darkened streaks on the abdomen or breasts *stria gravidarum*
   b. Low bacterial levels present in urine without discomfort *asymptomatic bacteriuria*
   c. Change in posture to keep balance during late pregnancy *lordosis*
   d. Change in blood pressure that causes lightheadedness when getting up *postural hypotension*
   e. Patchy darkened pigmentation on the face during late pregnancy *melasma*
   f. Darkened streak up center of abdomen *linea nigra*
   g. Number of times a woman has been pregnant *gravida*
   h. Acid indigestion *heart burn*

9-2 Hemodilution of pregnancy leads to the following signs in the woman:
   a. Slight elevation of BP in response to overload
   b. Decrease in Hct levels by the second trimester
   c. Supine hypotension in later pregnancy
   d. Reduction in pulse rate and increase in cardiac output

9-3 If at 34 weeks the client complains of flushed face, reddened palms, and nasal congestion, your counsel depends on knowledge of the following:
   a. These signs indicate increasing hypertension.

   b. All women do not get melasma, which will recede postpartum.
   c. This is an unusual complaint during pregnancy and needs follow-up.
   d. Symptoms result from increased peripheral circulation.

9-4 Rationale for use of the indirect Coombs' test during pregnancy may be best described by which of the following?
   a. Reveals the presence of maternal antibodies attached to the RBCs of an Rh-positive fetus
   b. Gives indication of the degree of jaundice that will occur in the infant at birth
   c. Indicates maternal antibody formation against Rh-positive fetal cells
   d. Measures fetal bilirubin level in the maternal system

9-5 Your anticipatory guidance during the first trimester is based on the understanding that:
   a. Pregnant women are eager to learn about growth and development.
   b. Nutritional balance is difficult to achieve during pregnancy.
   c. Pregnant women generally are anxious to follow health guidelines.
   d. Women may resent detailed questioning about their family situations and future plans.

9-6 Maria shows that she has understood your guidance about her skin changes when she states:

a. "This lotion is really working on those ugly stretch marks."

b. "I'm glad feeling so hot and sweaty will go away when the baby comes."

c. "I feel so strange with these marks on my face and body."

d. "Everyone comments on how good I look. I'm glad getting pregnant will change my future looks."

9-7 Changes in vital signs in the first trimester follow a recognized pattern. You would note problems if one of the following was present:

a. BP: 10/5 mm Hg below baseline

b. Pulse: 20 beats/min over baseline

c. MAP: 105 mm Hg

9-8 Jane S. would be demonstrating auto safety if at 28 weeks she told you that she always followed this pattern in the car:

a. Sat in rear seat and elevated her legs frequently

b. Fastened the lap belt below the bulge of the uterus

c. Adapted the shoulder belt so it did not touch the uterus

d. Used shoulder and lap belt during every ride

9-9 In the last trimester a pregnant woman should not wait for her regular appointment a week later to report one of the following:

a. Shortness of breath while climbing stairs with a load of laundry

b. Increased vaginal mucus that requires use of a vaginal pad

c. Bloated feeling and blurring of vision

d. Constipation with new hemorrhoids

9-10 During the last trimester, it is important to teach self-monitoring of which of the following?

a. Fatigue levels and interrupted sleep patterns

b. Patterns of edema in lower extremities

c. Heartburn and inability to take large meals

d. Changes in mild contraction frequency

Answer Key

9-1 a. Striae b. Asymptomatic bacteriuria c. Lordosis d. Postural hypotension e. Melasma f. Linea nigra g. Gravidity h. Heartburn 9-2 b 9-3 d 9-4 c 9-5 c 9-6 b 9-7 c 9-8 d 9-9 c 9-10 d

REFERENCES

American College of Obstetrics and Gynecology: Exercise during pregnancy and postnatal period. Home exercise programs, 4:1985, Washington, DC.

Alexander LL: The pregnant smoker: nursing implications, *J Obstet Gynecol Neonatal Nurs* 3:167, 1987.

Barry M, Bia F: Pregnancy and travel, *JAMA* 261:728, 1989.

Arneson S et al: Automobile seat belt practices of pregnant women, *J Obstet Gynecol Neonatal Nurs* 4:399, 1986.

Beischer NA, MacKay EU: *Obstetrics and the newborn*, ed 3, Philadelphia, 1993, Harcourt, Brace, Jovanovich.

Berg G et al: Low back pain during pregnancy, *Obstet Gynecol* 71:71, 1988.

Bernhardt JH: Potential workplace hazards to reproductive health, *J Obstet Gynecol Neonatal Nurs* 19:53, 1990.

Blackburn ST, Loper DL: *Maternal, fetal, and neonatal physiology*, Philadelphia, 1992, WB Saunders.

Blackwell R, Chang A: Video display terminals and pregnancy, *Br J Obstet Gynaecol* 95:466, 1988.

Brown E, Barglow P: Pseudocyesis: a paradigm for psychophysiological interaction, *Arch Gen Psychiatry* 24:221, 1971.

Brucker MC: Management of common minor discomforts in pregnancy. Part II. Managing minor pain, *J Nurse Midwifery* 33:25, 1988.

Brucker MC: Managing gastrointestinal problems in pregnancy, *J Nurse Midwifery* 33:67, 1988.

Brucker MC: Nonpharmaceutical methods for relieving pain and discomfort during pregnancy, *Matern Child Nurs J* 9:390, 1984.

Camann, WR, Ostheimer GW: Physiological adaptations during pregnancy, *Int Anes Cl* 28:2, 1990.

DeGrez SH: Bend and stretch, *MCN Am J Matern Child Nurs* 13(5):357, 1988.

Diamond FB: Patients' prenatal medical record precis, *J Obstet Gynecol Neonatal Nurs* 19:491, 1990.

Doshi ML: Accuracy of consumer performed in-home tests for early pregnancy detection, *Am J Public Health* 76:512, 1986.

Dougherty MC et al: The effect of exercise on the circumvaginal muscles in postpartum women, *J Nurse Midwifery* 34:8, 1989.

Engstrom JL: Measurement of fundal height, *J Obstet Gynecol Neonatal Nurs* 5:172, 1988.

Friedrick EG, Phillips LE: Microwave sterilization of Candida on underwear, *J Reprod Med* 33:1, 1988.

Harny M, McRone M, Smith D: Suggested limits to the use of hot tub or sauna by pregnant women, *Can Med Assoc J* 125:50, 1981.

Hytten FE, Leitch I: *The physiology of human pregnancy*, ed 2, Boston, 1972, Blackwell Scientific Publications.

Krozy R, McColgan J: Auto safety: pregnancy and the newborn, *J Obstet Gynecol Neonatal Nurs* 14:114, 1985.

Leviton A: Caffeine consumption and the risk of reproductive hazards, *J Reprod Med* 33:175, 1988.

Light HK, Fenster C: Maternal concerns during pregnancy, *Am J Obstet Gynecol* 118:47, 1974.

Little D, Billiar RB: Endocrine disorders, In Romney SL, ed. *Gynecology and obstetrics: the health care of women*, New York, 1975, McGraw-Hill.

McGuire L: Pain management, *NAACOG Update Series* 2:1, 1984.

McMurray RG et al: The effect of pregnancy on metabolic responses during rest, immersion and aerobic exercise in the water, *Am J Obstet Gynecol* 158:481, 1988.

Moses M: Healthworkers and reproductive hazards, *Birth* 14:153, 1987.

Nesler CL et al: Effects of supine exercise on fetal heart rate in the second and third trimesters, *Am J Perinatol* 5:159, 1988.

Parsley JE, Mellon MB: Exercise during pregnancy, *Am Fam Physician* 38:145, 1988.

Rook A et al: *Textbook of dermatology*, vol 1, Oxford, England, 1979, Blackwell Scientific.

Sala DJ et al: Maternal blood donation for intrauterine transfusion, *J Obstet Gynecol Neonatal Nurs* 21:365, 1992.

Samisoe AJ: Nausea and vomiting in pregnancy: a review, *Obstet Gynecol Rev* 41:422, 1987.

Samples JT et al: The dynamic characteristics of the circumvaginal muscles, *J Obstet Gynecol Neonatal Nurs* 5:194, 1988.

Sampselle CM: Changes in pelvic muscle strength and stress urinary incontinence associated with childbirth, *J Obstet Gynecol Neonatal Nurs* 19:371, 1990.

Samisoe G et al: Does position and size of the corpus luteum have any effect on nausea of pregnancy? *Acta Obstet Gynecol Scand* 65:427, 1986.

Schick-Boschetto B, Rose N C: Exercise in pregnancy, *Obstet Gynecol Surv* 47:10, 1991.

Schoenfeld A et al: Seatbelts in pregnancy and the obstetrician, *Obstet Gynecol Surv* 42:275, 1987.

Smith MSR, Edwards MJ, Upfold JB: The effects of hyperthermia on the fetus, *Devel Med Child Neurol* 28:203, 1986.

Thornton JG et al: Efficacy and long-term effects of antenatal prophylaxis with anti-D immunoglobin, *Br Med J* 298:1671, 1989.

Van Dinter MC: Ptyalism in pregnant women, *J Obstet Gynecol Neonatal Nurs* 20(3): 206, 1991.

Wallace AM: Aerobic exercise, maternal self-esteem and physical discomforts of pregnancy, *J Nurse Midwifery* 31:255, 1986.

Wallace AM, Engstrom JL: The effects of aerobic exercise on the pregnant woman, fetus, and pregnancy outcome, *J Nurse Midwifery* 32:277, 1987.

STUDENT REFERENCE SHELF

Diamond FB: Patients' prenatal medical record precis, *J Obstet Gynecol Neonatal Nurs* 19:491, 1990.
    Informative article on the use of prenatal record form and its effect on patient compliance regarding self-care activities.

Sampselle CM: Changes in pelvic muscle strength and stress urinary incontinence associated with childbirth, *J Obstet Gynecol Neonatal Nurs* 19:371, 1990.
    Results of study of pelvic musculature in maintenance of urinary continence and muscle relaxation as a consequence of vaginal birth.

Nutritional Guidelines during Pregnancy

KEY TERMS

Anorexia Nervosa
Body Frame
Bulimia
Complete Protein
Complex
 Carbohydrate
Epulis
Gingivitis
Hyperemesis
Hyponatremia
Lactase/Lactose
Pica
Ptyalism
Pyrosis

LEARNING OBJECTIVES

1. *Describe the caloric and nutritional requirements for pregnancy.*
2. *List nutritional problems created by use of fast foods.*
3. *Identify the point at which cultural differences in diet become dysfunctional.*
4. *Determine nutritional additions on the basis of a woman's weight gain pattern and dietary assessment.*
5. *Assist a client who is a vegetarian to plan her pregnancy diet.*
6. *Recognize possible presenting signs of pica, bulimia, and anorexia.*
7. *Describe the harmful effects of smoking, caffeine, saccharine, and alcohol on the client's nutritional health.*

Maternal Nutrition

Good nutrition before and during pregnancy builds a healthy fetus and protects the woman's own nutritional health. Fetal development from conception relies on nutrients in correct amounts (Figure 10-1). Because the first prenatal clinic visit usually occurs late in the fetal development timetable (less than 8 weeks), women need to prepare before pregnancy as well. Infants who weigh more than 5.5 lb (2.2 kg) have fewer problems after birth.

When women use alcohol, drugs, or cigarettes during pregnancy, their fetuses do not gain appropriately unless such activities stop and nutrition improves.

A great deal of attention has been placed on the correct weight gain during pregnancy. Women often have misconceptions about how much weight is appropriate. When patterns do not match the "average," anxiety can rise. Therefore weight gain patterns should be understood before a discussion of nutrients can be meaningful.

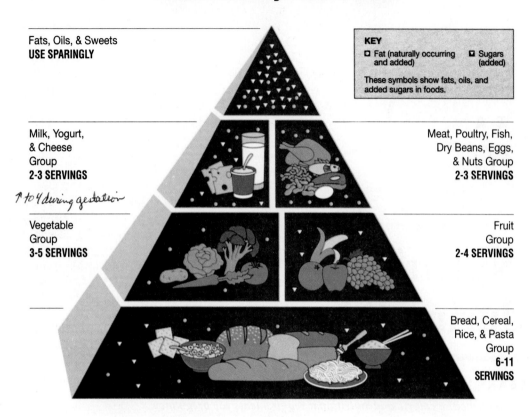

Food Guide Pyramid
A Guide to Daily Food Choices

Fats, Oils, & Sweets
USE SPARINGLY

KEY
□ Fat (naturally occurring and added) ▼ Sugars (added)
These symbols show fats, oils, and added sugars in foods.

Milk, Yogurt, & Cheese Group
2-3 SERVINGS

↑ to 4 during gestation

Meat, Poultry, Fish, Dry Beans, Eggs, & Nuts Group
2-3 SERVINGS

Vegetable Group
3-5 SERVINGS

Fruit Group
2-4 SERVINGS

Bread, Cereal, Rice, & Pasta Group
6-11 SERVINGS

FIGURE 10-1 The food pyramid includes guidelines for a healthy diet for individuals age 2 years and older.

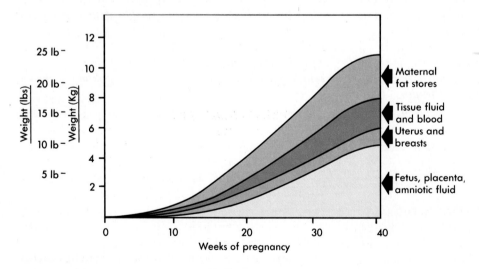

FIGURE 10-2 The components of weight gain in pregnancy. A weight gain of 25 to 35 lb is recommended. Note the various components total about 25 lb. (From Wardlaw GM, Insel PM: *Perspectives in nutrition*, ed 2, St Louis, 1993, Mosby.)

WEIGHT GAIN

Recommendations about weight gain in pregnancy have undergone significant changes in the past few decades. Gains used to be limited to about 14 lb because it was thought a smaller baby would have fewer birth-injury complications, the incidence of preeclampsia would be lessened, and the mother would have less weight to lose after the birth. With better obstetric management and because it is known that excessive weight gain does not cause preeclampsia, it is now recognized that inadequate weight gain poses a higher risk to the pregnant woman and her fetus. Inadequate weight gain may lead to low-birth-weight infants (see Table 10-7, Height-weight ratios).

TABLE 10-1   Distribution of Weight Gained during Pregnancy

BODY PART	WEIGHT (LB)
Breasts	1-1.5
Blood	3-4.5
Extra water	4-6
Uterus	2.5-3
Placenta	1.5-2
Amniotic fluid	2-3.5
Baby	7-8
Stores of fat	4-6.5
TOTAL	25-35

Modified from Dimperio D: *Prenatal nutrition: clinical guidelines for nurses,* White Plains, NY, 1988, March of Dimes Birth Defects Foundation, p 21. Reproduced with permission of the copyright holder and the author.

Therefore a gain of 25 to 35 lb over the prepregnancy level allows for the growth of the fetus and the maternal organs (Figure 10-2 and Table 10-1).

The rate of gain should not be linear; it should start gradually in the first trimester while the embryo is small, about 1 lb per month, then rise to about 1 lb per week in the second and third trimesters.

Other factors determine the amount of weight a woman should gain. Women carrying more than one fetus should be encouraged to gain liberally, 35 to 45 lb. Teenagers within 2 years of menarche are advised to gain about 5 lb more than mature women.

Underweight and Overweight Baselines

Women who are underweight must gain even more. In these cases the amount to be gained is based on the assessed nutritional status. Overweight women should gain an average of 15 to 25 lb. In studies of moderately and severely obese women, optimal perinatal outcomes occur when weight gain is limited to about 2 lb in the first trimester and two thirds of a pound per week thereafter (Brown, 1989).

The objective of dietary management is equal caloric intake and expenditure, thus preventing use of maternal fat stores. When maternal stores are mobilized, a state of *ketoacidosis* is produced. Studies have shown a high association of ketoacidosis with low birth weight and mental retardation (Catalano and Hollenbeck, 1992).

Weight Variations

Rapid fluctuations in the weight-gain pattern indicate that the client needs careful reassessment. Although there is cause for concern, this signal does not mean that the client is in danger, only that her status may have changed.

Weight loss. Many women experience weight loss from vomiting, particularly in early pregnancy. The loss is due to dehydration, which the nurse can address quickly by stressing increased fluid intake. A moderate weight increase followed by a weight loss can result from diuresis after water retention.

Poor weight gain. Inadequate weight gains occur in many women. Driven by a fear of "becoming fat," some do not eat properly. Others, because of economic circumstances or life-style behaviors, are undernourished for other reasons. Smoking has a detrimental effect on weight gain. Other substances that also cause poor weight gain are caffeine, alcohol, and drugs of abuse. Stressors of living, including increased family tension, high levels of activity, or even exposure to the cold, prevent adequate gain. In all instances of poor gain, contributing reasons must be assessed. Appropriate referrals should be made for counseling to modify detrimental life-style behaviors. If economic constraints exist, women should be referred to available food subsidy programs and other social services existing in the area.

Inadequate weight gain is a gain of 1 kg (2.2 lb) or less per month in the second or third trimester. A client may have an ideal weight for height at the onset of pregnancy but demonstrate insufficient weight gain during pregnancy.

Inadequate food intake cannot provide sufficient essential nutrients for mother and fetus. Some women worry about "losing their figures" and restrict their intake unnecessarily. They must understand that if sufficient calories are not provided for maternal and fetal growth, body proteins will be mobilized for calories. This would have detrimental effects on the fetus, particularly on brain formation because brain cell multiplication requires sufficient proteins. Dieting and fasting during pregnancy lead to more rapid and severe development of ketosis and hypoglycemia than in nonpregnant women. Ketosis is poorly tolerated by the fetus and can lead to neurologic impairment.

If women with inadequate weight gain appear for prenatal care only near the end of their pregnancy, it would be unrealistic to expect rapid weight gain to catch up with total desired weight. The goal for weight gain from this point of entry into care should be *double the weight gain* recommended for the particular gestational age, that is, 2 lb instead of 1 per week.

Sudden weight gain. By far the most common concern is a sudden weight increase. Before becoming alarmed, check the scale for balance and note whether the client is wearing heavy shoes or clothing. After the accuracy of the weight is established, determine whether the increase is the result of prior counseling to increase intake, to stop smoking, or to drink more liquids. A

Clinical Decision

A woman is 7 months' pregnant and has gained only 10 lb over her prepregnant normal baseline. What would you recommend for the remaining period of pregnancy?

physical assessment to rule out twins also is in order. Blood pressure (BP) measurement, edema assessment, and urine test strip analysis for proteinuria would indicate whether the woman is at risk for pregnancy-induced hypertension (PIH).

High weight gain pattern. Although they begin in the normal range, some women gain rapidly during pregnancy. A gain of more than 2 lb per week in the second and third trimesters is considered excessive weight gain. Again, a careful assessment must be made of each client (Box 10-1). In the assessment of these factors it is important to be sensitive to the client's perception of the weight gain. Some clients will fast, use diuretics or laxatives, or even avoid prenatal visits if they are worried about being weighed. Encouragement to avoid these practices and a supportive exploration of the cause of the gain with the client can be helpful. The client then may be able to plan her own intervention if it is needed.

If a client appears for prenatal care already having gained excessive weight for gestational age, it is unwise to restrict her caloric intake. Lowering calories to an unacceptable level results only in nutritional deficiencies for mother and fetus. Instead, the type of foods in her diet must be analyzed; a diet history will give insight into the problem. Goals for the remaining weight gain should be set according to the phase of pregnancy, i.e. at

BOX 10-1 Possible Causes of High Weight Gain Pattern

Excess calories
High fat/sugar intake
Infrequent, large meals
Low activity level
Emotional eating
Gain after weight loss early in pregnancy
Smoking cessation
Pica (e.g., laundry or cornstarch, ice)
Undetected multiple birth
Fluid retention

approximately 1 lb per week in second and third trimesters.

Many normal pregnancies have been marked by gains of 50 to 60 lb; in these instances some of the weight is attributed to a greater increase in the plasma volume, which results in hematocrit and hemoglobin levels in the low normal range and accompanying edema of the feet and ankles. Because their excess gain is due to fluid retention, these women need support and comfort measures rather than further limitation of calories.

Although edema occurs in normal pregnancies, it may be one of the signs of preeclampsia. It also may be caused by insufficient protein and calorie intake or by unrecognized cardiac disease. Assessment of these factors is necessary.

Normal Nutritional Requirements

Maternal nutrition should go beyond merely an adequate number of calories for the appropriate weight gain. Because the number of extra calories needed during pregnancy is not large (approximately 300 cal/day), "empty calories" from foods like potato chips, candy, and soda pop could fulfill the caloric requirement without providing needed nutrients. Emphasis on avoiding these foods and eating *nutrient-dense* foods can make a dramatic difference in nutrition. A balance between the food groups also is important for a well-rounded diet. Recommendations for nonpregnant women (shown in the food pyramid in Figure 10-1) should be compared with the increases recommended for pregnancy (Figure 10-3). Table 10-2 lists the functions and major sources of nutrients needed during pregnancy.

PROTEIN

Protein is needed for building and repairing all maternal and fetal tissue and specifically for the increase in blood volume and products, the growth of the placenta and fetus, and the formation of amniotic fluid. More than 20 different amino acids combine in different ways to form proteins. Eight *essential amino acids* are not synthesized by the body and must be supplied by diet. If a dietary protein contains all eight of the essential amino acids, it is a **complete protein.** Most complete proteins come from animal sources such as meat or milk. Most vegetable sources of protein are *incomplete* and require combination with another source that will supply the missing essential amino acids.

During pregnancy the American Dietetic Association (ADA) recommends at least four servings of milk or foods made from milk and three servings of meat or other protein foods each day. If carbohydrate or fat intake is insufficient, protein will be used for energy

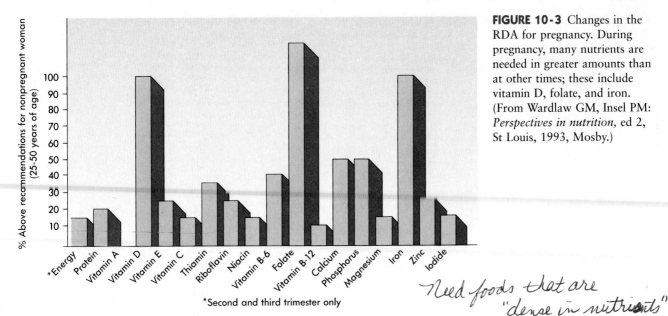

FIGURE 10-3 Changes in the RDA for pregnancy. During pregnancy, many nutrients are needed in greater amounts than at other times; these include vitamin D, folate, and iron. (From Wardlaw GM, Insel PM: *Perspectives in nutrition,* ed 2, St Louis, 1993, Mosby.)

Need foods that are "dense in nutrients"

instead of building tissue. This may be a problem especially for adolescents who have higher protein requirements because their bodies are still growing. The ADA recommends five servings of milk foods and three or four servings of protein foods every day for the pregnant adolescent (Box 10-2).

CARBOHYDRATE

Carbohydrates are the main sources of energy in the diet. Most carbohydrates should come from **complex carbohydrates** such as whole grain breads, cereals, and vegetables. These foods have the benefit of containing other nutrients, as well as fiber. Fiber intake helps to combat constipation, which is a frequent complaint in pregnancy. *Simple carbohydrates* should come from naturally occurring sources such as fruit and fruit juices rather than from sweets. Getting high-quality carbohydrate into the adolescent's diet may be a challenge. A discussion of better choices in fast foods may be more helpful than expecting a teenager to adhere to an ideal diet.

FAT

Fat has over twice the calories by weight as carbohydrates. In addition to supplying energy, fat provides essential fatty acids that are needed for myelinization of nerves and membrane synthesis. Fat also supplies and carries the fat-soluble vitamins A, D, E, and K. A fat-deficient diet is extremely rare in the United States; the more common problem is a high intake of fat at the expense of other nutrients. If a pattern of high weight gain seems to be linked with calorie intake, a diet history often reveals high fat choices.

VITAMINS

Vitamins help regulate the metabolism of carbohydrate, fat, and protein. Most vitamins need to be supplied daily in the diet inasmuch as they are not manufactured by the body. A balanced diet will supply most needed vitamins and minerals, with the possible exception of iron and folic acid. As a precaution against deficiencies, vitamin-mineral supplements sometimes are prescribed. It is important that the pregnant woman take only supplements designed for pregnancy use and appropriate to her nutritional needs because overdosage can be as harmful as a deficiency.

The *fat-soluble vitamins* A, D, E, and K are stored in the body, and thus large doses can be harmful. Megadoses of vitamins A and D have been shown to cause teratogenic effects. Excesses of this sort usually come from supplements rather than from diet. Vitamin A, which helps form and maintain skin and membrane tissues, is important in the mineralization of the fetal skeleton and in tooth bud formation. Some vitamin D can be produced by the body when skin is exposed to sunlight, but it is also readily available in fortified foods such as milk. Vitamin E helps maintain the structure of cell membrances and increases absorption of vitamin A. Vitamin K is necessary to form prothrombin for normal blood clotting. Deficiencies of A, E, and K vitamins are seldom seen.

Water-soluble vitamins are not stored in the body, and thus deficiencies are more common with these vitamins, that is, vitamin C and the B-complex vitamins—thiamin (B_1), riboflavin (B_2), niacin (B_6), folacin (folic acid), and B_{12}. Vitamin C helps to form collagen, which holds cells and body tissues together. Stress or infections increase the requirement for vitamin C, but megadoses are not advisable during pregnancy because cases of *rebound scurvy* can occur in the

TABLE 10-2 Functions and Sources of Major Nutrients

FUNCTIONS	SOURCES	FUNCTIONS	SOURCES
PROTEIN		**RIBOFLAVIN (VITAMIN B$_2$)**	
Builds and repairs all tissues	Meat, poultry, fish	Aids in use of oxygen and production of energy within body cells	Milk, cheese, ice cream
Helps build blood, enzymes, hormones, and antibodies	Eggs Milk, cheese Dried beans, peas Nuts	Promotes healthy skin, eyes, tongue, and lips	Enriched or whole-grain breads and cereals Meat (especially liver)
Supplies energy: 4 cal/g	Breads, cereals	Helps prevent scaly, greasy skin around mouth and nose	Eggs Green, leafy vegetables
CARBOHYDRATE		**NIACIN**	
Supplies energy: 4 cal/g	Breads, cereals	Aids in fat synthesis, tissue respiration, and use of carbohydrate	Peanuts, peanut butter Mcat (especially liver) Milk
Unrefined products supply fiber for regular elimination	Potatoes Dried beans, peas Corn Dried fruits (smaller amount in fresh fruit) Sugar, syrup, jelly, honey	Promotes healthy nervous system Promotes healthy skin, mouth, and tongue Aids digestion and fosters normal appetite	Enriched or whole-grain breads and cereals Beans, peas
FAT		**PYRIDOXINE (VITAMIN B$_6$)**	
Supplies energy: 9 cal/g	Shortening, oil	Aids in metabolism of protein	Meat, poultry, fish Whole-grain products
Supplies essential fatty acids	Butter, margarine, cream Salad dressing	Assists absorption of protein across intestinal wall	Legumes Potatoes, sweet potatoes Bananas
Provides and carries fat-soluble vitamins A, D, E, and K	Sausage, bacon Fat in meat	**VITAMIN B$_{12}$**	
VITAMIN A		Assists in protein metabolism, including DNA synthesis and red blood cell formation	Meat, poultry, fish Small amounts in dairy products and eggs (supplements are required for vegans)
Assists formation and maintenance of skin and mucous membranes, thus increasing resistance to infection	Liver Dark-green and deep-yellow (orange) vegetables	Functions in metabolism of fatty acids	
Functions in visual processes, promotes healthy eye tissue and eye adaptation in dim light	Deep-yellow (orange) fruits (e.g., peaches, cantaloupe) Butter, whole milk, cream Cheddar cheese	**PANTOTHENIC ACID**	
Helps control bone growth	Ice cream	Aids in transmission of nerve impulses	Meat
THIAMIN (VITAMIN B$_1$)		Functions in production of energy	Milk, cheese, eggs Whole-grain products
Promotes use of carbohydrate	Pork, other meats	Aids in synthesis of fatty acids and cholesterol	Legumes Peanuts
Contributes to normal functioning of nervous system	Eggs Enriched or whole-grain breads and cereals Dried beans, peas	Functions in the formation of hemoglobin	Broccoli Mushrooms Corn
Promotes normal appetite and digestion	Nuts Potatoes, broccoli, collard greens		Sweet potatoes

From Buckley K, Kulb N: *Handbook of maternal-newborn nursing*, New York, 1983, John Wiley; modified from Gazella JG: *Nutrition for the childbearing years*, Wayzata, Minn, 1979, Woodland; Green ML, Green JH: *Nutrition in contemporary nursing practice*, New York, 1981, John Wiley; National Dairy Council: *Nutrition source book*, Chicago, 1970, The Council.

TABLE 10-2   Functions and Sources of Major Nutrients—cont'd

FUNCTIONS	SOURCES	FUNCTIONS	SOURCES
BIOTIN		**CALCIUM**	
Assists in protein and carbohydrate metabolism	Organ meat	Helps build bones and teeth	Milk
Aids in synthesis of fatty acids	Egg yolk	Assists in blood coagulation	Yogurt
	Legumes	Functions in normal muscle contraction and relaxation	Cheese
	Peanuts		Sardines and salmon with bones
	Mushrooms	Functions in normal nerve transmission	Turnip, mustard, and collard greens
FOLACIN **(FOLIC ACID)**		Helps regulate the use of other minerals in the body	Kale
Assists in DNA synthesis	Dark-green, leafy vegetables		Broccoli
Aids transmission of nerve impulses			
Assists in maturation of red blood cells	Meat (especially organ meat	**PHOSPHORUS**	
	Nuts	Constituent of all body cells	Milk products
	Legumes	Regulates transport of chemicals into and out of cells; participates in energy production	Meat, poultry, fish
	Whole-grain products		Nuts
	Yeast		Whole-grain products
	Asparagus		Legumes
VITAMIN C **(ASCORBIC ACID)**		Participates in regulation of acid-base balance	
Aids in production of cementing materials that hold cells together, thus strengthening blood vessel walls, hastening healing of wounds and broken bones, and increasing resistance to infection	Citrus fruits	Aids in use of B vitamins	
	Strawberries	**IRON**	
	Cantaloupe	Combines with protein to form hemoglobin	Liver, other red meat
	Tomatoes	Functions as part of enzymes involved in tissue respiration	Eggs
	Broccoli, green peppers		Dried beans, peas
	Mango, papaya	Increases resistance to infection	Enriched or whole-grain breads and cereals
Aids in use of iron	Raw or lightly cooked greens and cabbage		Green, leafy vegetables
Helps regulate cholesterol level of blood			
VITAMIN D		**SODIUM**	
Aids in absorption and use of calcium and phosphorus, both of which are required for normal bone mineralization, muscle contraction, and conduction of nerve impulses	Fish liver oil	Participates in regulation of water balance	Table salt
	Milk fortified with vitamin D	Aids transportation of nutrients across cell membranes	Milk
	Sunshine on skin (nondietary)	Aids maintenance of acid-base balance	Meat, poultry, fish
			Eggs
			Green, leafy vegetables
		Participates in transmission of nerve impulses	Carrots
			Swiss chard
		Participates in muscle contraction	Celery
VITAMIN E			
Helps maintain integrity of cell membrane	Vegetable oils: corn, soybean, safflower, cottonseed	**POTASSIUM**	
"Spares" vitamins A and C		Participates in regulation of water balance	Meat, poultry, fish
		Required for protein formation	Whole-grain products
VITAMIN K			Legumes
Factor in blood coagulation	Green, leafy vegetables	Aids in converting glucose to glycogen	Prunes
	Pork liver		Leafy vegetables
	Eggs		Bananas
	Vegetable oils	Aids in transmission of nerve impulses	Oranges, grapefruits
			Tomatoes
		Aids in muscle contraction	Potatoes

BOX 10-2   Daily Minimum Food Intake during Pregnancy

Dairy products: 4 servings

- Provides calcium, vitamin D, riboflavin, vitamin A, and protein
- Serving size = 8 oz milk, 1½ cups cottage cheese or ice cream, or 1½-2 oz cheese

Protein foods: 3 servings

- Provides protein, B vitamins, and minerals
- 2 servings from animal source = 2-3 ounces meat, fish, or poultry
- 1 serving from vegetable source = 1 cup beans or ¼ cup nuts

Breads and cereal: 6 servings

- Provides B vitamins and iron (whole grains provide more B vitamins, additional minerals, and fiber)
- Serving size = ½ cup cereal or 1 piece of bread

Fruits and vegetables: 5 servings
Vitamin C sources: 1 serving

- Oranges, lemons, broccoli, bell peppers, strawberries, and greens
- Serving size = ½ cup, 1 piece, 6 oz juice

Leafy dark-green or deep-yellow vegetables: 1 serving

- Provides folic acid and vitamin A
- Includes asparagus, broccoli, Brussels sprouts, cabbage, and dark leafy greens (e.g., spinach and romaine lettuce), carrots, squash
- Serving size = 1 cup raw or 2.3 cups cooked (cooking destroys folic acid)

Other fruits and vegetables: 2 servings

- Provides vitamins A, B, and C and fiber
- Serving size = ⅔ cup, 6 oz juice, or 1 cup raw

From American Dietetic Association. Chicago, 1989, The Association.

neonate when it is cut off from high levels in the mother's blood at birth.

The B-complex vitamins function mainly as coenzymes, working with other enzymes in metabolic reactions in the body. *Thiamin* helps in carbohydrate metabolism, *riboflavin* and *niacin* in the metabolism of fat, carbohydrate, and protein, *folic acid* in DNA and RNA synthesis, and B_{12} in protein metabolism. Some studies (MRC Vitamin Study Research Group, 1991) have suggested that folic acid deficiency can cause defects in the development of the neural tube of the fetus. Women who have previously delivered babies with neural tube defects are at higher risk for having another baby with the same

problem. These women may be candidates for folic acid supplementation, a therapy that is now recommended (Mulinare et al, 1988).

MINERALS

Iron is a key mineral needed to maintain the well-being of the mother and fetus; specifically it is needed in the formation of hemoglobin, which carries oxygen to the cells. An increased intake is needed during pregnancy because of the increase in maternal blood volume, fetal blood formation, fetal iron stores for early infancy, and blood loss during delivery. Iron absorption from the diet, however, increases from the usual 10% to 20% to as high as 50% during pregnancy, and some iron is conserved with the cessation of menstruation. Even so, it is virtually impossible to meet the requirement for iron through diet without overeating. Consequently the National Research Council recommends an oral iron supplement of 30 to 60 mg/day (1989). Coffee, tea, milk, and calcium supplements decrease absorption of iron. Absorption is best if iron is taken at bedtime with citrus juice, but if it causes gastrointestinal upset, it may need to be taken with a meal.

The main function of *calcium* and *phosphorus* in pregnancy is to facilitate mineralization of the fetal skeleton and deciduous teeth. The fetus acquires most of the phosphorus and calcium in the last month of pregnancy, but if the woman is to have sufficient stores to meet the demand, it is important that she increase her intake during the entire pregnancy. If the mother's stores are inadequate, *demineralization* of her bones may occur to supply the fetus; this can contribute to osteoporosis later in life, particularly with frequent pregnancies. Some studies indicate that calcium supplements may lower blood pressure (Calcium supplementation, 1990), but their value in preventing pregnancy-induced hypertension is still controversial.

Iodine is a necessary component for the thyroid to regulate growth, metabolism, and reproduction. Iodine deficiency can cause retarded mental and physical development in the fetus. In areas where iodine content of the water is low, use of iodized salt provides adequate intake.

Zinc, a component of insulin, helps maintain the acid-base balance in tissues and is important in RNA and DNA synthesis. More attention has been paid to zinc after studies (Jameson, 1976; Soltan and Jenkins, 1982) showed that the rate of malformations and labor and delivery complications was higher in groups with zinc deficiencies. Meats and other protein foods have a fairly high zinc content; thus a diet with adequate protein intake should have adequate zinc. Because the safe upper limit of zinc supplementation has not been established, indiscriminate use of zinc supplements is not advisable.

mega doses of A & D Vit. also cause
birth defects.

Many women may think they are "ensuring" adequate nutrition by taking extra supplements. It is important for them to understand that self-medicating with megadoses of vitamins and/or minerals may harm their fetus and themselves. Even multivitamins should be specifically designed for prenatal use and discussed with the client's health care provider. The best source of vitamins and minerals, as well as other nutrients, is a varied, well-chosen diet.

Sodium

Because fluid retention increases in a normal pregnancy, a *slightly larger* amount of *sodium* is needed to maintain an adequate blood volume. Therefore severe restriction of sodium is not advisable inasmuch as it may cause *neonatal hyponatremia* (low blood sodium), as well as problems for the mother. Moderate intake of salt-seasoned and sodium-rich foods is appropriate during pregnancy. *Sodium intake should be 2 to 3 g/day,* a goal easily reached in most American diets (Worthington-Roberts and Brown, 1989).

FLUIDS

Water is a vital component of the nutritious diet. It aids in digestion, absorption of nutrients, excretion of wastes, and maintenance of blood volume. It also helps maintain body temperature. The pregnant woman should drink at least 6 to 8 glasses of fluid a day. The best choices are water, milk, and juices rather than soda pop with its empty calories and additives or caffeine-containing coffee and tea with their cream and sugar calories. A compromise may be more realistic when habits are ingrained. A woman may agree to use juice in sparkling water rather than soda pop, cut down on her caffeine intake, or drink milkshakes made with milk, ice, and fruit if plain milk does not appeal. *Limit Caffeine to 3 servings*

Some women may perceive herbal teas and remedies as "healthy" or at least harmless. Some, however, can induce labor, harm the fetus, or act as a diuretic or emetic. The effect of many herbal preparations simply is unknown. A moderate amount of mint or rose hip tea probably is safe, but more exotic preparations should be avoided. In general, it is wise to include a variety of fluids and cut down or eliminate substances that have little nutritional value or possible harmful effects.

Cultural Food Variations

Our culture has an impact not only on what we eat but how we think about food. Pregnancy is a time when many cultures advocate avoiding or including special foods. Some of these practices may be helpful, such as eating a traditional Chinese fish soup made for pregnant women that is high in calcium. Others may be problematic or *dysfunctional,* such as the belief of some Mexican-American women that they should avoid animal-protein foods during pregnancy. Other food preferences are *neutral* in that their use does not change nutritional balance.

Examples of these considerations are seen in the Hispanic culture, in which some foods are classified as hot or cold. It is believed that a person needs to maintain a balance between these two types to remain healthy. This can be a *neutral* food practice because there are many types of foods in both groups. Some Hispanic women avoid certain protein foods for fear of "marking" the baby. Alternative protein sources need to be found for them. Milk consumption often is low, with soda, fruit drinks, and coffee being preferred. Efficacious ways of increasing calcium intake would be to increase cheese intake or nonfat dried milk in preparing homemade tortillas (Kaufman-Kurzrock, 1989).

The Chinese diet during pregnancy may vary widely depending on the region of origin. One common *dysfunctional* practice is washing enriched rice before cooking, which should be discouraged because it causes loss of nutrients. Scanty milk intake also can be a problem, but soybean curd can be used in many ways and is a good source of calcium and protein. Vegetables commonly are stir-fried, which is an efficacious practice minimizing nutrient loss (Kaufman-Kurzrock, 1989).

Many Russian immigrant women state that they are given vitamins and told not to eat salt, oranges, or anything that might upset the baby. They are especially forbidden to eat any fat, particularly cream or sour cream because they believe these foods will give the baby a stomachache. They are encouraged to eat large amounts of cheese for calcium needs during pregnancy.

Table 10-3 summarizes some of the food preferences of various ethnic groups; these generalizations vary according to the woman's regional background and to the degree she has adopted a generic "American" diet. In assessing the diet of an ethnic group it is important to find out which foods from each of the food groups are acceptable to the woman and which beliefs influence her choices.

VEGETARIANS

Women who are vegetarians may need special help in obtaining a balanced protein intake. If they exclude only meat, they can obtain complete protein from dairy foods and eggs (Table 10-4). If they exclude eggs and even milk, more careful planning will be needed to obtain complementary protein from plant sources.

The woman should use calcium supplements and vitamin D, which should be in prescribed doses. Protein and iron come from legumes, seeds and nuts, and dark-green, leafy vegetables. Whole grain breads and cereals supply vitamin B_6, iron, and protein as well. Fruits and vegetables supply vitamins A and C and

TABLE 10-3 Cultural Food Patterns

MILK	MEAT	FRUITS AND VEGETABLES	BREADS AND CEREALS	POSSIBLE DIETARY PROBLEMS
NATIVE AMERICAN (MANY TRIBAL VARIATIONS; MANY "AMERICANIZED")				
Fresh milk Evaporated milk for cooking Ice cream Cream pie	Pork, beef, lamb, rabbit Fowl, fish, eggs Legumes Sunflower seeds Nuts: walnut, acorn, pine, peanut butter Game meat	Green peas, beans Beets, turnips Leafy green and other vegetables Grapes, bananas, peaches, other fresh fruits Roots	Refined bread Whole wheat Cornmeal Rice Dry cereals "Fry" bread Tortillas	Obesity, diabetes, alcoholism, nutritional deficiencies expressed in dental problems and iron-deficiency anemia Inadequate amounts of all nutrients Excessive use of sugar
MIDDLE EASTERN (ARMENIAN, GREEK, SYRIAN, TURKISH)				
Yogurt Little butter	Lamb Nuts Dried peas, beans, lentils Sesame seeds	Peppers, tomatoes, cabbage, grape leaves, cucumbers, squash Dried apricots, raisins, dates	Cracked wheat and dark bread	Fry many meats and vegetables Lack of fresh fruits Insufficient foods from milk group High consumption of sweetenings, lamb fat, and olive oil*
AFRICAN-AMERICAN				
Milk Ice cream Cheese: longhorn, American	Pork: all cuts, plus organs, chitterlings Beef, lamb Chicken, giblets Eggs Nuts Legumes Fish, game	Leafy vegetables Green and yellow vegetables Potato: white, sweet Stewed fruit Bananas and other fresh fruit	Cornmeal and hominy grits Rice Biscuits, pancakes, white breads Puddings: bread, rice	Extensive use of frying, smothering in gravy, or simmering Fats: salt pork, bacon drippings, lard, and gravies High consumption of sweets Insufficient citrus Vegetables often boiled for long periods with pork fat and much salt Limited amounts from milk group
CHINESE (CANTONESE MOST PREVALENT)				
Milk: water buffalo	Pork sausage† Eggs and pigeon eggs Fish Lamb, beef, goat Fowl: chicken, duck Nuts Legumes Soybean curd (tofu)‡	Many vegetables Radish leaves Bean, bamboo sprouts	Rice/rice flour products Cereals, noodles Wheat, corn, millet seed	Tendency of some immigrants to use large amounts of grease in cooking Limited use of milk and milk products Often low in protein, calories, or both Soy sauce (high sodium)

From Bobak IM: *Maternity and gynecologic care: the nurse and the family,* ed 5, St Louis, 1993, Mosby.
*Olive oil is all fat, with caloric but no other nutrient value.
†Lower in fat content than Western sausage.
‡Good source of protein and calcium.

TABLE 10-3 Cultural Food Patterns—cont'd

MILK	MEAT	FRUITS AND VEGETABLES	BREADS AND CEREALS	POSSIBLE DIETARY PROBLEMS
FILIPINO (SPANISH-CHINESE INFLUENCE)				
Flavored milk Milk in coffee Cheese: gouda, cheddar	Pork, beef, goat, rabbit Chicken Fish Eggs, nuts, legumes	Many vegetables and fruits	Rice, cooked cereals Noodles: rice, wheat	Limited use of milk and milk products Tendency to prewash rice Tendency to have only small portions of protein foods
ITALIAN				
Cheese Some ice cream	Meat Eggs Dried beans	Leafy vegetables Potatoes Eggplant, tomatoes, peppers Fruits	Pasta White breads, some whole wheat Farina Cereals	Prefer expensive imported cheeses; reluctant to substitute less expensive domestic varieties Tendency to overcook vegetables Limited use of whole grains High consumption of sweets Extensive use of olive oil* Insufficient servings from milk group
JAPANESE (ISEI, MORE JAPANESE INFLUENCE; NISEI, MORE WESTERNIZED)				
Increasing amounts being used by younger generations	Pork, beef, chicken Fish Eggs Legumes: soya, red, lima beans Tofu Nuts	Many vegetables and fruits Seaweed	Rice, rice cakes Wheat noodles Refined bread, noodles	Excessive sodium: pickles, salty crisp seaweed, MSG, and soy sauce Insufficient servings from milk group May use prewashed rice
HISPANIC, MEXICAN AMERICAN				
Milk Cheese Flan, ice cream	Beef, pork, lamb, chicken, tripe, hot sausage, beef intestines Fish Eggs Nuts Dry beans: pinto, chickpeas (often eaten more than once daily)	Spinach, wild greens, tomatoes, chilies, corn, cactus leaves, cabbage, avocado, potatoes Pumpkin, zapote, peaches, guava, papaya, citrus	Rice, cornmeal Sweet bread, pastries Tortilla: corn, flour Vermicelli (*fideo*)	Limited meats primarily due to cost Limited use of milk and milk products Large amounts of lard Abundant use of sugar Tendency to boil vegetables for long periods

Continued.

TABLE 10-3   Cultural Food Patterns—cont'd

MILK	MEAT	FRUITS AND VEGETABLES	BREADS AND CEREALS	POSSIBLE DIETARY PROBLEMS
POLISH				
Milk Sour cream Cheese Butter	Pork (preferred) Chicken	Vegetables Cabbage Roots Fruits	Dark rye	Sodium in ham, sausage, pickles High consumption of sweets Tendency to overcook vegetables Limited fruits, raw vegetables, meats
PUERTO RICAN				
Limited use of milk products Coffee with milk *(café con leche)*	Pork Poultry Eggs (Fridays) *Dried codfish* Beans *(habichuelas)*	Avocado, okra Eggplant Sweet yams Starchy vegetables and fruits *(viandas)*	Rice Cornmeal	Small amounts of pork and poultry Extensive use of fat, lard, salt pork, and olive oil Lack of milk products
SCANDINAVIAN (DANISH, FINNISH, NORWEGIAN, SWEDISH)				
Cream Butter Cheeses	Wild game Reindeer Fish (fresh or dried) Eggs	Berries Dried fruit Vegetables: cole slaw, roots	Whole wheat, rye, barley, sweets (cookies and sweet breads)	Insufficient fresh fruits and vegetables High consumption of sweets, pickled salted meats, and fish
SOUTHEAST ASIAN (VIETNAMESE, CAMBODIAN)				
Generally not taken Coffee with condensed cow's milk Plain yogurt Ice cream (rare) Soybean milk	Fish (daily): fresh, dried, salted Poultry/eggs: duck, chicken Pork Beef (seldom) Dry beans Tofu	Seasonal variety: fresh or preserved Green, leafy vegetables Yams Corn	Rice: grains, flour, noodles French bread "Cellophane" (bean starch) noodles	Fresh milk products generally not consumed Poultry/eggs may be limited Meat considered "unclean" is avoided Preference for a diet high in salt and pepper, as well as rice and pork High intake of MSG and soy sauce

minerals. The woman must adhere to amounts recommended in Table 10-5.

Copies of the table can be made available to vegetarian women, or cookbooks may be recommended; many vegetarians are motivated to achieve a healthy diet and may already have numerous resources. Low pregnancy weight and low weight gains can be problems in this group; thus high-energy foods can be recommended to help weight gain and to spare protein. Anemia also may be a problem for some women.

TABLE 10-4 Vegetarian Food Guide with Complementary Plant Protein Combinations

AMINO ACIDS DEFICIENT	COMPLEMENTARY PROTEIN FOOD COMBINATIONS
GRAINS	
Isoleucine	Rice + legumes
Lysine	Corn + legumes
	Wheat + legumes
	Wheat + peanut + milk
	Wheat + sesame + soybean
	Rice + brewer's yeast
LEGUMES	
Tryptophan	Legumes + rice
Methionine	Beans + wheat
	Beans + corn
	Soybeans + rice + wheat
	Soybeans + corn + milk
	Soybeans + wheat + sesame
	Soybeans + peanuts + sesame
	Soybeans + peanuts + wheat + rice
	Soybeans + sesame + wheat
NUTS AND SEEDS	
Isoleucine	Peanuts + sesame + soybeans
Lysine	Sesame + beans
	Sesame + soybeans + wheat
	Peanuts + sunflower seeds
VEGETABLES	
Isoleucine	Lima beans
Methionine	Green beans
	Brussels sprouts
	Cauliflower	+ Sesame seeds, Brazil nuts, or mushrooms
	Broccoli
	Greens + millet or rice

Modified from Lappe FM: *Diet for a small planet*, New York, 1971, Friends of the Earth/Ballantine.

TABLE 10-5 Modified Food Guide for Vegetarian Diets during Pregnancy

	RECOMMENDED SERVINGS PER DAY	
Food Group	Lacto vegetarian*	Lacto ovovegetarian+
Milk	5	5
Protein		
Eggs (2 = 1 serving)	0	1
Legumes	3	3
Nuts	1	1
Fruits and vegetables		
Vitamin C	3	3
Vitamin A	2	2
Other	4	3
Whole grain products	7	6
Others	1	1

From Bobak IM, Jensen MD, Zalar MK: *Maternity and gynecologic care: the nurse and the family*, ed 4, St Louis, 1989, Mosby.
Lactovegetarian: uses milk products but not eggs.
+*Lactoovovegetarian:* adds eggs to above.

 Clinical Decision

Mrs. Sharma is a vegetarian who does not eat eggs. What combination of foods should she eat to get enough complete protein in her diet if her main staple is rice?

LACTOSE INTOLERANCE

Many people have difficulty digesting **lactose** (milk sugar) because they lack a sufficient amount of the enzyme **lactase** in the small intestine. When milk or milk products are ingested and there is insufficient lactase, gas forms in the large intestine and causes abdominal cramping, diarrhea, bloating, and flatulence. Lactose intolerance is more common in Hispanic, African-American, Asian, Arab, and Native American populations. Because some women who say they cannot drink milk merely dislike it, it is important to determine whether they have the aforementioned symptoms. If a person merely dislikes milk, it can be incorporated in many ways such as the addition of powdered milk to casseroles or liquid milk to soups, custards, and other foods. The lactose-intolerant woman may find that she can tolerate small amounts of milk during pregnancy and some cheeses that are lower in lactose. Alternative sources of calcium can be supplied by legumes, nuts, dried fruits, and leafy, dark-green vegetables such as kale, cabbages, and turnip greens.

FAST FOOD

Fast food is available in almost every community in the United States, and many families visit fast food restaurants regularly. These habits are likely to continue throughout a woman's pregnancy and especially in the case of adolescent pregnancy. It is unrealistic to expect women to avoid fast foods totally; it may be more helpful to educate them about more nutritious fast food choices. For instance, a roast beef sandwich or plain hamburger rather than a superburger loaded with special sauce can mean 200 fewer calories and 5 teaspoons less fat. Choices that increase nutritional value include baked potatoes rather than french fries, fruit juice or milk rather than soda pop, frozen yogurt rather than cookies or pies, pizza rather than fried chicken, grilled items over fried, milk products over sweets, and ketchup and mustard instead of sauces. Because fast food consumption often has a strong social function for the adolescent, it is important that she feel comfortable making healthy choices and receive support and praise for doing so. She is preparing to make nutritional choices for her child as well; thus supportive education can go beyond the pregnancy.

Test Yourself

Of the following fast foods, pick the three most nutritious choices for a pregnant woman:
- Deluxe burger with sauce
- Grilled chicken sandwich
- Baked potato/butter
- French fries/ketchup
- Roast beef sandwich/mustard
- Fish fillet sandwich/sauce
- Frozen yogurt/granola topping
- Chocolate milkshake

Gastrointestinal Discomforts

In the middle of the second month of gestation, the woman begins to notice taste alterations. She has changed preferences for salty, sweet, and sour foods. Often she will not be able to tolerate coffee or heavy desserts. Some women state that this was a first indication of pregnancy.

NAUSEA

About 50% of women experience nausea during the first trimester. Although this is commonly called "morning sickness," the episodes are not limited to that time and can vary throughout the day. Some women report that it occurs regularly at certain times, for example, in the evening. This may be linked to their pattern of activity, such as working routines. In most instances the problem is not serious enough to compromise nutritional status. The woman should be assured that her nausea probably will stop by the end of week 13. *12th-14th week*

Acupressure is effective for treating nausea. Pressure is applied for 5 minutes every 4 hours while the woman is awake, or she can wear Sea-Bands, elasticized wrist bands with a button located over the P6 point (Figure 10-4). One is worn on each wrist (Beal, 1991; Hyde, 1989).

Client Teaching

Supportive treatment usually is sufficient. Nonpharmacologic interventions are preferable in relieving nausea; these include dry carbohydrate intake in the morning before arising; reducing fats, spices, and sweets in the diet; spacing intake throughout the day in small, frequent meals; drinking liquids between meals; and eating a high-protein snack before sleep. In addition, sodas, fruit juices, milk, and sour substances such as pickles help. Cold foods seem to be tolerated better than lukewarm foods.

She should be instructed to monitor her weight carefully. The need for self-care during the period of nausea can be a time for health teaching for the rest of pregnancy. A telephone number should be provided so that the woman's questions during this period can be answered. If there is danger of dehydration with persistent vomiting, the woman should be encouraged to drink electrolyte-containing fluids such as bouillon and juices, as well as to consult with her health care provider. A small percentage of women experience *hyperemesis*

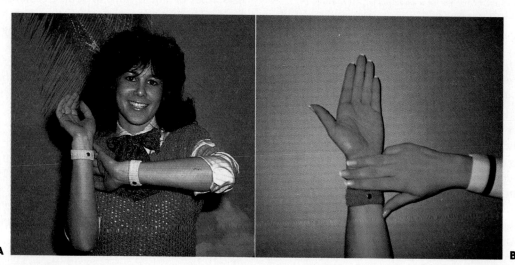

FIGURE 10-4 A, Woman wearing Sea-Band. **B,** Correct position for Sea-Band. (**A** Courtesy Sea-Bands of Solon, Ohio.)

gravidarum, that is, severe vomiting that requires medical intervention (see Chapter 24). Antiemetics are used when nonpharmacologic interventions fail to relieve nausea and vomiting and nutrition and hydration are compromised.

Antiemetics

The standard antiemetic, Bendectin, was removed from the market because of litigation. The same ingredients are available over the counter (OTC) in the form of doxylamine succinate and pyridoxine. For severe nausea, one of the following antiemetics may be prescribed but information on side effects and the benefit-to-risk ratio for teratogenesis (Brucker, 1988) must be included:

1. Scopolamine, transdermal skin patches *also*
2. Promethazine (Phenergan) *Tigan*
3. Prochlorperazine (Compazine) *Reglan*

A recent study (Sahakian et al, 1991) showed that oral doses of vitamin B_6 did not improve symptoms in women with mild to moderate nausea, but it significantly improved the condition in those with severe nausea, and it reduced vomiting in all the subjects.

> ### Test Yourself
>
> • What is the relationship of nausea to early pregnancy hormones? (See Figure 9-4.)

PTYALISM

The woman with **ptyalism** typically has a dry, swollen tongue, swollen salivary glands, irritated perioral skin, and speech difficulties. Interventions include small frequent meals, chewing gum, and use of oral lozenges. The woman should use mouthwash frequently and wipe her mouth with nonirritating tissue. She also should be questioned about pica (Horner et al, 1991; Van Dinter, 1991).

GINGIVITIS

Gingivitis, bleeding and tender gums, is related to increased peripheral circulation and will last for the rest of the pregnancy. **Epulis,** a vascular spongy outgrowth at the intersection of two teeth, may occur in some women but it regresses after birth. Self-care includes increasing vitamin C intake through fruits and vegetables and avoiding trauma to gums. Careful brushing and flossing are important. A visit to the dentist may reassure the mother.

HEARTBURN

Because of relaxed smooth muscle at the cardiac sphincter, the enlarged uterus may displace the stomach upward in the later part of pregnancy. There may be a slight hiatal hernia (5%) resulting in increased discomfort after meals.

Acid indigestion is **pyrosis** and may include burping and an acidic taste in the mouth. Heartburn results from regurgitation of stomach contents into the esophagus, where acids "burn" the lining. A number of nonpharmacologic remedies are available for these problems. In addition to the interventions for nausea, the woman should separate solid foods from liquids, not overfill the stomach, avoid rapid swallowing of cold liquids, avoid gastric irritants (such as coffee, alcohol, and smoking) and chocolate and very acidic juices, and recognize and limit gas-producing foods.

In addition, a change in body position is recommended; the woman should sit up for an hour after meals and sleep with a wedge under the mattress to raise her to the semi-Fowler's position. If these interventions do not seem to compensate, the health care provider may prescribe medication. The woman should be cautioned against taking OTC drugs such as Alka-Seltzer, soda bicarbonate, or citrate carbonate, all of which contain sodium in significant levels. Prescribed antacids contain combinations of magnesium and aluminum and/or simethecone (antiflatulant). Alone, magnesium causes diarrhea, and aluminum compounds cause constipation.

One way a father may help when discomforts of pregnancy reduce a woman's energy is by doing some of the meal preparation (Figure 10-5).

CONSTIPATION AND HEMORRHOIDS

Pregnancy is an appropriate time to teach health maintenance related to the intestinal tract. For instance, a high-fiber diet is known to be part of prevention of later colon cancer. The use of habit-forming OTC laxatives must be discouraged. Instead nonpharmaceutic interventions should be taught, including increasing daily

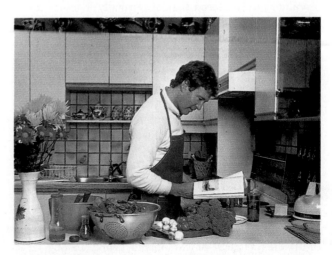

FIGURE 10-5 Nutrition is a family affair. (Courtesy Ross Laboratories, Columbus, Ohio.)

fluid intake to at least 8 glasses, increasing fiber and complex carbohydrates in the diet, increasing regular exercise (especially walking), drinking warm fluids in the morning, and establishing a regular stooling time. If medication is needed, the types prescribed may be bulk-forming agents or emollients. Stimulants or lubricants such as mineral oil should be avoided.

Test Yourself

- Why are some interventions similar for varicose veins and for hemorrhoids? Trace the way pregnancy may aggravate both problems.

Nutritional Risk Factors

A number of women are at nutritional risk because of life-style choices, poverty, adolescence, or eating disorders (Box 10-3). Severely underweight or obese women need evaluation for underlying medical problems (see Chapter 24).

SACCHARINE AND ASPARTAME (NUTRASWEET)

Saccharine is available in many foods today. London (1988) does not recommend its use during pregnancy because it passes freely to the fetus and has a very slow rate of clearance, thus causing accumulation in the fetus. In contrast, London shows that aspartame (NutraSweet) is safe to use in normal amounts because it also is found in foods as a variation of phenylalanine and aspartic acid. It is metabolized to form aspartate, phenylalanine, and methanol (which in turn breaks down to formaldehyde). Concern has been raised about this last metabolite, but it has been shown that the amounts rarely exceed that of normally ingested food. (A can of diet soda contains about the same amount of methanol as a banana.)

Research shows that aspartame is another dietary source of phenylalanine for people with phenylketonuria (PKU) and therefore is prohibited. London believes that aspartame is safe for use before and during pregnancy in reasonable amounts for non-PKU mothers. (See Chapter 24 for further discussion of the mother with PKU.)

CAFFEINE

Heavy caffeine use appears to affect fetal weight on a dose-response scale; the more caffeine, the smaller the fetus. Heavy users of caffeinated drinks in one large study had four times the risk of intrauterine growth-retarded infants (Fenster et al, 1991). Caffeine is found

---

BOX 10-3 Nutritional Risk Factors and their Significance

Adolescent
Increased nutritional needs, possible poor food habits

Frequent pregnancies or breast-feeding in past year
Depleted nutrient stores, especially iron and calcium

Overweight
Increased incidence of pregnancy complications; possible poor food habits

Underweight or poor weight gain
Increased incidence of pregnancy and neonatal complications; increased number of low-birth-weight infants

Chronic medical conditions (e.g., diabetes, PKU)
Need specially tailored diets to meet nutritional requirements/decrease complications

Complications of current pregnancy (anemia, hyperemesis gravidarum, preeclampsia, gestational diabetes)
Additional nutritional intervention needed for adequate nutrition

Dysfunctional dietary patterns
(pica, abuse of alcohol, drugs, tobacco)
May interfere with appetite and displace nutrients

Socioeconomic factors
(poverty, ethnic and language differences)
May interfere with ability to obtain nutritious food and accessibility to nutritious resources

Psychologic factors
(bulimia, anorexia, depression)
May have severe impact on food intake or absorption

---

in coffee and, along with theophylline, in tea, and with theobromine in cocoa. These chemicals have similar behavioral and physiologic effects (McKim, 1991). What most people do not realize is that there are many other foods and drinks with caffeine-like substances. Most colas today, including some clear-looking fluids like Mountain Dew, contain caffeine.

The warning about teratogenic effects was based on rat studies in which the equivalent of 80 cups of coffee were fed to pregnant rats. It seems reasonable to conclude that the usual adult intake cannot cause structural birth defects. The important point to remember is that caffeine half-life varies and has the longest duration in the last two trimesters (13 to 18 hours) so that a pregnant woman who continues her prepregnancy caffeine intake schedule may receive a cumulative dose because caffeine is being excreted so slowly. The *half-life* (when approximately half of the active drug is metabolized to be excreted) in the newborn is even longer, about 4 days. Thus asking about caffeine consumption is important for the admission interview at labor time. Some fetal heart arrhythmias have been attributed to maternal coffee intake just before labor. The newborn also may experience withdrawal from caffeine in the initial recovery days.

London (1988) has shown that maternal intake of the caffeine equivalent of three cups of coffee, cola, tea, or cocoa poses no risk. This information should be used to counsel the pregnant woman who may have no desire for coffee but who may be controlling her weight by drinking numerous diet colas.

SMOKING

There is a great deal of literature about the adverse effects of smoking on the human body. Chronic stress is placed on the fetus, probably from hypoxemia; evidence is seen in a higher-than-normal hemoglobin level at birth.

Severe changes occur in the inner wall cells of placental capillaries and major arteries. It has been suggested that the same cellular changes could be found in fetal vessels as well, with a potential for vascular problems in later life (Piriani, 1978). These vascular changes may account for placental insufficiency and reduced exchange of nutrients, oxygen, and carbon dioxide. In addition, there is the extra stimulation of nicotine. Finally, the mutagens in the maternal and fetal circulation may affect future reproductive outcome (Johnston, 1981). Reduced birth weight may be related to reduced maternal nutrition or to the vascular changes in the placental tissue.

The *fetal tobacco syndrome* includes weight reduction of 150 to 300 g and premature birth. Lowered mental scores may result. Some studies found that oral cleft lip or palate, inguinal hernia, and strabismus occurred more often in children of heavy smokers (Christianson, 1980). Women who smoke are more likely to use caffeine and alcohol (Aaronson and Macnee, 1989), and the combination may obscure the signs of each but increase the risk for poor fetal and newborn health.

✳ Self-Discovery

Analyze your daily intake of caffeine. How much do you take in and in which foods?

Prevention

Early in the pregnancy the woman should be taught the dangers of smoking, and the smoker should be encouraged to stop. If she cannot do so, she should cut back to no more than four cigarettes a day.

If the woman increases her nutritional intake but does not reduce cigarette number, the fetal effects persist. If she stops or reduces the number and eats well, the fetus will gain more than expected. In addition, passive smoke also affects the newborn and young infant.

ALCOHOL

Confusion about alcohol in pregnancy occurs because studies indicate different results. It is clear that heavy alcohol use (six or more drinks a day or a single binge in the first trimester) results in the *fetal alcohol syndrome (FAS)*, including overt signs of intellectual impairment with IQ as low as 40, neuromuscular disability, lag in growth, developmental delays, and facial characteristics recognizable at birth. These problems result from poor nutrition, as well as the additive effects of caffeine and nicotine inasmuch as most heavy alcohol users also smoke and drink coffee (Aaronson and Macnee, 1989). Ethanol primarily disrupts neural development, affecting migration of neural and nonneural brain cells (there may be large holes in the brain tissue). Alcohol also affects brain cell size, resulting in a smaller mass of tissue. Finally, it changes acid-base balance and metabolism (Barbour, 1990). (Newborn effects and care are discussed in Chapter 27.)

The Surgeon General since 1981 has advocated alcohol abstinence during pregnancy, and signs are posted everywhere alcoholic beverages are sold. This action has raised the public awareness, which is critical to modifying the problem. In the 1980s the FAS rate in this country was 1:800 among users of alcohol. In France and Sweden it was 1:300. Those countries have launched an intense drive to educate women about pregnancy and alcohol use.

Fetal Alcohol Effect

A more moderate use of alcohol has been associated with a variety of learning deficits, and the widespread alcohol use in this country may have contributed to the high level of learning disabilities seen in the school years. The group of neurologic factors that contribute to learning deficits from alcohol are labeled the *fetal alcohol effect (FAE)*. Box 10-4 shows the measurement of alcoholic drinks.

Prevention

Prevention education must begin before pregnancy. It is in the early weeks of development that the most severe damage occurs. Questions about use must be asked of

---

BOX 10-4   Alcohol Measurement

Single drink = 15 ml ($\frac{1}{2}$ oz) ethanol
= 12 oz beer
  4 oz wine
  1.2-oz 80-proof liquor
= Approximate amount nonpregnant body can metabolize in 60 min

---

BOX 10-5   Introductory Questions to Ask About Alcohol Use

How do you use alcohol?
Are you used to some alcohol every day?
Has your pattern of use changed over this year?
Has your pattern changed since you have known about the pregnancy?
Are you aware of why alcohol is restricted when you are pregnant?

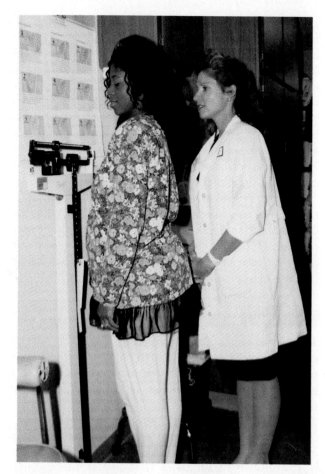

FIGURE 10-6 Weighing-in during a clinic visit. (Courtesy Marjorie Pyle, RNC, *Lifecircle*.)

every pregnant woman early in prenatal care. Box 10-5 presents nonthreatening questions to begin such conversations. It is important for the pregnant woman to know that structural defects that occur during the period of organogenesis cannot be reversed, but abstinence or a reduction in alcohol intake can bring a significant improvement in the size of the fetal brain cells. With improved nutrition, decreasing cigarette use, and abstinence from alcohol, the fetal brain has a chance to grow. (See Chapter 26 for discussion of care of the high-risk alcohol user during pregnancy.)

PREGNANT ADOLESCENTS ~~Read through →highrisk~~

As a group, pregnant adolescents tend to have poorer pregnancy outcomes than do older pregnant women. A mother who is younger than 15 years of age has twice the average risk of having a premature or low-birth-weight baby. Many adolescents enter pregnancy underweight and/or with diets deficient in iron, calcium, protein, vitamins A, D, B_6, and folic acid. Factors that influence the adolescent diet often include the desire to be slim, peer-group food practices, and irregular eating practices; more than 60% skip breakfast or have poor breakfasts. Fast foods and nonnutritious snacks may be mainstays of their diet. The teenager may not have total control of her diet if someone else does the cooking and shopping in her household (Figure 10-6). Substance abuse and bulimia

are more common in adolescents and may be hidden factors that influence diet. Because adolescent pregnancy is more common in low-income groups, economic problems may limit food choices.

In counseling a pregnant adolescent, it is important to remember that she is likely to be under a higher amount of stress than an older woman. She may not have the support of her family, the father of the baby, or her peer group. At a time when she is likely to be focusing on her own emotional development, she is confronted with the demands of becoming a parent. It is helpful to assess the impact these factors are having and to establish rapport in a relaxed atmosphere. Discovering what food she typically eats and likes, identifying any food groups lacking in her diet, and negotiating with her about adding needed nutrients are good starting points (Figure 10-7). Options for supplying breakfast may have to be "creative," such as a piece of pizza or a bowl of frozen yogurt. If a supportive relationship can be established, the teenager is more likely to ask questions or confide problems such as substance abuse or bulimia. Because it is unlikely that a

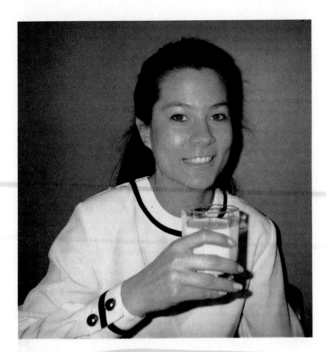

FIGURE 10-7 Three to four servings of milk products per day are recommended for pregnant adolescents.

nurse routinely will spend large amounts of time with the pregnant adolescent, it is appropriate to introduce her to support groups and education and family support programs in her community that may be able to meet more of her physical and emotional needs. A referral to WIC (the special supplemental program for women, infants, and children) should be initiated for those mothers whose low income limits their ability to buy food.

EATING DISORDERS

Bulimia

Bulimia, or a food binge followed by self-induced vomiting, is becoming more common, especially among adolescents. Because bulimic women tend to be near normal weight, they are more likely to be fertile than are anorexic women. The problem may not be evident because bulimic women tend to be secretive about their behavior and feel intensely guilty about it. In theory the greatest problem in addition to unbalanced nutrition is the detrimental biochemical environment that binging and vomiting creates for the fetus. In addition, bulimic women often abuse laxatives, which can cause malabsorption of nutrients. Their weight gain in pregnancy may cause panic so that they increase their episodes of vomiting. Some may be able to stop vomiting and purging but will continue to binge, gaining large amounts of weight.

Because bulimia is a complex and resistant problem, the nurse's primary intervention is detection of the prob-

lem and referral to an appropriate source for psychiatric help. Appealing to the bulimic woman to take care of herself may not be effective because she is already struggling with that issue. Education about the nutritional needs of the fetus and feedback on the baby's growth as indicated by fundal height measurements may help reinforce the need to provide the fetus with nutritional support. Undiscovered bulimia can be confused with hyperemesis gravidarum, but the distinction usually can be made during hospital management of a vomiting crisis. The person who truly wants to eat and gain weight will respond to physical interventions, whereas women with bulimia require psychologic intervention.

Anorexia Nervosa

Anorexia nervosa is characterized by rejection of food, extreme weight loss, and low metabolic rate. Because of the severe impact of anorexia on the body, fertility is reduced greatly. Women with anorexia rarely are able to conceive or carry a pregnancy. If a pregnant woman has had a borderline case of anorexia or a history of it, she could have special needs because of being underweight and having depleted stores of vital nutrients. She also may need psychologic support to eat appropriately inasmuch as her perception of her body's growth may be exaggerated.

Pica

Pica is a persistent compulsion to ingest unsuitable substances that have little or no nutritional value. Most women who have pica report craving clay, dirt, or laundry starch. Other substances include ice, burnt matches, gravel, charcoal, cigarette ashes, mothballs, antacid tablets, baking soda, coffee grounds, plaster, and pieces of the inner tubes of tires. Although the ingestion of clay and starch occurs more commonly in pregnant women who are African-American, live in rural areas, and have a family history of pica, the practice of pica is found in all regions, races, and economic groups. In addition to displacing needed nutrients, some pica substances may contain toxic compounds such as lead in wall plaster. Other complications have included dystocia from fecal impaction related to clay ingestion, parasitic infection from contaminated soil, and small bowel obstruction from excessive ingestion of laundry starch. In some cases pica has been associated with low birth weight and maternal and fetal death.

All pregnant clients should be screened for pica on initial assessment. Because iron deficiency is common among women who practice pica, they should be screened for anemia. Pregnant women who are anemic should be questioned about pica in case it was missed initially. The woman who practices pica will need education and counseling about the harmful effects of her habit, but first it may be helpful to determine her reasons for the practice. Many attribute their behavior to reasons based on superstition or custom that has been passed from mother to daughter.

Nursing Responsibilities

▶ ASSESSMENT

In assessing nutritional status, the measurement of height and weight and determination of **body frame** size provide a baseline for evaluating weight gain throughout the pregnancy. Body frame size can be determined by measuring wrist circumference (Table 10-6). A client may find it helpful to plot her weight gain on a grid as long as she is aware that real gains rarely will fall exactly on the recommended line every time. Figure 10-8 can be used to help the client understand her weight gain requirements. On this grid, zero is her ideal prepregnancy weight (PPW), which is obtained from the weight-for-height table (Table 10-7) and establishes her body frame in terms of her wrist circumference by the following steps:

- Put the weight numbers in column B.
- Put the ideal PPW at the zero on the grid.
- Fill in weight steps, adding 5 lb to the PPW for each of the lines up to the top of the grid from zero.
- Fill in weight loss of 5 lb each down from the zero (PPW) on the grid.
- Plot the woman's present weight at this visit, which requires knowing her week of gestation.

TABLE 10-6 Determination of Body Frame Size by Height and Wrist Circumference (Adult Female)

HEIGHT IN INCHES (WITHOUT SHOES)	WRIST CIRCUMFERENCE (INCHES)	MEDIUM FRAME (CM)
<63	$5\frac{5}{8}$-$6\frac{1}{4}$	14.3-15.8
63-65	$5\frac{7}{8}$-$6\frac{1}{2}$	14.8-16.3
66-67	$6\frac{1}{8}$-$6\frac{5}{8}$	15.3-16.8
68-69	$6\frac{1}{4}$-$6\frac{7}{8}$	15.8-17.3
70-71	$6\frac{3}{8}$-7	16.3-17.8
>71	$6\frac{5}{8}$-$7\frac{1}{4}$	16.8-18.3

Lower measurement = small frame.
Higher measurement = large frame.
With palm facing up, measure right wrist with insertion tape or nonflexible measuring tape distal to styloid process (toward fingers from wrist bone).

From Alton I, Caldwell M, editors: *Guidelines for nutritional care during pregnancy,* (HHS), Chicago, 1990, US Public Health Service Region V.

The new weight is plotted at each prenatal visit, or the woman may do this each week if she wishes. With this grid she can see her progress. It is important not to *scold* but to encourage by teaching and assessing her progress.

TABLE 10-7 Height and Weight for Women (Medium Frame)

HEIGHT	WEIGHT IN POUNDS (INDOOR CLOTHING, NO SHOES)			
	A (90%-100%)	B (101%-119%)	C (120%-139%)	D (140% AND OVER)
4'7"	<94	94-112	113-131	≥132
4'8"	97	97-115	116-135	136
4'9"	100	100-119	120-139	140
4'10"	103	103-123	124-143	144
4'11"	106	106-126	127-147	148
5'0"	109	109-130	131-152	153
5'1"	112	112-132	133-156	157
5'2"	116	116-137	138-161	162
5'3"	120	120-142	143-167	168
5'4"	124	124-147	148-173	174
5'5"	128	128-152	153-178	179
5'6"	132	132-156	157-184	185
5'7"	136	136-161	162-189	190
5'8"	140	140-166	167-195	196
5'9"	144	144-171	172-201	202
5'10"	148	148-176	177-206	207

Modified from Metropolitan Life Insurance Co, 1983.
Weight in column A is at or below the ideal. Weight in column B is considered 1% to 19% over the ideal, and column C is 20% to 39% over the ideal. Weight in column D is more than 40% over the ideal.

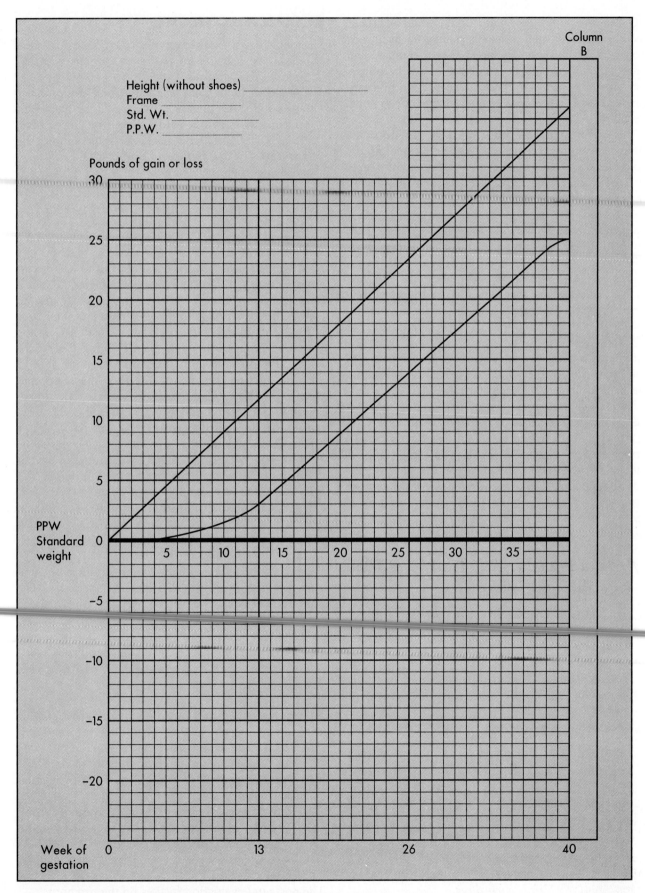

FIGURE 10-8 Chart for weight gain. (From Dimerio D: *Prenatal nutrition: clinical guidelines for nurses,* White Plains, NY, 1988, March of Dimes Birth Defects Foundation.)

Questions about intake and culture should be asked; food preferences and nondietary intake (pica) are important, as are special eating habits or routines. The home situation should be explored. Is there enough money to buy food? Are there adequate food preparation facilities? Does she have control over food selection?

The client should be questioned about intake of caffeine, alcohol, OTC medications, recreational drugs, and cigarettes. Her usual daily routine and activity level are important in planning to meet energy requirements for optimal weight gain.

A woman's physical appearance also provides clues about nutritional deficiencies; for instance, pallor, pale conjunctiva, and spoon-shaped, ridged nails may indicate iron deficiency. Many other signs of nutritional deficiencies often are nonspecific and thus are not reliable indicators by themselves. They must be confirmed with laboratory tests and diet history.

Screening Tests

Routine laboratory testing of hemoglobin and hematocrit levels is used to evaluate the woman's iron status. The hemoglobin level should be more than 11.5 g/dl and the hematocrit more than 34%. Urinary glucose and ketones also are measured frequently to screen for diabetes or insufficient intake; a glucose screen usually is performed at 24 to 28 weeks to test for gestational diabetes. Serum folacin, albumin, total serum protein, and vitamin B_{12} levels also may be measured as nutritional indicators. If test results are abnormal or there is high risk of a deficient nutritional status, more tests may be ordered to further evaluate the woman's condition.

$\bar{q}$ $\bar{c}$ 1° BS during gestation have ↑ risk for stillborn

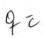 ### NURSING DIAGNOSES

Suggested nursing diagnoses include the following:
- Altered nutrition: high risk for more or less than body requirements
- Altered health maintenance related to life-style, socioeconomic, or age-related factors
- Knowledge deficit regarding pregnancy-related needs

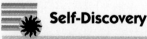 **Self-Discovery**

Use the nutrition assessment form in Figure 10-8 to analyze your diet this week. Are there elements missing? How much fluid do you regularly drink each day?

EXPECTED OUTCOMES

The following list provides samples of expected outcomes:
- Exhibits weight gain pattern consistent with expected parameters
- Identifies foods from each of the food groups in her diet and states plans for adding missing nutrients
- Hemoglobin and hematocrit levels remain normal
- States which nonpharmacologic interventions she will use for discomforts of pregnancy
- Seeks assistance from her health care provider if nonpharmacologic interventions fail to provide adequate relief

NURSING INTERVENTIONS

Each woman should work out additions to her diet to attain a pattern of healthy weight gain. Figure 10-9 is a sample dietary assessment form that she can use to analyze her diet. She should keep a record of intake for at least 3 days and check off what is missing from the four food groups. Although she may bring this record to the next prenatal visit, she should begin at once to add the missing ingredients. Together, the nurse and client may review the diet analysis at the visit and then continue to check on diet progress during each subsequent visit. Registered dietitians (RDs) are available for referral in some settings.

Women with socioeconomic problems may have a deficient diet because of lack of education or money. For this reason the women, infants, and children (WIC) federal supplemental nutritional program was established. The nurse should ensure that these women are enrolled during their first visit by initiating a WIC referral.

Table 10-8 includes the major topics that need to be taught to a pregnant woman. Usually a nurse or dietitian conducts a class and distributes literature. The nurse in prenatal care should be sure each woman receives information and then should assess the woman's understanding of how to achieve a balanced diet. Additional teaching points are included in Box 10-6.

EVALUATION

At each prenatal visit, evaluation takes place regarding appropriate dietary intake. The following questions may be asked in the process of evaluation.
- Was weight gain in a pattern appropriate to her status?
- Were her nutritional requirements met by adaptations in diet?
- Were there signs of anemia during pregnancy?
- Were gastrointestinal discomforts relieved without the use of OTC medications?
- Were referrals made for specialized nutritional requirements?

The postnatal evaluation focuses on the newborn:
- Was the infant of normal weight and development?

Dietary intake					Meat & meat substitutes	Milk & milk products	Breads & cereals	Vitamin C–rich foods	Dark green vegetables	Other fruits & vegetables	Other
Name _____											
Date _____											
Time	Place	Food	Amount	Preparation							
				Servings eaten							
				Servings recommended							
				Difference							

1. Is this the way you usually eat? Yes_____ No_____
2. If not, what is the difference?

FIGURE 10-9 Dietary assessment form. (Adapted from Buckley K and Kulb N: *Handbook of maternal-newborn nursing,* New York, copyright © 1983, John Wiley & Sons; and from Dimperio D: *Prenatal nutrition: clinical guidelines for nurses,* White Plains, NY, 1988, March of Dimes Birth Defects Foundation.)

TABLE 10-8 Nutritional Teaching Plan

TOPIC	GOALS	NURSING INTERVENTIONS
Desired weight gain for height	Woman will track her weight gain, will graph weekly weight. She will know causes of delayed or accelerated gain.	Record weight on chart and discuss rate of weight gain. Assess weight and nutrition during each visit.
Potential problems to be anticipated, including ptyalism, changes in taste, gingivitis, heartburn, nausea, flatulence, belching, constipation	Woman relates self-care steps to prevent or minimize each discomfort related to nutritional intake. She reports discomforts as needed. She follows directions for interventions. She denies use of OTC remedies.	Provide anticipatory guidance on self-care to prevent or minimize each of these discomforts. Emphasize avoidance of self-medication. Explain reason always to check with care provider before taking any medication.
Reasons for increase in specific food groups and nutrients	Woman states food groups and prepares a diet history to analyze her own diet.	Describe the reasons each group is needed. Assist her in diet analysis. Teach substitutions for limited budget. Refer her for nutrition counseling or supplemental food.
Danger to fetus of poor nutrition, smoking, and alcohol	Woman understands that basic fetal deficits may occur if she does not eat correctly or abuses alcohol or cigarettes.	Identify risk of low birth weight and prematurity. Inform of results of poor nutrition. Clarify woman's need to gain extra weight if unable to stop smoking.

BOX 10-6 Weight Control

The overweight client
- Eat regular, balanced meals.
- Avoid fried foods and concentrated sweets.
- Eat slowly (fast eaters often overeat).
- Choose fresh fruit for dessert rather than sweet desserts.
- Encourage low-calorie snacks.
- Drink water when thirsty.
- Set goals for weight gain.

The underweight client
- Review and stress basic nutrition principles.
- Suggest high-calorie, high-nutritional content snacks.
- Schedule five to six small meals a day.

KEY POINTS

- Adequate weight gain lessens the woman's chance of having a low-birth-weight infant who is at greater risk of morbidity and death than is an infant of normal weight.
- Prepregnancy weight influences the amount of weight a woman should gain during pregnancy.
- Excessive weight gain in pregnancy is not always due to excessive eating but may reflect increased body water.
- Megadoses of vitamins and minerals can be harmful to the fetus and should never be taken during pregnancy.
- Moderation and variety are key principles in achieving a healthy diet. Frequent small meals are preferable.
- A woman's diet may or may not follow the common practices of her ethnic group; she can learn to assess her own dietary needs.
- Morning sickness usually subsides by week 16; until then acupressure and vitamin B_{12} may be helpful.
- Pregnant adolescents typically are at higher nutritional risk because of poor food habits and emotional/environmental factors.
- Eating disorders increase risk, and interventions need to be specific and consistent.
- A woman might overcome the adverse effects of smoking and alcohol abuse by stopping their use and increasing balanced nutrition.

STUDY QUESTIONS

10-1 Select from the Key Terms list those that fit the following statements.
   a. Inability to digest milk is caused by an inadequate amount of *Lactase* in the small intestine.
   b. To have a balanced diet, *Essential* amino acids must be ingested.
   c. A common problem for vegetarians is getting enough *protein* and *iron* in their diets.
   d. A compulsion to ingest unsuitable substances during pregnancy is *PICA*.
   e. The fixed desire to remain thin by not eating is *anorexia*.
   f. Vomiting after eating large amounts is called _____ behavior. *Bulemic*

10-2 Which factors increase iron absorption?
   a. Pregnancy alone
   b. Milk and calcium supplements
   c. Taking iron supplement at bedtime
   d. Taking iron supplement with meals

10-3 Decide if the following statements are *true* or *false*.
   a. Self-medication with therapeutic vitamins and minerals is permissible in some situations. *F*
   b. Salt on foods and prepared foods with extra salt should be completely avoided during pregnancy. *F*
   c. If a woman gains the appropriate amount of weight for week of pregnancy, you can assume her nutrition is adequate. *F*
   d. Pregnant women should drink at least 6 glasses of fluid per day. *T*

10-4 If a woman experiences gastrointestinal discomforts, she should do the following:
   a. Lie on her left side after eating
   b. Take a mild antacid inbetween meals
   c. Assume a high Fowler's position when resting
   d. Eat 6 to 8 small meals instead of few large ones

Answer Key

True 10-4 D

10-1 a. Lactase b. Essential c. Protein, iron d. Pica e. Anorexia nervosa f. Bulimic 10-2 a, c. 10-3 a. False b. False c. False d.

REFERENCES

Aaronson LS, Macnee CL: Tobacco, alcohol, and caffeine use during pregnancy, *J Obstet Gynecol Neonatal Nurs* 194:279, 1989.

Aikins-Murphy P: Periconceptional supplementation with folic acid: does it prevent neural tube defects? *J Nurse Midwife* 37(1):25, 1992.

Alexander LJ: The pregnant smoker: nursing implications, *JOGNN* 17(3):167, 1987.

Barbour BG: Alcohol and pregnancy, *J Nurse Midwife* 35(2):78, 1990.

Beal MW: Acupressure and related modalities. II. Application to antepartal and intrapartal care, *J Nurse Midwife* 37(4):260, 1992.

Brown E: Improving pregnancy outcomes in the United States: the importance of preventive nutrition services, *J Am Diet Assoc* 89:631, 1989.

Brucker C: Management of common minor discomforts in pregnancy. III. Managing gastrointestinal problems in pregnancy, *J Nurse Midwife* 33:67, 1988.

Calcium supplementation prevents hypertensive disorders of pregnancy, *Nutr Rev* 50:233, 1990.

Carruth BR, Skinner D: Practitioners beware: regional differences in beliefs about nutrition during pregnancy, *J Am Diet Assoc* 91:435, 1991.

Catalano M, Hollenbeck T: Energy requirements in pregnancy: a review, *Obstet Gynecol Surv* 47:368, 1992.

Dawes MG, Grudzinskas JG: Repeated measurement of maternal weight during pregnancy: is this a useful practice? *Br J Obstet Gynaecol* 98:189, 1991.

Dimperio L, Mahan D: Influencing pregnancy outcomes through nutrition and dietary changes, *MMJ* 34:997, 1985.

Fenster et al: Caffeine consumption during pregnancy and fetal growth, *Am J Public Health* 81:458, 1991.

Horner RD, Lackey CJ, Kolasa K: Pica practices of pregnant women, *J Am Diet Assoc* 91(1):34, 1991.

Hyde E: Acupressure therapy for morning sickness, *J Nurse Midwife* 34(3):171, 1989.

Jameson S: Effects of zinc deficiency in human reproduction, *Acta Med Scand* (Suppl 593) 25, 1976.

Kaufman-Kurzrock L: Cultural aspects of nutrition, *Top Clin Nutr* 4(2):1, 1989.

London RS: Saccharine and aspartame (NutraSweet), *J Reprod Med* 33(2):17, 1988.

McKim EM: Caffeine and its effects on pregnancy and the neonate, *J Nurse Midwife* 36(4):226, 1991.

Merlin R: Understanding bulimia and its implications in pregnancy, *J Obstet Gynecol Neonatal Nurs* 21(3):199, 1992.

Mitchell C, Lerner E: Weight gain and pregnancy outcome in underweight and normal weight women, *J Am Diet Assoc* 89:634, 1989.

MRC Vitamin Study Research Group: Prevention of neural tube defects: results of the Medical Research Council vitamin study, *Lancet* 338:131, 1991.

Mulinare J et al: Periconceptional use of multivitamins and the occurrence of neural tube defects, *JAMA* 260:1341, 1988.

National Research Council, Food and Nutrition Board: Recommended dietary allowances, Washington, DC, 1989, National Academy of Sciences.

Newman V, Fullerton J: Role of nutrition in the prevention of preeclampsia: review of the literature, *J Nurse Midwife* 35:282, 1990.

Piriani BBK: Smoking during pregnancy: a review, *Obstet Gynecol Surv* 33:1, 1978.

Sahakian et al: Vitamin B_6 is effective therapy for nausea and vomiting of pregnancy: a randomized, double-blind placebo-controlled study, *Obstet Gynecol* 78:33-36, 1991.

Soltan MH, Jenkins MH: Maternal and fetal plasma zinc concentration and fetal abnormality, *Br J Obstet Gynaecol* 89:56, 1982.

Teffel M: Association between maternal weight gain and outcome of pregnancy, *J Nurse Midwife* 31:78, 1986.

Worthington-Roberts B, Brown J: Position of the American Dietetic Association: nutrition management of adolescent pregnancy, *J Am Diet Assoc* 89:104, 1989.

 ## STUDENT REFERENCE SHELF

Aaronson LS, Macnee CL: Tobacco, alcohol, and caffeine use during pregnancy, *J Obstet Gynecol Neonatal Nurs* 18(4):279, 1989. Review of the interaction between these three agents and effects on pregnancy and fetus.

Brucker C: Management of common minor discomforts in pregnancy. III. Managing gastrointestinal problems in pregnancy, *J Nurse Midwife* 33:67, 1988. Information and treatment of morning sickness, heartburn, constipation, and diarrhea during pregnancy.

Horner RD, Lackey CJ, Kolasa K: Pica practices of pregnant women, *J Am Diet Assoc* 91(1):34, 1991. A summary of current knowledge about pica practices during pregnancy that concludes pica is more prevalent than commonly believed.

Kaufman-Kurzrock DL: Cultural aspects of nutrition, *Top Clin Nutr* 4(2):1, 1989. A discussion of food classification systems and dietary patterns of various ethnic groups, including Hispanic, Chinese, and Filipino.

Van Dinter MC: Ptyalism in pregnant women, *J Obstet Gynecol Neonatal Nurs* 20:206, 1990. Discussion of ptyalism in pregnant women, including case studies and comfort measures.

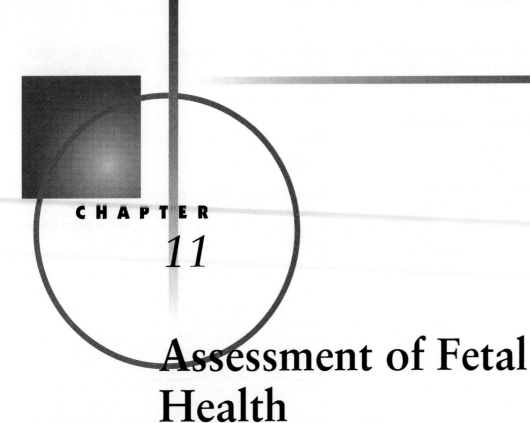

CHAPTER

11

Assessment of Fetal Health

KEY TERMS

Accelerations
Acoustic Stimulation
  Test (AST)
Alpha-Fetoprotein
  (AFP)
Amniocentesis
Biophysical Profile
  Score (BPS)
Chorionic Villus
  Sampling (CVS)
Contraction Stress
  Test (CST)
Electronic Fetal
  Monitoring (EFM)
Fetal Heart Rate
  (FHR)

Fetal Maturity
Fetal Well-Being
Fetoscopy
Growth Profile
Mammary Stimulation
  Test (MST)

Maternal Serum Alpha-Fetoprotein (MSAFP)
Nonstress Test (NST)
Reactivity
Surfactant
Transvaginal Sonography
Ultrasound

LEARNING OBJECTIVES

1. Describe fetal status in terms of well-being and maturity.
2. Select populations in need of multiple methods of fetal assessment.
3. Compare the uses of selected techniques of fetal assessment.
4. Relate the physical or psychologic effects these techniques have on the childbearing family.
5. Apply the nursing process to the care of the family undergoing fetal assessment.

The recent advances in fetal assessment and testing are comforting and disturbing. They can help couples increase their chances of having a healthy baby; yet the options they provide lead to difficult choices.

Highly technical methods of assessment can distance nurses from clients. The nurse can lessen that distance by remembering that thorough assessment begins with hands-on clinical skills such as listening

and touching. The ability to blend "high-touch" with "high-tech" will contribute to the client's comfort and well-being.

Basic assessment begins with assessment of maternal health and family history (see Chapter 9). Most clients are tested. In fact antepartum monitoring and ultrasonography have become a standard of care in most areas of the United States.

Nursing care includes thorough preparation and support of parents during this time. Therefore the nurse must be familiar with all methods of fetal assessment.

Fetal Well-Being and Maturity

Fetal health can be determined by fetal well-being and fetal maturity. **Fetal well-being** describes the fetus whose growth is appropriate for length of gestation and who has normal form and structure (morphology), metabolic functions, and adequate oxygenation and perfusion. **Fetal maturity** usually refers to pulmonary maturity, but neurologic, gastrointestinal, and metabolic maturity also are vital to survival after birth. Although prenatal care focuses on the prevention of prematurity, postmaturity also poses a threat to fetal and neonatal well-being.

Assessment of fetal maturity, or dating of the pregnancy, provides initial necessary information. Baselines for future evaluation of fetal growth and development will be established by several clinical methods.

FETAL MOVEMENTS

Historically, fetal movements have provided reassurance of fetal well-being to the pregnant woman and her health care practitioner. They provide the first subjective confirmation of pregnancy and still are used in the clinical estimation of gestational age. The fetus is capable of reflex movement from approximately week 7 of gestation, but fetal movements are not perceived as quickening until weeks 16 through 22.

Fetal movements are a sensitive alarm system in later pregnancy. These movements will decrease or disappear when the fetus is in trouble. No standard exists because of the wide range of normal movements. Each woman needs to sense her own fetus' pattern and evaluate movements against that pattern. Daily fetal movement counts now are being used worldwide because no cost is involved and results effectively reveal if the fetus is in jeopardy.

There are several patterns of counting. The woman is taught one pattern suitable to her life-style that she uses at a convenient time of day. One method requires counting for 60 minutes three times a day. Another method, the Cardiff method, requires a woman to begin at the same time every day and count 10 movements before she stops. The start and stop times are recorded. The following changes should be reported for follow-up nonstress testing and evaluation:

1. Less than 10 movements in 12 hours
2. Lack of movement for 8 hours
3. A sudden increase in violent movements, especially if followed by reduced movement

The woman should know that smoking can decrease fetal movements for more than an hour (Quigley et al, 1979), as well as decrease fetal breathing movements. Ultrasound use may increase movements. Objective assessment of fetal movements is included in the Biophysical Profile Score.

Biochemical Assessment

MATERNAL SERUM ALPHA-FETOPROTEIN

Maternal serum alpha-fetoprotein (MSAFP) testing is used to identify certain birth defects and chromosomal anomalies during the antepartum period. **Alpha-fetoprotein (AFP)**, produced by the fetal yolk sac and liver, enters the maternal circulation through the placenta and the amniotic fluid through fetal urine. Normally AFP is detectable in maternal serum at about 7 weeks of gestation and rises steadily to peak in the third trimester. Normal ranges exist for each week of pregnancy. All women should have serum testing performed at 16 to 18 weeks. Correct dating of the pregnancy is vital to interpret the significance of these levels. When serum levels are elevated or decreased, the fetus is examined by ultrasound, and the levels are rechecked. Fetal and maternal conditions related to abnormal AFP levels are listed in Box 11-1. *Serum levels vary weekly, important to know # of gestation*

When MSAFP levels are high, investigation for neural tube defects is achieved with ultrasound examination and analysis of amniotic fluid for acetylcholinesterase, an enzyme found in fetal spinal fluid. About 90% of anencephalic fetuses and 50% of those with open defects of the spine are identified by maternal serum screening followed by amniotic fluid analysis. If levels are low, the fetus may be affected with Down syndrome (trisomy 21).

Test Yourself

- Distinguish between fetal well-being and fetal maturity.
- Before alpha-fetoprotein is evaluated, it is important to consider _____ .

ESTRIOL AND HUMAN PLACENTAL LACTOGEN   *not used often anymore*

Maternal estriol measurements indicate fetoplacental function. The production of estriol is controlled in the fetus and metabolized in the placenta. Maternal serum and urine levels normally rise as pregnancy progresses and reflect the status of the fetoplacental unit.

Human placental lactogen (hPL) is a product of the placenta, whose increasing levels during pregnancy correlate with increasing fetal weight. These biochemical assays were used more often before ultrasound exami-

↑CHO diet may ↑ fetal activity to help assess fetal movement

must know exact weeks of gestation

nation was refined and the Biophysical Profile Score developed.

Biophysical Assessment
ULTRASONOGRAPHY

Ultrasound waves are intermittent sound waves at a frequency beyond the highest range of hearing. These waves are emitted by a transducer placed on the maternal abdomen. A clear gel is placed on the transducer before it is used to facilitate the transmission of these waves.

Types

Several kinds of ultrasound are used in obstetric evaluation; each produces a different type of image and therefore has different clinical applications.

A-mode uses pulse-echo information to move the tracing made on the oscilloscope upward in an amount proportional to the intensity of the echo. Thus A-mode will look like peaks and valleys from a baseline.

In *B-mode,* or brightness mode, the strength of the echo determines the brightness of the dots displayed on the screen, resulting in a two-dimensional image. Although the presence or absence of structures usually can be determined by B-mode ultrasonography, it is difficult to detect fine differences between them.

Gray-scale imaging relates echo amplitudes to varying intensities of gray, somewhat like a black and white television. Strong echoes are brighter, whereas less intense ones are a softer gray. Details of many placental and fetal characteristics become visible when this method is used (Figure 11-1).

If many serial gray-scale images are taken, they begin to run together in *real time* and show movement (much like the motion picture is a series of still photographs). Therefore the function of structures (such as fetal breathing movements and cardiac motion) also can be evaluated.

Risks vs Benefits

Ultrasonic examination appears to present little risk of injury to mother or fetus (Mole, 1986). There is very little client discomfort. Results can be seen immediately and further studies, interventions, or reassurance offered promptly.

Uses in the First Trimester

The early diagnosis of pregnancy by ultrasonic examination aids in the determination of the estimated due date (Box 11-2). Ultrasound also is used to determine the presence of an intrauterine device (IUD). For the client who has signs of an ectopic pregnancy,

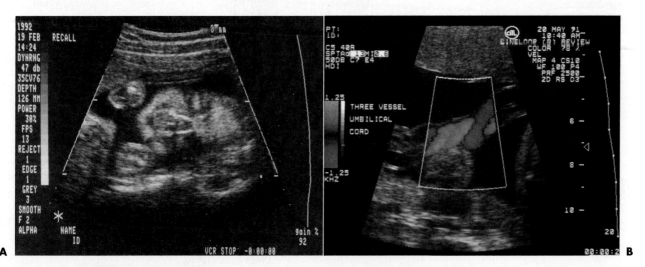

FIGURE 11-1 Two views of the fetus by ultrasonography. **A,** Fetal face (20 weeks). **B,** Umbilical cord (26 weeks). (Courtesy Advanced Technology Laboratories, Bothell, Wash.)

BOX 11-2   Ultrasonography Uses in the First Trimester

- Early confirmation of pregnancy
- Detection of an IUD
- Diagnosis of ectopic pregnancy
- Diagnosis of multiple gestation
- Assessment of placental location

BOX 11-3   Ultrasonography Uses in the Second and Third Trimesters

- Assessment of placenta
- Assessment of fetal morphology
- Assessment of fetal growth
- Visualization of fetus, placenta, and amniotic cavity during amniocentesis
- Assessment of fetal position and presentation
- Diagnosis of fetal viability
- Biophysical Profile Score

ultrasound offers confirmation for quick diagnosis and treatment. Clients who have had a previous pregnancy loss as a result of an ectopic implantation may be reassured by an early ultrasonic examination.

Diagnosis of multiple gestation is advisable because changes in the antepartum and intrapartum care of women with multiple fetuses can improve outcome. It is important also to know fetal size.

Assessment of placental location is vital if the client experiences vaginal bleeding. Location of a low-lying placenta may be made through ultrasound examination. The client will be monitored closely during pregnancy because the placenta may "move up" the uterine wall as the uterus grows or may remain in the lower segment, requiring cesarean delivery.

Uses in the Second and Third Trimesters

During the second trimester, assessment of the placenta to determine if placenta previa or separation has oc-

curred is advised for clients who experience vaginal bleeding (Box 11-3). Because ultrasound detects soft tissue location (in contrast to x-ray studies), placental condition may be assessed (Figure 11-2). The placenta also may be examined for **grading,** which is the detection of maturational changes caused by increasing calcification. Changes in the appearance of the placenta are noted in the following areas: the chorionic plate, placental substance, and basal layer. Grading is used by some in the Biophysical Score but has not proved of predictive value.

Assessment of fetal defects by ultrasound allows identification of congenital problems and thus helps the family make a decision about the management of the pregnancy. In addition, advances in neonatal intensive

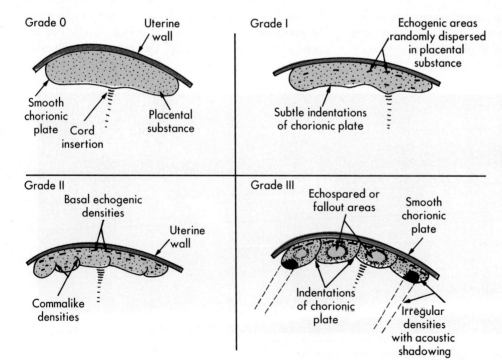

FIGURE 11-2 Placental grading demonstrates how the placenta ages. It can be used to assist in evaluating readiness or need for delivery. (From Grannum PA, Berkowitz RL, Hobbins JC: The ultrasonic changes in the maturing placenta and their relation to fetal maturity, *Am J Obstet Gynecol* 133:916, 1979.)

care have given many infants with congenital anomalies a chance for survival. Interventions that begin before birth can maximize these chances. Ethical, religious, and legal issues will influence the family's decision to continue or terminate the pregnancy (see Chapter 29).

Assessment of fetal growth is important because many maternal and fetal conditions can cause alterations. Because these conditions affect fetal well-being and oxygenation, as well as growth, their detection before fetal compromise is essential. If a fetus shows signs of growth retardation, further testing is done to assess its well-being. Serial ultrasonic examinations of fetal growth are more accurate than a single measurement. Several parameters of fetal physical growth should be examined and a **growth profile** determined. This consists of measurement of head and trunk size, soft tissue mass, length, weight, and proportions of body parts to one another.

1. For head size, head circumference (HC), biparietal diameter (BPD) and occipitofrontal diameter (OFD), and the ratio of the lateral ventricle to its cerebral hemisphere (lateral ventricular ratio [LVR]) may be used.
2. Trunk size may be determined through measurement of the anteroposterior and transverse abdominal diameters (APAD and TAD) and abdominal circumference (AC).
3. Soft tissue mass is assessed by measurement of the thigh circumference (ThC).
4. Early in pregnancy, length is measured by crown-heel (CH) or crown-rump (CR) length; later, femur length (FL) is used.

Ultrasound is a valuable adjunct to amniocentesis. Before ultrasound, amniocentesis was performed without direct visualization of the fetus, placenta, and amniotic cavity. Accidental trauma to the fetus, placenta, or umbilical cord was common. The addition of real-time ultrasound during amniocentesis has made it safer to aspirate amniotic fluid (see section on amniocentesis).

Diagnosis of fetal viability is important for the woman who reports decreased or absent fetal movements. She will need confirmation of fetal viability or death as soon as possible. Real-time ultrasonic examination of the fetal heart will immediately reveal the presence or absence of cardiac activity.

Doppler Velocimetry

Doppler ultrasonography, the basis of external fetal monitoring, has been applied to detecting the speed of flow through the umbilical vein and arteries. In *Doppler velocimetry* the systolic (S) rate of flow is compared with the diastolic (D). The normal S/D ratio should be at least 3:1 after 30 weeks' gestation (Gregor, Paine, and Johnson, 1991). If there is no diastolic end flow, im-

paired uteroplacental or umbilical circulation exists and the fetus is in jeopardy. A high ratio indicates preeclamptic changes in the placental vascular pressure (see Chapter 22). Doppler velocimetry is not performed routinely, but it is useful in conjunction with the BPS if complications are suspected.

Transvaginal Sonography

The technologic basis of **transvaginal sonography** is ultrasound, but the route is through the vagina with a probe that contains the sound wave source (Figure 11-3). It is aimed at the deep pelvic tissues and is especially useful early in pregnancy; detection of the amniotic sac is possible by 4 weeks and 3 days (Modica and Timor-Tritch, 1988). The transvaginal route allows the detection of ectopic pregnancy and is easier for the woman undergoing removal of ova for fertilization. When the uterus has grown out of the pelvic cradle, abdominal ultrasonography is used.

AMNIOCENTESIS

Amniocentesis is the collection of amniotic fluid and its cellular components for antepartum identification of birth defects and genetic diseases, fetal pulmonary maturity, evaluation of progress in pregnancies with isoimmunization, and therapy for polyhydramnios. When amniocentesis was initially performed in the 1930s, it was used to manage the fetus with Rh isoimmunization. Prenatal determination of fetal sex became possible in the 1950s by examination of cells found in amniotic

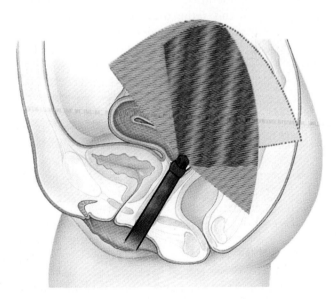

FIGURE 11-3 The major scanning planes of the transducer. *H*, Horizontal; *V*, vertical. (Redrawn from Modica M, Timor-Tritch: *J Obstet Gynecol Neonatal Nursing* 17:89, 1988.)

fluid. In 1966 the technique for culturing amniotic fluid cells was perfected and yielded enough cells for analysis of chromosomes and biochemical study.

Uses

Amniocentesis can be used for genetic studies. It is offered to families at risk for specific genetic disorders and birth defects (see Chapter 27). For this purpose, it is performed as early as 9 weeks, with ranges from 14 to 20 weeks for genetic testing during the second trimester of pregnancy. The results take 2 to 3 weeks because the sloughed fetal skin cells require time to grow in culture. This creates the very uncomfortable "tentative period" (Rothman, 1986) for the parents. Parent-infant attachment, which begins prenatally, is disrupted for the family who spends much time speculating about the test results and their choices; they must decide to continue or end the pregnancy if the results are abnormal (see Chapter 26).

Later, amniocentesis is performed to assess fetal status. Fetal pulmonary maturity indicates a rate of surfactant production adequate for pulmonary function. This state usually is achieved by week 35 of gestation, but the timing is variable.

Lung profile. Analysis of the lung profile is based on the lecithin/sphingomyelin ratio (L/S), phosphatidylglycerol (PG) levels, and desaturated phosphatidylcholine (DPC) levels.

Lecithin and sphingomyelin are phospholipids produced by the type II alveolar cells. The L/S ratio increases with gestation (Figure 11-4) and a ratio of 2:1 indicates lung maturity. There are several potential problems with this ratio; thus other parameters also must be measured. Meconium or blood in amniotic fluid alters the ratio. Despite a mature ratio in pregnancies complicated by diabetes, the neonate may still develop respiratory distress syndrome (RDS). In addition, a lag of several hours occurs before results are available.

Biologic maturation of surfactant production can be assumed when *PG*, also a pulmonary phospholipid, appears in amniotic fluid after week 35. Maternal diabetes or contamination of the amniotic fluid with blood or meconium does not influence the reliability of PG as a predictor of fetal lung maturity. Stressed fetuses, such as those whose mothers have pregnancy-induced hypertension and premature rupture of membranes (PROM), are less likely to develop RDS because lung maturity is accelerated in these fetuses.

Evaluation of fetal maturity also can be determined by amniotic fluid creatinine levels. *Creatinine* is excreted by the fetal kidneys when growth occurs. Creatinine amniotic fluid levels of more than 2 mg/dl reflect renal function and muscle growth.

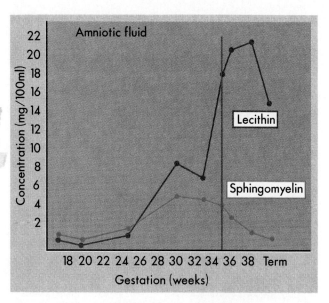

FIGURE 11-4 Levels of lecithin and sphingomyelin in amniotic fluid at increasing gestational ages. Note sharp rise in lecithin production at 35 weeks. (From Gluck L et al: Diagnosis of the respiratory distress syndrome by amniocentesis, *Am J Obstet Gynecol* 109:441, 1971.)

Amniocentesis can be used to evaluate pregnancies complicated by isoimmunization. As the excess unconjugated bilirubin produced by the affected fetus is only partially metabolized by the mother, much of it seeps into amniotic fluid, which is analyzed to determine the degree of fetal involvement (see Figure 28-18).

This method also can be used to treat effects of polyhydramnios. Unusual amounts of amniotic fluid are associated with specific fetal malformations. Polyhydramnios complicates pregnancy when excess amniotic fluid causes uterine overdistention with increased pressure on surrounding organs. Amniocentesis may be performed several times during pregnancy to drain excess fluid and thereby relieve pressure.

Amniocentesis Method

To undergo amniocentesis the client is instructed to wear comfortable pants and a top shirt; the pants will be only partially removed during the procedure. Written consent is obtained, and the woman is asked to empty her bladder. She is positioned in the supine position; a rolled towel is placed for slight lateral tilt to prevent supine hypotension. As required by policy, maternal and fetal vital signs are monitored. A prepackaged sterile tray contains necessary equipment.

An initial ultrasound scan is performed to confirm fetal viability and gestational age, to identify gross structural anomalies, and to locate the placenta or pockets of amniotic fluid in relation to the fetus (Figure 11-5).

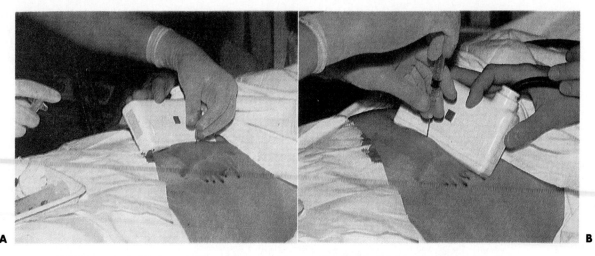

FIGURE 11-5 A, Under sterile conditions, a 10-cm, 20-gauge spinal needle is introduced through the abdominal wall into the amniotic cavity, under ultrasound guidance. **B,** As the needle stylet is removed, clear amniotic fluid slowly wells out and can be aspirated by a syringe. (From Al-Azzawi F: *Color atlas of childbirth and obstetric techniques,* St Louis, 1990, Mosby.)

1. A site for needle insertion is chosen to avoid the placenta and fetus and yield an adequate amount of amniotic fluid.
2. The maternal abdomen is prepared with the antiseptic, and the sterile drape is placed.
3. Local anesthesia is optional. A 3½-inch, 20-gauge spinal needle, attached to a 20-ml syringe, is inserted; when fluid begins to flow, the syringe is changed to avoid contaminating the fetal specimen with maternal cells.
4. About 20 ml of amniotic fluid is collected for analysis.
5. The client is informed that she will feel pressure as this is done.
6. The needle is withdrawn. Monitoring of maternal and fetal vital signs continues for about one-half hour.
7. The Rh D immune globulin (RhoGAM) is given to any mother who is Rh negative and not sensitized.

Risks

The client should know that she may experience cramping or local soreness. However, she should notify her physician or midwife if any of the following signs appear:

1. Leakage of amniotic fluid at the site or in the vagina
2. Localized or generalized signs of infection
3. Decreased or increased fetal movement (when amniocentesis is performed after 20 weeks)
4. Bleeding
5. Persistent uterine contractions

Spontaneous abortion is a complication of amniocentesis in 0.5% of women who undergo the procedure.

However, researchers do not know which abortions are procedure-induced and which are spontaneous.

CHORIONIC VILLUS SAMPLING

Chorionic villus sampling (CVS) is performed early (8 to 12 weeks) for identification of genetic disease. Because it is possible to culture the cells and analyze them more rapidly, this procedure greatly reduces the waiting time. Results are available in 1 to 2 weeks (Figure 11-6).

Method

By means of ultrasound a transcervical catheter is introduced, and 15 to 30 mg of chorionic villi are aspirated from several sites into a 20-ml syringe. When the procedure is completed, the Rh-negative client is given Rh D immune globulin prophylactically.

Risks   ↑ risk than in US

Complications of CVS are similar to those of amniocentesis and include amniotic fluid leakage, infections, bleeding, fetal death, and Rh isoimmunization. The abortion rate after CVS is reported to vary from 1.5% to 4.5% (Green et al, 1988; Pergament, 1986). Infection is a concern because the catheter must be passed transvaginally. The risk of infection seems to increase with the number of catheter passages needed to obtain the sample, leading some centers to limit this number to no more than three. A higher rate of failure and infection is seen in primigravidas because of more resistance to passage of the catheter. There also is the potential for diagnostic error during CVS, especially if maternal tissue is analyzed by error or if a multiple gestation is unnoticed.

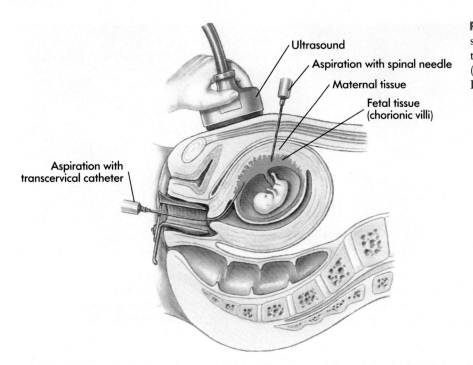

FIGURE 11-6 Chorionic villus sampling involves taking chorionic tissue for analysis of fetal problems. (Courtesy Medical and Scientific Illustration, Crozet, Va.)

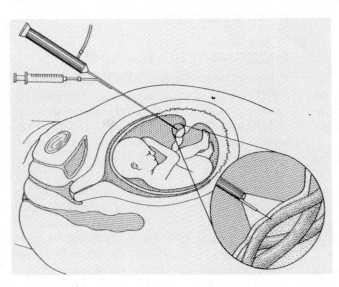

FIGURE 11-7 Fetoscopy has been used in the diagnosis of small fetal malformations (such as facial cleft or digital defects in families at risk from specific genetic syndromes), and for the visual guidance for fetal blood sampling, skin, and liver biopsy. (From Al-Azzawi F: *Color atlas of childbirth and obstetric techniques,* St Louis, 1990, Mosby.)

FETOSCOPY

Fetoscopy is a high-risk procedure for the visualization of the fetus. It has been replaced largely by ultrasound. Because of advances in technology the use of ultrasound has made fetoscopy safer when it is used for fetal blood and tissue sampling (Figure 11-7).

Fetoscopy, along with PUBS, is used to diagnose problems and treat the fetus in utero. Diagnosis may be obtained by direct visualization of fetal structures or analysis of samples of fetal tissue or blood.

Cordocentesis

Percutaneous umbilical blood sampling (PUBS) is a puncture of the umbilical cord (a *cordocentesis*) to obtain a blood sample while using ultrasound (Figure 11-8). It may be used to evaluate fetal blood components for diagnosis of anemias, blood incompatibility, and genetic problems. Also, a transfusion to the fetus is delivered through this route rather than into the peritoneal space.

Method

The cordocentesis begins with sonographic examination to locate the placenta and umbilical cord and to assess fetal growth and development. A flexible, small-bore "needlescope" (endoscope and needle) is passed through the maternal abdomen into the uterus and to the fetus or umbilical cord under ultrasonic guidance. Samples of

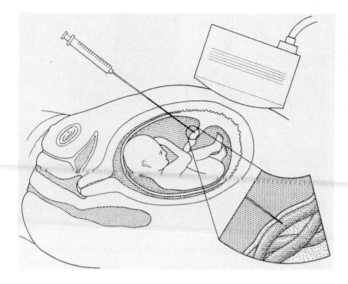

FIGURE 11-8 Cordocentesis has now superseded fetoscopy for fetal blood sampling and fetal blood transfusions. It is an outpatient technique performed with the mother under local anesthesia; the procedure-related loss is less than 1% (Nicolaides, Soothill, 1989). (From Al-Azzawi F: *Color atlas of childbirth and obstetric techniques,* St Louis, 1990, Mosby.)

fetal skin or blood are obtained for diagnosis of fetal genetic disorders. Intrauterine blood transfusion may be performed if the fetus is severely anemic as a result of blood incompatability. After the procedure is completed, the **fetal heart rate (FHR)** will be monitored to detect uterine contractions or fetal distress.

Risks

Infections, bleeding, and preterm labor occur in less than 1% of women who undergo cordocentesis.

Test Yourself

- How would you explain the use of ultrasound to a patient with first-trimester vaginal bleeding?
- What is meant by the "tentative period" of pregnancy?
- An L/S ratio of _____ : _____ is indicative of fetal lung maturity; however, this is not reliable in pregnancies complicated by _____ .
- Name five complications common to amniocentesis and chorionic villus sampling.

ELECTRONIC FETAL MONITORING

The introduction of **electronic fetal monitoring (EFM)** provided the opportunity to monitor continuous fetal response. Before its development, FHR monitoring was limited to sporadic auscultation, usually 30 seconds after the end of a contraction. Auscultation, however, cannot demonstrate periodic changes in heart rate patterns, baseline variability, objective assessment of uter-

ine activity, and other parameters. Many devices have been used as fetoscopes, including hollow, wooden, cone-shaped devices and regular and specialized stethoscopes.

Antepartum Monitoring

Antepartum fetal heart rate monitoring is now used for most women. In general, testing is not begun until the fetus is thought to be viable, at about 25 weeks of gestation. (See Chapter 14 for monitor use during labor.)

The **nonstress test (NST)** is used to identify the fetus who may not be adapting well to the intrauterine environment. Most tertiary centers perform an NST as part of the Biophysical Profile Score. Situations for which monitoring is recommended are found in Box 11-4.

During the NST the FHR is monitored for **accelerations in relation to fetal movements.** These accelerations are a sign of an intact central and autonomic nervous system.

Repeated monitoring by the same nurse or nurses in the NST unit allows the woman to establish a much-needed supportive relationship (Procedure 11-1). In addition, staff members familiar with subtleties of each individual's monitor strip will be better able to identify significant changes. A support person (family member or friend) may be present. Every effort is made to explain the procedure and its significance. In most centers, written consent is obtained.

Procedure 11-1 Nonstress Testing. Nonstress testing consists of the following steps:
1. The woman is asked to empty her bladder because confinement to bed or chair for at least 1 hour is probable. Fasting is not necessary; in fact, maternal hypoglycemia may adversely influence fetal activity.

BOX 11-4   Indications for Antepartum Monitoring

Maternal

- Maternal diabetes
- Maternal hypertension, essential or pregnancy in-duced
- Maternal collagen or vascular disease
- Drug use (therapeutic, tobacco, alcohol, or recre-ational)
- Poor uterine growth conditions
- Hemoglobinopathic conditions
- Isoimmunization
- Maternal heart disease
- Maternal renal disease
- Previous stillbirth
- Vaginal bleeding in second and third trimesters
- PROM
- Postterm pregnancy
- Premature labor indications
- Maternal age over 35

Fetal

- Intrauterine growth retardation
- Multiple gestation
- Oligohydramnios or polyhydramnios
- Assessment of fetus after amniocentesis
- Decreased fetal movement
- Placental perfusion or function problems

From NAACOG: *Electronic fetal monitoring: nursing practice competencies and educational guidelines,* Washington, DC, 1986, The Association.

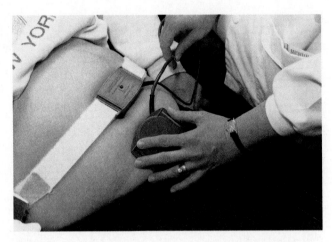

FIGURE 11-9 Beginning the NST by locating the best fetal heart sound. (Courtesy St. John's Mercy Medical Center, St. Louis, Mo.)

2. She may choose the semi-Fowler's with a lateral tilt or left lateral position; either will ensure adequate uterine blood flow.
3. Baseline maternal vital signs are obtained and reassessed regularly.
4. The tocodynamometer is placed over the *fundus* of the uterus. The ultrasound transducer is posi-tioned over the point of maximal impulse (PMI), which is determined by finding the shoulder of the fetus by Leopold's maneuvers (Figure 11-9). (See Figure 14-2 for points on the abdomen to obtain the FHT.)
5. The woman is asked to record fetal movements by pushing a button on a cable (similar to a call bell), which signals the monitor pen to mark the trac-ing. See placement of tocotransducer and ultra-sonic transducer in Figure 11-10.

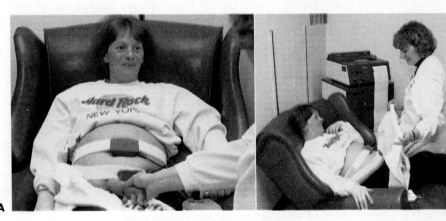

FIGURE 11-10 A, Applying acoustic stimulation to measure reactivity. **B,** Comfortable position for NST. (Courtesy St. John's Mercy Medical Center, St. Louis, Mo.)

Reactive nonstress test. A baseline FHR tracing is analyzed for baseline rate, changes, and variability in relation to fetal activity. The test is considered reactive if, over 20 minutes, there are two FHR accelerations, each of at least 15 beats/min, lasting at least 15 seconds, and occurring simultaneously with fetal movements. A reactive NST (Figure 11-11, *A*) is considered a good predictor of fetal well-being for 1 week, although in some centers a woman with multiple risk factors may be tested twice or three times a week.

Nonreactive nonstress test. Lack of fetal movement during the test may indicate fetal sleep. The nurse should attempt to rouse the fetus by gently manipulating the maternal abdomen (Figure 11-11, *B*). Fetal movements also may begin after maternal ingestion of fruit juice. The test period may be extended for an additional 20 minutes, or acoustic stimulation may be added. The healthy fetus who is not compromised by uteroplacental insufficiency will respond to these measures. Failure to elicit any FHR accelerations during the test may result from maternal drug use or fetal age of less than 32 weeks (this fetus may fail to exhibit accelerations because of immaturity of the central nervous system). If the fetus fails to fulfill the criteria for a reactive test, uteroplacental reserve must be further evaluated. Note also that NST results are considered in relation to other parts of the Biophysical Profile Score in many tertiary centers, and the decision to deliver the fetus will be based on the BPS. Figure 11-11, *B,* illustrates a nonreactive NST.

Acoustic Stimulation Test

Vibroacoustic stimulation—the **acoustic stimulation test (AST)**—by means of an artificial larynx sound has been used to stimulate the fetus who appears to be sleeping when the NST is performed. The sound is transmitted through the maternal abdomen and "wakes up" the fetus. According to the monitor record, within 5 minutes after the stimulus the fetus will show reactivity of two fetal heart accelerations of at least 15 beats/min lasting 15 or more seconds. Sometimes the acceleration continues for many more seconds. In many units the AST has largely replaced the longer NST. The test may take only 10 minutes, whereas the NST may take 30 to 60 minutes. Thus the AST may be more efficient in the physician's office or the antepartal testing area (Miller-Slade et al, 1991). Research is still in progress, however, to confirm that the abrupt sound will not cause hearing loss in the fetus.

Contraction Stress Test

When a borderline NST is recorded, some centers proceed to the next step, a **contraction stress test (CST).** or (OCT) oxytocin contraction stress test

An intravenous (IV) line is inserted, and increasing amounts of very dilute oxytocin are infused for a period long enough to cause three contractions within 10 minutes. This may take 1 to 2 hours. A positive CST reaction means that significant FHR changes, such as decelerations or bradycardia, result from poorer circulation to the placenta when the contractions occur. If the fetus cannot tolerate these mild contractions, intense labor would cause *fetal distress*, and the woman is scheduled for a cesarean delivery.

Mammary Stimulation Test

The basis of the **mammary** (or nipple) **stimulation test (MST)** is that such stimulus triggers release of oxytocin from the posterior pituitary. It also is called the breast stimulation test (BST). Oxytocin receptors in the uterus increase just before labor begins. Earlier, the client could be given oxytocin and contractions would not begin. The MST was developed on the basis of these factors. The test takes 20 minutes and requires no medication (see Chapter 21, MST).

A negative test reaction seems to provide a reliable prediction that the woman will not go into premature labor. This brief and inexpensive test is considered important because, as indicated in Chapter 21, home monitoring of premature labor is costly and considered to be one of the most important reasons for testing in the antepartal period. One reservation with use of this test is that in the event contractions become strong, endogenous oxytocin may not "switch off" as quickly as can be done with an IV flow.

BIOPHYSICAL PROFILE SCORE

The **biophysical profile score (BPS)** was developed by Manning and Platt in 1980 in an effort to identify the fetus in danger of death. The BPS consists of five items: four observations made during ultrasonic examination—fetal muscle tone, movements, breathing movements, and amniotic fluid volume—plus the results of the NST. Table 11-1 illustrates the scoring of the BPS.

Scores of 8 to 10 are considered *reassuring,* and repeat testing is indicated within the week. Scores of 5 to 6 are *equivocal* and require retesting within 24 hours. Scores of 4 or less are considered *abnormal and worrisome* and indicate the need for speedy delivery, especially because a score in the lower range rarely increases when the fetus is retested. Some medical centers add placental grading to the five original parameters in the BPS so that a perfect score is 12.

The BPS is an accurate predictor of a fetus in trouble (Gaffney et al, 1990). It can detect the development of intrauterine infection, and is performed to track onset of infection if preterm rupture of membranes occurs.

FIGURE 11-11 A, Reactive NST *(FM).* Arrows indicate fetal movement with acceleration. **B,** Nonreactive NST. No accelerations are seen. (From Fields LM, Haire MF, Troiano NH: *Current concepts in fetal monitoring,* Pleasantville, N.Y., 1987, PPG Biomedical Systems, Inc.)

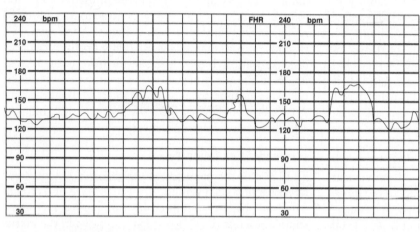

Fetal heart rate

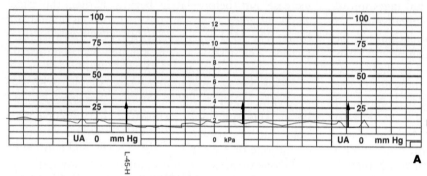

Uterine tonus

A

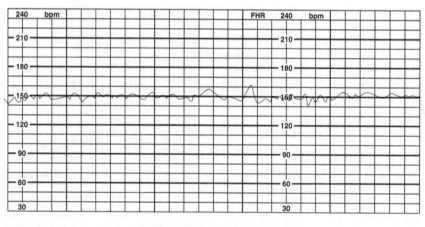

Fetal heart rate

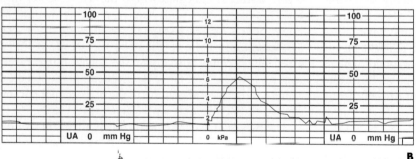

Uterine tonus

B

TABLE 11-1 Biophysical Profile Scoring

CRITERIA	SCORE 2	SCORE 0
Fetal muscle tone	One episode of flexion/extension of fetal spine, limbs, or hand in 30 min	Extremities in extension or slow return after slow extension
Fetal movements	Three gross movements/rolling in 30 min	Two or less gross movements
Fetal breathing	30 sec of continuous breathing within 30-min period	Absent respiratory effort or no episodes of >30 sec
Nonstress test	Two accelerations of 15 beats/min × 15 sec within 20 min	Nonreactive: <2 episodes poor or absent accelerations
Amniotic fluid volume	One or more pockets of fluid >2 cm vertically	Fluid pockets <1 cm or absent

From Manning FA et al: Fetal assessment based on fetal biophysical profile scoring. IV. An analysis of perinatal morbidity and mortality, *Am J Obstet Gynecol* 162(3):703, 1990.

Test Yourself

- Why is auscultation an unsatisfactory method of monitoring fetal heart rate patterns?
- Compare reactive vs nonreactive NST. What parameters would lead you to conclude that an NST was reactive or nonreactive?
- Name the areas assessed in the BPS.

Nursing Responsibilities

ASSESSMENT

Nurses manage NST and CST preparation and testing and may assist the physician with several other tests. In some settings, ultrasonography and BPS may be managed by nurses. The nurse must recognize *reassuring, borderline,* and *nonreassuring* results and report accurately to the physician. Legal problems can arise if the test is read incorrectly (see Chapter 14).

NURSING DIAGNOSES

A nurse involved with antepartal testing should consider the following nursing diagnoses:

- High risk for ineffective coping related to adverse findings
- Fear related to fetal health or illness
- Anxiety related to fear of the unknown and possible discomfort as a result of the procedure
- Risk for fetal injury related to hypoxia or specific invasive procedure

EXPECTED OUTCOMES

Because normal results of all fetal testing parameters do not always occur, families need to find healthy ways of coping with negative results and the decisions they must make based on those results. The following outcomes demonstrate the fulfillment of these needs.

1. Family members will support each other during this experience.
2. Client will demonstrate understanding of purpose and procedure of relevant assessment techniques.
3. Family members will express feelings about testing procedures, results, and their effects on the progress of the pregnancy.
4. Threats to fetal well-being will be recognized and their effects minimized.

NURSING INTERVENTIONS

Support for the woman undergoing testing is a major nursing intervention. Without exception, women will be anxious about the results of the test and will need to discuss their concerns.

The nurse will ensure that informed consent is obtained for any invasive procedure and will monitor vital signs before and after such procedures. Antepartal fetal monitoring requires that the nurse understand the physiology regulating fetal heart responses. The nurse will need to seek additional education to develop the competencies listed in Box 11-5.

The American College of Obstetricians and Gynecologists (ACOG) and the Nurses' Association of the American College of Obstetricians and Gynecologists (NAACOG) (now AWHONN) published a joint statement that describes practice competencies for nurses

BOX 11-5 Antepartum Electronic Fetal Monitoring

Nursing practice competencies

The nurse who will have responsibility for performing antepartum testing should first achieve and demonstrate competency in intrapartum fetal heart rate monitoring and subsequently complete an educational program to develop competency in antepartum electronic fetal monitoring. Before assuming responsibility for antepartum monitoring, the licensed nurse should be able to:

1. Describe antepartum testing criteria and indications for testing
2. Explain the purpose and procedure to the patient
3. Prepare the patient and apply external electronic fetal monitor
4. Recognize contraindications to the use of oxytocin or nipple stimulation
5. Conduct the prescribed antepartum test
6. Communicate the content of electronic fetal monitoring data for final interpretation in accordance with institutional policy
7. Document appropriate entries on the fetal monitoring strip chart and/or patient record
8. Terminate electronic fetal monitoring according to institutional policy/criteria
9. Communicate appropriate follow-up information to the patient

From NAACOG: *Electronic fetal monitoring: nursing practice competencies and educational guidelines*, Washington, DC, 1986. The Association.

involved in antepartum electronic fetal monitoring (Box 11-5).

▶ EVALUATION

The opportunity to evaluate supportive nursing interventions varies with the work setting.

- Are reactions of family members appropriate to situation and accepted by other members?
- Does the client verbalize concerns and ask questions?
- Were the fetal response and condition identified and potential injury minimized?

KEY POINTS

- Rapid growth has occurred in the technology of fetal assessment. Techniques valued today may later be abandoned for safer and more accurate tests.
- Effective fetal therapy is already being used in some centers.
- All women are tested for maternal serum alpha-fetoprotein (MSAFP) in mid-second trimester, with follow-up of amniocentesis if values are abnormal.
- Use of technologic advances may distance the woman from health care workers; therefore it is important to provide thoughtful interaction and explanations.
- Ultrasonography is a valuable tool to assess fetal breathing movements, maturity, defects, and general condition.
- The nonstress test is performed for every woman with any risk factor. It may be repeated as often as three times a week in high-risk situations.
- NST is part of the biophysical profile and can indicate when the fetus cannot survive labor.
- Nursing interventions can smooth the path for women who must have testing because the fetus is at risk.

STUDY QUESTIONS

11-1 Which Key Terms in this chapter are described by the following statements?
  a. Protein produced by the fetal yolk sac and liver that enters the maternal circulation through the placenta and the amniotic fluid through fetal urine _Alpha fetal Protein_
  h. Intermittent sound waves produced at a high frequency ____Ultrasound____
  c. Collection of amniotic fluid and its cellular components by needle tap _Amniocentesis_
  d. Fetal heart accelerations occurring with fetal movements during a measured period of monitoring ____Nons Stress Test____

11-2 At 36 weeks' gestation, Jane S. is instructed to count fetal movements for a period of time. She should count the first 10 fetal movements beginning at the same time each day and note:
  a. Where the baby is kicking her
  b. If position change makes a difference
  c. A change in strength and frequency of movements
  d. Fetal sleep periods

11-3 Mary's MSAFP was unusually elevated at 17 weeks. To what conditions might this be attributed?
  a. Fetal hypoxia
  b. Open defects of the spine
  c. Down syndrome
  d. Maternal hypertension

Answer Key

REFERENCES

Eden RD, Sokol RJ: Predicting prematurity: the mammary stimulation test, *Clin Perinatol* 19(2):291, 1992.

Ferguson JE et al: Transcervical chorionic villus sampling and amniocentesis—a comparison of reliability, culture findings, and fetal outcome, *Am J Obstet Gynecol* 163(3):926, 1990.

Grannum PA, Berkowitz RI, Hobbins JC: The ultrasonic changes in the maturing placenta and their relation to fetal pulmonic maturity, *Am Obstet Gynecol* 133:915, 1979.

Green JE et al: Chorionic villus sampling: experience with an initial 940 cases, *Obstet Gynecol* 71(2):208, 1988.

Gregor CL, Paine LL, Johnson TRB: Antepartal fetal assessment, *J Nurse Midwife* 36(3):153, 1991.

Leerentveld RA et al: Accuracy and safety of transvaginal sonographic placental localization, *Obstet Gynecol* 76(5):759, 1990.

Miller-Slade D et al: Acoustic stimulation-induced fetal response compared to traditional nonstress testing, *JOGNN* 20(2):160, 1991.

Modica MM, Timor-Tritch C: Transvaginal sonography, *JOGGN* 17(2):89, 1988.

Mole R: Possible hazards of imaging and Doppler ultrasound in obstetrics, *Birth* 13(special suppl):23, 1986.

Paul RH, Chez RA: Fetal acoustic stimulation, *Contemp Ob/Gyn* 17(2):123, 1988.

Pergament E: Chorionic villi sampling and its role in genetic diagnoses. In Rathi M, ed: *Clinical aspects of perinatal medicine,* vol 11, New York, 1986, Macmillan.

Policy statement: Maternal serum alpha-fetoprotein screening, *Am J Public Health* 81(2):241, 1991.

Quigley ME et al: Effects of maternal smoking on circulating catacholamines and fetal heart rate, *Am J Obstet Gynecol* 133(6):686, 1979.

Rothman BK: The *tentative pregnancy: prenatal diagnoses and the future of motherhood,* New York, 1986, Viking Penguin, Inc.

STUDENT REFERENCE SHELF

Davis L: Daily fetal movement counting, *J Nurse Midwife* 32(1):41, 1987. Instructions for a nontechnical method every mother can use.

Treacy B, Smith C, Rayburn W: Ultrasound in labor and delivery, *Obstet Gynecol Surv* 45(4)213, 1990. A review of the state of the art in ultrasound.

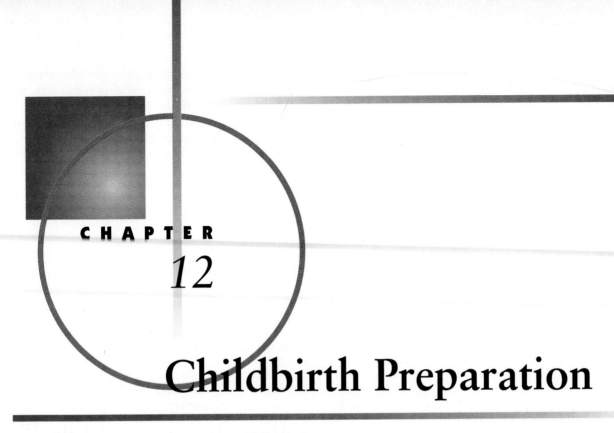

Childbirth Preparation

KEY TERMS

Birth Plans
Cues
Effleurage
Fear-Tension-Pain
  Cycle
Hypnosis
Locus of Control
Nonpharmacologic
  Analgesia
Open-Glottis Pushing
Valsalva's Maneuver

LEARNING OBJECTIVES

1. *Describe basic philosophy and concepts of preparation for childbirth.*
2. *Compare expectations placed on the laboring woman and her coach in selected methods of childbirth preparation.*
3. *Explain the rationale for neuromuscular conditioning for labor.*
4. *Demonstrate recommended exercises, relaxation techniques, and breathing patterns.*
5. *Relate the value of childbirth education to a couple's sense of control as they approach birth.*
6. *Summarize the role of the nurse as health teacher in preparation for birth.*

Childbirth Education

Preparation for the birth takes several forms. Because couples may not have a supportive extended family from which to learn, childbirth education assumes increased importance. Nursing interventions can change perceptions of the childbirth experience, even for an unprepared couple. It is important therefore that the nurse understand the support and teaching role in childbirth education.

The availability of formal programs of prenatal education is a rather modern phenomenon. Girls and boys have always been educated informally for their roles as parents. Depending on culture and family setting, this education varies in its positive and negative qualities. Because of the changes in family structure, the nuclear family does not have the support system of an extended family that includes mother and father, cousins, and aunts and uncles. Pregnant couples often seek preparation as they approach parenting without a clear notion of what it entails.

METHODS OF PREPARATION

The two major approaches to preparation for childbirth in the United States are the *psychophysical method* and the *psychoprophylactic method*. The psychophysical method evolved out of the natural childbirth movement in the 1940s and was founded on the writing and work of Dick-Read (Great Britain) and Thomas and Goodrich (United States). The program of education and

263

exercise is directed toward breaking the fear-tension-pain cycle. Expectant fathers are welcomed to class and are prepared for labor with their partners. Such courses frequently incorporate general prenatal education with specific techniques for comfort during labor. Many courses also add a postpartum class, requested by parents uncertain of their infant-care skills.

Preparation for childbirth provides the modern couple with the means to cope effectively with the stress brought about by the last weeks of pregnancy, the birth of the baby, and the early postpartum period. The psychophysical and psychoprophylactic methods (Table 12-1) are similarly based on the following three important areas:

TABLE 12-1 Comparison of Methods of Childbirth Preparation

| | PSYCHOPHYSICAL METHODS | | | PSYCHOPROPHYLACTIC METHODS (LAMAZE) | |
	DICK-READ	BRADLEY	KITZINGER	ADAPTED	CLASSIC
Rationale	Women negatively influenced by cultural conditioning and need to break fear-tension-pain cycle	Attempts to imitate other mammals' instinctive conduct in labor through intelligent reasoning	Mental and physical harmony produce a creative childbirth experience	Behavioral conditioning of mother produces reliable, constructive responses to demands of labor	Pavlovian conditioning raises threshold of pain by creating a zone of inhibition in cortex
Provision of support for mother	Medical labor attendants	Role of husband and physician central	Husband or significant other	Husband or significant other Medical labor attendant	Medical labor attendants, including a "monitrice" or specialized labor attendant
Prenatal physical exercise	Strenuous physical exercise thought inherent to preparing the body for labor	Rigorous exercise based on rationale of athletic qualities of labor	None specifically prescribed	Nonstrenuous program of physical fitness to increase comfort in pregnancy	"Body-building" exercise to prepare for "athletic event" of labor
Labor techniques	Create positive mental attitude Use of abdominal breathing for most of labor Use of panting	Imitation of sleep through position and use of abdominal breathing	Rhythmic breathing: slow to shallow as labor progresses	Rhythmic breathing: slow to shallow but not panting or rapid	Diaphragmatic breathing: slow and rapid; use of panting and vigorous blowing
	Passive relaxation exercise	Deep mental relaxation	Refined relaxation technique	Refined active relaxation and body awareness	Neuromuscular disassociation exercises
	Pushing technique	Pushing technique	Detailed pushing technique and exercise stressed	Detailed pushing technique	Pushing technique
Comments	Mystical overtones Diluted in practice by others from Read's original premise	Absolutes in methodology Domineering role of husband Role of techniques secondary	Adaptive approach to teach women to approach labor with confidence	Flexible but structured to integrate physical, emotional, and mental responses during labor	Often practical with rigid and dogmatic qualities

1. Accurate information to reduce anxieties and fears that accentuate pain
2. Acquisition of specific techniques of relaxation, muscular control, and respiratory techniques to reduce pain during labor
3. Creation and maintenance of a calm and supportive environment so the woman feels she can "go with" the process, using learned techniques when helpful

Maternity Center Association

The family-centered approach to preparation for birth was pioneered in New York by the Maternity Center Association. It focuses on alternatives to traditional medical settings for birth in its nurse-midwife–directed birthing center. The Maternity Center encourages physical and mental preparation for birth, including the inclusion of the expectant father; the creation of a warm, supportive environment during labor; and specific activities such as abdominal and chest breathing for the management of labor.

Bradley Method

Bradley (1974) based the method on his observations of animal behavior during birth. Most of the techniques for labor are derived from this "imitation of nature." Bradley describes these techniques as meeting the laboring mother's need for the following:

1. Darkness and solitude
2. Quiet
3. Physical comfort and relaxation
4. Controlled breathing
5. Closed eyes and the appearance of sleep

Bradley pioneered the rejection of the typically passive role for the expectant father. Instead, the partner acted as director of the woman's labor preparation and conduct. The emphasis on the partner may be interpreted by contemporary women as paternalistic and overbearing. Furthermore, pregnant women without traditional marital partners will feel excluded. The transference of the dominant male authority figure from physician to partner neglects in part the woman's need to take responsibility for her own behavior.

Kitzinger Method

In the writings of the British childbirth educator, Sheila Kitzinger (1980), a blurring of the distinction between psychophysical and psychoprophylactic methods is seen. Her program is structured to achieve a rhythmic coordination and harmony of the body during labor.

Kitzinger's approach advocates an elaborate system for relaxation that includes the father as a helper. The system was developed from the "method school" of acting and includes training in active relaxation. Although it does not claim to be part of an active conditioning process, it creates a new type of adaptive behavior for the mother. She uses breathing techniques, starting with slow breathing and progressing to shallow, rapid breathing for the final phase of labor. This approach is now merged somewhat in the next method.

Psychoprophylactic Method

Through the efforts of Marjorie Karmel and her book, *Thank you, Dr. Lamaze*, the Lamaze method became popular in the late 1960s. Lamaze (1972), working in Paris, applied Pavlov's classic conditioning techniques to the process of birth. Popularly known as the Lamaze method, psychoprophylaxis originally was a rigid and dogmatic approach. Today it is used less rigidly throughout the world; however, it is still *highly structured* and based on *conditioning, discipline,* and *concentration.* It is believed that the woman must undergo a period of disciplined training to substitute new responses to the stimulus of labor contractions. The support of a knowledgeable coach is recognized, and sound prenatal education is aimed at reducing psychic tension.

These methods incorporate what is referred to as **nonpharmacologic analgesia;** however, various types of anesthesia can be used as circumstances indicate. Criticism of these methods centers on the "structured, goal-oriented attitude that encourages couples to go into labor as into combat" (Noble, 1981).

Hypnosis

Hypnosis has been an effective approach to reduce the discomfort of labor, but it is not practical in hospital settings because it requires trained physicians and hypnotherapists to be available during the irregular schedule of childbirth. Through training in hypnosis the woman learns to enter a trancelike state, focusing on the therapist or on a prearranged self-hypnotic suggestion. It is possible to go through labor and birth, even by cesarean delivery, and to remain completely comfortable because this trance significantly reduces attention to outside stimuli.

Leboyer Method

During the 1970s, attention was given to Leboyer's method. Leboyer (1975) wanted to create a more satisfying birth experience through environmental changes. Although he did not advocate a new method of childbirth, he recommended the creation of a warm, human, and gentle environment for birth.

Leboyer sought to minimize what he considered to be the trauma of birth, and he appealed to the physician to take responsibility by eliminating unnecessary stimuli and encouraging the maternal-infant bond. One problem with the Leboyer method was neonatal delayed breathing caused by reduced stimulation after birth.

The Leboyer philosophy includes patience, emotional support, good communication, and education as integral parts of obstetric management. He emphasized a gentle, controlled delivery, specifically avoiding stress on the infant's craniosacral axis, suggesting that such stress interferes with the baby's well-being, particularly with initiation of breathing, and may cause irritability and other central nervous system problems. He advocated a gentle, warm water bath at birth to restore lost body heat, relax the infant physically, and thus place it in harmony with its environment.

Elements of Leboyer's approach have been integrated into many current popular methods of preparation. The emphasis, however, is on the physiologic and emotional needs of the mother and child at the birth rather than on prenatal preparation.

General Education

A few physicians teach childbirth classes as part of prenatal care. Most physicians who take the time to provide education for their clients find that there is a reduction in numbers of questions and a heightened sense of cooperation on the part of the couple. In fact, most prenatal classes are taught by nurses, either as part of a hospital-based program or as childbirth educators in private practice. General education uses most of the basic knowledge of the psychophysical method, but it may be much less structured.

EXPANDING SCOPE OF CHILDBIRTH PREPARATION

A large population of pregnant adolescents need prenatal and childbirth education. Their needs are based on their unique developmental requirements and social issues such as continuing education, economic support, and parenting skills. The traditional 6-week course for education is not adequate for these mothers. A number of research reports show that more extensive preparation is effective in reducing the fear-tension-pain cycle in adolescents (Hetherington, 1990; Slager-Ernest, Hoffman, and Beckmann, 1987).

For women delaying childbirth until their careers are established, childbirth preparation creates another kind of challenge. These women bring expectations that may or may not be realistic. They are accustomed to controlling and directing the details of their lives. Some are eager for the changes that parenting will bring; others are unrealistic about the demands of childbirth and parenting. Childbirth preparation classes afford a format in which these issues may be explored.

Sibling Classes

The number of classes for children to prepare them for the birth of the baby is increasing (Figure 12-1). The whole family attends, but the focus is on the child. It has been demonstrated that the use of a combination of techniques, such as charts, their own drawings, dolls, and

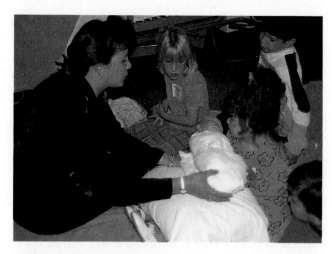

FIGURE 12-1 Siblings learn about infant care. (Courtesy Marjorie Pyle, RNC, *Lifecircle*.)

group activities, will keep children's interest. Films and stories may be used to enhance positive enjoyment and learning. Snacks are served. The brother or sister can ask questions and learn to anticipate the new rival with less apprehension (Spadt, Martin, and Thomas, 1990).

Breast-feeding Preparation

Women may elect to attend a class for breast-feeding preparation. Reading about breast-feeding and planning for it seem to support successful lactation. Women learn the benefits of early and frequent feedings and can insist on early access to the infant if they will not be in a labor-delivery-recovery (LDR) setting. They may share knowledge with the partner so he understands the process and does not feel left out.

> **Test Yourself**
> • Select three examples of social changes that have affected the scope of childbirth education.

NEED FOR A COACH

Practitioners of prepared childbirth have strongly advocated the active participation of the father as a labor coach. In situations in which the father is unavailable, a substitute is sought. The laboring woman wants desperately to help herself (which facilitates preparation) but also needs a caring person in her moment of emotional and physical vulnerability. The presence of a caring person knowledgeable about what should be done for support and control has a discernibly calming effect during this time of stress and challenge.

In studies of birth in which the husband was an active participant, the couple's relationship as partners and as parents was found to be enhanced. Each spoke

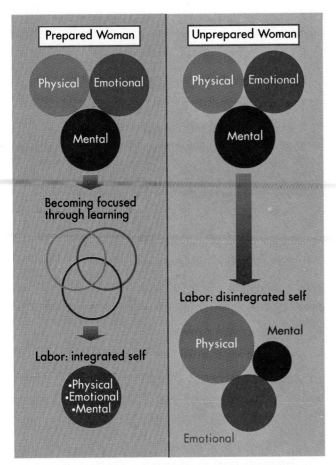

FIGURE 12-2 Results of childbirth education. Woman learns to integrate physical, emotional, and mental activity to remain focused and in control during labor. In the conditioning process, she substitutes learned responses to stimuli (contractions).

of the other in new appreciation; the bond seemed to be strengthened, and couples gained new perspectives on their marital and parenting roles. Objective, controlled studies demonstrate the validity of these observations (Westrich et al, 1991).

The anxieties of pregnancy are not limited to the pregnant woman but extend to her partner, thus creating a *pregnant couple*. Parent education in preparation for childbirth must deal with these anxieties. Such preparation seeks not only to present the partner with the same factual information as the woman but also to give him a sense of importance and relevance during the birth. He gains an appreciation of the physical effort of birth and the assurance that he, too, will be prepared to function in specific and definite ways as part of the team (Copstick et al, 1986).

"My boyfriend isn't sure if he wants to be with me when I have the baby. My sister said she would be my coach. When we went to birthing classes, I was afraid that I'd

have to choose between them. But the teacher welcomed them both. She made my boyfriend feel so much better, he's even saying he might come in the labor room with me."

The woman learns how to concentrate during labor. This response contrasts with that of the unprepared woman who remains out of focus, finds the physical responses to labor to be overwhelming, and becomes incapable of rational thought (Figure 12-2). The principles of training in basic athletic skills or learning a new subject apply to childbirth. In addition, training in relaxation and concentration has been shown to be beneficial in other medical areas (Mast et al, 1987). Through disciplined learning and applied technique, the prepared woman recognizes her responses and checks the inclination to panic; she works *with* the process of labor. She learns to minimize fatigue by reducing tension, fearful anticipation, and heightened perception of pain. Thus the need for analgesics, anesthesia, and obstetric interventions may be reduced. During birth the prepared woman works more efficiently and is able to cooperate with the powerful forces of the second stage.

Test Yourself

- What do you think of the following statements made by some teachers about the benefit of childbirth education?
- The mother is always able to cope with physical challenge of labor and thereby maintains control.
- Failure in labor that results in a cesarean birth is less common.
- The perception of pain is lessened by application of techniques.
- Self-esteem is fostered by a sense of being able to participate and manage self during labor.

EVALUATION OF CHILDBIRTH EDUCATION

Shearer (1990) states that despite prenatal classes it is the staff members who help or hinder the process:

In fact, attitudes and policies of labor and delivery personnel utterly swamp the effects of prenatal education. Bedside practices can make prenatal education appear to be effective, or to have made no difference, or to have actually caused harm to the patients. Obstetric staff do quickly ascertain the goals of patients admitted in labor (and the goals of their prenatal classes). The staff have their own feelings about various classes, consciously or not. Usually, they have discussed how much they will cooperate with patient's wishes, and which of their goals to promote, downgrade, or ignore. Regardless of how comparable or randomly chosen the class and no-class groups are in a study, obstetric management will completely dominate any effects of teaching. Bedside care can magnify or render meaningless—or even malignant—any prenatal training.

Studies of childbirth education effectiveness are difficult to evaluate with this random factor that is not acknowledged by most researchers. Two studies, for example, report different results: the physicians' study found no extra benefit (Sturrock and Johnson, 1990); the nurse's study found significant benefit (Hetherington, 1990).

SELECTION OF A HEALTH CARE PROVIDER

Parents-to-be may select their physician, clinic, and hospital on the basis of the cooperation of the health care providers in childbirth preparation. Most women desire the atmosphere of a family-centered maternity care unit as a continuation of their prenatal and labor education (Figure 12-3).

Until recently the outlook for the client who depended on a public hospital was bleak. She had no choices. The impersonal nature of many clinics, staffing procedures, and other policies made it difficult for the woman to be assured of a supportive situation or a sympathetic acceptance of the idea of prepared childbirth.

The nurse engaged in private or group practice as a childbirth educator is one of the most important sources for classes. Parents usually find an educator through referral by a friend or by their physician. If clinic care is

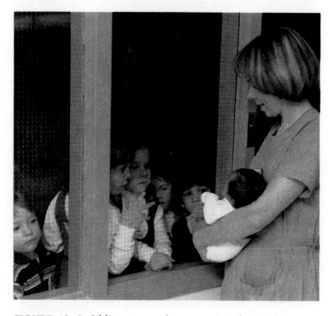

FIGURE 12-3 Siblings get a chance to visit the newborn nursery. (Courtesy St. John's Mercy Medical Center, St. Louis, Mo.)

selected, most now include childbirth classes. Unfortunately, classes may be as large as 40 to 50, with a dependence on videotapes or films as a substitute for more personal interaction with the nurse educator.

BARRIERS TO CHILDBIRTH EDUCATION

The barriers to preparation for childbirth and the woman's culture, education, attitude, family, and economic status must be considered. In certain cultural groups, the *lack of interest* by the woman's husband or family or their overt opposition to her interest is a strong enough factor to deter her consideration of childbirth preparation programs unless such preparation is an integral part of her prenatal care.

Other *cultural, social, temperamental,* or *maturational factors* influence the woman's involvement. Preparation for childbirth may violate sexual taboos, cultural expectations, or family structure. If the woman has unresolved conflicts about her sexuality, this pregnancy, or motherhood, she usually will not participate. A woman may be unaware of the availability of classes in her community and, lacking strong motivation, fail to seek such information. A single woman may hesitate to join a class because of her anticipation of criticism by others.

The woman may be *uninformed* about the basic concepts of childbirth preparation, especially if she is a member of a lower socioeconomic group. These particular deterrents need to be significantly modified by the accurate presentation of the purpose and availability of classes to the whole community.

Fatigue and other physical factors may seriously affect the woman's ability and motivation in seeking out and attending classes. If a woman's anxiety level is extremely high, she may avoid the counseling and education that would help her to cope.

Other factors are influential: classes must be made available at convenient times and locations for the couple, and the cost must be reasonable for all socioeconomic groups. Childbirth educators in private or group practice must make known their willingness to accept reduced fees if low-cost programs are not otherwise available. Costs range from free clinic classes up to $100 for six lessons by a private educator.

NURSING APPROACH

The central goal of parent education is the *reduction of anxiety and fear* through dissemination of accurate information (Box 12-1). When presenting factual information, the teacher directs the discussion to the level of the group. The direction and depth of information required may be assessed by a brief period of asking couples to share prior experiences or having the parents write a list of questions and concerns.

BOX 12-1   Objectives of Childbirth Education

- To minimize anxieties, correct misconceptions, and reduce fear by providing factual information about pregnancy, labor, and recovery
- To teach neuromuscular and respiratory skills to facilitate coping during labor
- To provide a framework of reference for the pregnant couple in which they may place their responses and concerns
- To create a setting within which parents may effectively use verbal and nonverbal communication
- To develop a relaxed, open group atmosphere conducive to learning and growing in self-awareness
- To promote informed consumerism

The content must be relevant and easily understood, with enough detail to give the couple an accurate and realistic picture of labor. Effective learning will take place if self-esteem is enhanced and anxiety is lessened by a positive approach (Figure 12-4).

Another goal of the educator is to *create informed and assertive consumers.* Too often the couple has been passive in the childbirth experience, allowing health care providers to do almost anything without questioning them. There still are many degrees of acceptance by those in the medical profession of the couple's involvement in the childbirth process; not all physicians welcome it. A couple should be encouraged to consult with their chosen physician about possible approaches and together make a tentative *birth plan* for labor, including potential use of analgesia or anesthesia.

Birth Plans

Helping couples create meaningful **birth plans** means a careful and reasoned exploration of traditional and nontraditional approaches to birth. The nurse must not place unreasonable expectations on the couple and must know the community and the likelihood of newer methods being used in local settings. Birth plans help the woman formulate a realistic view of the approaching events and can provide continuity in care when several health care persons are involved (Kitzinger, 1992).

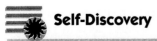

Self-Discovery

Create a birth plan for yourself.

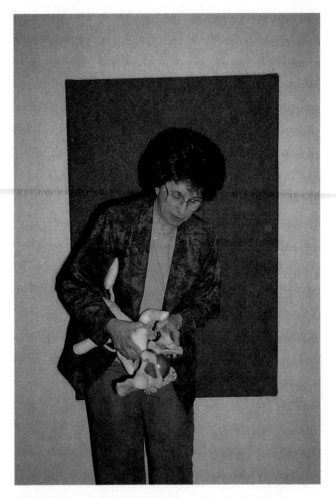

FIGURE 12-4 Childbirth educator demonstrates exit maneuvers for birth. (Courtesy Marjorie Pyle, RNC, *Lifecircle.*)

Partner's Skills

As the couple perfects neuromuscular and respiratory skills, childbirth educators provide opportunities for exploration of feelings, involving partners in nonthreatening ways. From the very first session the partner is introduced as the chief supporter and coach, and as the

Cultural Aspects of Care

"I was excited about going to prenatal classes, but as soon as I walked in I felt uncomfortable. I was the only black woman and the only one who had come to class alone. The instructor said that she would be my coach in class but then used me to show the class different things. I felt put on stage. The importance of the father's role in labor was stressed so much that, for the first time, I asked myself, "Am I really going to be able to do this alone?""

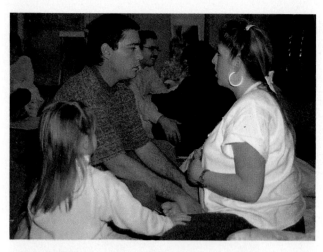

FIGURE 12-5 Learning relaxation exercises with the whole family. (Courtesy Marjorie Pyle, RNC, *Lifecircle*.)

class progresses, his importance in the process is emphasized. However, the educator should be sure to indicate that the coach can be someone other than the father and that women without partners are encouraged to choose a close friend or relative for that role.

In a more general way, childbirth educators encourage mutual respect for the roles of father and mother during the childbirth experience and foster the concept of birth as a family experience (Figure 12-5). Through this learning experience the partners become independent and cooperative and increase their self-esteem. **Locus of control** is not taken from them as they learn to manage a stressful situation. The result of childbirth preparation extends beyond the specific techniques used during labor. The family can be strengthened and emotional readiness for parenthood enhanced.

Content of Classes
INTRODUCTORY CLASS

During the first class (Box 12-2), group interaction is facilitated by making introductions that should be limited to simple information, including name, parity, due date, community, and hospital; describing occupations might divide the group along socioeconomic lines.

The educator makes general comments about the purpose of the course, presents realistic goals, and introduces basic concepts. Parents need to understand that they can establish their own goals as the class evolves.

Because the class is still a collection of persons and not yet a group, couples respond more readily to concrete and factual details. Pertinent information about conception and the trimesters of pregnancy is

enhanced by the use of visual aids. Discussion of fetal development and maternal changes reinforces the reality of the baby. The use of words such as "Now your baby's heart can be heard" helps the couple to identify their baby, particularly if it is their first. Comments such as "Many women feel very tired at this point" or "You may feel the need to talk over each detail" enhance maternal self-awareness.

Introducing physical conditioning exercises is appropriate to this first class. Couples are anxious to do something. These exercises increase the woman's sense of well-being and physical comfort during pregnancy. They are directed not toward the development of muscular strength but toward improvement of circulation, ventilation, body awareness, and posture. Exercise videotapes for pregnancy are available. (See Chapter 9 for restriction on exercise.)

Controlled relaxation is the foundation on which all other techniques are applied. As the woman begins to develop awareness of bodily changes, she learns how to be comfortable, to detect tension in her body, and to facilitate relaxation. Her partner begins to learn to detect tension in her by touch and observation. Together they concentrate on achieving the active (vs passive) relaxation necessary for control during labor. The partner is encouraged to touch and stroke her in ways to enhance relaxation and rest. Stroking always accompanies the verbal cue "relax" so that stroking itself soon becomes a signal for relaxation. Although jet hydrotherapy is not offered by many birth units, it too appears to be helpful (Aderhold and Perry, 1991).

Managing Pain

Childbirth education allows the woman alternatives to pharmacologic means to lessen pain. Pain is modified or inhibited when the person is able to have a specific focus of attention; when anxiety, fatigue, and muscle tension are reduced; and when there is an increase of controlled sensory input (see section on pain in Chapter 16).

As strategies, the woman may use light stroking (effleurage) by the coach or herself to create organized, controlled sensory input to relieve local irritability. When concentrating on the sensation at the skin, she may be able to disregard the more diffuse sensation from the pain fibers of the uterus or cervix. When the woman performs alternate activities such as breathing in specific patterns or relaxing in learned ways, she may further modify pain transmission. Mental rehearsal and imagery activate concentration and improve performance.

The woman is encouraged to respond to labor in a variety of ways. She may assume several positions, breathe as she is comfortable doing, and ask for assistance. It should be emphasized that the coach and staff members are available to assist her.

BOX 12-2   Sample Class Outline*

Introductory class

Introduce self and class participants.

Discuss basic purpose and goals of the course.

Present common terms.

Discuss highlights of conception, fetal development, maternal reactions, and physical changes.

Teach physical conditioning exercises and rationale:

  Tailor press

  Tailor stretch

  Tailor reach

  Pelvic tilt

  Bent-leg lift

  Perineal control (Kegel exercise)

Teach basics of controlled relaxation:

  Achieving comfort

  Facilitating relaxation

  Self-detection of tension and relaxation

  Coach's detection of tension and relaxation

  Role of touching and stroking to enhance relaxation

  Use of precise verbal cues

Intermediate classes

Practice relaxation techniques.

Introduce and develop the mechanism of labor.

Discuss related maternal reactions and emotional responses to the mechanism of labor.

Teach various labor techniques in which the couple needs to become proficient:

  Integration of controlled relaxation

  Rationale for respiratory techniques

  Rhythmic chest breathing: slow and modified rates

  Shallow chest breathing: combined with rhythmic chest breathing (modified rate) and rhythmic pattern of shallow breathing and short blows

  Open-glottis pushing

  Recognizing, preventing, and dealing with hyperventilation

  Expulsion techniques: overcoming fear of pushing, integrating controlled relaxation (especially perineal), using abdominal muscles effectively in directing pushing effort, correcting position to enhance the effort

  Managing back labor

Develop the couple's confidence and self-awareness.

Introduce couples to community resources (e.g., baby care classes, visiting nurse services, family planning services).

Acquaint couples with local hospital facilities and policies.

Concluding class

Complete review of mechanism of labor, maternal reactions, labor techniques, and partner's role.

Discuss immediate postpartum period:

  Physical recuperation

  Emotional responses

  Emotional needs

  Hospital facilities: recovery area, postpartum unit, nursery

Discuss newborn:

  Appearance at birth

  Care of infant in delivery room

  Characteristics of newborn during first few days

  Need for mother's physical contact

  Feeding, if pertinent to class needs

Discuss postpartum period at home:

  Physical changes

  Emotional needs and responses

  Simple exercises to improve muscle tone and sense of well-being

  Partner's needs and role

*The instructor uses visual aids, demonstration, questions and discussion, group participation, role playing, and tours in the class.

Test Yourself

Listed below are three factors that help diminish pain perception. An example is provided for each. List as many other actions as you can that would help a woman reduce pain sensations.

- Focused attention: Example—provide education that teaches mother to tune in to her body rather than yield to panic.

- Reduction of anxiety, fatigue, muscle tension: Example—provide consistent reassurance.

- Increased controlled sensory input: Example—woman or coach strokes abdomen.

INTERMEDIATE CLASSES

Building on the information and rapport of the introductory class, subsequent classes are expanded in a logical progression. Content is carefully structured to the interests of the couples, who need a clear understanding of what happens, how the woman will feel and react, how she can cope during each phase, and how her partner can support and direct her efforts.

In teaching the second stage, for instance, the instructor needs to be alert to the anxiety about and fear of giving birth. Attitudes toward sexuality, fear for safety, misconceptions, and inaccurate information contribute to these fears of pain and injury held by both partner and woman. The couple must gain an accurate

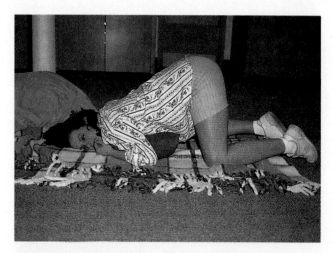

FIGURE 12-6 Knee-chest position is taught for changing infant position if necessary or if cord problems occur. (Courtesy Marjorie Pyle, RNC, *Lifecircle.*)

and positive understanding of the mechanism of birth and a realistic expectation about their ability to work with the birth process (Figure 12-6).

Test Yourself

• Identify three ways in which you can promote self-care during pregnancy and birth.

BREATHING TECHNIQUES

To enhance relaxation and remove the focus away from the contraction, breathing rhythms can be altered. Breathing normally is automatic; we do not think about breaths at all. To learn new techniques takes practice and interest in self-help. Starting with Dick-Read, childbirth education has taught various patterns for use during labor stages. Classic Lamaze technique has been modified by most teachers of psychoprophylaxis and includes the following basic aspects:

1. Chest breathing is said to diminish diaphragmatic interference on the uterine fundus and is used throughout. The woman feels as though she is breathing higher and higher in the chest as she progresses with the techniques.
2. A deep breath initiates and concludes each contraction. Also, the deep breath clears carbon dioxide and increases oxygen levels. This is an important signal for the woman and her coach. She has learned to relax consciously as she exhales this breath. These beginning and ending breaths make each contraction a single entity, as opposed to the sense of endless contractions.
3. A *focal point* increases the woman's concentration and diminishes distraction. It serves to direct her attention to dealing with the contraction constructively. The point of focus may change from time to time.
4. Verbal and nonverbal cues are used to indicate when the woman will use a breathing technique (e.g., "contraction begins . . . contraction ends"). At times these cues may be used by the coach during labor if the woman has become drowsy, tired, or uncertain about the actual onset of each contraction.
5. A comfortable position is important for effective relaxation and efficient respiration. The supine position will interfere with the progress of labor and cause undesirable intraabdominal pressure on the large blood vessels. The woman is encouraged to use a tailor-sitting, side-lying, or a more upright position in the bed or chair (Liu, 1989).

These techniques may be practiced in front of a mirror or with the partner timing the "practice" contraction. The couple should inform the nurse at the start of labor which sequences of breathing they have been practicing.

Early Phase

The first respiratory pattern the woman will use is *rhythmic chest breathing* at the slow rate of about eight breaths per minute. She inhales through the nose and exhales through the mouth; exhalation is stressed and slightly prolonged. In rhythm with the breathing, she can apply a circular stroke over the abdominal area, using her fingertips. Stroking may be done with one or both hands or by her coach. This type of breathing is continued as long as it is effective.

With the advance of dilation as the phase progresses, the woman also may need to progress in breathing activity. She modifies the rhythmic chest breathing by increasing the rate to 16 or 20 breaths per minute, continuing rhythmic stroking (Figure 12-7, *A*).

Active Phase

To deal with the intensity, the woman progresses to a combined pattern of modified rhythmic chest breathing and *shallow chest breathing*. She matches the increment and decrement with the rhythmic chest breathing pattern; she uses the lighter, faster shallow breathing for the acme. Rhythmic stroking is continued if she finds it soothing. As contractions demand, she may use shallow breathing for the entire contraction, permitting greater flexibility in rate and depth. When using this technique, she breathes lightly and evenly, inhaling and exhaling through her slightly opened mouth. The rate is just fast enough to ensure respiratory exchange (as opposed to simply moving tidal air) with minimal effort and depth of respirations (Figure 12-7, *B*).

Transition Phase

To handle this difficult period, a woman must use specific strategies. She uses a rhythmic pattern of shal-

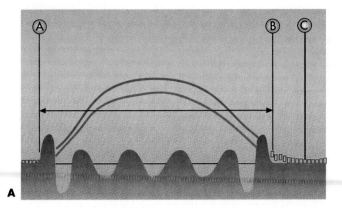

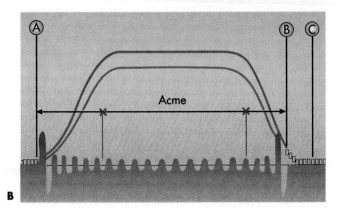

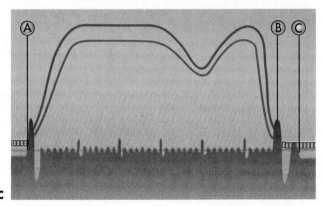

FIGURE 12-7 A, Latent phase contractions contrasted with rhythmic chest breathing. Duration (*A* to *B*) is 30 to 45 seconds; interval (*A* to *C*) is 10 to 5 minutes, and intensity is mild to moderate. Rhythmic chest breathing is at a rate of eight breaths per minute. Deep breath begins and ends each contraction. **B,** Active phase contraction contrasted with shallow chest breathing. Duration (*A* to *B*) is 50 to 60 seconds; interval (*A* to *C*) is 5 to 3 minutes, and intensity is moderate to strong with well-defined peaks. Shallow chest accelerated-decelerated breathing is matched to contraction intensity. **C,** Transition phase contraction. Duration (*A* to *B*) is 60 to 90 seconds; interval (*A* to *C*) is 2 to 3 minutes and intensity is strong with several peaks and rising tonus; shallow chest breathing is encouraged, alternating with blow (puff) breaths.

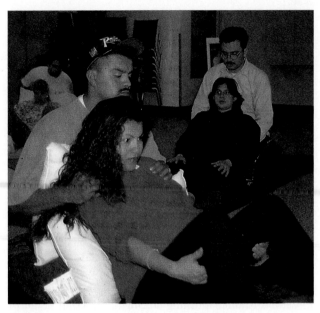

FIGURE 12-8 Practice with the pushing position during class. (Courtesy Marjorie Pyle, RNC, *Lifecircle.*)

low chest breathing with short puffs, which requires concentration and promotes a sense of control. The sequence usually is three or two breaths or one shallow breath, alternating with a puff. These patterns are altered in response to the intensity of each contraction. The pattern of one shallow breath and one puff is particularly useful in controlling intense peaks, sensations of pressure, or the urge to push (Figure 12-7, *C*).

Expulsion Phase

Technique focuses on controlled relaxation and voluntary bearing down. Recent research and studies have made it clear that expulsion techniques should avoid sustained breath holding. The woman learns to use her oblique abdominal muscles and a fixed diaphragm to bear down. By pushing as though she is going to quickly empty her bladder, she will direct her efforts through the vagina and not the rectum. Conscious release of the perineum reduces resistance to the head. Correct positioning into a **C** shape, whether semisitting or upright, will allow her to favorably influence the axis of the birth canal. The position of her body and legs influences the relaxation of the perineum, further reducing resistance to the baby's head as it emerges.

The woman learns to push during the peak of each contraction, permitting the contraction to build by taking two deep breaths. Then she is encouraged to bear down repeatedly, tuning in to her body (Figure 12-8).

To sustain the work, to increase the efficiency of that effort and the efficiency of her ventilation, and to avoid **Valsalva's maneuver,** she learns to use a series of breaths, holding for a moment to start the push and then bearing down vigorously as she exhales slowly; this is **open-glottis pushing.** She can say a word such as "push" or "out" or grunt to control the release of air as she maintains her pushing efforts. She may alternately hold her breath and bear down without the controlled exhalation as long as she avoids sustained breath holding.

Valsalva's maneuver. Holding breath and bearing down for more than 5 or 6 seconds is associated with a lowering in maternal blood pressure and a decrease in placental circulation. Like a domino effect, fetal pH and oxygen pressure (Po_2) decrease and carbon dioxide pressure (Pco_2) and fetal heart rate increase. Thus bearing down should be brief, accompanied by open-glottis pushing with air release (Roberts et al, 1987). Although this technique has been known since 1980, many units continue to insist that the woman do forceful sustained pushing during the second stage of labor. *Here is an area for nurse advocacy for the health of the laboring woman.*

CESAREAN BIRTH PREPARATION

When cesarean birth is expected, couples may attend classes that omit the emphasis on self-help during labor. Although preparation details may differ (Hassid, 1984), basics remain the same. Box 12-3 lists topics that are helpful to the couple.

Not all women take advantage of such classes, and the nurse will care for women who are unprepared or did not expect a cesarean birth. In these cases the list in Box 12-3 will be useful for teaching.

CONCLUDING CLASS

The couple's proficiency in technique and knowledge of labor must be reviewed and evaluated in the concluding class. The instructor can introduce material pertinent to the postpartum period. Couples need a basic awareness of the physical changes and emotional and social adjustments of the recovery period. They also need to be prepared for the "unfinished" qualities of the newborn, as well as its demands and needs. First-time parents

---

BOX 12-3 Teaching Topics for Cesarean Birth

- Reason for, safety, and risks of cesarean birth
- Couple's understanding of these reasons or their prior experiences
- Potential of vaginal birth after cesarean delivery
- Policies regarding cesareans, differing facilities, and costs
- Preparation before admission and procedures on admission
- Anesthesia choices and recovery process
- Couple's understanding of their choices
- Role of physician, anesthesiologist, nurse
- Signs of labor onset and what to do if early
- Actual cesarean procedure (films)
- Support role of partner before and after birth
- Parent-infant contact opportunities
- Recovery process, intravenous lines, catheters, pain management, fluids, food
- Relaxation responses that help—breathing, imagery
- Involution patterns and recovery expectations
- Discharge timing and choices
- Home care opportunities
- Managing at home
- Infant feeding choices, lactation support
- Neonatal care in delivery area, pattern of care in hospital
- Expected emotional response, integration of experience
- Possibilities of a cesarean support group

---

need to be aware that they will not suddenly be transformed into the romanticized image of parenthood but will grow into their new role.

Many primigravidas are unprepared for various aspects of physical recovery. A brief discussion of what to expect aids understanding of the physiology of the recovery period and provides a few practical suggestions for dealing with this recuperative period.

Because couples share in excitement and learning, new friendships may start. The childbirth educator often offers to hold a "reunion" at a reasonable time in the future.

KEY POINTS

- Information and support reduce the fear-tension-pain cycle of labor.
- The laboring couple functions best when they have discussed the birth plan with health care providers and feel a sense of trust.
- Effects of childbirth education may be diminished by unsupportive hospital personnel.
- Barriers to childbirth preparation should be recognized and arrangements made to facilitate classes for all women.

- Exercises and breathing practice develop a sense of self-care and foster self-esteem.
- Valsalva's maneuver can occur with incorrect bearing down; mother and fetus need protection by informed nurses.
- Those who plan a cesarean birth have as much or more need for prebirth preparation.

STUDY QUESTIONS

12-1

   a. A perineal exercise that strengthens perineal muscles is _____ .

   b. Control commands given to mother before a contraction are _____ .

   c. A breathing technique to enhance relaxation is _____

   d. A light stroking of woman's skin as a counterstimulus is _____ .

12-2 Which observation of the couple helps you make an assessment of potential coping skills?

   a. Expressions of anxiety

   b. The manner in which the couple interacts

   c. The skill demonstrated in performing learned techniques

   d. Comments about prior experiences

12-3 Select one important value of having a labor coach.

   a. The partner feels needed in the birth experience.

   b. Labor usually is shorter when the partner is present.

   c. The expectant mother retains a better sense of control.

   d. Less nursing attention is needed during labor.

12-4 Valsalva's maneuver will result in:

   a. Maternal dizziness

   b. Change in fetal acid-base balance

   c. Increased placental blood flow

   d. An extended second stage of labor

Answer Key   12-1 a. Kegel b. Cues c. Slow chest d. Effleurage 12-2 b, d 12-3 c 12-4 b

REFERENCES

Aderhold K J, Perry L: Jet hydrotherapy for labor and postpartum pain relief, *MCN* 16(2):97, 1991.

Beck N, Hall D: Natural childbirth: a review and analysis, *Obstet Gynecol* 52(3):371, 1978.

Bennett A, Hewson D, Booker E: Antenatal preparation and labor support in relation to birth outcomes, *Birth* 12(1):9, 1985.

Bradley R: Husband coached childbirth, New York, 1974, Harper & Row.

Carty EM, Tier DT: Birth planning: a reality-based script for building confidence, *J Nurse Midwife* 34(3):111, 1989.

Copstick SM et al: Partner support and the use of coping techniques in labour, *Psychosom Res* 30(4):497, 1986.

Hassid P: *Textbook for childbirth educators,* New York, 1984, Harper & Row.

Hetherington SE: A controlled study of the effect of prepared childbirth classes on obstetric outcomes, *Birth* 17(2):86, 1990.

Jimenez SL: Para dar la luz: reaching Hispanic women, Childbirth Instructor 2(2):42, 1992.

Johnsen NM, Gaspad ME: Theoretical foundations for a prepared sibling class, *JOGNN* 14(3):237, 1985.

Kitzinger S: *Pregnancy and childbirth,* New York, 1980, Penguin.

Kitzinger S: Birth plans, *Birth* 19(1):36, 1992.

Krutsky C: Siblings at birth: impact on parents, *J Nurse Midwife* 30(4):269, 1985.

Lamaze F: *Painless childbirth,* New York, 1972, Simon & Schuster.

Leboyer F: *Birth without violence,* New York, 1975, Alfred A. Knopf.

Lindell SG: Education for childbirth: a time for change, *JOGNN* 18(2):108, 1988.

Liu YC: The effects of the upright position during childbirth, *Image J Nurs Sch* 21(Spring):14, 1989.

Maloni JA et al: Expectant grandparents' class, *JOGNN* 16(1):26, 1987.

Noble E: Controversies in maternal effort during labor and delivery, *J Nurse Midwife* 26(2):13, 1981.

Roberts J et al: A descriptive analysis of involuntary bearing-down efforts, *JOGNN* 16(1): 48, 1987.

Shearer MH: Effects of prenatal education depend on the attitudes and practices of obstetric caregivers, *Birth* 17(2):73, 1990.

Slager-Ernest SE, Hoffman SJ, Beckmann CJA: Effects of specialized prenatal adolescent program on maternal and fetal outcomes, *JOGNN* 16(6):422, 1987.

Sosa R, Kennel J, Klaus M: The effect of a supportive companion on perinatal problems, length of labor and mother-infant interaction, *N Engl J Med* 303(11):597, 1980.

Spadt SK, Martin KR, Thomas AM: Experiential classes for siblings-to-be, *MCN* 15(3):184, 1990.

Stevens R: Psychological strategies for management of pain in prepared childbirth. I. A review of research. *Birth* 11(3):16, 1984.

Stevens R: Psychological strategies for management of pain in prepared childbirth. II. Study of psychoanalgesia, *Birth* 11(3):00, 1984.

Sturrock WA, Johnson JA: The relationship between childbirth education classes and obstetric outcome, *Birth* 17(2):82, 1990.

Westrich R et al: The influence of birth setting on the father's behavior toward his partner and infant, *Birth* 18(4):198, 1991.

Yeates DA, Roberts JE: A comparison of two bearing down techniques during the second stage of labor, *J Nurse Midwife* 29(1):3, 1984.

STUDENT REFERENCE SHELF

Mast D et al: Relaxation techniques: a self-learning module for nurses, *Cancer Nurs* 10(3):26, 1987. A student can learn these techniques to better support the woman in labor.

Spadt SK, Martin KR, Thomas AM: Experiential classes for siblings-to-be, *MCN* 15(3):184, 1990. Outlines an innovative approach for sibling preparation classes.

RESOURCES FOR EXPECTANT PARENTS

Teacher Preparation Courses

Psychoprophylaxis

Council of Childbirth Education Specialists
8 Sylvan Glen
East Lyme, CT 06333

Psychophysical

Maternity Center Association
48 E. 92 St.
New York, NY 10028

Parent-Teacher Groups

American Society for Psychoprophylaxis in Obstetrics (ASPO)
1523 L St. NW
Washington, DC 20005
International Childbirth Education Association (ICEA)
P.O. Box 5852
Milwaukee, WI 53220
National Association of Parents and Professionals for Safe Alternatives in Childbirth (NAPSAC)
P.O. Box 1307
Chapel Hill, NC 27514

UNIT
Three

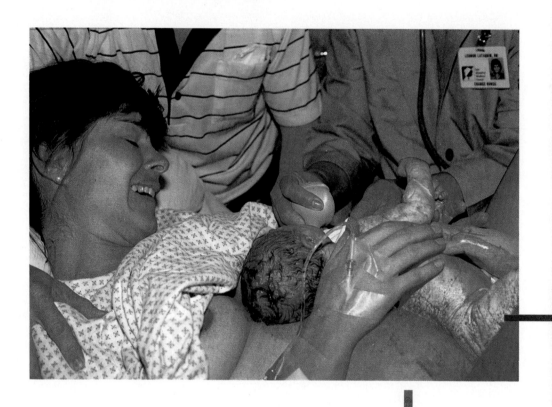

LABOR AND BIRTH

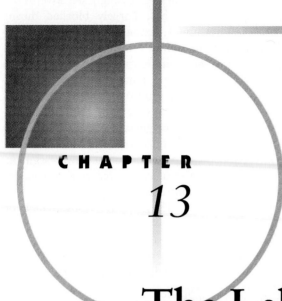

The Labor Process
and Nursing Care

KEY TERMS

Accoucheur
Active Phase
Breech Presentation
Cephalopelvic
  Disproportion
Chorioamnionitis
Descent
Dilation
Dystocia
Effacement
Engagement
Expulsion
Extension
External Rotation
Flexion
Gap Junctions
Hypertonic
  Contraction

Hyperventilation
Hypotonic Contraction
Internal Rotation
Latent Phase
Membranes
Molding
Occiput

Position
Presentation
Station
Tonus
Transition Phase
Triage
Vertex Presentation

LEARNING OBJECTIVES

1. *Compare observed labor process with the normal labor curve.*
2. *Relate physiologic conditions of the labor process to fetal responses.*
3. *Alter nursing interventions to observed fetal or maternal responses during labor.*
4. *Use appropriate terms and abbreviations in documenting labor progress.*
5. *Describe how a therapeutic relationship may be established with the laboring couple.*
6. *Identify important strategies for comfort and control to be used by the woman and her coach.*
7. *Develop nursing care plans that integrate principles of conservation of energy, integrity, and self-care during labor.*

Labor is the process by which the uterus expels or attempts to expel the fetus, placenta, and amniotic sac. It is accomplished by rhythmic contractions of the uterus. Anatomic landmarks of the uterus important during labor are shown in Figure 13-1. Pressure against the cervix created by the fetus and amniotic sac results in effacement and dilation of the cervix, which allow passage of the fetus from the uterus through the cervix and birth canal and into the extrauterine environment. To accomplish this process, there must be coordination among the "powers," "passage," and "passengers." The powers are the uterine contractions. The passage is the

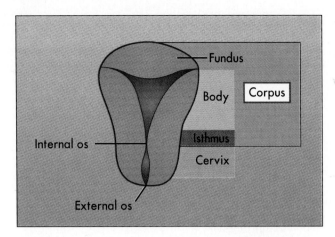

FIGURE 13-1 Anatomic landmarks of uterus important during labor.

bony pelvis, cervix, vagina, and introitus. The passengers are the fetus, amniotic sac, umbilical cord, and placenta. Normal labor requires that the powers be sufficient to expel the fetus, that the passage be of adequate size to allow descent and expulsion of the fetus, and that the passengers be of average size and in positions to allow negotiation of the passage during labor.

The Powers

The uterus provides the force necessary to expel the fetus. Effective contraction of the uterus leads to changes in the cervix necessary for delivery.

UTERINE CONTRACTIONS

Normally the uterus begins to contract effectively 280 days after the last menstrual period (LMP) or 266 ± 8 days after ovulation and fertilization. However, irregularities in the menstrual cycle make precise calculation of gestational age difficult. Amniotic fluid studies and ultrasonography can be used to more accurately determine gestational age of the fetus and the estimated date of birth (EDB, or EDD).

Contractions supply the involuntary or *primary* power for birth. During the last stage of labor the woman must add, by pushing down, the voluntary or *secondary* powers to complete the birth.

The muscles have a unique structure that provides the ability to contract from the fundus down and, in a mesh-like fashion, to constrict the numerous blood vessels that cross the muscle to enter the placenta. The lower uterine segment, in contrast, is stretched by the pressure of the fetus and fluids and does not rhythmically contract in the same way. This allows the fetus to descend smoothly.

After birth the empty uterus rapidly reduces its size by contraction. The myometrium thickens and the fundus moves, within a few minutes, from just under the diaphragm to below the umbilicus.

Uterine muscle becomes increasingly sensitive to oxytocin as birth approaches. Largely blocked during pregnancy by hormonal action, oxytocin levels rise slightly as labor approaches. Prostaglandins also affect contractions: increased amounts have been found in amniotic fluid as labor nears. Finally there are pacemakers in the myometrium; groups of these pacemakers trigger rhythmic contractions (see Initiation of Labor).

Uterine contractions originate in the fundus, the location of the highest concentration of muscle cells. The contraction then spreads into the lower segment. The contractility of the uterus increases as pregnancy progresses. Mild contractions occur infrequently throughout pregnancy. These contractions, which do not change the cervix, are short in duration and occur irregularly. During the last month of gestation, they increase in frequency and may occur every 10 to 20 minutes. They can be palpated by an observer but usually are not experienced as discomfort by the mother. If measured by a tocodynamometer, they rarely exceed 20 mm Hg or last longer than 60 to 80 seconds. During late pregnancy, these contraction patterns, which also are known as *Braxton Hicks contractions,* may be misunderstood for preterm labor.

Effective contractions provide the powers with which to efface and dilate the cervix and then, with maternal pushing efforts, expel the fetus and placenta. Each contraction has three parts: an increment (increasing intensity), an acme (peak), and a decrement (decreasing intensity). Note in Figure 13-2 the increment is steep and rapid, whereas the decrement is more prolonged and gradual. The contraction is a bell-shaped curve, with a steeper slope during increment. A relaxation phase (decrement) lasts for two thirds of contraction. Resting tone (lowest intramniotic pressure between contractions) amounts to 10 mm Hg. The area above 10 mm Hg is considered an active pressure area. Pain threshold is intrauterine pressure above which contraction is painful, about 10 to 15 mm Hg over resting tone. As labor progresses, the **tonus** or resting tone may begin to rise.

The degree of relaxation between contractions is very important because it allows the fetus and uterine muscles to recover from the stress of the contraction. During the *interval* or *resting phase* the uterus and placenta refill with blood, allowing for the exchange of oxygen, carbon dioxide, and nutrients at the placenta. A uterus does not relax sufficiently between contractions when there are **hypertonic** contractions. This contraction pattern is abnormal and may result in fetal hypoxia or a rapid, uncontrolled delivery. If the uterus is unable to contract strongly enough to be effective, it is in **hypotonic** labor. Abnormally slow or nonprogressive labor pattern is called **dystocia**. If the uterus is incapable of the necessary powers to allow progress of labor, the result is a prolonged labor phase caused by uterine dysfunction.

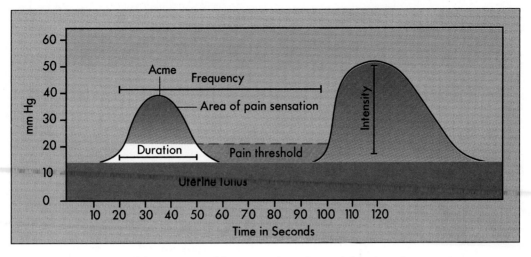

FIGURE 13-2 Measurement of frequency, intensity, and duration of contractions.

Contractions may be monitored by palpation of the fundus, by external monitoring, or by internal pressure catheter. Contractions must be assessed for frequency, intensity, and duration (see Figure 13-2). *Frequency* is the time from the beginning of one contraction to the beginning of the next, usually recorded in minutes. Strength or *intensity* is the force of the contraction and is recorded as mild, moderate, or strong. *Duration* is the time from the beginning to the end of a contraction, usually recorded in seconds. The nurse notes this information when the woman is in active labor and assesses contractions to identify a pattern of effective contractions. Although external monitoring gives only an approximation, contractions are recorded as mild, moderate, or strong contractions by palpation or by monitor readings as follows:

By Palpation	By Internal Monitor
Mild	Under 40 mm Hg
Moderate	40-70 mm Hg
Strong	Over 70 mm Hg

CERVICAL CHANGES

Effective contractions lead to progressive changes in the cervix. With each contraction the cervix draws slowly and progressively up into the lower uterine segment. This shortening and thinning of the cervix is called **effacement.** The force of the contractions, with the pressure of the presenting part and amniotic sac, causes cervical **dilation** (opening). There is a difference in primigravid and multigravid effacement and dilation (Figure 13-3). A primigravida's cervix usually must efface *before* significant dilation begins, whereas in the multigravida, both effacement and dilation can occur at the same time.

The cervix itself must be ready for labor. Normally it is firm, resembling the consistency of the tip of one's nose. For labor to be effective, it must be soft or "ripe," partially dilated and effaced, and tipped forward or anteriorly in the vagina. These changes normally occur during the weeks before the onset of labor.

The progress of effacement and dilation is assessed by internal vaginal examination. These examinations

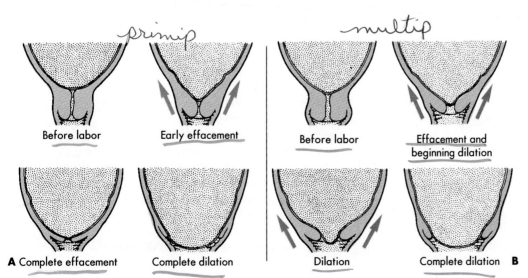

primip   *multip*

A Complete effacement   Complete dilation   Dilation   Complete dilation **B**

Before labor   Early effacement   Before labor   Effacement and beginning dilation

FIGURE 13-3 Degrees of effacement and dilation. **A,** Primigravida. **B,** Multigravida. (Used with permission of Ross Laboratories, Columbus, Ohio 43216. From Clinical Education Aid: *The phenomena of normal labor,* © Ross Laboratories.)

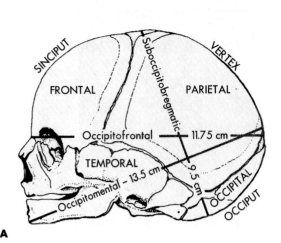

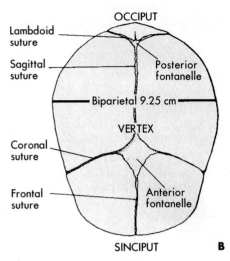

FIGURE 13-4 Fetal skull. **A,** Side view. B, Vertex view. (Used with permission of Ross Laboratories, Columbus, Ohio 43216. From Clinical Education Aid: *The phenomena of normal labor,* © Ross Laboratories.)

should be performed only as needed. Strict asepsis must be maintained to avoid introduction of bacteria into the birth canal.

The Passengers

The passengers are the fetus and the placenta. Various fetal factors, including lie, attitude, presentation, position, and station, are assessed during labor.

THE FETUS

To negotiate the maternal passageway, the fetus must fit through the bony pelvis. The fetal head is the largest, least compressible, and most common presenting part. It consists of seven bony plates separated by suture lines. These bony plates, which are soft and not totally ossified, may change position slightly, resulting in molding. Molding allows the fetal head to adapt to the shape of the bony pelvis (see Chapter 18).

The presenting diameter of the fetal head varies greatly, depending on the degree of its flexion or extension. Ideally the head should be flexed, chin on the chest; thus the smallest diameter, the **suboccipitobregmatic,** comes first. Note the position of this diameter in Figure 13-4.

Lie

Lie is the relationship of the long axis of the fetus to the long axis of the mother. Until the ninth month the fetus has had room to move in the uterus and has taken a variety of positions. During the last few weeks of pregnancy as the fetus approaches the maximum size and the amount of amniotic fluid decreases, the lie becomes stabilized. In 99% of pregnancies at term the fetus exhibits a longitudinal lie. The infant in Figure 13-5 is in a longitudinal lie. If the fetus is sideways, the lie is transverse.

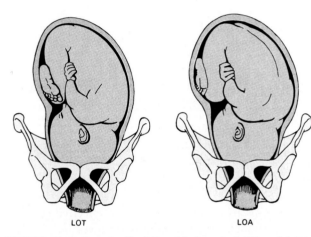

LOT   LOA

FIGURE 13-5 Longitudinal lie with fetus in LOT and LOA positions. (Used with permission of Ross Laboratories, Columbus, Ohio 43216. From Clinical Education Aid No. 18, © Ross Laboratories.)

Attitude

Attitude refers to the position of fetal body parts in relation to themselves. The fetus commonly assumes the "fetal position," with the back curled, head flexed, and legs folded on the abdomen. The arms are at the sides or are flexed and crossing the chest.

Presentation

Presentation refers to that portion of the fetus coming first to the pelvic inlet. There are three major *presentations:* vertex, breech, and **shoulder.** The incidence of these presentations is 95% vertex, 3.5% breech, and 0.5% shoulder (Oxhorn, 1986). The presentation determines the *presenting part,* the part of the fetus closest to the cervix, and that can be felt by the examining finger during vaginal examination. Presentations other than vertex may result in a prolonged labor or a cesarean delivery.

Position

Position refers to the relationship between a point of reference on the presenting part and the four quadrants of the maternal pelvis. The point of reference in a cephalic presentation is the **occiput;** in a face presentation, the chin (**mentum**); and in a breech presentation, the **sacrum.** The fetus is commonly in the left occiput transverse (LOT) position at engagement and rotates to left occiput anterior (LOA) as it descends through the pelvis. This means that the occiput of the fetus is directed toward the mother's left abdominal surface as the fetus descends through the birth canal. Figure 13-5 shows the fetus in an LOA position. There are six possible positions for each of the presentations, which are demonstrated on the pelvic model (Table 13-1).

Fetal position and presentation can be assessed by abdominal palpation, vaginal examination, and ultrasonography. Figure 13-6 indicates the suture lines that would be palpated vaginally with a fetus in an LOA position. Figure 13-7 illustrates other positions of the fetal head. Abdominal palpation is performed by using Leopold's maneuvers. Any variation in position, lie, or presentation can adversely affect the progress of labor. More attention has been directed toward changing position of the fetus by maternal positioning. An occiput transverse (OT) or occiput posterior (OP) position can be influenced by maternal positioning; standing, kneeling, leaning on hands and knees, or using the lateral Sims position may help to attain an occiput anterior (OA) position (Roberts, 1984). There is a trend toward increased use of the external version (turning) to change breech presentations to vertex and thus facilitate vaginal delivery (see Malposition).

Test Yourself

If you palpate a soft, irregular mass in the fundus and firm irregularities on the right lower anterior side of the abdomen, what would the position of the fetus be?

TABLE 13-1 Possible Variations in Position

PRESENTING PART	FETAL POINT OF REFERENCE	MATERNAL RELATIONSHIP
Vertex	Occiput (O)	Anterior or posterior (A or P)
Face	Mentum (M)	and
Brow	Brow (B)	Right or left side (R or L)
Buttocks (breech)	Sacrum (S)	or
Feet	Sacrum (S)	Transverse (T)
Shoulder	Scapula (Sc)	

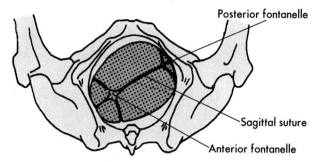

FIGURE 13-6 Position of suture lines and fontanelles in LOA position.

Station

Station refers to the relationship of the presenting part to the ischial spines of the pelvic midplane (Figure 13-8). When the presenting part is at the level of the ischial spines, it is said to be at a 0 station; this is **engagement.** Levels above the spines are designated in centimeters by negative values, −1, −2, −3. Levels below the spines are designated by positive values, +1, +2, +3, +4, down to the pelvic floor. A presenting part that does not descend to 0 station is called *floating.* If during labor the presenting part fails to descend, a cesarean birth will be necessary.

Station is important when determining and comparing the rate of descent with normal rates (see Figure 13-12). An *arrest of descent* can be detected, which usually indicates **cephalopelvic disproportion (CPD).** If stations do not progress, operative birth is chosen.

AMNIOTIC FLUID

Membranes, or the amniotic sac, normally remain intact until middle or late labor. The surrounding fluid will equalize pressures on all parts of the fetus. A pocket of fluid, the *forewaters,* cushions the presenting part and is considered a protection from the pressures exerted by the cervix and uterine muscle.

The amniotic sac or membranes may rupture spontaneously (**SROM**) before or during labor or be artificially ruptured (**AROM** or **ARM**) by a physician or midwife after the presenting part is well engaged (at 0 station) and active labor has been established. If the break is high, there may be only a trickle of fluid during a contraction. If there is a question about whether the membranes have ruptured, Nitrazine paper is used; if amniotic fluid is present, the paper turns dark blue because amniotic fluid is more alkaline than vaginal fluids. A microscopic test also may be performed by making a smear of the fluid and then observing for *ferning,* a fernlike crystallization of sodium chloride.

When membranes rupture, the fetal heart rate should be checked. If the rupture is accompanied by a gush of fluid and the head is not well engaged, the umbilical

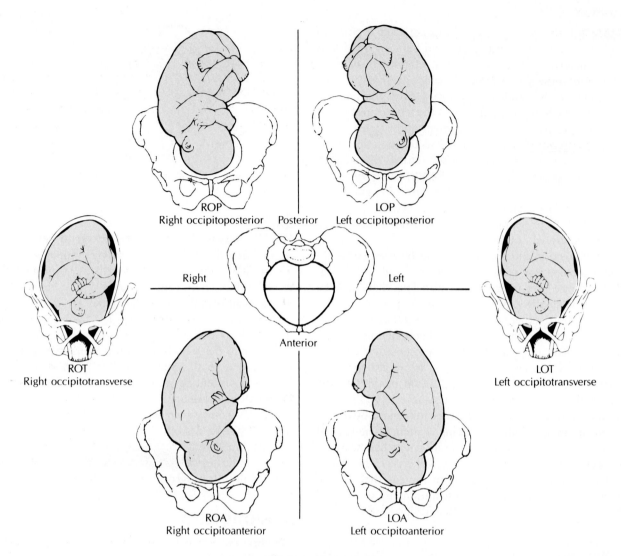

ROP
Right occipitoposterior   Posterior   Left occipitoposterior
LOP

Right

Left

ROT
Right occipitotransverse

LOT
Left occipitotransverse

Anterior

ROA
Right occipitoanterior

LOA
Left occipitoanterior

Lie: Longitudinal or vertical
Presentation: vertex
Presenting part: occiput
Attitude: complete flexion

FIGURE 13-7 Examples of fetal vertex (occiput) presentations in relation to front, back, or side of maternal pelvis. (Modified from Iorio J: *Childbirth: family-centered nursing,* ed 3, St Louis, 1973, Mosby.)

cord may be washed downward and be compressed between the presenting part and the cervix. If the membranes are ruptured artificially (ARM or AROM) by the physician, the fetal heartbeat should be checked before and after the procedure.

The amniotic fluid should be observed for color, odor, and amount. Normally it is a clear, straw color, with flecks of *vernix caseosa,* the creamy substance on the fetal skin. If it is brownish green, it indicates the presence of *meconium* caused by a relaxation of the fetal anal sphincter. Note the color and consistency of the fluid that contains meconium to determine whether it is thick or thin, dark or light green, or looks "old" or

"new." Meconium-stained fluid at the introitus is considered normal in a breech presentation because of pressure on the baby's abdomen, which causes stooling. If the fluid is yellow, it indicates the presence of bilirubin. If any blood is present, it usually indicates hemorrhage (very rare).

Amniotic fluid has a characteristic odor. A foul-smelling odor may indicate an infectious process, chorioamnionitis. The normal amount of amniotic fluid at 36 to 38 weeks is 800 to 1000 ml, and it decreases until term. *Polyhydramnios* and *oligohydramnios* may indicate congenital anomalies in the fetus (see Fetal Distress, Chapter 14).

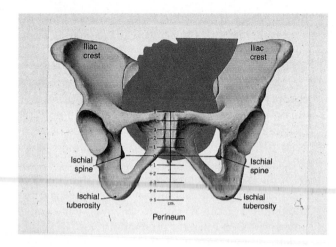

FIGURE 13-8 Station in relation to descent of fetal head. (Used with permission of Ross Laboratories, Columbus, Ohio 43216. From Clinical Education Aid: *The phenomena of normal labor,* © Ross Laboratories.)

Test Yourself

- What are the reasons for not rupturing membranes early in labor?

UMBILICAL CORD

Normally the umbilical cord floats in the amniotic fluid around the fetus. It may, however, become compressed against the fetal body during contractions, resulting in fetal hypoxia. If the fetus is monitored, this compression appears as variable decelerations in the fetal heart rate pattern. A change in the maternal position may relocate the cord and alleviate cord compression. The cord may prolapse through the cervix and into the vagina when membranes rupture before the presenting part is engaged (see Fetal Distress, Chapter 14).

PLACENTA

The placenta is essential to the well-being of the fetus in the uterus. Any dysfunction affects fetal status during labor. Placental perfusion and oxygenation are always reduced during contractions. Transient fetal hypoxia is normally overcome by a healthy placenta as it refills after a contraction. Placental problems are discussed with Fetal Distress.

The Passage

The pelvis is the bony ring through which body weight is distributed to the lower extremities. It consists of the sacrum, coccyx, and two innominate bones. The innominate bones are joined to the sacrum by the sacroiliac joints; the sacrum and coccyx are joined by the sacrococcygeal joint, and the innominate bones are joined together in front by the symphysis pubis. Anatomic landmarks important during assessment of the adequacy of the pelvis are the ischial spines and the ischial tuberosities. There appears to be very little flexibility in the pelvic joints; however, because ligaments are made more stretchable by *relaxin,* some flexibility in the pelvis is possible during pregnancy and birth.

PELVIS

The pelvis is divided into the true and "false" sections at the linea terminalis. The false pelvis, although essential to support abdominal organs, is of no obstetric significance. The true pelvis is the bony birth passage. For a vaginal delivery, this passage must be of adequate size and shape to allow the movement of the fetus.

Each pelvis is classified according to the shape of the inlet (Figure 13-9). The gynecoid pelvis is ideal for birth. The platypelloid shape allows the fetus to enter only in an OT position because the anteroposterior diameter is too short. The android pelvis, similar to a male pelvic shape, forces the fetal head to engage in an OP position because of *cephalopelvic disproportion* (lack of fit). The anthropoid shape tends to result in an OP position. These positions usually result in long labor and a delivery with forceps or require cesarean birth.

Diameters

The pelvis is divided into the inlet plane, midpelvic plane, and outlet.

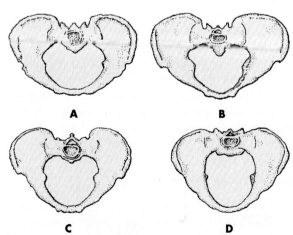

FIGURE 13-9 Types of pelves. **A,** Platypelloid. **B,** Android. **C,** Gynecoid. **D,** Anthropoid. (Redrawn from Ullery JC, Castallo M: *Obstetric mechanisms and their management,* Philadelphia, 1957, FA Davis Co.)

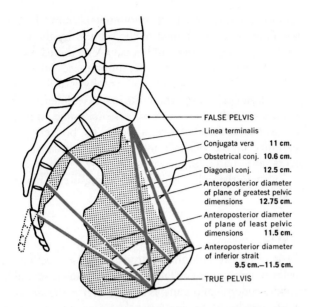

FALSE PELVIS
Linea terminalis
Conjugata vera   11 cm.
Obstetrical conj.   10.6 cm.
Diagonal conj.   12.5 cm.
Anteroposterior diameter
of plane of greatest pelvic
dimensions   12.75 cm.
Anteroposterior diameter
of plane of least pelvic
dimensions   11.5 cm.
Anteroposterior diameter
of inferior strait
                    9.5 cm.—11.5 cm.
TRUE PELVIS

FIGURE 13-10 Diameters of pelvic planes. (Used with permission of Ross Laboratories, Columbus, Ohio 43216. From Clinical Education Aid No. 18, © Ross Laboratories.)

The inlet plane is assessed by the diagonal conjugate, obstetric conjugate, and conjugate vera (Figure 13-10). The *diagonal conjugate* is the most significant measurement and is measured during vaginal examination by placing the tip of the middle finger on the sacral promontory and then marking where the symphysis pubis touches the index finger. If the measurement is at least 11.5 cm, the pelvic inlet is of adequate size.

The midpelvic plane can be assessed only by x-ray examination. In Figure 13-9 the planes of greatest and least pelvic dimension reflect this plane. Inadequacies may be suspected if the *ischial spines* are prominent (Figure 13-10), if the pelvic side walls are narrow, or if the curve of the sacrum is shallow. The interspinous diameter (usually 10 cm) is the smallest diameter which the fetus must accommodate. The sacrum, coccyx, and ischial spines can be palpated by the examiner's fingers. The coccyx should be movable.

The plane of outlet is assessed by measurement of the transverse diameter, the distance between the ischial tuberosities. A measurement of 8 cm or greater is considered adequate. The pubic arch must allow passage of the fetal head as it extends during birth. The angle of the arch should be at least 90 degrees.

Mechanisms of Labor

To negotiate the bony pelvis the fetus must go through the mechanisms of labor or the *cardinal movements*. The mechanisms of labor for the LOA position are illustrated in Figure 13-14. Follow the steps as you read.

1. First, the presenting part must become **engaged**, or descend to enter the true pelvis. The part (head or breech) descends in a transverse position so that the largest diameter of the pelvis will accommodate the largest diameter of the head.
2. This **descent** will be measured in stations.
3. The head also flexes as a result of the resistance encountered. **Flexion** must occur for the other mechanisms to follow, and flexion is maintained until the last step when the head extends.
4. Next the head, to pass the ischial spines, must rotate 45 degrees to the right or left from that transverse position. **Internal rotation** is a crucial step and may take some time to accomplish. When the part has rotated, the fetus is said to be in a left occiput anterior (LOA) (or right occiput anterior [ROA]) or a left occiput posterior (LOP) (or right occiput posterior [ROP]) position. If it has not yet completed rotation, it is still in a left occiput transverse (LOT) (or right occiput transverse [ROT]) position. In Figure 13-11 the fetus is in an LOA position after internal rotation. The part again rotates to bring the occiput or sacrum in alignment with the anterior or posterior center point of the pelvic outlet.
5. The head then extends under the symphysis. **Extension** allows it to negotiate the pelvic arch. It is at this point that the infant's scalp or buttocks are seen at the vaginal opening.
6. **External rotation** involves two movements. After the head is delivered, it turns to realign with the shoulders, which are still in the transverse diameter of the pelvic inlet. The movement also involves the rotation of the shoulders to an anteroposterior position so that they may emerge from the vaginal opening.
7. **Expulsion** or birth of the rest of the baby occurs as the anterior shoulder moves just under the symphysis pubis. The posterior shoulder should be delivered carefully to prevent perineal tearing, and then the anterior shoulder and the rest of the body should follow easily.

To accomplish these *maneuvers*, proper coordination of the *passengers, passage,* and *powers* must exist. If the presenting part is too large or the lie is transverse, engagement cannot occur. If the position is OP, the head does not apply equal pressure on the cervix and labor is slowed. If contractions are too weak or irregular, the force does not propel the fetus through the pelvis. If the pelvis is too small, the fetus cannot negotiate the passage (see Dysfunctional Labor).

Initiation of Labor

Initiation of contractions is still not completely understood. It is a crucial research topic because of the rate of premature labor. If all the trigger mechanisms were known, therapy could be aimed to cut the loop at one point.

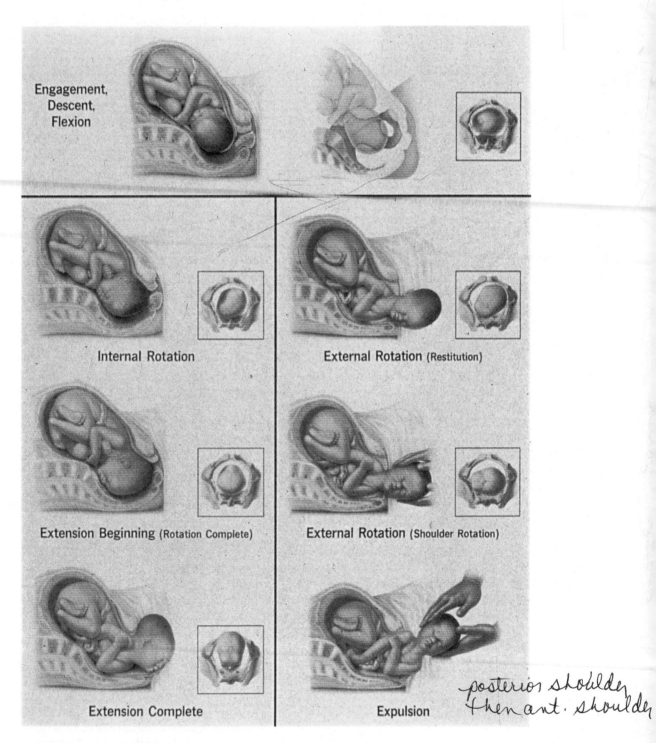

Engagement, Descent, Flexion

Internal Rotation

External Rotation (Restitution)

Extension Beginning (Rotation Complete)

External Rotation (Shoulder Rotation)

Extension Complete

Expulsion

posterior shoulder then ant. shoulder

FIGURE 13-11 Mechanisms of labor in vertex position (LOA). (Used with permission of Ross Laboratories, Columbus, Ohio 43216. From Clinical Education Aid No. 12, © Ross Laboratories.)

CERVIX

Preparation for labor begins at about week 34 as the cervix very slowly starts to "mature" or to "ripen," becoming less hard and unyielding. Until labor, it holds in the contents of the uterus so that it is firm, long, and directed toward the posterior part of the vagina. The cervix *cannot contract;* that is, it can only become softer, more spongy, and more yielding so that during labor it may be stretched to such a remarkable degree. Because it is composed of 85% connective tissue and only 15% smooth muscle surrounded by a gel-like matrix of proteoglycans (Challis, 1989), once dilation begins, it will not close again.

Under the control of a changing ratio of estrogen to progesterone and prostaglandin (PGE_2), structural changes begin in the isolated strands of smooth muscle. This effect may be seen in use of PGE_2 as a gel applied to the cervix to prepare it for labor (see Induction of Labor in Chapter 15).

In addition, this cervical *compliance* (yielding, softening, effacement) increases abruptly *during* labor. Changes begun in the few weeks before labor onset will speed up once labor has begun. Consistency will resemble an overstretched rubber band, and only after birth will the cervix slowly close up.

MYOMETRIUM

The myometrium has two qualities: (1) *elasticity,* which allows it to stretch, maintain tone, and then shrink after birth and (2) *contractility,* which allows it to shorten and lengthen in a synchronized pattern only during birth so that force may be applied to expel the fetus. Before labor, as already noted, contractions are mild, irregular, and nonsynchronized. To be coordinated or work together (to be synchronized), **gap junctions,** or cell-to-cell communication points, must develop between the smooth muscle cells. This process apparently functions—with increased calcium ion flow, cellular adenosine triphosphate (ATP), and increased mitochrondria—to suddenly boost the energy in the muscle cells. Communication is almost instant. As pacemakers signal a contraction, a wave of tightening—beginning at the top—goes over the whole uterus.

These gap junctions gradually increase in size and number during the last weeks of pregnancy and then develop rapidly *during labor.* The length of latent labor varies from woman to woman and is believed to be the time needed for gap junction formulation, oxytocin receptor enhancement, and collagen changes (Steinman, 1991). Once preparation has begun, it is very difficult to stop the process. For instance, it is almost impossible to stop preterm labor once the cervix reaches 3 to 4 cm dilation (see Chapter 21).

Theories. Labor onset is thought to be a complex combination of a number of factors working together. The following factors are based on reports by Blackman and Loper (1992), Huzar and Naftolin (1984), and Steinman (1991).
1. *Genetic* factors have a role, perhaps in influencing hormonal levels and patterns of labor.
2. An increase in availability of *estrogen* and a decrease in availability of *progesterone* in the myometrium is present. (Progesterone suppresses uterine contractions.) Estrogen fosters gap junctions, increases oxytocin receptors, and stimulates prostaglandin production. Some estrogen originates in the fetal adrenals so that fetal hormonal activity helps to trigger labor onset.
3. *PGE_2* contributes to cervical changes and *PGF_2* to contractions and formation of gap junctions. These prostaglandins increase calcium ion flow in the cells, which will strengthen contractions. Prostaglandins come from the placenta, fetal membranes, and the uterus. The effect of prostaglandin may be seen in the fact that antiprostaglandin agents such as aspirin and indomethacin will delay labor onset.
4. *Oxytocin* receptors increase 100 to 200 times by term. Thus oxytocin effectively stimulates labor in full-term pregnancies but has less effect earlier.
5. *Relaxin* is present throughout pregnancy and probably works with progesterone to block uterine activity. Its role during labor is unclear, but it may be involved with connective tissue changes.
6. Uterine distention contributes in some way.

EFFECTIVE (TRUE) LABOR

The onset of labor usually is equated with the onset of regular contractions experienced by the mother. Evaluations in the last weeks of pregnancy show that some effacement and dilation of the cervix almost always take place before true labor begins. This period used to be called *false labor* but is an integral part of the process, so the term *prelabor* is now used. Few women enter effective labor without some dilation. Those who have not achieved adequate dilation usually have a potential labor problem or have come to the labor room too soon. A client, unaware of contractions, may report for routine appointment and be found to have a cervix almost fully effaced and partially dilated.

Readiness for labor is the key factor in how long the body will take to accomplish the work of the first stage of labor. Some of the work of getting ready for labor manifests with characteristic signs.

Early Signs

Braxton Hicks contractions. One to two weeks before the onset of labor, Braxton Hicks contractions become more frequent, occurring every 15 to 20 minutes, and they increase in intensity and duration, averaging 20 mm Hg and 60 to 80 seconds. As these early contractions become better coordinated, they aid in *ripening*, that is, preparing the cervix for labor.

Lightening. Approximately 10 to 14 days before the onset of active labor, *lightening* or *engagement* occurs in the nullipara. This settling of the fetus into the pelvic cavity is characterized by relief from pressure in the upper part of the abdomen and by renewed pressure on the pelvic organs, with increased urinary frequency. The decrease in fundal height may be very noticeable; people often say that "the baby dropped." This descent usually does not occur in the multipara until after the onset of active labor (Box 13-1).

Increased pressure. Although the earliest sign for a nullipara may be lightening, other women experience increasing pressure sensations throughout the pelvic area 1 to 2 weeks before labor. Multiparas particularly complain of perineal or groin pressure. A characteristic "pregnancy waddle" can be observed as a woman walks. One to two days before the onset of labor there may be a weight loss of 1 to 3 lb and varying energy levels.

Bloody show. Several hours before labor a thick strand of mucus is expelled, the *mucous plug*. This may be mixed with slight amounts of blood and has been called *bloody show*; it indicates dilation of the cervix and is equated with the onset of effective but early labor.

Effacement in primigravida

STAGES OF LABOR

Labor is divided into three stages. The first stage is from onset to full effacement and dilation of the cervix. The second stage lasts until the descent and complete birth of the baby, and the third stage lasts from the birth of the baby until complete delivery of the placenta. Some add a fourth stage, the period during repair of any

surgical incisions and the immediate recovery 1 to 2 hours after the delivery of the placenta.

First Stage

The first stage traditionally is divided into latent, active, and transition phases.

Latent phase. The **latent phase** extends from the beginning of effective labor (progressive effacement and dilation) until 3 cm dilation has been achieved. Often the start of latent labor is not known so that measurements of duration are only approximate. Contractions become increasingly intense, more regular, and more frequent, starting about 15 to 20 minutes apart and progressing to 4 to 5 minutes apart. This sequence is equivalent to approximately four an hour, increasing to 10 to 12 per hour. Duration is 30 to 40 seconds, and intensity is mild to moderate.* *avg 6-9 hrs, Not to exceed 20 hrs. Cervix begins to efface & dilate, but no fetal descent.*

Active phase. **Active phase** labor extends from dilation between 3 and 8 cm. Contractions are more regular, more intense, and more frequent. Although labor patterns show some variation, active labor contractions are 3 to 5 minutes apart, last 50 to 75 seconds, and are moderate to strong in intensity. During this phase cervical dilation should occur rapidly, or be *accelerated*.

Transition phase. **Transition phase** is the most difficult period, during which the cervix opens the last 2 cm, from 8 to 10 cm. Painful, intense, erratic contractions occur every 2 to 3 minutes with an intensity that the woman finds very difficult. The tonus rises, and there seems to be little relief from the painful, frustrating sequences. Intense contractions persist for 75 to 90 seconds. As the cervix is stretched the last inch, small capillaries may break and vaginal fluids may appear as bright red. However, active bleeding or clotted flow should not occur. As the phase ends, dilation rate *decelerates*.

Friedman's Phases

Friedman (1985), on the basis of dilation progress, divided labor into only two phases, *latent* and *active* (Figure 13-12). His latent phase extends from the onset of labor to the beginning of active dilation. Friedman divides the active phase of labor into three parts, an *acceleration phase*, the *phase of maximum slope*, and a *deceleration phase*. Table 13-2 compares the classic divisions of labor with those of Friedman.

BOX 13-1   Early Labor Signs

- Increase in contraction rate to more than 4-5/hr
- Contraction rate intensifies with walking
- Feeling of heaviness in pelvis
- Diarrhea
- Ruptured membranes
- Increase in vaginal mucus. Expelling the thick strand of blood-tinged mucus (bloody show)

---

*Intensity and duration here are determined by abdominal palpation so that the nurse may teach the client to palpate her uterus. Add approximately 15 seconds to the figures for the more sensitive monitoring tracing of contraction duration from resting tonus.

Friedman's study indicates the time for the latent phase for the nullipara to be from 8 to 10 hours but not more than 20, and that for the multipara to be 3 to 5 hours but not more than 14. In assessing the progress of dilation, however, the use of *centimeters per hour,* rather than total number of hours, makes possible early recognition of labor problems. During active dilation, the nullipara averages 3 cm/hr and at least 1.2 cm/hr, whereas the multipara averages 5.7 cm/hr and not less than 1.5 cm/hr. A graph of a client's labor (Figure 13-13) provides a much clearer picture of labor progress than do separate recordings. Note that the normal pattern is an S-shaped curve; note also the normal curve of descent. Any significant variation in the shape of the patterns reflects difficulty that requires further assessment.

This model of labor timing has been one of the contributing factors in the increased cesarean rate. Each woman has a different pattern, and Friedman's graph is *only an average.* In a number of cases the graph has been used too literally and a small delay was used as an indication of operative delivery.

Nurse-midwives do not use the labor curve rigidly, and as long as progress is being made and baby and mother are responding well, labor is continued.

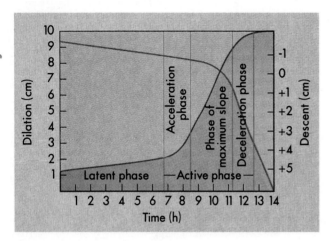

FIGURE 13-12 Friedman's labor curve and divisions of labor. (From Friedman E, Greenhill JP: *Biological principles and modern practice of obstetrics,* Philadelphia, 1975, WB Saunders.)

TABLE 13-2   Comparison of Classic Labor and Friedman's Phases

CLASSIC DESCRIPTION	FRIEDMAN'S PHASES
FIRST STAGE	
Latent (0-3 cm)	Latent (0-2 cm)
Active (3-8 cm)	Active (3-10 cm)
Transition (8-10 cm)	Acceleration (3-4 cm)
	Maximum slope (5-8 cm)
	Deceleration (9-10 cm)

Second Stage

The major function of the second stage of labor is *descent.* Friedman defined the normal limits of descent to guide recognition of early problems. This guide is for normal presentations uncomplicated by malposition or other problems. For the nullipara whose birth canal has not been previously distended, the fetus can be expected to descend at least 1.5 cm/hr but in most cases at 3 cm/hr. In the multipara the fetus usually progresses faster than 2.1 cm/hr and most often at about 5 cm/hr. The average duration of second stage for the multipara is 30 minutes to 1 hour and 1 to 2 hours for the nullipara. The second stage usually does not exceed 3 hours.

To accomplish descent, the resistance of the vaginal canal must be overcome. The pelvic floor, composed chiefly of the levator ani muscles and fasciae, must be displaced downward and outward by the fetal head.

FIGURE 13-13 Graphic labor record.

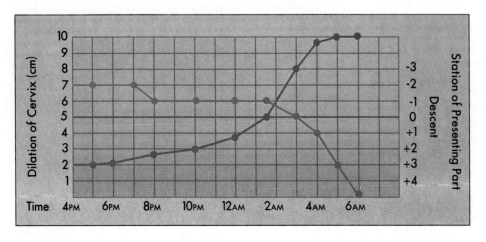

Clinical Decision

Mary F., a 26-year-old primipara, was admitted with her husband at 10 PM. Her status on evaluation was membranes ruptured at 6 PM; contractions every 5 minutes, 40 seconds, mild-to-moderate intensity; cervix 4 cm, 75% effaced, bloody mucus observed; and vertex presentation, at –1 station. Your assessment of Mary's labor would be consistent with which phase of labor?

At 2 AM Mary's contractions are strong, occurring every 3 minutes and lasting 60 seconds. Vaginal examination shows dilation of 5 cm, but vertex is still at –1 station. Use the following graph to chart her progress.

At 4 AM Mary is comfortable after regional anesthesia, but her station is 0 and dilation is still at 5 cm. According to your graph of Mary's progress, if unchanged at 5 AM, what would this indicate?

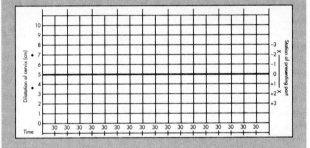

The resistance is variable and can be evaluated during vaginal examination. The folds (rugae) of the vagina form a lining membrane for the canal. The fascial layers are thinned as they stretch, making vaginal tissue susceptible to tears. The client must add voluntary expulsive efforts during contractions to achieve the pressure needed for this process.

Third Stage

The main function of this stage is placental separation and expulsion. Immediately after the birth of the infant the uterus should contract firmly around the placenta. The site of placental attachment becomes smaller than the placenta, causing separation, descent, and expulsion of the placenta and membranes. In most instances, by 1 to 5 minutes after delivery, there will be indications that the placenta has separated and moved into the lower segment and vagina.

1. The uterus becomes smaller and spherical.
2. There is a slight gush of blood from the vagina.

3. The umbilical cord lengthens by several inches.
4. The uterus may rise in the abdomen because the separated placenta displaces it upward.

Chapters 14 and 15 complete the discussion of fetal assessment during labor and care during the second, third, and fourth stages.

Universal Precautions

Because blood and body fluids are known to be reservoirs for hepatitis and the human immunodeficiency virus (HIV), exposure is a special hazard for health care personnel in obstetrics (see Chapter 25 for complete discussion). During labor, universal precautions must be observed consistently. Gloves must be used for any contact with body fluids, and double gloving is required for nurses who scrub for cesarean section or perform vaginal examinations. Waterproof gowns, masks, and hair and eye coverings are used for splash exposure. Actually, the best line of defense is good hand-washing technique. Violations of universal precautions are registered at approximately 48% in labor areas (Ginsberg, 1990), even though these precautions are reviewed regularly for all staff members. The current rate of HIV conversion to positive status per needle stick or cut is 0.5%, that is, 1 in 200 incidents. For hepatitis B virus (HBV) it is 30% to 70% (Ginsberg, 1990). Fortunately, vaccination is now available for HBV, and every person who works in this area should be immunized (Box 13-2).

Nursing Responsibilities

Chapters 13, 14, and 15 discuss nursing responsibilities during labor, intrapartal fetal monitoring, and birth. Because care changes from hour to hour during this process, nursing responsibilities are summarized at the end of each phase. Nurses working in the labor unit share in a dynamic and significant human experience. Modern technologies and knowledge of the impact of birth interventions demand a high level of technical competence. The capacity to assist and encourage mothers and their support persons during labor is equally important.

Women today seek positive birth experiences that are physically safe and emotionally gratifying. Women not

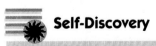

Self-Discovery

Observe your own performance on the unit regarding use of universal precautions. How do you feel about the restrictions?

BOX 13-2   Universal Precautions to Reduce Risk of HIV-HBV and Other Blood Pathogen Transmission in Obstetric Care

- Body fluids to which universal precautions apply
  - Known to transmit HIV or HBV infection
    - Blood, semen, vaginal secretions
    - Other secretions that are visibly bloody
    - Amniotic fluid
  - Unknown risk of transmission of HIV or HBV
    - Cerebrospinal, synovial, pleural, peritoneal, or pericardial fluid
    - Tears and saliva
- Body fluids to which universal precautions do not apply
  - Risk of transmission of HIV or HBV is extremely low or nonexistent
    - Feces, nasal secretions, sputum, sweat, tears, urine, and vomitus.
    - Some of these secretions represent potential sources for other pathogens, and recommendations for prevention of transmission are available.
    - Breast milk is a rare source of perinatal transmission but is not implicated in transmission to health care workers. Health care workers may wish to wear gloves if they have frequent exposure to breast milk.

Precautions

- Use appropriate barrier precautions to prevent skin and mucous membrane exposure when contact with blood or bodily fluid from *any* client is anticipated.
  - When caring for all clients, gloves should be worn for:
    - Contact with blood (venipuncture, finger stick, intravenous insertion, changing perineal pads, chux, linen)
    - Contact with bodily fluids (changing saturated pads, chux, linen, clothing after rupture of membranes)
    - Contact with mucous membranes (vaginal examination)
    - Contact with nonintact skin
    - Handling items soiled with blood or bodily fluids (soiled pads, chux, bedding, clothing)
- Gloves should be changed after contact with each client and between client contacts.

- Medical gloves (vinyl or latex sterile surgical or non-sterile examination gloves) should not be washed and reused. Washing with surfactants may enhance penetration of liquids through undetected holes in gloves.
- Masks, protective eyewear, or face shields should be worn during procedures that commonly cause splashes of blood or bodily fluids onto mucous membranes of mouth, nose, or eyes.
  - Vaginal or cesarean birth
  - Cutting umbilical cord between infant and placenta
  - Possible artificial rupture of membranes under pressure
- Fluid-resistant gowns or aprons should be worn during procedures likely to cause splashes of bodily fluids.
  - Persons performing or assisting with vaginal or cesarean births
  - Artificial rupture of membranes
- Gowns and gloves should be worn by health care workers handling placenta or infant until blood and amniotic fluid have been removed from infant's skin by bathing
  - Gloves should be worn for care of umbilical cord after delivery
- Removal of infant nasopharyngeal secretion at delivery should use mechanical suction (not by De Lee).
  - Resuscitation should use resuscitation bags or other ventilation equipment.
- Gloves torn or punctured by needle stick or other injury should be removed and replaced as promptly as possible.
- Precautions should be taken to prevent injury from needles and surgical instruments.
  - Needles should not be recapped, bent, broken, or removed from disposable syringes.
  - After use, needles, scalpel blades, and other sharp items should be placed in puncture-resistant containers for disposal.
  - Surgical instruments should be carefully cleaned to avoid injury.

Modified from Centers for Disease Control (CDC): Recommendations for prevention of HIV transmission in health care settings, *MMWR* 36(suppl):2S, 1987; CDC: Update: universal precautions for prevention of transmission of human immunodeficiency virus, hepatitis B virus and other blood-borne pathogens in health care settings. *MMWR* 37(24):377, 1988.

---

prepared in childbirth techniques may be assisted and coached by nurses but may find control more difficult to achieve.

A number of problems may occur during labor. Nursing assessment must determine each couple's needs as they approach this experience that is filled with meaning, feeling, and anxiety. Nursing action focuses on supportive hospital environments and addresses the physical, medical, emotional, and social needs of the woman, infant, and partner. Nursing measures that promote physical comfort reinforce the other skills and techniques the woman has learned. Pertinent nursing

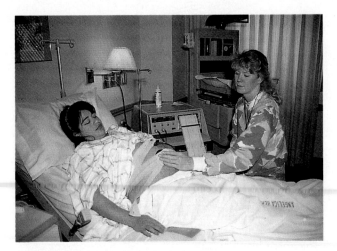

FIGURE 13-14 Admission to the labor area includes orientation and usually a period of time for contraction and fetal heart monitoring. (Courtesy Marjorie Pyle, RNC, *Lifecircle.*)

diagnoses may be selected for each couple who begins labor (Box 13-3).

Levine describes four basic principles of nursing management that apply to the birth experience. They are *conservation of energy, structural integrity, personal integrity,* and *social integrity.* These principles serve as a framework for determining an appropriate nursing care plan during all stages of labor, facilitating nursing assessment, planning, implementation, and evaluation.

CONSERVATION OF ENERGY

Poor appetite, difficulty with digestion, interference with sleep patterns, general physical discomforts, and the overall physical demands of pregnancy cause many women to experience fatigue during the final weeks of pregnancy. The application of skills of controlled relaxation, comfort positions, appropriate activity, rest periods, and modifications in daily life play important parts in decreasing fatigue and reducing the depletion of the woman's energy.

Pregnant women in difficult socioeconomic circumstances may enter labor without adequate rest, nutrition, prenatal education, and preparation; these women are at greatest risk for energy depletion.

Position for Labor

The woman's position during labor can affect physical comfort and the physiologic processes of birth. Traditionally, each culture has promoted a position for labor and birth (see box: Cultural Aspects of Care). In this country until the last few years the position has been recumbent: supine with slightly elevated head and shoulders. With the changes spearheaded by nurse-midwives, gradually the medical profession has accepted alternate positions; many physicians, however,

---

BOX 13-3 **Problems Leading to Nursing Diagnoses**

- Fear related to lack of knowledge or prior negative experiences
- Ineffective individual or family coping related to the couple's youth, prior negative experiences, or problems during labor related to unresolved stress
- Impaired verbal communication related to inability to understand English or medical terminology; misunderstanding may lead to heightened anxiety. On occasion the woman may be deaf.
- Fluid volume excess related to lack of control of intravenous fluids or too much infused fluid before regional or general anesthesia. These iatrogenic problems should not occur.
- Anxious questioning related to prior experience in labor
- Altered nutrition; e.g., if the woman is not allowed clear oral fluids, hypoglycemia may arise during a long labor.
- Sleep-pattern disturbance related to a long latent period and a long labor
- An ineffective breathing pattern in women who have difficulty with labor breathing techniques, or had no prenatal classes
- Labor pain which is always present, degree depending on the status of the mechanisms of labor.
- Caregiver role strain in companion, related to a long or difficult labor

Examples of outcomes

- Will be able to cope with anxiety and stress during each phase of labor.
- Uses appropriate techniques for the physical discomforts and tension of labor.
- Coach gives appropriate support throughout labor.
- Exhibits impaired maternal and fetal perfusion and metabolic balance.
- Verbalizes understanding of the process through which she is going and the reasons for any interventions.
- The couple exhibits positive attachment behaviors with the newborn infant.

---

insist on the lithotomy position during labor and birth. Table 13-3 compares the advantages and disadvantages of selected positions for labor and delivery.

Research has shown that the upright position—high Fowler's, sitting in chair, or ambulating during active labor—shortened the phase of maximum slope (4 to 8 cm) by an average of 90 minutes (Roberts et al, 1984). Although changes in pain perception or fetal outcome did not occur, contractions were more efficient, intense, and frequent. In addition, dilation possibly was speeded because of the effects of gravity. Such a finding should

TABLE 13-3 Positions for Labor

POSITION	
ADVANTAGES	**DISADVANTAGES**
RECUMBENT	
Supine	
Convenient for fetal monitoring, vaginal examination, treatments, and palpating contractions; familiar resting position	Decreases strength of contractions. Increases risk of supine hypotension; increases length of labor (Liu, 1989)
Lithotomy	
Facilitates a standing or sitting position for physician; exposes perineum widely for vaginal examination; used for fetal monitoring; helpful in hemorrhage, emergency	Increases venous return and central blood volume when legs higher than heart. Adverse effects: tachycardia, increased blood pressure.
Left lateral	
Comfortable for woman; more intense, less frequent contractions (Roberts et al, 1984). Prevents vena caval compression. Allows birth in relaxed position for woman; reduces potential for perineal lacerations	More difficult to obtain consistent fetal heart rate; longer labor than upright position (Roberts et al, 1983)
UPRIGHT	
High Fowler's, In chair, Ambulating	
Facilitates efficient and more intense contractions (Aderhold and Roberts, 1991); cervical dilation assisted by gravity effect	May need position change as woman gets fatigued; fetal monitor tracing more difficult to obtain

be implemented into standard labor nursing practice (Figure 13-15).

Use of hydrotherapy, with the woman in flotation for 15 to 20 minutes at intervals during labor, also seems to facilitate labor, whether through relaxation or position changes. The woman's position in the tub may be leaning on hands and knees, resting in a side-lying position, or floating with abdomen down (Aderhold and Perry, 1991).

The woman should be encouraged to be ambulatory as long as possible (Box 13-4). The use of comfort devices such as rocking chairs, birthing beds, and hydrotherapy conserves energy and promotes healthy labor.

Because "failure to progress" is a leading reason for cesarean births, nursing measures that conserve energy, prevent fatigue, encourage the efficiency of the process, and encourage the woman's stamina are important.

Fluids

In the earliest periods, mothers are instructed to drink clear liquids frequently and to eat simple foods such as tea, gelatin (a liquid), Popsicles (a liquid), and toast and jelly. After labor is well established, liquids usually are continued. Fluids by mouth, especially fruit juices, help the woman to maintain appropriate colloid osmotic pressure. In general, babies have fewer problems with hy-

poglycemia, jaundice, and weight loss when the mother had adequate liquids during labor (Keppler, 1988).

Although in some settings nothing by mouth during labor is still the fixed rule (Broach and Newton, 1988), more physicians and most midwives in hospitals encourage fluids. (See Chapter 16 for reasons that fluids remain controversial.) When intravenous fluids are given, Ringer's lactate is the solution of choice. Care must be taken with the flow rate because a too-rapid infusion may result in circulatory overload. The exception is the increased intravenous rate used before a regional anesthetic. The rate is changed and monitored by the anesthesiologist. The normal rate of flow is 125 ml/hr. Some units use only a heparin lock for intravenous access if there should be hemorrhage. Birthing centers encourage oral fluids during labor.

Communication

During the inevitable stress of labor the woman may seem to regress to a more dependent state. She will be sensitive to indifferent or negative interpersonal exchanges. Often she may not talk about it until the infant is born. The nurse can set a positive tone for the labor experience simply through an introduction, asking her the name she prefers to use, and orienting her carefully to the space she will occupy. Establishing interpersonal

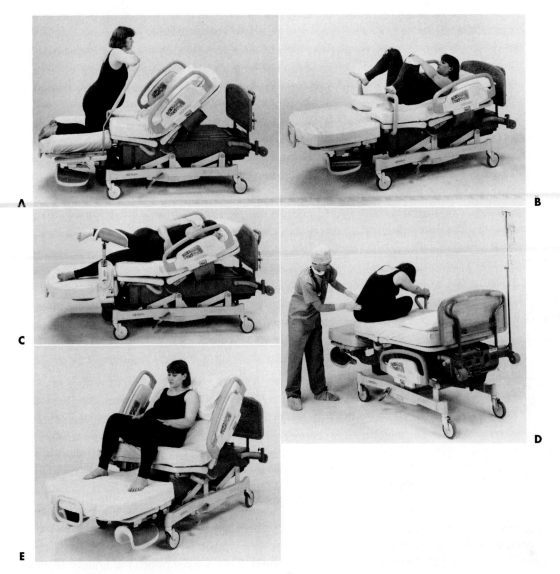

FIGURE 13-15 The birthing bed facilitates a variety of labor and birth positions (A-E). (Courtesy The Affinity Bed, Hill-Rom, Batesville, Ind.)

BOX 13-4   Appropriate Activity During Labor for Low-Risk Mothers

- Early labor: ambulating; upright
- Active labor: ambulating, if desired; if in bed, upright, lateral; sitting
- Bed rest after rupture of membranes unless fetal head is well engaged and danger of cord prolapse is negligible
- Second stage: sitting, semisitting, squatting, left lateral

trust is important because the woman is vulnerable in an entirely new way for the hours of labor and birth (see the box on p. 298).

Providing the woman with information and interpreting labor data and treatments also help her conserve energy. She gains a perspective on labor that reduces anxiety. Words of *encouragement, affirmation,* and *validation* diminish fatigue.

CONSERVATION OF STRUCTURAL INTEGRITY

The nurse assesses the woman's physical condition, the progression of labor, and the baby's condition. Obser-

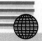 **Cultural Aspects of Care**

The transcultural committee at our hospital learned that 84 Kurdish refugees from northern Iraq would be settling in the area. Members educated themselves about Kurdish cultures and the Muslim faith and held workshops for the staff to prepare them should the Kurds need hospital services. Consequently, when a Kurdish mother arrived with her own midwife for her first hospital experience and her ninth birth, personnel made every effort to accommodate her customs. There were only female attendants, including a female translator, and the mother chose to deliver the baby in the hands and knees position to which she was accustomed. She also kept her head and the infant's head covered at all times.

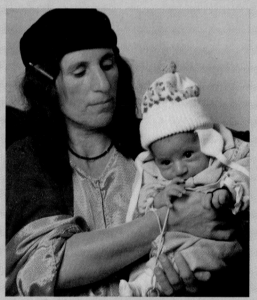

(Courtesy The Idaho Statesman, Boise, Idaho.)

vation of the woman's responses and interactions is extremely valuable. The woman's care takes precedence over "the machines." If her condition is being monitored, however, the nurse also should be skillful in manipulation of electronic monitoring equipment and interpretation of data. Caring for the physical condition of the woman involves careful execution of procedures so they do not interfere with the woman's or infant's physical integrity.

During the second stage, maternal positions also are important in maintaining *structural integrity*. In particular, there is concern about the effect of position on the maternal perineum. Anatomically favorable positions help to eliminate lacerations and reduce the need for an episiotomy (Johnson, Johnson, Gupta, 1991).

 Cultural Aspects of Care

Hispanic mother

In my family, when you hurt, you make noise. Every time I moaned or cried out in labor, the nurse offered me pain medication. When I refused, she'd tell me to use the breathing I'd learned in class to help me stay in control. Making noise *was* my way of staying in control.

She also kept asking my mother and sisters to leave the room. She didn't understand that this birth wasn't just happening to me, it was happening to my whole family. I needed them with me.

CONSERVATION OF PERSONAL INTEGRITY

During labor the woman may experience achievement and self-control or a sense of loss of control, anxiety, and fear.

The nurse remains alert to expressions of concern and anxiety through verbal and nonverbal behavior, remembering that "routine" nursing care is quite unique to the couple. The woman needs reinforcement and support to use the adaptive response to labor she has learned. She is experiencing the "real thing," and her application of techniques may need interpretation and validation. Therefore the nurse should inquire about the type of prenatal education the woman received.

The partner also requires accurate information, clarification, and guidance. The couple should be appropriately involved in decision making. They also seek validation of their efforts and their perceptions of labor. Interpersonal skills that support the couple in labor through respectful affirmation of their self-worth, preservation of human dignity, and regard for the individual—plus practical guidance—are as important as technical skills and medical expertise.

CONSERVATION OF SOCIAL INTEGRITY

Instead of directing the woman and controlling all aspects of management and environment, the nurse and the physician should balance care and interventions with participation by the expectant mother and her partner. Parents need this receptiveness.

Changes in the attitude toward parental decision making are shown by the extent to which parents have become involved in formulating birth plans. For example, types of birth, including indications for surgical interventions, procedures, partner involvement, and strategies to reduce the need for surgical interventions, are discussed during prenatal education classes. The nurse is in a position to promote the parents' positive responses during childbirth through education and encouragement during labor.

SUPPORT DURING LABOR

Results of studies indicate that women have various levels of need for support during labor (Mackey and Lock, 1988). Women expecting minimal nursing involvement were those who had prepared for labor and whose partners were actively involved. These women saw the nurse's role as being competent at technical tasks, monitoring, and evaluating labor progress. They viewed the nurse as a source of information, someone who would provide support in the following ways:

1. Respect their wishes
2. Let them do what they wanted
3. Leave them alone with the partner
4. Not interrupt during a contraction

In the same study, other women expected a high degree of nurse involvement. These women had less need to manage their labors and more need for the physical presence of the nurse, including use of comfort measures, touch, support for the father, and frequent affirmation that they were "doing a good job" (Mackey and Lock, 1989).

How do you know which woman in labor needs extensive support? Birth plans help identify that person. Direct discussion of the woman's need for assistance is the best way to communicate. Another support study found that nurses in a Toronto study spent only 9.9% of their shifts in supportive care (McNiven et al, 1992). Supportive care included physical care, emotional support, instruction, and information and advocacy. All other direct and indirect care activities took 81.4% of the time. These included physical assessments, performing or assisting with techniques, documenting care, and all other non–patient-related activities on the unit. Hodnett and Osborn (1989) also found that women received very little support during labor. Nurses tend to spend time on technologic tasks and activities that derive from medical functions. Sometimes it seems that obstetric technology results in an engineering approach that views the client as a complex machine. It is easy to get caught up in the mechanistic view of labor. In contrast, support by means of caring behavior—through nursing acts, demeanor, and conduct that convey a sense of well being and security for the patients helps the client to feel cared for (Malinowski, Pedigo, Phillips, 1989).

Touch is one aspect of support that has been extensively studied by Weaver (1990), Penny (1979), Kintz (1987), and others. In her study Weaver (1990) defined touch as "physical contact, usually made with the hands, in a transactional activity within a nurse-patient relationship." The following conclusions were drawn.

1. Touch is an essential strategy in the nurse-patient relationship in obstetric nursing.
2. Touch is potentially a powerful modality for receiving and giving messages.
3. Touch is used by nurses within an interactive framework based on experience and sensitivity.
4. In the nurse–laboring client relationship the nature of touch is sincere and inherently reciprocal—that is, the use of touch includes elements of giving and receiving (reciprocity).
5. The use of touch can be a learned competency, acquired through socialization, experience, and role modeling.
6. Negative aspects of the nurse-client relationship usually result in withholding of nurse-initiated touch.

Although much has yet to be learned, we know that during the labor period women need "to be sustained by another human being, to have relief from pain, to have a safe outcome for self and fetus, to have attitudes and behaviors accepted and to receive bodily care" (Mackey and Lock, 1988). On this basis, nurses can develop better supportive behaviors in labor nursing, knowing that support is a learned behavior that can be observed and practiced and that can contribute toward improved job satisfaction, as well as better client care.

Admission to Labor

When a client comes to the hospital labor area, the initial assessment takes the form of a quick overview of essential points to ascertain any urgent problems. This is a form of triage that determines priorities in care (Angelini et al, 1990) (Box 13-5). To prioritize care, the following information is needed:

- When labor started
- What is the current contraction pattern
- When, or if, membranes ruptured
- Baseline vital signs and fetal heart rate
- Woman's parity, type of prenatal care, and birth plan
- Any presenting problems affecting progress in labor

Usually the external fetal heart monitor is attached to obtain a short tracing as a baseline reading. Findings are documented on the admission form (Figure 13-16).

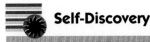

Self-Discovery

Note four ways you could build interpersonal trust with a woman and her partner during the labor experience.

BOX 13-5   Orientation for Maternal-Infant Care during Labor and Birth after Criteria-Based Performance Evaluation

Labor care: admission through triage

Determines priorities (triage) with clients in preparation room

Obtains complete admission history and nursing physical assessment

Uses fetal monitoring equipment accurately, detecting abnormalities

Reviews prenatal care data, including significant points in admission notes

Detects high-risk conditions requiring immediate medical attention: notifies physician or midwife and checks response time

Initiates an individualized nursing care plan

Communicates effectively with woman and her companion

Introduces self; uses woman's preferred name at all times

Explains sequence of admission procedures; gives supportive instructions if woman to wait for admission

Documents all care and treatments

Uses universal precautions in all care

After the initial overview, the nurse gathers data from the prenatal chart that is on file in most units. If not, the nurse notifies the physician's office or clinic of the woman's arrival and the need for chart information.

PHYSICAL EXAMINATION

While the nurse performs or assists with the obstetric examination, conversing with the woman, instructing her in breathing and relaxation technique (see Chapter 4), and gentle, careful explanation of findings are important.

Unless labor is advancing rapidly, external assessments take place before the vaginal examination. The chest is auscultated for signs of alterations in breath sounds or upper respiratory infections. Breast size and nipple condition are observed, and the height of the uterine fundus and contours of the abdomen are noted. Because examination of the fetal presenting part often is puzzling, Leopold's maneuvers are used to determine fetal position. The position of the fetal head is determined—whether it is angled to the right or left of the mother's anterior or posterior plane.

Vaginal Examination

The vaginal examination is an important procedure to assess progress of cervical dilation, fetal descent, and pelvic adequacy. Unfortunately, it also may provide a route by which ascending infection is speeded. Even with aseptic technique, vaginal bacteria will be tracked up into the cervical canal. Therefore examinations must be kept to a minimum and performed quickly. After AROM or SROM in active labor the number of times a "vaginal" is done should be minimized and each examination documented. If a later infection of endometrium develops, quality assurance and the infection control team may track the relationship of number of examinations with onset and severity of maternal or newborn infections (See Chapter 25).

Vaginal examinations are *never done* when there is frank vaginal bleeding, known low placental location, or early rupture of membranes. A sterile speculum examination may be performed in these cases to visualize the vagina and cervix and to test the fluids for spontaneous rupture. (Follow the steps for preparation as discussed in Chapter 4.)

Once the sterile, lubricated, gloved hand is inserted in the vaginal canal, it must not be removed until the assessment is completed. Because findings during the contraction must be compared with positions during the resting phase, the duration of the vaginal examination may seem long to the woman.

The *Bishop score* may be used to determine readiness for labor or early phase of labor. After the vaginal examination a score of 0, 1, 2, or 3 is given for each of the following:

- Consistency of the cervix (firm to soft)
- Position of the cervix (posterior to anterior)
- Effacement of cervix (up to 80% effaced)
- Dilation of cervix (up to 5 cm)
- Station of presenting part (from floating down to +2)

A total score of less than 5 to 7 indicates that labor is not yet effective, and the client should be instructed carefully about signs and phases of labor and sent home to wait further effective labor.

PROCEDURES FOR "WALK-INS"

Women without prenatal care may arrive at the labor area. Often they are immigrants who lack fluency in English and have not sought care because of fear, cost, or cultural reasons.

This client may be advanced in labor on admission. The concept of *triage* will come into focus inasmuch as assessment detects advanced labor with potential complications. Each assessment step must be documented.

Assessment and support take on an intensity because of time constraints and need for information. First, an interpreter may be needed, a role that the partner may be able to fill. In addition to the usual admission steps, the physician performs a complete physical examination to determine the presence of any impending obstetric or medical complications. Blood is sent to the laboratory for screening for sexually transmitted infec-

City Hospital Center
Labor Admission Record

Date of admission: _____ Time: _____

Reason given _____

MD exam by _____ Time: _____   Addressograph

_____

OB History

Parity _____ EDO _____ Wks pregnant _____ Maternal age _____

Any medical problems? _____

_____ Hepatitis B _____

Allergies: _____ Drug use history _____ STD history _____

Explain extent use of drug: Cigarette _____ Cocaine _____ Alcohol _____ Other _____

_____

Physical Assessment

TPR _____ BP _____ Fetal heart rate status _____

Initial vaginal exam: Cx _____ Eff. _____ Station _____ Presentation_____

Contraction status: _____ Onset? _____ for VDAC? _____

Membrane status: _____ SROM time/date _____ Fluid color _____

Admitting Screening

Blood type: _____ See clinic chart _____ Rubella status _____

Baseline CBC _____ (last prenatal)

Blood sent for: Type/x-match ___ CBC _____ Hepatitis _____ VDRL _____ Other _____

Urine spec. for Albumin _____ Glucose _____ Ketones _____ WBC _____ Other _____

Straight catheterization: Y/N Urinalysis _____ Albumin _____ WBC _____ C&S _____

Other admitting procedures: Ultrasound: Position _____ Placenta _____

_____

Additional observations _____

Support System

Primary language spoken _____ English? Y/N

Preferred name during labor _____ Birth companion _____

Requests tubal? Y/N Consent on chart? _____ General consent: signed/witnessed. _____

                                    Interpreter needed Y/N

Personal effects (specify): With pt _____ Sent with family _____

To labor room at: _____ Room # _____

Signature: _____

FIGURE 13-16 Labor admission record.

PROCEDURE 13-1   Vaginal Examination

Step one: Examine the perineal area. Look for signs of health, intact skin, proportions, and signs of inflammation or infection on perineum. Note any fluid leaking or bloody show; note any strong odor to fluids, as well as color and consistency. Note any scars indicating episiotomy or prior perineal surgery.

Step two: Apply sterile lubricating jelly to a sterile latex glove, and part the labia to slip the first two fingers into the vagina. Direct fingers to the back of the vagina and move fingers up to contact the cervix. The opposite hand is placed over the abdomen, palpating and, during a contraction, pushing down slightly in the direction of the perineum (Figure 13-17). Assess the cervix for the following criteria

Position: Is the cervix directed toward posterior, midposition, or anterior?

Consistency: Is the cervix firm, medium, or soft?

Effacement: Recorded as a percentage as follows:

%	Result
Not begun	2 cm long and thick
25	1.5 cm long and softened
50	1 cm long and very soft
75	0.5 cm long
100	Feels very thin; ready to be pulled up into the lower uterine segment

Dilation: Recorded as a range up to 10 cm (fully dilated); measurement is approximate and depends on the examiner's finger size.

Dilation (cm)	Result
Closed or fingertip	Cannot insert fingertip into canal
2	1 fingerwidth can be inserted into canal
3-4	2 fingerwidths
4-5	3 fingerwidths
5-6	Finger moves easily from side to side of fetal presenting part before touching cervix
7-8	Cervix is felt like a low smooth ridge surrounding the curve of the presenting part
8-9	Ridge of encircling cervix is stretched taut, with more vaginal bleeding as capillaries are broken in the cervix
9-10	Cervix flat, almost pulled up around presenting part; may still be felt as an anterior or posterior rim or "lip"
Complete	Cervix cannot be felt as fetal part slips through, enters vagina, descends through stations

Station: Assess the level of descent of the presenting part by locating the ischial spines on either side of the canal and assessing the relative location of the fetal part to these spines (see Figure 13-11).

Step three: Explain findings to woman, and make her comfortable after examination procedure is concluded.

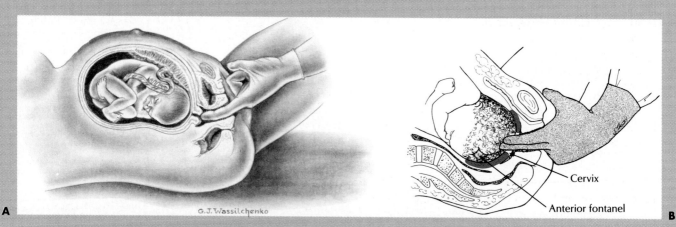

FIGURE 13-17 Vaginal examination. **A,** Undilated, uneffaced cervix; membranes intact. **B,** Palpation of sagittal suture line. Cervix effaced and partially dilated. (From Bobak IM, Jensen MD: *Maternity and gynecologic care: the nurse and the family,* ed 5, St Louis, 1993, Mosby.)

• • •

OPTIONAL ACTIVITY: Write a sample nursing note correctly documenting the performance of this procedure.

tions, hepatitis B, anemia (hemoglobin and hematocrit values), Rh antibodies, rubella antibodies, and white blood cell and platelet counts. Sometimes women who have not had prenatal care are abusing drugs, and signs of use must be noted (see Chapter 26). Special care with universal precautions must be used in these cases.

PLANNING CARE

As the nurse plans and provides care, the plan's effectiveness is measured against the degree to which self-care is accomplished; nursing actions assist in moving the woman and coach toward responsible actions, and the family becomes increasingly confident.

Realistic care incorporates modern technologic realities and the family's growth. Throughout the labor process, the nurse's actions should be directed toward supporting and encouraging the efforts by the woman and her partner that facilitate and preserve physical, mental, and emotional integrity. With nursing assistance the woman's self-care ability must be encouraged. Independence and participation in decision making should be promoted despite medical therapies or technology that may take away such a sense of control. The nurse determines the presenting nursing diagnoses and begins the care plan for the woman's stay in the unit. (See Care Plans.)

The Latent Labor Phase

The latent phase extends from the beginning of effective dilation to 3 cm. Contractions begin to be effective because they progress in frequency from about 3 to 4 per hour to 10 to 12 per hour (20 minutes apart progressing to 4 to 5 minutes apart). The contractions may not be sensed as painful, but as the phase progresses, the woman may have to begin the pattern of slow chest breathing. Contractions are mild at first with an acme below 35 mm Hg, increasing to moderate, or acme between 50 and 60 mm Hg as measured by the tocotransducer (Figure 13-18).

CHARACTERISTICS

Cervical changes become evident during this period because contractions will almost complete effacement and bring dilation to 3 cm. Usually the presenting part gradually moves deeper into the pelvis. The rupture of membranes does not profoundly influence labor in the early phase.

MOOD

The woman's reactions vary. She is comfortable; she may be excited, ambivalent, or anxious. Her mood parallels the ambivalence of the first trimester. Her

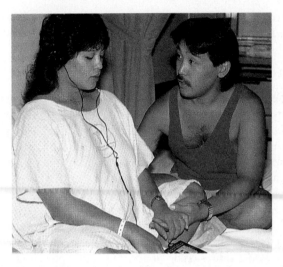

FIGURE 13-18 Any comfortable position may be assumed in active labor. Music and the coach encourage concentration. (Courtesy Marjorie Pyle, RNC, *Lifecircle*.)

confidence in herself and her coach is reinforced as she begins to apply techniques appropriately.

The unprepared woman's perception may be drastically altered by anxiety. Relaxation and self-directed activities may be difficult because concern for her own and her baby's well-being increases. As a result, perception of contractions may be felt as more acute pain.

COMFORT MEASURES

The prepared couple should be encouraged to view the woman's work during labor as a close parallel to that of a long-distance runner or swimmer. After warm-up, the race is begun. Runners pace themselves with controlled effort, coordinated muscular effort, and rhythmic breathing patterns.

At the beginning of the early phase, the woman may continue diversional activities, interspersing them with rest periods. She should urinate often to prevent bladder distention and interference with labor. Her diet usually is restricted to liquids that will sustain her for labor. If she awakens with mild contractions, she should be encouraged to get up, take a warm shower and a cup of tea, and then try to sleep. If she is unduly apprehensive, she can use controlled relaxation.

She takes a deep breath as the contraction begins, relaxes her body completely as she exhales, concentrating on the contraction. She may breathe normally as she permits the contraction to work. If needed, she can begin controlled breathing activities.

COACH

The woman needs the coach during the latent phase to indicate caring and concern. The coach supports and encourages the woman by assisting, reinforcing, directing, and clarifying.

NURSING APPROACH

The nurse who is available for consultation during the earlier phases of labor can offer suggestions about technique, aid in maintaining the couple's self-confidence, and validate their appraisal of labor. The nurse also can interpret instructions from the physician in a positive and supportive manner.

Unless membranes rupture early, educated parents should stay at home in the latent phase of labor. Being admitted and put to bed may slow labor. Therefore the nurse should encourage activity during this phase. If the woman does come in and the active phase has not yet begun, she may be sent "walking" in hospital corridors and should not be put to bed in a recumbent position. (One birthing center sends the woman in this phase out for a meal at a local restaurant. Walking and eating use up the hour or two she needs to move into active labor.)

If they have come to the hospital too early, the couple should not be sent home with an abrupt dismissal. The nurse can underscore the need for rest and the maintenance of fluid balance and energy reserves and remind them of the nature of the labor process. The couple at this point see themselves as amateurs and appreciate specific directions relevant to their needs.

Vital Signs during Labor

The nurse should always be aware of baseline readings obtained from the last prenatal visit rather than the labor admission chart, because the woman may be excited on admission. The *pulse* rate should be considered in terms of excitement, impending fever (pulse rises first), or alteration in cardiac output related to blood volume or drugs. Maternal tachycardia also may influence the fetal heart rate (see Chapter 14).

The *blood pressure* is perhaps the most significant indicator of maternal cardiovascular status (see Chapter 9). It is abnormal for any young woman to have a diastolic pressure above 80 mm Hg. Therefore if a comparison of pressures with the baseline readings for the last trimester reveals an elevation—even if not above 80 mm Hg—further assessment includes checking the urine for albumin. Blood pressure during labor is taken only with the woman in a lateral position or with a wedge tilt to the side to avoid supine hypotension. It is recorded on the flow sheet, including the position of the arm on which the reading was taken. Each unit has a protocol for timing of vital signs. Usually temperature, pulse, and respiration are obtained every 4 hours unless there is an elevation of temperature. Blood pressure is taken every 4 hours in early labor, every hour when active labor begins, and every 30 minutes in second-stage labor.

Temperature can begin to rise for several reasons during labor. First, the woman may have not received adequate fluids and may be dehydrated. A urine concentration check will establish this condition. If membranes have ruptured more than 8 to 12 hours before the onset of labor, it is possible to have ascending infection, with inflammation of the chorion and the uterine endometrium. (See Chapter 25 for discussion.) The temperature will rise slowly. Any temperature above 99.0° F should be checked more frequently (Table 13-4). Finally, if epidural anesthesia is used, there may be an elevated temperature (see Chapter 16).

Bladder Care during Labor

The bladder is checked for fullness every 2 hours, and the woman is encouraged to void. A full bladder delays descent of the fetus, and pressure on the full bladder may injure the tissue. There is a standing order for straight catheterization if two hourly specimens show a lower than normal output. Concentrated urine indicates dehydration. There are many reasons for fluid loss, mainly diaphoresis and more rapid respiratory loss related to breathing patterns.

On occasion, with the use of an epidural anesthetic, the woman is not be able to void and a Foley catheter is placed. This catheter *should be removed before the pushing phase of labor* because the inflated ballon may traumatize bladder tissue. It also causes discomfort and inhibits pushing efforts. The bladder should be emptied by straight catheterization just before application of forceps or if the fetal head is having difficulty descending when the bladder is palpated during late second-stage labor. This catheterization is routinely performed by the **accoucheur** (obstetrician or midwife).

Before a cesarean, a Foley catheter is placed to empty the bladder and minimize risk of surgical trauma. The lower uterine segment is attached to the bladder by

---

TABLE 13-4   **Vital Signs during Labor/Birth**

		CERVICAL PROGRESS	
Sign	Latent	Active	Second Stage
Blood pressure	q4h	q2-1h	q30-10min
Fetal heart rate	q1h	q30min	q10min
Check monitor	q1h	q15-30min	q5-10min
Temperature	q4h	q4h	q4h
If elevated	q1h	q1h	q1h
Pulse	q4h	q2-4h	q2-4h
Respirations	q4h	q4h	Not done pushing

Follow unit protocol. Record signs on flow sheet and, if fetal monitoring in place, on strip chart.

fascia; it must be dissected away before the incision into the uterus is made. If the bladder is not empty, there is danger of cutting into it during surgery.

Monitoring intake and output. It is important to understand why intake and output recording is necessary during labor. First, activities of labor lead to *dehydration,* which is revealed by dry mucous membranes, slight elevation of temperature, and dark concentrated urine. Second, fluid restrictions in some units or liberal oral fluids in others will change the normal voiding patterns. Intravenous fluid *overload* is a key iatrogenic (treatment-caused) problem in labor, especially if epidural anesthetics are used. Third, a full bladder hinders descent of the fetus, and pressure may injure the urethra and bladder tissues. All of these problems are avoided by careful monitoring, with appropriate interventions by the nurse.

Checking the urine during labor. On admission, each woman is requested to void so that urine may be checked for albumin, ketones, glucose, and leukocytes. Because of the vaginal fluids, this must be a midstream, clean-voided specimen. The key indicator of problems is the presence of urinary albumin, which will affect treatment during labor. If the leukocyte count is too high, a straight catheterization may be ordered to obtain a specimen for culture and sensitivity. Counts greater than 100,000 colonies/mL indicate bacteriuria. Unless blood in the urine is marked, its presence usually is believed to result from red blood cells in the bloody show. Ketones and glucose are checked on admission, and later, if the woman has diabetes, capillary glucose will be used to follow her blood glucose levels. Ketones are checked on each voiding because their presence is not unusual with a normal serum glucose (see Chapter 24).

SUMMARY OF NURSING RESPONSIBILITIES

When the client and partner come to the unit, courteous greeting and settling into the waiting area are essential. They need to understand that they may have come too early because of excitement. The nurse performs the initial evaluation; in some settings the physical examination is done by the medical personnel.

1. Obtain prenatal history; ask about immediate events such as onset of labor, status of membranes, bloody show.
2. Assess phase of labor and condition of woman, obtain vital signs, and perform physical assessment, including Leopold's maneuvers.
3. With external fetal tocodynamometer and ultrasound transducer, run a monitor strip for a period of 10 minutes. This enables assessment of contraction strength and frequency, as well as fetal heart responses to contractions.

4. By means of vaginal examination, assess station, cervical status, and condition of external perineal tissues.

The nurse decides if the woman is in active labor or if there are reasons for her to stay. If not, she should be given careful instructions about activities within the next few hours and how to know when to return. Once the decision is made about admission, further steps are taken.

1. Continue with admission activities after determination of status. Complete nursing history. Attach the mother's identification band.
2. Ensure that blood is drawn for admission tests, usually complete blood cell count, type and crossmatch (kept for use by blood bank if needed), plus any other specimen as ordered by individual physician. Some units use a heparin lock for drawing blood and administering needed intravenous fluids.
3. Note where woman's belongings are placed.
4. Assist couple to settle into the labor room. Establish a relaxed atmosphere. Explain equipment, orient them to routines of vital signs, checking monitors, and physician's visits.
5. Determine couple's birth plan, type of childbirth preparation, and expectations for nurse involvement in support. Assure them that you will be flexible in your interventions for support.
6. Promote comfort by showing them positions to assume during labor, where to obtain ice chips, and how to use comfort equipment.
7. Evaluate couple's response to this phase of labor. Document all findings.

The Active Labor Phase:

The active phase includes a period of accelerated, progressive dilation with well-defined contractions at frequent intervals and a *transition* period immediately before complete dilation.

 Clinical Decision

Mary and Jim arrive in the labor unit at 4 AM for their first birth. She has had mild labor for 6 hours. They had two classes but did not find time to practice consistently. Mary is anxious; Jim looks "blank" and wants to be with Mary but looks as if he does not know what to do. How would you work to smooth the transition into their being a "laboring couple"?

At the midpoint of cervical dilation, 5 cm, contractions become strong and more consistent in interval and duration, with shorter rest intervals. This phase demands the total concentration of the laboring woman and the encouragement of those attending her if she is to remain confident.

CHARACTERISTICS

The cervix is effaced further while rapid dilation of 4 to 8 cm occurs. The dilation may plateau or seem to stop at 5 cm, but this phase is short.

MOOD

The woman's confident, talkative mood is replaced quickly by an intense, total absorption in labor. As this phase continues and fatigue increases, the woman's confidence begins to waver; she requires active supportive measures.

The unprepared woman may exhibit a disorganized pattern of behavior. Apprehension increases, and sentences become fragmented. She may become irritable, unable to cope if left alone, and beg to be "put to sleep."

COMFORT MEASURES

The woman must now direct her conscious efforts to controlled relaxation. She becomes aware of the importance of concentration as she deals with contractions (Figure 13-19).

Back Labor

A woman may experience "back labor" because of a posterior position of the fetus or a focus of tension. While using appropriate breathing techniques, she should direct her concentration on releasing tension, specifically in the sacrum, perineum, buttocks, and thighs. She avoids lying on her back; her coach applies firm *counterpressure* to the sacral area. The partner should not *rub* the skin; over the hours of labor the skin will become irritated. Some women find relief by having cold or warm compresses applied to the sacrum or by doing the *pelvic rock exercise,* rounding the back and tilting the pelvis forward.

Hyperventilation

If a woman begins to hyperventilate, a respiratory imbalance of decreased carbon dioxide (CO_2) levels will develop. She must rebreathe exhaled air from a small paper bag or cupped hands, which usually corrects the imbalance and relieves the symptoms of **hyperventilation,** including dizziness, light-headedness, and tingling.

COACH

The need for coaching increases with the active phase. As contractions heighten and occur more frequently, the woman's perspective becomes distorted. She needs to be reminded to take one contraction at a time. Her coach helps her to focus on the contractions by counting off each 15-second interval with the contraction.

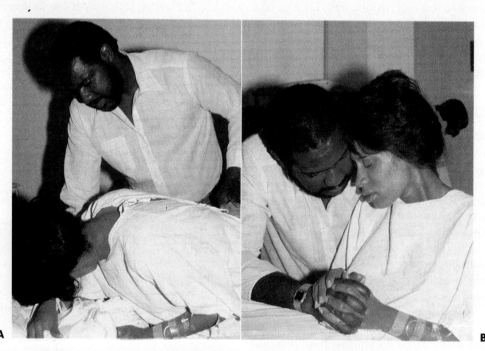

A   B

FIGURE 13-19 As labor becomes more intense, (**A**) backrubs and (**B**) emotional support are crucial to coping. (Courtesy Marjorie Pyle, RNC, *Lifecircle.*)

NURSING APPROACH

Although the couple has learned various skills, discomfort still occurs. Ensure that the couple understands medication, anesthetics, and other obstetric techniques that may be indicated for the birth. If they have not attended class, explain so the partners may discuss options.

In observing labor and reactions, the nurse must rely on the woman's judgment of her comfort. She may appear to be in distress when actually she is concentrating and working hard. Note that cultural variations may significantly change labor responses. Comments such as, "You're working very hard," "Having a baby is hard work. You're doing a good job," or "That contraction was not easy, but you managed it" underscore appreciation of the work of labor and the effectiveness of her efforts.

The unprepared woman needs special encouragement. Ideally, provision should be made for a nurse to remain with her, on a one-to-one basis, which often is not possible because of staffing limitations. The woman needs to be informed of her progress and the baby's condition in terms she can understand. The nurse's direct and positive manner and use of simple terms can help the woman with relaxation and breathing techniques.

SUMMARY OF NURSING RESPONSIBILITIES

The active phase of labor requires the nurse to be increasingly involved. As the phase progresses, fetal responses may change and the woman's coping abilities are tested. In addition to continuing the supportive care of the first phase, the nurse performs the following functions:

1. Monitors woman's responses by checking vital signs, observing contractions by palpation or tocodynamometer, and noting changes in show or rupture of membranes
2. Monitors progress of cervical dilation and fetal descent, remembering to avoid frequent vaginal examinations after membranes rupture
3. Assesses fetal responses to phase of labor, checks heart tones in relation to contractions, and documents every hour, as protocol requires
4. Maintains woman's hygiene for comfort and asepsis; observes vaginal fluids for any changes during this phase
5. Promotes positions of comfort, supports coach in using comfort measures, and notes mood changes and coping abilities
6. Interprets labor progress to couple and affirms their coping abilities
7. Assists with analgesic or regional anesthetic administration if needed
8. Monitors intake and output
9. Evaluates nursing interventions and makes necessary modifications
10. Documents all findings

Active Phase: Transition Period

As cervical dilation nears completion, the woman enters the most intensive and demanding part of the first stage. Fatigue, the inconsistency and discomfort of contractions, and the intensity of labor make self-control difficult.

Most of this period is in the *pelvic phase,* as the fetus begins its descent through the pelvis in preparation for entry into the birth canal. Internal rotation is occurring.

CONTRACTIONS

Intervals shorten to 3 to 2 minutes; there is little rest, and tonus may rise. Contractions build rapidly into very strong peaks, which last about two thirds of each contraction. The monitor printout may show intensity to 100 mm Hg or more. The contraction also subsides quickly, but the woman often feels as though they never completely disappear. Her body is being bombarded with stimuli, and she is highly sensitized. Multiparas may experience multiple peaks.

CHARACTERISTICS

With contractions forcing the baby deep into the pelvis and against the cervix, the cervix now dilates fully, from about 8 to 10 cm. This produces a heavy show because more cervical capillaries rupture. The presenting part may cause strong sensations of pressure in the rectum, back, groin, or perineum. A woman may feel as though she is going to have a bowel movement and may call for a bedpan.

 Clinical Decision

Sara is in the accelerated period of the active phase. She was admitted at 4 cm of dilation and is now at 6 cm. This is her first pregnancy, and she is progressing at a rate of about 1 cm/hr. She and her husband, Rick, have participated in childbirth preparation classes, but they have begun to call for you frequently. Describe four appropriate interventions.

MOOD AND PHYSICAL REACTIONS

The woman becomes agitated and intense during this period. The physiologic changes of labor and fatigue make her irritable, discouraged, panicked, and restless. Her reactions are like those of a marathon runner "going against the wall" at the 19 to 20 mile point. She finds it difficult to cope with contractions; relaxation during the brief rest intervals is almost impossible without special strategies. She may sweat profusely, become chilled, or alternate between these reactions. She may be nauseated and briefly vomit. Her legs may tremble and cramp. She may feel overwhelmed and discouraged; she wants to give up. Her perspective is severely distorted.

COMFORT MEASURES

To assist efforts to relax between contractions, restore respiratory balance, and foster a sense of well-being, the woman uses the rhythmic chest breathing at its slowest rate, eight breaths per minute, during the brief intervals and puff-blows in rhythms of 4-1, 3-1, 2-1, and 1-1 during the contractions.

Effleurage is irritating and distracting during the advanced phase, but the woman may find relief in supporting the lower abdominal area with her hands. The coach may hold her hand, embrace her, or give counterpressure to the lower back (Figure 13-20). Position changes may be helpful.

COACH

Coaching must be specific and direct. The woman's reactions frequently require active and continual direction. The coach may have to touch the abdominal area lightly to help her discern the absence of a contraction. Verbal and nonverbal communication is very important to her ability to remain in control.

NURSING APPROACH

The woman's need for reassurance intensifies. The nurse continues to interpret progress of labor through vaginal examinations, monitoring readings, palpation, and observation. The woman must not be left alone at this phase. At the same time, preparations for the birth phase need to be organized. The couple needs to know when and if the woman will be moved to another room for the birth. In an LDR room, the nurse will already have checked supplies and equipment so there will be no interruption of nursing support. The infant's condition is checked every 10 minutes as a minimum standard of care, although documentation is not required so often. The nurse remains alert to sudden changes in the position and station of the presenting part, particularly with multiparas, in whom dilation may progress dramatically from 8 to 10 cm in a few minutes.

SUMMARY OF NURSING RESPONSIBILITIES

1. Assess the woman's condition and the progress of the phase of labor.
2. Assess fetal response to accelerated labor every 10 minutes.
3. Observe for signs of fetal distress.
4. Maintain perineal hygiene and a dry underpad.
5. Take appropriate action in assisting physician or midwife.
6. Ready the birthing room.
7. Evaluate woman's responses to interventions.
8. Support partner as he or she helps with breathing and coping activities.
9. Document all observations.

Appendix 5 lists many of the competencies nurses working in this area will need to develop. Table 13-5 summarizes all the phases of labor. A sample care plan for vaginal birth follows.

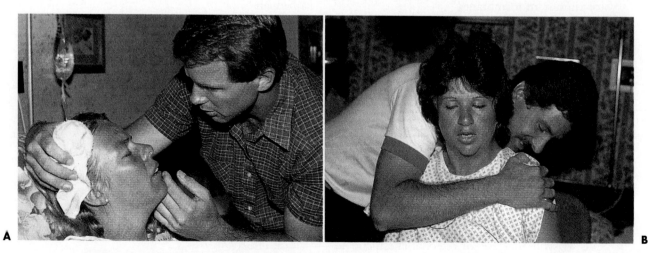

FIGURE 13-20 Transition is the most difficult phase. **A,** A cold washcloth helps. **B,** The coach offers support. (Courtesy Marjorie Pyle, RNC, *Lifecircle*.)

TABLE 13-5 Labor Summary*

PHASE	RECOMMENDED COPING TECHNIQUES	COACHING
LATENT: EARLY *Duration:* Nullipara, 8.6-20 hr*; multipara, 5.6-14 hr* *Contractions:* Mild to moderate, 30-45 sec long, 20-10 min, then 10-5 min apart, more regular *Work:* Effacement and dilation to 3 cm *Mood:* Talkative, comfortable, excited, ambivalent	Conserve energy. Call physician; emphasize degree of comfort. Take clear fluids as permitted. As necessary: use controlled relaxation. For control, use rhythmic chest breathing: slow rate at 8 breaths/min and modified rate at 16-20 breaths/min.	Time contractions; note progress every hour. Support her efforts. Help with relaxation. Monitor her breathing techniques. If at home, help with organizing household; assist general relaxation. Notify obstetrician/midwife.
ACTIVE: ACCELERATED *Duration:* Average 2-3.5 hr *Contractions:* Strong, 50-60 sec, 5-3 min apart *Work:* Dilate from 3 to 8 cm *Mood:* Very intense, concentrated; if membranes break, contractions increase in strength	Conserve energy. For control, use controlled relaxation, combined breathing pattern (rhythmic chest or shallow). If necessary, use shallow, accelerated-decelerated with contraction. Usually go to hospital. Take sips of water or ice chips, if allowed.	"Count down" contractions. Use mouth rinses, cool cloth to woman's hands and face. Touch and stroke her arms and legs. Talk to her; encourage her efforts. Remind her that labor is intermittent. Monitor her breathing.
ACTIVE: TRANSITION *Duration:* 20-60 min but not more than 2 hr for primipara *Contractions:* Erratic, intense, 60-90 sec, 3-2 min apart *Work:* Dilate 8-10 cm *Mood:* Irritable, discouraged, overwhelmed *Physical sensations:* nausea, vomiting, chills, trembling, profuse sweating, pressure sensations, difficulty in relaxing	Use controlled relaxation. Use shallow breathing: pant-blow 3/1, 2/1, 1/1 as contraction demands. Use for rectal pressure: 1/1 pant-blow rhythm. Use for urge to push: repeated blows. Use rhythmic chest breathing between contractions.	Give specific directions. Insist that she take one contraction at a time. Remind her that baby is almost here. Encourage her. Monitor her breathing. If she uses repeated "blowing" or has the urge to push, summon nurse.

*This pattern reflects an average labor for a first birth. Duration of contractions is determined here *by palpation;* the maternal tocotransducer may indicate a longer duration. *TENS,* Transcutaneous electrical nerve stimulation.   *Continued.*

TABLE 13-5 Labor Summary—cont'd

PHASE	RECOMMENDED COPING TECHNIQUES	COACHING
Special considerations		
Hyperventilation: Tingling, dizzy, light-headedness, apprehension, out of rhythm	Rebreathe exhaled air between contractions, or hold breath for 8-10 counts.	Monitor her breathing. Correct technique—mark cadence, breathe with her.
Back labor: Strong discomfort in small of back; difficulty in relaxing; contractions erratic; increase in tension	Prevention: keep breathing lightly and rhythmically. Lie on side. Focus on progressive relaxation throughout each contraction. Warm or cold compresses; TENS. Constant pressure to small of back.	Talk through contractions. Apply counterpressure. Stroke. Encourage her.
SECOND STAGE		
Duration: Multipara 20-60 min; nullipara, primipara up to 120 min	The harder the push, the better it feels.	Coach efforts: in, out/in, out/in, hold, relax key areas, push (count slowly to 10), push while releasing air (repeat); several deep breaths at end of each effort.
Contractions: Rhythmic, strong, 90 sec, 2-4 min apart	Use expulsion technique.	
Work: Descent and birth of baby	If instructed to stop pushing at birth of head, use pant-blow.	
Mood: Refreshed, sense of work, cooperative		Change positions as she desires.
Physical: Vaginal fullness, pressure in rectum; burning, stretching		
Episiotomy: painless, "unzipped"		
THIRD STAGE		
Delivery of placenta: 10-30 min	Push as directed.	Enjoy baby together.
Contractions: Moderately strong	Enjoy baby.	Praise her efforts.
Mood: Thinking of baby		
Work: Placenta expelled		

NURSING CARE PLAN • Labor

CASE: With no formal preparation for labor, Jenny M, a primipara, was admitted to the labor area at 11 PM. All lab and physical exam parameters were normal. Membranes ruptured at 10 PM, with normal characteristics. Bill, her spouse, remained throughout labor and birth but was very anxious. She was apprehensive until an epidural was begun at 5 AM. Baby girl Joanna born at 7:30 AM, Apgar 9-9, weight 7 lb, midline episiotomy, moderate bleeding, and recovery normal. Discharge plan in 24 hours.

ASSESSMENT

1. No preparation for labor or birth plan, routine prenatal care.
2. 19-year-old primipara, ruptured membranes 1 hour prior to admission.
3. Active labor, normal FHT
4. Prenatal weight gain average, lab parameters normal.
5. Partner and client apprehensive.

NURSING DIAGNOSES

1. Knowledge deficit regarding anticipated events secondary to lack of preparation.
2. Anxiety (moderate) r/t lack of preparation, tension, parity.
3. Pain (varying degrees) r/t deficit in self-management techniques, progressive labor.
4. Ineffective breathing patterns for labor r/t lack of preparation.

EXPECTED OUTCOMES

1. Couple express satisfaction with labor and birth experience.
2. Couple participate as much as possible in decision making and will voice concerns.
3. Mother and infant exhibit effective adaptation to birth stressors.

NURSING INTERVENTIONS

1. Establish a relaxed atmosphere, orient to labor room and staff.
   Provide anticipatory guidance and status reports.
   Assist partner with supportive interventions.
   Explain intake and output parameters.
   Encourage expression of anxious feelings.
2. Continue assessment of progress of labor and compare with fetal responses.
   Monitor for restlessness, crying, pain behaviors.
   Assist with epidural analgesia administration and monitor vital signs.
   Relate TPR to time of ruptured membranes.
   Monitor for ineffective bearing down.
3. Individualize instruction for coping strategies.
   Teach breathing and relaxation methods.
   Assist couple with comfort measures.
   Affirm positive coping behaviors.

EVALUATION

1. Did Jenny use effective methods for coping with fear, tension, and pain?
2. Did partner and nursing support help her and affirm self-esteem?
3. Did mother and infant exhibit uneventful course of labor?

KEY POINTS

- Alterations in the powers and the passage may change the processes of normal labor.
- An intact amniotic sac may cushion the fetal head and prevent ascending infections.
- There are several theories of how labor begins. Causes of preterm labor, however, are largely unknown.
- Women should be taught signs of preterm labor and effective labor, as well as when to seek evaluation of cervical status.
- The phases of the first stage have distinct characteristics. Timing, however, may vary widely.
- Universal precautions are mandatory when handling blood and body fluids. Labor is a high-risk area for health care personnel.

- Nursing management of labor includes conservation of physical energy and personal, structural, and social integrity.
- Position in labor facilitates or hinders the labor process, and the nurse is responsible for promoting good positioning.
- Fluids usually are permitted in labor unless a complication is present inasmuch as epidural anesthesia is much more commonly used than is general anesthesia.
- Support for the woman in labor takes several forms depending on the birth plan and process of labor, but the process is always important to the couple.
- Competency in labor nursing care is mandatory. Serious legal implications accompany lack of knowledge in this area.

STUDY QUESTIONS

Choose the Key Terms that fit the following definitions:

13-1 a. Changes in the infant's head shape as a result of birth pressure: *molding*
b. Relationship of a fixed point on the fetus to the quadrants of the maternal pelvis: *position*
c. Cervical changes that allow dilation to progress: *effacement*
d. The opening up of the cevix: *dilation*
e. When *CPD* occurs, the rate of descent is arrested
f. An imbalance of oxygen and carbon dioxide because of rapid breathing: *hyperventilation*
g. Selecting the actions that take priority in a crisis situation: *triag*

13-2 For a primigravida with adequate pelvic measurements, match the description of labor progress with the appropriate phase of labor in which the signs occur.

Signs of progress

a. Mild contractions occurring about 10 minutes apart, lasting 40 seconds, cervix 2 cm dilated, partial effacement: *Latent*
b. Contractions building into intense peaks every 2 to 3 minutes, cervix 8 cm dilated and effaced: *transition*
c. Strong contractions occurring 4 to 5 minutes apart, lasting 60 seconds, cervix 6 cm dilated: *active*

Phase of labor

(1) Latent phase
(2) Active, accelerated phase
(3) Active, transition phase

13-3 To determine the duration of contractions, you should measure the time interval between:
a. The beginning of a contraction and the acme of that contraction
b. The acme of a contraction and the end of the same contraction
c. The beginning of a contraction and the end of the same contraction
d. The beginning of a contraction and the beginning of the next contraction

13-4 At the end of the first stage of labor, an increase in show primarily results from:
a. Placental bleeding
b. Small tears in the vaginal mucous membranes
c. Capillary bleeding from the final stretching of the cervix
d. Onset of minor clotting deficiency as labor ends

13-5 Contractions were noted at 3- to 4-minute intervals and at 50 mm Hg pressure on the monitor record. This describes contraction:
a. Intensity and duration
b. Frequency and interval
c. Duration and frequency
d. Frequency and intensity

13-6 Effacement is the process by which the cervix is:
a. Opened to its widest diameter
b. Pulled up into the lower uterine segment
c. Freed of the mucous plug
d. Forced to move into the upper vagina

13-7 The rationale for waiting until the head is well engaged to rupture membranes includes two reasons below:

a. To ensure that a small amount of amniotic fluid is left in the uterus to lubricate the birth canal

b. To speed the labor process after being sure the fetus is flexed

c. To prevent prolapse of the cord with a gush of fluid

d. To cushion the fetal head as long as possible

13-8 Ann and Joe have not attended class for their second child. As transition progresses, Ann becomes very anxious, hyperventilates, and cries out that this labor is much worse than the first. Joe is upset and turns to you for help. Your first response should be:

a. "Tell me what happened in your first labor."

b. "Calm yourself, Ann; your rapid breathing may make the baby distressed."

c. "Ann, I can see that you are really making progress. I'll stay to help Joe help you."

d. "Do you want pain medication at this point?"

13-9 Ann's hyperventilation needs nursing intervention. You would:

a. _____

b. _____

c. _____

13-10 The first stage of labor is considered to have ended when:

a. Regular 3-minute contractions have been established.

b. The membranes have been ruptured.

c. The cervix is completely effaced and dilated.

d. Pushing is an overwhelming need.

Answer Key

13-1 a. Molding, b. Position, c. Effacement, d. Dilation, e. Cephalopelvic disproportion, f. Hyperventilation, g. Triage 13-2 a (1), b (3), c (2) 13-3 c 13-4 c 13-5 d 13-6 b 13-7 c and d 13-8 c 13-9 a. Reinforce correct breathing, b. Instruct in brief rebreathing of expired air, c. Support Joe in helping Ann regain control 13-10 c

REFERENCES

Aderhold KJ, Perry L: Jet hydrotherapy for labor and postpartum pain relief, *MCN* 16(2):97, 1991.

Aderhold KJ, Roberts JE: Phases of the second stage of labor, *J Nurse Midwife* 36(5):267, 1991.

Andrews CM, Chrzanowski M: Maternal position, labor and comfort, *Applied Nurs Res* 3(1):7, 1990.

Angelini DJ: Nonverbal communication in labor, *Am J Nurs* 78:1221, 1978.

Angelini DJ et al: Toward a concept of triage for labor and delivery: staff perceptions and role utilization, *J Perinat Neonatal Nurs* 4(3):1, 1990.

Bergstrom L et al: "You'll feel me touching you, sweetie": vaginal examinations during the second stage of labor, *Birth* 19(1):10, 1992.

Birch E: The experience of touch received during labor: postpartum perceptions of therapeutic value, *J Nurse Midwife* 31(6):270, 1986.

Blackman ST, Loper DL: Maternal, fetal, and neonatal physiology, Philadelphia, 1992, WB Saunders.

Broach J, Newton H: Food and beverages in labor, Part I: Cross-cultural and historical practices, *Birth* 15(2):81, 1988.

Buck GM et al: Labor and delivery events and risk of sudden infant death syndrome (SIDS), *Am J Epidemiol* 133(9):900, 1991.

Caldeyro-Barcia R: Influence of maternal position on time of spontaneous rupture of the membranes, progress of labor, and fetal head compression, *Birth Family J* 6(1):7, 1979.

Challis JRG: Characteristics of parturition. In Creasy RK, Resnik R, editors: *Maternal-fetal medicine: principles and practice,* Philadelphia, 1989, WB Saunders.

Chapman L: Searching: expectant fathers' experiences during labor and birth, *J Perinatal Neonatal Nurs,* 4(4):21, 1991.

Collings B: Role of nursing in labor and delivery, *JOGNN* 15(5):412, 1987.

Cumminski KC et al: Induction of labor with pulsatile oxytocin, *Am J Obstet Gynecol* 163(6):1868, 1990.

Elkington KW: At the water's edge: where obstetrics and anesthesia meet, *Obstet Gynecol* 77:304, 1991.

Fenwick L: Birthing: techniques for managing physiologic and psychologic aspects of childbirth, *Perinat Neonat* 5:8, 1984.

Friedman E: Failure to progress in labor. In Queenan J, editor: *Management of high-risk pregnancy,* Oradell, NJ, 1985, Medical Economics Books.

Ginsberg R: Occupational exposure to bloodborne pathogens: the new OSHA regulations, Pediatr AIDS & HIV infect:fetus to adolescent 2(1):37, 1990.

Hazle N: Hydration in labor: is routine intravenous hydration necessary? *J Nurse Midwife* 31:171, 1986.

Hedstrom L, Newton N: Touch in labor: a comparison of cultures and eras, *Birth* 18:181, 1986.

Hill WC et al: Let's get rid of the term Braxton Hicks contractions, *Obstet Gynecol* 75(4):709, 1990.

Hodnett E, Osborn R: Effects of continuous intrapartum professional support on childbirth outcomes, *Res Nurs Health* 12:289, 1989.

Huzar G, Naftolin F: The myometrium and uterine cervix in normal and preterm labor, *N Engl J Med* 311:571, 1984.

Jennings B et al: Use of prostaglandins in nurse-midwifery practice, *J Nurse Midwife* 34(3):137, 1989.

Johnson N, Johnson VA, Gupta JK: Maternal positions during labor, *Obstet Gynecol Surv* 46(7):428, 1991.

Kennel J et al: Continuous emotional support in a US hospital: a randomized controlled trial, *JAMA* 265:2197, 1991.

Keppler AB: The use of intravenous fluid during labor, *Birth* 15(2):76, 1988.

Klaus M et al: Effects of social support during parturition on maternal and fetal morbidity, *Br Med J* 293:585, 1986.

Kilpatrick SJ et al: Characteristics of normal labor, *Obstet Gynecol* 74(1):85, 1989.

Kintz D: Nursing support in labor, *JOGNN* 16(6):126, 1987.

Klein RDP et al: A study of father and nurse support during labor, *Birth* 8(3):161, 1980.

Liu Y: The effect of maternal position during labor, *Am J Nurs* 74:2205, 1974.

Liu Y: The effects of the upright position during childbirth, *Image: J of Nurs Scholarship* 21(1):14, 1989.

Lupe P, Gros T: Maternal upright posture and mobility in labor, *Obstet Gynecol* 67:727, 1986.

Mackey MC, Lock SE: Women's expectations of the labor and delivery nurse, *JOGNN* 17(6):505, 1988.

Malinowski JS, Pedigo CG, Phillips CR: *Nursing care during the labor process*, Philadelphia, 1989, FA Davis.

May L, Ditolla K: In-hospital alternative birth centers, *MCN* 9:48, 1984.

McNiven P, Hodnett E. O'Brien, Pallas LL: Supportive women in labor: a work sampling study of the activities of labor and delivery nurses, *Birth* 19(1):3, 1992.

Metzger BL, Therrien B: Effect of position on cardiovascular response during the Valsalva maneuver, *Nurs Res* 39(4):200, 1990.

Mynaugh PA: A randomized study of two methods of teaching perineal massage: effects on practice rates, episiotomy rates and lacerations, *Birth* 18(3):153, 1991.

NAACOG: *Standards for obstetric, gynecologic, and neonatal nursing*, Washington, DC, 1986, The Association.

Nodine P, Roberts JA: Factors associated with perineal outcome during childbirth, *J Nurse Midwife* 32(3):123, 1987.

Oxhorn H: *Human labor and birth*, ed 5, New York, 1986, Appleton-Century-Crofts.

Penny, K: Postpartum perceptions of touch received during labor, *Res Nurs Health* 2:9, 1979.

Roberts JA: Factors influencing distress from pain during labor, *MCN* 8(1):62, 1983.

Roberts JA et al: The effects of maternal position on uterine contractibility and efficiency, *Birth* 10:243, 1983.

Roberts JA et al: Effects of lateral recumbency and sitting on the first stage of labor, *J Reprod Med* 7:477, 1984.

Shields D: Nursing care in labor and patient satisfaction, *J Adv Nurs* 3:535, 1978.

Sosa R et al: The effect of a supportive companion on perinatal problems, length of labor and mother-infant attachment, *N Engl J Med* 303(11):597, 1980.

Steinman G: Forces affecting the dynamics of labor, *J Rep Med* 36(12):868, 1991.

Stewart P et al: Posture in labour, *Br J Obstet Gynaecol* 96(11):1258, 1989.

Ventura SJ: First births to older mothers, *Am J Public Health* 79(12):1675, 1989.

Weaver DF: Nurses' views on the meaning of touch in obstetrical nursing practice, *JOGNN* 19(2):157, 1990.

 STUDENT RESOURCE SHELF

Albers LL et al: Birth settings for low-risk pregnancies—an analysis of the literature, *J Nurse Midwife* 36(4):215, 1991. Helpful analysis of the many settings for birth.

Kennel J et al: Continuous emotional support in a US hospital; a randomized controlled trial, *JAMA* 265:2197, 1991. The United States is the only country that has until recently kept women from having support ad lib during labor. Now the physician team that studied bonding goes a step further to find the benefits of support so that the mother has emotional energy to bond with her infant.

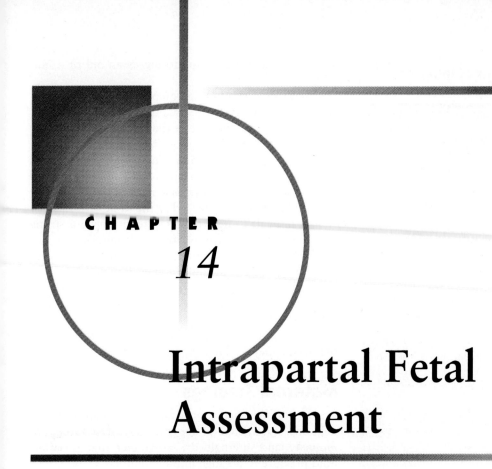

Intrapartal Fetal Assessment

KEY TERMS

Accelerations
Amnioinfusion
Artifact
Asphyxia
Baseline Rate
Beat-to-Beat
 Variability
Bradycardia
Cord Compression
 (CC)
Decelerations
End-Stage Variables
Fetal Distress
Fetal Electrocardio-
 graphy
Meconium Aspiration
 Syndrome (MAS)

Nonreassuring
 Pattern
Nuchal Cord
Ominous Pattern
Periodic Heart Rate
Prolapse
Questionable Pattern

Reassuring Pattern
Resting Tonus
Sinusoidal Pattern
Tachycardia
Uteroplacental
 Insufficiency (UPI)

LEARNING OBJECTIVES

1. *Recognize when fetal monitoring should be used.*
2. *Describe fetal physiologic responses to labor.*
3. *Differentiate between reassuring and nonreassuring fetal heart rate patterns.*
4. *Recognize normal and abnormal patterns of uterine activity.*
5. *Relate nursing interventions to physiologic factors underlying selected patterns.*
6. *Describe documentation of fetal assessments according to protocols.*
7. *Explain uses of monitoring and fetal assessment tests to the laboring woman and her support person.*

During the birth process the fetus is passive and wholly dependent on its environment for survival. Simultaneous measurement of fetal heart rate and uterine contractions allows detection of the fetus unable to withstand the stress of labor.

Fetal heart rate monitoring is now commonly mandated during active labor in most hospital birth units. Some units require that the client be monitored constantly after admission. Factors that *require* continuous monitoring are a premature or postmature fetus, abnormal fetal heart rate tracing or labor pattern, early rupture of membranes, meconium-stained fluid, and chronic problems such as diabetes or hypertension.

A more flexible protocol will specify monitoring on the woman's admission until a satisfactory normal tracing has been obtained and then remonitoring at set intervals. This flexible procedure allows the client to find a position of comfort or to ambulate. If she decides to return to bed for a time, the monitor can be reapplied. These variations in policies may influence whether the woman perceives fetal monitoring as an aid or a hindrance to labor.

If ultrasonic monitoring equipment is not available, the fetal heart rate must be auscultated. The frequency for listening to the fetal heart rate is determined by the stage of labor and the presence of risk factors. It should be assessed at least every 30 minutes, increasing to 15 minutes as the active phase of labor progresses, and then every 5 to 10 minutes during the second stage of labor. Monitor recordings should be checked at the same intervals.

It is difficult to hear the fetal heart during a strong contraction, but when electronic monitoring is not available, the examiner must obtain a 30-second reading during decrement and another 1 minute later for comparison. This provides information about fetal response to the contraction.

Box 14-1 summarizes the potential benefits and risks of intrapartum monitoring, including the consideration that its use may tend to dehumanize the birth experience.

Maternal Tracings

Tracings of maternal contractions are obtained by two methods, externally by *tocotransducer* or *tocodynamometer* and internally by a catheter that transmits fluid pressure to a gauge in the monitor.

METHODS

Tocotransducer

The tocotransducer is a spring-loaded device for external monitoring that is applied with an elastic belt around the woman's abdomen over the fundus. As a contraction builds, increasing pressure is transmitted from the uterus through the maternal abdominal wall to the spring mechanism. The "toco" sends the signal to the recorder, which traces a continuous record of contractions as they occur (Figure 14-1, *A*).

Intrauterine Catheter

Internal pressure is obtained when there are indications for accurate assessment of the pressure on the fetus. The cervix must be dilated and membranes ruptured before internal monitoring is possible. The catheter is passed through the cervix and along the presenting part into the uterine cavity (Figure 14-1, *B*). The increasing intrauterine pressure that occurs during a contraction is transmitted through the catheter to the recorder, which traces a continuous record of contractions as they occur. The system must be calibrated and the catheter freely placed within the uterus.

INTERPRETING MATERNAL TRACINGS

The maternal part of the fetal monitoring record is obtained externally or internally. The monitor pen records

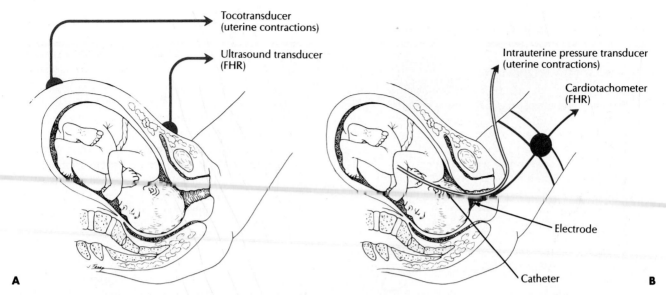

FIGURE 14-1 Intrauterine pressure monitors. **A,** External noninvasive fetal monitoring with tocotransducer and ultrasound transducer, with ultrasound transducer placed below umbilicus and tocotransducer placed on uterine fundus. **B,** Internal fetal monitoring with intrauterine catheter and spiral electrode in place (membranes ruptured and cervix dilated). (From Bobak IM, Jensen MD: *Maternity and gynecologic care,* ed 5, St Louis, 1993, Mosby.)

uterine contractions on the lower tracing of the graph paper. The intrauterine baseline pressure, or **resting tonus,** is read where the pen traces between contractions. Normal resting tonus varies with the stage of labor; it is less than 5 mm Hg in the latent stage, less than 12 mm Hg in the active stage, and less than 20 mm Hg in the second stage of labor. The duration and intensity of the contractions need to be assessed (Figure 14-2). Internal monitoring of the client facilitates the most accurate assessment of all three factors. The frequency of contractions (time from the beginning of one until the beginning of the next) and the duration of each (time from the beginning to the end of any one contraction) can be assessed through external monitoring. The intensity, or strength of contractions, however,

cannot be accurately assessed by the tocotransducer because it senses only the pressure transmitted from beneath it. This pressure may increase for reasons other than uterine contractions (for example, maternal muscle tension during movement or coughing or fetal movement). Therefore clients in need of accurate intrauterine pressure monitoring will have a transcervical catheter placed.

It is important to remember that the tocotransducer cannot completely replace hands-on assessment. Often a mother states that her contractions are stronger than those seen on the monitor. Although her perceptions may be inaccurate (especially if she is a primipara), they require evaluation. Contractions that seem stronger than what the recording shows should be palpated, as

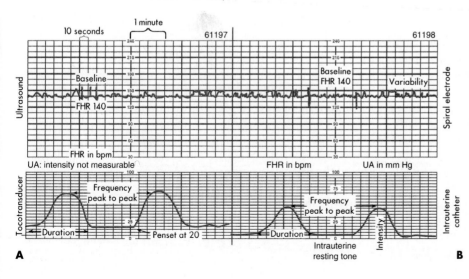

FIGURE 14-2 Display of FHR and uterine activity on monitor strip. **A,** External mode: ultrasound and tocotransducer are the signal sources. **B,** Internal mode: spiral electrode and intrauterine catheter are the signal sources. Other significant information is supplied. (From Tucker SM: *Pocket guide to fetal monitoring,* St Louis, ed 2, 1992, Mosby.)

BOX 14-2 Intrapartum Electronic Fetal Monitoring

Nursing practice competencies

To function independently in the use of intrapartum electronic fetal monitoring, the licensed nurse should be able to:

1. Explain the use of the electronic fetal monitor to the patient and her support person(s)
2. Choose the appropriate electronic fetal monitoring method based on hospital policy or procedure
3. Apply external transducers and adjust the electronic fetal monitor accordingly
4. Describe the limitations of information produced by external transducers
5. Prepare the patient, set up equipment, and complete connections for fetal electrode and intrauterine pressure catheter
6. Calibrate the monitor for the use of the intrauterine pressure catheter
7. Identify artifacts and technically inadequate tracings and take appropriate corrective action
8. Obtain and maintain an adequate fetal heart rate and uterine contraction tracing
9. Interpret uterine contraction frequency, duration, strength, and baseline resting tone as appropriate based on monitoring method, and determine if abnormal findings are present
10. Identify baseline fetal heart rate, baseline variability, and the presence of periodic changes and determine if findings are reassuring or nonreassuring
11. Implement appropriate nursing intervention based on electronic fetal monitor findings
12. Identify the clinical situations based on electronic fetal monitor findings in which immediate physician notification is appropriate
13. Communicate the content of electronic fetal monitoring data, its interpretation, and resulting nursing intervention in written and verbal form in an appropriate and timely manner
14. Document appropriate entries on the electronic fetal monitoring strip chart and patient record
15. Demonstrate appropriate maintenance of electronic fetal monitoring equipment

From NAACOG: *Electronic fetal monitoring: nursing practice competencies and educational guidelines*, 1986, Washington, DC, The Association.

should those accompanying a labor pattern that does not seem to correlate well with the tracing.

The American College of Obstetricians and Gynecologists (ACOG) and NAACOG (AWHONN) have published a joint statement describing practice competencies for nurses involved in intrapartum electronic fetal monitoring (Box 14-2). To achieve competency in fetal-maternal monitoring requires that a nurse seek continuing education.

Fetal Tracings
PLACENTAL FUNCTIONS

The placenta functions for the fetal lungs (respiratory functions) and kidneys and gastrointestinal tract (nutritional and renal functions) and provides an interface between fetal and maternal circulations. Placental nutritional functions have been evaluated throughout pregnancy by serial examination of fetal growth, either clinically or through ultrasonic assessment. Placental renal (excretory) functions can be seen indirectly by the volume of amniotic fluid and by the fact that waste products are carried to the maternal circulation for excretion. Placental respiratory functions are evaluated through electronic fetal heart rate monitoring. Several factors can affect placental function and therefore fetal oxygenation.

Mild fetal asphyxia accompanies normal labor because of the effect of uterine contractions. This is commonly referred to as the *stress of labor*, with the fetal heart rate referred to as the *fetal response*. The healthy fetus with a functioning placenta copes well; in fact this mild asphyxia is one factor that stimulates the neonate's first breath (see Chapter 18).

Disturbances in fetal/placental circulation can affect the fetal central nervous system and myocardium. The heart in both the fetus and the adult is controlled by the interaction of the sympathetic and parasympathetic nervous systems. Several situations that occur during intrauterine life cause characteristic changes in fetal heart rates.

Causes of Functional Changes

Insufficient uterine blood flow or **uteroplacental insufficiency (UPI)** may be caused by maternal hypotension, pathologic conditions of the uterine arteries, or hypertonic labor patterns. A common and easily correctable reason for UPI is compression by the heavy uterus of the maternal great vessels (aorta and vena cava). This is why the supine position is not recommended during pregnancy. Especially during labor, when there are normal periodic interruptions in placental circulation with uterine contractions, this position must be avoided.

Changes in placental function also may be caused by viral disease, hypertension with calcification of maternal vessels in the placenta, which can lead to abruptio placentae, placenta previa, or maternal diabetes mellitus.

Interruptions in umbilical blood flow may result from reduced flow because of compression of the umbilical cord caught between the fetus and uterine wall or around a fetal part or because of a short cord or a knot in the cord. As the infant descends through the pelvic canal, the cord tightens and blood flow is restricted. Variable decelerations indicate **cord compression (CC)**.

METHODS

Intrapartum monitoring may be performed externally (indirectly) or internally (directly). As in all maternal-fetal monitoring, a fetal heart rate tracing and a maternal tracing are recorded as the pattern of uterine contractions.

Tracing Fetal Responses to Labor

Fetal tracings are obtained by two methods: Doppler ultrasound and **fetal electrocardiography.** (Doppler monitoring is discussed in Chapter 11.)

Doppler ultrasound. Doppler ultrasound (external) monitoring requires the use of an ultrasonic transducer applied to the maternal abdomen and held in place with an elastic belt or tape. The transducer is placed over the area yielding the clearest fetal heart sounds. Figure 14-3 illustrates the various points at which to auscultate the fetal heart. These points vary with fetal position.

Because the thin layer of air between the transducer and the maternal abdomen hinders the transmission of sound waves, ultrasound jelly is placed on the transducer before it is positioned. The transducer emits high-frequency sound waves, which strike fetal cardiac valves and then bounce back to the transducer at frequencies that vary with the movement of the valves.

The signals are interpreted by the transducer and changed into an audible sound that varies with the part of the fetal circulation struck by the ultrasound beam. Monitoring of cardiac valve activity produces a sharper, clearer sound, whereas umbilical, placental, or fetal aortic flow produces a softer "whoosh." If the beam of ultrasound misses the valves but strikes the apex of the heart, umbilical cord, or aortic blood flow, it may still be possible to record the fetal heart rate.

The monitor also analyzes the *intervals between cardiac cycles* and interprets each interval in relation to a full minute of time, yielding a digital readout of a rate that will change from **beat to beat.** A written tracing is made of the trend of fetal heart rate changes and this **beat-to-beat variability.**

Direct fetal electrocardiography. To obtain a direct fetal electrocardiogram (FECG) by internal monitoring, the cervix must be dilated at least 3 cm and membranes ruptured. An internal fetal electrode (IFE) is a thin, spiral needle that will be attached in the subcutaneous tissue of the presenting part (Figure 14-4). A grounding circuit is attached to a small metal leg plate to which electrocardiographic gel is applied before placement on the mother's thigh. In this way a direct tracing of the fetal cardiac cycle may be recorded without interference from maternal or fetal movement. The FECG is valid for recording beat-to-beat variability and is used when impending fetal distress requires a more accurate readout than that obtained by ultrasound.

INTERPRETING FETAL TRACINGS

The nurse should develop a system of interpretation that provides a comfortable approach, for example, starting with observation of the fetal heart tracing and then interpreting the maternal tracing before putting the two together. The monitor pen records the fetal heart

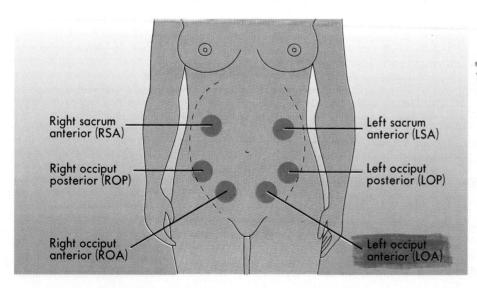

Right sacrum anterior (RSA)

Left sacrum anterior (LSA)

Right occiput posterior (ROP)

Left occiput posterior (LOP)

Right occiput anterior (ROA)

Left occiput anterior (LOA)

FIGURE 14-3 Position at which fetal heart tones are best heard varies with fetal position. The nurse should try to listen over the fetus' back. (From Hamilton PM: *Basic maternity nursing,* ed 6, St Louis, 1989, Mosby.)

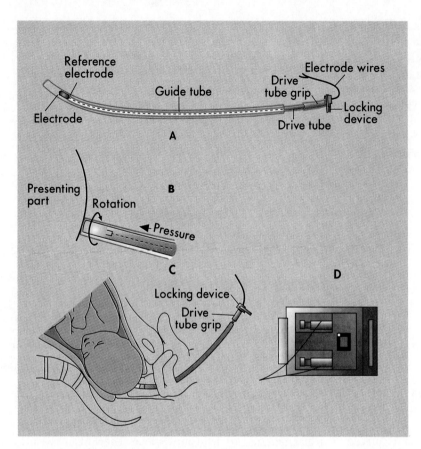

FIGURE 14-4 Fetal heart rate monitor. **A** to **C,** Spiral electrode used for internal fetal heart rate monitoring. **D,** Attached to leg plate. (Courtesy Corometrics Medical Systems, Inc.)

rate on the upper tracing of the graph paper. Note the markings on the tracing paper in Figure 14-2.

Baseline Rate

The nurse looks first at the fetal tracing when there are no uterine contractions. These are called *baseline changes.* The *baseline fetal heart rate* is the average rate during 10 minutes of monitoring (Figure 14-5). This

average rate decreases with increasing gestational age because of maturation of the parasympathetic nervous system. Thus one would expect a higher baseline rate for a premature infant than for a full-term infant.

As discussed earlier, the normal fetal heart beats somewhere in a range of 120 to 160 beats/min. Each fetus has its own baseline rate, as can be seen when there is a twin pregnancy. The normal rate may change during labor in response to stress and adverse factors (Box 14-3). Figure 14-6 illustrates fetal **tachycardia** and **bradycardia.** Table 14-1 lists reasons for baseline rate changes.

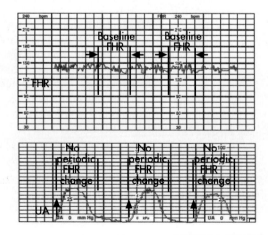

FIGURE 14-5 Baseline FHR is identified between uterine contractions. (From Tucker SM: *Pocket guide to fetal monitoring,* ed 2, St Louis, 1992, Mosby.)

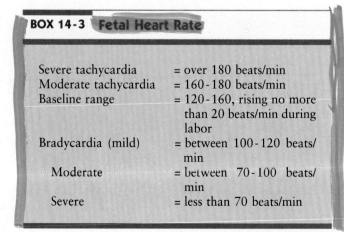

BOX 14-3	Fetal Heart Rate
Severe tachycardia	= over 180 beats/min
Moderate tachycardia	= 160-180 beats/min
Baseline range	= 120-160, rising no more than 20 beats/min during labor
Bradycardia (mild)	= between 100-120 beats/min
Moderate	= between 70-100 beats/min
Severe	= less than 70 beats/min

Fetal Tachycardia   Fetal Bradycardia

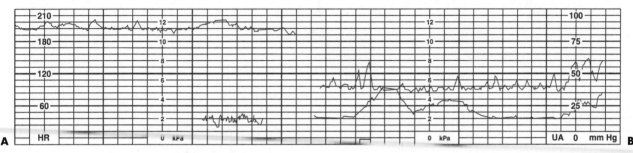

FIGURE 14-6 A, Fetal tachycardia. B, Fetal bradycardia. (From Fields LM, Haire MF, Troiano NH: *Current concepts in fetal monitoring,* Pleasantville, NY, 1987, PPG Biomedical Systems, Inc.)

Bradycardia. If the umbilical cord is occluded or the placenta is compressed during uterine contractions, fetal baroreceptors react to the increase in fetal arterial blood pressure and cause fetal bradycardia. Increased intracranial pressure (which may develop late in labor), interruption of blood supply, or direct pressure to branches of the vagus nerve also can cause bradycardia. Asphyxia and acidosis are other causes of bradycardia (Figure 14-6).

Prolonged bradycardia is associated with acidosis, which decreases responsiveness to resuscitative measures. Infants depressed from analgesic or anesthetic medications that have crossed the placental barrier tend to have lower cord blood–oxygen levels, to be more acidotic, and to respond more slowly or need resuscitation. The choice of medications and the timing and dosage are therefore extremely important (see Chapter 16).

Tachycardia. The cause of tachycardia may be sympathetic stimulation related to breathing movements or pressure applied to fetal parts other than the head, mild fetal asphyxia, maternal drug use, intrauterine infection, maternal temperature elevations, and fetal auditory stimulation (see Figure 14-6). A rising baseline during labor signals concern because an elevation of baseline of more than 20 beats/min indicates *beginning tachycardia* even though the actual number may be in the normal range. Often, for instance, this mild tachycardia begins before signs of elevated maternal temperature.

Test Yourself

• Compare fetal tachycardia and bradycardia for the following:
  Rate limits
  Etiologic factors
  Clinical significance
• Describe a reassuring fetal heart pattern.

Beat-to-Beat Variability

The interaction between sympathetic and parasympathetic stimulation causes quickening and slowing of the fetal heart rate. This change can occur from one beat to the next, causing **beat-to-beat variability.** These changes indicate fetal well-being. The *baseline variability* is the irregularity of the entire fetal heart rate tracing. It is important to look for baseline changes in rate or variability that have occurred during 10 minutes of tracing.

Baseline variability. The baseline variability may be short or long term; however the changes are interdependent and therefore should be considered together. *Short-term variability* is seen as the monitor pen records the intervals between one heartbeat and the next, which usually varies from two to three beats per minute; it gives the monitor tracing small spikes.

Long-term variability is seen as the monitor pen records wavelike fluctuations in fetal heart rate that contain the short-term spikes. These rhythmic changes do not occur from one beat to the next but instead occur from two to six times per minute. Variations in variability are described as follows:

Range*	Assessment
0-2	No variability
3-5	Minimal variability
6-10	Average variability
11-25	Moderate variability
>25	Marked variability

*In beats/min.

A comparison of variabilities is shown in Figure 14-7.

It is difficult to assess variability during Doppler ultrasound (external monitoring) because of **artifact** (interference with transmission or reception of the signal). Therefore loss of variability during external tracing is especially significant.

Sinusoidal patterns. **Sinusoidal patterns** have a snake-like appearance, with alternating small accelerations

TABLE 14-1   Baseline Fetal Heart Rate Changes

CAUSES	RATIONALE
TACHYCARDIA	
Fetal	
Prematurity	Immaturity of the parasympathetic nervous system
Infection	Increased fetal stress
Arrhythmias	Disturbed cardiac innervation
Hypoxia (mild or chronic)	Sympathetic stimulation
Anemia	Sympathetic stimulation
Hyperactivity	Reactivity of cardiac control center
Maternal	
Fever	Increased maternal metabolic rate and fetal oxygen need
Anxiety	Placental transfer of maternal catecholamines
Medications	Beta$_2$-sympathomimetics (ritodrine, terbutaline) stimulating fetal beta$_2$-receptors
	Parasympatholytics (atropine, scopolamine) inhibiting vagal response
Hypothyroidism	Placental transfer of thyroid-stimulating hormone, which simulates fetal thyroid function
BRADYCARDIA	
Fetal	
Acute hypoxia	Depression of cardiac center
Congenital heart block	Rhythm disturbance
Beta-blocking drugs (used in local and regional anesthesia or propranolol)	Blocks beta-receptors
DECREASED VARIABILITY	
Fetal	
Prematurity (less than 32 weeks)	Immaturity of parasympathetic response
Congenital anomalies	Central nervous system malformation
Fetal sleep	Normal response for 15-20 min
Hypoxia and acidosis	Depression of cardiac control center
Tachycardia	More sympathetic than parasympathetic stimulation, therefore less "flip-flop" between the two
Maternal	
Drugs: magnesium sulfate (MgSO$_4$)	Depressed central nervous system
(Atropine, phenothiazines)	Blocked parasympathetic response, which contributes to variability
INCREASED VARIABILITY	
Fetal	
Mild hypoxia with normal pH	Increased fetal adrenergic response

and decelerations centering around the baseline. There may be little or no fetal movement, and short-term variability is decreased. This pattern frequently is seen in severely anemic or asphyxiated fetuses and is thought to be the direct result of damage to the cardiac control center. This pattern also may be caused by a maternal dose of alphaprodine (Nisentil). The fetus with a sinusoidal heart rate pattern needs immediate attention.

Test Yourself

• The interaction between the parasympathetic and sympathetic nervous systems causes the fetal heart rate to slow and quicken. This is reflected in the monitor strip as _____ .

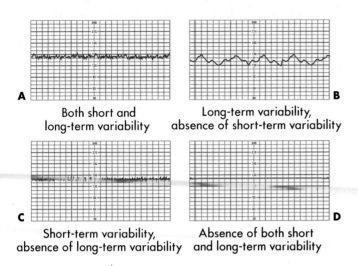

A — Both short and long-term variability

B — Long-term variability, absence of short-term variability

C — Short-term variability, absence of long-term variability

D — Absence of both short and long-term variability

FIGURE 14-7 *A–D,* Variations in short- and long-term variability. (Modified from Tucker SM: *Pocket guide to fetal monitoring,* ed 2, St Louis, 1992, Mosby.)

Periodic Changes

Next, **periodic heart rate** changes in the fetus are examined. These are short-term changes, lasting from a few seconds up to 10 minutes, usually occurring *with* uterine contractions or fetal movement. During these periods, fetal heart rates provide data to assess status, because with additional stress of contractions or movement, heart rates may show reassuring or **nonreassuring signs.**

Accelerations. Fetal heart rate accelerations usually are associated with fetal movement. These are transient elevations that may rise 5 to 15 beats/min from the baseline, stay elevated for several seconds to minutes, and then return to the baseline rate. Accelerations indicate that the cardiac control center in the medulla is functional; the rise in heart rate seen with fetal movement is similar to a rise after physical activity. Accelerations with fetal activity may be less marked in a premature fetus. The presence of accelerations with fetal movement is a *reassuring* sign and the basis of the nonstress test (NST) (see Figure 11-12, *A*).

Decelerations. Fetal heart rate decelerations may indicate fetal distress or may not be significant. **Decelerations** are classified (Hon and Quilligan, 1967) as early, late, and variable, or types I, II, and III. The differences in the three are related to their *shape* and *timing* in relation to uterine contractions (Figure 14-8).

Early decelerations. Early decelerations (type I) result from a *vagal response to head compression,* often after rupture of membranes or during the second stage of labor. They have a smooth, U-shaped form and *begin and end when the contraction begins and ends.* The lowest point of the deceleration occurs at the highest point of intensity of the contraction. For this reason, they are said to "mirror" contraction shape (Fig. 14-8, *A*). Almost always during early decelerations, the fetal

heart rate is within the normal range of 120 to 160 beats/min. These decelerations do not indicate fetal distress; in fact, the fetus is showing healthy reactivity to head compression. These decelerations are seen most commonly during advanced labor. When fetal distress occurs, fetal heart decelerations will be *late* in relation to the contraction, a result of reduced uteroplacental perfusion (Figure 14-8, *B*). Or there may be variable decelerations caused by cord compression, which inhibits flow to the fetal system (Figure 14-8, *C*). (These changes are discussed in the section on fetal distress.)

Fetal Distress

The fetus sends a signal that its environment is lacking nutrients or oxygen; this reaction is **fetal distress.** Fetal distress may be *chronic,* occurring during the course of pregnancy, or become *acute,* usually occurring during labor but also when the woman is deprived of oxygen (with poorly administered anesthesia or a bleeding complication). The classic description of a distressed fetus included abnormalities of the heart rate and meconium in the amniotic fluid. These signs are now recognized as later signs of deepening distress. Fetal monitoring capabilities and fetal blood sampling have made early diagnosis more precise.

The stresses of labor and delivery may leave the infant poorly equipped for the major adjustments that must be made. The following risk factors require close follow-up:

1. Rupture of membranes more than 12 to 24 hours before birth or maternal hyperthermia
2. Anything that might reduce maternal blood pressure and therefore diminish blood supply to the placental circulation, including a drug reaction, reaction to conduction anesthesia, supine hypotension, or hemorrhage

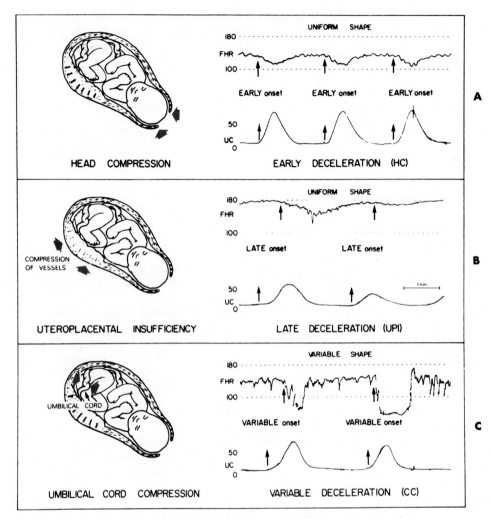

FIGURE 14-8 Mechanisms of fetal heart rate patterns. **A,** Head compression *(HC),* usually observed only during transition and second stage. **B,** *UPI,* present when blood flow to fetus is compromised. **C,** *CC,* returning to normal heart rate only when pressure is relieved. (From Hon EP: *An introduction to fetal heart monitoring,* Hartford, Conn, 1968, Harty Press.)

3. Any indication of hypertonic or ineffective contractions
4. Any fetal response outside of normal ranges
5. Occlusion of the cord by any cause

FETAL RESPONSES TO HYPOXIA

Fetal distress is a sign of increasingly poor tolerance to the stress of labor. This stress is imposed by contractions, during which the blood flow to the placenta is basically stopped. If there is sufficient reserve in the fetus, the 60- to 90-second period without "new oxygen" is not harmful and the fetus recovers quickly in the rest period when oxygen freely circulates to the maternal-fetal placental transfer points (Figure 14-9).

Remember, good fetal oxygenation is shown by a fetal heart rate between 120 and 160 beats/min and not more than 20 points change in baseline rate during labor, while maintaining good beat-to-beat variability. During any contraction the fetus will demonstrate the ability to maintain its normal heart rate. When distress occurs, the heart rate will change in the following ways. Decelerations occur from baseline: these may be brief, with a slow recovery, or they may persist in bradycardia. Loss of normal long- and short-term variability in heart rate (a flat rate) often is accompanied by increasing tachycardia. Without intervention the fetus in distress will become increasingly acidotic and when born may be slow to recover, may be injured by asphyxia, or may die.

The Meaning of Meconium

In utero meconium passage is seen only after 34 weeks of gestation and therefore is considered a maturational sign. Although it often accompanies fetal hypoxia, term infants may pass meconium without having been asphyxiated. A baby in breech position usually passes meconium during the descent phase. Hypoxic stress may cause the diving reflex, with shunting of blood away from the gastrointestinal tract and toward vital organs such as the brain and heart. Dilation of the anal sphincter and peristalsis follows.

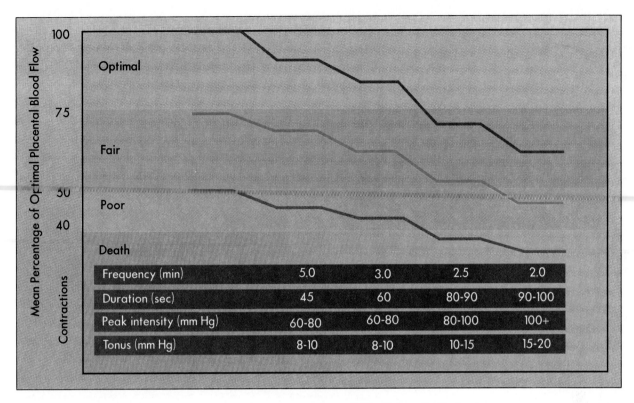

FIGURE 14-9 Effect of myometrial contractions on mean placental blood flow (PBF). As the duration and frequency of contractions increase, PBF progressively decreases. Even mild contractions may cause fetal distress or death when PBF is poor. (After Spencer, 1989.)

About 11% to 22% of all babies have meconium in the amniotic fluid at birth (Weitzner et al, 1990). Not all of these infants will be distressed at birth. Meconium is a *sign, not a cause,* of fetal distress. The visually black feces (Figure 19-13) are full of bilirubin, which when diluted have a strong yellow-green color. The concentration of meconium is directly related to the volume of amniotic fluid. Assessment of the characteristics of meconium-stained fluid is critical because thick meconium is more likely to cause respiratory problems in the newborn. The readings are subjective unless a "meconium crit" is performed (Weitzner et al, 1990). Amniotic fluid is collected and spun in a centrifuge, and readings are obtained as for hematocrit readings.

    <4 g/dl ml = Thin: dilute brownish fluid

    4-9 g/dl ml = Moderate: yellowish brown fluid, not clear

    >9 g/dl ml = Thick: pea-soup consistency

If an asphyxiated fetus takes deep gasping breaths before birth, stimulated by hypoxia, the meconium-stained fluid can be aspirated into the lower portion of the lung and, if it is thick, can partly obstruct airways.

Meconium aspiration syndrome (MAS) may lead to further cardiorespiratory problems (see Chapter 28).

The Meaning of Asphyxia

Asphyxia is the metabolic state of hypoxia, hypercapnia, and acidosis. The cycle of events leading to fetal asphyxia begins with the lack of oxygen (O_2) and excess build-up of carbon dioxide (CO_2). This may occur because the balance of production and elimination of CO_2 is upset. CO_2 must be released across the placenta to the mother and oxygen taken up: the O_2 and CO_2 *gradient* between mother and fetus is greatly affected by alterations in placental perfusion, exchange across the placenta, or maternal hypoxemia. Respiratory acidosis begins first as CO_2 increases. As oxygen levels fall, further energy production converts from aerobic to anaerobic paths, causing lactic acid to accumulate. The result is a mixed respiratory and metabolic acidosis. (Study Figure 14-10 to see how at a certain point in the sequence, lactic acid begins rising rapidly, with pH dropping quickly. See Chapter 28 for resuscitation of the asphyxiated infant. Normal and low pH levels are listed in Box 14-4.) Further management of labor varies with the progress of labor and other fetal or maternal conditions. Operative delivery will be arranged quickly to prevent further damage in an asphyxiated infant.

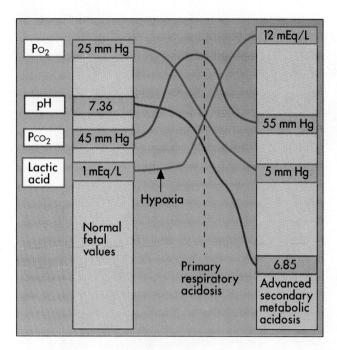

FIGURE 14-10 A sample pattern of fetal blood gases, pH, and lactic acid with fetal distress caused by hypoxia. (After Spencer, 1989.)

BOX 14-4   Fetal pH Range

Normal: more than 7.25 (mild asphyxia normally accompanies labor)
Borderline: 7.20-7.25
Severe acidosis: 7.19 and below
Potential death: 7.00 and below

Table 14-2 shows changes in umbilical artery and the resultant acidosis scores associated with birth Apgar scores. Whenever a fetus is distressed, the physician is obligated to check pH from the fetal scalp and make a decision regarding method of birth. A pH value must be obtained from the cord blood as well.

Cord pH values should be obtained on every newborn who has been subjected to extra labor stress and had any difficulty maintaining its normal heart rate, on every baby of a high-risk pregnancy, and every infant with an Apgar score below 7 at 1 minute. Blood should be obtained from the umbilical artery, which is more

TABLE 14-2   Umbilical Artery pH Compared with Apgar Score

	APGAR SCORE			UMBILICAL ACIDITY SCORE		
	CLIN. SCORE	CLINICAL STATE		ACIDITY-SCORE (UA)	˙UA PH ACT	CLINICAL CHARACTERIZATION
Normal	10	optimal		10	>7.35	optimal
	9		vigorous	9	7.30–7.34	acidity
	8	still normal		8	7.25–7.29	still normal
	7			7	7.20–7.24	
Pathologic	6	slightly		6	7.15–7.19	slight
	5			5	7.10–7.14	
	4	moderately	depressed	4	7.05–7.09	moderate
	3			3	7.00–7.04	acidosis
	2			2	6.90–6.99	
	1	severely		1	6.80–6.89	severe
	0			0	<6.80	

Ua, Umbilical artery. From Spencer JAD, editor: *Fetal monitoring*, Philadelphia, 1989, FA Davis.

difficult to puncture because arteries are smaller, but the blood here gives a truer picture of the newborn's status. The cord arterial pH is 0.05 to 0.07 below that of the umbilical vein pH.

Lactate levels. Lactate is a result of anaerobic metabolism; first CO_2 rises, then O_2 levels fall. Lactate is thought to build up after CO_2 levels rise and to be more damaging. The pH levels are the result of combined elevated lactate and hypercapnia (Persson et al, 1992). A new dry strip test similar to Dextrostix has been developed to assess fetal or cord blood lactate levels. Testing lactate levels may be used along with the pH to decide on the depth of the asphyxia in the fetus or newborn.

Test Yourself

- What is the lower limit for normal fetal blood pH?
- Describe how poor placental perfusion can cause fetal acidosis.

Fetal Scalp Blood Sampling (Procedure 14-1)

Another technique for diagnosis of fetal distress was needed when it was found that sometimes with variable or late decelerations the fetus was indeed not acidotic. Analysis of fetal blood for pH reveals whether the fetus is acidotic. Blood can be obtained by making a small puncture in the fetal scalp (or breech). The amniotic membranes must already be ruptured and the cervix partially dilated. Indications for fetal blood pH measurements are as follows:

1. Severe late or variable decelerations with poor return to baseline
2. Poor beat-to-beat variability, bradycardia, or tachycardia
3. Thick meconium with oligohydramnios

UTEROPLACENTAL INSUFFICIENCY

Late decelerations (type II) are deceptively subtle. The form is similar to that of the early decelerations: smooth and U-shaped. However, *the timing is different.* A late deceleration starts when the contraction is at its height, peaks when the contraction is almost over, and does not return to baseline until well after the contraction has ended. It resolves *late.* Again, the fetal heart rate most often stays within the normal range. Late decelerations are caused by *UPI* (see Figure 14-7, *B*), which may occur in the following instances:

1. Complicated pregnancies in which placental abnormalities such as infarctions or calcifications are present

2. Labor patterns with intense contractions occurring less than 2 minutes apart
3. Hypertonic contractions lasting more than 90 seconds in active labor and 120 seconds during the transition phase
4. Maternal hypotension from vena cava syndrome
5. Epidural or general anesthesia that decreases blood pressure and uteroplacental perfusion

It is common to see late decelerations, a rising baseline rate, and decreased baseline variability together because hypoxia depresses the cardiac control center in the medulla. The presence of late decelerations is always *ominous* and necessitates immediate investigation about the cause and appropriate interventions to increase fetal oxygenation.

Interventions for Late Decelerations

When signs of distress related to uteroplacental insufficiency appear, assessment must reveal the possible causes. Because blood supply may be affected on the maternal or fetal side, the examiner looks first for the most common causes:

- Maternal hypotension, with or without low blood volume, which may be caused by
  —Vena caval compression
  —Dilation of lower extremity vessels after epidural or spinal anesthesia
  —Bleeding, hidden or overt, that depletes blood volume
- Hypertonic uterine contractions from excessive response to oxytocin or naturally hypertonic contractions in later labor
- Poor placental perfusion related to placental abnormality such as preeclampsia, hypertension, diabetes, premature separation of placenta, or inadequate placental size that causes intrauterine growth retardation (IUGR) or birth defects

On the basis of the signs, interventions must be directed to correct causes, beginning with the least complicated interventions and observing responses of the fetal heart.

1. Change position in bed: vena caval compression by the heavy uterus can occur in lithotomy, supine, semi-Fowler's, and a slight right or left lateral tilt. Turn her completely to the left or right side. Sometimes sitting up or getting on hands and knees can be helpful.
2. Increase main-line Ringer's lactate solution if the problem could be a low blood volume related to anesthesia or bleeding. Be sure to note exactly when and how much fluid is given during this period.
3. At the same time, observe the monitor and the character of the contractions. Are they hypertonic for the stage of labor? Is oxytocin infusing in a

PROCEDURE 14-1 Fetal Scalp Blood Sampling

The woman must be in position so that the physician can visualize the fetal part through the cervix. Care must be taken to avoid mixing maternal blood or air with the specimen because it will influence the results (Figure 14-11). After the procedure, careful observation of the amount of vaginal bleeding (source may be fetal scalp) will be important.

1. Explain reasons for procedure.
2. Position: lithotomy position is very uncomfortable and may contribute to vena caval compression, so left-lying position also may be used.
3. Maintain fetal monitor record during procedure.

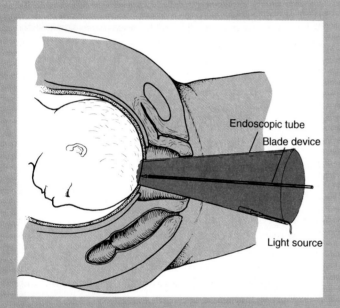

FIGURE 14-11 Fetal blood sampling. (From Tucker SM: *Pocket guide to fetal monitoring,* ed 2, St Louis, 1992, Mosby.)

4. Sterile kit contains:
   a. Long heparinized capillary tubes
   b. Conical endoscope
   c. Long cotton swabs with bactericidal solution
   d. Long dry cotton swabs
   e. Silicone ointment or spray
   f. Long plastic rod with small blade to nick scalp
5. Provide a light source if not with kit, plus the following:
   a. Sterile gloves
   b. Small basin with ice if blood tubes must be transported to a laboratory
6. Physician inserts endoscope into vagina, visualizes fetal scalp or breech through a dilated cervix, washes with solution, and sprays on or applies silicone to facilitate forming a bubble of blood. Small cut in the scalp is made and blood collected in heparinized tubes. The puncture site is cleansed, and pressure is applied to stop bleeding (scalp is highly vascular).
7. Endoscope is removed and woman positioned comfortably while attendant obtains pH reading (plus $Paco_2$ and Pao_2 if required).
8. Maternal blood may also be sent to laboratory to determine if a base deficit has occurred.

Risks include the following:

1. Breaks in fetal skin integrity, especially if the woman has an infection or sexually transmitted disease. Hepatitis or HIV transfer may be promoted (Ross and Dickason, 1992).
2. Scalp bleeding, unless pressure is applied carefully to the scalp nick.
3. Procedure may need to be repeated as labor progresses. This scalp injury needs afterbirth assessment and care.

• • •

OPTIONAL ACTIVITY: Write a sample nursing note correctly documenting the performance of this procedure.

secondary line? If contractions are strong and oxytocin is infusing, turn off the intravenous (IV) pump to stop the flow.

4. Begin, according to protocol, oxygen by mask set at 8 to 10 L/min. Women are mouth breathers during labor; thus nasal oxygen usually is not used. (Some physicians do not use oxygen freely, believing that it does not change the uptake significantly.)

5. Check maternal blood pressure and pulse to correlate with recent activities such as regional anesthesia and examinations.

6. Notify the physician or midwife of the incident and results of interventions. Document time of notification and response on chart and monitor strip. If late decelerations do not improve as a result of interventions, the physician or midwife must check fetal pH levels and plans may begin for cesarean "rescue" operation.

VARIABLE DECELERATIONS: CORD COMPRESSION

Variable decelerations (type III) look different from early and late decelerations and often look different

Clinical Decision

Karen T. has been in labor for 4 hours. The cervical dilation is now 6 cm and the following is seen on the fetal monitoring strip.

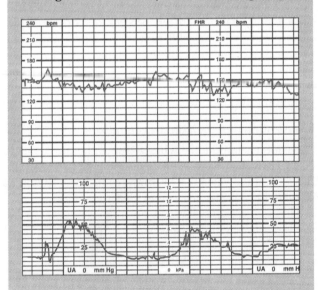

What would you do next?

from each other. The fetal heart rate decreases sharply, stays down for a *variable* number of seconds, and then usually returns to baseline as sharply as it descended (Figure 14-7, C).

Occlusion of the umbilical cord first causes the heart rate to increase; the fetus with normal placental oxygen reserve compensates with tachycardia. As the occlusion progresses, it interrupts blood flow through the umbilical arteries, causing an increase in peripheral resistance. Stimulation of fetal carotid sinus and aortic arch baroreceptors follows; parasympathetic fibers then cause the fetal heart rate to decrease.

Although an occasional variable deceleration is benign, repetitive decelerations are serious and indicate a fetus who may become increasingly hypoxic and acidotic. A *late component* may start to appear, during which variable decelerations fail to return to baseline until after the contraction has ended. There may be loss of baseline variability as the fetal cardiac control center is depressed further. The rule of 60's is used to determine ominous cord compression (Box 14-5).

Second-Stage Variables

Variables often are seen toward the end of labor after rupture of membranes, when cord compression accompanies fetal descent and expulsion. Then they are called **end-stage variables**. About 90% of labor patterns show variable decelerations in the second stage. Some are significant; most are not. If, however, variables have begun in the first stage, they may become progressively worse. (Study Figure 14-12 to note the various patterns seen in the second stage of labor when head compression plus descent may be aggravated by the expulsive pushing efforts of the mother.)

Types 0 to 1 are considered normal because the baseline is maintained between contractions.
Type 2 shows progressive bradycardia added to cord compression and is an ominous sign.
Type 3 is ominous because the peaks you see are really accelerations above a bradycardic baseline; the infant will enter a state of severe acidosis rapidly.
Type 4 shows a normal heart rate, which is followed by a rapidly falling bradycardia and loss of beat-to-beat variability, and is very serious.

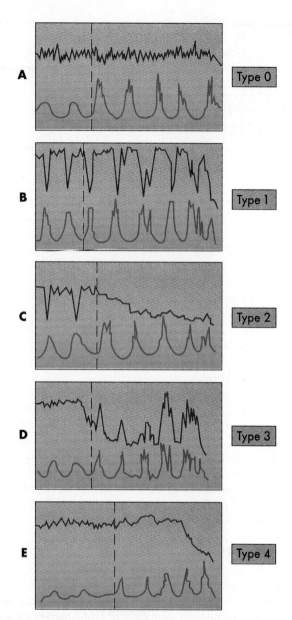

FIGURE 14-12 Melchior classification of second stage FHR. The recording is at the rate of 1 cm to 1 min. **A**, Type 0: Normocardia—no decelerations. **B**, Type 1: Normocardia between contractions—presence of decelerations. **C**, Type 2: progressive bradycardia, with or without decelerations. **D**, Type 3: Bradycardia and accelerations. **E**, Type 4: Normocardia followed by bradycardia (sudden or progressive). (After Melchior, 1976. From Spencer JAD, editor: *Fetal Monitoring*, Philadelphia, 1989, FA Davis.)

Causes

Variable decelerations are a result of compression of the umbilical cord and may be caused by a number of precipitating events.

1. Cord is caught between fetus and uterine wall.
2. Cord around fetal neck, arm, shoulder, or other part is being pulled tightly as fetus descends in labor (**nuchal cord**).

3. There is a true knot in the cord that is tightened during labor.
4. Occult (hidden) or frank (obvious) **prolapse** of the cord occurs through the cervix.
5. There is pressure on cord because of insufficient amniotic fluid (oligohydramnios).
6. Fetus is growth retarded and has a deficient amount of Wharton's jelly to cushion the cord.

Long or short cord. Knots or loops in the cord occur if the cord is excessively long (>100 cm). During labor these knots may be pulled tighter or if looped around the neck (nuchal cord), the cord becomes stretched and narrowed as the fetus goes through descent.

A short cord (<32 cm) also is likely to show signs of traction, with narrowed umbilical vessels during descent. *End-stage variables* result from these types of changes, as well as from pressure against all parts of the cord during the second stage. Remember, if *recovery to baseline* occurs after the contraction, the fetus is not considered in jeopardy with variable decelerations. If, however, the patterns resemble that in Figure 14-12, *C-E*, or are accompanied by a late component or continuing bradycardia with no recovery and poor beat-to-beat variability, the fetus requires rescue and intervention must be prompt (Roberts, 1989).

Cord Prolapse

When the cord lies beside the presenting part or below it, the pressure of the head or buttock will pinch off circulation (Figure 14-13, *A*). *Cord prolapse* will result in varying degrees of cord compression (CC) and variable decelerations or in complete loss of heart rate. Complete CC occurs most frequently with premature rupture of membranes when the fetal presenting part is not engaged or when there is a footling or complete breech presentation. Fifteen percent of cord prolapse cases occur at home with rupture of membranes, and these carry a high risk of fetal death. First there is a change in fetal heart rate and a lack of fetal movements. A vaginal inspection might show the bluish shiny cord protruding through the cervix.

Interventions for Variable Decelerations

Prevention is important. When artificial rupture of membranes (AROM) occurs, the fluid should be released very slowly and the vaginal area inspected at once. Monitoring should continue before and after the procedure.

If variable changes begin, position change must be tried first to relieve pressure.

1. Use the lateral Sims position first. Rotate to the other side if no effect is achieved. If the cord is not through the vagina, it may be between the internal os and the head.
2. Then a knee-chest position may help to move the fetus off the cervix. Because this position is diffi-

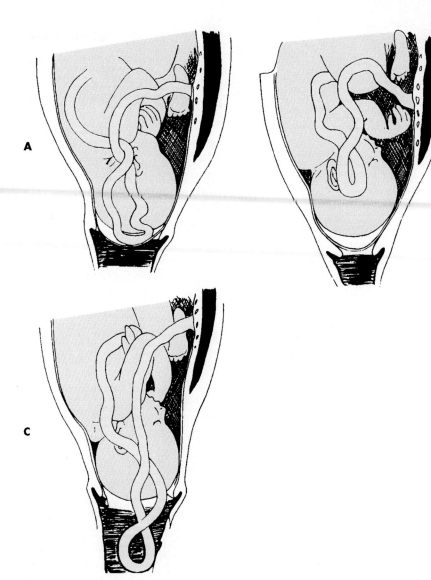

FIGURE 14-13 Prolapse of cord. **A,** Partial (trapped beside presenting part). **B,** Hidden. **C,** Complete, demonstrating cord visible in vagina.

cult to assume during labor, a modified Trende-lenburg position can be tried.

3. If the cord is prolapsed and visible in the vagina, the only recourse is to put on a sterile glove and manually push the presenting part off the cord so that circulation can continue while preparations are made for emergency cesarean delivery.

4. Some units report that inserting a Foley catheter and instilling 500 ml into the bladder while hold-ing the fetal head off the cord will push the fetus up in the uterus and relieve pressure long enough for surgery (Beischer and MacKay, 1986). Of course the surgeon would not use a low incision near the distended bladder.

5. Continue monitoring with FECG clip. (Position may prevent obtaining a contraction pattern.)

6. Use appropriate interventions for late decelera-tions also; administer oxygen by mask and stop oxytocin flow.

If prolapse is not the cause of variable decelerations, a simple position change, as noted in the preceding list, may solve the problem. Should the baseline return to normal and the decelerations improve, no further action may be required. As labor progresses, however, these variables may recur.

Amnioinfusion (Procedure 14-2). When there is less am-niotic fluid than normal, the cord may be compressed (see Chapter 7 for normal volumes). If variable decelerations are not improved by other interventions, **amnio-infusion**—instilling a warmed sterile normal saline solu-tion into the uterine cavity by catheter—can have a ben-eficial effect. In one series it reduced the rate of cesarean deliveries from 22% to 3% in those with distress from variable decelerations (Nagoette et al, 1985). Usually the physician and nurse work together in this procedure.

Preparation for amnioinfusion must be accomplished quickly once the need arises. The woman needs a

PROCEDURE 14-2   Amnioinfusion

- Place client in side-lying position.
- After a vaginal examination, monitoring by FECG is begun if not already established.
- After clearing IV tubing of air with 1000 ml normal saline, run tubing through a blood warmer.
- Attach a connector to the intrauterine pressure probe and clear the air.
- Insert probe gently through cervix into a pocket of amniotic fluid (around and above presenting part) located by use of ultrasound.

- Infuse saline at 15-20 ml/min until the CC decelerations stop; give no more than 800 ml, which takes approximately 1 hour.
- Observe contraction pressure, fetal heart tone, and maternal blood pressure carefully.
- Ultrasound may be used to evaluate fluid volume before and after procedure, or a second intrauterine pressure catheter is inserted to measure pressures.
- Support woman during a tense time, when many tubes and wires are inserted into her vagina.

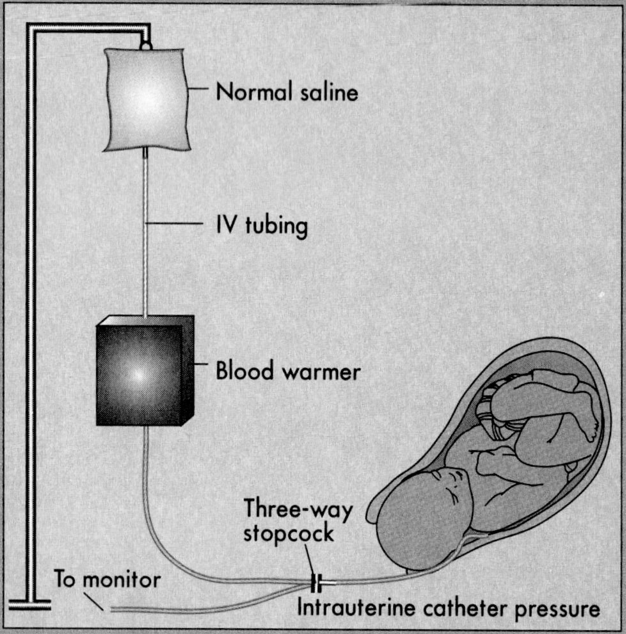

FIGURE 14-14 Amnioinfusion

● ● ●

OPTIONAL ACTIVITY: Write a sample nursing note correctly documenting the performance of this procedure.

careful explanation of the procedure and its objectives. In addition, many units ask the woman to sign an informed consent (Figure 14-14).

The purpose of managing fetal nonreassuring responses at any level is to support placental perfusion to the fetus. Thus, if one pictures the flow directions, the rationale for these corrective interventions will be logical. The procedures, which involve more than one nurse, must be performed rapidly. Therefore it is helpful to think of steps as simultaneous.

The nurse also will be checking the fetal heart rate for improvement. If an internal electrode has not yet been placed, it should be accomplished as soon as possible. At the same time the woman needs explanations about what is occurring and why so that she may cooperate.

> **Test Yourself**
>
> • If you were working alone, list the logical sequence of actions you would choose in response to moderately severe late decelerations.

SUMMARY OF PATTERNS

Reassuring patterns provide information that indicates the adequacy of fetal oxygenation and perfusion. The baseline rate is considered normal between 120 and 160 beats/min. Remember that baseline variability can be truly assessed only during internal monitoring; an average of 6 to 10 beats/min is considered normal. Normal periodic changes include accelerations with fetal movements and early decelerations during the later phases of labor. The nurse's intervention for reassuring patterns is to continue observation.

Questionable patterns signal possible alterations in fetal oxygenation or perfusion. The baseline rate may be near the upper or lower limits of normal. *Mild bradycardia* (100 to 120 beats/min) may be normal if no other problems are present and the baseline heart rate has not changed significantly. *Mild tachycardia* may be related to prematurity, fetal arrhythmias, perinatal infection, chronic or mild fetal hypoxia, maternal or fetal anemia, maternal fever, anxiety or hyperthyroidism, or administration of beta-sympathomimetic or parasympatholytic drugs to the client.

Increased baseline variability (over 25 beats/min) is associated with maternal and fetal movements but may be an early sign of fetal malposition or cephalopelvic disproportion (CPD). Finally, *variable decelerations* may be considered questionable patterns if the fetal heart rate drops no lower than 80 beats/min for less than 30 seconds, variability remains normal, and there is no late component or significant change in baseline rate.

Ominous patterns indicate significant alterations in fetal oxygenation or perfusion; these usually are mixed or show several configurations. *Bradycardia* is especially worrisome when associated with late decelerations, variable decelerations, or loss of variability. *Decreased baseline variability* (less than 3 to 5 beats/min) may be related to maternal drug administration (meperidine and other analgesics, magnesium sulfate), fetal sleep, prematurity, anomalies of the central nervous system, or fetal tachycardia or hypoxia. Decreased variability is always a warning sign if not explained by medications or fetal sleep-wake patterns.

> **Test Yourself**
>
> • Describe three ominous findings on the strip chart.

Nursing Responsibilities during Fetal Monitoring

The nurse is the primary manager of fetal monitoring. Skill in interpretation of patterns and regulating equipment is expected. Hospital units must educate and evaluate the nurse's competency in recognition of borderline and ominous fetal heart rate patterns. Nurses also need to take initiative and seek out continuing education in this area. The rate of lawsuits that involve use or misuse of the fetal monitor reinforces the nurse's need to know the documentation requirements.

DOCUMENTATION TO AVOID LIABILITY

One half of the recent malpractice claims in the United States involved the use or misuse of electronic fetal monitoring (EFM). Cases include failure to monitor in labor and just before birth or failure to respond correctly to the tracing results, especially to perform a cesarean delivery to interrupt fetal distress (Herbst, 1992). Failure to monitor or respond correctly indeed may not have happened, but someone neglected to write down the findings. It should be kept in mind that, according to legal statute, "If it is not written, it was not done." The importance of documentation is heightened because cases may come to court 5 to 10 years later; no one can remember details for so long. Thus nurses must take special care in documenting observations. There is a bedside flow sheet for noting the usual points: vital signs, contraction characteristics, amniotic fluid status, and vaginal examinations and findings about cervix status and station, as well as fetal heart rate and reactivity. Treatments, medications, and anesthesia also are noted in written form in several places. In careful

TABLE 14-3 Correct Documentation for Fetal Strip and Maternal Chart

NURSE/PHYSICIAN ACTIVITY	CLIENT ACTIVITY
Vaginal examinations and result	Change of position
Artificial rupture of membranes	Spontaneous rupture of membranes (SROM)
IV therapy	Bedpan use
Oxytocin rate	Vomiting
Other medication dose/rate	Oral intake
External/internal transducer change	Pushing
Epidural	Vital signs
Oxygen begun/ended	
Procedures	

Identify each strip with name, age, parity, membrane status, cervix status, and station and when started or continued (give strip identification [ID] number).

Clinical Decision

Asha S. is a 32-year-old primigravida in early labor. Your admission assessment reveals that her membranes have been ruptured for 17 hours, cervix is 2 cm dilated and 70% effaced, and contractions are irregular. She has chronic hypertension; admission BP is 170/90. Describe the risk factors for fetal distress and how they may manifest in the fetal heart rate tracing.

recording, most of this information also will be noted on the monitor strip but in an abbreviated fashion. Table 14-3 shows information required on the strip. Legally the strip should be able to stand alone as a record of the fetal response to labor. The nurse already knows that this is true about the client's chart, and the strip is an important part of the chart.

Each unit has a protocol for fetal monitoring management. On newer monitors, automatic entries are printed on the strip and times are printed with each entry. Otherwise, the nurse must remember to include the time for an entry. The bedside chart and the strip need to show evidence of at least one entry every 30 minutes, even if just an initial on the strip of a client who is in an early phase.

If there is *artifact* and a poor FHR signal, that also should be noted. Sometimes it is difficult to obtain an adequate external fetal heart reading for an obese patient. Contraction characteristics, as well as variability and periodic changes, that appear on the strip must be described on the flow sheet. In this legal climate, documentation

is essential to the practice of "defensive nursing." It is also important to list times of physician notification and response. When the physician does not respond promptly, nursing actions should be included. The nurse who notes inadequate physician response or intervention is legally required to report to a superior—a nurse supervisor or attending physician—to obtain satisfactory follow-up. A number of nurses have been involved in lawsuits because they did not follow through in securing adequate help for the fetus in distress.

 ASSESSMENT

The nurse gathers information from the prenatal history and physical assessment that accompanies the family, as well as personal assessment, and determines the following:

1. Whether the client has had prior experience with antepartum or intrapartum fetal monitoring
2. The client's parity and previous fetal losses and whether they were close to term or during labor
3. Whether the couple or woman has attended preparation for childbirth classes
4. Whether there are factors that place this pregnancy at risk (prematurity or postmaturity, intrauterine growth retardation, hypertension, diabetes mellitus, or other chronic conditions) and how they might affect the fetus's ability to withstand the stressors of labor
5. Whether the maternal vital signs are within normal limits
6. Whether the baseline fetal heart rate and variability are within normal range
7. Whether there are any periodic changes in fetal heart rate, including decelerations or accelerations; whether they are associated with maternal medications, fetal movement, or changes in maternal position; and their significance

NURSING DIAGNOSES

Examples of nursing diagnoses include the following:
1. Maternal anxiety related to fetal health or prior experience
2. Altered tissue perfusion in fetal/placental unit related to maternal condition or cord compression

EXPECTED OUTCOMES

1. Couple will be kept informed and will participate in decision making.
2. Fetal injury will be avoided or minimized by prompt interventions.

NURSING INTERVENTIONS

The nurse maintains as natural a birthing setting as possible during intrapartum monitoring. The woman should be encouraged to ask questions and to remain mobile as long as possible. The nurse keeps the family informed of all changes and proposed interventions in as timely a manner as possible and allows them to have input when possible. The mother should not be separated from her support person, even when problems arise, and childbirth techniques should be reinforced.

Nursing interventions should always minimize the potential for fetal hypoxia while maintaining the woman's comfort and sense of control. Simple measures such as avoiding the supine position can prevent fetal distress.

The nurse observes the monitor tracing every 15 to 30 minutes and records findings on the strip chart and the bedside chart. When ominous patterns begin, the nurse tries various interventions and notes response. Differences in opinion about significance of findings may occur among personnel; consultation should be sought. The fetal condition may change quickly, and all staff members must be ready to intervene as needed. When a depressed fetus is to be delivered, persons who are skilled in newborn resuscitation must be present at the birth (see Chapter 28).

EVALUATION

To evaluate outcomes during fetal monitoring the nurse asks questions such as the following.
1. Did the couple participate in decision making? Was anxiety kept to a minimum by information and support?
2. Was fetal perfusion maintained as evidenced by fetal heart rate? Was delivery accomplished before any injury had been sustained?

KEY POINTS

- Monitoring contractions and fetal status during labor is a standard of care in most settings.
- If EFM is not used, auscultation must be performed on the same schedule.
- Nurses have the management responsibility in most settings for application of the monitor, reading and reporting patterns, and documenting findings.
- Adequate placental perfusion underlies a normal tracing. The nurse looks for causes of interrupted flow that results in uteroplacental insufficiency.
- Cord compression is a mechanical problem, and many times relief comes by position or amnioinfu-

sion. Otherwise the infant with severe cord compression must be delivered as quickly as possible.
- Levels of fetal acidity govern rates of recovery in the transition period. Assessment of acidity is the physician or midwife's responsibility.
- In every case the care giver's responsibility is to prevent asphyxia or to rescue the infant if a hypoxic environment is uncorrectable.
- Maintain communication to support the couple because interventions may be abrupt and anxiety-producing.

STUDY QUESTIONS

14-1 Choose the Key Terms that fit the following definitions:

a. A result of cord compression during labor: _____ *Variable deceleration*

b. Range of fetal heart rate within 1 minute: _____ *Short term variability*

c. The average rate during 10 minutes of fetal heart rate monitoring: _____ *Baseline heart rate*

d. Fetal heart rate less than 120 beats/min: _____ *Brady.*

e. Fetal heart rate more than 160 beats/min: _____ *Tachycard.*

f. Pattern caused by fetal head compression and stimulation of the vagus nerve: *early deceleration*

g. Pattern caused by uteroplacental insufficiency: _____ *late deceleration*

14-2 Ms. P. has been admitted to the labor and delivery unit in labor. External monitoring is begun. Choose four parameters assessed when you read the maternal tracing.
   a. Interval of contractions
   b. Frequency of fetal movements
   c. Resting tonus
   d. Intensity of contractions
   e. Duration of contractions
   f. Reaction of fetus to labor

14-3 Choose four parameters assessed when you read the fetal tracing.
   a. Baseline rate
   b. Response to fetal movements
   c. Intensity of maternal contractions
   d. Periodic changes
   e. Baseline variability

14-4 In the descent phase, when the monitor suddenly begins to show variable decelerations during each contraction, the nursing intervention should be to:
   a. Change pushing position to a side-lying position and observe response
   b. Call the physician at once
   c. Call the anesthesiologist
   d. Coach for more effective pushing

14-5 The only valid method of assessing fetal heart rate beat-to-beat variability is via direct fetal electrocardiography. True/False

14-6 Which procedure may be used to correct variable decelerations caused by cord compression as a result of oligohydramnios?
   a. Amnioinfusion
   b. Cesarean section
   c. Maternal overhydration
   d. Stimulation of labor

Answer Key

14-1 a. Variable deceleration b. Short-term variability c. Baseline heart rate d. Bradycardia e. Tachycardia f. Early decelerations g. Late decelerations 14-2 a, c, d, e 14-3 a, b, d, e 14-4 a 14-5 true 14-6 a

REFERENCES

Beischer NA, MacKay EV, editors: *Obstetrics and the newborn*, ed 3, Philadelphia, 1993, WB Saunders.

Blackburn ST, Loper DL: *Maternal, fetal, and neonatal physiology*, Philadelphia, 1992, WB Saunders.

Dauphinee JD: Antepartum testing: a challenge for nurses, *J Perinat Neonatal Nurs* 1(1):29, 1987.

Eganhouse DJ: Electronic fetal monitoring: education and quality assurance, *JOGNN* 20(1):16, 1991.

Galvin BJ, Van Mullen C, Broekhuisen FF: Using amnioinfusion for relief of repetitive variable decelerations during labor, *JOGNN* 18(3):222, 1989.

Harvey CJ: Interpreting the electronic fetal monitor, *J Nurse Midwife* 34(2):75, 1989.

Haubrich KL: Amnioinfusion: a technique for the relief of variable decelerations, *JOGNN* 19(4):299, 1990.

Herbst AL: Medical professional liability and obstetric care: the Institute of Medicine report and recommendations, *Obstet Gynecol* 75(4):705, 1989.

Hon E, Quilligan EJ: The classification of fetal heart rate. II. A revised working classification, *Conn Med* 31:779, 1967.

Johnson N et al: Fetal monitoring with pulse oximetry, *Br J Obstet Gynecol* 98(1):36, 1991.

Melchior J et al: Le rythme cardinal foetal pendant l'expulsion de l'accouchment normal, *Sociêté Franc Med Pêrinat* 6:225, 1976.

Miyazaki PS, Nevarez F: Saline amnioinfusion for relief of repetitive variable decelerations: a prospective randomized study, *Am J Obstet Gynecol* 153(3):301, 1985.

Nagoette MP et al: Prophylactic intrapartum amnioinfusion in patients with preterm premature rupture of membranes, *Am J Obstet Gynecol* 153:557, 1985.

Persson LNB, Shimojo N, Westgren M: Fetal scalp and umbilical artery blood lactate measured with a new test strip method, *Br J Obstet Gynecol* 99:3067, 1992.

Picard F et al: The validity of fetal heart rate monitoring during the second stage of labor, *Obstet Gynecol* 72(5):746, 1988.

Roberts JE: Managing fetal bradycardia during second stage labor, *MCN* 14(6):394, 1989.

Ross T, Dickason EJ: Nursing alert: vertical transmission of HIV and HBV, *MCN* 17(4):192, 1992.

Small ML et al: Continuous pH monitoring in the term fetus, *Am J Obstet Gynecol* 161(20):323, 1989.

Spencer JAD, editor: *Fetal monitoring*, Philadelphia, 1989, FA Davis.

Tucker SM: *Pocket guide to fetal monitoring*, ed 2, St Louis, 1992, Mosby.

Weitzner JS et al: Objective assessment of meconium content of amniotic fluid, *Obstet Gynecol* 76(6):1143, 1990.

STUDENT RESOURCE SHELF

Gregor CL, Paine LL, Johnson RB: Antepartum fetal assessment, *J Nurse Midwife* 36(3):153, 1991. A good overview of the techniques involved in assessment.

Roberts JE: Managing fetal bradycardia during second stage of labor, *MCN* 14(6):394, 1989. Interpretation of end-stage variables, with suggestions for descriptions and management.

Treacy B, Smith D, Rayburn W: Ultrasound in labor and delivery, *Obstet Gynecol Rev* 45(4):213, 1990. This journal regularly prints review articles that bring together the state of knowledge about a specific care issue.

The Birth Process and Nursing Care

KEY TERMS

Accoucheur
Bearing-Down
  Efforts (BDEs)
Caput Succedaneum
Cephalhematoma
Cesarean Birth
Crowning
Dystocia
Episiotomy
Forceps
Hypertonic
  Contraction
Induction
Laceration
Open-Glottis Pushing
Reorganization

Uterine Inertia
Vacuum Extraction/
  Ventouse

Vaginal Birth After
  Cesarean (VBAC)
Valsalva's Maneuver

LEARNING OBJECTIVES

1. *Compare the management of normal birth with birth in an unexpected location.*
2. *Relate principles of conservation of energy and integrity to the second stage of labor.*
3. *Explain the rationale for choosing different positions for birth.*
4. *Explain the rationale for using specific breathing methods for labor and birth.*
5. *Identify additional safety precautions necessary when labor is induced.*
6. *Anticipate the need for operative interventions.*
7. *Discuss the pros and cons of episiotomy use.*
8. *Recognize why women often harbor feelings of guilt and failure for months after surgical birth experiences.*
9. *Recognize the variety of cultural responses to the stress and pain of childbirth.*

The Second Stage of Labor

With full dilation, the forces of labor focus on descent. The baby must pass through the dilated cervix, maneuver through the pelvic outlet, then distend the vagina, pass through the perineal muscles and labia, and emerge. Controlled and efficient voluntary bearing down by the woman contributes to an effective and safe delivery. **Bearing-down efforts (BDEs)** add about 40 lb of pressure to the uterine contraction work. The expulsive action of the uterus, the woman's sense of renewal, and prior instruction enable her to be an effective and active assistant.

The erratic quality of contractions now changes to a more rhythmic pattern; strong, lasting 90 to 100 sec-

---

BOX 15-1 Second-Stage Phase Boundaries

Phase 1 Latent—resting

From complete dilation until the urge to bear down becomes frequent and rhythmic.

Phase 2 Active—descent

Onset of rhythmic BDEs until crowning. The presenting part will become visible in the middle of this phase.

Phase 3 Transition—perineal

Crowning until the birth of the baby.

Modified from Aderhold KJ, Roberts JE: Phases of the second stage of labor, *J Nurse Midwifery* 36(5):267, 1991.

---

onds with well-defined rest periods. The intervals may be 2 to 4 minutes apart and the woman may fall asleep briefly between contractions.

The second stage of labor has been divided into three phases that reflect the three phases of the first stage of labor. Aderhold and Roberts (1991) have published numerous articles from their *Phases of the Second Stage of Labor* study indicating correct ways of working with women during the second stage. Recognition of these subdivisions of the second stage may change traditional care. The study identifies the accompanying nursing care (Box 15-1). Since three phases of the first stage are accepted, it should not be difficult for care givers to recognize these three second-stage phases, although perhaps less clearly defined and happening more rapidly. These phases need different interventions.

PHASE ONE: EARLY OR LATENT PHASE

Similar to the mood of latent labor, this period follows the time of full dilation of the cervix. There can be a dramatic shift from the agitation of transition to a calm, a lull, when the woman may drop off to sleep briefly. Contractions occur less frequently and are not as strong or painful. This phase may be thought of as a period of **reorganization** as the body prepares for expulsion. During the 10 to 30 minutes, let her rest. She also may complain of backache and leg ache and be anxious during this time. The care givers should not force the woman to push as soon as full dilation is reached (as is the current practice in many settings).

PHASE TWO: DESCENT OR ACTIVE PHASE

This phase has often been taken for the start of the second stage, but it is the active phase of descent of the presenting part through the vagina. The woman has an urge to push rhythmically with each contraction, bearing down and perhaps making grunting noises. The woman will cooperate now, feeling a sense of progress. Pushing or bearing down must follow the dictates of her own urges, unless she has been given an epidural anesthetic. See Chapter 12 for ways to avoid the adverse effects of **Valsalva's maneuver.**

Approximately halfway through the descent phase, the presenting part may be seen at the vaginal opening (introitus). Then as she is cheered on, BDEs become stronger. The woman is focused and may need to change position frequently. During this phase the care giver should offer sips of water, a cool washcloth, and position changes to refresh her for the last phase.

Gradually the labia separate until the fetal scalp is seen. Between contractions the fetal head is forced back by the elasticity of the muscles of the pelvic floor. After a few contractions, the labia flatten with distension, and the head maintains the perineal opening during the relaxation phase; this is **crowning.** *Crowning* means that the presenting part stays visible when the contraction is over (Figure 15-1).

PHASE THREE: THE PERINEAL PHASE

This phase is short, approximately 5 to 12 minutes. The perineum begins to bulge, the anal area dilates, and stool may be expelled. Contractions are frequent and intense. Women worry about "ripping open" and ask frequently about their progress. Preparations for the birth go on. For a multipara, this phase may be only one or two contractions. Emotional intensity parallels the transition phase of the first stage. A partner directly involved will be of great help during these few minutes. Women can get "out of control," crying out and feeling panicked. They need direct statements about when to push and when to breathe in pant-blow breaths.

BIRTH

The skin over the perineum glistens as it is stretched to its limit. If there is adequate elasticity and dimensions, the occiput progresses, with the head in flexion, until the largest area is encircled. The occiput emerges, and then, by extension of the head, the face and chin slip out over the perineum.

Delivery of the head should not be hurried. If progress seems too fast to adequately stretch the perineum, the mother can be coached to pant rather than push during contractions. The physician or midwife may then ask her to exert some pressure between contractions to ease the head out under better control. Forcible pressure must never be put on the head to restrain its progress (Figure 15-2).

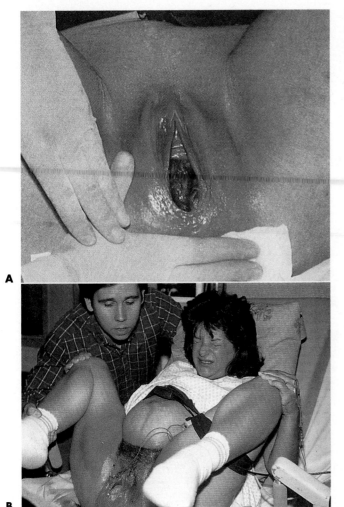

A

B

FIGURE 15-1 **A,** Crowning. **B,** Bulging of the perineum seen here just before birth. (**A** from Al-Azzawi F: *Color atlas of childbirth and obstetric techniques,* St Louis, 1990, Mosby. **B** Courtesy Marjorie Pyle, RNC, *Lifecircle.*)

As soon as the head emerges, the nose and mouth are cleared of mucus and amniotic fluid to prevent aspiration when the infant first breathes. The physician feels for the cord. If it is wrapped around the neck, an attempt is made to slip it over the head. If this cannot be done, it is clamped and cut. Usually the anterior shoulder advances to the pubic arch, which acts as a pivot. Then the posterior shoulder moves forward over the perineum. The anterior shoulder will be lodged just at the upper vaginal opening, and, while watching the perineum carefully and applying steady pressure, the midwife delivers the posterior shoulder. The rest of the body slips out easily.

There are differences of opinion regarding whether the cord should be cut before or after draining the residual volume of blood to the fetus. The prevailing opinion is that this extra blood increases the likelihood of hyperbilirubinemia in the neonatal period (see Chapter 28). Therefore the baby is held at the level of the perineum until cord pulsation has ceased or the cord is clamped in two places and cut between the clamps. A baby held too high above the perineum may transfuse blood back into the placenta and be anemic with a low blood volume during the recovery period.

MOOD

The irritability, discouragement, and agitation that marked the final hour of the first stage disappear at full dilation and the beginning of the woman's cooperative efforts. It is important that the woman be prepared for the sensations that accompany expulsion so she can put them in proper perspective. These include distension of the vaginal tissue (increasing pressure on the perineum), rectal pressure, and absence of the perception of the contraction itself with the pushing effort.

The father's encouragement to sustain the immense pushing effort is very important. Although she becomes oblivious to peripheral activity, she is susceptible to confusion if conflicting directions are given or several people attempt to direct her. The unprepared woman may completely lose control. She may utter loud screams at the peak of the contraction. She frequently is unable to follow directions unless they are simple and repeated.

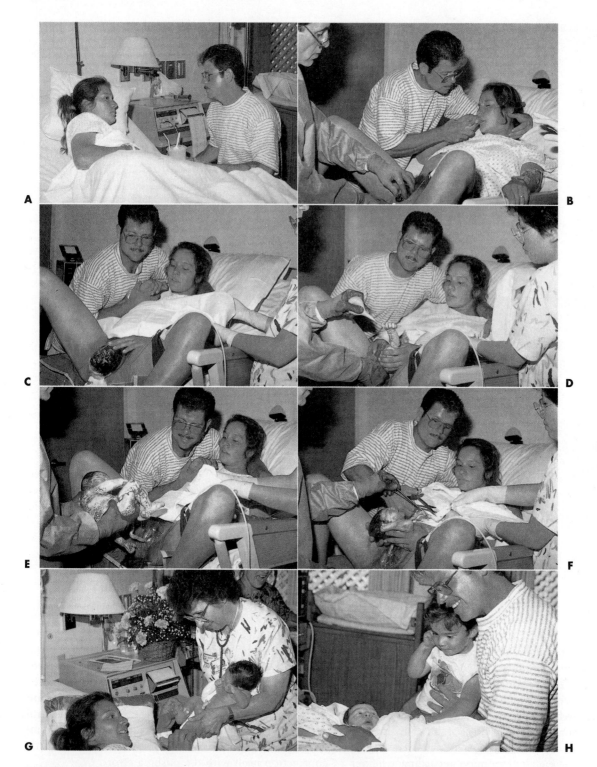

FIGURE 15-2 A, Woman chooses side-lying position between contractions; coach facilitates relaxation. Note monitor. **B,** Second stage of labor; vertex presentation. **C,** Delivery of head. **D,** Mother supports infant while physician clears nose of mucus with bulb syringe. **E,** Infant fully delivered. **F,** Nurse and physician assist as father cuts clamped cord with infant supported on mother's abdomen. **G,** Cleansed and with identification bands in place, newborn is returned to mother. **H,** Sibling is encouraged to become acquainted with new family member. (Courtesy Marjorie Pyle, RNC, *Lifecircle.*)

Cultural Aspects of Care

Ritual circumcision

Women who have migrated from parts of Africa north of the equator or from parts of the Arab world may have been ritually circumcised to sexually desensitize them (Lightfoot-Klein, 1991). This involves removal of the clitoris, and/or infibulation (removal of inner layer of labia majora) with a flap of skin pulled down over the urethra, with a median scar. Health care personnel working with these women need an understanding of the requirements for cutting the skin flap—where to incise if an episiotomy is necessary and how to resuture. Catheterization, if necessary, is difficult but possible. It is done by gently raising the flap with one finger. Lightfoot-Klein's article is mandatory reading for personnel in contact with ritually circumcised women.

COACH

The father's presence at the birth can be a profound experience for the new parents and makes them aware of parenthood as a mutually shared effort. The partner remains at the woman's side, speaking directly into her ear, if needed. He has learned the correct pushing technique to encourage her efforts. During practice and in delivery, use cue words, such as *Breathe—In, out; in, out; hold* (your breath); *relax* (key areas, such as jaw, mouth, and perineum; push out (use the abdominal muscles; push out through the vagina, while releasing air and grunting).

Repeat the sequence several times for each contraction and slowly count to help her sustain pushing for up to 6 to 8 seconds at a time. Between contractions, encourage her to relax by speaking in soothing tones, stroking, or using a cool cloth.

The woman will appreciate anything to increase her comfort, such as wiping her face, giving her ice chips, or adjusting the birthing bed to a higher position. It is impossible to push effectively when lying supine.

During the second phase, the coach may also assist in placing a warm, wet towel over the perineum to relax the tissues, or an ice compress may be placed over the clitoris during crowning to reduce the pain.

Test Yourself

• As a coach during the second stage, Joe could use which comfort measures for Ann?

NURSING APPROACH

By recognizing the mother's progress through the phases of the second stage and changing interventions as needed, the nurse backs up the father or coach. It is important to control the number of people giving directions to the woman. Too many voices confuse her. Only one person should take the lead, with turns taken by another. The woman should not be left alone to push. If the second phase lasts more than an hour, the coach will be fatigued and needs comfort, too, with explanations.

Positioning is most important. One cannot push in the supine position. The birthing bed has many settings (Figure 15-3), or the woman may assume a hands and knees posture, especially if the fetus is in a posterior position (see Figure 15-10). Squatting or holding on to a bar (if the setting includes such equipment) has been used by some women. Squatting is the usual birthing position for women in many developing countries. It opens the passage as widely as possible. In Europe, many births are in the side-lying position. Pushing can be done effectively in this position; the upper knee may be held by the coach. The side-lying position may slow descent but appears to relax the perineum, thereby reducing the need for an episiotomy (Gardosi et al, 1990).

Positioning for the third phase had been routinely in the lithotomy position, with the legs higher than the trunk and head. This is incorrect and should be altered to a moderate semi-Fowler's position, with the knees and legs lower than the heart. When the legs are put high into the leg holders, approximately 2000 ml of blood are autotransfused into the central system, increasing cardiac workload (Odent, 1990). Since BDEs also affect cardiac function, a woman with hypertension or cardiac problems will be compromised by such a position (if hemorrhage occurs, the head may, of course, be lowered [Odent, 1990]). With a birthing bed it is possible to adjust the legs in a number of positions (Figures 15-4 and 15-5).

Throughout the second stage, the fetus is monitored, with observation every 10 minutes as a standard of care. This must be continued until birth. In units where the woman is moved to a delivery room, this means using a portable Doptone to obtain FHR, which must then be documented correctly.

SUMMARY OF NURSING RESPONSIBILITIES

1. Assess the phases of the second stage, changing comfort measures as indicated.
2. Observe fetal responses every 10 minutes and notify accoucheur of any adverse changes. Be alert to the emergence of end-stage variables. Document findings.

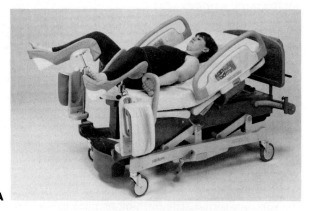

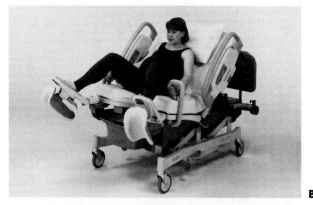

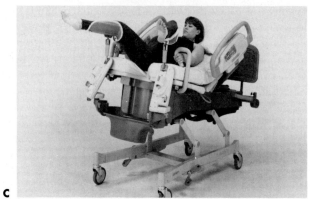

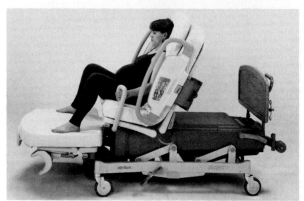

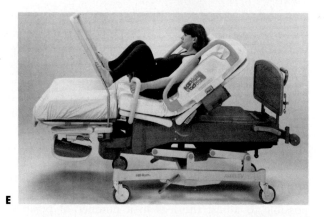

FIGURE 15-3 A-E, Birthing bed allows various positions for pushing and birth. (Courtesy the Affinity Bed, Hill-Rom, Batesville, Ind.)

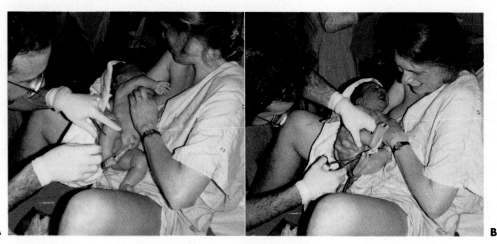

FIGURE 15-4 A, Wet newborn as cord is clamped. Note skin tone and mother's birthing bed position. B, After first clamp is applied, note collapsed white cord. Hands and feet are still bluish. What is the Apgar score on this infant? (Courtesy Brian Hopewell.)

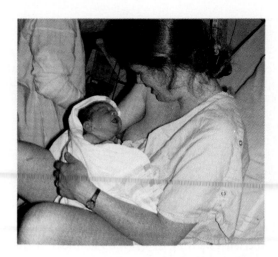

FIGURE 15-5 First look at the infant. Note the reddish blue color of the crying newborn's face. This infant has little skin pigment, so underlying color shows through clearly. (Courtesy Brian Hopewell.)

3. Position the woman for effective BDEs.
4. Support the coach in giving verbal instructions to push or rest.
5. Maintain a safe environment.
6. Protect self and staff with universal precautions for body fluids.
7. Maintain hygiene and fluids and encourage voiding. Catheterize if bladder is full and the mother is unable to void.
8. Prepare birth equipment.
9. Explain each step of the activities: position, monitoring, and preparations for the birth.
10. Evaluate the woman's response to interventions.
11. Assist physician or midwife during the birth.
12. Fill in all records of the birth and condition of the baby.

Test Yourself

- List the signs of each phase of the second stage of labor.

Third Stage

The placenta, after completing its intricate life-sustaining function, separates from the wall of the uterus after it contracts. The uterus, now considerably smaller, assumes a globular shape. The placenta is expelled as the mother pushes for the last time. The physician may ask her to bear down to deliver the placenta. If she is anesthetized, fundal pressure may be exerted. Controlled cord traction may be used to facil-itate delivery after separation has occurred. (Cord traction and fundal pressure must be performed with great care to avoid inversion of the uterus and avulsion of the cord.) As the placenta delivers, it presents the shiny fetal side, Schultze mechanism, or the rough maternal side, Duncan mechanism. The Schultze mechanism is more common. The only significance to this observation is that the Duncan mechanism may be associated with complications such as retained membranes (Figure 15-6).

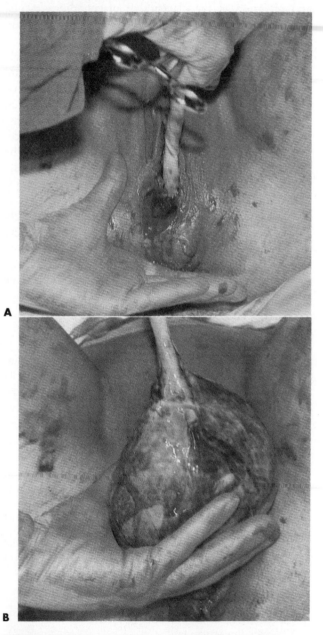

FIGURE 15-6 Placental delivery with slight controlled traction. **A,** The woman pushes the placenta out of the uterus into the vagina by controlled bearing down. **B,** Afterward all parts and membranes must be inspected. (From Al-Azzawi F: *Color atlas of childbirth and obstetric techniques,* St Louis, 1990, Mosby.)

After the placenta is delivered, it must be inspected to be certain that no segments or membranes have been left in the uterus. Medications such as oxytocin 20 U in lactated Ringer's may be routinely given intravenously in hospitals after the delivery of the placenta to aid uterine contraction and decrease the risk of hemorrhage. However, nipple stimulation or breast-feeding adequately stimulates oxytocin release from the posterior pituitary for normal births.

Complications of the third stage include hemorrhage and retention of the placenta or placental fragments. Risk factors associated with these complications are listed in Box 15-2. In cases in which separation is delayed or does not occur, there may be considerable bleeding. If there is a delay in separation of the entire placenta or if the placenta is incomplete, the placenta or fragments must be manually separated and removed with care and with meticulous asepsis. The client must be anesthetized while it is removed because the procedure is very painful. A light general anesthesia must be available. Then the cervix and vagina must be carefully inspected for lacerations so that they can be repaired if necessary to prevent further blood loss.

A placenta does not have to be removed immediately if there is no danger to the mother. In a setting where there is no anesthetic or intravenous fluids, manual removal is dangerous. Putting the infant to the mother's breast provides the necessary stimulation for uterine contraction in most cases.

MOOD

After the birth of the baby, the mother may be exhilarated and talkative, despite the length or intensity of the labor and delivery. She feels very close to the father; she reaches out physically and emotionally for her baby. Her prevailing reaction is one of elation, tempered by the new responsibility of parenthood. Other mothers may be exhausted and not have the energy to reach out. This may be a temporary effect or may be a sign of future difficulty with bonding, especially if the parents react negatively to the sex of the infant.

BOX 15-2   Risk Factors Associated with Complications of the Third Stage

- Dysfunctional uterine activity during labor (hypotonic contractions)
- Extended oxytocin induction
- Overdistension of the uterus
- Dehydration
- Exhaustion
- Full bladder

Cultural Aspects of Care

Certain Asian and Islamic cultures feel that a male child is preferable to a female child. If the mother has several girls already, and gives birth to another girl, she may be unable to look at the infant because she feels ashamed of not producing a "man child." (Later, you may be able to explain to her that the husband solely determines the sex of the infant. It is likely that she will not believe this, however.)

If she is not given the opportunity to hold her baby, she experiences strong deprivation and loss. Most progressive hospitals make sure this opportunity is provided, even for cesarean births, to diminish the loss and increase her feeling of well-being.

More women are asking to breast-feed immediately after delivery. The infant's sucking reflex is very strong at this point, although the baby may just lick the nipple. Nursing seems to create strong maternal bonds with the infant, an important aid to the newly delivered mother (Figure 15-7).

SUMMARY OF NURSING RESPONSIBILITIES

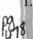

1. Do Apgar score at 1 and 5 minutes. Monitor adjustment and immediate adaptation (discussed in full in Chapters 18 and 19).
2. With the infant under a warmer or on the mother's abdomen, clear air passages with small suction bulb (for alternate suctioning, see Chapter 19).
3. Assess the mother's immediate condition. If she is stable, spend the first few minutes preparing the baby for an extended visit with its parents.
4. Apply plastic clamp to the cord, and cut off the excess. Wrap the infant warmly. *Leave long cord for any distressed infant*
5. Identify the infant with the mother by your unit's method.
6. Encourage both parents to hold and become acquainted with the infant.
7. Wait for placental separation. Administer ordered medication.
8. Check maternal vital signs.
9. Document events while physician or midwife is completing sutures of episiotomy, if present.
10. After all procedures are completed, make the woman comfortable with dry clothing, perineal pad, and linens. Adjust position. Provide nourishment. (Some units monitor recovery for an hour before offering fluids.)
11. Encourage family interaction if the infant's condition is stable. The mother may experiment with breast-feeding.

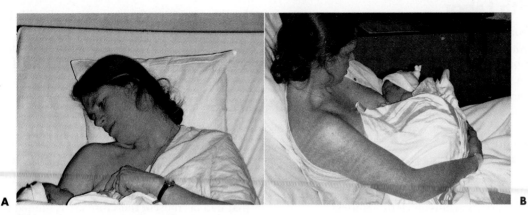

A   **B**

FIGURE 15-7 A, First breast-feeding. Note "en face" position. **B,** Note head covering and extra blankets to keep the infant warm. (Courtesy Brian Hopewell.)

Fourth Stage   *1-4 hrs*

The first hour after delivery is a critical period for the mother. The blood vessels and myometrium are intertwined in such a way that natural ligatures are created when the uterus contracts. Observations every 15 minutes must be made to see that firm contraction of the fundus is maintained to prevent hemorrhage. The uterus is palpated to assess the degree of contraction. The fundus should be firm, at the level of the umbilicus or below, and in the midline. The perineal pad and bed pad are observed for lochia, color, clots, and amount. Normally the lochia is bright red and may contain small clots. The amount should not saturate more than one pad in an hour. The perineum and episiotomy (enlargement of the vaginal opening), if present, should be inspected for hematomas and swelling. An ice pack should be routinely applied to the perineum to decrease swelling and alleviate discomfort.

During the hour after placental delivery, the physician or midwife repairs the episiotomy and any lacerations that may be present, using a local anesthetic. The mother's general condition is observed, particularly in regard to bleeding. The placenta is examined to ensure that it was delivered intact.

The major complication of the fourth stage is hemorrhage. Hemorrhage from the placental site is controlled by contraction of the uterus. Anything interfering with the normal contraction of the uterus, including a full bladder, may result in hemorrhage. Displacement of the uterus upward or laterally indicates a full bladder. The client should be encouraged to void and if unable to do so may have to be catheterized. If the fundus is not firmly contracted (boggy), it may be gently massaged until it becomes firm. The presence of a well-contracted uterus, but with large clots and excessive bleeding, may indicate soft tissue lacerations caused by the trauma of delivery or retained placental fragments. If lacerations are suspected, the client may need to be returned to the delivery room for inspection and repair of the lacerations. If retained placental fragments or membranes are suspected, they must be manually removed. (See Chapter 17 for discussion.)

Clinical Decision

Examine this picture. Which nursing interventions could improve the parent-infant acquaintance just after birth?

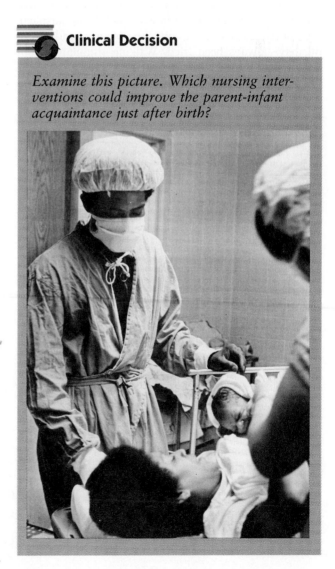

Assistance with Labor

Although normal labor is experienced by a majority of women, 30% to 40% receive some type of medical intervention to assist birth. Women need to be aware of the possibility that a problem could develop during labor. To gain cooperation and reduce anxiety, full explanations are considered helpful and should be part of informed consent. Too often, however, when the problem and treatment are announced, the client's natural alarm is silenced by guilt-producing statements such as "Don't you want to help your baby?" or "If we don't do this, you and your baby will be in trouble." Labor nurses must protect the parents against such thoughtless statements.

STIMULATION OF CONTRACTIONS

Stimulation of uterine contractions requires careful control and monitoring to allow the procedure to be useful. Under ordinary circumstances, the blocks to uterine contractility in pregnancy are very effective. Progesterone blocks the effect of oxytocin; therefore it is often difficult to start labor "from scratch." Nonpharmacologic methods, including exercise, enemas, and castor oil, have always been tried. Walking stimulates labor after it has begun; an enema in early labor clears the lower intestinal tract and may slightly stimulate contractions. More recently, amniotomy or artificial rupture of the membranes (ARM) was tried, but rupturing the membranes early placed the mother at risk for ascending infection.

Uterine activity is started (*induction*) or when inadequate contractions are present, labor may be intensified (*stimulation*).

For induction, the processes of prelabor, which normally take several weeks, must be effected in a few hours. These changes are movement of the head into the pelvic inlet to engagement, stretching of the lower uterine segment and upper vaginal wall, and softening (ripening) of the cervix. The cervix is evaluated by the Bishop score to check its readiness. The client goes through the same work of labor but over a shorter period. Thus the total pressure needed to dilate the cervix completely and to cause descent and expulsion of the fetus is the same as for spontaneous labor, but the contractions may be *more intense, more frequent, and longer in duration.*

There should be medical indications for induction. The FDA prohibits induction merely for convenience, "baby by appointment." The reasons for medical induction are mainly fetoplacental insufficiency caused by preeclampsia, hypertension, diabetic or renal disease, prolonged pregnancy of more than 41 weeks, mild antepartum hemorrhage, intrauterine fetal death, intrauterine growth retardation, and Rh sensiti-

zation. All other reasons for induction should be questioned.

Labor may be stimulated when uterine contractions are inefficient after labor has begun. The method for stimulation is similar to that for induction.

Prostaglandin Use

Prostaglandins E_2 and F_2 (PGE_2; PGF_2) are normal body hormones active in initiating and sustaining labor. Uterine sensitivity increases as labor approaches. The half-life of prostaglandins is short, but prostaglandin use for induction of labor resulted in adverse effects in the high oral doses that had been used; therefore use is limited to situations without a viable fetus, such as late abortion or in cases of intrauterine death. In these cases vaginal suppositories of PGE_2 (dinoprostone 20 mg) are used.

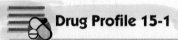

Drug Profile 15-1

Prostaglandin E_2, Prostin gel
Action
Cervical effacement, mediates changes in connective tissue. Primes the cervix for induction when cervix less than 2 cm and 50% effaced.

Uses
Reduces required oxytocin dose, length of induction and labor. Apparently safe for use with vaginal birth after cesarean (VBAC) inductions.

Informed consent
Not yet FDA approved. Woman must sign specific consent.

Dosage and routes
Prostaglandin E_2 in 10 ml Tylose gel in syringe. Keep frozen. Thaw by hand warmth before insertion to the surface of the cervix. May be held in place by a diaphragm.
Or, 0.5 to 5 ml gel placed into cervical canal by small catheter attached to syringe containing gel (less common method). Reapply every 4 to 6 hours for 2 days.
Or, PGE_2 vaginal suppository, 20 mg placed into posterior fornix of vagina every 3 hours until birth of an intrauterine fetal death; only used for a death in utero.

Side effects/adverse reactions
Rare hypertonic contractions, with fetal distress. Remove diaphragm and gel, swab vagina with gauze sponge. May need tocolysis. Oxygen and position change to support fetal oxygenation. *Nausea, diarrhea* may be treated with Compazine, Kaopectate.

Cervical application of *low-dose* PGE_2 gel works effectively to ripen (thin and soften) the cervix in preparation for induction with oxytocin. Its use reduces the needed time and total dose of oxytocin for induction (Jennings et al, 1989). There appear to be no adverse effects with low doses. However, hypertonic contractions occur rarely with the gel. In this situation, the vagina is swabbed with gauze, and tocolysis may be needed (see Drug Profile 15-1 for description).

Oxytocin Use

Oxytocin is a normal body hormone synthesized in the hypothalamus and secreted from the posterior pituitary (see Drug Profile 15-2). Its effect is blocked by progesterone. As labor approaches, contractions are strengthened in direct proportion to the decrease in progesterone from the aging placenta. When present in the body, oxytocin is inactivated by *oxytocinase*, making its half-life 10 to 12 minutes in early pregnancy and 1 to 6 minutes in late pregnancy.

Oxytocin receptors are found in the myometrium and mammary epithelium. These myometrial receptors increase during the first stage of labor. Naturally occurring amounts during labor are about 2 to 3 mU/min (Darwood, 1989). Based on this physiology, to prevent adverse effects, oxytocin is administered in dilute amounts during labor. Oxytocin receptors become saturated within about 40 minutes of the start of the infusion (Brodsky and Pelzar, 1991). With excessive doses uterine muscle fibrillation, uterine hyperstimulation with reduced oxygen to the fetus, and fetal distress occur. Maternal blood pressure may fall, and pulse with hypotension and tachycardia occurs (Spielman et al, 1988). You need to remember:

- Very few clients tolerate oxytocin-augmented contractions and remain in control in the true Lamaze sense. Therefore some analgesia will be needed.
- Oxytocin sensitivity depends on the number of receptors and varies markedly from person to person, and from phase to phase of labor.
- The setup, observation, and maintenance of a problem-free infusion fall within nursing measures, but the obstetrician usually is responsible for beginning the intravenous infusion and for titration of the dosage (which includes remaining with the client for a sufficient period after each change in rate or dosage to ensure a problem-free administration). The physician must be on call for unexpected problems.
- An infusion pump as a piggyback addition to a plain infusion must control the rate of flow. Insertion of secondary line must be as near the primary point of insertion as possible.
- Labor may be substantially shortened and may move toward delivery more rapidly than expected.

Drug Profile 15-2

Oxytocin during labor and birth
(Pitocin, Syntocinon)

Action
Naturally produced hormone secreted by posterior pituitary, blocked by progesterone until approaching labor. Acts on receptor sites in myofibrils of uterus and myoepithelial cells in breast, to cause contractions and the let down reflex stimulated by infant sucking on nipple. Inactivated by *oxytocinase*, short half-life during labor allows safe IV use if regulated carefully and diluted × 1000 ml isotonic fluid.

Dosage/route
Stimulation/induction labor: 1 ml (10 U) diluted in 1000 ml Ringer's lactate or NS by secondary line through IV pump. Begin at 0.5-1.0 mU/min. Incremental doses of 1 mU every 20-30 min are titrated with maternal response of contraction pattern. Never more than 20 mU/min.
Prevention postbirth hemorrhage: 10-20 U in 1000 ml Ringer's lactate at no more than 250 ml hr, or IM; *not both.* Rarely IV; very slow push and must be diluted with IV fluids.

Side effects/adverse effects:
Hypotension with too rapid infusion or push. *Tachycardia.* **Hypertonic contractions** cause placental perfusion, cause fetal distress.

Precautions
Maternal: Because of antidiuretic effect of oxytocin, high doses of oxytocin will cause oliguria, *fluid overload.* Observe for arrhythmias, water intoxication, poor output, nausea, vomiting, headache, hypotension. Follow I&O, vital signs.
Fetal: May promote *hyperbilirubinemia* in high maternal labor doses. If fetal distress occurs, turn off pump at once.

Therefore close observation and use of the fetal monitor are mandatory.
- Because labor accelerates, there will be more pressure on the presenting part, less recovery time between contractions, and a greater possibility of fetal distress. Therefore the fetal heart rate monitoring strip must be evaluated regularly.

The starting dose for oxytocin now has been markedly reduced because PGE_2 is almost always used to prepare the cervix, thus avoiding a long infusion time with oxytocin. The American College of Obstetricians

and Gynecologists (ACOG) recommendations (1991) are for the following:
- Begin with 0.5 to 1.0 mU/min
- Observe fetal and maternal responses
- Increase dose every 30 to 60 minutes by 1 to 2 mU/min until desired contraction rate, which is
  —Frequency 2 to 3 minutes,
  —Intensity between 40 and 90 mm Hg,
  —Duration between 40 and 90 seconds, and
  —Resting tone <15 to 20 mm Hg.

There are other protocols, and each unit must have one; all should now include lower doses as recommended to avoid adverse effects of this powerful drug. At a certain point, additional increase in dose is useless because it is now known that the uterine muscle can use only a certain dosage.

Increasing the dose beyond that point is inappropriate and may be dangerous. In addition, sensitivity changes during later labor, and doses should be decreased as desirable contractions continue. In this way adverse effects can be avoided. The desire to "speed things along" solely for the benefit of the physician is not acceptable. This concept is dangerous. The dose must be *titrated* with the woman's responses, not with the clock. *More is not better* in this case. *Warning signs* of adverse effects include:
- Contractions more frequent than every 2 minutes
- Intensity over 75 to 90 mm Hg
- Duration more than 90 seconds
- Resting tone over 20 mm Hg
- Fetal tachycardia, bradycardia, or altered beat-to-beat variability

In the event of adverse response, discontinue the piggyback flow by turning off the pump (remember the short half-life). Intervene as described in Chapter 14 with position changes, oxygen by mask, and increase in mainline fluids; observe results of interventions. Notify the obstetrician or midwife of your actions and the client's responses (see Chapter 14). Terbutaline as a *tocolytic* may be used in some cases when hypertonus persists (see Chapter 21).

When labor is augmented later in the first stage or in second stage, the same guidelines apply.

Test Yourself

There is a concentration of 20 U oxytocin in 500 ml of IV fluid. The order reads: Increase infusion to 3 mU/min. For the patient to receive this amount, set the rate for:
_____ mL/min or _____ mL/hour.

DYSFUNCTIONAL LABOR

Several factors may contribute to dysfunctional labor and birth. The quality of contractions and the fetal position and size in relation to the pelvic canal may be major causes of difficulty in the birth process.

Uterine dystocia occurs when labor contractions are ineffectual, erratic, or unable to do the work of dilating the cervix or causing fetal descent. Dysfunctional labor patterns are described as follows:

1. A *prolonged latent phase* lasts for more than 20 hours in a nullipara or more than 14 hours in a multipara. If the latent phase is truly prolonged (the mother was not admitted during the prodromal phase), reasons underlying the delay may be an unready cervix and ineffective power in the hypotonic contractions.

2. *Prolonged active labor,* slower rates of cervical dilation or fetal descent may result from malpositions, ineffectual contractions, or CPD. If second stage descent problems are present, position changes may improve progress. For instance, the supine position forces the fetal head to move against gravity, up and over the pelvic outlet. For this reason, birthing chairs and beds and a high Fowler's or semisitting position may facilitate descent.

3. *Hypertonic contractions* may occur in labor. The same work of labor is required to dilate the cervix and cause fetal descent. If contractions are **hypertonic** (that is, stronger and longer than expected for the phase of labor), labor may progress rapidly to a precipitate birth, or labor may be prolonged. In any case, the uterine muscle will be exhausted, and postbirth bleeding is possible. The oxygen supply to the infant may be diminished during labor with potential fetal perfusion problems.

4. *Arrest of the head* may occur during late active transition just as the deceleration phase (second stage) should begin. The head in this case is too large to rotate through the ischial spines and appears to be "stuck on the spines" in the OT position. The cervix may be fully dilated, but the station remains at –1, 0, or +1.

5. *Arrest of the shoulders* may occur with a large baby during the second stage. As dilation is completed, the fetal head rotates and enters the vagina. The mother may push effectively, but the head does not move farther down the canal. A prolonged second stage (protracted descent) lasts more than 3 hours for a nullipara and more than 1 hour for a multipara. It is extremely important to ascertain whether this type of fetopelvic disproportion is the problem. If the head has descended, but the shoulders are unable to follow, the amount of molding of the fetal head and the body size will be estimated. Sometimes the mother becomes exhausted from pushing and simply cannot push a large baby the last few inches. Then even forceps or operative delivery is difficult.

For operative delivery to occur when the head is firmly lodged, the head must be pushed back up the birth canal to be extracted from the lower uterine

PROCEDURE 15-1   Induction

- Set up solution of 1000 ml Ringer's lactate or normal saline solution. Add 10 U (1 mL) oxytocin. Flush secondary line tubing and thread through IV pump changers. Label IV bag with dose, date, and time.
- Insert secondary line into IV tubing close to main-line insertion site.
- Calculate flow rate, remembering there are 1000 milliunits (mU) in 1 unit of oxytocin. Use the following formula for 0.5 mU/min starting dose:

$$\frac{0.5 \text{ mU}}{1 \text{ min}} \times \frac{1 \text{ U}}{1000 \text{ mU}} \times \frac{1000 \text{ mL}}{10 \text{ U}} = 0.5 \text{ mL/min}$$

- Initiate the secondary oxytocin flow after evaluating contractions and fetal heart rate, and the initial procedures in the protocol are completed.
- Medical reasons are determined and documented by the physician.
- A baseline monitor strip is obtained, evaluated, and documented.
- Begin with the lowest dosage; evaluate at 15 and 30 minutes after initial dose.
- Each increase in dosage by the physician must follow step-by-step increment. Never skip a step.

- Check the bedside monitor for at least 20 minutes to evaluate the response. When effective labor is reached, stop increments.
- Reduce increments or stop the pump at any sign of UPI, CC, or reduced variability.
- The resident or attending physician must be on call in the maternity unit.
- Documentation on strip includes times of start, each increase, and stop; also record examinations and results, procedures, position changes, and maternal activity interfering with tracing. Record maternal vital signs on the routine schedule.
- Documentation on progress record includes times of start, each increase, and stop and all examinations, procedures, position changes, and maternal activity interfering with tracing, as well as the time the physician was notified of any changes and time of response.
- Observe the monitor strip and record observations q 30 minutes.
- Check maternal BP every hour.

●   ●   ●

OPTIONAL ACTIVITY: Write a sample nursing note correctly documenting the performance of this procedure.

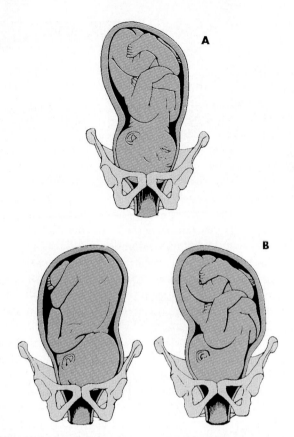

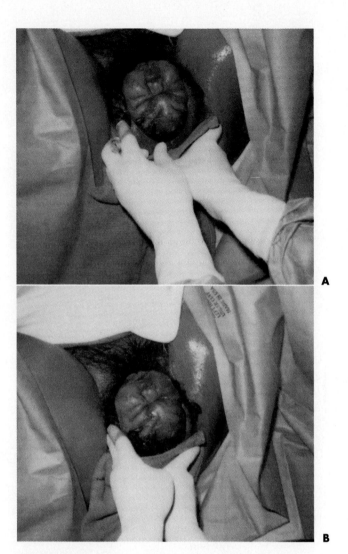

FIGURE 15-8 A, Brow presentation. B, Face presentation. (Used with permission of Ross Laboratories, Columbus, Ohio 43216, from Clinical Education Aid: The phenomena of labor, © Ross Laboratories.)

FIGURE 15-9 A and B, Unusual vaginal birth of a face presentation. Note how edematous the face is. Several days will elapse before edema and bruising will resolve. (Courtesy Marjorie Pyle, RNC, *Lifecircle*.)

incision. To do this, one physician inserts a sterile gloved hand into the vagina and firmly pushes while another physician pulls the infant's shoulders and body from the uterus, a potentially stressful delivery for mother and fetus.

6. *Dystocia* may occur with malposition of the head. When flexion has not occurred as expected, a persistent *brow or face presentation* may result (Figure 15-8, A). The infant cannot be delivered with a brow presentation because the largest diameter of the head will be coming through the birth canal. When hyperextension rather than flexion has occurred at engagement, the face is the presenting part (Figure 15-8, B).

Because the face presents a smaller diameter than the brow, it could be delivered, but trauma to facial tissues and the extreme backward molding of the occiput are potentially injurious to the fetus. Face presentation is initially difficult to diagnose because the face becomes

edematous and may be confused with the buttock of a breech presentation. These infants are almost always delivered by cesarean birth (Figure 15-9).

Occiput Posterior Position

When the vertex presentation changes to a posterior position during internal rotation, the birth will be prolonged. A larger arc of 180 degrees must be crossed over the sacral curve, rather than simpler extension under the symphysis. The woman experiences considerable back pain and may feel that her coccyx is being "sprained." Some women will experience difficulty cop-

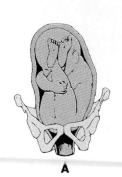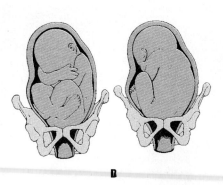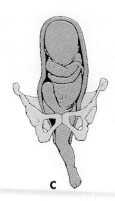

FIGURE 15-10 Breech presentation. **A,** Frank breech. **B,** Complete breech. **C,** Incomplete breech or footling. (Used with permission of Ross Laboratories, Columbus, OH 43216, from Clinical Education Aid: The phenomena of normal labor, © Ross Laboratories.)

A   B   C

ing with this position without analgesia and/or transcutaneous electric nerve stimulation (TENS) and a great deal of emotional support (see Chapter 16). Maternal positions are key factors in labor management.

> **Test Yourself**
>
> A multipara has been in the second stage, pushing for 1 hour. The baby is in occiput posterior position and is still at +1 station. What do the findings indicate?

Breech Presentation

When engagement of the buttocks takes place, it may occur in three ways (Figure 15-10):

1. Frank breech, in which the thighs are flexed and knees are extended so the feet are beside the head
2. Complete breech, in which the infant appears to be sitting cross-legged
3. Incomplete or footling breech, in which one leg is extended so the foot is the leading part

Breech presentations can be delivered vaginally (Figure 15-11), but they carry a higher risk. A preterm or the second or third infant of a multiple pregnancy will often present in this way. Small infants are not as difficult to deliver as larger infants (>8 lb). The larger infant may have shoulder or head dystocia because the cervix may allow the body to protrude before full dilation. The head then becomes trapped by the tight cervical rim. In addition, there is a higher rate of cord prolapse, PROM, trauma to the infant, and fetal distress.

Until cesareans were done more frequently for breech deliveries, a mortality of 10% to 20% was related to these mechanical problems. The overall incidence of breech presentation is about 3% to 4%.

Management. More than 75% of breech presentations are delivered by cesarean methods. Presentation is usually settled in the last few weeks before birth. A number of centers are reporting success with maternal positions that facilitate fetal turning. The knee-chest position or being on hands and knees with the abdomen hanging loosely has been demonstrated to reduce pressure on the fetus and allow turning, even when amniotic fluid is somewhat diminished (Figure 15-12).

Internal version (changing fetal position) is not done today because of the potential for trauma to the mother and fetus. External version may be tried at 37 to 38 weeks by several methods in the fetal evaluation unit. An NST is performed first. The woman is placed in Trendelenburg position, and by gentle pressure the head is pushed toward the pelvis while the breech is pushed toward the fundus. Powder is used on the woman's skin to smooth the movement of the examiner's hands. After the version, an NST is done and the fetus is observed for responses. In approximately half of such cases, fetuses remain in vertex position, whereas the others move back to breech or lodge in a transverse presentation, requiring cesarean delivery (Beischer and MacKay, 1993).

Assistance with Birth
EPISIOTOMY

An episiotomy is a surgical incision made into the perineal area to enlarge the introitus for the birth of the infant. The most frequently used incision is made midline between vaginal introitus and anus (Figure 15-13, *A*). The rationale for a midline episiotomy is that because less tissue is incised, there is subsequently less discomfort, and recovery is more rapid. A mediolateral incision (Figure 15-13, *B*) may be indicated when a forceps delivery is required or when there is a posterior fetal position, a breech birth, or a very large infant. More tissue is cut, but potential extension into the anal sphincter is avoided.

Only since the 1920s has routine use of an episiotomy been practiced. Today such routines are questioned because many studies have shown that

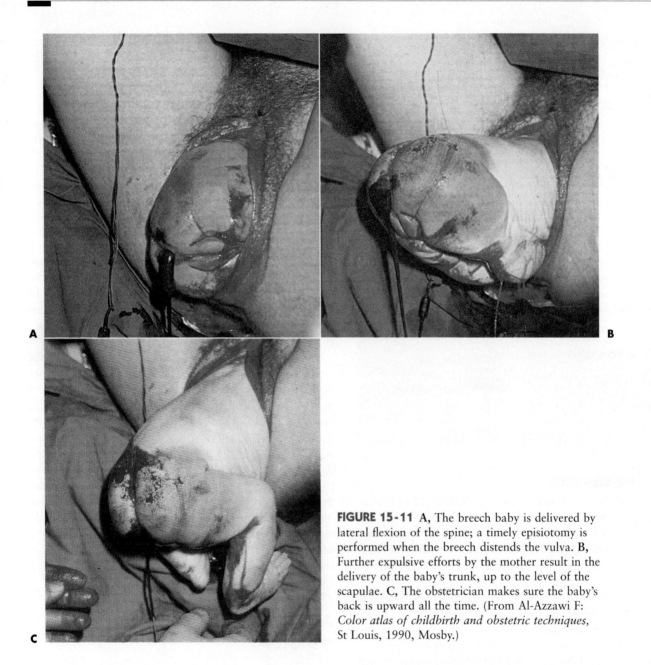

A

B

C

FIGURE 15-11 A, The breech baby is delivered by lateral flexion of the spine; a timely episiotomy is performed when the breech distends the vulva. **B,** Further expulsive efforts by the mother result in the delivery of the baby's trunk, up to the level of the scapulae. **C,** The obstetrician makes sure the baby's back is upward all the time. (From Al-Azzawi F: *Color atlas of childbirth and obstetric techniques,* St Louis, 1990, Mosby.)

supposed benefits may indeed be adverse to women's future perineal integrity.

There is little evidence to support the routine use of episiotomy to *prevent perineal trauma;* in fact, recent studies demonstrate that incidence of third- and fourth-degree lacerations was increased in women who had midline episiotomies (Thorpe and Bowes, 1989; Bromberg, 1986). The use of episiotomy to *prevent over-stretching of perineal muscles* with later development of marked relaxation that allows prolapse of bladder or rectum (cystocele or rectocele) with accompanying incontinence has been questioned. One large study found perineal muscle function to be related to regular exer-

cise done by the individual and not to method of delivery (Gordon and Logue, 1985).

Delivery position is a factor and incidence is higher with the lithotomy, and lower in Sims position. It is more routinely done by physicians than by midwives. The use of anesthesia, either epidural or pudendal, raises the incidence of episiotomy as well, perhaps reflecting the difficulty of delivery. There is a suggestion that informed consent be obtained specifically for this surgical procedure because the result of poorly performed or timed episiotomies can be lifelong perineal dysfunction. See Box 15-3 for risks and benefits (Bromberg, 1986).

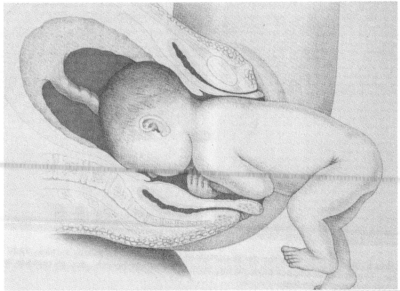

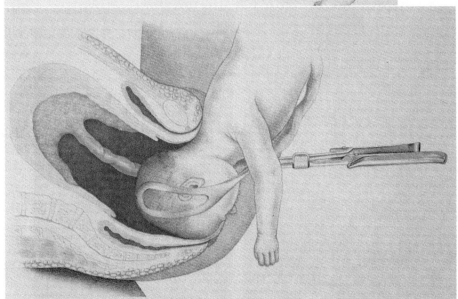

FIGURE 15-12 Breech delivery. **A,** When infant's back is upward, a towel is wrapped around the body. **B,** Piper's forceps may be applied to the after-coming head and used to initially pull downward, and then slowly and gently upward; the head is born. (From Al-Azzawi F: *Color atlas of childbirth and obstetric techniques,* St Louis, 1990, Mosby.)

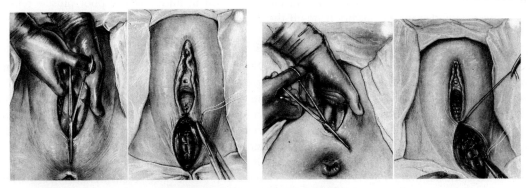

FIGURE 15-13 **A,** Anatomic location of midline episiotomy. **B,** Anatomic location of mediolateral episiotomy. (From Willson JR et al, eds: *Obstetrics and gynecology,* ed 8, St Louis, 1987, Mosby.)

BOX 15-3   Risks and Benefits of Episiotomy

Risks

- Blood loss up to 300 ml
- Potential for hematoma
- Infection
- Potential for poor repair
- Sexual dyspareunia (60%) lasting up to 6 months
- Temporary loss of libido
- Healing accompanied by moderate to severe pain
- Higher risk of third- or fourth-degree laceration if midline.

Benefits

- If done before tissue overstretched, possible benefit
- Reduces pressure on fetal head in last phase
- Useful with forceps or malpositions of fetus
- Easier to repair: more regular scar than a jagged laceration of same degree

BOX 15-4   Types of Lacerations

Perineal lacerations

First-degree:

Skin, mucous membrane of posterior fourchette and proximal vagina

Second-degree:

Muscles and fascia up to anal sphincter, plus above tissues

Third-degree:

Laceration of above tissues continuing through anal sphincter

Fourth-degree:

In addition to above tissues, torn anterior rectal wall

Sulcus tear

Folds of the vagina torn, often over the ischial spines

Periurethral tear

Tissues around the urethra torn, sometimes the urethra itself

Cervical tear

Any degree, from small shallow tears to deep lacerations through entire cervix into lower uterine segment

Uterine tear

Usually in lower uterine segment, which is thinner during later pregnancy; especially possible if multifetal gestation, site of placenta previa, or precipitate labor

LACERATIONS

Lacerations of the perineum and vagina may occur with or without an episiotomy. These lacerations are classified as first, second, third, and fourth degree. Box 15-4 describes the types of lacerations that may occur and their locations. Lacerations may result in excessive bleeding and the development of hematomas (see Chapter 21). Episiotomies and lacerations are repaired with chromic sutures, which dissolve several weeks after delivery.

Avoiding Lacerations

An episiotomy may be thought of as a second-degree laceration (Box 15-4). Even a carefully conducted, slow birth with full maternal cooperation may result in first- or second-degree lacerations around the vaginal opening or near the urethra (sulcus tear). Position has been found to be important; those positions with relaxed perineum have the lowest incidence. In addition, women who had practiced Kegel exercises and perineal massage in preparation for birth and were able to relax that muscle group had better outcomes (Gordon and Logue, 1985). The accoucheur can, during the last phases of second stage, gently massage the lower perineal tissue, stretching the opening. Finally, a slow, controlled exit of the fetus allows an intact perineum in most cases. A woman with this type of birth is capable of getting up and walking to the bathroom or chair without pain or discomfort. Contrast that recovery with one who has had extensive suturing, swelling, and pain, who cannot even sit comfortably for several days, and who has dysuria and painful bowel movements.

The importance of protection of the perineum becomes evident when it is shown that third- and fourth-degree lacerations result in unnecessarily poor muscle tension at the anus because of scar tissue (Box 15-5).

Nursing Responsibilities

1. During labor, reinforce the process of labor and how to push.
2. Position the woman for best perineal outcome and monitor bearing down efforts to coordinate with her own involuntary urge to push (Nodine and Roberts, 1989).
3. Offer warm compress to the perineum during BDEs and an ice pack to clitoris during crowning.
4. Advocate for side-lying or semi-Fowler's position with legs positioned so tension on the perineum is avoided.

BOX 15-5 Measures To Avoid an Episiotomy

- Allow woman to follow own urge to push.
- Encourage perineal relaxation during pushing.
- Apply hot compresses to perineum.
- Tell woman to avoid pushing during crowning.
- Apply ice compress to clitoral area during crowning.
- With sterile gloved hand, massage perineum and stretch vaginal opening gently.
- Modify birth position to side-lying or semisitting in birthing chair. If in stirrups, do not hyperextend but hold legs; lower legs at birth to reduce tension on obstetric perineum.

5. Legs should be lower than the heart and not hyperextended at the hip. For care after birth, see Chapter 17.

FORCEPS DELIVERY

Assisted delivery may require the use of forceps to shorten the second stage of labor. If there are complications such as ineffective bearing down efforts caused by the anesthetic or by fatigue, if there are malpositions, or if the baby is large, forceps will be an effective way to assist in the birth. If there is fetal distress, the last phases of labor will be shortened by use of forceps.

Forceps are curved metal blades shaped to grasp the head of an infant in a way that allows the physician to apply controlled traction (Figure 15-14). Forceps deliveries are classified as low forceps or midforceps. A *low forceps* delivery is performed when the head is on the perineum; the forceps are used to extend the head. A *midforceps* delivery is done to rotate the head from an LOA or ROA to an OA position. The head is at the level of the ischial spines and may have an arrest of internal rotation. This delivery is difficult and can be traumatic to the mother and infant. The mother *must be anesthetized* to tolerate a midforceps delivery because the pressure created is intense. High forceps deliveries are no longer performed. If the head is unengaged, a cesarean birth is the method of choice. Box 15-6 lists indications for the use of forceps.

Before forceps can be applied, several requirements must be met. The cervix must be fully dilated, the head must be engaged, the position of the head must be known, the pelvis must be adequate to allow passage of the infant, and the membranes must be ruptured. After the forceps are applied to the head, pressure is applied in a downward direction to bring the head under the symphysis pubis. As the head rotates around the pubic bone and crowns, the forceps are gently removed and the rest of the birth is accomplished (Figures 15-15 and 15-16).

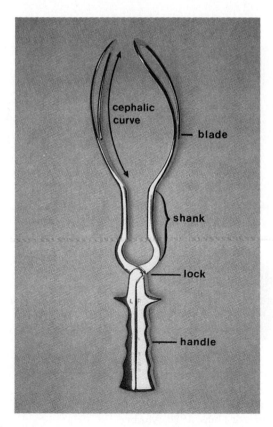

FIGURE 15-14 Parts of the obstetric forceps (Neville-Barnes). (From Al-Azzawi F: *Color atlas of childbirth and obstetric techniques*, St Louis, 1990, Mosby.)

BOX 15-6 Indications For Use of Forceps

Fetal problems
- Arrested descent
- Arrested rotation
- Abnormal presentation
  - Face or brow
  - Breech (forceps for head)
- Fetal distress in late second stage
- Preterm infant (to protect fragile head)

Maternal problems
- Uterine inertia in late second stage
- Inability to push effectively resulting from exhaustion, regional or general anesthesia, mild CPD, or poor position for pushing
- Chronic disease requiring the least possible stress during delivery (for example, cardiac, chest disease, and hypertension)

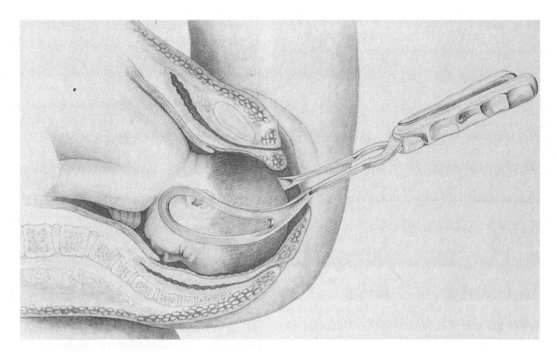

FIGURE 15-15 Forceps correctly applied to the head. Note relation of curve of pelvis to curve of forceps. (From Al-Azzawi F: *Color atlas of childbirth and obstetric techniques,* St Louis, 1990, Mosby.)

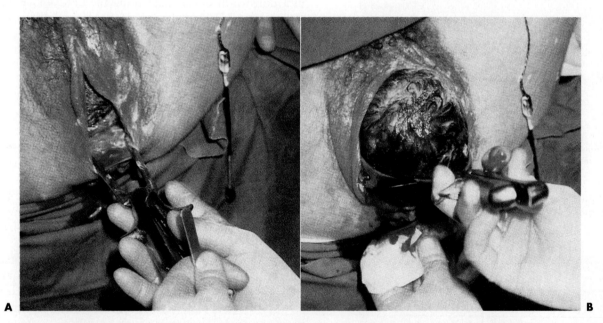

A   B

FIGURE 15-16 A, The mother is encouraged to bear down with the onset of the following uterine contraction, and simultaneous traction is applied on the fetal head. **B,** During delivery of the head, the perineum is supported with a gauze pad, holding it back and preventing further distension; at the same time, traction is directed upward away from the perineum. (From Al-Azzawi F: *Color atlas of childbirth and obstetric techniques,* St Louis, 1990, Mosby.)

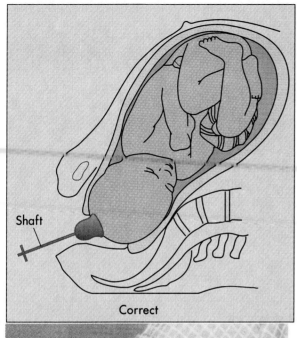

Shaft

Correct

A

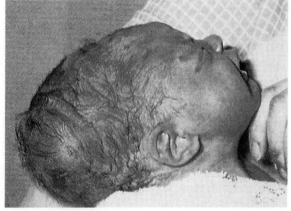

B

FIGURE 15-17 Vacuum extraction. **A,** Position. **B,** The chignon is seen in profile; it usually disappears within 24 to 48 hours. (**B** from Al-Azzawi F: *Color atlas of childbirth and obstetric techniques,* St Louis, 1990, Mosby.)

Complications of forceps deliveries may include injury to the cervix, vagina, rectum, and bladder.

Risks

There may be additional severe pain for the woman if anesthesia is partial. Soft tissue injury for the fetus is not uncommon. Forceps marks may leave bruised areas over cheekbones that heal quickly. More serious damage to the facial nerve, with resulting facial palsy, may occur from pressure on the facial nerve. The skull may sustain a fracture in very rare cases of midforceps trauma.

VACUUM EXTRACTION/VENTOUSE

A safer alternative to forceps birth is a soft vacuum extraction (VE) cup made of pliable plastic (Silastic,

Mitivac). Vacuum from a suction pump is used after the cup has been placed on the presenting part. Usually the infant is delivered with three to four pulls. Sometimes during pulling the cup detaches and must be reapplied again. If undue suction should be used, the cup falls off the vertex. This procedure, called **ventouse,** is common in Europe as a substitute for forceps. It has not yet gained extensive use in this country (Figure 15-17). The procedure is indicated in failure to rotate, arrest or delay in the second stage, fetal distress, borderline CPD, and maternal indications for a shortened second stage (that is, cardiac disease, respiratory disease, and severe hypertension). The prerequisites to its use are a vertex presentation, ruptured membranes, no presence of CPD, and completely dilated cervix.

Risks

Vacuum extraction allows for safe rotation of the fetal head, whereas with forceps deliveries undue traction can result in injury to the head. Neonatal findings with VE are **caput succedaneum,** which is scalp edema and bruising in a circular area under the cup. This raised edematous area usually resolves within 24 to 48 hours, but bluish or reddened areas may darken and take several days to resolve. **Cephalhematomas** (bleeding between periosteum and bone that does not spread across the bony plate) may develop in the first few hours after birth and are more common with VE (6% to 15%) than forceps birth (Dell, Lightler, and Planché, 1985).

Cesarean Birth

The goal for operative birth is the same as that for vaginal birth—the safe delivery of a healthy infant. Cesarean birth is a safer procedure today than in prior decades. Women are usually awake with epidural anesthesia. Their partners sit at the head of the bed and both see the infant at birth. However, surgical procedures and anesthesia always entail risk; in a large survey the risk was four times that of a vaginal birth (USDHHS, 1981). Both have very low mortality today, but morbidity of 5% to 10% in operative delivery is higher than it should be. Wound, urinary, or uterine infections continue to be problems. Hemorrhage is at a higher rate (see Chapter 21), and trauma to bladder and bowel with some developing later adhesions must be avoided by better surgical technique. Finally, pulmonary or vascular emboli and rarely clotting defects (disseminated intravascular coagulation [DIC]) can occur.

Neonatal problems with elective (scheduled) surgery center around two outcomes: (1) preterm birth if assessment of gestational age was inaccurate and the infant is delivered too early, and (2) problems caused the term infant by a birth without labor. Normal labor appears to prepare the infant for adequate respiratory effort; more infants have respiratory difficulty after a cesarean than after a normal vaginal delivery. In emergency situations, the stressors are those causing the crisis, and the infant's condition may be poor as it is rescued from the intrauterine environment.

INCIDENCE

Cesarean birth accounts for 25% to 35% of births in the United States today. One third are repeat cesareans. In some high-risk tertiary centers the rate is even higher because of more complicated labors. This means that two in five of your clients will have surgical births.

This increase, from about 5% in 1965, is the result of a number of factors. First, problems can be identified earlier by means of ultrasound and fetal testing. Second, Friedman's computerized labor pattern has led physicians to declare that delay in labor can be reasons for surgical birth from "failure to progress." How stringently the average labor pattern is followed affects the rate of cesareans in a particular unit. However, the labor grid is only an *average,* not a rigid pattern. Often a cesarean section can be avoided by good consistent bedside coaching. When a woman is pressured to "perform" to a clock, only adverse responses occur. Midwives have found that not using the curve, provided all else is progressing and the fetal heart rate is in a good range, can result in a normal vaginal birth (Cosner and deJong, 1993).

Third, the concern about malpractice suits has led obstetricians and gynecologists to be more cautious. Herbst (1989) states that 70% of OB/GYNs have had at least one suit, often with no fault on their side. This experience is a painful one for the physician and breeds careful responses. Issues related to legal suits are discussed further in Chapter 30. Herbst states that major factors include (1) a breakdown in communication and respect between the patient and the physician (remember, angry people sue) and (2) that a client can have unreasonable expectations for a healthy infant even when she has been told the truth about the infant's condition; people have sued for genetic defects. For these and other reasons, in approaching an operative delivery, the client must be fully informed about the benefits and risks and sign the consent only after she indicates understanding of the reasons for the surgery.

INDICATIONS

The surgery may be planned as an elective procedure or done as an emergency just before or during labor when it is evident that the infant will not tolerate vaginal birth. The abdominal route is chosen when additional hypoxic stress must be prevented, when pelvic dimensions are inadequate, or when some pathologic condition is causing excessive maternal or fetal distress. Box 15-7 lists indications for cesarean birth. Emergency cesareans are performed for complications such as placenta previa, premature separation of the placenta, developing severe infection of the uterus, inadequate labor, and fetal distress developing during labor. Surgery is planned when:

- Prenatal testing indicates there is disproportion between the fetal size and the pelvic canal
- There are malpresentations such as breech
- Multiple fetuses are in poor position
- It is known that the placenta is located so as to cause severe bleeding before or during labor (placenta previa)
- Severe hypertension or diabetes exists
- Fetal jeopardy is shown by prenatal assessment

BOX 15-7 Indications For Cesarean Birth

Delay in labor
- In preparatory period: No response to oxytocin, postmaturity
- In active phase: Arrest of dilation, prolonged active phase, or uterine inertia
- In descent phase: CPD, cervical dystocia, uterine inertia

Abnormal presentations
- Brow, mentum, poor flexion of head, occiput posterior position in a primipara
- Transverse position
- Breech position, especially in primigravida

Fetal distress
- Chronic: Poor environment demonstrated by high-risk pregnancy
- Acute: During labor severe changes of UPI, CC, and loss of fetal heart tone or falling pH

Maternal illness
- Placental dysfunction, placenta previa, abruptio placentae, herpes progenitalis (active)
- Diabetes if uncontrolled
- Chronic hypertension, severe preeclampsia
- Cancer of cervix or uterine fibroids
- Repeated stillbirths for no known cause
- Elderly primigravida with other problems

Previous cesarean delivery
- Usually repeat if incision on uterus is classic. Allow labor with careful observation if first incision is into the lower uterine segment.

BOX 15-8 Examples of Criteria For Trial of Labor For VBAC

- Previous cesarean with low transverse uterine incision
- No CPD or fetal complications
- Fetal size under 4000 g
- Physician or midwife in constant attendance
- Continuous fetal monitoring during active labor
- Uterine pressure gauge for monitoring contractions if oxytocin used

Finally, in about a third of cases, cesareans are repeated. It is on this rate that emphasis is being placed. It is safe practice for a number of these women to have a vaginal birth after having had a cesarean (VBAC) (Box 15-8).

TYPES OF INCISIONS

The type of uterine incision is determined by the fetal presentation and by the conditions of surgery. It is important to realize that the type of abdominal incision does not indicate the type of uterine incision. The woman should be informed because one of the first questions asked after an unexpected cesarean is "Do I always have to have surgery for other children?" Only by checking the type of uterine incision can a correct response be given.

An abdominal incision to approach the uterus may be a *vertical* one with a subumbilical or midline incision. Or, a *transverse* incision may be made through skin, muscle, and fascia, usually at the crease just above the mons pubis (Figure 15-18). A uterine incision can be *classic* where the upper segment is incised, or it can be a *lower uterine incision* through the less muscular, more inactive portion of the uterus. This lower uterine incision may be transverse or vertical with the advantages of less bleeding and less tissue repair. However, to reach the lower uterine segment, the bladder must be dissected away because it is attached by fascia to the site. Later it must be resutured. (You can see why a Foley catheter is used to deflate the bladder and how it is possible to nick the bladder during surgery.) Figure 15-19 shows sutures on a vertical incision of the uterus.

Once the incision is made, the physician inserts a hand to grasp the presenting part (Figure 15-20) and pulls. Suction must be available to clear the oropharyngeal airway. (Figure 15-21 shows the prepared setup for cesarean delivery.) Once the infant is out of the uterus, the cord is clamped in two places and cut, and the infant is given to the pediatrician and circulating nurse for immediate care. The placenta is then extracted manually and checked that all pieces are intact. The

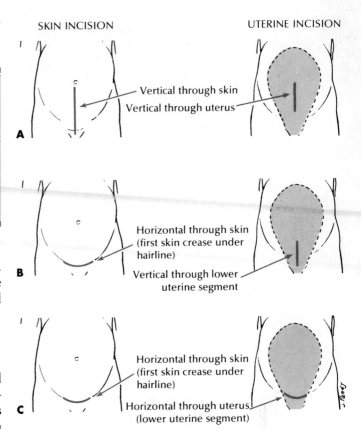

FIGURE 15-18 Cesarean delivery: skin and uterine incisions. **A,** Classic vertical incisions. **B,** Low cervical incision. **C,** Low cervical incision of skin and uterus. (From Bobak IM, Jensen MD: *Maternity and gynecologic care: the nurse and the family,* ed 5, St Louis, 1993, Mosby.)

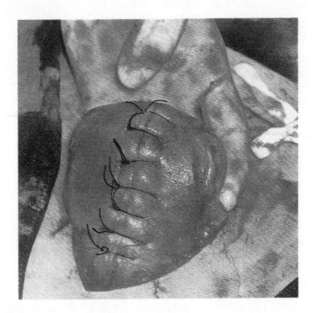

FIGURE 15-19 Suture on vertical uterine incision. (From Al-Azzawi F: *Color atlas of childbirth and obstetric techniques,* St Louis, 1990, Mosby.)

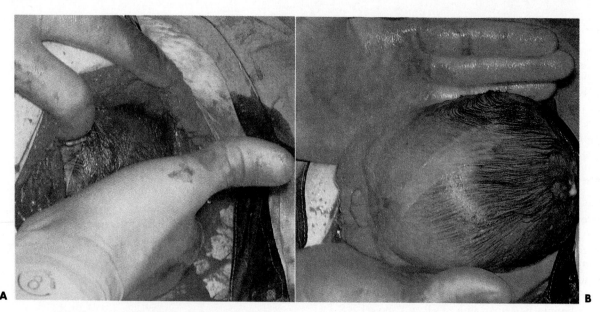

A   B

FIGURE 15-20 Cesarean section delivery. **A,** The surgeon's right hand is inserted under the fetal head, which is levered out through the uterine wound. The baby's nostrils and mouth are cleared by suction as soon as the head is delivered. **B,** The rest of the baby is delivered by the application of traction on the baby's head. The cord is clamped and cut between two artery forceps and the baby passed to the attending pediatrician. (From Al-Azzawi F: *Color atlas of childbirth and obstetric techniques,* St Louis, 1990, Mosby.)

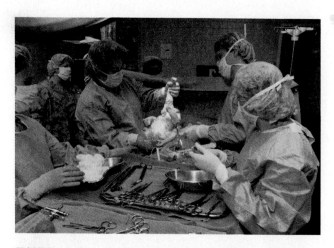

FIGURE 15-21 A newborn infant, delivered through a lower abdominal incision. (Courtesy St John's Mercy Medical Center, St Louis, Mo.)

uterus is massaged and shrinks rapidly. Absorbable sutures are placed from the inner to outer layers (see Figure 15-19) and the fascial, muscle, and skin layers are closed.

Some women have cesarean hysterectomies. The reason may be related to excessive hemorrhage—a lifesaving reason, or the woman may have known that this final step will be taken because she has multiple myomas (fibroids) or carcinoma and this will be the last birth she has planned.

VAGINAL BIRTH AFTER CESAREAN (VBAC)

A vaginal birth after cesarean may be considered in every case, but especially if the surgery was a result of unforeseen causes such as prolapse of the cord, or fetal distress, or where there is an adequate pelvis but the previous infant was very large. If the woman has no pathologic problems or constricted pelvic bony structure, she should be able to go through the labor process (Box 15-8). The major concern is that the scar tissue on the uterus will not be flexible enough to withstand contractions and thus has the possibility of separating from the muscle. Scar separation, if it occurs, may be insidious, or in rare cases a rapid "unzipping" might happen. For this reason, some physicians hesitate to allow VBAC for women who had vertical incisions into the upper segment of the uterus. Since today the majority of incisions are lower uterine, VBAC will become much more common (Taffel et al, 1991).

ACOG (1991) has produced guidelines and with the National Institutes of Health has encouraged physicians and midwives to allow a trial of labor to every prior cesarean case. Each hospital unit formulates a protocol to be followed. These procedures include presence of a physician or midwife during the labor, fetal and uterine monitoring, and extremely careful use of oxytocin and/or Prostin gel.

Observations must be made for fetal distress that may indicate uterine problems, signs of uterine scar separation such as an irregular change in contractions or uterine outline, increased vaginal bleeding, and poor labor progress. The woman needs much support and help if the trial is not successful. There has been a varied response; when physicians are committed to VBAC, more occur. Graham (1984) found that 60% of women with previous cesareans were able to deliver vaginally. Other studies show a rate of 20% to 40%.

PREPARATION FOR OPERATIVE BIRTH

Parents need to be aware of the possibilities of planned or emergency cesareans during labor. For planned surgery, preparation includes a conference with the anesthesiologist and a tour of the surgical and recovery areas (see Chapter 12 for prenatal teaching plan). The client needs to know the types of treatments that will be used (Box 15-9). She should arrange for the presence of her partner in the delivery room. In any case, he should be present until the time of surgery and directly after to experience some of the excitement of the birth (Figure 15-22). Regional anesthesia is used for planned cesareans almost universally; the mother is awake and may converse with her partner, who is at her shoulders.

When a woman is to have a cesarean after labor has been in progress, she depends much more on the nursing staff for meeting her health care needs. Nursing care moves from a supportive, teaching role to a partially or wholly compensatory focus. You must expect that the mother and her partner will experience some (Donovan and Allen, 1977) or all of the following:

1. Relief if the labor was long, difficult, and painful
2. Anxiety and fear that something will happen unexpectedly to the mother or infant as a result of surgery
3. Guilt related to the woman's behavior during labor or any activity in the weeks before

---

BOX 15-9 Topics for Preoperative Preparation For Cesarean Birth

Process of preparation and procedures
   Blood work
   Skin prep
   Bladder care
   Intravenous line
Anesthesia choice discussed with anesthesiologist
   Additional questions answered by nurse
Presence of partner and when both will see infant after birth
Postoperative self-care: demonstrate techniques
   Cough and deep breathing methods
   Splinting/supporting incision
   Positioning for sleep, breast-feeding infant
   Becoming ambulatory
   Isometrics
   Pain and other medications
Process of involution and self-care in home recovery

---

4. Anger directed, in general, at the childbirth educator for not giving a more complete understanding of the possibility of cesarean, at the physician for a possibly perceived lack of communication, or sometimes at the infant for being too small, being too big, or causing its mother such trouble
5. Bewilderment, sadness, or loneliness, feelings of failure, frustration, and regret because of a lost normal experience
6. Helplessness and dependence robbing parents of their sense of control

These feelings may continue well into the first year. Use these potential problems to indicate nursing diagnoses for the couple. See Chapter 17 for further discussion.

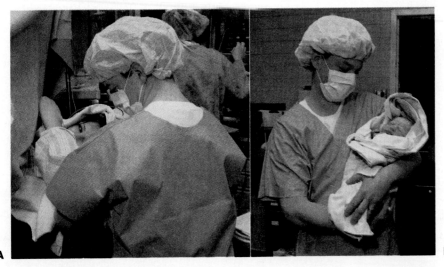

FIGURE 15-22 **A,** Parents' first look at the new baby during the cesarean. **B,** Father-infant bonding is important. (Courtesy St John's Mercy Medical Center, St Louis, Mo.)

A   B

NURSING CARE PLAN • Assisted Surgical Birth

Case: Angela M., Para 1-0-0-1, and her partner, Bruce, have been in the LDR since midnight. Their birth plan indicates no analgesia and an early discharge. Contractions slowed and oxytocin drip was started to stimulate labor. At 10 AM when cervix was 6 cm and station +1, an epidural was started. Five hours later station was still +1 and dilation was 8 cm. However, variable decelerations with a late component appeared and progressed despite interventions. Because fetal pH showed falling readings and there was a maternal temperature of 100° F, a cesarean was indicated.

ASSESSMENT DATA

1. Childbirth education classes taught possibility of cesarean.
   Parents anxious about fetal status.
   Support by partner is positive.
2. Position and station indicate delayed descent, signs of distress.
   Possible factors leading to infection.

3. Epidural in place, effective analgesia. Oxygen by mask.
   Hydration adequate as shown by output.
   Oxytocin stopped because of variables. Positioned on left side.

NURSING DIAGNOSES

1. Knowledge deficit regarding anesthesia, postoperative care.
2. High risk for reduced fetal and maternal perfusion related to anesthesia and evidence of maternal complications.

3. Anxiety and fear for self and infant related to surgical procedure.
4. Altered self-esteem related to not following birth plan.

EXPECTED OUTCOMES

1. Fetal and maternal perfusion maintained.
2. Infection prevented or controlled by interventions.
3. Effective coping skills used to reduce anxiety.

4. Adjustment after birth to fact of surgical birth progresses normally.

NURSING INTERVENTIONS

1. Maintain side-lying position, oxygen by mask.
   Monitor vital signs every 30 minutes.
   Record maternal fluid intake and response to regional anesthesia.
   Encourage voiding, insert Foley catheter before surgery.
   Monitor recovery for infection, bleeding, change in vital signs.
2. During preparations for cesarean section maintain continuous monitoring of heart rate and contractions.
   Assist with fetal blood sampling. Monitor newborn for scalp injury.

3. Assess if couple understands the reasons for surgical intervention.
   Encourage verbalization of feelings. Use positive reinforcement of coping strategies.
   Ensure that support person remains with her during preparation and in delivery room.
4. Use positive reinforcement of cesarean as an alternative birthing method.
   Focus on infant's need for safe birth.
   Encourage bonding activity after birth.
   Diffuse any anger by answering all implied or frank questions.

EVALUATION

1. Was maternal and fetal perfusion maintained adequately?
2. Did the mother tolerate surgery without complications?

3. Was infant healthy? Apgar scores above 7?
4. Was self-esteem maintained despite birth plan? Does Angela understand there may be lingering negative feelings during the first year?

Be especially aware that anxiety inhibits the couple's ability to understand information. They should not go into the recovery period without a clear grasp of the reasons for the decision to operate. This will be accentuated if they were prepared only for an unmedicated vaginal birth.

The results of these feelings may be loss of self-esteem and emotional distress, which are discussed in depth in Chapters 17 and 26. Explanations and support may reduce the intensity of the sense of loss (see Nursing Care Plan). Emphasize positive care of the infant. Enable attachment as soon as possible after birth. Assure the parents that the staff are monitoring the condition of the infant and mother. And finally, explain everything before performing preparatory procedures.

Unexpected Birth

Any birth occurring outside a planned, prepared environment is considered unexpected. Before the emphasis on home births, an emergency delivery was considered any delivery outside the delivery room of a hospital. Today many births take place in alternative settings, with preparation, supervision, and backup provisions if complications occur.

Unexpected birth occurs when labor progresses rapidly, usually in less than 4 hours; often this birth is referred to as a *precipitous* delivery. Women who deliver this way generally fall into three groups: those with unusually rapid preterm labor, those with rapid progressions through stages of term labor and a high threshold for pain, and those who are uninformed or do not understand ways to seek help (for example, women with a language barrier, a terrified teenager, or one who is mentally retarded). For these women, psychosocial problems or environmental problems may complicate care. Unexpected birth may occur at home, in a clinic, in the hospital, in transport, or in a public place. Birth en route to the hospital may be caused by external events, such as traffic jams and car breakdown. Health personnel must be informed about steps of support and care during emergency delivery.

BIRTH IN A DISASTER SETTING

Birth during an emergency or disaster may result when the pregnant woman is sequestered in a shelter or marooned in an isolated place. If birth is in a disaster setting, everyone usually protects the woman and infant. Follow the basic guidelines, remembering that the recovery care must include fluids for mother and infant. If there is no way to sterilize a knife, select the cleanest material to tie and cut the cord. Monitor mother and newborn for thermoregulation, fluid balance, and nutri-

tion. See Box 15-10 for information to record after the birth.

BIRTH IN A PUBLIC PLACE

The environmental setting dictates what is available to aid in a delivery. For example, in a public place, soda may be available as a fluid to use for rinsing hands and the perineum. The following interventions apply to a public place and may be modified for other settings:

1. Labor *always* progresses through a step-by-step pattern to delivery. In many emergency cases, progress is merely more rapid through phases than in normal labor.

2. Panic in the woman and the assistants must be avoided. The most knowledgeable person should take charge. Send volunteers for equipment and help. Maintain a calm atmosphere. Get the woman to focus, helping herself by correct breathing and position.

3. Cooperate with the natural forces of labor because skill in manipulation or instruments are absent. Do not do vaginal assessments of dilation. External signs are clearly recognizable. Position the woman to facilitate delivery: a semisitting or squatting position to push, and a Sims position or semisitting for delivery. Position to allow space at the perineum to manipulate the shoulders during the final moments of birth.

4. The infant must be protected against respiratory dysfunction and cold stress; anticipate and fulfill fluid and nutritional needs of the mother and infant.

5. Put the infant to the nipple to stimulate oxytocin release. Skin-to-skin contact, with the baby covered by the woman's clothing, helps to prevent chilling.

BOX 15-10   Information To Record

- Fetal position and presentation
- Color and any unusual odor of the amniotic fluid
- If the cord was around the neck; number of loops
- Time of delivery of entire body
- Estimate of Apgar score
- Resuscitation efforts
- Condition of infant
- Sex of infant
- Time of placental birth and appearance, with amount of bleeding
- Woman's condition: interventions to control bleeding, condition of perineum

Nursing Responsibilities
▶ NURSING DIAGNOSES

Although nursing diagnoses are not formulated in this emergency, think through which would apply.

1. Fear related to setting, lack of preparation, loss of control.
2. High risk for altered tissue integrity and infection related to trauma of birth.
3. High risk for altered maternal-fetal perfusion related to rapid birth.
4. Ineffective thermoregulation related to environmental temperature.
5. High risk for altered oxygenation of newborn if adequate assistance is not available.

▶ EXPECTED OUTCOMES

1. Woman is cooperative and responsive to nursing assistance.
2. Completes uneventful birth of a viable infant.
3. Infant exhibits consistent body temperature between 97° and 98° F.

▶ NURSING INTERVENTIONS

In making a decision about the timing of birth, determine your options. Evaluate the location. Enlist someone to get help, someone to control a potential crowd, and someone to get equipment. Suggested types of equipment are listed below.

For cleansing the mother	Water with dishwashing liquid, or wipe down with underclothes
For padding or protection during delivery	Newspapers (unused), when in a public space, large plastic bags, old sheets, towels, shower curtain
To clear infant's airway	Ear bulb syringe, meat basting syringe, and manual milking of nose and throat
For the cord (if no help available)	Strong yarn, new razor blade, scissors or knife (flame sterilized) (only if no help to be available)
To warm the baby	Mother's clothes, skin-to-skin contact, blanket, towel, sheet, clean newspapers, padded box
To feed the baby if no help available	Milk powder, bottle, nipple (if not breast-feeding)
Fluids for the mother	Any available

Follow Figures 15-23 and 15-24 to note the hand positions for the delivery of the head and shoulders.

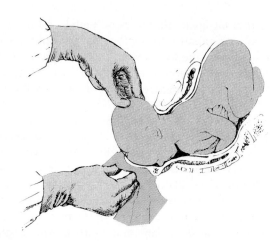

FIGURE 15-23 Assistance may be needed if head does not extend smoothly (Ritgen's maneuver). Exert hand pressure downward on occiput with forward pressure applied to obstetric perineum, just between vaginal and anal openings. Feel for chin, and exert forward pressure on it through perineal tissue. For emergency delivery, use article of mother's clothing (cleanest material available) because skin will be slippery. (From Willson JR: *Altas of obstetric technic,* ed 2, St Louis, 1969, Mosby.)

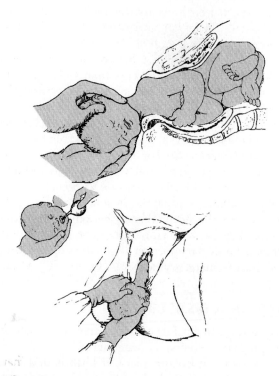

FIGURE 15-24 Baby's head is gently directed downward to help in partial delivery of anterior (upper) shoulder to "park" it under the symphysis pubis. Then proceed with delivery of lower shoulder by pulling up on the head. (From Willson JR: *Atlas of obstetric technic,* ed 2, St Louis, 1969, Mosby.)

When the birth occurs in a health care facility, a birthing pack is available for precipitous birth. When birth is outside a facility, you must use what is prepared or available.

For the delivery process, follow the mechanisms of labor. It is most important to provide a controlled birth. Have the woman pant so she does not push until you direct her to push. To avoid a laceration, if sterile gloves are available, massage the perineum, with first finger inside the vagina, helping to stretch out the labia. When the head crowns, support the perineum with gentle back pressure to prevent lacerations. If the head has difficulty emerging, use the Ritgen maneuver (Figure 15-23).

When the head emerges, the amniotic sac will usually rupture if it has not already. If it does not, puncture it and remove membranes (the caul) from the infant's face so breathing may start. Check for loops of the umbilical cord around the neck. Slip the loop over the head and pull the slack to slip it over the shoulder. If the cord is tight and needs to be clamped while in place, use the two clamps provided in the delivery kit and cut between those clamps. *If there is no equipment,* gently stretch the cord to slide the loop over the head.

Wipe any blood and mucus off the face using towels or the woman's clothing. Clear the mouth of mucus with a cloth over fingers or a suction bulb if available. "Milk" the nose and throat by applying moderate stroking pressure on the throat in the direction of mouth if no suction equipment is available. In the same way, gently squeeze and expel mucus from the nose.

Delivery of the shoulders proceeds by first pulling the anterior shoulder under the symphysis pubis and then carefully easing the posterior shoulder out by gently pulling up on the head. An assistant may apply gentle but steady pressure on the fundus if the shoulders seem difficult to deliver. The slippery body will quickly follow. Grasp the body firmly, supporting the head and trunk with one arm. The infant must be immediately dried off and should be placed on the woman's abdomen with the head in a slightly dependent position to drain mucus. Protect the infant from cold by drying and covering the infant and have the woman hold him securely. Observe respirations, color, and activity. You should estimate an Apgar score for later report (Box 15-10).

Do not rush to tie and cut the cord. Because the infant's first breath will close fetal circulation, the cord *does not* have to be tied and cut if no sterile equipment is available. If no help will be forthcoming, the cord may be cut after it has been tied when the knife or razor blade has been cleaned, if ties are available.

The placenta will be ready for birth in a few minutes. You will see a gush of blood preceding lengthening of the cord at the vagina. It is appropriate to wait up to an hour for separation of the placenta. The infant should be put to the breast to lick or suck the nipple while waiting for separation. When the uterus rises up into a globular shape and the cord lengthens at the vagina, ask the woman to push down to give birth to the placenta.

Have a newspaper ready to catch the placenta; wrap it after you briefly examine it for missing pieces. Then ask the woman to rub her fundus. Continue the infant at her breast to stimulate oxytocin release. Save the placenta for complete examination if the woman is to be transferred to a health care facility.

Assess the state of the perineum. If lacerations have occurred, obtain ice if possible; wrap it in plastic and then newspaper or piece of clean sheeting and place it at the perineum to assist with hemostasis. Watch the uterus for atony and assess the amount of bleeding. Obtain assistance as necessary to move the woman for observation and follow-up care.

An unexpected birth can be a pleasant, successful experience or a frightening one for the woman and attendant. The person in charge makes the difference. If the birth occurs at home, the infant may be bathed in a gentle warm water bath while the family gathers around to enjoy the new baby. Remember the predictability and naturalness of the event while remaining alert for evidence of problems.

▶ EVALUATION

The results of the unexpected birth would be safe if:
- No injury occurred to mother or infant.
- The woman was supported during the process.
- Assistance was obtained for any problems.
- Recovery of mother and infant proceeded normally.

KEY POINTS

- The nurse's attentiveness to the client means that she will be often at the bedside to support the coach and see that ability to cope and progress of BDEs are maintained.
- Clients who have an attentive nurse have less tendency to lose control and thus be unable to cooperate during the second stage of labor.

- Induction is truly difficult for the woman because of anxiety about labor, fatigue because of the extended labor, and more intense discomfort related to oxytocics.
- Induction is unique in that the aim is to begin labor in the active phase, i.e., contractions of 2 to 3 minutes apart lasting 30 to 50 seconds.

- The Friedman graph describes the so-called average labor; some women progress faster, many in a normal slower pattern.
- Bearing-down efforts need not begin as soon as the cervix is dilated fully. Instead, allow the reorganization of the first phase and follow the woman's own involuntary BDEs. Remember to prevent the Valsalva maneuver and adverse effects of extended breath-holding.
- Position in labor and for birth is a crucial nursing responsibility and promotes an intact perineum.
- Discuss caput, cephalhematoma, and head molding with the new parents when ventouse or forceps have been used, to allay fears of deformity.
- Assisted birth takes many forms, with the goal of an active, viable infant.

- Clients prepared for cesarean birth recover faster with less guilt and sadness. Those who have emergency intervention often grieve over the lost normal birth and wonder what they did wrong in the process. This grieving lasts well into the first year; client may benefit from counseling.
- VBAC is now considered for all repeat cesareans unless there are accompanying complications, CPD, and/or a vertical uterine incision.
- When birth takes place in public places or during a disaster, the mother and infant must be protected from injury, infection, cold, stress, and hemorrhage. The most knowledgeable person should take charge.

STUDY QUESTIONS

Match key terms with the statements below.

15-1
  a. The vaginal opening shows the fetal head between contractions _____ . *Crowning*
  b. There is delayed descent requiring assistance with birth _____ . *Aystocia*
  c. A tear results from the extreme stretching of the perineum _____ . *Laceration*
  d. Blood pressure falls and fetal perfusion is affected by _____ . *Valsalvas Maneuver*
  e. A pushing technique that fosters good oxygenation of the fetus *Open glottis*

15-2 Ann needs instruction on the breathing pattern for second stage pushing. This breathing is correct when the following is done during a contraction.
  a. Holds breath and pushes toward vagina, releasing air at 30 seconds, repeating until contraction is over.
  b. Pushes down at the diaphragm, holding breath for as long as possible during contraction.
  c. Inhales and pushes down while very slowly releasing air, repeats every 15 seconds for duration of contraction.
  d. Pushes down ad lib, as if to defecate when she feels the involuntary urge to push.

15-3 A woman, para 0-0-2-0, is bearing down with contractions. The nurse notes caput at the introitus. After calling for assistance, the next most appropriate action would be:
  a. Ask the woman to pant with the next contraction, prepare for transfer to delivery room.

  b. Tell her to stop pushing while you prepare for the birth.
  c. Turn her on her left side.
  d. Stay with her, providing reassurance.

15-4 Descent, flexion, internal rotation, and extension allow normal birth. These movements are designed to:
  a. Shorten the second stage of labor.
  b. Ease the passage of infant through birth canal.
  c. Allow smallest presenting diameter to pass through first.
  d. Allow the infant to be born in an occiput position.

15-5 Why is it safe to use oxytocin (Pitocin) for induction when protocols for its use are followed?
  a. There are several effective antagonists that may be administered.
  b. Fetal heart rates do not respond to oxytocin.
  c. The drug follows a physiologic pattern even if too much is given.
  d. Rapid metabolism results in a very short half-life.

15-6. Match the phase of second stage labor with the signs listed below.
  a. Contractions change character, become regular, 3 to 5 minutes apart
  b. Anus bulges, perineum distends
  c. Fetal part may be seen at introitus, even between contractions
  1. Phase one
  2. Phase two
  3. Phase three

Phase one, b. Phase three, c. Phase two
15-1 a. Crowning b. Aystocia c. Laceration d. Valsalva's maneuver e. Open glottis 15-2 c. 15-3 d. 15-4 c. 15-5 d. 15-6 a.

REFERENCES

American College of Obstetricians and Gynecologists: *Induction and augmentation of labor.* In Technical Bulletin 157, Washington DC, 1991, ACOG.

Aderhold KJ, Roberts JE: Phases of the second stage of labor, *J Nurse Midwifery* 36:267, 1991.

Akhoury HA et al: Oxytocin augmentation of labor and perinatal outcome in nulliparas, *Obstet Gynecol* 78:227, 1991.

Avery MD, Burket BA: Effect of perineal massage on incidence of episiotomy and perineal laceration in a nurse-midwifery service, *J Nurs Midwifery* 31:128, 1986.

Beischer NA, MacKay LV: *Obstetrics and the newborn*, ed 2, Sydney, 1993, Harcourt, Brace, Jovanovich Group.

Bergstrom L et al: "You'll feel me touching you, sweetie": vaginal examinations during the second stage of labor, *Birth* 19(1):10, 1992.

Blackman ST, Loper DL: *Maternal, fetal, and neonatal physiology*, Philadelphia, 1992, WB Saunders.

Brodsky PL, Pelzar EM: Rationale for the revision of oxytocin administration protocols, *J Obstet Gynecol Neonatal Nurs* 20:440, 1991.

Bromberg M: Presumptive maternal benefits of routine episiotomy: a literature review, *J Nurse Midwifery* 31:121, 1986.

Brown ST et al: Characteristics of labor pain at two stages of cervical dilation, *Pain* 38:289, 1989.

Caldero-Barcia R: Influence of maternal position on time of spontaneous rupture of membranes, progress of labor and fetal head progression, *Birth Family J* 6:7, 1979.

Chalmers JA, Chalmers I: The obstetric vacuum extractor is the instrument of choice for operative vaginal delivery, *Br J Obstet Gynaecol* 96:505, 1989.

Combs CA et al: Prolonged third stage of labor—morbidity and risk factors, *Obstet Gynecol* 78:893, 1991.

Cosner RK, deJong E: Physiologic second-stage labor, *Am J Maternal Child Nurs, MCN* 18(1):38, 1993.

Cucco C et al: Maternal-fetal outcomes in prolonged pregnancy, *Am J Obstet Gynecol* 161:916, 1989.

Davis-Floyd R: Routines and rituals in childbirth: a new view, *NAACOG Update Series* 5:1, 1986.

Darwood MY: Evolving concepts of oxytocin induction of labor, *Am J Perinatol* 6:167, 1989.

Dell DL, Lightler SE, Plauché WC: Soft cup vacuum extractions: a comparison of outlet delivery, *Obstet Gynecol* 71:624, 1985.

Donovan B, Allen RM: The cesarean birth method, *J Obstet Gynecol Neonatal Nurs* 6:37, 1977.

Flamm BL et al: Vaginal birth after cesarean delivery—results of a five-year multicenter collaborative study, *Obstet Gynecol* 76:750, 1990.

Friedman F: Failure to progress in labor. In Queenan J, ed: *Management of high-risk pregnancy*, Oradell, NJ, 1985, Medical Economics Books.

Galvan B et al: Obstetric vacuum extraction, *J Obstet Gynecol Neonatal Nurs* 16:242, 1987.

Garfield RE et al: Increased myometrial responsiveness to oxytocin during term and preterm labor, *Am J Obstet Gynecol* 161:454, 1989.

Gardosi J et al: Alternative positions in the second stage of labour, randomized controlled trial, *Br J Obstet Gynaecol* 96:1290, 1990.

Gordon H, Logue M: Perineal muscle function after childbirth, *Lancet* 2:123, 1985.

Goyert GL et al: The physician factor in cesarean birth rates, *N Engl J Med* 320:706, 1987.

Graham A: Trial of labor following previous cesarean section, *Am J Obstet Gynecol* 149:35, 1984.

Green JR et al: Factors associated with rectal injury in spontaneous deliveries, *Obstet Gynecol* 73(Part I):732, 1989.

Hagadorn-Freathy A S et al: Validation of the 1988 ACOG forceps classification system, *Obstet Gynecol* 77:356, 1991.

Hanagan WC: Tentorial hemorrhage associated with vacuum extraction, *Pediatrics* 85:534, 1990.

Herbst AL: Medical professional liability and obstetric care: the Institute of Medicine report and recommendations, *Obstet Gynecol* 75:705, 1989.

Jennings B et al: Use of prostaglandins in nurse-midwifery practice, *J Nurse Midwifery* 34(3):137, 1989.

Klein-Kaye V et al: The use of fundal pressure during the second stage of labor, *J Obstet Gynecol Neonatal Nurs* 19:511, 1990.

Knauth D: Effect of pushing techniques in birthing chair on length of second stage of labor, *Nurs Res* 35:49, 1986.

Laube D: Forceps delivery, *Clin Obstet Gynecol* 29:286, 1986.

Laufer A et al: Vaginal birth after cesarean section: nurse-midwifery management, *J Nurs Midwifery* 32:41, 1987.

Lightfoot-Klein H et al: Special needs of ritually circumcised women patients, *J Obstet Gynecol Neonatal Nurs* 20:102, 1991.

MacKay SM, Roberts JE: Second stage of labor: what is normal? *J Obstet Gynecol Neonatal Nurs* 14:101, 1985.

Mahomed K et al: External cephalic version at term—a randomized controlled trial using tocolysis, *Br J Obstet Gynaecol* 98:8, 1991.

McKay S, Roberts J: Second stage labor: what is normal, J Obstet Gynecol Neonatal Nurs 14(2):101, 1985.

Myers SA et al: A successful program to lower the cesarean-section rates, *N Engl J Med* 319:1511, 1988.

Nurses Association of the American College of Obstetricians and Gynecologists: *OGN Nursing Practice resource: the nurse's role in the induction/augmentation of labor*, Washington DC, 1988, NAACOG.

Nodine PM, Roberts JE: Factors associated with perineal outcome during childbirth, *J Nurs Midwifery* 32:123, 1989.

Odent MR: Position in delivery, *Lancet* 335:1166, 1990.

Oxhorn H: *Human labor and birth*, ed 5, New York, 1986, Appleton-Century-Crofts.

Paine LL, Tinker DD: The effect of maternal bearing-down efforts on arterial umbilical cord pH and length of the second stage of labor, *J Nurse Midwifery* 37(1):61, 1992.

Pitkin RM: Once a cesarean, *Obstet Gynecol* 77:939, 1991.

Roberts J et al: A descriptive analysis of involuntary bearing-down efforts, *J Obstet Gynecol Neonatal Nurs* 16:48, 1987.

Rosen MG et al: Vaginal birth after cesarean—a meta-analysis of morbidity and mortality, *Obstet Gynecol* 77:465, 1991.

Schifrin BS et al: Labor's dysfunctional lexicon, *Obstet Gynecol* 74:121, 1989.

Spielman FJ, Herbert WNP: Maternal cardiovascular effects of drugs that alter uterine activity, *Obstet Gynecol Surv* 43(9):516, 1988.

Taffel SM et al: 1989 U.S. cesarean section rate steading—VBAC rate rises to nearly one in five, *Birth* 18(2): 73, 1991.

Thorpe JM, Bowes WA: Episiotomy: can its routine use be defended? *Am J Obstet Gynecol* 160(Part I):1027, 1989.

Varney H: *Nurse-midwifery*, Boston, 1987, Blackwell Scientific.

US Department of Health and Human Services: *Cesarean childbirth*, Bethsada, MD, 1981, National Institutes of Health.

🔬 STUDENT RESOURCE SHELF

Dundes L: Evolution of maternal birthing position, *Am J Public Health* 77:636, 1987.
A review of how birth has been handled in various decades.

Metzger BL, Therrien B: Effect of position on cardiovascular response during the Valsalva maneuver, *Nurs Res* 39:198, 1990.
Answers the questions about pushing techniques.

Perinatal Guidelines for Drugs and Anesthesia

KEY TERMS

Action
Acupressure
Acupuncture
Analgesia
Anesthesia
Benefit-to-Risk Ratio
Cricoid Pressure
Effect
Endorphin
Enterohepatic
 Recycling
Epidural
Equigesic Dose
Equilibrium
Half-Life (t½)
Informed Consent
Ionization
Membrane Barriers

Minimum Effective
 Concentration
 (MEC)
Nociceptors
Patient-Controlled
 Epidural Analgesia
 (PCEA)

Saturation
Somatic Pain
Time-Dose Interval
Transcutaneous
 Electric Nerve
 Stimulation (TENS)
Visceral Pain

LEARNING OBJECTIVES

1. *Describe medication risks in relation to the phases of pregnancy and lactation.*
2. *Correlate physiologic changes of pregnancy with medication absorption and excretion patterns.*
3. *Identify the significant membrane barriers regulating medication passage to the fetus and newborn.*
4. *Relate the precautions of medication and anesthesia use during the transitional period of labor.*
5. *Explore alternatives to analgesic use during labor.*
6. *Describe nursing interventions when drugs are used because of altered comfort.*
7. *Explain medication precautions necessary during lactation.*

Drugs and Pregnancy

Most women are aware of questions about medication use during pregnancy, but "taking a pill" is a habit for many when they have symptoms such as a headache, fatigue, or an allergy. In addition, many women do not understand that alcohol and nicotine are adverse drugs.

We use the word *drugs* to mean prescription, nonprescription medications, chemicals, and additives in food and the environment.

Nurses administer medication and are counselors for women regarding drug effects. To provide safe care, nurses should know medication basics as a result of their pharmacology study and apply this knowledge to the welfare of the woman and the fetus. A thorough understanding of the adverse effects of drugs during the phases of pregnancy is, of course, important.

The physiologic changes of pregnancy affect a woman's response to medications. Physiologic changes in hormonal levels, body water, fatty tissue, albumin levels, and increased blood volume influence medication distribution and use. Changes in kidney function influence excretion rates. Mechanisms that regulate placental drug transfer and, after delivery, movement of agents across the membranes separating maternal blood and breast milk are particularly relevant to the pregnant woman and her infant.

The nine months of pregnancy should be viewed as a constantly changing, complex interaction between the woman and fetus. Most drugs taken in by the mother cross the placenta, achieving **equilibrium,** a state of balance, in the fetus and woman. In some cases there may be a higher concentration in fetal circulation than in maternal circulation. Unbound drugs of low molecular weight cross easily. Molecular weights over 1000 usually prevent the drug molecule from crossing; examples are insulin and heparin.

The first Collaborative Perinatal Project (Neswander and Gordon, 1973) studied the histories of 53,000 women from a number of large hospital centers and found that each woman used at least four different drugs while pregnant. Some used as many as nine. Because of the publicity generated from the findings, a general awareness of the potential for adverse effects has developed. Today many women avoid most medications during pregnancy; others are apprehensive about taking any at all. A large number of uninformed women, however, still self-medicate.

The most commonly used drugs are analgesics, antacids, antibiotics, antiemetics, antihistamines, diuretics, iron and vitamin supplements, sedatives, alcohol, and cigarettes. Over-the-counter (OTC) medications are a serious concern because of the variable doses women take; too often the OTC drug has been on the home medicine shelf and is outdated. Inadvertent ingestion of environmental pollutants also may affect both the woman and the fetus. (See Chapter 27 for discussion of teratogenic effects of these substances.)

BENEFIT-TO-RISK RATIO

The **benefit-to-risk ratio** determines if the benefit to the woman or fetus is greater than the risk of a worsening maternal condition or fetal compromise because of the medication or the mother's illness. Table 27-7 lists the FDA categories for drug labeling to indicate risk during pregnancy.

INFORMED CONSENT

All women who need to receive prescribed drugs during pregnancy should give their **informed consent.** They should understand the benefit-to-risk ratio and agree to be medicated. It is a violation of the woman's rights to withhold this information from her or to be unsure that she understands the language in which the information is given. Lawsuits may be initiated because the woman is angry over violation of her right to know how a drug may affect her infant (see Chapters 27 and 30). A current example is the drug isotretinoin (Accutane). More than 1000 severe birth defects and many miscarriages have been reported as a result of women taking the drug during the first trimester.

Drug Absorption

Drug absorption is modified during pregnancy. The mechanisms of diffusion, facilitated diffusion, active transport, filtration, and pinocytosis cause the drug molecule to be moved across body membranes as they do in nonpregnant states.

ABSORPTION ACROSS BODY MEMBRANES

A drug must be absorbed to reach its site of action. Absorption usually involves penetration through a membrane made of lipid (fat) and protein molecules containing small pores through which water and some water-soluble substances can move. The degree of **ionization** of a drug influences its ability to be absorbed and excreted. *Fat-soluble* medications tend to be nonionized and are absorbed easily. *Water-soluble* medications tend to be ionized and less easily absorbed. Drugs can be altered to become more or less ionized when in a pH environment different from their own. Acid drugs become more ionized in an alkaline pH such as the small intestine. Alkaline drugs become more ionized in an acidic environment such as the stomach or duodenum.

Figure 16-1 shows a schematic drawing of the way drugs move across membrane barriers. Each molecule of drug is headed for its specific receptor site. Note the different "shapes" indicating different bonding into different tissues; note also the electrical (ion) charges.

Membrane barriers to consider during pregnancy are the placental barrier, the blood-brain barrier, and, during lactation, the blood-milk barrier.

Placental Barrier

The placental barrier is not a barrier but is rather like a sieve. It is made up of the chorionic cells that line the villi in the placenta. The thickness diminishes from 25 to 2 mμ during pregnancy, meaning that permeability increases as the fetus approaches birth. Usually,

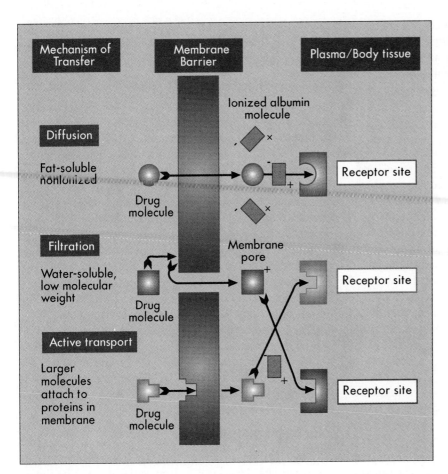

FIGURE 16-1 How medications cross body membranes. (Modified from Dickason EJ, Schult MO, Morris EM: *Maternal and infant drugs,* New York, 1978, McGraw-Hill.)

within minutes of maternal intake of a drug, the free, unbound portion of the drug crosses over to the fetus. Technical measurements of maternal/fetal ratios are given with one as the maternal measurement, for example, 1:0.8. The ratio indicates that proportionately the fetus has 80% of the mother's serum level. Most drugs, except those of high molecular weight, cross easily depending on the gradient, that is, the difference in concentration of the drug in the mother compared with the fetus.

Blood-Brain Barrier

The blood-brain barrier is the lipoid (fatty) sheath of myelin around the capillaries and nerves of the brain that separates brain tissue from extracellular fluid (ECF). It has no pores and because capillaries are covered with a tight lipoid sheath, lipid-soluble, non-protein bound drugs have the greatest possibility of entering the brain tissue. Anoxia and trauma alter the permeability of the blood-brain barrier, a point important to remember for high-risk infants.

During fetal life a higher proportion of blood flow is distributed to the fetal brain. The results can be seen in the effects of opioids and barbiturates, which concentrate in higher amounts in the fetal brain than in the maternal brain. This is one of the reasons for depressed responses if birth is too close to maternal sedative intake.

Because the myelin sheath develops gradually, the degree of permeability is related to gestational age; that is, the younger the fetus, the more easily drugs may enter the fetal brain. Because of this increased permeability, a preterm infant is more affected by maternal sedation than a full-term infant.

Blood-Milk Barrier

The blood-milk barrier follows the same principles as the blood-brain barrier. (See Medication Excretion in Breast Milk.)

ABSORPTION THROUGH THE GASTROINTESTINAL TRACT

Absorption of a medication taken orally is affected primarily by the dose and form (e.g., liquid, tablet, spansule, enteric coating), gastrointestinal motility, presence and type of food in stomach, and the pH of the stomach, duodenum, and intestine. Medication taken together or with certain foods may enhance or inhibit absorption; for instance, ferrous compounds are inhibited by milk and enhanced by citrus juice.

During pregnancy the digestive tract changes in many ways. Reduced formation of hydrochloric acid leads to slower absorption when a drug needs an acid environment. In addition, slower gastric emptying delays movement if absorption is only in the duodenum or intestine.

PARENTERAL ABSORPTION

During pregnancy, circulation time is faster, blood volume and cardiac output are increased, and renal clearance is faster. If medications are injected intravenously, they always *must be diluted and injected slowly.* A bolus is required for only a few drugs. All intermittent infusions should follow the time schedule and be diluted with at least the minimum amount indicated by the manufacturer. Drugs that are continuously infused maintain an almost equal serum level on both sides of the placental barrier. Therefore when a medication is continuously infused, the level in the fetus may be higher than levels when the drug is given orally or by intermittent infusion.

DERMATOMUCOSAL ABSORPTION

During pregnancy, all *mucous membranes have enhanced blood supply* so drugs are absorbed more quickly than in the nonpregnant state. In the United States, there has been concern about povidone-iodine preparations occasionally used for vaginal examinations during labor. Iodine is absorbed across the mucous membrane; because of this, another lubricant should be used. The agent always should be washed off the skin because some clients are allergic to this substance.

Lung alveolar membrane has a very rapid rate of absorption because it is thin and its rich blood supply is augmented during pregnancy. Depending on the size of the aerosol particles, medication will be delivered to nasal passages, trachea, or smaller airways. Because of augmented circulation to the lung tissue and some hyperventilation during pregnancy, *use of general anesthetic gases results in more rapid induction of anesthesia.*

Bioavailability: Distribution and Metabolism

Many factors influence how long the drug will affect the fetus before being returned to the maternal circulation to be metabolized and excreted by the mother. These factors are tissue and protein binding, the state of ionization of the drug, the pH of the fluids and acidity of the drug, and the half-life of the drug.

HALF-LIFE

Half-life ($t\frac{1}{2}$) is the time period in which half the absorbed dose is metabolized or made inactive. Knowl-

edge of the medication's half-life especially affects the timing of doses during transition, labor, and the newborn period.

Minimum Effective Concentration

One way to measure medication absorption, distribution, and metabolic rate is by determining the level of **minimum effective concentration (MEC)** in the blood. Doses should be given at intervals close enough to maintain the correct MEC but not close enough to let the concentration enter the toxic range; in addition, the dosage should not be too low or infrequent and thus made ineffective. *Rapidly metabolized medications must be given at closer intervals.* Some medications (e.g., oxytocin) require continuous intravenous infusion to be very effective because of a half-life of 3 to 6 minutes. Other drugs such as magnesium sulfate have a very narrow therapeutic range and without careful monitoring may easily reach toxic levels.

Medications that are highly tissue or protein bound take longer to reach the MEC and may need to be given only once or twice a day. Such drugs may need a "loading" dose to bring the client up into the MEC more quickly (Figure 16-2).

PROTEIN BINDING

To be effective, a drug must be free to move to its receptor site. However, a drug molecule may be linked to an albumin molecule or to nucleoproteins, blood erythrocytes, globulins, or lipoproteins.

Most bound drugs are linked to an albumin molecule by ionic bonds (Figure 16-3), which may easily be reversed. Only a *free drug molecule*—that is, unbound—will be able to move to the receptor site. Binding of a drug molecule is limited by the available number of albumin molecules and by the specific binding sites available for that drug (Koch-Weser and Sellers, 1976):

Unbound drug + Albumin = Drug-albumin complex

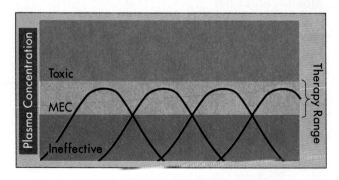

FIGURE 16-2 Minimum effective concentration (*MEC*) is achieved by giving drug at specific intervals determined by its rate of metabolism.

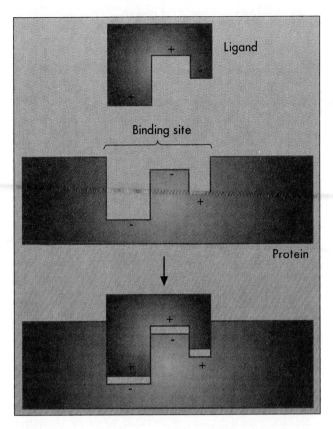

FIGURE 16-3 Complementary shapes of ligand and protein binding site determine the chemical specificity of binding.

When all binding sites are filled up with the drug, the rest of the free molecules seek the receptor sites and cause *effects*. The binding of the drug is limited by the numbers of albumin molecules, and the ionic bonds may be easily reversed. Medications poorly soluble in water (lipophilic, "loving fat," or hydrophobic, "hating water") are often highly protein bound and unable to move to the site of action. These medications have a long half-life and are excreted slowly. However, there is constant binding and unbinding and movement to and from the receptor site and to the liver for metabolism before excretion by the kidney. Only 5% to 20% of many drugs will be left unbound at one time; for example, chlorothiazide is 95% bound, and nafcillin is 90% bound. In these cases, higher doses may be needed to obtain initial action. A loading dose may be ordered to obtain enough free drug to be active.

During pregnancy there appears to be increased competition for protein-binding sites because plasma albumin is decreased and estrogen and progesterone are strongly protein bound. In addition, metabolic sources of energy are altered to conserve carbohydrates, and fatty tissue metabolism is increased, resulting in a rise in free fatty acids, triglycerides, cholesterol, and phospholipids, all of which are carried in the plasma attached to proteins. If such sites are not readily available for binding drugs during pregnancy, a larger percentage of the drug will be free to move to receptor sites or to cross the placental barrier. The classic example is the change in insulin needs as pregnancy progresses.

TISSUE BINDING

Medications may have an affinity for other body tissues such as bones, hair, nails, and adipose tissue. Tissue binding may lead to storage of large amounts of the drug, and *saturation* in that tissue must be reached before there is free drug to attach to receptor sites. When a drug is discontinued, tissue deposits give up their share slowly, causing a persistence of drug effect (e.g., sedatives and hypnotics that leave a "hangover" because of slow release). Pregnancy, because of increased fatty tissue, may cause a persistent effect of tissue-bound drug.

Biotransformation

Medications produce their effects by combining with enzymes or cell components. This interaction produces a chain of specific biochemical and physiologic changes for a given medication. The initial result of the interaction is the **action**, and the result of that action is the **effect**. The action precedes and produces the effects. The effects might be far from the site of action.

Drug action usually is terminated by metabolism and excretion or by leaving the receptor and moving to other tissues. Some medications are inactivated on the first pass through the liver; others are metabolized much more slowly because of protein and tissue binding. This delay may cause problems for the fetus. According to Koch-Weser and Sellers (1976):

It is well worth recalling that metabolism of drugs and other foreign chemicals may result in metabolites which have equal, greater or different pharmacologic activity and may produce compounds that are harmful to fetal tissue.

The microsomal portion of the liver produces many of the enzymes active in medication metabolism. These enzymes may be induced or stimulated, resulting in faster metabolism, or they may be inhibited, thus slowing metabolism. *Certain functions of the microsomal portion of the liver are further slowed* during pregnancy, which delays metabolism of some medications. In addition, the gallbladder becomes hypotonic in response to the effect of estrogen. There is a delayed excretion of bile, with increased possibility of the formation of gallstones.

The metabolic process continues until the drug is completely altered into an active metabolite or into an inactive product. The process works toward making the drug molecule *more water soluble* (hydrophilic) *with weaker ionization* and thus less able to bind to protein, to cross membranes, or to be reabsorbed by the kidney.

METABOLISM IN THE PLACENTA

The placenta has a role in metabolism, especially of endogenous hormones (e.g., androgen to estrogen, maternal cholesterol to pregnenolone and then to progesterone). Drugs that compete in the placenta for metabolic activity may alter steroid production enough to interrupt the function of important hormones that control fetal development (Gray and Yaffe, 1986).

EXCRETION

The major route of excretion is the urine, but drugs also are excreted through bile to feces, as well as in saliva, respired air, and sweat. Medications not completely metabolized may be excreted through bile into the intestine and then are reabsorbed into the circulation to pass a second time through the liver. This **enterohepatic recycling** is responsible for the delay in the excretion of many medications in the newborn.

An increase of 50% in renal circulation occurs by the second trimester. The rate is altered by body position; the supine position reduces blood flow to the renal arteries. In addition, the glomerular filtration rate is increased even more (70%) during pregnancy, a factor that appears to allow increased excretion of waste products without changing the urine volume. Because of increased circulation to the kidney, easily excreted drugs may be lost from the body more quickly than in the nonpregnant state.

Of interest is that a medication may be excreted by the fetus into amniotic fluid. It will slowly diffuse back across the amnion. It may also be swallowed by the fetus and may accumulate in amniotic fluid. For example, penicillins have been found in higher amounts in amniotic fluid than in maternal or fetal blood.

Test Yourself

- Which types of drugs move most easily across membrane barriers?
- If drugs are in equilibrium on both sides of the placenta, what does this mean?

Transition Precautions

During pregnancy, the woman's body handles drug metabolism and excretion for the fetus. If labor begins while the mother has an active, free drug in her system, depending on the time of birth in relation to her last dose, the infant may be born with nearly the maternal serum level; it then must metabolize this amount on its own.

In the transition period of labor and birth, doses should be spaced in relation to expected time of birth. The half-life is compared with the expected time of birth to determine when the medication (usually analgesia) should be given. This is the **time-dose interval.**

If the woman receives medications by continuous intravenous infusion for a complication, levels at birth will be almost equal in mother and baby. In this case, one looks for delayed infant responses to drugs during recovery.

Medication Excretion in Breast Milk

BLOOD-MILK BARRIER

The blood-milk barrier is difficult to cross by active transport and diffusion. Increased circulation to the breast and variation in milk production, however, make it difficult to predict the amount of medication that will enter the breast milk.

Fat-soluble, nonionized medications enter breast milk easily. Water-soluble medications of low molecular weight may enter milk by filtration through spaces between alveolar epithelial cells. Only free drug molecules, unbound in maternal plasma, are able to enter the milk. Levels in maternal serum affect levels in the milk.

The pH of milk ranges between 6.9 and 7.0, which is slightly more acidic than plasma; therefore basic drugs pass more easily than acidic ones. Additional factors make it difficult to determine how much of the medication is ingested by the baby. The volume of milk taken at a feeding varies during 24 hours. Colostrum is secreted in a range of 10 to 40 ml in 24 hours, and in one large study, milk production at the seventh day of lactation averaged only 400 to 500 ml/24 hours (Hytten, 1976). Thus, the low volume of milk in the first week reduces potential intake during recovery. In addition, some drugs may return to the maternal system, some are metabolized in the alveolar cells themselves, and some are bound to milk proteins and, although taken in by the infant, are not absorbed or are destroyed in the baby's gastrointestinal tract (Figure 16-4).

In general, only 1% to 2% of the maternal dose reaches the milk. This percentage is only a fraction (less than 0.5%) of the standard doses of the same medica-

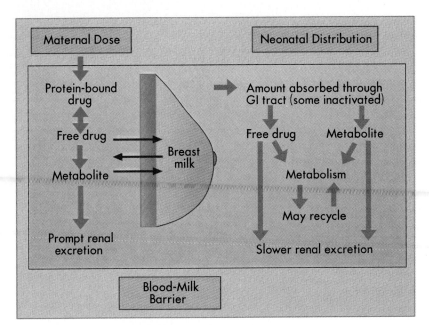

FIGURE 16-4 Drug distribution through breast milk.

tions prescribed for infants in the high-risk nursery or pediatric units (Rivera-Calimlim, 1987).

Interest in medications in breast milk is heightened because the number of lactating women is increasing. In the past, studies have used case reports or only small samples, but current ability to obtain sophisticated measurements should allow researchers to be more specific about medications that must be avoided. For the status of specific drugs, see Appendix 4.

TIME-DOSE INTERVAL

Careful timing of maternal doses may help to reduce medication concentrations in milk. There are differing opinions about when to administer the medication so that peak effects do not coincide with the full breast. The following schemes are recommended on the basis that a baby breast-feeds for about 60 minutes and that most milk is taken in the first 10 minutes on each breast.

1. Some authorities suggest giving oral doses at the beginning of a session. Absorption time to peak is about 20 to 40 minutes, depending on the medication. Most of the milk will have been taken before the medication reaches the barrier.
2. Berlin (1991) and Rivera-Calimlim (1987) suggest that all medications be given just after a feeding session.
3. Intravenous and intramuscular doses should be given just after a feeding session. By the parenteral route medication reaches the MEC more quickly and usually is metabolized and excreted before the next feeding.

4. If a medication is highly protein bound and given every day (such as digoxin or methadone) or passes in larger amounts into breast milk, timing the dose after morning or late afternoon feeding has been suggested (Berlin, 1991); this allows at least 4 hours before the next feeding, or formula may be substituted at the next feeding.

SAFETY PRINCIPLES

A number of authors recommend the following principles in regard to medication and lactation.

1. No medication should be prescribed for a pregnant or lactating woman unless it is necessary for her health or the health of her baby. If medication is used, the most effective medication with the fewest side effects should be selected (American Academy of Pediatrics Committee on Drugs, 1983).
2. The drug with the shortest half-life should be used and the smallest doses given (Rivera-Calimlim, 1987).
3. Most medications of low molecular weight are found in breast milk in low doses (1% to 2% of maternal dose), depending on frequency of dose

 Clinical Decision

Jane is taking a drug orally twice a day for hypertension. When should she take her doses in relation to her 1-month-old infant's nursing periods?

and the amount and characteristics of the medications. Therefore, the amount reaching the baby is very small.

4. Most medications usually are not hazardous, even though found in milk, because they are metabolized in alveolar cells or are destroyed in the baby's gastrointestinal tract. (Exceptions are listed in Appendix 4.)

5. If a woman was taking medication on a regular basis during pregnancy, the fetus received a much higher dose because medications cross the placental barrier more efficiently.

6. Medications given by continuous intravenous infusion are more concentrated in breast milk than medications intermittently given orally or intravenously because of higher maternal serum levels.

7. If there is a question about adverse effect, the level of the drug in the baby and other laboratory evaluations may be measured.

8. A lactating woman should always consult her physician before taking medication.

9. Breast-feeding is considered to be so valuable to the infant that special care should be taken not to deny its possibility because of a short-term intake of a drug on the caution list.

Pain During Labor

Two different kinds of pain occur during labor. **Visceral pain** generally is experienced during active dilation and is related to cervical stretching and uterine contraction intensity. **Somatic pain** is related to pressure on and stretching of the birth canal as descent occurs. There is overlapping of sensations, but observation of a woman in labor reveals changes in her expression of pain sensations.

VISCERAL PAIN

Pain may be transmitted slowly (through unmyelinated fibers) and felt as dull, diffuse, persistent, or aching sensations. Pain sensations conveyed through myelinated fibers travel more rapidly and are perceived as sharp, localized sensations. During the first stage of labor the nerve impulses enter the sympathetic chain at L1 to L5 and then travel to the posterior roots of the tenth, eleventh, and twelfth thoracic nerves and up the spinal cord to the thalamus (Figure 16-5).

There also may be referred pain through the dermatomes of the same nerves. Pain is felt in the skin, thighs, lower back, and hips, as well as "hot" spots of generalized aching. Some of this pain is pressure induced; some may be caused by fatigue and hypoxia of the uterine muscle. During labor, areas of referred pain change location. If labor is prolonged, uterine fatigue factors may increase pain sensations.

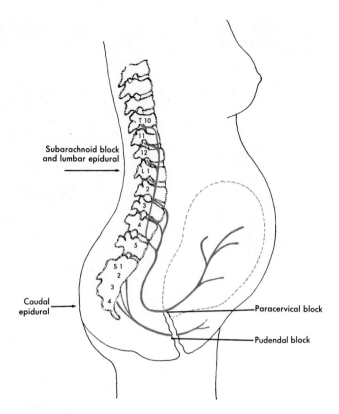

FIGURE 16-5 Pathways of pain during labor. (Courtesy Abbott Laboratories.)

SOMATIC PAIN

Somatic pain usually begins during the transition phase because descent is speeded. The pressure of the fetus on the cervical, vaginal, and perineal tissues is intense. First felt as a need to bear down, this sensation may become overpowering. These pain sensations travel primarily via pudendal nerves through the dorsal roots of the second, third, and fourth sacral nerves.

Pain is felt when the contraction intensity rises 15 to 20 mm Hg above the resting tonus (Figure 16-6). Therefore one looks for pain at intensities above 25 mm Hg pressure on the monitor strip. (External monitoring does not give a completely accurate picture of the actual intensity of the contraction. Sometimes the mother appears not to be in effective labor and yet is having painful contractions.) There should be less discomfort during rest periods. If there is continuing acute discomfort, the problem should be investigated.

PHYSIOLOGIC FACTORS

Stress produces a rise in cortisol and catecholamine levels. All nurses have observed anxious women who are tense, restless, and frightened. Hypertension, hyperventilation, and increased oxygen use may occur during severe stress. For these reasons the nurse uses supportive measures that modify pain.

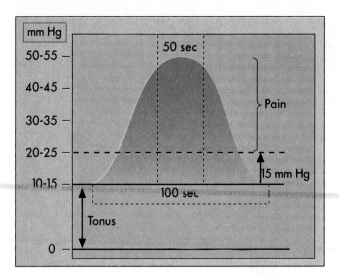

FIGURE 16-6 Pain is felt when the contraction pressure rises 15 mm Hg above resting tone.

Some stress is beneficial because it stimulates endogenous opioids, mainly β-endorphin. Just before labor, endogenous **endorphin** levels normally rise. If the woman enters labor at term, is knowledgeable about the procedures and process, and is accompanied by a support person, she often can tolerate labor fairly well and may not request analgesia. Plasma β-endorphins (endogenous morphines) are natural analgesics.

PAIN THRESHOLD

A high pain threshold may be explained by somewhat increased endorphin levels. Cahill (1989) found that β-endorphin plasma levels rose slightly during labor but not to the degree of increased pain as reported by women in labor. She suggests that β-endorphins did not eliminate but blunted the perception of pain.

Illness and fatigue lower a person's pain threshold, and cultural expectations seem to affect a person's perception of pain and pain behaviors. Cultural responses may override "normal" pain responses; some women are taught to be stoic, others to cry out. Nurses must not impose their cultural assumptions on their clients. Rather, **Loeser's model of pain** (1982) may help the nurse support a woman in labor. Loeser uses four parameters for pain analysis: nociception, pain, suffering, and pain behavior. **Nociceptors** are free nerve endings that generate pain impulses. Therefore the term **nociception** indicates the causative factors for pain impulses. Use of this model requires consideration of the following factors during pain assessment:

1. *Nociception:* What are the physiologic causes that initiate pain signals? Assess the phase of labor and any abnormality in progress or position. Is the pain visceral or somatic?
2. *Pain:* What is the client's description of what she feels? Subjective: have her describe location and intensity; objective: check changes in vital signs, intensity of contractions, and restlessness.
3. *Suffering:* What are her responses to pain and the significance she attaches to it? Is she angry, upset, grim, guilty, stoic, or crying? What is her emotional response to the pain?
4. *Pain behaviors:* How does she act? How does she express tension? What brings her relief?

The nurse might provide an outline of the body similar to those in Figure 16-7 and ask the woman to point to where it hurts and how. Then comfort measures can be specific.

RESPONSES TO LABOR PAIN

Pain studies have shown changes in pain intensity and location during labor (Figure 16-7); these changes vary from hour to hour. In addition, Melzack et al (1984) found the following:

1. A correlation exists between history of severe menstrual pain and more pain in the first and subsequent labors.
2. Childbirth preparation tends to allow a woman to cope, to remain in control, and thus able to describe her pain as more manageable, even though it may be as intense as that experienced by an unprepared woman.
3. Usually primiparas complain of more painful labors than do multiparas. If, however, a woman weighs more than usual and has a larger baby than expected, pain levels are higher.
4. Finally, there is no correlation of pain levels with duration of labor unless fatigue occurs.

Melzack et al (1984) used the McGill pain questionnaire (Figure 16-8) to determine levels of pain sensation during labor.

It is difficult to assess the level of pain from observation because people respond differently to altered comfort. According to Moore (1983), responses to labor-related pain may be influenced by the following factors:

1. Usual level of anxiety and responses to stress
2. Feelings of self-worth and femininity
3. Significance of pregnancy (welcomed or not)
4. Feelings passed on to the woman by her mother
5. Experience with a previous childbirth
6. Anxiety over risk factors or illness
7. Degree of education and preparation for childbirth
8. Actual progress through labor phases
9. Presence of a support person
10. Perceived support of health care personnel

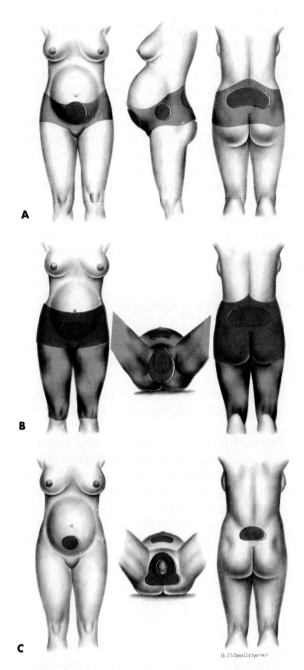

G.J.Wassilchenko

FIGURE 16-7 There are changing areas and intensities of pain sensations during labor. **A,** Early labor. **B,** Transition. **C,** Late labor and birth. (From Bobak IM, Jensen MD: *Maternity and gynecologic care: the nurse and the family,* ed 5, 1993, Mosby.)

McGill Pain Questionnaire

Client's Name_____
Date_____Time_____

1	Flickering	___	11	Tiring	___
	Quivering	___		Exhausting	___
	Pulsing	___			
	Throbbing	___	12	Sickening	___
	Beating	___		Suffocating	___
	Pounding	___			
			13	Fearful	___
2	Jumping	___		Frightful	___
	Flashing	___		Terrifying	___
	Shooting	___			
			14	Punishing	___
3	Pricking	___		Gruelling	___
	Boring	___		Cruel	___
	Drilling	___		Vicious	___
	Stabbing	___		Killing	___
	Lancinating	___			
			15	Wretched	___
4	Sharp	___		Blinding	___
	Cutting	___			
	Lacerating	___	16	Annoying	___
				Troublesome	___
5	Pinching	___		Miserable	___
	Pressing	___		Intense	___
	Gnawing	___		Unbearable	___
	Cramping	___			
	Crushing	___	17	Spreading	___
				Radiating	___
6	Tugging	___		Penetrating	___
	Pulling	___		Piercing	___
	Wrenching	___			
			18	Tight	___
7	Hot	___		Numb	___
	Burning	___		Drawing	___
	Scalding	___		Squeezing	___
	Searing	___		Tearing	___
8	Tingling	___	19	Cool	___
	Itchy	___		Cold	___
	Smarting	___		Freezing	___
	Stinging	___			
			20	Nagging	___
9	Dull	___		Nauseating	___
	Sore	___		Agonizing	___
	Hurting	___		Dreadful	___
	Aching	___		Torturing	___
	Heavy	___			
				PPI	
10	Tender	___	0	No pain	___
	Taut	___	1	Mild	___
	Rasping	___	2	Discomforting	___
	Splitting	___	3	Distressing	___
			4	Horrible	___
			5	Excruciating	___

FIGURE 16-8 McGill Pain Questionnaire. Categories of pain: Sensory, 1 to 10; Affective, 11 to 15; Evaluative, 16; Miscellaneous, 17 to 20. Rank the value for each word based on its position in each category. Sum of rank values = pain rating index (PRI). Index of present pain intensity (PPI) is based on scale of 0 to 5. (From Melzack R: Severity of labor pain: influence of physical as well as psychologic variables, *Can Med Assoc J* 30(3):580, 1984.)

Clinical Decision

Jenny is in labor and experiencing a considerable amount of discomfort. Choose the word from the Loeser model of pain to describe each of the following:
a. Jenny is restless, moaning, and turning from side to side.
b. She has been recently examined and is 7 cm dilated; contractions occur every 3 minutes and last 70 seconds. Station is +1.
c. She cries out and says, "My tail bone is breaking!"
d. She clings to her partner's hand, saying "Don't leave me!"
Answer: (a) Pain behaviors. (b) Nociception: pain from visceral and somatic causes during transition. (c) Pain description. (d) Suffering expressed in need for presence of significant other.

Cultural variations in response to labor pain include loud crying, which some women believe to be important in showing the partner how difficult the process is. The nurse should not be misled about the phase of labor and the pain intensity (see Cultural Aspects of Care).

NONPHARMACOLOGIC METHODS OF PAIN RELIEF

Transcutaneous Electric Nerve Stimulation

Transcutaneous electric nerve stimulation (TENS) during labor has been used in some settings on a research basis (Grim and Morrey, 1985). It is commonly used in Canada and Europe. The emphasis on continuous fetal

Cultural Aspects of Care

Crying During Labor
Some Indian women cry throughout labor. In India, men were never in the room but nearby. Here the partner may be at the bedside, perhaps against his real inclination and cultural values. (Remember, he needs support and explanations of the labor process.) The opposite extreme is found in some Asian women who control crying or any sound, although their pain may be intense. The father may refuse to be at the bedside, because birth is thought to be exclusively women's territory.

monitoring may have limited its adoption for labor in this country. TENS does not interfere with monitoring unless used at a high intensity. Careful observation of the record indicates when electric impulses may be distorting the record (Miller-Jones, 1980).

TENS is effective with chronic pain by stimulating release of β-endorphins. It allows the client to control the level of stimulation, which helps her to cope. The physical therapist is familiar with the machine and can be asked to instruct the nursing staff in its use. Clients oriented before labor to its use are more comfortable with it (Figure 16-9).

One pair of electrodes is applied to either side of the spine at T12-11 for uterine pain in the first part of labor. For later labor and transition, the electrodes may be moved to S2 to S4. For the second stage the electrodes may be kept at the sacral level and another pair applied suprapubically. TENS is said to have the analgesic effect of 75 to 100 mg of meperidine. It is more effective in active labor than in transition, according to one study (Augustensson et al, 1977). Most women using the technique stated that they would reuse it for a subsequent labor. Because it is especially effective for back pain, it may be the choice for a labor when the fetus is in a posterior position.

Acupressure and Touch

The use of touch in a purposeful way to bring reassurance or reduce pain sensation has been used in varying childbirth methods. *Effleurage* is an accepted method of alternative sensation. Touch as a means of reassurance has been used by placing a hand on the fundus of the uterus while questioning the woman about her feelings and sensations. A great deal more research is needed in this area (see Chapter 13). Bodden (1986) has used a

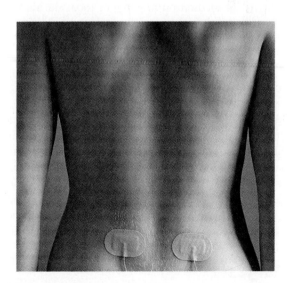

FIGURE 16-9 One site for TENS electrode placement during labor. (Courtesy 3M HealthCare, Minneapolis, Minn.)

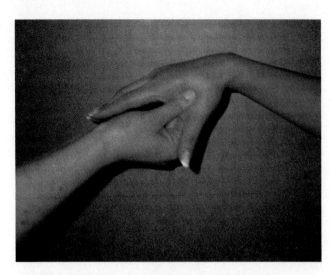

FIGURE 16-10 Site of acupressure point for labor contractions as used by Bodden (1986).

form of **acupressure** during labor contractions to obtain additional endorphin response and relief of painful sensations (Figure 16-10).

Acupuncture and Asian Medicine

Acupuncture is a branch of Asian medicine. In Asian cultures, pregnancy and birth are considered normal activities for the healthy woman, and difficulty with any aspect is considered a sign of imbalance. A practitioner of Asian medicine seeks to find the underlying imbalance in the woman's energy through a wide range of diagnostic skills and then selects the modality for restoration of balance.

Asian medicine appears to be especially effective in cases of functional as opposed to structural pathologic conditions.

The use of meditation to enhance focus during labor has been helpful to many women. Those women from cultures familiar with meditative techniques should be encouraged to prepare themselves to use this method for pain relief. In China, fetal position has been changed through the use of a heat technique called *moxibustion* (Beal, 1990).

Although not in common use in this country, *acupuncture* may be used to augment or lessen labor contractions and provide some analgesia. In China, cesarean delivery has been conducted under acupuncture analgesia. After delivery, many women consider Oriental herbs essential for restoring strength and helping with lactation difficulties. The woman who relies on these modalities during recovery should be supported.

Analgesia

All opioids cause approximately the same analgesic effect in **equigesic doses**. Respiratory depression may occur in the woman and baby. The effect of large doses may cause reduced fetal movements and poor beat-to-beat variability as seen on the fetal monitor. These drugs pass easily to the fetus and more readily pass the blood-brain barrier. *The younger the fetus, the more it will be depressed.*

Drugs are chosen for labor **analgesia** on the basis of their duration of action so that the time-dose interval may be better controlled before delivery. The timing of analgesics in labor is important. The drug should be given at least 3 to 4 hours before delivery to allow metabolism and excretion. The time of birth is difficult to predict, and as a result the baby occasionally is born with most of the maternal dose in its system. In this case a narcotic antagonist may need to be given to the infant to reverse respiratory depression. Naloxone (Narcan) is the drug used currently.

OPIOID ANALGESICS

Morphine

Morphine is the analgesic whose effectiveness in alleviating pain is the standard against which synthetic narcotics are measured. This classic drug is effective as a central nervous system depressant. It raises the pain threshold and depresses cough and respiratory centers. It may, however, trigger the vomiting center. Morphine is administered through the epidural catheter for postoperative analgesia, but is not given IM during labor because effective doses depress the infant's respiratory center.

Meperidine

Meperidine (Pethidine, Demerol) acts in many ways like morphine, although it is less effective in relieving severe pain (see Drug Profile 16-1). It has equally depressant effects on respirations at equal analgesic doses. It depresses fetal activity and slightly increases the frequency and duration of contractions (Zimmer, Divon, and Vadasz, 1988). In Zimmer and colleagues' study, *short-term heart rate variability* was reduced during the baseline period. Within a half hour the tracing appeared "flatter"; less variability and reactivity were noted.

Meperidine works best on *visceral pain* and has a slight relaxant effect on intestinal and vascular smooth muscle. Hypotension and nausea tend to occur, especially when it is given intravenously. Postural hypotension and tachycardia also may occur, and voiding may be inhibited.

Meperidine has been studied extensively. Its time-dose interval is clear; intravenous onset is 2 to 3 minutes and peaks at 1 to 1½ hours. Only low doses should be used during labor because in high doses meperidine depresses newborn respirations. In addition, the higher levels of the metabolite *normeperidine* linger for extensive periods in the infant. Brackbill (1974) reported that for the larger maternal doses given then,

Drug Profile 16-1

Meperidine HCl (Pethidine, Demerol)
Action

Depresses pain impulse transmission at the spinal cord via opioid receptors. Works best with visceral pain. Slight relaxant effect on intestinal and vascular smooth muscle. Half-life is 1 to 2 hours. Time-dose interval is important when used in labor. Drug almost always is given with antianxiety agent.

Dose/route

SC or IM if no IV, 25 to 50 mg with promethazine (Phenergan). In labor with IV use 5 ml saline to dilute, and give slow IV push over 4 to 5 minutes. Promethazine 12.5 to 25 mg added to dose.

Side effects/adverse effects

Labor dose: hypotension, dizziness, confusion, headache, euphoria; nausea/vomiting, blurred vision; rash, diaphoresis, flushing. Respiratory depression may occur in neonate but rarely in woman. Narcan is antidote.

Precautions

Addictive with other narcotic agents, recreational drugs, alcohol, sedatives, general anesthesia. Check monitor carefully for signs of contractions or fetal distress, because woman may go to sleep. Use side rails.

metabolites in the infant were present for more than 1 month after birth. These metabolites seem to depress neurologic adaptation. Responses to the Brazelton scale were altered in infants who received high levels of this medication. In children with learning disabilities, studies have been unable to isolate long term meperidine effects from the adverse effects of acidosis and hypoxia.

If doses are timed correctly to enable the drug to be almost completely metabolized and excreted by the mother before birth, meperidine may be useful during labor. Some women do not react to it well, however. If the woman gets more restless and does not obtain adequate relief, further doses of the drug are not given, and an alternate analgesic is used such as an epidural injection.

Fentanyl

Fentanyl (Innovar or Sublimaze) is a narcotic analgesic similar to meperidine. It has a shorter onset and duration of action than meperidine. It is commonly used now as part of the epidural dose. If respiratory depression occurs, Narcan is the antagonist.

Alphaprodine

Alphaprodine (Nisentil) has been used during labor because of its shorter onset (10 minutes) and duration of action (2-3 hours) when given subcutaneously or intramuscularly. There is no difference in duration when it is given intravenously. Two problems should be noted with this drug. When low doses are given intravenously (20 mg), there may be an *increase in fetal heart rate variability* for about 30 minutes. If higher doses are used intramuscularly (40 to 60 mg), a *sinusoidal fetal heart rate* pattern, which lasts for about 1 hour, has been noted.

NONNARCOTIC ANALGESICS

Butorphanol

Butorphanol (Stadol) is used commonly in this country. A nonnarcotic analgesic (mixed agonist-antagonist) with a duration of effect of 3 to 4 hours, crosses the placental barrier but does not cause excessive residuals in the baby because metabolites are inactive (see Drug Profile 16-2).

Pentazocine

Pentazocine (Talwin Nx) is an agonist-antagonist, nonnarcotic analgesic used for postoperative pain. A few centers use it during labor because it crosses the placenta less readily, and respiratory depression is about half that of morphine and meperidine. This drug is an analgesic and a narcotic antagonist, with about 2% the

 Drug Profile 16-2

Butorphanol tartrate (Stadol)
Action

Depresses pain impulses by interacting with spinal cord opioid receptors. A nonnarcotic, mixed agonist-antagonist analgesic. Widely used for labor pain because metabolites are inactive in fetus. Half-life is 2½ to 3½ hours. Crosses placenta and milk barriers. Time-dose interval is important. Narcan is antidote.

Dose/route

IM 2 mg (deep injection) q3-4h or IV 1 mg q3-4h. Dilute IV dose with normal saline (NS) and give slow push as contraction subsides.

Side effects/adverse effects

Nausea/vomiting, clamminess. Rarely headache, dizziness, lethargy, palpitation, slow pulse; rash.

Precautions

Increases effects of other narcotics, sedatives, skeletal muscle relaxants, alcohol. Check I&O, vital signs, fetal responses. Use side rails.

effect of naloxone. Thus it may reverse the effect of concurrently administered narcotics. Central nervous system effects include analgesia and respiratory depression. Large doses cause cardiovascular effects of tachycardia and some hypertension. Duration is 1 to 3 hours intramuscularly and 2 to 5 hours orally.

ANTIANXIETY AGENTS

Antianxiety agents are used during labor to calm the client and to potentiate (increase the strength of) analgesic effects. When combined, the analgesic dose may be reduced *at least by half.* Several of these medications also have an antiemetic effect. Because these drugs cross the placenta, the infant may have reduced muscle tone and a slightly lower temperature and respiratory rate. In small doses, however, no lasting effect has been recognized in the newborn infant (see Drug Profile 16-3).

OPIATE ANTAGONIST: NALOXONE

Naloxone (Narcan) is the only medication used as an antagonist to the depressing effects of narcotic analgesics (see Drug Profile 16-4). It lacks the morphinelike

 Drug Profile 16-3

Tranquilizers as adjuncts to analgesics
Promethazine (Phenergan)

Dosage: 25-50 mg IM, onset 15-20 min, duration 3-4 hr. 25 mg IV, onset 3-5 min, duration 2-3 hr.
Maternal effects: Antihistamine action adds extra sedation with narcotic; potentiates narcotic, allowing lower doses; stimulates respiration; decreases nausea and vomiting; some disorientation and hypotension; possible tachycardia; no effect on labor progress.
Fetal effects: CNS depression: equilibrates with maternal level within 15 minutes of intravenous solution; transitional effects depend on dosage.

Diazepam (Valium)

Dosage: 5-10 mg IM, onset 10-15 min, duration 5-7 hr. 5-10 mg IV diluted in 5 ml normal saline given over 5 min, onset 2-3 min, duration 5-6 hr. Might be used by anesthetist if a difficult assisted vaginal birth.
Maternal effects: Not used during labor, but may be given IV during delivery only. Potentiates any analgesic. Not recommended if mother is breastfeeding in early recovery period.
Fetal effects: Will concentrate in fetus. Higher doses (>30 mg) affect thermoregulation in newborn up to 1 week. Observe vital signs during recovery.

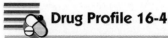 **Drug Profile 16-4**

Naloxone (Narcan)
Use with epidural narcotics

Action

Narcotic antagonist reverses respiratory depression of narcotics. Used when epidural morphine or other narcotics used. Also used for neonatal respiratory depression (see Chapter 28). Has 1-hour effectiveness; respiratory depression may recur.

Dose/route

Maternal: 0.1-0.2 mg IV, repeat q2-3 min × 2 as necessary. IV, IM, or SC.
Neonatal: 0.01 mg/kg into umbilical vein at birth. Repeat q2-3 min × 3.

Side effects/adverse effects

Maternal hypertension, tachycardia with high dose. Pulmonary edema if preexisting cardiovascular (CV) problems or other CV drugs are in use. Nausea/vomiting. Delay lactation until narcotics and Narcan out of system.

Precautions

Be sure client is not using other drugs of abuse. Reversal may be abrupt with tremulousness, sweating, nausea and vomiting, tachycardia, hypertension.

qualities that other antagonists show. It acts to combat central nervous system and respiratory depression. Some units have given the woman a dose just before birth. Others give the depressed newborn 0.01 mg/kg intramuscularly or through the umbilical vein. The dose may be repeated while resuscitation is being carried out. The neonate should be observed carefully for a return of depression as much as 6 to 8 hours later because its metabolism is more rapid than that of the analgesics.

Naloxone also reverses signs of drugs such as heroin or cocaine for a short time. In these infants, severe withdrawal signs may be observed later, which should be kept in mind when giving immediate care to the newborn (see Chapters 19 and 28).

Anesthesia

Anesthesia is a condition of lack of pain, with or without loss of consciousness. Anesthetics may provide local or regional numbness, with loss of sensation to pain, or they may result in general muscle relaxation and loss of sensation and consciousness because of varying degrees of central nervous system depression.

Because the maternity client presents special considerations for anesthesia, a prepared anesthesiologist should be on staff in birth centers. In a national survey (Gibbs et al, 1986) a wide variation in obstetric anesthesia practice was identified. Complete anesthesia coverage is not available in many smaller centers. Because births are unscheduled, it is not always possible to have an obstetric anesthesiologist present.

General anesthesia places a maternity client at much more risk than does regional anesthesia because of the potential risk of aspiration of stomach contents during induction and recovery. In fact, aspiration and its results are causes of maternal mortality. A woman entering the birth area may have heard about problems with anesthesia. Her concerns should not be dismissed; rather, every effort should be made to be sure that she understands what medications she is receiving.

The nurse who works in the birth area needs to be particularly aware of types of anesthesia; expected and adverse reactions; and the roles of anesthesiologist, nurse anesthetist, obstetrician, and midwife. In addition, full recognition of the nurse's role and responsibilities in preparation for and care of the mother during and after anesthesia is vital.

LOCAL ANESTHETICS

Chemicals used as local anesthetics have the suffix, *-caine,* in their names. Preparations such as lidocaine, mepivacaine, dibucaine, and bupivacaine are *amides,* which are metabolized slowly and are protein bound and yet may slowly cross the placental barrier. *Esters*—procaine, chloroprocaine, tetracaine, and cocaine—are metabolized swiftly and are not commonly used. Local anesthetics are used in lower concentrations and in smaller doses for birth than in other operative situations because the fetus may be affected, depending on the rate of transfer across the placenta. Adverse effects in the infant are inhibited muscle tone and responsiveness, with metabolites continuing in the infant's system for long periods (Abboud, 1985).

Adverse Maternal Reactions

Local anesthetics cause varying degrees of vasodilation. Depending on the location and concentration of the medication, *hypotension,* which can be severe unless measures are taken to prevent it, can occur. Mild reactions include dizziness, palpitations, and headache. If the solution enters the circulation in significant amounts, excitement, apprehension, tachycardia, disorientation, tremors, and rarely, convulsions may occur. The fetus may show bradycardia. Some few persons have hypersensitivity ranging from allergic dermatitis to bronchospasm and anaphylactic reaction. Because of these possibilities, a *test dose* is always given before

administration of the full dose, and the smallest effective amount is chosen. The client always should be asked about prior experiences with local anesthetics in her dental office.

Infiltration

Local infiltration provides a pain-free area for episiotomy or repair of lacerations. A few minutes for absorption must be allowed before the procedure begins. The woman will sense the tugging and pulling of surrounding tissue and will expect to feel pain. A simple explanation may help her to relax during suturing.

REGIONAL ANESTHESIA

Local anesthetics may be injected to block a group of nerves leading to a region of the body. Medication is injected into or around a nerve pathway or at the plexus of the nerve.

Pudendal Block

The pudendal block provides effective regional anesthesia for the second stage of labor and delivery. The pudendal nerve plexus lies just above and behind the ischial spines, and the nerve itself supplies sensation to the whole perineal area. A block eliminates most of the *somatic pain* of tissue pressure and stretching, but the woman will still feel the *visceral pain* of contractions and still is able to bear down. The block must be done 5 to 10 minutes before delivery to gain the full effect. If time is not sufficient, the delivery will be painful, but suturing will be painless. Pudendal block usually is sufficient for low forceps delivery but not for more extensive manipulation. A pudendal block is administered by the midwife or obstetrician (Figure 16-11). *fetal effects*

Because the area is vascular, anesthetic absorption may slightly affect vital signs. There is no limitation on movement after delivery. The anesthetic should wear off in less than an hour. Observe for bladder distention because some lingering anesthetic effect may inhibit voiding during the immediate recovery period.

> **Test Yourself**
> • Pudendal block results in effective anesthesia for which parts of the reproductive tract?

EPIDURAL ANESTHESIA

There are two approaches to epidural anesthesia. Medication can be injected by lumbar or caudal approaches. The term epidural is applied to either approach, but

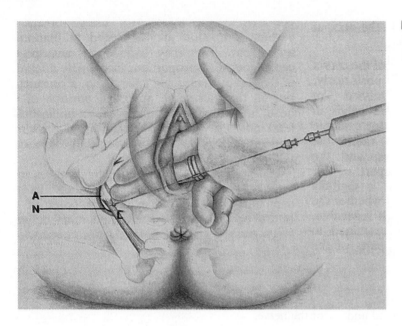

FIGURE 16-11 Pudendal block. (From Al-Azzawi F: *Atlas of childbirth and obstetric techniques*, St Louis, 1990, Mosby.)

lumbar epidural is more commonly used. The epidural (extradural) space runs the length of the spine and is located between the dura mater and the periosteal layer (Figure 16-12). Because this space contains connective tissue and fat, obese women are given a lower dose. There are blood vessels in the space, and the veins running through this space are slightly dilated from the increased blood volume. As a result, during pregnancy *less* medication must be used, and there is a slightly greater risk of injecting one of these vessels.

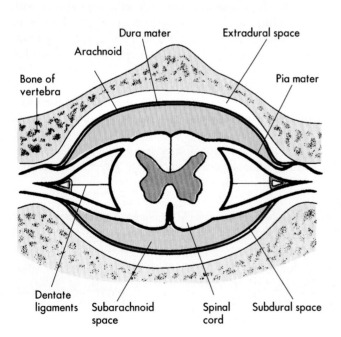

FIGURE 16-12 Cross-section through spinal cord and its membranes. (From Luciano D, Vander AJ, Sherman JH: *Human anatomy and physiology*, New York, 1983, McGraw-Hill.)

The anesthetic fluid should encircle the dura mater, affecting the nerves as they exit to the lower body. Just after the fluid is inserted, positioning is critical to promote its movement in the correct directions. If there are malformations in this area, a client may get a one-sided or partial effect. There may be an inadequate block, a unilateral block, or just one "spot" left unanesthetized. The woman should be informed of these possibilities. In addition, if manipulation is required to extract a baby, the mother may feel pressure and equate it with pain. This sensation can be compared with a tooth being pulled.

Depending on the dosage, epidural administration may be used for analgesia during labor or for anesthesia for vaginal or cesarean birth. If a cesarean delivery is needed, the anesthetic must circulate high enough to affect thoracic nerves at T6-7, and a larger dose will be administered than is usual for labor analgesia.

Lumbar Epidural Block

The lateral position may be used for an epidural block. The neck and knees are slightly flexed. The lumbar area remains fairly flat, not rounded as in a spinal tap. The client must be able to breathe freely and stay absolutely still during the puncture. The sitting position is used when the anesthesiologist prefers it. In this position the woman supports her feet on a chair. The hands should be resting on the thighs or on an over-bed table, a position that is difficult to hold when in labor (see Figure 13-15, *D*).

The lumbar epidural is approached at the L4-5 interspace between the spinous processes. The technique is more difficult than a spinal tap; avoiding puncturing the dura mater takes special skill. Because a short but wider gauge needle is used, if the dura mater is punctured there is more loss of spinal fluid than with a subarachnoid block technique. With a **continuous epidural** the needle is withdrawn when the thin catheter is located properly and the catheter is taped in place with a strip of tape up the back and over the shoulder (Figure 16-4). Additional doses are given through an entry port at the end of the catheter.

Caudal Epidural Block

The client must be in a lateral position. The injection is made through the opening in the lower end of the sacrum into the sacral cornua (see Figure 16-13). The anesthesiologist inserts a long needle into the caudal space and administers a test dose of medication. The client is observed for untoward response, and then the full dose is administered slowly and the needle withdrawn. Because of the extent of the caudal space, more medication is required for this route than for the lumbar epidural route. However, the technique is easier than the lumbar route. A continuous caudal block may be established after inserting a catheter into the space, which is taped in place; smaller doses can be administered at intervals. A caudal block may be administered after the active phase of labor has begun.

Nursing responsibilities. Epidural anesthesia is very effective for labor and vaginal and operative birth. The woman with epidural anesthesia is comfortable, unstressed by pain, and is awake and aware at birth, able to see and hold her infant and initiate breast-feeding. This is a valuable benefit for the woman and her partner.

Major complications are uncommon; yet the nurse should be prepared to assist when problems arise and to participate in monitoring and assessment after administration. Because of vasodilation at first, hypotension is always expected because of blood "pooling" in the legs. With hypotension, perfusion to the fetus is reduced;

therefore the following preventive measures always precede epidural administration.

1. A loading dose of intravenous fluid to support blood volume (500 to 1000 ml within 30 minutes) is regulated by the anesthesiologist.
2. Turn off any oxytocin drip during administration.
3. Prevent vena caval compression by correct positioning. Then follow directions of anesthesiologist regarding position change after the first test dose; then a therapeutic dose or further doses are given.
4. Monitor BP every 2 to 3 minutes after test dose and every 5 to 10 minutes until the woman is stable. *Never position hypotensive pt in trendelenburg position d/t poss paralysis of respiratory nerves.*
5. Monitor the fetal heart rate to note fetal response.
6. Document on monitor strip and nursing chart the time of start and finish of procedure and the doses administered, including client and fetal heart responses to doses and increments.

Depending on the dose during labor, the mother may not sense bladder distention and be unable to void. Therefore bladder status is monitored, and if usual methods to promote voiding are ineffective, a straight catheterization should be performed. The bladder should be emptied before delivery, especially if forceps will be used. If a Foley catheter is used, it must be removed before bearing-down efforts become strong because the balloon may traumatize the bladder.

Depending on the dose, the bearing-down reflex may be numbed, and the mother may not push effectively during the second stage. A low forceps delivery may be required. Therefore epidural doses usually are timed so that *somatic feeling* is present during this stage. If the woman is able to participate in pushing, she may have a longer second stage with an epidural but should be able to deliver without forceps.

Serious early complications. Subarachnoid (total spinal) injection into the spinal fluid of the larger epidural

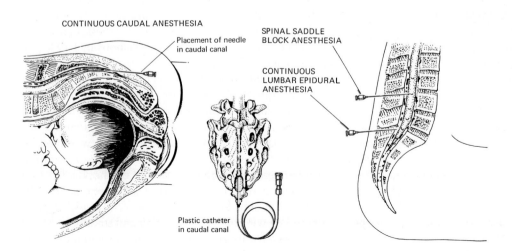

CONTINUOUS CAUDAL ANESTHESIA

Placement of needle in caudal canal

SPINAL SADDLE BLOCK ANESTHESIA

CONTINUOUS LUMBAR EPIDURAL ANESTHESIA

Plastic catheter in caudal canal

FIGURE 16-13 Caudal and lumbar epidural anesthesia and saddle block. (Used with permission of Ross Laboratories, Columbus, Ohio 43216. From *Clinical Education aid no. 17,* © Ross Laboratories.)

dose may cause unconsciousness, apnea, bradycardia, and cardiac arrest. Indications during *test doses or early in the injection are slurred speech* (notice that the anesthesiologist always asks the mother to talk during the injection), respiratory and pulse changes, and severe hypotension. Subarachnoid injection is an emergency, and cardiopulmonary resuscitation (CPR) is performed with ventilator support.

Later complications. Headache is not common after epidural administration. When it occurs, it often is related to poor technique; if the dura mater is punctured with the large-bore needle or the epidural catheter is withdrawn before any anesthetic is given, the loss of spinal fluid may cause a "spinal" headache. These clients used to be kept in a supine or side-lying position for 6, 8, 12, or 24 hours after administration. The client with a postpuncture headache may be instructed to follow the same regimen. Research, however, indicates that strict adherence to the flat position does not alter the incidence of headache (Albright et al, 1986). Effective treatment has been an epidural blood patch (5 to 10 ml of the woman's blood inserted into the puncture site). This acts as a "plug" to stop any more leakage. In addition, extra intravenous fluid (2000 to 3000 ml) and analgesics as needed help the client as the fluid pressure returns to normal. Sometimes a tight abdominal binder is requested. Without treatment the client may complain of the headache for up to 1 week. This interrupts recovery and infant bonding. Therefore it is important to be alert to the first signs of this reaction.

Other reactions. On rare occasions a hematoma may occur in the epidural space. If the mother has a bleeding disorder or platelet levels are below 150,000/mm^3, epidural administration should not be done.

Infection is a possibility without absolute asepsis; if the client is already septic, epidural injections are not administered.

In very rare instances a piece of the catheter may break off, usually when it is being removed. To avoid this problem the catheter is removed slowly by the anesthesiologist and then checked to see that it is intact. The nurse should remember to document removal of an intact catheter on the nursing notes.

Epidural and Intrathecal Analgesia

Epidural narcotics are instilled into the epidural space and then diffused through the dura mater to the cerebrospinal fluid (CSF) to attach to the opiate receptors on the dorsal horn of the spinal cord (Nicholson, 1990). Morphine, meperidine, fentanyl, and sufentanil are in current use. The analgesic effects usually are sufficient for the first half of labor. To handle the pain of the second half of labor, many women need combined doses of a local anesthetic and a narcotic. The most common combination is fentanyl with bupivicaine. The combination reduces the total requirements for the analgesic.

Some units provide small premeasured, self-regulated doses with a bedside pump. *Patient-controlled epidural analgesia (PCEA)* has been shown to be safe and to reduce narcotic and local anesthetic (usually bupivicaine) doses by as much as 40% to 50% (Nicholson, 1990), compared with women required to wait for their "top up" dose given after pain returns.

A newer use for morphine is as a postepidural "morphine wash." A small dose is inserted into the epidural catheter before withdrawal. Alternatively, morphine can be administered in small amounts into the intrathecal space with use of a spinal needle.

Morphine applied locally to the spinal nerves through an epidural catheter provides effective analgesia for 16 to 24 hours after surgery. Analgesia given through the epidural route is effective, allowing the mother to move freely after cesarean delivery. It promotes her recovery and her ability to pay attention to her infant. If the low dose is used, there are few side effects.

Side effects of epidural opiates. *Pruritus* may occur in about 50%, and the client should be observed for urticaria. Diphenhydramine (Benadryl) or naloxone (Narcan) may be ordered to relieve the symptoms. Because *nausea and vomiting* accompany transition labor, the phase should be observed in relation to the timing of the medication. The physician may order an antiemetic. *Urinary retention* is to be prevented for any laboring woman, and bladder distention and voiding frequency and amount should be monitored. After the birth naloxone may be given per order for inability to void.

Delayed respiratory depression is a serious side effect; thus 24-hour monitoring of respiratory rates is mandatory after epidural morphine. Lethargy and a respiratory rate under 10 per minute should be noted. Other central nervous system depressants are not given without a specific order from the anesthesiologist, and naloxone 0.4 mg is the antidote (Nicholson, 1990) (see Drug Profile 16-4).

Epidural administration calls for frequent assessment of vital signs, fetal heart rate, bladder distention, and assistance and coaching for pushing during descent of the fetus. After the birth, the nurse monitors vital signs, assesses bladder distention, and determines when feeling and motor tone have fully returned to the extremities. Skin temperature of the legs should be checked because vasodilation recedes as the local anesthetic wears off; both legs should be equal in temperature. Blood pressure, taken with the woman sitting and standing, should be assessed for its ability to maintain normal levels. The

NURSING CARE PLAN • Epidural Anesthesia

CASE: Anna M., para 0000, is reluctant to have an epidural since she attended a Lamaze childbirth preparation class. Her first stage of labor has now lasted 15 hours, and the cervix is 6 cm dilated. She is exhausted. Her physician explains the benefits to her and she agrees.

ASSESSMENT DATA

1. Current gestational age
2. No recent use of drugs or alcohol
3. Response to dental anesthetics
4. No prior injury of or defects in spinal area
5. Level of knowledge about epidural
6. Preanesthetic vital signs, fetal heart rate
7. Informed consent
8. Intake and output, IV fluid within last hour
9. Laboratory reports, especially WBC, platelet counts

NURSING DIAGNOSES

1. Pain related to phase of labor
2. Anxiety related to administration and process of anesthesia
3. At risk for altered tissue perfusion related to hypotension/bradycardia secondary to regional anesthesia
4. Altered urinary output related to lack of voiding sensation

EXPECTED OUTCOMES

1. States her understanding of what epidural anesthesia will do for her and understands basic benefit-risk ratio.
2. Manages her anxiety and verbalizes when she needs a dose.
3. Does not show signs of decreased tissue perfusion during the epidural.

NURSING INTERVENTIONS

1. Collect pertinent prenatal history. Ask specific questions.
2. Provide further explanations of benefits and risks, if she does not understand. Allow questions from both partners.
3. Assess level of anxiety about anesthesia and birth.
4. Assess level of perceived pain by observing behaviors, asking.
5. Monitor vital signs before and frequently after initiation of epidural.
6. Monitor fetal response and labor progress. Position to prevent vena caval compression.
7. Monitor intake; especially note IV fluids for hydration. Slow rate as soon as amount is absorbed.
8. Compare output with intake to prevent overload. Note bladder fullness, encourage voiding or, as necessary, do straight catheterization.

EVALUATION

1. Does epidural analgesia relieve labor pain without affecting fetal or maternal tissue perfusion?
2. Does Anna express confidence in her decision to have an epidural? Does she indicate feelings of failure at not completing labor without medication?
3. Do her circulatory and urinary functions remain normal?

client should not ambulate until full control has returned, usually 4 to 6 hours. Postural hypotension is a common problem during early recovery.

SUBARACHNOID BLOCK

Spinal anesthesia provides a subarachnoid block that erases motor tone and feeling below the block level. It is now used only for operative delivery. Because its technique is similar to that of a spinal tap, it may be performed by the obstetrician or nurse anesthetist. There are two types, saddle and spinal block; both are used less frequently today than epidural anesthesia (Figure 16-14).

Saddle Block

Low spinal administration is called a *saddle block* because the parts of the body come in contact with a saddle are some of the parts anesthetized. Because a saddle block usually does not stop contractions, it can be administered during the second stage of labor and provides anesthesia from L5 to S5 for descent and delivery. It may be used for a forceps delivery, but visceral pain still may occur, depending on the dose. A modified saddle block provides anesthesia from T10 to S5 and complete pain relief during delivery for the perineum and contractions, but it is not high enough for cesarean delivery.

The client is in a sitting position with the lower portion of her back rounded, feet supported, and forearms on her thighs or the over-bed table. Puncture into the dura mater is made at the L4-5 interspace with a long, small-gauge needle. CSF has been tapped when fluid drips back through the needle. Hyperbaric solution of the anesthetic (mixed with a glucose solution so

it is heavier than CSF) is inserted and the client is kept in a sitting position for 1 to 3 minutes to allow the anesthetic to settle downward in the spinal fluid. The client is assisted by two persons to lie supine with her neck flexed on a pillow. There should always be a lateral tilt to her lower back (with a small pillow or wedge) to prevent vena caval compression.

Spinal Block

A cesarean birth performed with lower uterine incision requires anesthesia for at least 60 to 90 minutes. Sensory levels to T6-7 should be anesthetized. Without an indwelling catheter, additional medication cannot be added if surgery takes longer than expected. Therefore, as with an epidural, concentrations of medication are chosen carefully for their duration of effect. Spinal block for cesarean delivery is accomplished in the same way as saddle block, but the client may be placed in the side-lying position for needle insertion. Her lower back should be rounded. She must stay absolutely still during the injection. A higher volume of local anesthetic is inserted. Recovery is slower, and adverse reactions are more possible. A spinal anesthetic is administered just before surgery to block uterine activity.

Adverse reactions. Adverse reactions are similar to those of epidural administration in some ways. Because of vena caval compression, hypotension always occurs and is more severe than with an epidural injection. Positioning after the injection is in a lateral tilt. A preload of intravenous fluids is administered to prevent lowered blood pressure.

Allergic reaction to the medication or occurrence of a high spinal are rare. Postpuncture headaches sometimes occur and are treated as already described. In very rare

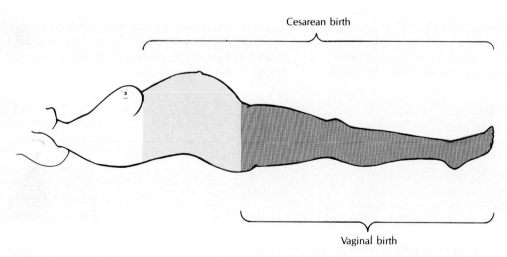

Cesarean birth

Vaginal birth

FIGURE 16-14 Level of anesthesia required for vaginal delivery and cesarean section. (Used with permission of Ross Laboratories, Columbus, Ohio 43216. From *Clinical Education aid no. 17,* © Ross Laboratories.)

instances the cord itself may be injured from too-deep or rough needle injection. In the recovery period, voiding may be a problem; most women after cesarean delivery have an indwelling catheter for 12 hours.

Nursing responsibilities. Nursing interventions are similar to those of epidural interventions after cesarean delivery. Return of sensation and postural hypotension is monitored, and position and fluids are managed to reduce the incidence of postpuncture headache. The inability to void may continue into recovery; therefore the nurse monitors for bladder distention and bleeding.

GENERAL ANESTHESIA

In effective concentrations, general anesthetics cause unconsciousness by depression of the central nervous system. Uterine muscle becomes relaxed, which can be beneficial when hypertonic contractions are present but may be a problem that can precipitate hemorrhage after delivery. General anesthesia is used in smaller centers when an anesthesiologist is not available for epidural administration, when there is an emergency delivery and no time for another approach, when regional anesthesia is contraindicated (e.g., for hemorrhage, infection, bleeding disorder, or a neurologic problem in the spinal area), when there are no contraindications, and when the woman requests it.

General anesthetics are given by the intravenous route or by inhalation. In some countries, certain inhalants are used in low doses for labor analgesia. The mother uses a hand-held inhaler. When she is sleepy, the mask falls away from her face so that she does not receive significant doses. This method usually is not used in this country.

Because the anesthetic in the doses needed for surgery passes quickly into the fetal circulation and depresses the fetal respiratory center, the induction must be rapid. The time-to-birth interval is important and usually is kept under 8 minutes. All principles of medication transfer across the placenta apply to anesthesia by this route. There is a search for anesthetic agents that work effectively and do not transfer easily.

Balanced Anesthesia

To prevent newborn depression, several agents in low doses are used; an intravenous dose of thiopental or ketamine is accompanied by a muscle relaxant and inhalation of anesthetic gas.

Nitrous oxide. Nitrous oxide has been used for more than 100 years. It provides rapid analgesia. With oxygen it may be sufficient for vaginal delivery. The effect on the fetus is related to the length of analgesia. Within 15 minutes the equilibrium across the placenta is ap-

proximately 87%. With extended analgesia the infant may be depressed and hypoxic. Therefore anesthetic administration for vaginal delivery must be timed as carefully as that for operative delivery.

Nitrous oxide has shown a teratogenic property in rat offspring when given during early gestation. Health professionals must be aware that there may be reproductive effects of chronic exposure to this gas.

Halogenated agents. Agents such as halothane, enflurane, and isoflurane have a smooth induction and stimulate less vomiting than other agents. Effective anesthesia occurs at low levels, as well as rapid excretion and recovery. These agents have not replaced all others in obstetrics because of their relaxant effect on smooth muscles. A number of studies on bleeding after delivery, including that of Gilstrap et al (1987), conclude that women who received halogenated agents had significantly greater postpartum anemia as measured by reduced hemoglobin and hematocrit measurements and the need for transfusions. The nurse notes the type of anesthesia each client receives and observes for amount of postanesthetic bleeding.

Ketamine. Ketamine induction is pleasant and rapid. Fetal equilibrium occurs within minutes of intravenous injection. Deep analgesia may be obtained quickly, and recovery is rapid. For this reason it can be used just before difficult manipulation in a vaginal delivery.

Ketamine also relaxes bronchial smooth muscle and is a good choice for clients with asthma. The risk of vomiting also is reduced. The cardiovascular stimulation of this medication raises the blood pressure 10% to 15%, and uterine blood flow is increased. Therefore it often is chosen if the fetus is distressed or maternal hypotension is a factor. This drug is not used in hypertensive states.

During recovery the woman may have unpleasant dreams as she awakens and may be restless. If anesthesia has been deep, she should be watched for vomiting and aspiration during recovery.

Thiopental sodium. Thiopental sodium is a short-acting barbiturate used for induction (in 30 seconds) but is not itself an analgesic. It must be used with a muscle relaxant, usually succinylcholine, and nitrous oxide or a halogenated anesthetic. An endotracheal tube is necessary. Hypotension will be evident and vena caval compression must be avoided by use of a lateral tilt position. Recovery is smooth, with little nausea and vomiting.

Prevention of Hazards: Fluid during Labor

For all general anesthesia, the woman is at risk because of *vomiting and aspiration*. These hazards lead to most of the deaths from general anesthesia. Aspiration of acidic contents of the stomach occurs if the woman vomits while her gag and cough reflexes are partially or completely anesthetized. The result is irritation to the lungs and possible respiratory arrest, cardiopulmonary changes, and death. In rare cases an inability to pass the endotracheal tube causes the woman to suffer from anoxia. In many of these cases the women were markedly obese.

The pregnant woman always is at risk for pulmonary aspiration. Thus determination of the interval from the time of the last meal until general anesthesia is unnecessary because all women in labor have slowed emptying of stomach contents. The woman who has fasted before elective cesarean has nearly the same stomach volume as the woman undergoing emergency cesarean (Albright et al, 1986). The woman who has received meperidine or another opioid analgesic is at much higher risk because her stomach emptying is markedly delayed by these drugs (Box 16-1).

About 80% of obstetric units allow clear, nutritious fluids and ice chips during labor to provide energy and comfort and are addressing the problem of aspiration in a different way. Before operative delivery under general anesthesia, the woman should receive a clear antacid such as sodium citrate (Bicitra or Alka-Seltzer Effervescent, two tablets in 30 ml water) just before induction. If the cesarean is scheduled, histamine blockers such as ranitidine (Zantac) are effective, given orally 2 hours before surgery. Suspensions of aluminum, magnesium, or calcium are more harmful than helpful; if aspirated, the particles damage the lungs. The goal is to raise the gastric pH above 2.5. The best protection from aspiration of stomach contents because of vomiting during induction is the use of **cricoid pressure** during tracheal intubation.

A nurse may be asked to apply pressure to the *cricoid cartilage*, pressing it to the cervical vertebrae to close the esophagus during intubation (Figure 16-15). Pressure should be *maintained or increased* if the client begins to vomit. The anesthesiologist will direct the nurse's action here. After the endotracheal tube is in place and the cuff inflated, the woman is protected from aspiration.

After the birth, the infant is observed for signs of respiratory depression. The mother has no awareness of the birth or of the infant until she has recovered. Depending on the dose, the period of recovery may be 1 or 2 hours, with lingering drowsiness lasting up to 8 hours.

After surgery the client is observed for vomiting and positioned to prevent aspiration. Her head and shoulders should be turned to the side, and she requires close observation during waking. Recovery is gradual, depending in part on her body size and the dose received. Protection from injury is a priority because restlessness is typical during emergence. Because pain perception is

---

BOX 16-1   Steps to Decrease Risk of Pulmonary Aspiration during Induction of General Anesthesia

- Neutralize stomach contents by administering a clear antacid (for example, sodium citrate 5 minutes before induction).
- Preoxygenation: the effects of the physiologic changes of pregnancy on the respiratory system cause the parturient to desaturate faster than the nonpregnant client.
- Use a rapid-acting barbiturate (thiopentone) and a depolarizing muscle relaxant (succinylcholine) to induce unconsciousness and facilitate tracheal intubation by muscle relaxation.
- Immediately on administration of these drugs, apply cricoid pressure (Sellick's maneuver) by a trained assistant.
- Intubate the trachea and inflate the cuff to seal the airway.
- Check to ensure that the endotracheal tube is properly positioned before releasing cricoid pressure.

From Douglas MJ: The case against more liberal food and fluid policy in labor, *Birth* 15(2):93, 1988.

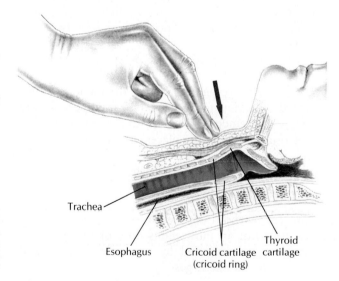

FIGURE 16-15 Technique of applying pressure on cricoid cartilage to occlude esophagus prevents pulmonary aspiration of gastric contents during anesthesia induction. (From Bobak IM, Jensen MD: *Maternity and gynecologic care: the nurse and the family,* ed 5, St Louis, 1993, Mosby.)

distorted, clients may complain of a great deal of pain. Analgesics are given in one-half doses during immediate recovery because of the potential for hypotension. Vital signs are monitored frequently. Smooth muscle may be relaxed; therefore postural hypotension is a possibility, as is hemorrhage. All women have difficulty voiding after general anesthetics.

Test Yourself

- List three reasons for and three against oral fluid intake during labor.

Nursing Responsibilities

Because the nurse understands the effects of drugs, the care plan should include observation and assessment of medication effects on clients and teaching preventive care. The following steps can be taken to increase awareness and improve assessment and intervention.

1. Include education about medications in antepartum and postpartum classes, as well as for every lactating woman.
2. Explain the benefit-to-risk ratio for questionable medications.

3. Counsel all mothers about nonpharmacologic methods for alleviating minor discomforts of pregnancy and recovery.
4. Encourage women to take childbirth classes to help to reduce medication levels during delivery, and support the educated mother in her attempts to cope with labor and delivery.
5. During the interview and assessment of the mother, include a record of any incidental nonprescription or prescription medications taken before labor.
6. Inform nursery nurses of transitional medications that might affect the newborn during recovery. Inform them about timing and level of analgesia and anesthesia.
7. Increase your ability to assess the newborn for normal behavioral responses. Records must be more descriptive during the newborn period if long-term behavioral effects of drugs are to be evaluated.
   a. Note iatrogenic factors affecting responses.
   b. Be alert for delayed excretion, cumulative effects, and altered physiologic states when noting medication effects.

When these steps are taken, it should be possible to provide informed nursing support to any woman during pregnancy or recovery and to discover subtle signs of medication influence on the infant.

KEY POINTS

- Pregnancy changes protein and tissue binding so that more drug may be free to seek receptor sites. Women note more sensitivity to drugs as a result.
- Membranes are porous to most substances so that levels of drug become equal on both sides of the placental barrier, and with some exceptions also cross the blood-brain and blood-milk barriers.
- A woman's serum drug level during late labor is crucial in evaluating newborn signs of drug effects.
- Transfer through the blood-milk barrier is affected by the pH of milk, volume at each feeding, and metabolic breakdown in tissue or the newborn's gastrointestinal tract. Only fractions of the maternal dose reach the newborn, compared with neonatal standard doses.
- Nurses should teach lactating women to space drug intake when it is necessary so that the lowest level is in the milk just before a feeding.

- Pain during parturition and after birth needs serious attention with nonpharmacologic analgesia emphasized.
- Nurses should not withhold analgesia, because pain interrupts mother-baby acquaintance.
- Patient-controlled analgesia administered intravenously or by the epidural route results in less demand for analgesics and higher client satisfaction.
- Pain thresholds vary widely as do pain behaviors. Cultural differences are seen clearly in labor responses.
- Epidural anesthesia with local anesthetics or with addition of fentanyl is a widely used anesthesia for vaginal or cesarean birth.
- General anesthesia places the woman at risk of aspiration; therefore a clear antacid must be given before and cricoid pressure applied during intubation.

STUDY QUESTIONS

16-1. Choose terms from this chapter to complete the following definitions.
   a. Lipoprotein membrane between maternal and fetal circulation _____
   b. The fatty sheath of myelin around capillaries and nerves of the brain _____
   c. The limited amount of drug molecules that may attach to a specific type of protein in maternal circulation _____
   d. The measurable period of time in which half of a drug dose is metabolized and excreted _____
   e. Pain originating from smooth muscle and felt as dull and diffuse is from _____ fibers. Sharp and referred pain is from _____ fibers.

16-2. Pudendal block produces anesthesia for which parts of the body?
   a. Lower uterine segment and cervix
   b. Vagina and entire perineum
   c. Uterus, cervix, bladder, and rectum
   d. Parts affected by the perineal nerve

16-3. Which types of drugs move more easily across membrane barriers?
   a. Hydrophilic, ionized drugs
   b. Low molecular weight, protein-bound drugs
   c. Lipophilic, partially ionized drugs
   d. Fat-soluble, nonionized drugs

16-4. If equilibrium of a medication is present in maternal and fetal circulations, the following is true:
   a. The drug accumulates in higher levels in the fetus than in the mother.
   b. An adverse effect will occur in the fetus.
   c. The fetus will be more affected by the drug than the mother.
   d. The ratio of free medication is the same on both sides of the placenta.

16-5. Which of the following situations would result in the highest level of drug in the newborn?
   a. Mrs. J., who has an infection, is being given ampicillin 2 g, q6h by piggyback IV. Her last dose was 4 hours before birth.
   b. Mrs. K., because of high blood pressure, is receiving an IV with magnesium sulfate, 2 g/hr, by infusion pump.
   c. Mrs. L. received Demerol and Phenergan 3 hours before birth.

16-6. After the first test dose of medication has been inserted into the epidural catheter, the client must be observed for:
   a. Allergic responses
   b. Hypertonic contractions
   c. Accidental injection into dural or intrathecal spaces
   d. Headache and nausea

16-7. After the therapeutic dose of a epidural anesthetic has been injected, you must observe for which of the following?
   a. A change in contraction rate and intensity
   b. Complaints of thirst and increased anxiety
   c. Vasodilation resulting in hypotension
   d. Increase in bloody show with possible rupture of membranes

Answer Key

16-1 a. Placental membrane, b. Blood-brain barrier, c. Bound drug, d. Half-life, e. Unmyelinated, myelinated, 16-2 b 16-3 d 16-4 d 16-5 b 16-6 a 16-7 c

REFERENCES

Abboud TK: The neonatal neurobehavioral effects of mepivacaine for epidural anesthesia during labor, *Anesthesia* 63(9)A:449, 1985.

Albright GA et al: *Anesthesia in obstetrics: maternal, fetal, and neonatal aspects,* ed 2, Boston, 1986, Butterworth.

American Academy of Pediatrics Committee on Drugs: The transfer of drugs and other chemicals into breast milk, *Pediatrics* 72:291, 1983.

Augustensson L et al: Pain relief during delivery by transdermal electrical nerve stimulation, *Pain* 4:50, 1977.

Beal MW: Acupuncture and related treatment modalities. II. Applications to antepartal and intrapartal care, *J Nurse Midwife* 37(4):260, 1990.

Beeley L: Drugs and breastfeeding, *Clin Obstet Gynecol* 13(2):245, 1986.

Berlin M: Effects of drugs on the fetus, *Pediatr Rev* 12(9):282, 1991.

Bodden C: Relief of labor pain by acupressure, master's thesis, Garden City, NY, 1986, Adelphi University.

Brackbill Y et al: Obstetric meperidine usage and assessment of neonatal status, *Anesthesiology* 40:116, 1974.

Briggs GC, Freeman RK, Yaffee SJ: *Drugs in pregnancy and lactation,* ed 2, Baltimore, 1986, Williams & Wilkins.

Bulham JAJ: Guidelines for drug therapy during lactation, *JOGNN* 7(1):65, 1986.

Cahill CA: Beta-endorphin levels during pregnancy and labor: a role in pain modulation? *Nurs Res* 38(4):200, 1989.

Dawood MY, Ramos J: Transcutaneous electrical nerve stimulation (TENS) for the treatment of primary dysmenorrhea, *Obstet Gynecol* 75(4):657, 1990.

Ferrante FM et al: Patient-controlled epidural analgesia: demand dosing, *Anesth Analg* 73:547, 1991.

Gaston-Johannson F, Fridh G, Turner-Nowell K: Progression of labor pain in primiparas and multiparas, *Nurs Res* 37(2):86, 1988.

Geden EA et al: Effects of music and imagery on physiologic and self-report of analogued labor pain, *Nurs Res* 38(1):37, 1989.

Gibbs CP et al: Obstetric anesthesia: a national survey, *Anesthesiology* 65:298, 1986.

Gilstrap LC III et al: Effect of type of anesthesia on blood loss at cesarean section, *Obstet Gynecol* 69(3):328, 1987.

Gray DG, Yaffe SJ: Prenatal drugs. Symposium on Learning Difficulties, 1986, Johnson & Johnson, New Brunswick, NJ.

Grim LC, Morey SH: Transcutaneous electrical nerve stimulation for relief of parturition pain; a clinical report, *Phys Ther* 65(3):337, 1985.

Hawkin DF: *Drugs and pregnancy,* ed 2, New York, 1988, Churchill Livingstone.

Koch-Weser J, Sellers EM: Binding of drugs to serum albumin, *N Engl J Med* 294(6):311, 1976.

Loeser J: Concepts of pain. In Stanton-Hicks M, Boss R, editors: *Chronic low back pain,* New York, 1982, Raven Press.

Melzack R et al: Severity of labor pain: influence of physical as well as psychologic variables, *Can Med Assoc J* 30(3):580, 1984.

Miller-Jones CMC: Transcutaneous nerve stimulation in labour, *Anaesthesia* 35:372, 1980.

 STUDENT RESOURCE SHELF

Stampone D: The history of obstetric anesthesia *J Perinat Neonat Nurs* 4(1):1, 1990. A review of the progress in pain management during labor and birth.

Moore ML: *Realities in childbearing,* Philadelphia, 1983, WB Saunders Co.

Neswander KR, Gordon M: *The women and their pregnancies: the Collaborative Perinatal Study of the National Institute of Neurologic Disease and Stroke,* Philadelphia, 1973, WB Saunders Co.

Nice FJ: Can a breast-feeding mother take medication without harming her infant? *MCN* 14(1):27, 1989.

Nicholson JR: Nursing considerations for the parturient who has received epidural narcotics during labor and delivery, *J Perinat Neonat Nurs* 4(4):14, 1990.

Olsson G, Parker G: A model approach to pain assessment, *Nurs 87* 5:52, 1987.

Rivera-Calimlim L: The significance of drugs in breast milk, *Clin Perinatol* 14(1):51, 1987.

Zimmer EZ, Divon MY, Vadasz A: Influence of meperidine on fetal movements and heart rate beat-to-beat variability in the active phase of labor, *Am J Perinatol* 5(3):197, 1988.

17

The Recovery Process and Nursing Care

KEY TERMS

Engorgement
Episiotomy
Fundus
Involution
Latching-On
Let-Down Reflex
Letting Go
Lochia
Postpartum
  Depression
Puerperium
Rooting Reflex
Sucking Reflex
Taking Hold
Taking In
Uterine Atony

LEARNING OBJECTIVES

1. State major components of involution in postpartum recovery.
2. Determine the client's need for knowledge supplementation.
3. Instruct the postpartum client in self-care during recovery.
4. Describe appropriate care for alterations in patterns of recovery.
5. Contrast vaginal and surgical birth in relation to self-care needs.
6. Evaluate effectiveness of nursing interventions for postpartum families.
7. Recognize expected psychologic responses of the new mother, noting deviations from normal.
8. Identify factors that initiate, maintain, or interfere with successful breast-feeding.

Recovery Process

Dramatic changes begin to occur in a woman's body systems as soon as a baby is born; the processes that occurred during pregnancy are reversed. Some systems undergo only minimal reversal, whereas others undergo extensive changes. For example, more pregnancy and involutional changes occur in the cardiovascular and reproductive systems than in the respiratory system. Within 6 weeks the woman's body will revert to her prepregnant physical status.

Whether the new mother and her family view this period as a positive or a negative time depends in part on the nurturing received during the hospital stay. The nurse can do much to influence the new mother through the teaching and caring she receives and through affirmation of her parenting skills and abilities.

INVOLUTION OF REPRODUCTIVE ORGANS

Involution is the process whereby the pelvic reproductive organs, particularly the uterus, return to their prepregnant size and position. This period also has been referred to as the recovery, postpartum, postnatal, or postdelivery period, or the **puerperium.** All women who deliver an infant must pass through this recovery period.

The recovery period usually is considered to last from immediately after the delivery to the sixth week (42 days). After delivery the woman is cared for in the postpartum unit until discharged and is instructed to return in 6 to 8 weeks to her physician or clinic for a checkup. By this time most of her pelvic organs have returned to their prepregnant position and approximate prepregnant size. Many women, however, do not feel recovered from pregnancy and birth in 6 to 8 weeks and may require a longer period.

Uterus

At delivery the woman's uterus weighs approximately 1000 g (2.2 pounds), and by the end of puerperium, it will have returned to its prepregnant weight of 60 g (2 ounces). The uterus can return to its prepregnant weight and shape because muscle cell size increased during pregnancy although the number of cells remained basically the same. During recovery the protein cytoplasm of the muscle fibers undergoes catabolic or autolytic changes that cause a reduction in cell size. The products of this process are carried off in the urine as nitrogenous waste.

Immediately after delivery, the very hard, round, contracted uterus lies midway between the symphysis pubis and the umbilicus. Within hours of delivery it rises to the level of the umbilicus or slightly above it. The uterus begins its descent into the pelvic cavity on the first postpartum day. It diminishes rapidly in size, weight, and position until the tenth day, when it may be palpated at or below the level of the symphysis pubis (Figure 17-1). Throughout the postpartum period the firm and contracted uterus should be found in the midline.

Because uterine blood vessels and the uterine muscles are intertwined, a tourniquet action prevents bleeding or hemorrhage from the open blood vessels at the placental site when the uterus contracts. After delivery the uterus contracts on its own unless there is interference; for example, placental fragments keep the uterus from contracting. Occasionally, because of overdistention from multiple gestation, a large fetus, or an exhausted uterine muscle, a uterus may contract poorly.

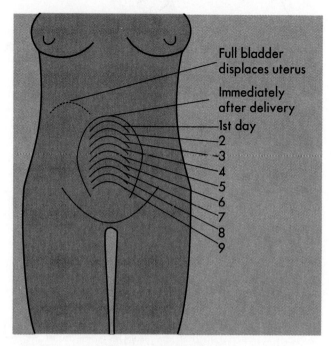

FIGURE 17-1 Postpartum descent of uterus into pelvic canal.

Uterine atony, failure of the uterus to remain firmly contracted, can lead to postpartum hemorrhage.

A full bladder is a major cause of uterine atony. Because of change in intraabdominal pressure after delivery and volume of intravenous (IV) fluids, the bladder becomes easily distended, pushing the uterus up and to the side (generally the right). The uterus must be able to contract to stop the bleeding from the placental site; therefore a soft, "boggy" uterus, out of the midline and above the umbilicus, is a strong indicator that the bladder is full.

Lochia. After delivery the decidual lining of the uterus sloughs off as **lochia.** This discharge contains blood, decidual tissue, epithelial cells from the vagina, mucus, bacteria, and occasionally fragments of membranes and small clots. Its odor is fleshy but not offensive (as menstrual discharge can be).

The lochia, which is red and bloody during the first stage, is called *lochia rubra (rubra* meaning red). This phase lasts 1 to 3 days and initially may contain a few small blood clots. The next stage is termed *lochia serosa;* it lasts 5 to 7 days, is serosanguineous, and is reddish pink to brown. The third and final stage is called *lochia alba.* It is white (primarily because of leukocytes) and lasts 1 to 3 weeks (Blackburn and Loper, 1992). The color of lochia indicates healing of the placental site. By 6 weeks the placental site usually has healed from the inner epithelial surface outward as the necrotic area covering the placental site sloughs off

TABLE 17-1 Lochial Characteristics

	RUBRA	SEROSA	ALBA
Color	Bright red; bloody	Pink-brown	Creamy white
Clots	Small clots	No clots	No clots
Odor	Slightly "fleshy"	No odor	No odor or stale body odor
Length	1-3 days	5-7 days	1-3 wk

and is replaced with new, healthy cells. This process prevents placental scarring. Otherwise, after a few pregnancies the inside lining of the uterus would be full of scar tissue, making it unsuitable for further implantation. Table 17-1 lists lochial characteristics.

Return of menses. The exact mechanism responsible for resumption of the menstrual cycle is not fully understood. With the drop in estrogen and progesterone levels after placental separation, however, the menstrual cycle is reestablished. In general, it takes longer for nursing mothers than nonnursing mothers to resume their cycles. The speed with which a woman resumes menses depends on whether she is breast-feeding, if she is feeding at night, and if she is relying completely on breast-feeding or merely supplementing her infant's diet. Cycles can begin in lactating mothers as early as 8 weeks or as late as 14 months after delivery. If the mother is breast-feeding and not supplementing the infant's diet, menses may resume by 4 to 8 months (Lethbridge, 1988).

The cycle may begin in the nonlactating mother as early as the fourth to sixth week, although the average time is 6 to 8 weeks. Menses resumes in most nonlactating mothers by the third month (Blackburn and Loper, 1992). The first menstrual cycle usually is anovulatory; in other words, menstruation occurs before the body produces and expels mature ova. A few cycles may pass before menses resume their prepregnant rhythm and length. Precautions against conception, however, should always be taken.

Cervix

Whereas the upper part of the uterus after delivery is firm, hard, and contracted, the lower uterine segment and cervix remain loose, thin, and stretched. The cervix also may appear edematous and bruised from the delivery and may have some tears or lacerations. It will admit the entire hand for several hours, making manual examination of the uterus possible. By the first postpartum day, however, the cervix has sufficiently narrowed

and regained its normal consistency to admit only two fingers. The parous cervix does not (will never again) look like the nonparous cervix. The external os, which previously resembled a dimple, now resembles a slit or smile, and any lacerations to the cervix during delivery may leave scar tissue.

Vaginal Canal

The vaginal canal has been stretched to accommodate the delivery of the fetus and placenta. The external vaginal orifice or introitus appears jagged and irregular in shape after delivery. Tears may occur as a result of delivery, particularly if it was very rapid or uncontrolled. Occasionally, a hematoma may develop as a result of descent and delivery. The usual places for the development of hematomas are the introitus, vaginal wall at the ischial spines, and the episiotomy site. Any woman who complains of severe or excessive perineal pain or sensitivity should be carefully assessed for hematomas. *instruct Kegal exercises*

In a few weeks the introitus will be sufficiently healed for resumption of sexual relations, although the vagina may be dry until hormonal balance is restored.

Perineum

After delivery the muscles of the floor of the perineum are stretched, swollen, and often bruised. Some tears may be extensive, invading the deeper levator ani muscles. The type of episiotomy will be noted in the client's record (see Chapter 15).

During pushing and the delivery of the fetal head, the straining and pressure on the lower bowel often cause the extrusion of internal hemorrhoids. After delivery, however, they reduce in size and can be manually reinserted into the rectum. Hemorrhoids present during the pregnancy also shrink. Surgical reduction after delivery rarely is necessary.

Ovaries

The ovaries have been inactive during the last two trimesters of the pregnancy. Because of the drop in the placental hormone level, however, the body gradually resumes its prepregnancy menstrual cycle. *recurrancy period 6-8 wks pp*

Breasts

Depending on whether the mother decides to breast-feed or bottle-feed, the breast responds accordingly. If she determines to breast-feed, the stimulation of the baby's sucking will release prolactin, causing the breast to produce milk (Figure 17-2). As the blood and lymph surge into the breast in anticipation of milk production, the breasts enlarge and swell, becoming very firm and warm around the third postpartum day.

If there is no stimulation by the infant, the breasts, which had been prepared for breast-feeding during

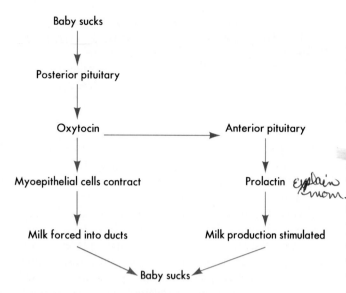

Baby sucks

↓

Posterior pituitary

↓

Oxytocin → Anterior pituitary

↓   ↓

Myoepithelial cells contract   Prolactin

↓   ↓

Milk forced into ducts   Milk production stimulated

↘   ↙

Baby sucks

FIGURE 17-2 Let-down reflex is triggered by the infant's sucking.

pregnancy, will recede in size back to their prepregnancy state. Nonnursing mothers also experience fullness and **engorgement.** (See nursing care for treatment of engorgement.) Lactation physiology and methods are discussed in a special section in this chapter.

CARDIOVASCULAR FUNCTION

Some of the most dramatic changes in the puerperium occur in the cardiovascular system. During pregnancy the blood volume increases by 30% to 50% over the prepregnancy volume. After delivery, however, there is no need for excess blood volume, and drastic shifts occur in body fluids. During birth and placental delivery, the woman loses approximately 300 to 500 ml of blood (up to 1000 ml during cesarean birth). This loss depletes a portion of the additional fluid (Combs et al, 1991).

The blood from the pelvic region returns to the general circulation, and the extracellular fluids that accumulated during pregnancy return to the circulating blood for excretion. Additional fluid will be lost through diuresis and diaphoresis.

Heart Rate and Blood Pressure

During pregnancy the heart rate increases up to 15 beats/min over the prepregnancy baseline, and the stroke volume increases to handle the increased blood volume. After delivery, however, the heart rate decelerates, at times reaching as low as 40 to 60 beats/min. Therefore, if an *increase* in pulse rate is noted, a secondary cause, such as hemorrhage, infection, thrombosis, anxiety, or excitement related to the delivery, should be explored.

During labor the blood pressure may fluctuate; it may rise during contractions or when the woman pushes or experiences pain. It also may fall because of supine hypotensive syndrome, regional anesthesia, or hemorrhage. It should, however, return to normal after delivery, unless complications such as pregnancy-induced hypertension (PIH) have occurred.

Although the delivery may have been uncomplicated, orthostatic hypotension may occur because of fluid shift and decreased intraabdominal pressure. (See Chapter 22 for discussion of hypertension.)

Blood Values

Hemoglobin and hematocrit. Hemoglobin and hematocrit levels may fluctuate during the immediate postpartum period, especially if blood volume has been diluted with a large amount of intravenous fluids or an excess of blood has been lost during delivery. Hematocrit values may be altered from prenatal blood values, depending on several factors, including the following:

- The amount of intravenous fluids received during the intrapartum period
- The amount of blood loss at the time of delivery
- The amount of perspiration during labor and delivery
- An elevated temperature during delivery
- Fluid shift from extravascular tissues to the general circulation

After the first day, the fluid shift from extravascular tissues into the vascular compartment may depress the hematocrit level because of this dilution. If levels dropped on the first postpartum day, a repeat evaluation is obtained. If the client lost a considerable amount of blood during delivery, laboratory values should be periodically checked at the same time every day because hemoglobin and hematocrit levels tend to fluctuate during the day, being slightly higher in the morning than in the afternoon (Table 17-2).

White blood cells. The normal white blood cell count when the woman is not pregnant is between 5000 and 8000/mm^3. The count rises during late pregnancy and labor and can reach levels of 18,000/mm^3. This count is within normal limits for pregnancy and immediate recovery. Levels fall quickly to 6000 to 10,000/mm^3 and to normal levels by 4 to 7 days. Therefore persistent elevation indicates infection (Blackburn and Loper, 1992).

An increase in the granulocytes, particularly neutrophils (which are polymorphonuclear [PMN] cells), causes the increase in white blood cells. Neutrophils, which normally constitute more than half of the white blood cell profile, increase in the body in response to inflammation, pain, anxiety, stress, and labor and delivery; protect against invading organisms, engulfing them

TABLE 17-2 Postpartum Laboratory Values

	NORMAL	ABNORMAL
Temperature	97°-100.4° F (36.2°-38° C)	≥100.4° F (38° C) after first 24 hr
Pulse	50-80 beats/min (may drop to 40 beats/min)	Tachycardia because of hemorrhage, thrombosis, infection, dehydration, fever, medication, anxiety, excitement with respiratory difficulty
Respiration	16-24/min	↑ with respiratory difficulty
Blood pressure	Pregnancy levels; orthostatic hypotension as a result of fluid shifts and lower intraabdominal pressure	↑ PIH, hypertension, delivery excitement ↓ because of hypovolemia from anesthesia or hemorrhage
Red blood cells (RBC)	3.75-5 million/mm³; gradual ↑ to prepregnancy levels	↓ because of hemorrhage or ↑ IV fluid
White blood cells (WBC)	10,000-18,000/mm³	↓ 10,000/mm³ or ↑ 20,000/mm³ may indicate a problem
Hemoglobin (Hb)	11.5-14 g/dl	Blood loss of 500 ml decreases Hb 1-1.5 g/dl*
Hematocrit (Hct)	32%-42%	Blood loss of 500 ml decreases Hct 3% to 4%*
Platelets	↑ during recovery	↓ HELLP syndrome, lupus
Fibrin	↑ during immediate recovery to normal by 3-5 days	↓ bleeding related to DIC
Urine		
Output	↑ 3 L/day	Concentrated urine
Glucose	↑ lactosuria	Check for diabetes if glycosuria
Blood urea nitrogen (BUN)	↑ because of catabolism	

Data from Blackburn and Loper, 1992.
HELLP, Hemolysis, elevated liver enzymes, and low platelet count.
*American Association of Blood Banks: *Blood transfusion therapy: a physician's handbook,* Arlington, Va, 1983, The Association, p. 8.

through phagocytosis; and débride the decidual tissues of dead cells during the healing process.

Red blood cells. The red blood cell count actually increases during pregnancy, but because of a greater increase in plasma volume, these values appear to drop slightly. During recovery the red blood cell count gradually returns to prepregnancy blood values.

Platelets and fibrin. Platelet and fibrin levels are elevated during recovery and may contribute to formation of a thrombus (see Chapter 22).

RESPIRATORY FUNCTION

After delivery and during recovery the respiratory rate should not noticeably change. However, the respiratory system should be assessed regularly during the immediate recovery period. Because the enlarged uterus no longer presses upward on the diaphragm, women find breathing easier. If, however, the woman received inhalation or general anesthesia, extra precautions should

be instituted because of the possibility of vomiting, with aspiration or congestion. Lung sounds should be assessed by auscultation.

RENAL FUNCTION

The hormones (particularly progesterone) that caused ureter dilation are no longer present. Dilated ureters require a longer period than the rest of the urinary tract structures to return to the prepregnancy condition. The enlarged uterus no longer compresses the bladder, causing frequency. Instead, as a result of decreased intraabdominal pressure and relaxed abdominal muscles, the capacity of the bladder increases. It may fill to 1000 or 1500 ml without discomfort.

Retention of urine may result because of stretching of the perineal floor, with accompanying bruising and edema of the trigone and urethral meatus. During labor and delivery, the fetus places pressure on the bladder, particularly if it is full. Regional anesthesia may temporarily diminish sensations from the bladder, contributing to urinary retention. Because a full bladder can lead to a

normally we do not release > 800-1000 cc urine from bladder @ 1 time, however immed p.p. its Ø unusuall to have but if need to straight cath, do pause before full emptying.

relaxed uterus and subsequent hemorrhage, the nurse must assess the bladder regularly during the recovery period and encourage and assist the client to void. q̄ 2-4°

Body water in the extravascular spaces and excess blood volume from the pregnancy are eliminated rapidly. By the second postpartum day, diuresis and polyuria occur. Up to 3 L of urine are eliminated daily for a few days. This physiologic condition should be explained to the client. Within a week, she will return to her prepregnancy voiding pattern because diuresis diminishes and the muscle tone of the bladder returns.

Glycosuria, primarily caused by the presence of lactose, may occur during the puerperium. Also, as a result of catabolic changes taking place in the uterus, nitrogenous waste may appear in urine. These are physiologic changes during involution.

GASTROINTESTINAL FUNCTION

After the delivery of the placenta and cessation of placental hormones, the gastrointestinal tract begins to revert to its prepregnancy peristaltic and digestive activities, condition, and tone. After delivery, women generally are hungry or thirsty and want to eat or drink something light (e.g., juice, toast, or tea). The type of analgesia or anesthesia and the delivery route influence when the client may have her first oral intake. Many units wait 1 hour to monitor recovery and then provide fluids ad lib. No woman should be given oral fluids or food until she has recovered from general anesthesia. After initial adjustment, however, she may request extra portions of food. By discharge, most women have regained their usual appetite.

Most recovering women do not have a bowel movement until a few days after delivery. The reasons are varied. The woman may have had diarrhea at the onset of labor and no food intake for up to 24 hours (or more). An enema may have been given during early labor. Fear of pain with the episiotomy while straining for a bowel movement poses a barrier. Painful hemorrhoids also may delay the first bowel movement. Because so many women experience this delay, it has become standard practice in many hospitals to order stool softeners the first few days after delivery. If a woman has not had a bowel movement by the third day, an enema or a suppository may be prescribed. The speed with which her bowels become regulated will depend on her daily activities, diet (adequate roughage and fluid), activity (including exercises), and schedule.

Weight Loss and Nutrition

Although diuresis and diaphoresis provide mechanisms for reduction of body water, fat deposits intended for lactation remain. If the mother breast-feeds, these deposits are slowly metabolized in the first 3 to 5 months and she should lose weight gradually. If she bottle-feeds,

these fat deposits must be lost by calorie reduction and exercise.

The recovery diet should follow the same guidelines as the pregnancy diet, with a gradual reduction of dairy products from four to two servings (if not breast-feeding) and a gradual reduction of protein foods from three to two servings. Avoiding concentrated sweets facilitates weight reduction. Severe caloric restriction cannot provide sufficient nutritional supply to replace calcium, iron, protein, or vitamin stores that may have been reduced during pregnancy. When oral contraceptives are used, additional nutrients such as folic acid, vitamin B_6, and, to a lesser extent, riboflavin, thiamine, and ascorbic acid appear to be indicated. (See Chapter 5 for discussion.) Exercise is discussed later in this chapter.

Typically 10-15# is lost = infant, placenta, fluid 5# diuresis & perspiration

INTEGUMENTARY FUNCTION

After delivery the changes that occurred in the skin of the pregnant woman begin to recede. The hormones, particularly the melanocyte-stimulating hormone that caused pigmentational changes, have been eliminated. Not all changes will completely disappear. The striae gravidarum or stretch marks, for example, will turn a silvery color and fade, but many women have them indefinitely. The linea nigra and the darkened areola fade, but in some women faint traces remain. Melasma disappears unless excessive pigmentation occurred.

Palmar erythema because of increased circulation and estrogenic influence also subsides. Accelerated hair and nail growth slows down. Many women complain after delivery that their hair falls out "by the handful." Actually hair growth has entered a resting phase, and the additional hair that grew during pregnancy is just being shed. In a few months, hair and nail growth will return to prepregnancy patterns. Spider nevi also recede during the postpartum period and urticarial rashes usually subside.

MUSCULOSKELETAL FUNCTION

Immediately after delivery the woman may be fatigued or even exhausted. The labor position and pushing techniques may leave arms, neck, shoulders, and perineal muscles sore and aching.

Under the influence of relaxin the pelvic joints, particularly the symphysis pubis, may separate slightly during labor and delivery. After birth the ligaments and cartilage begin to ease back into the prepregnancy position; as a result, some women feel pain and discomfort in this area. Eventually this pain, described as a "pinching," subsides. A few women have severe pain and difficulty in walking for a short time.

During pregnancy, labor, or delivery some women may experience a separation of the vertical, central abdominal muscle group (the rectus abdominis muscles). This is called *diastasis recti abdominis (diastasis,* meaning separation). If this occurs before or during delivery, pushing may become difficult or impossible because these muscles help to push the baby through the birth canal. In general, no particular treatment is indicated for this condition, but restoration of the muscles may be prolonged. The abdominal wall is somewhat relaxed for all women in the first few weeks of puerperium.

Shivering

Many clients experience transient trembling after delivery. Several theories concerning this shivering have been proposed. These include exhaustion from the strenuous activities of labor and delivery, the sudden decrease in intraabdominal pressure, the sudden and complete withdrawal of placental hormones, and reaction to the small transfusions of fetal blood or amniotic fluid that may have entered maternal circulation during placental separation. The cool environment of labor rooms and room-temperature IV fluids are a major cause of chilling. This trembling and chill usually are not associated with an elevation of temperature (Harper et al, 1991).

Reassure her & encourage relaxation.

Exercise *do provide supportive care — blankets, do & allow to hold infant while trembling*

After delivery the client gradually may resume exercising in the same way she exercised during the prenatal period. She should be cautioned not to exercise too strenuously at first but to pace her activities. Frequent walking is one of the best exercises; when women were confined to bed for extended periods after delivery, many complications such as hypostatic pneumonia, thromboses, and emboli occurred. For this reason, encourage ambulation and exercise soon after delivery. In addition, Kegel exercises for perineal muscles are continued into the recovery period.

Test Yourself

- Refer to Chapter 10 to review the amount of weight that is related to the amniotic fluid (1 L) and extra plasma in the circulation (35%). When a woman asks how much weight she should lose by the end of the first week, the nurse should check the client's weight to see how much she has lost, ascertain the following factors, and calculate early weight loss related to the infant, amniotic fluids, and diuresis:
  —Infant's weight, 7 lb
  —Woman's prepregnancy weight, 130 lb
  —Woman's weight at the time of labor, 175 lb
  —What weight is to be expected?

ENDOCRINE FUNCTION

Placental hormones are abruptly reduced at delivery. Estrogen and progesterone no longer affect the blood vessels, ureters, intestinal tract, and reproductive tract. It takes several weeks, however, for all these structures to regain muscle tone and proper function. Full restoration of normal bowel functioning may take a few weeks, and urinary tract changes may require a month.

After delivery, prolactin production is taken over entirely by the anterior pituitary gland. The impetus for prolactin excretion is nipple stimulation. Otherwise the hormone is not secreted.

Stimulation of the breast during breast-feeding also induces the release of oxytocin, which causes the milk to be released from the breasts by the action known as the let-down reflex. At the same time oxytocin causes strong contractions of the uterus, the afterbirth pains.

Other endocrine glands—the thyroid and adrenal glands and the pancreas—return to their prepregnancy size and activity within a few weeks of delivery.

↑ afterbirth pains c̄ ↑ parity (more births, more birth pains)

INFECTION

The skin is the first line of defense against infection. Any break in that barrier by surgery or trauma can result in pathogenic invasion. Signs of infection may be subjective, for example, a woman's complaint of severe, unexpected pain, malaise, or chills. Often the signs are objective, such as the presence of fever or abnormal tissue. If any discharge occurs, always send a specimen for a culture and sensitivity test and notify the physician for follow-up care. Antibiotics should not be administered *until* the culture is obtained but may be administered before results are received. Culture and sensitivity results are necessary for the definitive diagnosis of an infection.

Fever

An elevation of temperature in the first 24 hours after delivery may be caused by dehydration, excitement, fatigue, chilling, and blood loss. The temperature may be as high as 38° C (100.4° F), which is within normal limits. If the temperature remains elevated after the first day, however, the cause must be found and treated. Infection should be considered, especially if there is a history of premature rupture of the membranes, hemorrhage, a long or traumatic labor and delivery, or a preexisting infection. A thorough assessment of the woman's condition provides data about the source of the problem.

Most often, low-grade fever accompanies engorgement of the breasts. The infant is not separated from the mother when she has a fever, unless specifically directed by the physician. Because the infant and mother usually have the same bacterial and viral agents, nothing is usually gained by isolation (see isolation precautions in Chapter 25).

Test Yourself

Fill in the normal findings in the first 24 hours after delivery.
- White blood cell count _____
- Lochial color and amount _____
- Temperature (oral) _____
- Appetite _____
- Fatigue level _____
- Emotional mood _____

Psychosocial Adjustments
BONDING

[handwritten: occurs during 6wk recovery period]

Post partum can be viewed as a time of transition from nonparenthood to parenthood. (See Chapter 20 for further discussion.)

Parent-infant attachment that leads to the bonding depends in part on the infant's responsiveness. The baby's response reinforces the parents and encourages them to continue interaction. The result is a stable bond between the infant and parents that will endure despite any separations. *Bond formation* is an outgrowth of reciprocal attachment stimulus-response and affectional ties that help form a coordinated, constructive social relationship. The nurse can only infer that bonding is progressing satisfactorily through observation of attachment behavior (i.e., behaviors that serve to maintain contact and demonstrate affection toward the baby) (Figure 17-3). Examples of this behavior include kissing, fondling and cuddling, and holding the infant in the en face position to maintain eye contact.

[handwritten top of right column: Rubins stages of maternal devel.]

MATERNAL DEVELOPMENTAL TASKS

Rubin (1975a) delineated several stages or phases that the new mother goes through during recovery; these include **taking in, taking hold,** and **letting go.** After the delivery the mother is exhausted and needs rest and sleep. During the first or second day, she will be *taking in* all the experiences of labor and delivery and may become introspective and contemplative. She may ask many questions regarding the labor and delivery experience and worry about her condition and her infant. Her physical needs and deficits of nourishment, rest, and comfort must be met by a caring nursing staff; then the new mother will be able to care for the needs of her baby. *Taking hold* describes the period when the mother attends to the infant's care needs, the role changes to come, and her own recovery needs. During this phase women usually are eager to learn how to care for themselves and their infant.

[handwritten: 2-3rd d. pp]

During recovery the mother also must *let go* and view the infant as a separate person. Some women have difficulty accomplishing this task, and if it is not resolved, psychologic problems could ensue. A mother may have great difficulty letting others assist with care of the infant, for example, or an overprotective mother may not allow herself to go out if a baby-sitter is needed. She still is attached to the child because she views it as an extension of herself. Because this behavior is not evident in the hospital stay, the clinic nurse or pediatric staff members could identify this unresolved task. Occasionally, professional psychologic help may be necessary.

[handwritten: not resolved. This process is needed for mother & infants benefit.]

SELF-ESTEEM NEEDS

All persons need *self-esteem;* it underlies personal satisfaction and effective functioning. It is the extent to which an individual believes herself to be capable, worthy, successful, and significant. Self-esteem depends on maintenance of control over self and achievement of expectations. In adulthood, individual expectations are

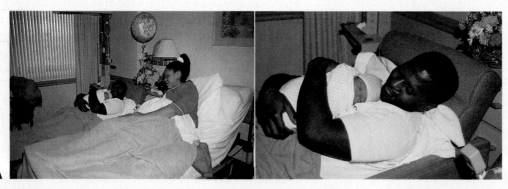

FIGURE 17-3 A, Getting acquainted in the labor-delivery-recovery and postrecovery (LDRP) room where mother and father have time with their new baby. **B,** Father may stay overnight in an LDRP setting. (Courtesy Marjorie Pyle, RNC, *Lifecircle.*)

affected by demands from the common group, society, or culture and are experienced as roles. During pregnancy these roles take on new meaning, and emphasis is placed on responsibilities toward the growing child. Studies show that women set psychologic tasks to carry out, especially during labor and delivery. In a study by Tribotti et al (1988), role performance was selected as a leading concern of women after birth. The congruence or lack of congruence between the idealized self and the actual self determines feelings of self-worth and self-esteem. Childbirth is a crisis event, an emotional milestone. The woman, already in a state of disequilibrium, is vulnerable to self-criticism and to anything that may be perceived as criticism from others. A woman who has planned for and expects to give birth in a controlled situation with her partner feels disappointment, anger, sadness, guilt, and failure when she is unable to achieve this goal.

In today's society, in which a great emphasis is placed on active participation in and control over life experiences, many couples desire the "ideal" childbirth experience, which includes a prepared and well-controlled labor and delivery, sharing with the baby's father, and no medication (Carty and Tier, 1989). When a woman who planned birth without medication and with minimal assistance experiences a labor that deviates from normal and then requires medication, anesthesia, or forceps or cesarean delivery, she often feels that she has failed. The outcome may be some degree of shame and decreased self-esteem.

The husband or partner is undoubtedly the most important influence in the woman's self-satisfaction. His reactions to her performance greatly affect her self-esteem, and if she senses disappointment from him because he was unable to participate or be present at his child's birth, she feels less "successful."

POTENTIAL FOR MOOD CHANGES

The first few days after delivery—even up to 10 or 14 days—could be considered a period of "normal" crisis and disequilibrium, especially for the first-time mother (Rubin, 1977). It is a time of transition, readjustment, reappraisal of roles, added responsibility, excitement, fatigue, and recovery from pregnancy, labor, and delivery. Relationships are strained. It rarely is a time of peace and tranquility because the new family attempts to establish boundaries, functions, schedules, and roles (Figure 17-4).

Many new mothers (and even new fathers) experience "the blues" or postpartum depression. **Postpartum depression** can be divided into the following categories, depending on the severity of symptoms manifested by the mother—whether she has postpartum blues or postpartum psychosis.

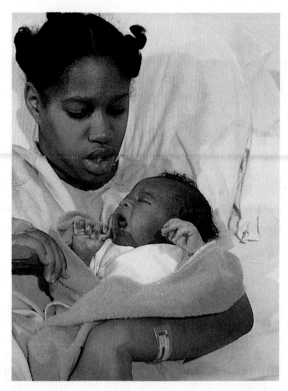

FIGURE 17-4 If the young mother is tense and the baby is crying, feeding times may seem a disaster. This situation requires intervention. (Courtesy Concept Media, Irvine, Calif.)

Inform mom to expect this & it will pass.

The "baby blues," or third-day blues, is considered to be a normal mild, transient mood disturbance lasting a few days or more (Selby et al, 1980). Changes in mood coincide with the drop in the hormones estrogen and progesterone, which reach their lowest level on those days.

Other causes of postpartum blues in addition to the drop in hormone levels have been suggested; these include lack of sleep during the first month of recovery, the demand of additional responsibilities, and discomforts of infection or pain. Several studies have examined the reasons for postpartum blues according to maternal responses. Some of the reasons given by mothers included worries about the baby, difficulties involving breast-feeding, homesickness, and pain, but many could give no reason for their depressed feelings. *moody, crying, anger, inable to concentrate*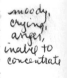

Postpartum depressed feelings are characterized by one or more of the symptoms listed in Box 17-1. Depending on the source cited, the incidence of postpartum blues ranges between 50% and 70%.

Postpartum Psychosis

The severe form of postpartum depression is postpartum psychosis or puerperal psychosis. This depression is characterized by acute psychotic behavior characteristic

BOX 17-1   Symptoms of Postpartum Depression

Irritability
Restlessness
Crying spells
Sleeplessness
Anger directed at family members, including the
    infant
Anxiety
Inability to concentrate
Moodiness

of affective, schizophrenic, or organic disorders. It manifests suddenly sometime within the first 6 months of recovery; 45% of women who manifest behaviors do so within the first 2 weeks of delivery (Herzog and Detre, 1976). It occurs in approximately one or two of every thousand mothers. Clients at risk include women with a history of psychiatric disorders, primigravidas, and women displaying anxiety and neuroticism during pregnancy. Postpartum psychosis probably results from a combination of factors. As with the postpartum blues, the leading causative factor is the drop in the level of the hormones estrogen and progesterone. Other factors are the change in roles, added responsibilities and hostilities toward family (baby, partner, other children) (Selby et al, 1980), and physical problems such as infection and sleep-cycle disturbances (Cox, Holden, Sagovsky, 1989).

As with any psychiatric disorder, the actions of the client are exaggerated. For example, the mother experiencing postpartum blues may express irritability, moodiness, and hostility but not to the degree that the mother developing a psychosis might. The exaggerated and often prolonged periods of irritability, hostility, labile behavior, ineffective coping mechanisms, withdrawal, and inappropriate responses to the baby, herself, or her family should indicate that she is experiencing more than just postpartum blues. The health and well-being of the baby and the mother must be safeguarded in this instance. Professional help, not merely emotional support, comfort, and encouragement, is needed. When hospitalization is required, every attempt should be made to keep the mother-infant relationship intact while caring for both parties.

Education seems to prevent or reduce the incidence of postpartum depression. The best results were obtained when the partner attended classes, when resources (personal and social) are mobilized in the early puerperium, and outside interests are maintained.

Women need to be prepared for childbirth and the transition to motherhood roles, and families need to be prepared and assisted in making the transition from hospital to home. Rooming-in is a way of introducing the mother and father to their new responsibilities and roles while under the supervision of professional care givers (Selby et al, 1980).

A questionnaire such as the one in Box 17-2 has been helpful for women to recognize their own moods and to seek help when depressed.

Implications of Early Discharge

Just 40 years ago a woman was hospitalized for 7 days after birth. Recovery was called *confinement*. Over the years, however, health care personnel have realized that early return to normal activities is the best course for uncomplicated births. Today, going home in 24 hours is not unusual, and a 2.7 day stay for vaginal birth and 4.3 days for cesarean birth is a diagnosis-related group (DRG) standard. (Home care is discussed in Chapters 20 and 26.)

Early discharge limits the time the woman has to listen, to learn, and to practice self-care. Consequently nurses begin discharge teaching at the first postpartum check—reinforcing, expanding, and evaluating its effectiveness until the woman goes home. Written instructions assume new importance. Because there are too many impressions in these first few hours after birth, the woman may not remember instructions. Many units follow up by a telephone call in the next day to see how the parents are managing. Such follow-up is especially appreciated by the parents.

Nursing Responsibilities

Whether the woman has had a spontaneous vaginal delivery, assisted delivery, or a surgical delivery, certain aspects of care are universal. These common factors are the focus of this section. (Needs specific to individual mothers with complications are discussed in later sections.)

The woman in recovery is a person at risk; she is vulnerable in many ways. Physical stability must be ensured and a positive client-nurse relationship established so she can be assisted in her developmental tasks of parenting and maintaining self-esteem.

▶ **ASSESSMENT**

The transfer from the labor and delivery area does not end the recovery process. The critical phase of recovery necessitates accurate observations, nursing history, and physical assessment to allow formulation of appropriate nursing diagnoses and an effective plan of care.

BOX 17-2   Edinburgh Postnatal Depression Scale (EPDS) (Department of Psychiatry, University of Edinburgh)

Name:
Address:
Baby's age:
*As you have recently had a baby, we would like to know how you are feeling. Please **underline** the answer which comes closest to how you have felt in the past 7 days,* not just how you feel today.

Here is an example, already completed.

I have felt happy:

Yes, all the time
Yes, most of the time   No, not very often
No, not at all

This would mean: "I have felt happy most of the time" during the past week. Please complete the other questions in the same way.

In the past 7 days:

1. I have been able to laugh and see the funny side of things
   As much as I always could
   Not quite so much now
   Definitely not so much now
   Not at all

2. I have looked forward with enjoyment to things
   As much as I ever did
   Rather less than I used to
   Definitely less than I used to
   Hardly at all

*3. I have blamed myself unnecessarily when things went wrong
   Yes, most of the time
   Yes, some of the time
   Not very often
   No, never

4. I have been anxious or worried for no good reason
   No, not at all
   Hardly ever
   Yes, sometimes
   Yes, very often

*5. I have felt scared or panicky for no very good reason
   Yes, quite a lot
   Yes, sometimes
   No, not much
   No, not at all

*6. Things have been getting on top of me
   Yes, most of the time I haven't been able to cope at all
   Yes, sometimes I haven't been coping as well as usual
   No, most of the time I have coped quite well
   No, I have been coping as well as ever

*7. I have been so unhappy that I have had difficulty sleeping
   Yes, most of the time
   Yes, sometimes
   Not very often
   No, not at all

*8. I have felt sad or miserable
   Yes, most of the time
   Yes, quite often
   Not very often
   No, not at all

*9. I have been so unhappy that I have been crying
   Yes, most of the time
   Yes, quite often
   Only occasionally
   No, never

*10. The thought of harming myself has occurred to me
   Yes, quite often
   Sometimes
   Hardly ever
   Never

Instructions for users

1. The mother is asked to underline the response which comes closest to how she has been feeling in the previous 7 days.
2. All 10 items must be completed.
3. Care should be taken to avoid the possibility of the mother discussing her answers with others.
4. The mother should complete the scale herself, unless she has limited English or has difficulty with reading.
5. The EPDS may be used at 6-8 weeks to screen postnatal women. The child health clinic, postnatal check-up, or a home visit may provide suitable opportunities for its completion.

From Cox JL, Holden JM, Sagovsky R: *Br J Psych* 150:782, 1989.

The Edinburgh Postnatal Depression Scale (EPDS) has been developed to assist primary care health professionals to detect mothers suffering from postnatal depression: a distressing disorder more prolonged than the 'blues' (which occur in the first week after delivery) but less severe than puerperal psychosis.

The validation study showed that mothers who scored above a threshold 12/13 were likely to be suffering from a depressive illness of varying severity. Nevertheless the EPDS score should *not* override clinical judgment. A careful clinical assessment should be carried out to confirm the diagnosis. The scale indicates how the mother has felt *during the previous week,* and in doubtful cases it may be usefully repeated after 2 weeks. The scale will not detect mothers with anxiety neuroses, phobias, or personality disorders.

*Response categories are scored 0, 1, 2, and 3 according to increased severity of the symptom. Items marked with an asterisk are reverse scored (i.e., 3, 2, 1, and 0). The total score is calculated by adding together the scores for each of the 10 items. Users may reproduce the scale without further permission providing they respect copyright (which remains with the *British Journal of Psychiatry*) by quoting the names of the authors, the title and the source of the paper in all reproduced copies.

Clinical Decision

> *Your client Susan tells you that she is most troubled about two of the postpartum concerns you had not thought to discuss with her. She feels that social isolation and loneliness are her chief concerns after going home. How will you begin your conversation about these concerns, and what assistance might there be for her?*

Initial Observations

First impressions of a client provide the nurse with a good idea of how she is recovering from childbirth. Establishing physical stability is critical. Two factors easily noted are general appearance and presence of pain. The client's color reflects circulation and perfusion. Observe her for pallor, flushing, or cyanosis and note general responsiveness. Is she extremely fatigued, unusually quiet, or very excitable or anxious? Does she look comfortable, or is she in distress?

An intravenous line still may be in place when a woman is admitted to the postpartum unit, and its patency must be ensured. Note the type of solution, any medications added, amount left in the bag, and the rate of flow and assess the insertion site for irritation or infiltration. If the woman has had surgery, a Foley catheter will be in place. If she is at risk for phlebitis, there may be an alternating pressure device or elastic stockings on her legs; check for placement of the sleeves and wrappings and for the functioning of the pump.

In addition to physical findings, the nurse notes whether the client is alone or accompanied, and if so, by whom. Is support evidenced, does the mother speak about the baby, or is she very concerned over her own welfare?

Although far from thorough, this initial admission assessment gives basic information and can provide direction for possible problems and areas for further investigation.

Physical Assessment

As soon as possible after admission to the postpartum unit, the woman's stability is determined, which provides a base for further evaluation. The following factors are checked:

1. *Vital signs.* Take pulse, respiration, and blood pressure to assess normal blood volume and recovery. Temperature is taken to ensure that the woman is not dehydrated and to rule out infection.
2. *Involution.* For vaginal delivery, check the fundus level and tone to determine adequate uterine

contraction and descent. For cesarean delivery, check the dressing, including its condition and presence of bleeding.

3. *Abdomen.* Check for distention, softness or firmness, rigidity, and tenderness. Check also for the presence or absence of bowel sounds after general anesthesia or cesarean delivery.
4. *Bladder.* Palpate for emptiness or fullness and distention. Observe whether a Foley catheter is in place.
5. *Breasts.* Determine whether they are soft or firm or tender or nontender; ask the mother if she is planning to breast-feed.
6. *Perianal area.* Observe the perineal pad for amount and color of lochial discharge, noting unusual odor or presence of clots; check for intact sutures along the line of episiotomy: any bleeding, edema, ecchymosis, or pain; and observe the anus for repaired lacerations or hemorrhoids.

With initial physical assessment completed, the nurse can determine whether the woman can be left comfortably and safely, which will provide time to complete data collection.

Nursing History

Depending on the institution, information can be obtained from a history taken on admission to labor and delivery or a second interview during the postpartum period. Necessary background data include the following:

1. Type and time of delivery
2. Anesthesia and medications received during labor and delivery
3. Present gravidity and parity; blood type and Rh factor
4. Status of baby
5. Chosen method of feeding the baby
6. Significant past medical and surgical history
7. Allergies, including medication, food, and environmental conditions
8. Medications taken on a regular basis
9. Diet, including medical, religious, or cultural limitations
10. Social, occupational, and economic factors that may affect the woman's recovery and parenting
11. General educational background for this experience, including prepared childbirth
12. Classes attended
13. Home situations that will affect recovery and parenting, including whether she will have help with the baby or need to climb stairs after a difficult or surgical delivery

Chart Review

The final source of pertinent data is the chart itself. Use it to verify any previously obtained information and obtain additional facts about the labor and delivery before planning care. Check the physician's orders in terms of activity, diet, medications, intravenous infusion orders, and any special treatments or procedures (e.g., administration of rubella or Rh immune globulin injections). The antepartum chart usually contains laboratory data, including the woman's blood type and Rh factor, serologic tests, and rubella titer.

▶ NURSING DIAGNOSES

The nurse identifies specific self-care needs or deficits appropriate to each postpartum woman and formulates nursing diagnoses that focus on the woman's problems. These diagnoses will be the basis for the plan of care that should reflect her physical, emotional, and developmental needs.

Some nursing diagnoses are universal to every woman, regardless of type of delivery. These include the following:

1. High risk for fluid volume deficit related to uterine atony, retained placental fragments, or bleeding
2. High risk for infection (uterine, perineal, incisional) related to type of birth
3. Pain related to type of incision
4. Knowledge deficit regarding parenting, hygiene, or recovery process related to prior experience
5. Constipation related to anesthesia, diet, medication, or pain
6. Urinary retention related to periurethral edema from delivery

In other instances the type of delivery or other special circumstances necessitate formulation of diagnoses to meet specific needs. After a complicated birth or cesarean delivery, a woman may exhibit needs related to the following diagnoses:

1. Altered tissue perfusion (phlebitis) related to immobility
2. Situational low self-esteem related to childbirth difficulties
3. Altered parenting related to disappointment or discomfort

It is interesting to note that the nurse and client may focus on different problems. It saves time for the nurse and the new mother to sit down and discuss priorities. A study by Tribotti et al (1988) found significant variations in concerns, which changed day by day during recovery. The five nursing diagnoses recovering women most frequently selected in the early period were as follows:

1. Alteration in comfort (pain)
2. Potential for growth (family coping)
3. Alteration in body fluids (fluid volume excess or deficit)
4. Impaired physical mobility
5. Sleep pattern disturbance

TABLE 17-3 **Nursing Diagnoses Most Often Identified by Women (n = 231)**

	PERCENTAGES	
DIAGNOSIS	**CESAREAN** (n = 115)	**VAGINAL** (n = 116)
Alteration in comfort	91.3	82.6
Impaired mobility	85.2	47.8
Sleep pattern disturbance	73.0	57.4
Alteration in bowel elimination	65.2	47.8
Anxiety	57.0	33.9
Activity intolerance	41.7	17.4
Self-care deficit	37.4	7.8
Fear	35.7	20.0
Potential for injury	16.5	7.0
Alteration in health maintenance	15.7	7.0
Ineffective breathing pattern	13.9	1.7
Social isolation	13.9	5.2
Ineffective family coping	13.0	5.2

From Tribotti S et al: Nursing diagnoses for the postpartum woman, *JOGNN* 17(6):410, 1988. All responses are significant at $p \leq 0.05$. (Nursing diagnoses, NANDA, 1987.)

These women focused on their bodily changes at first. After cesarean birth, these physical changes assumed an even greater importance. By 25 to 72 hours after birth, women were concerned about altered sleep patterns and facing the future. By 73 to 96 hours after birth, many more diagnoses were selected by the participants (an average of 9 each). Table 17-3 lists some of the differences between vaginal and cesarean births, and Table 17-4 lists differences between primipara and multipara concerns.

▶ EXPECTED OUTCOMES

Because of the short stay, the nurse usually will be able to evaluate only short-term achievement during the short hospital stay. Therefore outcomes need to be brief, with referral for problems that cannot be quickly resolved. Reasonable expectations include the following outcomes:

1. Fluid balance restored as evidenced by stable vital signs, lochial flow, and hydration
2. No signs of infection during recovery
3. Reestablishment of normal elimination patterns
4. Comfort achieved
5. Attachment begins with signs of bonding
6. Performs self-care appropriately
7. Demonstrates basic infant care and feeding techniques
8. Apparent availability of family support
9. Talks about birth experience and evidences positive self-esteem

TABLE 17-4 Selected Nursing Diagnoses

	PERCENTAGES	
DIAGNOSIS	PRIMIPARAS (n = 118)	MULTIPARAS (n = 113)
Lack of knowledge	47.5	20.9
Alteration in health status	5.8	17.4
Social isolation	4.2	15.7
Ineffective family coping	5.8	13.9
Ineffective breathing pattern	5.0	12.2

From Tribotti S et al: Nursing diagnoses for the postpartum woman, *JOGNN* 17(6):410, 1988. All responses are significant at *p* ≤ 0.05.

▶ NURSING INTERVENTIONS

During all recovery care certain critical elements must be observed (Box 17-3), and adherence is assumed in good nursing practice.

Involution Check

The postpartum "check" is first performed on the woman's admission to recovery, whether in a labor-delivery-recovery (LDR), a labor-delivery-recovery and postrecovery (LDRP), or postpartum unit. At regular intervals in the next days it is repeated. During the first hour, uterine and lochial checks are performed every 15 minutes and then every 1 to 2 hours for the next 4 hours. If all signs show expected progress, checking is decreased to every 8 hours until the woman is discharged.

Fundus check. An assessment of the uterus is performed after vaginal and cesarean birth (Procedure 17-1).

Palpate the abdomen to locate the **fundus** or top of the uterus by pressing in and down with the side of the palm (Figure 17-5). Describe the descent by measurements in *fingerbreadths* from the umbilicus (one fingerbreadth measures 1 cm).

In the surgical birth, palpation generally may be omitted when there is a vertical incision to avoid pressure on tissue and incision lines. Checks are part of protocol. Perform them gently, approaching from the sides to the midline for a woman with a low segment incision.

The uterus should be firm in consistency, comparable to a grapefruit. A fundus that is hard to find or one that is soft or boggy signifies inadequate contraction, and hemorrhage could occur. If the fundus is firm at the midline and at the expected level and if lochia is the appropriate color and amount, the nurse accurately documents these data. If, however, the fundus is soft or boggy, gentle massage is applied by rotating the cupped hand over the fundus until it feels firm. Vigorous massage or kneading should be avoided because it may overstimulate the uterus and cause it to become more fatigued and thus decrease contractility.

While palpating the fundus, inspect the perineal pad and bed pad. Lochia may be increased as "old" clots or lochia pooling in the vagina is expelled by pressure. On the other hand, a boggy or relaxed fundus may indicate excessive bleeding. Note if the fundus becomes firm, and measure the amount of blood on the pads after palpation. The fundus should be located in the midline. If it is to the side, the bladder is assessed for distention, which is the usual cause of an atonic uterus. After the bladder is emptied, the location and firmness are determined again.

Discharge teaching. Explain the procedure and why it is important for the fundus to be firm. Show the woman how to palpate the fundus, and teach her how to massage it to improve uterine contractility in the first few days (see Figure 17-5).

Lochia. Lochia is observed for amount and color. The terms *rubra, serosa,* and *alba* describe if the flow is bright red, pinkish brown (serosanguineous), or whitish. Describing amount is more difficult. The terms ***scant, moderate,*** and ***heavy*** (large) describe the amount. Descriptions are based on the number of pads used in 1 hour and the saturation of the pad. Ask the woman who might have discarded a pad to describe the flow in terms of usual menstrual amounts. In the initial recovery period, lochial flow is normal if no more than two pads are saturated within the first hour (the bed pads should be checked as well). As involution continues, the flow decreases to one pad per 2 to 4 hours in the next 8 hours and then will be comparable to menstrual flow (Moore, 1983).

Objective evaluation of flow is important in cases of abnormal amounts. A "flow chart" is kept and amounts charted. Remember that for every 500 ml blood lost,

---

BOX 17-3 Critical Elements: Maternity Care

- Use latex gloves when there is contact with blood or other body fluids. Universal precautions are considered an essential part of maternity care.
- Explain before and after a procedure.
- Encourage participation in self-care.
- Provide privacy by pulling curtains and draping appropriately.
- Support parents during hospital stay.

PROCEDURE 17-1   Involution Check

- Assess that the client has an empty bladder, and ask when her pad was last changed.
- Have client lie supine, if possible.
- Put on nonsterile gloves.
- Locate fundus with palm of hand.
- Cup hand, and place lateral side of hand slightly above fundus.
- Place your second hand above the symphysis pubis to support and stabilize the uterus during palpation.
- Gently, but firmly, press into abdomen toward the spine and then slightly downward toward the perineum until a mass is felt in the palm of the hand. At the same time, note the degree of contraction.
- Measure the number of fingerbreadths at which the fundus is felt below the umbilicus. In general, fingerbreadth measurement should correspond to the number of days after delivery.
- With gloved hand, check perineal pad for color and amount of lochia.
- Explain results to the woman, and encourage her to perform the check herself.
- Offer perineal care, if needed, and provide a clean pad.

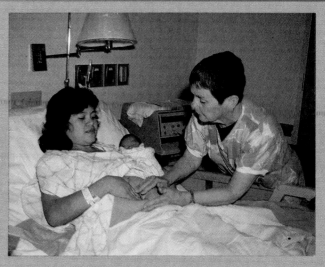

FIGURE 17-5 Demonstrating the fundal check. The woman should feel the fundus and learn to rub it at intervals in the first days. (Courtesy Marjorie Pyle, RNC, *Lifecircle*.)

● ● ●

OPTIONAL ACTIVITY: Write a sample nursing note correctly documenting the performance of this procedure.

the hematocrit will fall 3% to 4% and hemoglobin 1.0 to 1.5 g/dl (Combs et al, 1991). A more standardized approach measures the size of the lochial stain or the weight of the pad. Absorbency of the pad will affect measurements; the type of pad in use in each unit should be tested. Luegenbiehl et al (1991) determined that for one pad type, scant lochia was a stain less than 2 inches long with a volume of less than 10 ml. A large lochial flow was seen on a pad with greater than a 6-inch stain and with more than 50 ml volume. (Weight of 1 g of blood equals approximately 1 ml of blood.)

In addition to noting amount and color, characteristics are evaluated to determine whether they are appropriate for the time of recovery. Any change in pattern or unusual characteristic should be noted. If the fundus is firm and there is too much lochia, the physician should be notified. Constant trickling of oxygenated blood (brighter red) may mean an unrepaired arterial laceration or a clotting defect. Assessment of lochia is important for the woman after cesarean delivery. It is common to see a gush of lochia when the woman gets out of bed for the first time. Fluid has collected in the vagina during sleep. Reassure her and provide an extra disposable bed pad to catch the "drip" until she gets to the bathroom.

When lochial flow is excessive or suddenly increases, check for a change in the client's activity level (e.g., excess straining, lifting, or walking). If a fundal check and uterine massage do not produce a firm fundus, oxytocic agents such as methylergonovine maleate (Methergine) may be indicated. If unusual lochial color or odor is found, obtain a specimen for a culture and sensitivity test, check vital signs, and notify the physician for medical follow-up care.

Discharge teaching. Describe the usual sequence of lochial changes. Instruct the woman in the warning signs: resumption of heavy bleeding after lochia serosa begins, clots passed in the lochia, or any unusual or unpleasant odor to the flow.

Oxytocic use during recovery. To stop excessive blood flow after birth, oxytocin doses of 10 to 20 units (U) may be given intramuscularly (IM) or in an IV solution of 1000 ml Ringer's lactate to run at 125 ml/hr. If the bag has less than 500 ml at the time recovery begins, a new bag of fluid should be started to prevent too concentrated an infusion.

The main side effect is an *antidiuretic effect* (a partner hormone from the posterior pituitary is vasopressin, an antidiuretic hormone). Therefore during an infusion with oxytocin the total fluid intake must be carefully watched and checked hourly with output. Repeatedly, it has been noted that doses over 20 U/ 1000 ml fluid in 8 hours result in *oliguria.* When the

solution is changed to an isotonic, plain solution, diuresis immediately begins to occur. Water intoxication also has resulted if the dose has been given in large amounts of IV solution. Signs are elevated BP and headache.

Ergot derivatives. Two members of the oxytocic family may be used after birth for bleeding. Ergonovine maleate (Ergotrate) 0.2 mg may be given orally or intramuscularly. The half-life is 3 to 4 hours; thus the drug is *never* given before the baby is born. Because the uterus is capable of contracting without any drug, intervention should not be excessive. When there is frank hemorrhage uncontrolled by oxytocin, ergonovine maleate or methylergonovine maleate (Methergine) may be given (see Chapter 21). Both drugs have a hypertensive effect and are administered only if the maternal blood pressure is in the normal range. Ergonovine maleate particularly causes systemic and pulmonary hypertension and is therefore much less commonly used today (Ergotrate).

Infection. A perineum that has undergone the trauma of an episiotomy or a laceration is at risk for infection from the proximity to fecal material and the potential growth medium that lochial bleeding provides. Once infected, the tissue allows pathogens to travel into the vagina and even to the uterus itself (see Chapter 25).

Visual inspection of the perineum for signs of infection is important. Elevated temperature and complaints of severe pain are clues that an infection may be developing. An abdominal incision should be examined carefully after the initial dressing is removed.

The abdomen is palpated for distention or rigidity, and an involutional check is performed to rule out complications. The incision is inspected for signs of bleeding, hematoma, or infection. The woman should be assisted to turn to a more comfortable position, such as side lying, to decrease tension on the sutures.

If the client becomes febrile, the incision is reassessed. If infection occurs, warm soaks or irrigations with peroxide and saline may be indicated, with frequent sterile dressing changes. Support of the client during this time is vital; the treatment should be explained, and she needs help to cope with another interruption of the childbirth experience; this problem also may affect her self esteem.

Perineal care. Perineal hygiene is essential in preventing infections. The client is instructed to use lavage each time she voids or defecates, first cleansing with the aseptic solution if used by protocol and then with plain warm tap water to rinse. Teach her to cleanse at the front, moving toward the anus to prevent the spread of fecal organisms to the vaginal area. Soft wipes instead of regular toilet tissue should be provided, and the client should use a front-to-back single-tissue wiping technique. "pat dry"

Discharge teaching. Beginning with the first perineal care after birth, explain how to perform the correct

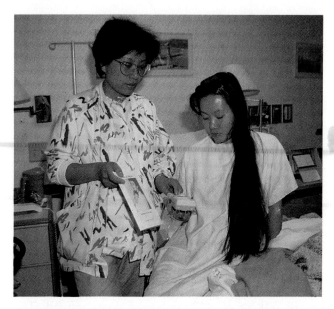

FIGURE 17-6 Teaching perineal care before the first time out of bed. (Courtesy Marjorie Pyle, RNC, *Lifecircle*.)

technique. She should continue perineal care until the perineum heals and lochia ceases (Figure 17-6). It should be emphasized that perineal pads should be applied and removed in a front-to-back direction. Hand washing before and after is reinforced as essential in prevention of infection. Suggest that the woman inspect her perineum and episiotomy by means of a mirror. A woman may feel uncomfortable handling her own genitalia because of personal or cultural factors. Providing a mirror may help to assess the perineum (see Incisional Pain: Episiotomy).

Output

Bladder distention is assessed with each involutional check, and output records are kept during the first 24 hours. When the woman ambulates on her own to use the bathroom independently, provide a pan that will fit under the seat and instruct her to report voiding so volume may be measured. She should be taught always to fill the bottles to the same level so the amount of water used in the lavage may be subtracted from the total urine output.

 Clinical Decision

If your client has a morning fever of 101.4° F 30 hours after birth, what assessments must take place before notifying the physician?

Early specimens always are mixed with lochia. A clear-voided specimen must be obtained if there are any questions regarding urine color and clarity, if there is cloudiness or unusual color, if the client becomes febrile, or if there are signs of dysuria or frequency. A specimen is sent for culture and sensitivity testing and the physician notified for medical follow-up care. The only way to obtain a clear, sterile specimen is by means of straight catheterization.

If the woman is unable to void, increase fluid intake and ambulation. Running tap water, using a sitz bath to relieve edema and relax the sphincter, and applying ice to the suprapubic area are aids to urination.

There will be a standing order to relieve distention by straight catheterization once. After that, the physician is notified and an indwelling Foley catheter is inserted and attached to a closed gravity drainage system. Although the general rule is to allow no more than 800 ml of urine to drain at one time, this is not as critical in the postpartum woman, who has been able to withstand increased intraabdominal pressures from a gravid uterus and a full bladder and has already experienced a sudden decrease in pressure with delivery. Therefore slowly drain the initial 800 ml, leave the catheter in position, and clamp for a few minutes. Continue draining until the bladder is completely emptied.

Constipation also is a potential problem. The intestinal musculature, already relaxed by progesterone, responds further to anesthesia and analgesia and becomes more sluggish. In addition, fear of pain from a perineal laceration, episiotomy, or hemorrhoids and the inconvenience of sharing bathroom facilities may inhibit normal bowel movement. Change in diet and activity also plays a part.

The abdomen is visually inspected for distention, palpated for firmness or rigidity, and auscultated for the presence of bowel sounds, especially after surgical delivery. The woman is asked if she is able to pass flatus rectally or feels the urge to defecate. Encourage her to increase fluid intake and recommend ambulation to enhance peristalsis. Stool softeners and laxatives are administered as ordered. If these measures fail, an enema or suppository may be needed.

Pain

Any complaint of pain requires a nursing response. Because pain is subjective, assess the level of pain by asking for a description on a numerical scale, with the lowest number indicating absence of discomfort. Observe the woman's *pain behaviors* as well (see Chapter 16). Location and kind of pain are determined—sharp, burning, throbbing, aching. Precipitating factors are identified. Pain unrelieved by standard interventions usually indicates complications, and the physician is notified for follow-up.

Contractions. Strong contractions of the involuting uterus are called *afterbirth pains.* Cramping is increased when the uterus has been distended, for example, with a very large infant or a multiple pregnancy. For the first hours after birth an infusion that contains oxytocin to improve muscle contraction may be used. Breast-feeding contributes to these cramping pains because sucking stimulates oxytocin release from the pituitary. Reassure the woman that uterine contractions are a normal part of recovery from childbirth and that they last for only a few days. She can lie prone with a small pillow or rolled towel under the middle of her abdomen. The cramping may worsen initially because of pressure on the uterus, but she should soon notice relief.

Incisional pain: episiotomy. Most women who have had an episiotomy or vaginal lacerations will experience some degree of pain during immediate recovery after the local anesthetic effect wears off. Assess any changes in the suture line by putting on a pair of gloves and using a light to inspect the perineum. Observe also for hemorrhoids, anal fissures, and unrepaired surface vaginal tears. The external labia are carefully observed during the inspection, and note if touching the area elicits more pain. The acronym *REEDA* describes findings:

- **Redness,** inflammation around wound
- **Edema** of surrounding tissues
- **Ecchymosis** around area (includes evaluation for hematoma)
- **Discharge** from wound
- **Approximation** of skin surfaces

Inspection ensures an accurate description.

Discharge teaching. Techniques of sitting can decrease pain. Instruct her to tighten the buttocks and perineum before sitting to alleviate pulling on the area. Encourage her to take rest periods in bed with her feet elevated. The use of Kegel exercises to increase blood circulation to the area and to tighten perineal muscles can be reinforced. The woman should be able to demonstrate these comfort measures before discharge.

Abdominal incision pain. The low, transverse "bikini" incision usually is less painful than a vertical incision. Some pain, however, is related to an incision. A distended abdomen will cause pressure on suture lines and increase pain sensation.

The woman is taught to support the incision while moving and to *splint* by holding her hand or a pillow over the incision during deep breathing and coughing. A binder may be ordered to provide extra support for an obese woman or during recovery from cesarean birth. It should be applied when the client is supine or in a low Fowler's position.

Women with an abdominal incision should learn postoperative self-assessment: checking wound REEDA and noting temperature elevation or localized, unresolving pain.

Pain management. Pharmacologic management after cesarean birth has improved in the last few years. Long-acting epidural narcotic analgesia will last up to 24 hours (see Chapter 16). If this is not available, meperidine (Demerol, Pethidine) is given at doses of 75 to 100 mg, depending on body weight, and administered IM every 3 to 4 hours. Patient-controlled analgesia (PCA) is used in some centers. An IV solution containing a narcotic is inserted as a secondary line into the mainline setup. Programmed by pump to deliver small bolus injections, this arrangement allows a woman to have the dose as she needs it. Safety features built into the pump prevent accidental overdose, and a record is kept of the number of doses infused. The stepdown is to Percocet or Percodan and then usually oral acetaminophen as needed, 600 to 900 mg every 4 hours. By the third or fourth day a woman should be mainly free from pain except for soreness on moving, and acetaminophen may keep her comfortable.

Cold compresses are applied as soon after birth as possible and for the first 24 hours to prevent and decrease edema and to diminish local sensation. Commercial cold packs may be used, or an examination glove can be filled with crushed ice, tied shut, and wrapped in a paper washcloth. Never apply cold packs directly against skin without a barrier in between. Cold packs should be left in place only for about 20 minutes and removed for a period before reapplication. Sustained vasocontriction from cold can cause tissue damage and is not advisable.

After cold is used in the first period, warm, moist heat is offered by providing the woman with her own sitz bath kit. She is taught to fill it with comfortable warm water, place it on the toilet seat, and sit in it, adding warm water to keep the desired temperature. Provide topical analgesic creams or ointments or pads such as Tucks.

Breast Discomfort

At delivery the breasts, which are soft and not tender, secrete colostrum. Milk flow will occur about the third or fourth day. Sudden breast fullness and firmness or engorgement precede this milk flow.

Nonlactating engorgement. Show the woman how to use ice packs to decrease fullness and pain and emphasize that these packs should never be placed directly on the skin but wrapped in a washcloth to prevent tissue burns. Discourage expression of milk manually or by pump. Although expression may seem to give relief initially, it actually stimulates milk production and causes the discomfort to last longer. The woman should be advised to wear a well-fitting brassiere at all times. *24/d*

If a woman asks for medication to "dry up" the milk, explain that such medications usually are not given. Some physicians prescribe antilactation drugs, most commonly bromocriptine mesylate (Parlodel) (Drug Profile 17-1). However, engorgement may recur after medication is discontinued. Therefore all women need to know how to care for engorgement. (Further discussion relating to the lactating woman follows in a later section.)

Activity

Rest. The amount of energy expended during labor and birth leaves the new mother in great need of rest. Often women fall asleep during a quiet recovery. Others are so excited that they find it impossible to relax and sleep. After the initial period of elation and stimulation, encourage the woman to use relaxation techniques to calm herself. Although sleep may not seem very important to the new mother, she will become fatigued if she does not set regular times of rest. Fatigue adversely

Drug Profile 17-1

Bromocriptine mesylate (Parlodel)
Action

Ergot derivative. Inhibits prolactin release by activating certain dopamine receptors. Used in infertility, endometriosis, and Parkinson's disease. Used to prevent breast fullness and engorgement post partum. Engorgement may return when drug course is completed.

Dosage/route

PO, 2.5 mg tablet bid with a meal for 14 to 21 days. Must begin dose within the first 4 hours after birth.

Side effects/adverse effects

Closely monitor after first dose for allergic response, hypotension. Transient hypotension, dizziness, nausea. During second week, hypertension, headache, blurred vision may begin and must be reported.

Precaution

Not used in hypertensive condition; may increase action of antihypertensive medication. Not given to client with allergy to ergot derivatives. Alcohol, oral contraceptives should be avoided.
Use barrier contraceptives because of the high incidence of premature ovulation.

affects milk production, interferes with learning, can precipitate depression, and can lower her self-esteem. Care should be planned so that the new mother can rest while she is in the recovery unit. If the baby is rooming-in (LDRP), encourage the partner in helping her rest. Discuss with her the ways she can get rest in the home situation, for example, limiting visitors at first, encouraging helpers to do the nonbaby care tasks, and disconnecting the telephone during feeding or nap times. She will miss sleep at night, so she should plan to nap when the baby does. The nurse can emphasize to the partner the importance of rest while encouraging him to assist with baby and mother care.

Exercise. After delivery the client may gradually resume exercising in the same way she exercised during the prenatal period (Figure 17-7). She should be cautioned not to exercise too strenuously at first but to pace her activities. Frequent walking is one of the best exercises; when women were confined to bed for extended periods after delivery, many complications such as hypostatic pneumonia, thromboses, and emboli occurred. For this reason, ambulation and exercise are encouraged soon after delivery. In addition, Kegel exercises for perineal muscles should be continued into the recovery period.

Gentle isometric stretching exercises may begin after birth. For the next few days, abdominal strengthening exercises, such as arm and leg lifts, and flexing to touch the chin to the chest start the process of returning to the woman's prepregnant condition. Sit-ups are delayed for a few weeks. (Box 9-1 presents guidelines for exercise during the postpartum period, and Figure 17-7 demonstrates typical exercises to regain contours.)

Sexuality and Contraception

Sexual intercourse usually is restricted until the perineum (in a vaginal delivery) and uterus have completely healed. Traditionally healing was considered accomplished by 6 weeks, but it is probably adequate at 2 to 4 weeks. After that time generally no physical contraindication to the resumption of normal sexual activities is indicated. Often, however, fear of pain from an episiotomy or laceration, discomfort from breast stimulation in the nursing mother, or abdominal tenderness after a cesarean delivery may inhibit new parents (Reamy and White, 1985).

The topic of sexual relations is introduced as early as possible in the postpartum period, and before discharge the couple's expectations and understanding of potential problems are assessed. The nurse discusses methods of relieving discomfort during intercourse, such as the use of water-soluble lubricants or plain vegetable oil to decrease perineal trauma and vaginal dryness. The mother needs to be reassured that it is normal to

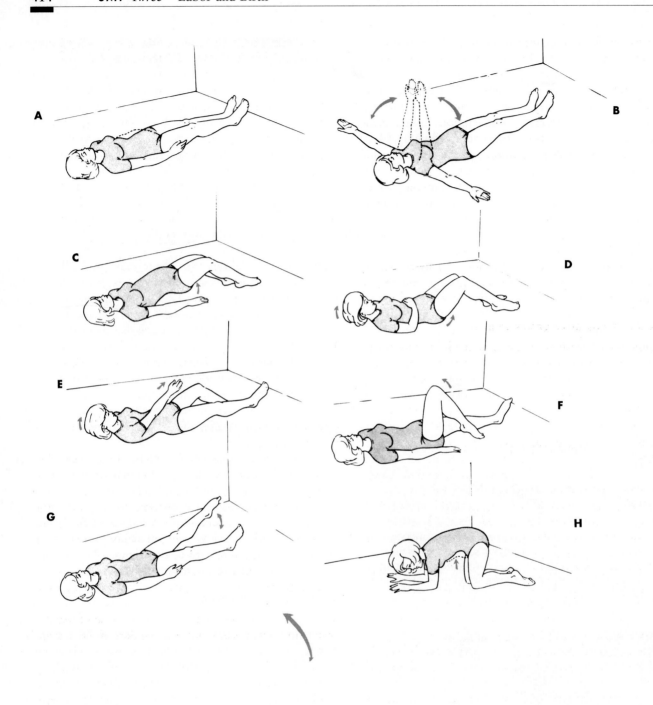

FIGURE 17-7 A-H, Postpartum exercises to regain muscle strength and improve posture.

experience strong contractions during orgasm. The nursing mother should be told that stimulation of full breasts may be uncomfortable, may cause some leaking, and will be less bothersome if "planned" after a feeding rather than before. (The couple should be encouraged to try various positions that lessen pressure on the perineum, abdomen, and breasts, and that are more comfortable.)

The couple also should be encouraged to express their feelings about another pregnancy and how they plan to prevent it. Facts about the return of menstruation and ovulation are reviewed. The parents may be worried about another pregnancy but unsure of an appropriate method of family planning. Because birth control often is planned around the menstrual cycle, the woman should understand that she may not have her first menses for 4 to 6 weeks if she is not nursing and for as long as 4 months if she is not supplementing breast-feeding.

Condoms with foam or gel are useful when lactating. The breast-feeding mother should not use combined oral contraceptives because lactation hormones and the milk supply may be affected. Because the cervix and vagina are enlarged after delivery, an old diaphragm may not fit properly and therefore will be ineffective and must be refitted. Natural family planning, which involves interpretation of the cycle and mucous secretions, is not always possible until hormone levels have stabilized and several cycles have occurred. The only contraceptive choice in the immediate postpartum period may be the use of a condom with foam or gel, doubling the amount until involution is complete (see Chapter 5).

Special Needs after Cesarean Birth

Although *childbirth* is the main factor in planning care for all postpartum women, the mother who has had a cesarean birth has special needs related to her surgery and will require additional nursing considerations. After surgical birth the woman requires affirmation to reinforce her confidence and feelings of self-worth.

The stress of childbirth is worsened when a woman is unprepared for a surgical procedure; additional anxiety, pain, and frustration, or loss of self-esteem result. In the recovery period some women state that they have little memory of the details of the surgical birth, especially if it was unexpected or an emergency. The nurse can arrange a time to review the experience with the new mother with questions such as the following:

- Tell me what you understand about what happened during surgery.
- Did you feel that you had unanswered questions?
- What could the nurses have done to make things easier for you?

Listen to the woman's feelings about her experience and encourage her to recount her perceptions and express excitement, pride, sadness, regret, anger, or disappointment. There may be elements of the grieving process as she copes with the perceived loss of an active birthing experience. In the recovery period, the nurse emphasizes the woman's individuality and ability as a new mother. As she talks about her cesarean delivery, the focus should be on achievement and the birth of her baby.

Postpartum "blues" are seen more often after surgical delivery because she is hospitalized longer than other mothers. The nurse assesses for excessive reactions and refers her for counseling if her coping mechanisms do not appear adequate. Follow-up care by telephone or home care visits is planned, and the mother is prepared for the fatigue and discomforts the

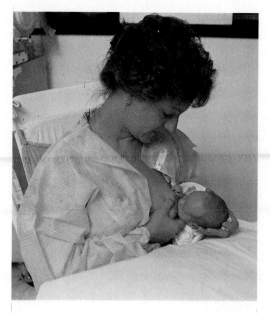

FIGURE 17-8 The mother may go to the NICU to feed a stabilized preterm infant. Note supporting the baby's chin to assist in sucking strength. (Courtesy Ross Laboratories, Columbus, Ohio.)

new mother often feels at home and on her own with the new infant.

A father also needs to discuss his experience. The nurse offers understanding of the disappointment or even anger that he may feel and encourages communication with his partner to foster mutual support. Emphasize the importance of his role as successful father, especially if the mother is unable to fully participate in infant care because of pain or limited mobility.

Complicated births often result in compromised infants who require special care in a neonatal intensive care unit (NICU). To the new parents, this causes additional stress and a sense of loss because of fear for their baby's well-being and interruption of the normal bonding process. Encourage and assist them to visit the nursery to see, touch, and participate as much as possible in care of their baby (Figure 17-8). If this is not possible, act as liaison between the parents and the NICU nurses to relay information about the infant's condition and progress.

Respiratory needs. Discomfort from a surgical incision, especially a classic or vertical incision, and abdominal distention interfere with the mother's normal respiratory pattern. To prevent increased abdominal pressure, she avoids deep breaths and coughing, which result in decreased tidal volume, decreased air exchange, and accumulation of bronchial secretions. Complications that can arise are atelectasis and pneumonia.

As soon as possible, explain pulmonary exercises, assisting the woman to as high a Fowler's position as she can tolerate and offer her a pillow to hold across her abdomen while she coughs. Gentle pressure supports the abdominal musculature, decreasing pain and relieving anxiety that "the stitches will rip."

"Ladder" breathing or "huffing" before coughing is useful and an incentive spirometer will be ordered. These devices encourage deep breathing by having the client use her breaths to make a ball or gauge move. The deeper the breath, the more the ball rises, and the client can see results and work at her own pace, increasing respirations gradually as tolerated.

Pain medication is offered before beginning respiratory therapy, with the explanation that it will help the woman with the activity. After an IM injection the wait is 15 minutes and after oral analgesics half an hour to allow for adequate absorption and action. Auscultate the lung fields before and after treatment to assess patency and air flow.

Recovery from anesthesia. Chapter 16 details care of the person recovering from anesthesia. During the initial assessment the type and duration of anesthesia are noted. Some women will be groggy and confused as they awaken from general anesthesia. They may have been in labor a long time before the decision for cesarean birth was decided, and fatigue will be a major factor in their recovery. When an epidural has been planned for and understood, women may have a very smooth recovery period. Other women after regional block anesthesia feel heaviness in the legs and have difficulty when first out of bed. The newly recovering woman should never get up alone and should sit on the side of the bed for a period to prevent orthostatic hypotension.

Circulation. After a complicated or surgical birth, ambulation may be difficult. When muscular activity is decreased or absent, venous return is decreased and stasis may occur. A state of increased viscosity from fluid losses and the temporary elevation in clotting factors in the immediate period have already occurred; these factors predispose the woman to the formation of phlebitis and thromboembolism (see Chapter 22).

The initial assessment reveals a history of or risk for thrombophlebitis or varicose veins. If complications require bed rest for even 1 or 2 days, preventive care includes isometric exercises and active range of motion. Be alert for complaints of pain in the legs; examine extremities for warmth, redness, and swelling, and assess for *Homans' sign* (Figure 17-9 and Procedure 17-2).

Obviously, the best prophylactic treatment plan calls for helping the woman walk as soon as possible.

For the client unable to ambulate early, leg movement, isometric exercises, and turning are encouraged.

Antiembolism stockings are applied to give support to the vein walls and thus aid blood flow. After cesarean or complicated deliveries, the woman may enter the unit with a counterpressure mechanical pump. The pump, connected to bandages or plastic sleeves over thromboembolic disease (TED) stockings, provides intermittent inflation to apply pressure needed to assist venous return. The nurse checks the settings, verifies the functioning of the system, and reassures the woman about the sensations she may experience.

Discharge teaching. Isometric exercises are initiated during early recovery. The woman can elevate her legs at home when sitting and avoid crossing her legs while lying or sitting. Describe signs of phlebitis and emphasize the need to report any evidence to the physician.

Delayed peristalsis: gas pains. Intestinal peristalsis can be decreased by the action of anesthetics, analgesics, altered food intake, and change in activity level. After a cesarean delivery, for example, it may take 24 hours for motility in the small intestine to resume and 3 to 5 days for complete function in the large intestine to return. Air and the breakdown of old materials in the colon produce flatulence and distention and thus pain and incisional discomfort because of increased pressure.

Small sips of water and ice chips may be allowed until bowel sounds are heard, and then the ordered diet is advanced slowly. The woman avoids iced and carbonated drinks that may increase flatulence. Early and frequent ambulation is encouraged to stimulate normal peristalsis. If a medication such as simethicone is ordered prophylactically, the client is instructed to chew the tablets thoroughly before swallowing.

Gas pains generally occur on the third postoperative day. The woman is advised to lie on her right side and to turn frequently to facilitate passing gas. The nurse may place a rectal tube to decompress the lower bowel or administer a Harris flush (return-flow enema) as ordered. The use of analgesics that further slow peristalsis is discouraged.

▶ EVALUATION

Evaluating outcomes within the short stay for birth must be directed toward the preparation for going home.

1. Have vital signs stabilized? Is involution pattern normal?
2. Can she demonstrate accurate self-assessment and care?
3. Does she exhibit confidence and competence in infant care?
4. Are there needs for referral?
5. Can she describe infant needs for nutrition, rest, sleep, activity, and safety? Have the parents obtained a car seat for going home?

PROCEDURE 17-2   Checking Homans' Sign

- Have the client lie supine.
- Gently flex her foot while straightening her knee.
- If she experiences pain in the calf, document a positive Homans' sign and seek medical follow-up care.

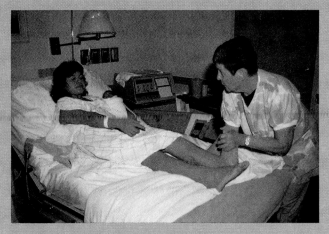

FIGURE 17-9 Checking Homans' sign for any woman who is not ambulatory in the first few hours. (Courtesy Marjorie Pyle, RNC, *Lifecircle.*)

● ● ●

OPTIONAL ACTIVITY: Write a sample nursing note correctly documenting the performance of this procedure.

6. Has she received follow-up literature and instructions in all areas of self-care, including family planning?

Learning Infant Feeding
FORMULA FEEDING

Emphasis today is placed on breast-feeding, and the nursing mother receives encouragement, support, and assistance. The woman who chooses to bottle-feed has many needs as she begins caring for and satisfying her baby (Figure 17-10). If there is an apparent lack of understanding about how to do it, a young mother will become quickly frustrated if her baby does not respond to her efforts or is unsatisfied after a tense feeding time.

The mother is encouraged to ask questions and express concerns. Is she comfortable holding, offering the bottle to, and bubbling the baby? The nurse stresses the importance of cuddling and eye contact during the feeding and observes for signs of attachment in her feeding behaviors. It should be reinforced that the *method* of feeding is not as important as the mother's and baby's satisfaction with the experience.

It is important not to appear judgmental of the woman who does not wish to nurse or who becomes frustrated with infant feeding. Those with low self-esteem often feel the baby "does not like me" if the infant is sleepy at feeding time or slow to suck. The new mother needs positive reinforcement for her ability to decide how she wishes to feed her child and to learn the best ways to do so.

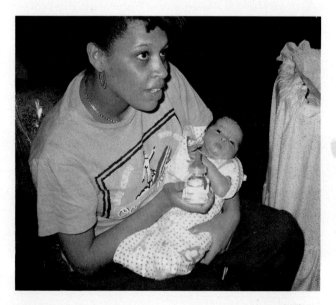

FIGURE 17-10 Bottle-feeding raises many questions for new mothers. She will need assistance with her awkward position. (Courtesy Camille Bodden.)

BENEFITS OF BREAST-FEEDING

In recent decades the popularity of bottle-feeding over breast-feeding has led to a gap in knowledge. Mothers and grandmothers cannot instruct their daughters in the art of breast-feeding, although there is increasing awareness that it is good for the baby.

Breast-feeding provides a unique bonding experience for mother and child. It stimulates most of the senses, and close body contact allows the baby to recognize its mother's smell. The baby also can feel and hear the sound of her heartbeat, which is similar to the intrauterine environment.

Breast-feeding can and should be a satisfying experience for both mother and baby. The nurse needs to be prepared to support the decision to breast-feed. By acknowledging anxiety and frustration, offering needed assistance and direction, and praising successes the nurse aids in *empowering* the new mother to overcome the possible difficulties that will be encountered in the first few weeks. *Typically takes 3 wks for nursing patterns to be estab. Supplement is discouraged during this time*

The scientific approach to breast-feeding is a relatively new field, one that is constantly evolving. Thus some older theories and protocols, such as limiting time on the breast at first, must be *unlearned* so that an improved approach may be used. It often is difficult to make changes in policy or in habits. By introducing new findings with confidence, the nurse can assist in improving care for breast-feeding women.

Before going home, the woman must have a basic understanding of the mechanism of lactation. She needs to know self-care, including breast care, adequate nutrition, fluids and rest, and sources of support from other women or organized groups such as La Leche League.

Immunologic Benefits

Human milk is a biochemically unique substance perfectly adapted to the infant's needs. Colostrum is available to the baby for the first 2 to 3 days of life. It contains antibodies, depending on the maternal titers of antibodies, against organisms such as *Staphylococcus, Salmonella,* poliovirus, influenza virus, *Bordetella pertussis, Escherichia coli,* and others. The newborn has immature antibody response until about 6 weeks of age. Without the protection of the antibody system the baby is vulnerable. In addition, before the system functions well in the gastrointestinal tract, large molecules of protein can reach the intestinal tissues of the formula-fed baby and be absorbed into the circulation, producing an immune response and predisposing the baby to an allergy to cow's milk. It has been estimated that 5% to 6% of all infants are sensitive to cow's milk (Halpern, 1977). This allergy can cause eczema, vomiting, diarrhea, diaper rash, and upper respiratory tract infections.

In the breast-feeding baby, however, the intestine is coated with immunoglobulins that were in the colostrum. Human milk has low allergenicity and contains a factor that promotes growth of *Lactobacillus bifidus,* which produces lactic and acetic acids in the gastrointestinal tract. These acids turn the stool acidic and provide additional protection against the growth of enteric infections. The formula-fed baby has a more alkaline stool that does not have the same protective effect.

Nutritional Benefits

Breast milk contains a proper amount of nutrients for an infant. There is a lower solute load and more unsaturated fatty acids. Proteins and fats are more easily digested, and carbohydrate content is appropriate for growth. When an infant is breast-fed, problems caused by poor sanitation, lack of refrigeration, ignorance, or illiteracy are avoided. Finally, for the baby, adequate protein intake is available even in a diet-deficient environment.

Maternal Physiologic Benefits

Breast-feeding benefits not only the infant. There are also physiologic benefits for the mother. Nipple sucking by the breast-feeding infant stimulates the release of oxytocin from the posterior pituitary, which in turn causes the uterus to contract. Each time the infant nurses, the uterus contracts, hastening the descent of the uterus back into the pelvic cavity. The contraction of the uterus also reduces the possibility of postpartum hemorrhage, which can result from a relaxed uterus.

Breast-feeding requires the expenditure of a great deal of energy by the mother to produce milk, thereby helping the mother lose weight and return to her prepregnancy weight sooner.

MATERNAL NUTRITION DURING LACTATION

The nutritional status of the mother has no direct relation to the nutritional quality of breast milk. Instead, if nutritional intake is inadequate, there will be *less milk* but its quality remains stable. A lack of fluid intake also leads to reduced production of milk.

Human milk is very different from cow's milk in composition; all formulas must be modified to be as similar as possible to human milk (Table 17-5). A remarkable characteristic of human milk is its variation in concentration during the day. In addition, fore milk (available at the start of feeding) varies from hind milk (available at the end). Hind milk contains four to five times more fat than fore milk.

Levels of protein fat and carbohydrates are in the following ranges (Bertino, 1981):

Protein	0.6-1.5 g/dl
Fat	2.1-3.3 g/dl
Carbohydrates	6.9-7.2 g/dl (lactose)
Water	87%-95%

TABLE 17-5 Contrast between Human and Cow's Milk Concentrations

	HUMAN	COW
Calories	Higher	Lower
Protein	Lower	Higher
Fat	Higher	Lower
Carbohydrates	Higher	Lower
Calcium	Lower	Much higher
Phosphorus	Lower	Higher
Iron	Low	Only trace
Sodium	Lower	Higher
Potassium	Lower	Higher
Vitamin A	Higher	Lower

Calories

During the first 2 weeks, an average of 600 to 650 ml/day is produced. As the baby matures, production rises to about 950 to 1000 ml/day. The mother uses 30 calories for every 30 ml of milk produced (there are 20 calories in 30 ml of breast milk). Stored maternal fat provides an extra 100 to 150 kcal per day for milk production in these first 3 months. Therefore at first, the woman should add 500 calories to her baseline prepregnancy diet. After her weight has returned to its former level, she needs to take in about 750 calories over baseline (more if she is undernourished) to maintain caloric requirements for lactation.

Protein

Lactation requires an increase in protein of 15 to 20 g over baseline. During lactation the woman takes the same milk requirements (4 cups of whole milk), which will provide all the extra calories, protein, and calcium required for lactation. If the woman does not like milk or is sensitive to it, other sources of protein and calcium can be used. The nurse should encourage her to include alternative sources in her diet.

A thin or malnourished woman may use extra milk to supply her increased protein and calcium intake. Protein needs may pose a problem for vegetarians (see Chapter 10 and Table 10-3). Many vegetarians allow protein increases when they understand the importance of the increase.

Other Nutrients

Consumption of citrus fruits, vegetable oils, and leafy, green vegetables satisfies the increased need for ascorbic acid, iron, vitamin E, and folic acid. Dark-green and yellow vegetables provide vitamin A. The breast-feeding mother may continue to take prenatal vitamins.

Fluid Intake

Because the lactating woman produces 900 ml or more of milk, she should receive at least that amount of extra

TABLE 17-6   Nutritional and Fluid Intake during Lactation

FOOD	AMOUNT FOR ADULT
Milk	4 cups (5-6 cups for teenager)
Meat/meat substitutes	2 servings
Vegetables	2-3 servings
Fruits	2-3 servings
Breads	6 servings
Fluids	6-8 cups in addition to milk (noncaffeinated and water)

fluid through her normal intake. The importance of fluids to a new mother should be stressed. See Table 17-6 for fluid and nutritional recommendations.

Precautions

A mother often asks whether she should omit any foods. There is no physiologic basis for avoiding certain foods, such as curry, garlic, or chocolate. Foods tolerated by the mother generally are tolerated by the baby. If there is a question about a food, the health care provider may advise omitting it on a trial basis.

Alcohol, too, is secreted in milk. Empiric data indicate that a small glass of wine or a light beer is unlikely to affect the nursing baby and in a tired mother may assist the let-down reflex by increasing relaxation. Excess alcohol, however, may inhibit milk ejection. Larger quantities of alcohol have a dose-response effect. (See Chapter 28.)

Smoking should be curtailed or eliminated during lactation. Passive smoking has been recognized as a major health problem, especially for young infants, because of rapid absorption through the lungs. Smoking also reduces the volume of milk produced by affecting the release of prolactin and oxytocin.

Caffeine in large quantities can cause the mother and infant to be jittery, wakeful, and irritable. Caffeinated beverages (coffee, tea, soda) should be limited to two servings a day. (See Chapter 16 for a complete discussion of drugs and lactation.)

Test Yourself

- What factors inhibit adequate lactation?
- How much fluid over baseline does a lactating woman need and why?
- What are the dietary recommendations for lactating adolescents?

PREPARATION OF BREASTS

No special preparation of breasts is necessary. There is no need to toughen the nipples by rubbing, rolling, or applying alcohol. In fact, these measures can irritate, injure, and dry the tissue. In addition, nipple stimulation may cause increased contractions during the last trimester (see Chapter 11). Colostrum that may ooze from the nipples in the last trimester may be washed away or rubbed into the nipple as a lubricant. Manual expression of colostrum is not necessary.

Breast size and nipple size vary widely and are not important to breast-feeding. The woman should be reassured that milk supply depends not on breast mass but on the alveoli in the breast. Small, flat nipples are not a problem if the infant can latch on. To assess this, the woman can press the thumb and index finger into the breast behind the nipple. If the fingers can grasp the nipple, the baby will be able to do so. Nipples that appear inverted often respond to pressure on the areola

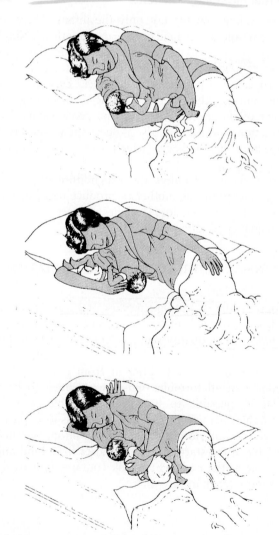

FIGURE 17-11 Three positions for nursing. Note infant's position in relation to mother. (From Fogel CI, Woods NF: *Health care of women,* St Louis, 1981, Mosby.)

while the infant sucks. Breast shields (a small dome and rubber nipple that fits over the areola) occasionally may be used. Only rarely do inverted nipples prevent lactation. Care must be taken not to allow too great a pressure that could injure the tissue.

INITIATION OF FEEDING

Breast-feeding should be initiated as soon as possible after delivery. After the placenta is delivered and the mother is comfortable, the baby can be put to the breast for a few minutes (see Figure 15-7). The infant may nurse enthusiastically or may just lick the nipple and not suck at all; however, this skin-to-skin contact is an intense bonding experience for a woman and her child. The mother and baby should not become chilled. A radiant warmer, if available, can be placed over the delivery table or in the recovery room.

Positions for Nursing

Common positions are the "madonna hold" with the baby cradled in an arm, the "football hold" in which the mother's arm supports the baby's head and back and the infant's body and legs are to the side and behind

the mother, or side lying with the mother and infant facing each other (Figure 17-11). Side lying may be most comfortable for the woman who has had an episiotomy or a surgical birth.

Latching-on, the ability of the baby to grasp the nipple, is the single most important aspect of breast-feeding. Regardless of position the baby must be lined up with the mother's body so that the head is directly in front of the breast and the nipple within easy reach (Figure 17-12). Pillows can be used to obtain this position. If necessary, the mother supports her breast with four fingers under and the thumb on top. Neither the baby's head nor the breast should be moved to the side, or the neck will be extended, hyperextended, or turned, interfering with swallowing and also creating traction on the nipple tissue. With correct positioning the nipple is simply guided to the baby's open mouth for **latching-on** (Figure 17-13, *A*).

Sucking and Swallowing

The **sucking reflex** is developed by week 34 of gestation, although small infants may become easily fatigued. Because sucking involves compression of the nipple and areola between the tongue and palate, the mouth must

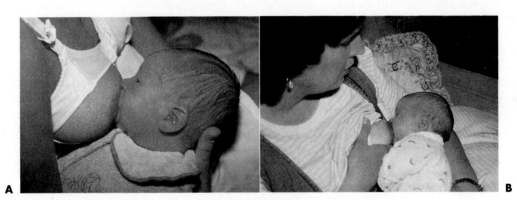

FIGURE 17-12 A, Football hold. Note correct "fish-mouth" position of the baby's lips so that nipple and areola are pulled forward into the mouth. **B,** Madonna hold. Note placement of mother's hand. (Courtesy Marjorie Pyle, RNC, *Lifecircle*.)

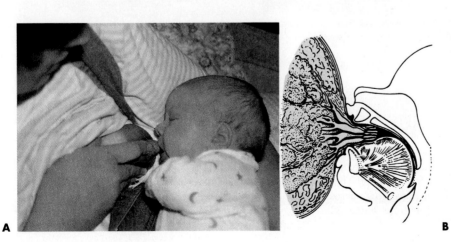

FIGURE 17-13 A, The nipple is guided into the baby's mouth. **B,** Its position should be located above the tongue and toward the hard palate. (**A** from Marjorie Pyle, RNC, *Lifecircle*; **B** from *Clinical education aid, no. 10,* Columbus, Ohio. © Ross Laboratories; used with permission.)

be open enough and the tongue positioned at the bottom of the mouth along the lower gum. The mouth must cover the nipple and at least 1 inch of the areola as well. This amount of breast tissue must be within the mouth so that the lactiferous sinuses can be compressed (Figure 17-13, *B*).

Swallowing is assessed after the first attempts at latching-on. Swallowing should be quiet and rhythmic, quicker at first, and slowing as the ejection of milk increases. Sucking or smacking noises or milk dribbling from the lips indicates incorrect attachment. The baby should be repositioned.

Timing of Feedings

Hungry babies should be fed on demand, usually every 2 to 3 hours at first. This means that newborns have feedings 8 to 10 times a day. The method of assessing intake is to examine the voiding and stooling pattern. If the baby wets clear urine and has soft, often pasty yellow stools, intake usually is sufficient (see Chapter 19). Hospital routines have interfered with lactation when babies were brought to the mothers every 4 hours. With rooming-in, the woman is free to observe signs of hunger and to respond. When the baby is sleepy or seems disinterested at first, gentle stimulation, unwrapping, or talking may awaken the infant to eat. To feed well, breast-fed infants must be awake and interested.

Length of feeding sessions no longer is limited. Traditionally women were told to limit early feedings to 2 to 3 minutes on a side, building up time gradually. Because it takes at least 5 minutes of sucking to trigger the let-down reflex in first-time mothers, limiting the time is self-defeating. The nipples will not become sore if the baby is correctly positioned and therefore not "chewing on the nipple." Instead the mother learns to recognize signs of satisfaction in the infant—slowing down in sucking and swallowing and finally falling asleep.

The mother who has had a cesarean birth or is very tired will need help in changing sides during feeding. Pillows can make both comfortable, and perhaps a raised side rail can be used as a handle for turning.

Bubbling

Bubbling or burping the baby should be performed before the feeding to eliminate air in the stomach that might displace milk or cause it to be spit up. Often the baby has been crying or sucking the fist and swallows air this way. If the baby sucks correctly, less air is swallowed. Usually women find it easiest to bubble the baby halfway through the feeding, while changing sides, or when the infant appears to slow down (Figure 17-14). Small amounts of undigested milk may be regurgitated (spit up) with the bubble. This is different from vomiting of partially digested milk.

Supplemental Feedings

Supplemental feedings adversely affect the establishment of the mother's milk supply. Therefore newborns should not be given supplemental feedings of glucose water or formula unless indicated by the medical condition of the mother or baby. In some states, withholding of supplementation for breast-feeding infants is mandated by state health policies. Early supplementation also may cause "nipple confusion" and result in the baby's refusal to breast-feed. Mothers are strongly encouraged in the initial establishment period of 2 to 3 weeks to only breast-feed until the milk supply is stable.

A   B   C

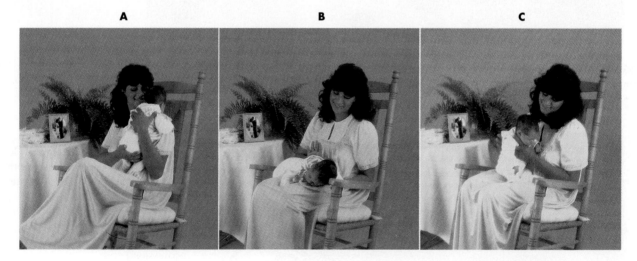

FIGURE 17-14 Once or twice during a feeding, the infant may need to be burped or bubbled by patting or rubbing the back for a minute. The three positions for burping the baby are upright against mother's shoulder (**A**), face down across her lap (**B**), and upright on her lap as she supports the head and chest with her hands (**C**). (Courtesy Ross Laboratories, Columbus, Ohio.)

VARIATIONS FOR MULTIPLE BIRTHS

A mother who breast-feeds twins will find that she has enough milk. Two babies sucking provide a tremendous stimulus to the breasts, and milk production increases accordingly. The mother will need to greatly increase her fluid and caloric intake and be particularly aware of her own nutritional needs. Twins can be fed at the same time or alternately (Figure 17-15). If fed together, the mother will need initial help in positioning the babies.

Breast-feeding twins can be easier to manage than bottle-feeding them. Once a routine is established, nursing the two together can actually be simpler because both are satisfied at the same time. Many variations are of course possible. A number of mothers use both breast and formula, feeding the hungriest first on the breast, then giving a bottle to the next. Some mothers change in the middle of the feeding, one hand giving a bottle to one while breast-feeding the other because it is awkward to feed both at the breast at the same time.

CESAREAN BIRTH

Initially, breast-feeding can be more difficult after a cesarean delivery. With regional anesthesia the mother should be encouraged to nurse as soon as she feels able, within several hours of delivery. After general anesthesia the mother and baby will be groggy and, in the baby's case, this grogginess may last several days. The nurse will need to spend time waking the baby up and getting the mother into a comfortable position; she will probably be most comfortable in a side-lying position. She needs help in switching the baby from one breast to the other. Leaving the bed rails up can give her something on which to hold as she turns over.

COMMON PROBLEMS

Discomfort: Breast Fullness

The two human mammary glands are designed to provide enough milk to feed more than one infant. Because most women have only one baby at a time, there is an overabundance of milk, especially in the first 10 days. When the milk "comes in" about the third postpartum day, fullness occurs. Lactation specialists now differentiate between *fullness* and its more severe state, *engorgement*. Nurses often still refer to this first fullness as engorgement. Breasts are full, heavy, and uncomfortable. The mother usually can alleviate this fullness by nursing the baby frequently (q 2 to 3 hours) to empty the breasts, wearing a supportive brassiere, and applying warm compresses before feeding. Because milk supply works on a demand basis, once lactation has been established, the amount produced will decrease to the amount the growing baby needs.

Engorgement

Engorged breasts will look swollen and shiny. They feel hot, heavy, hard, or lumpy and may leak a little milk. The nipple recedes into the engorged breast, making it harder for the baby to latch on. The mother will complain of tenderness and pain in the breasts and nipples.

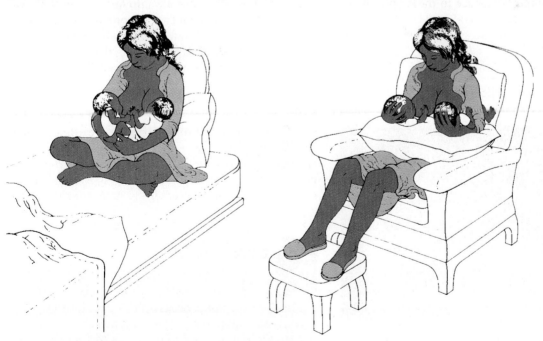

FIGURE 17-15 Positions for nursing twins. (From Fogel CI, Woods NF: *Health care of women,* St Louis, 1981, Mosby.)

Engorgement is a result of insufficient emptying of the alveoli because of poor sucking or infrequent or inadequate nursing. With milk back-up, clogging of ducts can occur and cause a predisposition to mastitis or breast abscess. If the baby cannot suck sufficiently to empty the breast, then milk needs to be expressed from the breast either by hand or with a pump (Figure 17-16). *Sore nipples* are caused by poor latching-on as a result of incorrect positioning, poor tongue placement, or traction on the nipple. Sore nipples are directly related to the pressure on the nipple incorrectly placed in the baby's mouth. To prevent problems the following directions are helpful to the new mother.

- Express a few drops of milk before putting the baby to the breast.
- Make sure the baby is properly fixed on the breast and is sucking on the areola.
- Remember, the reflex takes several minutes to operate in the new nursing mother.
- Nurse in different positions so the pressure of suction affects a different portion of the nipple.
- Avoid pulling the baby off the breast; break the suction first.
- Expose the nipples and let them air dry for at least 10 minutes after feeding; the longer the better. Apply a few drops of breast milk to the nipples before drying to aid in the healing process.
- Keep nursing pads and bras dry at all times. Remove any plastic linings.
- Avoid using soap on the nipples, instead apply pure lanolin or vitamin E oil.
- Apply cold compresses or ice to the nipples if the pain is severe.

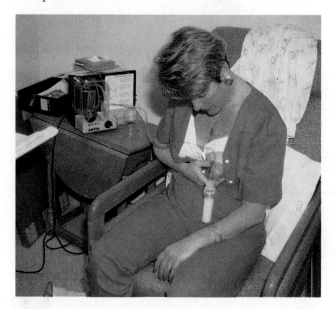

FIGURE 17-16 A hand-operated breast pump is useful for working mothers and for alleviating breast fullness. (Courtesy Marjorie Pyle, RNC, *Lifecircle*.)

Plugged Ducts

If undue pressure is applied to the breast, as from a poorly fitting brassiere or pressure of the baby's chin during nursing, stasis can occur in a duct. The water content of the milk there is absorbed by the tissue, leaving a thick viscous substance that irritates the tissue. Inflammation occurs as a response (noninfective mastitis).

Mastitis

Mastitis is a bacterial infection of the connective tissue surrounding the breast glandular tissue and is not an infection of the glands or ducts themselves. The means by which bacteria gain entrance and colonize the tissue around the mammary gland are unknown. Sore, inflamed, or cracked nipples are thought to precipitate mastitis. Most likely, bacteria shared between the infant's oropharynx and the maternal areola gain entrance through small cracks or fissures within the areola and cause infection. *Staphylococcus aureus*, group A and B streptococci, or other skin or mouth flora generally are believed to cause mastitis.

Infective mastitis occurs infrequently in 0.8% to 2.5% of lactating women. Symptoms usually occur within the first 2 weeks after birth, with another peak 5 to 6 weeks later. Delay of more than 24 hours in initiating antibiotic treatment may contribute to abscess formation.

Signs. Women with mastitis usually note breast tenderness or pain localized to one specific area. In addition, general malaise, fever often higher than 101° F, increased pulse rate, and local erythema and warmth may be present. Complaints of flulike symptoms in the postpartum or breast-feeding woman should always

  Clinical Decision

Ada S. has been eager to prove that she is a good mother and breast-fed her baby for long periods. Her nipples are now red and bleeding. Which strategies should be included in her plan of care and why?

initiate evaluation for some type of postpartum infection. Catecholamines released in response to pain may inhibit the let-down reflex and disturb breast-feeding. Symptoms usually improve within 36 to 48 hours of antibiotic treatment.

Clinical management. Care includes antibiotic therapy, analgesia, education, and support for continued breast-feeding. Antibiotic choices include oral dicloxacillin, cephalosporin, or erythromycin if the woman is allergic to penicillin (Lewis and Hurden, 1988). Continuation of breast-feeding is strongly encouraged by use of both the affected and unaffected breasts. There appears to be no additional risks to the newborn inasmuch as the bacteria causing the infection probably are part of the newborn's normal oropharyngeal flora.

Although mastitis is not a contraindication to breast-feeding, an *abscess* is. The baby should not nurse on the affected side but may continue on the unaffected side. The abscessed breast can then be emptied by pumping until the infection is resolved. The mother should be instructed that the full course of antibiotic therapy must be completed, usually 10 to 14 days.

The best way to treat these conditions is to be sure the breasts are empty after each feeding. The woman can assist this process by taking a warm shower or applying warm compresses before feeding and gently massaging the breast. Severe discomfort may be relieved by lying in a hot bath on the affected side and allowing the breast to float. Milk may then be expressed into the hot water. Because of edema associated with mastitis and abscess, milk flow will be impaired and increased sodium content in the milk may taste unpleasant to the infant. Even though the affected breast is offered to the infant, it may be refused; a breast pump is then used to empty the breast (Figure 17-16).

Maternal Illness

In the past the mother was not allowed to breast-feed if her temperature had become elevated over 100.4° F in the previous 24 hours. Today, on the basis of the understanding that dehydration, fatigue, and early healing processes may elevate temperatures in the first 24 hours, most infants are at the breast as soon as is feasible. Colostrum contains helpful antibodies, and the infant may have already been exposed in utero to the mother's early signs of an infection. Only in the presence of active tuberculosis, hepatitis B, human immunodeficiency virus (HIV), chickenpox, or high fever of unknown origin is breast-feeding interrupted. (See Chapter 25 for isolation precautions for mother and infant.) Urinary tract, respiratory tract, or local infections are not indications to stop, especially if treatment with antibiotics has begun. Nursery staff personnel, however, need to know the current temperature and

condition of the mother and take precautions to avoid the spread of infection to other babies in the nursery. Other conditions interfere if the mother is unable to care for herself or the baby because of recent anesthesia, pain, or weakness.

SPECIAL PROBLEMS WITH INFANTS

Jaundice

Approximately 50% of newborns normally develop visible jaundice during the first week of life (see Chapter 17). In fewer than 1% of breast-feeding mothers, a factor that inhibits the metabolism of bilirubin is secreted in milk. The jaundiced infant who is breast-feeding may be further affected by *pregnanediol*, a compound in the breast milk formed by the reduction of progesterone. The level of jaundice may rise above normal but appears noninjurious. To rule out breast-feeding as the cause of jaundice, a physician may ask the mother to discontinue breast-feeding for 48 hours to allow the level to fall. In this case the mother may continue to pump her breast to maintain supply. It is extremely rare that jaundice will be an indication to discontinue lactation (see Chapter 28 for discussion).

In fact some researchers believe that because of increased stooling, bilirubin levels actually drop more quickly in breast-fed infants than in those bottle-fed or supplemented with formula or water. If the baby receives adequate fluid by nursing, there is usually no need to interrupt breast-feeding (Lemons et al, 1986).

Preterm Infant

Infants weighing less than 1 kg have no sucking reflex. In general, preterm infants are able to suck and swallow by about week 34 of gestation (Lemons et al, 1986). The energy required, however, often is too great, and they still may require gavage feeds (see Chapter 28). Some discussion continues about whether breast milk at the early period in the third trimester is totally sufficient, although it is more easily digested and can prevent necrotizing enterocolitis (NEC) (Beckholt, 1990).

The breasts are fully developed for lactation by the end of the second trimester, and the mother who has delivered prematurely can produce an adequate amount of milk for her baby. The nurse encourages the mother of a baby not yet able to nurse to express her milk by use of an electric breast pump, showing her how to massage her breasts before expressing milk. Her milk supply will become established, and the expressed milk can be fed by tube or bottle to the baby. Expressing her milk not only provides the baby with the best possible nutrition but can be a source of comfort and bonding for the mother who has been physically separated from her child and feels helpless (see Chapter 28).

DISCHARGE PLANNING

Breast-feeding usually is only barely established during the 2 or 3 days that the mother and infant are in the hospital; the mother has the support of the hospital staff members and their assurance that her baby is doing well. When she goes home, however, she may be very much on her own and can easily lose confidence in her ability to feed her baby. Feelings of self-doubt may be fostered by relatives and friends who ask whether the baby is getting enough milk. "Not having enough milk" is the most common reason for failure in breast-feeding.

Some maternity areas employ a lactation clinical specialist who distributes literature and holds individual or small-group instruction sessions. If not, the nurse in recovery takes on this responsibility. Be sure to refer her for assistance and WIC food supplements as needed. Lactating women qualify for additional help and instruction through the WIC program.

In many areas, home care services are available to a mother when it has been determined that she needs follow-up care or is discharged early. Breast-feeding coordinators and clinicians may follow up with new mothers by telephone. Finally, the mother is encouraged to seek out other women who have breast-fed successfully. If a mother has no support in the home, she may contact La Leche League, an organization dedicated to promoting breast-feeding. By telephone and through local group meetings, support and advice are available to new mothers. To find a local group a woman may write to La Leche League International, P.O. Box 1209, Franklin Park, IL 60131-8209; telephone 1-312-455-7730.

The Family after Birth

Family processes always undergo alterations with the childbirth experience. Whether this baby is the first or is joining other siblings, changes in roles, routines, and priorities are a challenge to all family members. Understanding their concerns and encouraging participation in the restructuring of the family unit facilitate successful transition.

FATHERS

Traditionally the father was an observer during the intrapartum period. Not only was he an inactive participant in the birth event, he was not permitted in the delivery area. After the birth, care and feeding were considered the domain of the mother, and the father was left to distribute cigars and make telephone calls. Today the picture is very different. Most fathers choose to be a vital part of the process as coach during birth. With increased societal emphasis on shared parenting and the recognition of paternal bonding, many fathers

are active in care giving and enjoy the closeness it brings (Figure 17-17).

Almost universally, hospitals have eliminated visiting restrictions for fathers; there is an open visiting policy. Fathers may claim their babies at the nursery to take to the mothers' rooms, are involved in baby care classes, and are instructed with the mothers. Fathers also should be involved in discharge planning (Figure 17-18) because they are essential in early care at home.

GRANDPARENTS

Most grandparents are delighted at the arrival of a new family member, particularly if it is the first grandchild.

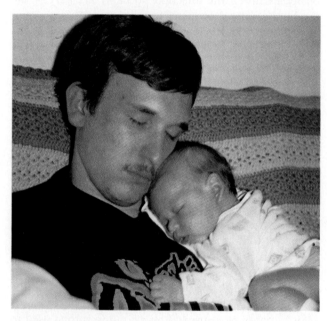

FIGURE 17-17 Father and son tired out but together. (Courtesy Eric Schult.)

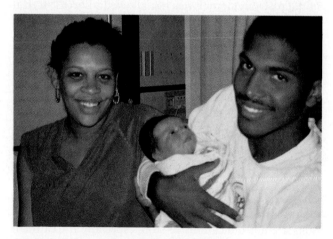

FIGURE 17-18 Early involvement of young fathers builds confidence. (Courtesy Camille Bodden.)

They have been following the pregnancy and are anxious to see the child.

The emotional and comforting support offered by grandparents during pregnancy and birth is finally being recognized by health care personnel. Grandparents are allowed in some labor suites and are encouraged to visit the postpartum units because they are in a position to offer help and guidance as needed.

A special bond often develops between grandparent and grandchild. Special memories are formed as the grandparents do their best to spoil the child, often giving him or her things and time not available when their own children were young. It is as if they have been given a second chance at child rearing, with all the pleasures and joys and none of the responsibilities (Figure 17-19).

Despite all the joys and pleasures of having the grandparents around, conflicts sometimes can arise regarding child-rearing practices. If the new parents do not agree in their views of child rearing, the grandparents may step in to offer advice, even when it is not desired. They may force their opinions on the inexperienced parents and evoke guilt if advice is refused. Therefore ground rules for the raising of a child must be set down by the new parents so that conflict is reduced. Once the grandparents take over rearing tasks, it may be hard to reestablish the parents as the primary care givers. Grandparents are a rich source of knowledge, but their knowledge must be available without the young parents relinquishing authority. This task must be worked out early within the family structure. When the new parent is an adolescent, the task is more difficult (see Chapter 8).

SIBLINGS

The arrival of a new addition to the family has a profound effect on the other members, including children (Figure 17-20). The way in which the siblings are prepared before the birth may help to determine whether they will adjust to and accept the new baby (Box 17-4 and see Chapter 12). In LDRP settings siblings visit freely.

Parents must realize that children often regress in their behavior. The 4-year-old child may begin to wet in bed at night, and the 3-year-old child may want to suck at the breast with the new baby. These situations have to be handled sensitively so the older child does not feel guilty because of the regressive behaviors. A special time with the child each day may restore confidence and security, and some lactating mothers have found that letting the toddler nurse allows him to realize that it is no "big" request and thus soon forgets about it. Each family has to work out its own way of handling sibling rivalry to suit the specific situation. Every child experiences feelings of rivalry when a new infant enters the family system.

Home Care

Self-care is no longer a philosophic issue but a practical and real need. The nurse cannot possibly continue to monitor everything through the recovery phase but must instead teach the new mother to understand the

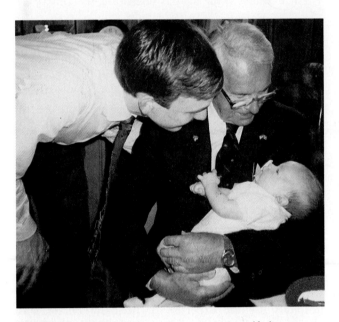

FIGURE 17-19 Three generations meet. Grandfather, son, and new grandson. (Courtesy Eric Schult.)

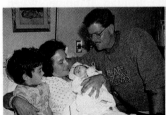
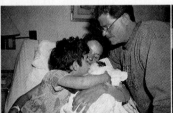
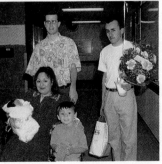

FIGURE 17-20 A and B, Sibling takes time to warm up to the new intruder. **C,** Ready for going home. (Courtesy Marjorie Pyle, RNC, *Lifecircle.*)

BOX 17-4   Caring for Siblings

Before the baby comes
- Include the child in activities preparing for the event.
- Plan with the child where the child will stay during mother's hospitalization. If staying with a neighbor or relative, he might stay the night as a "dry run" before the expected due date.
- Be aware that children can misinterpret; parents should be matter-of-fact and positive about the impending hospitalization.
- If the older child will be going into a new bed, make the transfer as early in pregnancy as possible.
- If possible, begin toilet training well in advance of the new baby's arrival. Otherwise, delay toilet training until the older child is accustomed to the new baby.
- Consider buying (and wrapping) inexpensive items and storing them for use when gift-laden visitors arrive for the newcomer.

When the baby arrives
- Try to understand that the older child needs to express his continued dependency and need for attention. Gentle and frequent explanations of the positive aspects of "growing up" help to prevent regressive behavior.
- When guests arrive with gifts for the baby, give the older child the tucked-away surprises at intervals and allow him or her to pull the wrappings from the baby's gifts, especially if the youngster is 2 or 3 years old.
- Consider giving the child a special gift when the baby is brought home from the hospital, specifying it as the newcomer's "thank you" for making everything ready for him.
- Remember that older children still need physical attention, including snuggling, rocking, and hugging. This extra assurance helps to convince the child that love can be expanded to fit two or three or more children.
- Let the child "help" with the baby; this helps him to feel important. However, do not overdo it to the point that he feels like "I'll never get to play again."
- Prevent any anger or hurt that might be displaced onto the baby.
- If there is a change in the expected plan for the newborn, deal with the older child's fears realistically. For example, if the baby is premature, try to have a picture taken to show to the older child.
- Take advantage of books that express the message of the problems the older child experiences in living with the new arrival; examples include *Peter's Chair* and *A Baby Sister for Frances* (Harper & Row, Inc.) and *The Very Little Girl* and *The Very Little Boy* (Doubleday).

Modified from Kappleman M: *What your child is all about*, New York, 1974, Reader's Digest Press.

Let Father carry new infant in house so mom can greet other sibling

processes of recovery and how to evaluate her successful progress.

Physically, within the first 24 hours, a woman should be capable of caring for herself as evidenced by her ability to palpate her fundus and recognize that it is firm, recognize the amount and type of lochia, use aseptic technique for perineal care, recognize signs of infection or complications, monitor and evaluate urine output and bowel function, and assess changes in breasts as the milk supply begins and deal with these changes depending on her method of feeding. She also must be able to perform tasks related to the care of her infant.

Nursing follow-up after discharge must become the norm rather than the exception. The nurse will be called on to assess and continue teaching after the woman goes home. This may be achieved by telephone or in person through classes and support groups. Because of early discharge, nursing follow-up care in the home may become routine. Innovative programs are being developed to compensate for shortened hospital stays. In one such program, Empire Blue Cross encourages early maternal discharge by offering three home visits during the first week by an approved nurse if the woman is discharged within the first 24 hours after birth. In this way the woman who chooses to go home early still receives professional assessment, planning, and care within the privacy and comfort of her home. Some hospitals use the expertise of perinatal nurses who alternate working in the home and hospital on a rotating basis. This nurse meets the client on her first postpartum day, checks charts, receives physician orders, and plans to meet the woman at home. When making the home visit, the nurse is able to assess the situation and the needs of the mother and neonate. Women's response to both in-home visits and follow-up telephone calls is very positive (Williams and Cooper, 1993) because it gives them an opportunity to seek information, validates their experience, and permits them to obtain help when they are at home alone without the constant support of hospital personnel and services.

NURSING CARE PLAN • Recovery from Birth

Case: Mary, age 18, g1, P0, and Leonard, age 20. Estimated date of birth (EDB) 6/8/93. Rupture of membranes (SROM) 5/18/93 22 hours before birth. Normal spontaneous delivery (NSD) of a 5 lb 10 oz female 37-week infant. RML episiotomy and third-degree laceration. Admitted to recovery room; vital signs (VS) 99.8/80/22, BP 104/68. Complains of "pain in the bottom—a lot." Social history—worked at local fertilizer plant until delivery. Plans to return to work. Husband is truck driver—out of town often. Attended two childbirth preparation classes with sister who also accompanied her to hospital and stayed with her through delivery. Nutritional history—ate out often at fast-food restaurants (mainly French fries and hamburgers) but as a result of prenatal guidance added more fruits and vegetables to diet. Cut smoking from 2 packs/day to 1 pack/day. Drank beer with co-workers after work a few nights per week.

ASSESSMENT DATA

1. Social history
   Nutritional history
   Knowledge of parenting

Infant feeding plan: breast or bottle
Role expectations, partner support

NURSING DIAGNOSES

1. High risk for fluid volume deficit R/T blood loss secondary to uterine atony
2. High risk for infection R/T impaired skin integrity
3. Pain related to episiotomy and third-degree laceration
4. Knowledge deficit: postpartum recovery self-care related to inexperience
5. Altered nutrition: less than body requirements for postpartum recovery related to inadequate food intake and poor eating habits
6. High risk for altered parenting related to family structure and support and parental employment

EXPECTED OUTCOMES

1. Fluid balance maintained
2. Episiotomy/lacerations heal without difficulty
3. Experiences minimal discomfort.
4. Attains an adequate knowledge base of self-recovery to monitor progress and report warning signs of infection promptly.
5. Modifies eating habits to consume adequate nutrients.
6. Reports adequate support system for self, husband, and infant; evaluates workplace and work schedule for maximum benefit for self and infant.

NURSING INTERVENTIONS

1. Assess involution, vital signs, and sign of recovery.
2. Discuss process of recovery and signs and symptoms of postpartum infection. Give telephone number to report problems.
3. Discuss nonpharmacologic as well as pharmacologic modalities for pain relief.
4. Ensure basic self-care and infant care skills have been demonstrated.
5. Obtain complete nutritional and diet history. Describe nutritional requirements of postpartum; work out with client a diet plan that will encourage compliance. Refer to nutritionist if necessary.
6. Explore sources of support, enpower client to find help; make referrals to appropriate agencies as needed. Encourage client to look realistically at work schedule with partner and support persons.

EVALUATION

1. Did she monitor self-care and report problems promptly?
2. Did she report relief from pain?
3. Does she demonstrate self and infant care skills?
4. Is she eating a proper, adequate diet as evidenced by appropriate weight, adequate healing from delivery, and adequate milk production?
5. Has she reported adequate support, and are her work environment and schedule conducive to parental and infant health and well-being?

KEY POINTS

1. Every body system returns to the prepregnancy state by reversing the unique developments during pregnancy.
2. Childbirth places stresses on the new mother and entire family, and support networks may determine whether these stresses are easily resolved.
3. Monitoring of involution, vital signs, pain, and infection is essential in the early postpartum period.
4. Facilitating the mother's self-care and her care of the infant is the major goal of postpartum nursing care.
5. Nursing responsibilities include assisting the woman in developmental tasks and in achieving beginning satisfaction in the parenting role.
6. Support and teaching enable most women who choose breast-feeding to be successful and lessen the chances of problems or complications.
7. Women who give birth by assisted or surgical methods may need more support to maintain self-esteem.
8. Use of nursing process assists the nurse in identifying focus areas for effective and appropriate care for the childbearing family.

STUDY QUESTIONS

17-1 Choose an appropriate key term to fill in the blanks of the following statements.
   a. Through _____ the body returns to its prepregnant state. *involution*
   b. The fluids from the lining of the uterus are called _____ . *Lochia*
   c. The beginning of outward interest in her baby and surroundings occurs when a new mother starts _____ . *Taking hold*
   d. The _____ is the 6- to 8-week period of immediate recovery after birth. *puerperium*
   e. Intense discomfort in the incompletely emptied breasts is due to _____ *engorgement*
   f. Milk will not be ejected properly until the _____ reflex occurs. *let down*

17-2 May H. is a 33-year-old primipara, gravida 3, para 1 vaginal birth. She gave birth to a healthy, full-term baby girl 3 hours before your assessment. An intravenous solution of Ringer's lactate, with 20 units of Pitocin added, is infusing at 100 ml/hr. During initial postpartal check, you note that her pad is soaked and has multiple small clots. Choose the first nursing interventions for Mrs. H:
   a. Giving and explaining perineal care and placing a new pad.
   b. Calling her physician to report lochia change.
   c. Performing a fundal check and ensuring the patency of the intravenous solution.
   d. Taking no measures because this condition is common with multigravid women.

17-3 Mrs. H.'s fundus is found to be one finger-breadth above the umbilicus and deviated to the right. What is your assessment?
   a. This position is normal for this involutional period.

   b. This position is a sign of early postpartum hemorrhage.
   c. This position indicates that the client's bladder is probably full.
   d. This position indicates that there is a tilted uterus.

17-4 Which of the following indicates need for further assessment during the first 24 hours after delivery?
   a. White blood cell count of 18,000/mm^3
   b. Scant lochia rubra
   c. Thirst and fatigue
   d. Temperature of 100.4° F

17-5 Vital signs are taken frequently during the immediate postpartum period because:
   a. The standing order indicates frequent checks.
   b. Early hemorrhage is best detected by changes in vital signs.
   c. Most recovery problems can be detected through assessment of vital signs.
   d. Vital signs may change rapidly throughout the immediate postpartum recovery period.

17-6 Which of the following lochial patterns should the mother report?
   a. Bright red discharge with a small clot on the first recovery day
   b. Serosanguineous discharge on the fourth day
   c. No lochia on the third day
   d. Yellowish white mucus on the fourteenth day

17-7 Kegel exercises are helpful in the recovery period because they:
   a. Tone up the upper thigh muscles.
   b. Relieve lower back pain caused by the delivery position.
   c. Relieve the pain of breast engorgement.

d. Strengthen the perineal muscles and promote healing of the episiotomy.

17-8 In addition to sufficient infant nursing, to ensure adequate milk supply during lactation the woman should:

a. Avoid salty foods and eat balanced meals.

b. Drink at least 12 cups of fluid per day.

c. Drink at least 1 quart of fruit juice a day, in addition to required milk intake.

d. Increase vegetable and complex carbohydrate intake.

17-9 The client is experiencing breast engorgement on the third postpartum day. Select the appropriate nursing intervention to relieve the pain for this mother who is not breast-feeding.

a. Encourage Kegel exercises.

b. Suggest that she breast-feed temporarily to relieve engorgement.

c. Apply warm soaks to her breasts or have her take a warm shower to relieve congestion.

d. Apply a firm bra and ice packs to her breasts.

17-10 Immediately on arrival of a new mother to the postpartum unit, you should:

a. Assess bonding between parents and newborn.

b. Verify identification bands with chart information.

c. Assess involution, comfort, and intravenous solution patency.

d. Check orders for activity, diet, and medications.

17-11 Mary C., gravida 1, para 1, gave birth to a term boy by cesarean delivery because of unexpected fetal distress. She has seen the infant for a brief visit the first evening. She complains frequently of incisional and gas pains, is tearful and fatigued, and has general malaise. What is the first nursing diagnosis that must be addressed?

a. Pain

b. Activity intolerance

c. Knowledge deficit regarding infant

d. Altered parenting (bonding)

17-12 Which statement by Mary would indicate that she was struggling with maintaining self-esteem?

a. "I should have followed the breathing patterns better during labor."

b. "I'm really angry that this happened."

c. "I couldn't have gone through this alone. Jim stayed."

d. "I wish it could have been a natural birth."

Answer Key

17-1 a. Involution, b. Lochia, c. Taking hold, d. Puerperium, e. Engorgement, f. Let-down, 17-2 c 17-3 c 17-4 b 17-5 d 17-6 c 17-7 d 17-8 b 17-9 d 17-10 c 17-11 a 17-12 a

REFERENCES

Bertino JS: The pharmacology of human milk, *Birth* 8(4):19, 1981.

Beckholt A: Breast milk for infants who cannot breastfeed, *JOGNN* 19(3):216, 1990.

Blackburn ST, Loper DL: *Maternal, fetal, and neonatal physiology,* Philadelphia, 1992, W B Saunders.

Briggs GC, Freeman RK, Yaffe SJ: *Drugs in pregnancy and lactation,* ed 2, Baltimore, 1986, Williams & Wilkins.

Brooten D et al: Early discharge and special transitional care, *Image J Nurs Sch* 20(2):64, 1988.

Carty EM, Tier DT: Birth planning: a reality-based script for building confidence, *J Nurse Midwifery* 34(3):111, 1989.

Combs CA, Murphy EL, Laros RK Jr: Factors associated with hemorrhage, *Obstet Gynecol Surv* 46:362, 1991.

Cox JL, Holden JM, Sagovsky R: The Edinburgh postnatal depression scale, *Br J Psych* 150:728, 1989.

Donovan B: *The cesarean birth experience,* Boston, 1977, Beacon Press.

Evans CT: Description of a home follow-up program for childbearing families, *JOGNN* 2:113, 1991.

Fortier JC: The relationship of vaginal and cesarean birth to father-infant attachment, *JOGNN* 2:128, 1988.

Gay JT, Edgil AE, Douglas AB: Reva Rubin revisited, *JOGNN* 6:394, 1988.

Gillerman H, Beckham MH: Postpartum early discharge dilemma: an innovative solution, *J Perinat Neonatal Nurs* 5(1):9, 1991.

Halpern SR: Development of childhood allergy in infants fed breast, soy, or cow milk, *J Allergy Clin Immunol* 51:139, 1977.

Hampson SJ: Nursing intervention for the first three postpartum months, *JOGNN* 2:116, 1989.

Harper R et al: Observations on postpartum shivering phenomenon, *J Reprod Med* 36(11):803, 1991.

Hawkin DF, editor: *Drugs and pregnancy,* ed 2, New York, 1988, Churchill Livingstone.

Herzog A, Detre T: Psychotic reactions associated with childbirth, *Dis Nerv Syst* 37:229, 1976.

Kearney MH et al: Breastfeeding problems in the first week postpartum, *Nurs Res* 39:90, 1990.

Lemons P et al: Breast feeding the premature infant, *Clin Perinatol* 13(1):111, 1986.

Lethbridge DJ: The use of breastfeeding as a contraceptive, *JOGNN* 1:31, 1988.

Lethbridge DJ et al: Validation of the nursing diagnosis of ineffective breastfeeding, *JOGNN* 1:57, 1993.

Lewis PJ, Hurden EI: Breastfeeding and drug treatment. In Hawkins DF, ed: *Drugs and pregnancy,* New York, 1988, Churchill Livingstone, Inc.

Little B, Billiar RB: Endocrine disorders. In Romney SL, editor: *Gynecology and obstetrics: the health care of women,* New York, 1975, McGraw-Hill.

Luegenbiehl D et al: Standardized assessment of blood loss, *MCN* 15(4):241, 1991.

McGregor JA, Christiansen FB: Treatment of obstetrics and gynecologic infections, with an emphasis on beta-lactamase–producing organisms, *J Reprod Med* 33(suppl 6):591, 1988.

Minchin M: Positioning for breastfeeding, *Birth* 16(2):67, 1989.

Moore ML: *Realities in childbearing,* Philadelphia, 1983, WB Saunders.

Niebyl JR et al: Sporadic (non-epidemic) puerperal mastitis, *J Reprod Med* 20:97, 1978.

Reamy K, White S: Sexuality in pregnancy and the puerperium: a review, *Obstet Gynecol Surv* 40(1):1, 1985.

Rhode MA, Barger MK: Perineal care then and now, *J Nurse Midwifery* 4:220, 1990.

Rook A et al: *Textbook of dermatology,* vol 1, Oxford, England, 1979, Blackwell Scientific Publications.

Rosner AE, Schulman SK: Birth interval among breastfeeding women not using contraceptives, *Pediatrics* 86:747, 1990.

Rubin RA: Maternal tasks in pregnancy, *Matern Child Nurs J* 4(3):143, 1975.

Rubin RA: Maternity nursing stops too soon, *AJN* 10:1680, 1975.

Rubin RA: Binding-in in the postpartum period, *Matern Child Nurs J* 6(2):67, 1977.

Selby JW et al: *Psychology and human reproduction,* New York, 1980, Free Press.

Shrago L, Bocar D: The infant's contribution to breastfeeding, *JOGNN* 3:209, 1990.

Starr G: Prevention of nipple tenderness and breast engorgement in the postpartal period, *JOGNN* 17(3):203, 1988.

Swartz MK: Primary care and differential diagnoses of the newborn, *J Nurse Midwifery* 37(2):185, 1992.

Tribotti S et al: Nursing diagnoses for the postpartum woman, *JOGNN* 17(6):410, 1988.

Weiss ME, Armstrong M: Postpartum mothers' preference for nighttime care of the neonate, *JOGNN* 4:290, 1991.

Williams LR, Cooper MK: Nurse-managed postpartum home care, *JOGNN* 1:25, 1993.

Wilson JR, Carrington ER: *Obstetrics and gynecology,* ed 9, St Louis, 1991, Mosby.

STUDENT RESOURCE SHELF

Evans C: Description of a home follow-up program for childbearing families, *JOGNN* 20(2):113, 1991. Early discharge of the mother and her infant has made postpartum follow-up at home a necessity. The reasons for this need and the response of a model program are discussed in this article, emphasizing the importance of telephone communication between the new mother and nursing staff members along with in-home visits by the nurse.

Luegenbiehl D et al: Standardized assessment of blood loss, *MCN* 15(4):241, 1990. In an effort to make the measurement of postpartum lochial flow more consistent and objective, nurses were taught to assess lochia by recording cubic centimeters of blood stain on a perineal pad and by weighing pads and recording in milliliters. Accuracy of postpartal blood loss increased significantly.

Shrago L, Bocar D: The infant's contribution to breastfeeding, *JOGNN* 19(3):209, 1990. Difficulties with breast-feeding often are attributed solely to the mother's discomfort or ineptness. These authors share what they have learned about helping the *infant* learn to nurse more effectively and successfully.

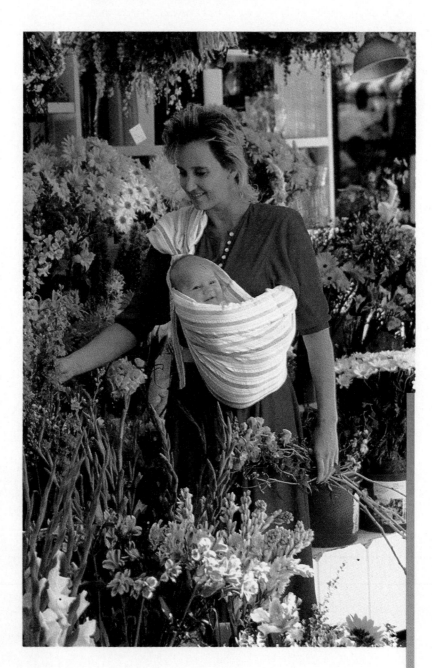

NEWBORN CARE

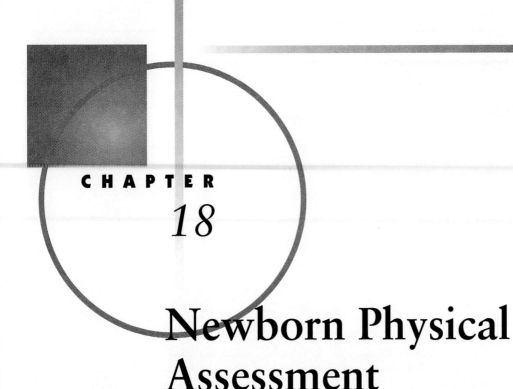

CHAPTER

18

Newborn Physical Assessment

LEARNING OBJECTIVES

1. *Identify components of the neonatal health history and physical assessment.*
2. *Determine risk status of neonate based on data from prenatal history and intrapartum progress.*
3. *Describe major physiologic changes in transition to extrauterine function.*
4. *Distinguish between normal and abnormal structure and function for full-term neonates.*
5. *Describe normal neonatal behavior patterns.*
6. *Explain the purpose of gestational age assessment.*
7. *Recognize physical characteristics of preterm, postterm, small-for-gestational age (SGA), and large-for-gestational age (LGA) infants.*
8. *Determine gestational age using size, weight, and specific developmental characteristics.*

Newborn infants usually are considered to be tiny and powerless, completely dependent on others for life. Although this is true as far as obtaining food and water, it is not so regarding basic life processes. Within 1 minute of birth the normal newborn adapts from a dependent fetal existence to an independent one, capa-

---

BOX 18-1   Neonatal Health History

Date _____ Infant _____
Date of delivery _____ Sex _____
Time of delivery _____ Age (in hours) now _____

Prenatal data

Maternal age _____ Blood type and Rh _____
Indirect Coombs' _____ EDB via dates _____
EDB via ultrasound _____

Previous obstetric history

Parity (explain all items) _____
Previous pregnancies:

Date	Gestational age	Sex	Weight	Delivery	Complications

Complications of this pregnancy

Preeclampsia _____ Hypertension_____
Diabetes (class) _____ Bleeding _____
Viral/bacterial infection _____
Environmental teratogens _____
Drug use _____
Over the counter _____ Alcohol _____
Prescription _____ Cocaine _____
Heroin _____ Methadone _____
Other _____

Results of fetal testing

AFP assay _____
Ultrasound _____ Amniocentesis _____
NST _____ BPS _____

Intrapartum data

Onset of contractions _____
Rupture of membranes (ROM) _____ When? _____
Bloody _____ Meconium stained _____ Foul smell _____
Abnormalities of maternal vital signs _____
Medications during labor _____
Anesthesia/analgesia _____ Time last administered _____
Fetal monitoring (external/internal) _____
Fetal distress _____ Fetal pH _____
Length of stages of labor: First _____ Second _____ Third _____

---

ble of oxygenation and carrying on life processes. Understanding and appreciating this transition are vital to the assessment of the newborn.

This chapter is organized by body systems and reviews techniques for assessing the normal transition to extrauterine function. For information on the high-risk infant and several of the problems mentioned here, refer to Chapters 27 and 28.

The nurse frequently is the first health care provider who has contact with the neonate. In some birth settings it can be as long as 24 hours before a physician is required to examine a new baby. These first hours are crucial because multiple organ systems are making the transition from intrauterine to extrauterine functions. The nurse requires the skill to identify the baby who is having difficulty so that proper therapy can be instituted. The use of universal precautions with barriers such as gloves until the newborn has the first bath is important to protect both nurse and client from communicable diseases.

Physical Assessment

Neonatal physical assessment is similar to adult assessment; that is, the same methods of data collection are used. A major focus will be on assessment of growth

BOX 18-1 Neonatal Health History—cont'd

Delivery

Time _____ Route _____
Reason for operative delivery _____

Resuscitation

Apgar score: 1 minute _____ 5 minute _____
Suction _____ Whiffs of O_2 _____
Positive pressure _____ Via mask/endotracheal tube _____
Length _____
Time of first spontaneous breath _____
Medications _____

Other

Voided in delivery room _____ Stool _____
Breast-fed _____ Bonding time _____
Observations of bonding behavior _____

In nursery

Time of transfer to nursery if applicable _____
First temperature _____ Placed in warmer/Isolette _____
Eye prophylaxis _____
Vitamin K _____ Time _____ Location _____

EDB, Estimated date of birth; *AFP,* alpha-fetoprotein; *NST,* nonstress test; *BPS,* biophysical profile score.

and development. The object of the assessment is to identify any alterations in health status that would make adjustment difficult. A list of warning signs follows each system. These are assessment findings that necessitate interventions, discussed further in Chapter 28. Health history is a prelude to assessment; therefore the neonatal health history (Box 18-1) should be completed before beginning the physical examination. History of the pregnancy and birth helps focus on specific risks that may be present.

Usually physical assessment is begun with the head and proceeds downward. Infants are stimulated by physical assessment and may lose heat quickly when undressed. Therefore the order of the examination has been changed to minimize heat loss and to enlist the infant's cooperation. Attention is given to prenatal development; developmentally related body systems are reviewed at the same time. In addition, the examiner notes differences in behaviors and vital signs during the early periods of reactivity.

GENERAL EXAMINATION

The nurse begins with a thorough but quick scan of the infant (Figure 18-1), looking for overt signs of difficulty for which immediate intervention is necessary. These manifest as abnormalities in vital signs, color, tone, movement, and size. The following questions provide a focus for the procedure.

Vital Signs

Are the vital signs—temperature, heart rate, respiration, and blood pressure— within normal limits?

Temperature. An axillary temperature can be taken with minimal disturbance by gently slipping the thermometer into the axillary space. Figure 19-8 illustrates the correct placement of an undressed baby. Rectal temperatures are not routinely taken because the vagus nerve is stimulated, and there is risk of

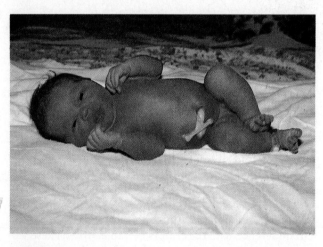

FIGURE 18-1 Healthy newborn. (Courtesy Marjorie Pyle, RNC, *Lifecircle.*)

rectal perforation. Thermogenesis is discussed under Metabolic Control later in this chapter. Normal ranges of axillary temperatures are 36.1° to 36.5° C (97.0° to 97.7° F.)

Heart rate. An apical heart rate of 110 to 160 beats/min should be heard on the left side of the chest near the nipple, and the examiner may listen for less than 1 minute and multiply appropriately. For alterations in heart sounds, see discussion of cardiorespiratory system.

Respiration. The irregularity of respirations requires counting for a full minute. A range of 30 to 60 breaths/min is normal. The rate is irregular and abdominal, with a possibility of brief (less than 3 to 5 seconds) periods of pause or apnea. Some otherwise healthy infants may show tachypnea during the first hour as excess lung fluid is absorbed. The examiner listens for the quality of breath sounds at each midaxillary line.

Blood pressure. Initial readings are taken with the Doppler device (Dinomap) on an arm and a leg and compared (see Figure 18-6, *B*). In the first 3 days the range is from 75/45 to 50/30, with an average of 65/41. If there is a reading above or below these levels, further evaluation of blood volume is done.

Color

The infant's color should be pink, with the exception of hands and feet.

Acrocyanosis (peripheral cyanosis) (Figure 18-2) is normal in the first 12 hours of birth. Later it may be a sign of difficulty controlling temperature or glucose. The rest of the body and mucous membranes should be pink. The examiner looks especially during feedings to see if the infant's mouth becomes bluish.

Measurements

The weight and length, as well as head and chest circumferences, should be consistent with the estimated gestational age.

The examiner needs an infant scale and paper barrier, a paper tape measure, and a growth chart. The head circumference is measured (Figure 18-3) from occiput to forehead and the chest circumference is measured (Figure 18-4) at the level of the infant's nipples. Length is measured by stretching the paper tape measure under the infant from tip of head to sole of foot. A very active infant can be positioned with the head touching the top of the crib and one leg gently extended. This distance can then be marked and measured.

Compare the infant's birth weight, length, and head circumference with the criteria in Table 18-1. These values can be plotted on a growth and development chart

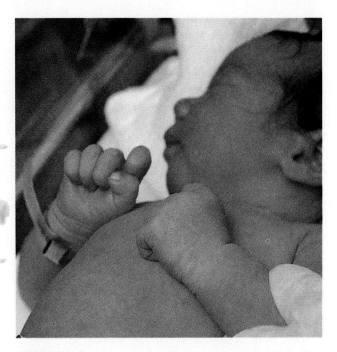

FIGURE 18-2 Acrocyanosis of hands in newborn. (From Seidel HM et al, eds: *Mosby's guide to physical examination,* ed 2, St Louis, 1991, Mosby.)

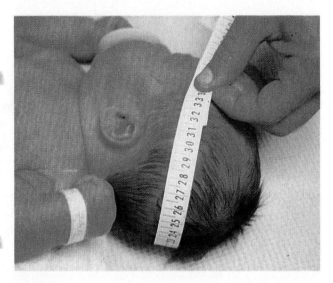

FIGURE 18-3 Appropriate placement of the measuring tape to obtain the head circumference. (From Seidel HM et al, eds: *Mosby's guide to physical examination,* ed 2, St Louis, 1991, Mosby.)

(see Figure 18-28) after gestational age assessment is completed. The range in weight is from 2500 to 4000 g. Measurements of length range from 44 to 55 cm. Head circumferences average from 33 to 35 cm, with chest circumference always 1 to 2 cm less. If the chest is larger than the head, the infant should be closely observed for **microcephaly.** A head circumference less than the 10th

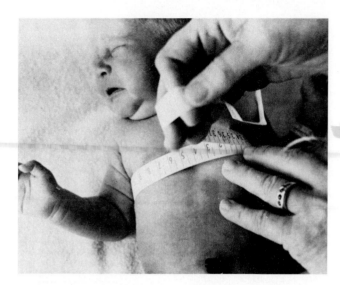

FIGURE 18-4 Measuring chest circumference. (Courtesy John Young.)

percentile indicates microcephaly associated with congenital malformations and infection. A head circumference greater than the 90th percentile indicates **macrocephaly,** caused perhaps by hydrocephaly. Some infants whose parents are constitutionally large or small may exceed or fall short of these limits, but the measurements should not fall in widely divergent percentiles. For ex-

ample, an infant whose weight and height fall within the 75th percentile should not have a head circumference in the 25th percentile. If the infant's head is greatly molded, the head and chest circumferences may be equal until the molding resolves. Remeasurement within 3 days is advised (Table 18-1).

Movement and Tone

After assessing measurements, consider the following questions.

> *Does the infant move all four extremities and return to a symmetric position of flexion?*
> *Does any motion seem limited or hypotonic in comparison with the other body parts?*

Note especially birth injuries or anesthesia effects on muscle responses. A hypotonic infant also may have acidosis, hypoglycemia, hypothermia, or congenital problems (see Chapter 27).

Behavioral State

Assess the behavioral state in terms of the following questions.

> *Is the cry appropriate?*
> *Does the infant seem interested in the environment?*
> *Is the transition from sleep to wake a smooth one?*

Because the behavioral state will influence assessment, it is important to relate the infant's period of reactivity to

TABLE 18-1 Normal Term Newborn Measurements

VALUE	NORMAL RANGE	VARIATIONS
Weight	2500-4000 g	Average is 3400 g (7½ pounds).
Length	44-55 cm	Average is 50 cm (20 inches); because molding of head can influence this value, remeasure before discharge.
Head circumference	32-37.5 cm, average 33-35 cm	Check molding of head.
Chest circumference	1-2 cm less than head circumference	Breast engorgement or molding of head can influence this ratio.
Axillary temperature	36.1°-36.5° C (97.0°-97.7° F)	Environmental temperature extremes, sepsis, and altered neurologic function can cause hypothermia or hyperthermia.
Respirations		
Rate	30-60 breaths/min	Respirations may be relatively tachypneic (rate over 60) during first hour but should not rise.
Quality	Easy, abdominal, without use of accessory muscles	Infant may have period of grunting, flaring, and retractions during first hour.
Apical pulse	110-160 beats/min	Rate of 100-120 is normal during sleep but should accelerate with stimulation; rate over 160 common with increased activity and crying.
Blood pressure (taken in arm and leg)	Systolic 50-75 mm Hg	Hypotension may mean low blood volume.
	Diastolic 30-45 mm Hg	Should be equal in upper and lower extremity.

BOX 18-2   Periods of Neonatal Reactivity

First phase (30-60 min)

Active, alert

Eyes open, gazing

Active rooting, sucking

Vital signs labile: rapid irregular heart rate and respirations, may have rales, grunting, retractions, flaring nares

Activity labile: observe for tone, symmetric movement

First sleep (2-4 hr)

Quiet sleep, no interest in feeding

Stabilized vital signs

Onset of bowel sounds

Second reactivity period (4-10 hr after birth)

Infant awake and alert

Rooting and sucking strong

Variable vital signs with mild cyanosis

Mottling, increased mucus

Passage of meconium and urine

Clinical Decision

Fill in the following data for a full-term infant you observe, and then compare with the normal ranges in Table 18-1. Is the infant deviating from normal?

Activity level (active, quiet and alert, sleeping) _____

Apical heart rate _____

Respiratory rate _____

Axillary temperature _____

Weight _____ *Length* _____

Head circumference _____

Chest circumference _____

Abdominal circumference _____

Movement of extremities _____

these questions (Box 18-2) to the findings. Although a "yes" answer to the seven questions under Vital Signs, Color, Measurements, Movement and Tone, and Behavioral State does not guarantee an uneventful recovery, it indicates that the infant is in no immediate distress. The following warning signs may indicate a need for intervention:

- Axillary temperature less than 36.1° or over 37.2° C (97° or over 99° F)
- Heart rate less than 110 or over 160 beats/min (if asleep may fall to 100 or if active may rise to 180)
- Respiratory rate less than 30 or over 60 breaths/min (may rise transiently if active)
- Cyanosis other than acrocyanosis (*hands & feet only*)
- Jaundice
- Periods of apnea lasting over 15 seconds
- Lack of movement and responsiveness
- Hypotonic or hypertonic position
- Lack of interest in the environment
- Birthweight <5 pounds or >9 pounds
- Head circumference less than the 5th percentile
- Large or small for gestational age

Cardiorespiratory System

The respiratory and cardiovascular systems are considered together because of their obviously related functions, importance to survival, and proximity during assessment.

NORMAL TRANSITION: RESPIRATION

The First Breath

There are several stimuli to breathing. During vaginal delivery, the infant's thorax is first compressed and then rapidly reexpands, or recoils. This draws in a small amount of air. The comparative cold of the extrauterine environment, the bright lights, noises, pressure on the infant's body, and sensation of weight from the addition of gravity all stimulate the newborn to take a deep gasping breath.

Mild asphyxia (hypercapnia, hypoxia, and acidosis) normally accompanies labor and delivery (see Chapter 14). Mild asphyxia is a chemical stimulant to respiratory control centers in both the adult and newborn. Animal studies show that animal fetuses that are warm and submerged will not breathe despite this chemical stimulus but will take a first breath when they are exposed to the cooler environment. There are implications here for alternative birth practices that attempt to extend the intrauterine environment after birth. Several newborn deaths related to home underwater birth have been documented. These infants were submerged for up to 1 hour, with the parents thinking that the infant "enjoyed" the water (*Birth* 18:2, 1991).

Establishment of Respiration

An adequate supply of *surfactant* is needed if normal respirations are to continue. In its absence, alveoli collapse with each exhalation, and there is no residual volume. With each breath the preterm infant must try to inflate lungs that are collapsed. The tremendously increased respiratory effort soon leads to respiratory failure. This is the basis of respiratory distress syndrome (RDS) (see Chapter 28).

Once respirations are established, the range will be between 30 and 60/min and will be irregular in rate, rhythm, and depth. The face and trunk will have a pink tone, although the extremities may still show a bluish color.

As the infant breathes, the partial pressure of oxygen (Po_2) in the blood increases, whereas the partial pressure of carbon dioxide (Pco_2) decreases. As acidosis resolves, blood pH approaches adult values. The pulmonary blood vessels, constricted in fetal life, dilate in response to the increased oxygen levels and allow a dramatic increase in blood flow to the newborn lungs. The results of normal transition occur as follows.

1. Surfactant production is maintained.
2. Residual volume is established.
3. Physiologic acid-base balance continues.
4. Blood flow to the lungs is increased.
5. Vital signs are within normal limits.
6. A pink, oxygenated color is evident.

NORMAL TRANSITION: CARDIOVASCULAR

Transitional Circulation

Fetal circulation should be reviewed before transitional circulation is studied.

Changes that occur during the transition from fetal to newborn circulation are closely linked to changes in the respiratory system. These changes are caused by the alterations in systemic and pulmonary pressures that result from the first deep breath and the establishment of respirations. Therefore, clamping the umbilical cord does not cause the reversal from fetal to adult circulation. Circulatory patterns will change from fetal to newborn even if the infant is born unattended and the cord is not clamped immediately after birth (see Unexpected Birth, Chapter 15). Figure 18-5 illustrates the following description of transitional circulation.

1. The infant's first breath raises the Po_2, which causes the pulmonary arterial blood vessels to dilate and allows blood to flow freely to the lungs. Now the pulmonary blood pressure is decreased.
2. The *umbilical arteries* constrict in response to increased Po_2 levels, and the cord is cut.
3. Circulation through the *umbilical vein* ends.
4. As the *ductus venosus* closes, the systemic blood pressure rises.
5. These changes in pressures cause blood flow through the ductus arteriosus to reverse its direction, thus changing one of the right-to-left shunts. The ductus arteriosus then constricts (also in response to increased Po_2 levels), preventing blood flow through it by the end of the first day. It will later become the ligamentum arteriosum.
6. Because of increased blood flow to the lungs, there must be increased flow from the lungs

through the pulmonary veins and to the left atrium.
7. The increased pressure of this blood against the *foramen ovale* forces it to close against the interatrial septum. This reverses the other right-to-left shunt. (The site of the old foramen ovale will later become the fossa ovalis.)
8. These allow blood to flow to the newborn lungs for gas exchange and return to the heart for distribution to the body. All fetal vessels, first functionally and then anatomically, adapt to adult circulation by atrophy (Table 18-2).

The rate of the neonatal heart will be relative to the fetal heart rate but will gradually become slower. The rate continues to be irregular in rate and rhythm, but variability also decreases. The rate responds to stimuli as did the fetal heart rate. The results of normal transition are as follows:

1. Decrease in pulmonary blood pressure *with* resultant increase in pulmonary blood flow.
2. Closure of the foramen ovale.
3. Constriction of the ductus arteriosus.
4. End of flow through umbilical vein.

Failure of this transition is a life-threatening disorder, *persistent fetal circulation (PFC)* or *persistent pulmonary hypertension of the newborn (PPHN)*, which is reviewed in Chapter 28.

Assessment

Inspection. The infant is observed at rest and during activity. The examiner looks for skin color and symmetric expansion of the chest. The infant's color should be pink centrally, but there still may be acrocyanosis. Bulging of the chest may indicate that air is trapped in the pleural space below (pneumothorax). The respiratory rate is counted by watching the lower portion of chest and the abdomen rise and fall (watching the cord can be helpful) for a full minute because the neonate's normal irregular pattern of respiration will cause the total to be inaccurate if the counting is discontinued before 60 seconds have lapsed. Although respirations range from 30 to 60 breaths/min (Table 18-1), there may be changes according to state and period of reactivity. The quality of respiration is assessed by noting retractions or nasal flaring. **Retractions** are caused by use of accessory muscles of respiration and are seen as inspiratory "pulling in" of the chest wall above and below the sternum (suprasternal and substernal retractions) and between and below the ribs (intercostal and subcostal retractions). Recognition of retractions as mild, moderate, or severe requires practice. When nasal flaring is present, the nares seem to dilate with each inspiration, indicating that the fluid that fills the lungs during fetal life has not yet been absorbed or that more serious difficulties in extrauterine adjustment may be present (see Figure 28-7).

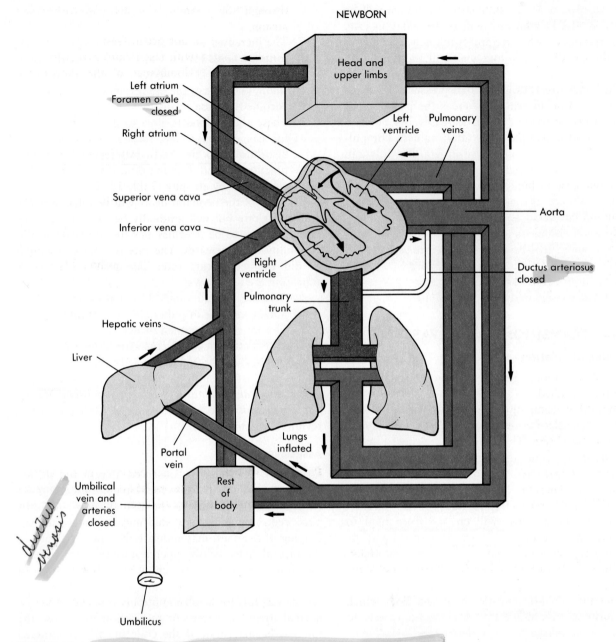

FIGURE 18-5 Transitional circulation in the newborn. (Courtesy G David Brown.)

TABLE 18-2 Anatomic Changes in the Fetal Structures after Birth

FETAL STRUCTURES	INFANT STRUCTURES	RANGE IN WHICH CHANGE IS COMPLETED
Foramen ovale	Fossa ovalis	Several weeks to 1 yr
Ductus arteriosus	Ligamentum arteriosum	Several weeks to 1 yr
Ductus venosus	Ligamentum venosum of the liver	1-2 mo
Umbilical arteries	Lateral umbilical ligaments	2-3 mo
Umbilical vein	Ligamentum teres of the liver	2-3 mo

The presence of meconium staining of the skin, nails, and cord should be noted. This staining may be associated with respiratory distress if meconium aspiration has occurred during labor. While assessing respiratory status, the examiner notes the number and spacing of the nipples and the presence of **gynecomastia,** or breast engorgement. A few infants may have extra nipple tissue, that is, supernumerary nipples. The apical impulse or point of maximal impulse (PMI) also may be seen.

Auscultation. The best place to listen to breath sounds is at the midaxillary line, but all lobes should be examined. An equal amount of air entry on each side of the chest should be heard. Scattered *rales* (sounds of moisture within the lungs) are considered normal during the first few hours of life, especially in the infant delivered by surgical intervention. There should be no stridor or noise during inspiration. *Grunting* is an abnormal expiratory sound heard as the infant forcibly exhales against a closed glottis to keep the alveoli from collapsing. It may be possible to hear this grunting without a stethoscope. It is a warning of respiratory distress.

The examiner concentrates on the heart sounds, auscultating the entire cardiac region. One pattern is to begin at the apex, found on the infant at the *point of maximal impulse* where the pulse is best felt. The PMI is found just to the left of the midclavicular line at the fourth intercostal space. This point is higher than in the adult because the neonatal heart lies in a more horizontal position. The examiner works from the apex, up the left sternal border, toward the base of the heart and then listens along the right sternal border, turning the infant over and listening between the scapulae.

The normal neonatal heart rate ranges from 110 to 160 beats/min, but a rate of 100 may be observed when the infant is at rest, and a rate of 170 to 180 may occur during periods of activity. If a rate of less than 110 is heard, stimulating the infant to cry should make the rate rise. Although neonatal heart rates have variability similar to fetal heart rates, obvious irregularities in the cardiac rhythm should not occur. Gestational age also influences heart rates (with faster rates earlier in gestation) because of the dominance of the sympathetic nervous system.

The next focus is the quality of heart sounds and the presence of extra sounds. S_1 and S_2 are the first and second heart sounds. S_1 is heard when the atrioventricular valves (mitral and tricuspid) close, and S_2 occurs when the semilunar valves (aortic and pulmonary) close. The "lub-dub" sounds are S_1 and S_2, respectively. The time between S_1 and S_2 is *systole*, and the time between S_2 and S_1 is *diastole*.

In evaluating heart sounds, a separate and distinct S_1 and S_2 should be heard, usually with no extra sounds during systole or diastole. The sounds should be easy to hear (i.e., it should not seem as though the heart is far from the stethoscope). However, "closeness" of heart sounds to the chest wall is a parameter that can be assessed accurately only with experience. A good order to use when auscultating the heart is as follows.

1. Count the rate, noting its regularity and variability with the infant's activity.
2. Locate the place where the sounds are best heard in the chest.
3. Differentiate between S_1 and S_2.
4. Decide if there are extra sounds.

Palpation. Brachial pulses are palpated at the antecubital space and the femoral pulses bilaterally along the inguinal ligament halfway between the iliac crest and the symphysis pubis (Figure 18-6, *A*). Their relative rates and volumes should be equal.

Percussion. Percussion of the neonatal chest generally is not undertaken because any questions concerning the size and condition of organs are investigated by radiographic or ultrasonic examination.

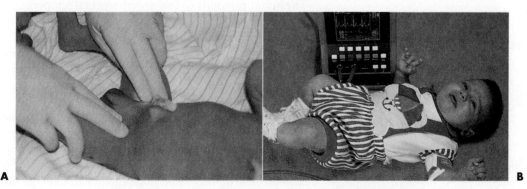

A   **B**

FIGURE 18-6 **A,** Palpating femoral pulses. **B,** Baby blood pressure is taken on each extremity. (Here an older baby is used for illustration.) (**A** courtesy Marjorie Pyle, RNC, *Lifecircle.* **B** courtesy Dinamap Plus Blood Pressure Monitor and Disposa-Cuff Blood Pressure Cuff.)

Cardiorespiratory warning signs require intervention:

- Sustained heart rate <110 or >180 beats/min
- Respiratory rate <30 or >60 breaths/min
- Central cyanosis
- Apnea for more than 15 seconds
- Muffled heart sounds or heard shifted to right
- Cardiac murmur
- Unequal breath sounds

Test Yourself

- Recall the changes in fetal circulation shunts after birth.
- Why should you count respirations for one full minute?
- Describe two variations in breath sounds.

Metabolic Control
HEAT TRANSFER

The newborn enters an environment at least 20° to 25° F cooler than core body temperature. Unless the infant is protected against heat loss, deep body temperature can drop 0.5° to 2° C (0.9° to 3.6° F) within 5 to 10 minutes of birth. Thermal receptors are present on the body surface, with many on the face. When they are triggered, the response is peripheral vasoconstriction. The head, 20% of the body surface, is wet at birth and difficult to dry completely. Because most of the heat loss is through evaporation and radiation, drying is a priority. Use of radiant overhead warmers has significantly reduced initial heat loss. Incubators also are useful to control heat loss from convection.

The **temperature gradient** is the difference between the skin and the environment (external gradient) or between the core of the body and the skin (internal

Clinical Decision

Of the following findings after your assessment of a 3200 g full-term newborn boy, which should be reported?
- *Heart rate of 140 beats/min during sleep, which rises to 160 when the infant cries*
- *Pink with blue hands and feet when crying*
- *Brachial pulses that feel much fuller in volume than femoral pulses, which are barely palpable*

gradient). Temperature control in the newborn is influenced primarily by this temperature gradient.

When ambient temperature falls in the adult, increased metabolism raises internal or core temperature by means of involuntary high intensity, rhythmic shivering, and voluntary muscle activity. This muscle activity is *physical thermogenesis*. However, the newborn infant can use only chemical thermogenesis. Chapter 7 describes a special form of fat, brown adipose tissue (BAT), that is deposited during fetal life. Newborns produce body heat by increasing their metabolic rate and by metabolizing this tissue. They do not shiver. A decrease in ambient temperature stimulates production of norepinephrine, which increases brown fat metabolism. This response is impaired when an infant has hypoxia or if lipid stores are already depleted. Certain drugs also can block this response. During BAT metabolism, oxygen is consumed and fatty acids and glycerol are produced. Newborns are vulnerable despite these mechanisms because (1) there is a large skin surface to body weight ratio, which promotes a more rapid loss of heat from the core to the skin surface, and (2) the presence of substantial layers of white fat as additional insulation depends on gestational age and birth weight.

Extremes of environmental temperature, therefore, will stress the infant. This may lead to *overheating*, which will cause an elevated body temperature, vasodilation with flushed skin, and tachypnea as the infant tries to dissipate the extra heat. For this reason an infant should never be left unattended under a radiant warmer without a continuous *servomechanism* for temperature feedback. These devices monitor the skin temperature and change the heat output as needed to maintain the set temperature.

More commonly the environmental temperature will be too low and initiate the adverse effects termed cold stress.

Cold Stress

The infant responds to low environmental temperatures with peripheral vasoconstriction, which leads to increased anaerobic metabolism and acidosis. Initially, peripheral vasoconstriction will make the skin temperature drop while the core temperature is maintained. Later, core temperature will fall. Neonatal cold stress is discussed in Chapter 28.

One goal of nursing care is maintenance of a *thermal neutral environment* in which heat production (measured as oxygen consumption) is minimal, yet core temperature is within the normal range. Infants cared for in such an environment need not expend extra energy nor consume extra oxygen to maintain normal internal temperature. Although this may not make a tremendous difference to the healthy, full-term infant, the added stress can be disastrous for the sick infant.

GLUCOSE AND CALCIUM

Maintenance of adequate blood glucose levels is vital because of the brain's dependence on glucose for energy; lack of glucose may cause tremors, seizures, and permanent neurologic damage. Maintenance of serum calcium levels also is necessary for normal neuromuscular function; low calcium levels may cause tremors, tetany, and seizures. Abnormally increased calcium levels are rare in the neonate.

Glucose is needed for the increased energy demands that occur after delivery. The newborn infant must breathe and maintain body temperature. The infant's movements also are more vigorous than those in utero. At birth, glucose levels are maintained by glycolysis of hepatic glycogen and gluconeogenesis. These prenatal stores will be the primary source of energy until feedings are well established.

Large amounts of glucose infused during labor may result in fetal hyperinsulinemia with a postnatal rebound hypoglycemia. For this reason glucose is usually not infused during labor (Hazle, 1986). There also may be transient neonatal tachypnea, hyponatremia, and elevated bilirubin levels when fluid intake during labor has not been carefully regulated (Keppler, 1988).

Several factors influence neonatal calcium metabolism and increase the risk for hypocalcemia. At delivery, maternal calcium supplies end. Levels of hormones that control calcium metabolism are low at birth. In addition, the fetus that is stressed in utero also is at high risk for hypocalcemia. (For treatment, see Chapter 28.)

Results of a normal transition show serum glucose levels in the normal range of 50 to 100 mg/dl and calcium in the normal range of 7 to 8 mg/dl. A difficult transition may manifest in several ways. Tremors are most commonly seen, but *lethargy, tachypnea, pallor,* and *cyanosis* also are common signs of hypoglycemia or hypocalcemia. It is important to anticipate metabolic imbalances in infants who are especially at risk: those who are small or large for gestational age, infants of diabetic mothers (IDM), and premature and postmature infants.

Warning signs of poor metabolic control are as follows:

1. LGA, SGA, IDM, preterm, or postterm infants
2. Temperature less than or above normal range
3. Tremors, tachypnea, pallor, cyanosis
4. Glucose <50 mg/dl
5. Calcium <7 mg/dl

Integumentary System

The integumentary system is the next system to be evaluated as the nurse continues to undress the infant. The information obtained from assessing this system often is related to the integrity of other systems (e.g., skin color provides information as to the health of the cardiovascular and hematologic systems).

NORMAL TRANSITION

At birth the skin and its structures are exposed to the dry, colder extrauterine environment. Any vernix that remains is absorbed. Therefore skin commonly becomes dry and may crack at the ankles and wrists. The term infant's skin normally will peel within 2 days of birth; peeling before that time is not normal. **Desquamation** (peeling) over the entire body is a classic sign seen in the postmature infant.

If the infant is chilled, *cutis marmorata,* which is a mottled or marbled appearance over the body, may be observed. It is caused by dilation of the small blood vessels, not an expected reaction to chilling (Figure 18-7, *A*). It usually is seen only during early infancy but may persist longer in infants with certain congenital problems. The *harlequin sign* is a phenomenon seen only in the newborn infant, more often in those of low birth weight. The infant who is lying on one side will become bright red over the dependent half of the body and very pale over the half that is superior. There is a definite line of demarcation between the two colors, which will reverse sides if the infant's position is reversed. This sign is benign and lasts a short while.

Pigmentation is genetically determined and influenced by the extrauterine environment. After birth, when the infant is exposed to light, the skin of black infants will continue to darken. About 90% of all infants of black, Asian, or Latin origin will have **mongolian spots,** which result from the deep dermal infiltration of melanocytes. These flat, irregularly shaped, pigmented lesions are seen most commonly over the lumbosacral region. They vary in size (some may be quite large) and color from gray-blue to blue-black. With age these lesions appear to fade but actually become less obvious as the overlying skin loses its transparency. After age 4, these mongolian spots may seem to have disappeared (Figure 18-7, *B*).

The most common skin variation seen during the transition period is **erythema toxicum** (Figure 18-7, *C* and *D*). The cause of this is not known, but its appearance has alarmed the mothers of many full-term infants. These pale yellow to white pustules and papules with reddened bases usually erupt first on the trunk but then may spread to the entire body, with the exception of soles and palms. The lesions disappear spontaneously within hours to days after their appearance.

Many full-term infants are born with **milia,** or epidermal inclusion cysts (Figure 18-7, *E*). These small white or yellow papules are commonly found on the nose, chin, and forehead. When they appear on the palate or gums, they are called *Epstein's pearls.* Both types disappear early in infancy. Sweat may be retained in small, noninflammatory vesicles called **miliaria.** These also are seen over the forehead, as well as the neck and diaper area. Because this condition usually

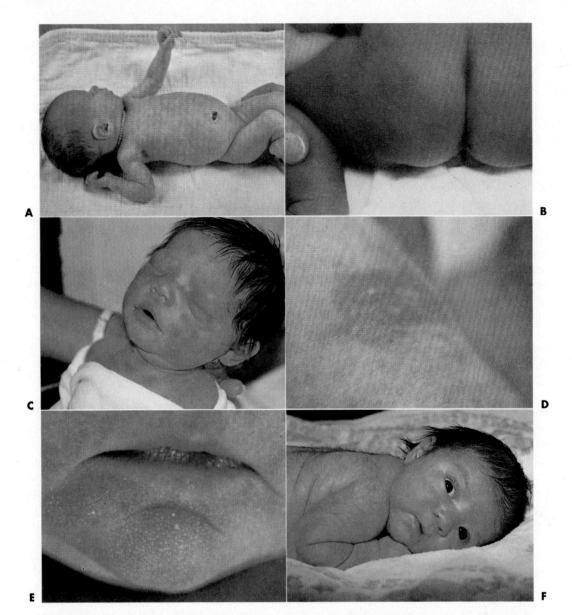

FIGURE 18-7 Skin characteristics of the newborn. **A,** Skin mottling. **B,** Mongolian spots. **C,** Early observations of skin show newborn rash and swollen eyelids. **D,** Erythema toxicum. **E,** Milia. **F,** Hair distribution. (**A, D,** and **E** courtesy Mead Johnson; **B** from Seidel HM et al, editors: Mosby's guide to physical examination, ed 2, St Louis, 1991, Mosby; **C** and **F** courtesy Marjorie Pyle, RNC, *Lifecircle.*)

occurs in infants who live in a hot, humid environment, cooling and drying the infant will cause the vesicles to resolve.

ASSESSMENT

Inspection of the integumentary system takes place during the examination of other systems. It is presented here to provide guidance for the balance of the examination.

The skin color is observed in natural light. If this is not possible, the examiner should recognize that fluo- rescent light tends to alter true color. Skin thickens as gestational age increases; therefore the less mature in- fant's skin is more transparent.

The pigmentation, which ranges from pale to dark brown, is assessed. Mucous membranes should have underlying pink tones, and no cyanotic changes should be seen with crying or activity. Acrocyanosis and mottling occur early but may be abnormal if they persist. The examiner notes whether the infant is pink or has **pallor** (pale pink or white underlying tone) or **plethora** (ruddy, purplish color). The skin of the forehead or abdomen is blanched by applying finger pressure momentarily and observing the return of color (capillary filling), which should be prompt. This is an indication of perfusion. The presence of jaundice also is noted.

It is important to examine the entire skin surface, including the neck and inguinal and axillary folds. At term, vernix caseosa is found only in these deep skin folds. Skin *turgor,* an indication of adequate intrauterine growth, is examined by gently pinching a fold of skin on the abdomen or thigh. Any edema or extra folds of skin also are noted.

The quality and distribution of *hair* are important parts of both gestational age assessment and evaluation of the infant at risk for genetic disease. Unusual patterns and distributions of hair growth are associated with some genetic syndromes (e.g., Cornelia de Lange syndrome). In addition, certain racial groups have heavier hair distribution at birth (Figure 18-7, *F*). Lanugo is fine, downy hair that covers the back, shoulders, and forehead of a preterm infant and is present on the shoulders at term. Nail growth increases with gestation; nails will have grown to the end of the fingers at term and past the fingertips after term. The skin thickens and begins to peel (*desquamation*) if the infant is postmature.

The examiner looks for birth marks, skin injuries, and meconium staining and gently *palpates* masses for consistency, tenderness, and return of color noting whether a reddened lesion blanches with pressure, which indicates a vascular connection. Tiny red spots that do not blanch with pressure may be **petechiae** or microhemorrhages within the skin, possibly caused by pressure during birth. Another cause, thrombocytopenia, can be life threatening but is also a sign of congenital infection. Oval reddened areas (forceps marks) may be observed on the cheeks of infants whose delivery has been assisted with forceps. Most of these marks gradually disappear.

Some integumentary structures are subject to prenatal stimulation by maternal hormones. One manifestation is secretion of a colostrum-like fluid ("witch's milk") by the breasts during the neonatal period, which is seen in both male and female infants.

Other structures also may appear to mature early. Occasionally a tooth may erupt during fetal life and be seen at birth (natal teeth). It is almost always a prematurely erupted deciduous tooth rather than an extra, or supernumerary, one. An attempt is made to save the tooth, if possible. Before the infant is discharged, however, a loose tooth is removed to prevent possible aspiration.

Nevi are genetic changes in the skin. There are many types of nevi; some spontaneously disappear and others do not. Within each of these groups are two other subdivisions: *telangiectatic,* or flat, and *hemangioma-*

tous, or raised. Salmon patch or strawberry hemangiomas are flat, pale pink, irregularly shaped lesions called "stork's bites" when found at the nape of the neck (Figure 18-8). About 50% of all white newborns have a simple hemangioma either on the sacrum, the back of the neck, the face, or eyelids. These are small at birth, then grow, and eventually disappear. Although they fade with age, parents may express concern when they are first noticed. Nevus flammeus, or port-wine stain, is seriously disfiguring and most often found on the face; unfortunately, this does not disappear. Giant hemangiomas are larger and raised; these can be dangerous if they trap platelets and thereby lower the amount of circulating platelets (Figure 18-9).

Most skin lesions are harmless, although they usually are a source of concern to parents who naturally hope for the perfect infant. Parents need to know which of

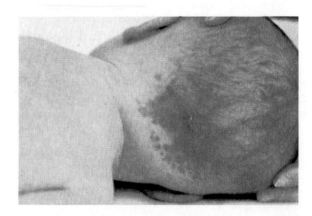

FIGURE 18-8 Nevus at nape of neck, "stork's beak" mark. (Courtesy Mead Johnson.)

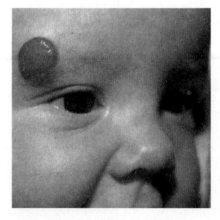

FIGURE 18-9 Giant hemangioma in infant. (From Seidel HM et al, eds: *Mosby's guide to physical examination*, ed 2, St Louis, 1991, Mosby.)

these will disappear spontaneously and which need treatment. Common skin lesions described in the following list are *warning signs of integumentary system problems* (Box 18-3):

- Long nails and desquamation indicating postmaturity

- Thin, translucent skin with abundant vernix and lanugo, indicating prematurity
- Pallor, possibly caused by hypothermia, anemia, sepsis, or shock
- Cyanosis, possibly caused by cardiorespiratory disease, hypoglycemia, polycythemia, sepsis, or hypothermia
- Petechiae, possibly caused by thrombocytopenia, sepsis, congenital infection, or pressure sustained during delivery
- Plethora, possibly caused by polycythemia
- Meconium staining, possibly caused by intrauterine asphyxia
- Abnormal hair distribution (unrelated to gestational age) or extra skin folds, possibly associated with genetic syndromes
- Poor skin turgor associated with intrauterine growth retardation and hypoglycemia
- Large (cavernous) hemangiomas, which may trap platelets within their borders and cause thrombocytopenia
- Bullae or pustules, possibly caused by staphylococcal infection

---

Test Yourself

- Describe how the neonate responds to a drop in ambient temperature.
- List the signs of cold stress.

Gastrointestinal System
NORMAL TRANSITION

For the first 15 minutes to ½ hour after birth (first period of reactivity), the healthy, full-term infant will be alert and eager to suck—this is the ideal time to initiate breast-feeding. Newborn gastric capacity at term is about 10 to 20 ml. Although the stomach will not empty completely during the first few hours of life, this is not a concern because the breast-feeding infant will consume only a small amount of colostrum.

The suck-swallow mechanism that has been functioning prenatally further matures after birth to prevent aspiration. The result of this maturation is the rapid opening of the epiglottis during swallowing and closing during respiration. The *cardiac sphincter* between the esophagus and stomach in the newborn infant frequently is less than fully functional; therefore reflux of gastric contents into the esophagus and upward into the pharynx may occur (**regurgitation**), which increases the possibility of aspiration. This especially may occur during the second period of reactivity from about the second to sixth hour after

---

BOX 18-3 Common Neonatal Skin Lesions

Nevi
Hemangiomas (developmental vascular abnormalities)
Flat (telangiectatic) hemangiomas: Salmon-pink color and easy to blanch; found at nape of neck, eyelids, and forehead; fade within 1 year
Nevus flammeus (port-wine stain): Red to black in color; if found on face along trigeminal nerve tract, may be associated with cerebral vascular malformation
Raised and giant (cavernous) hemangiomas: Bright red to reddish blue in color; tend to increase in size after birth; cavernous type may trap platelets, causing thrombocytopenia

Pigmented lesions
Mongolian spots: Gray to blue; found on lumbosacral area in black, Asian, and Native American infants; fade in first few years of life
Café-au-lait spots: Small, brown patches; if more than six are present or any are larger than 4 × 6 cm infant may have neurofibromatosis; with aging these may undergo precancerous changes

Erythema toxicum
Maculopapular rash that may include small pustulelike lesions containing sterile fluid and eosinophils (white cells indicative of an allergic response rather than infection); found on the trunk and face; fades within a few days

Milia neonatorum
Epidermal cysts containing keratogenous material; look like whiteheads found over the nose and chin; fades within a few days

Miliaria
Retention of sweat in unopened exocrine glands causing clear vesicles on the face, scalp, and perineum; resolve in a few days if environmental heat and humidity are not extreme

Bullae
Blister over 1 cm in diameter

Pustules
Small lesion containing pus; may be signs of staphylococcal infection; needs to be differentiated from erythema toxicum

---

delivery when the infant demonstrates variability in several areas of adjustment to extrauterine life. It is also during this time that the infant may become "mucousy," or have difficulty with mucus secretions. The infant may gag or choke, and it may be necessary to clear the airway by changing the position or by suctioning any secretions.

Bowel sounds can be heard as the first period of reactivity ends. Meconium usually is passed during the second period of reactivity, although it may occur in utero or at delivery.

There are several congenital defects that affect the gastrointestinal system. Early general assessment may detect if there is an *imperforate anus*. With feeding, lack of an intact esophagus would immediately cause an infant to choke. (See Chapter 27 for full discussion of the *tracheoesophageal fistula*.)

ASSESSMENT

Inspection

The abdominal wall should be free of defects. The cord is observed for color and amount of Wharton's jelly. Umbilical cord changes should be consistent with the age in days; it will blacken and become dry within 2 to 3 days. An umbilical hernia may be present. This mass protrudes more when the infant cries and is seen more commonly in black infants. The abdominal girth is measured just above the umbilicus. The rectum should be patent, and meconium should be passed within 24 hours. Some meconium-filled loops of bowel may bulge through the abdominal wall until this occurs.

Auscultation

The examiner always auscultates for bowel sounds before palpating the abdomen because bowel motility can be affected by palpation. Bowel sounds should be present several hours after birth (see Box 18-2).

Palpation

Palpation of the newborn abdomen requires gentle firmness. It should be done at least 2 hours after a feeding. The entire abdomen is palpated in a systematic manner, noting masses. The liver should be evaluated for size by palpation from the right iliac crest up to the right costal margin until the lower liver edge is felt to slip against the fingers (Figure 18-10) to 1 to 3 cm below the right costal margin. The spleen tip may be felt at the left costal margin.

There should be no masses, but the examiner may feel some loops of bowel. There may be *diastasis* or separation of the rectus muscles, which feels like softness in the midline between the two bands of rectus muscles.

Observation of any of the following *warning signs for the GI system* requires intervention:

- Obvious defects in the abdominal wall, possibly gastroschisis or omphalocele
- Single umbilical artery associated with congenital, especially renal, anomalies

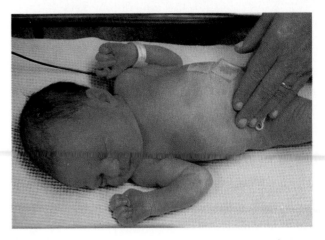

FIGURE 18-10 Positioning to examine infant's abdomen to palpate liver. (From Seidel HM et al, eds: *Mosby's guide to physical examination*, ed 2, St Louis, 1991, Mosby.)

- Meconium stained or shriveled umbilical cord associated with intrauterine growth retardation or perinatal asphyxia
- Imperforate anus, which may be associated with a tracheoesophageal fistula or esophageal atresia
- Hepatosplenomegaly (enlarged liver and spleen) associated with congenital infections and hemolysis
- Flat or scaphoid abdomen, which may be associated with a diaphragmatic hernia (congenital defect in which abdominal contents are in the thorax)
- Failure to pass meconium stool within 24 hours
- History of polyhydramnios during pregnancy
- Masses anywhere in abdomen

Genitourinary System
NORMAL TRANSITION

Renal

The removal of the placenta at birth ends the neonate's dependence on the maternal kidneys for renal function. The quality of renal function in the term infant generally is adequate for the infant's needs. However, the ability of the newborn kidney to adapt to stress is limited. This deficiency improves during the first week of life and continues to mature to adult levels as infancy continues. During the neonatal period, urine composition changes from dilute (specific gravity 1.004 to 1.010) to more concentrated as renal function matures. By 2 months of age the infant's urine has a strong odor and the specific gravity of adult urine.

Adrenal

The normal fetus responds to the stress of labor and delivery with secretion of catecholamines, which cause fetal heart rate accelerations and help to mobilize hepatic glycogen for energy in the immediate neonatal period.

ASSESSMENT

Kidneys and Bladder

The quantity of amniotic fluid is the first clue that the kidneys are functioning. After birth the infant should void within the first 24 hours. The first voiding is easy to miss because newborn urine is quite dilute and may not be noticed in the excitement immediately after birth. Newborns then void frequently, wetting six to eight diapers a day. If measured, the normal infant's output of urine is 1 to 3 ml/kg of body weight per hour. The kidneys are palpated bimanually (using both hands). The examiner, supporting the infant's lumbar region from below, palpates the flank deeply to the spine just under the costal margin.

Female Genitalia

The examiner assesses the configuration of the labia and hymen and notes the placement of the urinary meatus and rectum and the length of the perineum, as well as the size of the clitoris and labia, which vary with gestational age.

In the full-term female, the labia almost completely cover the clitoris (Figure 18-11). There should be no fusion of the labia; hymenal tags (small tags of mucous membrane extending from the vagina) are not significant. A white mucous discharge, sometimes streaked with light pink blood (**pseudomenstruation**), often is present and is the result of withdrawal of maternal hormones for a few days after birth. The labia may be edematous and darker than usual in response to birth pressure and maternal hormones.

Fused labia, clitoral hypertrophy, and placement of the urinary meatus anterior to the clitoris are signs of sexual ambiguity (see Chapter 27). With prematurity, there are widely spaced labia majora and a large clitoris. Bulging of the hymen may be caused by the pressure of fluid behind an imperforate hymen.

Male Genitalia

The examiner inspects the penis for correct placement of the urinary meatus (Figure 18-12), which should always be at the tip of the penis. The scrotum is observed for color, size, and rugae (deep wrinkles), which vary with gestational age. The scrotum is larger and covered with rugae close to term. The color is dark because of the passive transfer of maternal hormones. After a breech delivery the infant may have bruising and edema of the genitalia, which resolves after several days, but gross abnormalities should not occur. (See Figure 18-27 for gestational age assessment.)

The examiner palpates the testes by blocking the inguinal canal with one finger while gently palpating the scrotum with a thumb and forefinger. The fullness of the scrotal sac is noted. By 36 weeks each testis should have descended into the scrotum and is palpated separately. Each should be smooth, about 1 cm in diameter, and freely movable. The testes may retract into the inguinal canal if the infant is cold.

Male infants frequently have erections, which also may surprise new parents. Infants have been observed engaged in pelvic rocking. The possibility of infantile sexual reactions is disturbing to some. Cutaneous sensation, however, is the first sensory capability to develop and remains a major source of sensory input during the neonatal period.

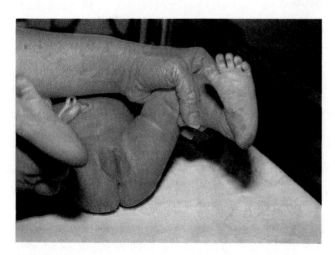

FIGURE 18-11 Female genitalia. (Courtesy Marjorie Pyle, RNC, *Lifecircle.*)

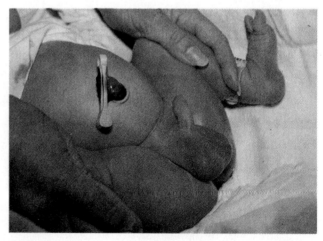

FIGURE 18-12 Male genitalia. (Courtesy Marjorie Pyle, RNC, *Lifecircle.*)

The following conditions are *warning signs of genitourinary system problems:*

Female and male
- Oligohydramnios
- Mass palpated in abdomen
- Defects of the abdominal wall
- Failure to void within 24 hours

Female genitalia
- Clitoral hypertrophy
- Fused labia
- Abnormal placement of the urinary meatus

Male genitalia
- Hypospadias (urinary meatus opening on ventral surface of penis)
- Epispadias (urinary meatus opening on dorsal surface of penis)
- Micropenis
- Bifid or split scrotum (not fused in midline)
- Scrotal masses
- Hydrocele (fluid within scrotal sac)

Test Yourself

- Why should you press on the groin to block the inguinal canal when palpating the scrotum?
- What is the significance of the whitish pink vaginal discharge in a newborn girl?

Hematologic System
NORMAL TRANSITION

At birth the hematologic system is infused with oxygen. The relatively low oxygen tension of umbilical venous blood is replaced with the higher oxygen tension now supplied by the lungs via the pulmonary artery. Adjustment from a fetal to adult state of function occurs gradually. Observations focus on the ability of this system to carry oxygen, rid itself of its fetal hemoglobin load, and maintain normal coagulation.

Hemoglobin vs Hematocrit

The normal term infant has a blood volume of about 80 ml/kg of body weight. Hematocrit values will range from 45% to 65% if drawn from a vein or artery; because of the normally sluggish peripheral circulation, it will be higher if a capillary sample is examined. Hemoglobin levels are about one third of total hematocrit; that is, an infant whose hematocrit value is 60% will have a hemoglobin level around 20 g/dl. Within the first few days, the red cell mass decreases from a prenatal 5 to 6 million/mm^3 to a more adult level of 4 to 5 million/mm^3. This extra red cell destruction contributes to the bilirubin load to be metabolized (Figure 18-13).

Blood volume is affected by birth technique. If the neonate is held above the level of the placenta before the cord is clamped, enough blood can flow back into the placenta from the infant to produce anemia. If the baby is held below the level of the placenta, or if the cord is squeezed along its length toward the infant ("milked"), there will be enough extra blood transfused to cause *polycythemia*. Because each condition is dangerous, it is recommended that the infant be held level with the placenta until cord clamping is accomplished.

The function of hemoglobin is the same in fetal and adult life. Adequate growth and metabolism cannot proceed without a constant supply of oxygen. The infant's ability to provide this depends on the concentration of oxygen in the air, the level of pulmonary maturity, adequate cardiac output, adequate volumes of blood and hemoglobin, and ability of the blood to carry and deliver oxygen to the tissues. The concentration of oxygen in the blood (Po_2) and the ability of the blood to carry oxygen (determined chiefly by the amount and type of hemoglobin) contribute to oxygen saturation. Normally between 96% and 98% of hemoglobin is

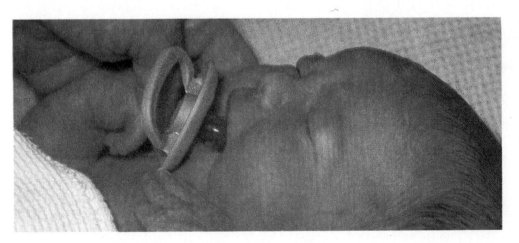

FIGURE 18-13 Ruddy color of newborn. (From Seidel HM et al, eds: *Mosby's guide to physical examination,* ed 2, St Louis, 1991, Mosby.)

saturated with oxygen. During fetal life, oxygen is supplied via umbilical venous blood flow in a concentration far lower (Po_2 is 30 mm Hg) than that which is normal during extrauterine life. Thus fetal oxygen saturation must still be kept in the normal range, although less oxygen is available. The following adaptations have evolved in the human fetus to allow for this.

1. Total hemoglobin concentration is increased (15 to 20 g/dl vs 11 to 13 g/dl in the adult).
2. Red cell mass is increased in the fetus to 5 to 6 million/mm³.
3. Fetal hemoglobin has a high hemoglobin-oxygen affinity (hemoglobin-oxygen binding).

The increased affinity of fetal hemoglobin for oxygen makes it harder to detect hypoxia by observing cyanosis in the neonate, because a greater amount of hemoglobin is associated with oxygen at any Po_2. This concept is illustrated by the hemoglobin-oxygen dissociation curve (Figure 18-14).

Bilirubin

Bilirubin is produced when the heme portion of the hemoglobin molecule is catabolized. The destruction of 1 g of hemoglobin yields 35 mg of bilirubin. Bilirubin is produced in the reticuloendothelial system and is bound to albumin, a plasma protein, for transport to the liver. In the liver, two acceptor proteins remove the bilirubin from the circulation. The bilirubin at this point is *indirect*, also called unconjugated or fat soluble. When bilirubin is not conjugated, it is available for diffusion across cell membranes. Conjugation, the most important step in bilirubin metabolism, occurs in the liver. Conjugation is a process by which fat-soluble, indirect bilirubin is converted to a water-soluble substance called conjugated, or *direct*, bilirubin. Bilirubin must be metabolized in this way to be excreted (see Chapter 28). If the metabolic process is delayed, high levels of bilirubin (or **hyperbilirubinemia**) will produce jaundice or yellow discoloration of the skin and sclerae. More important, high levels of indirect bilirubin are toxic to the brain and will produce kernicterus.

Jaundice

At birth most infants, even those severely affected with intrauterine hemolytic disease, will not have jaundice. The situation quickly changes, however, when the maternal system is no longer available for metabolism of bilirubin. Jaundice is not apparent until the serum bilirubin level rises above 5 mg/dl of blood and should not develop until the infant is more than 24 hours old. The timing of its appearance is influenced by the factors that produced it. The large hemoglobin load is one factor contributing to the frequency of physiologic jaundice because unconjugated bilirubin produced prenatally is easily carried across the lipid-rich cell membrane of the placental endothelium and transported to the maternal liver for metabolism and secretion into bile. It is then excreted via the mother's small and large intestine.

Coagulation

The newborn infant's bowel is sterile at birth and thus does not support the normal production of vitamin K until adequate food and bacteria are in the intestine. Because vitamin K will not be produced before adequate food intake has occurred, parenteral administra-

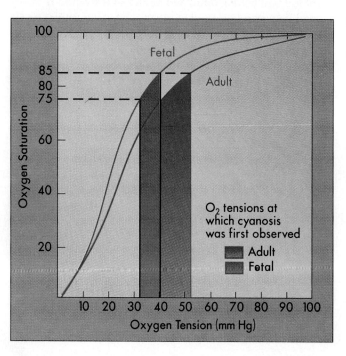

FIGURE 18-14 Hemoglobin-oxygen dissociation curve. (From Klaus M, Fanaroff AA: *Care of the high-risk neonate,* ed 3, Philadelphia, 1986, WB Saunders.)

tion of vitamin K soon after delivery is an established way of correcting this lag in production. Most term neonates are deficient in factors II, VII, IX, and X. These deficiencies are even more prevalent in the premature infant. It may take weeks to several months for the neonate to develop adult levels of clotting factors. The normal newborn, however, has adequate platelets for hemostasis.

ASSESSMENT

The examiner integrates assessment of the hematologic system with that of the skin, eyes, gastrointestinal, and cardiorespiratory systems. In natural light the infant's skin tone is observed for pallor, plethora (ruddy color caused by a high hematocrit level), and jaundice. Firmly pressing the skin over the forehead, sternum, or calf, the examiner looks quickly for the first color in the pressed spot. If it is yellow, it indicates jaundice. In infants with brown skin it may be necessary to look at the mucous membranes and sclera of the eye. Jaundice proceeds from head to foot in a cephalocaudal direction as bilirubin levels rise, although the sclera become yellow last. Thus this examination provides some idea of the severity of the hyperbilirubinemia, but a serum level always should be established for confirmation. (Box 18-4 shows normal levels by newborn age.) Palpation of the liver and spleen aids the assessment because enlargement of these organs often accompanies newborn hemolytic disease. The examiner also checks the maternal and neonatal blood types and indirect and direct Coombs' test results (see Chapter 9). (A full discussion of treatment is found in Chapter 28.)

Small red spots that *do not blanch* with pressure are *petechiae* (microhemorrhages within the skin). Large bruises (areas of ecchymosis) called *purpura* also may be present on the face of an infant whose cord was around the neck or on areas of pressure during the birth process (vertex or breech). These bruises may indicate thrombocytopenia, which must be investigated.

Warning signs of hematologic system problems are as follows:
- Pallor
- Plethora, hypoglycemia (associated with polycythemia)
- Jaundice
- Hepatosplenomegaly
- Petechiae or purpura not over pressure area
- Thrombocytopenia

Immunologic System
NORMAL TRANSITION

Although developed prenatally, the immune system begins to function sluggishly at birth. The normal full-term newborn will experience exposure and colonization with an endless number of organisms. Infection should not develop. Whether infection occurs is a function of the infant's own immunity, the presence of IgA and other immune factors found in breast milk, and the hand-washing diligence of the neonatal staff. Sepsis has been called the "great pretender" because its signs and symptoms are so varied in the neonate. Chapter 28 presents techniques for careful observation of signs of sepsis so that treatment may be started promptly. (See Chapter 7 for the immunoglobulins that may protect the infant.)

ASSESSMENT

The examiner observes the infant for pallor, cyanosis, jaundice, lethargy or irritability, and poor or shrill cry, with special attention to an infant with the following risk factors:
1. Low birth weight
2. Prematurity regardless of birth weight
3. Birth more than 24 hours after rupture of membranes
4. Mother a known hepatitis B carrier, drug user, or lacking in prenatal care

A complete blood cell count, culture of blood, cerebrospinal fluid, and urine may be ordered for infants at risk for sepsis.

The following *warning signs pertain to immunologic system problems:*
- "Doesn't look right"
- Foul-smelling amniotic fluid
- Maternal fever during labor
- Pallor/cyanosis/lethargy/petechiae
- Respiratory distress
- Hypoglycemia
- Hypothermia

BOX 18-4   Neonatal Laboratory Values

Hemoglobin: 13.5-21 g/dl
Hematocrit: 45%-65% (central)
Red blood cells: 4-6 million/mm^3
White blood cells: 10,000-30,000/mm^3
Platelets: >100,000/mm^3
Total serum bilirubin:
First 24 hr: <5 mg/dl
Second 24 hr: <10 mg/dl
Third 24 hr: <12 mg/dl
   Decreases thereafter
   No jaundice after the first week

Clinical Decision

You observe that a 36-hour-old baby delivered by cesarean birth 26 hours after rupture of membranes is not feeding well. There is no change in temperature or stooling pattern from normal. What is the possible significance of this finding? What else should you check to add to assessment data?

Head and Neck

Examination of the head, ears, eyes, nose, and throat, as well as special senses, will precede neurologic assessment because the condition of these structures often is a sign of the integrity of the neurologic system. Many anomalies of the head and neck are associated with neurologic dysfunction.

ASSESSMENT

Head

The head is inspected from all sides for size, shape, and evidence of trauma. **Molding** may be present with vaginal or cesarean delivery. If the fetus has been in the breech position, the vertex may be flattened and the occiput prominent.

The condition of the scalp and cranial bones is considered. If internal fetal heart rate monitoring or fetal blood sampling was performed during labor, lacerations of the scalp may be present. Occasionally an infant delivered by cesarean birth sustains a scalp laceration during incision of the uterus. The quality of the hair also is noted; premature infants have woolly hair, whereas the hair of full-term infants is soft and silky.

The examiner palpates the head from the frontal bone, following the suture line to the diamond-shaped anterior fontanelle, then along the coronal suture, and next along the sagittal suture to the triangle-shaped posterior fontanelle (Figures 18-15 and 18-16). The occiput is palpated, and the assessment continues laterally to the parietal bones until the entire skull has been examined. If there is molding, the suture lines may be overriding, or there may be only a small space between the cranial bones. Premature closure of one or more sutures (*craniosynostosis*) retards brain growth and causes the skull to develop an odd shape.

Fontanelles should feel soft and flat. The normal anterior fontanelle measures 2 × 3 cm and closes about 18 months after birth. The posterior fontanelle is much

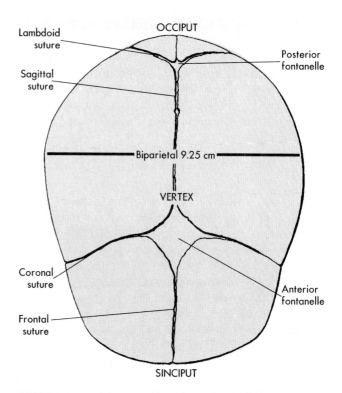

FIGURE 18-15 Anterior and posterior fontanelles. (Used with permission of Ross Laboratories, Columbus, Ohio 43216. From *Mechanisms of normal labor,* © Ross Laboratories.)

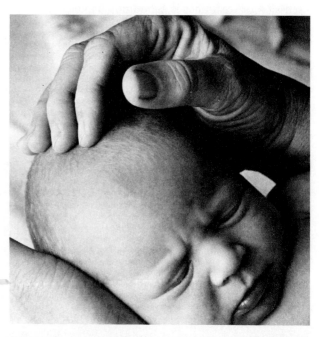

FIGURE 18-16 Palpating anterior fontanelle. (Courtesy John Young.)

smaller and closes by the fourth month. Abnormally large fontanelles may be a sign of hydrocephaly, osteogenesis imperfecta, or congenital hypothyroidism. Unusually small fontanelles also may be normal or associated with microcephaly.

During birth the head is subjected to pressure from the forces of labor. The sutures and fontanelles provide space for movement of these bones during labor and delivery, causing temporary *molding* of the fetal head (Figure 18-17). If, however, the transitional stage of labor is excessively long, the pressure of the ischial spines on the fetal parietal bones may cause subperiosteal bleeding, or **cephalhematoma.** Pressure on the presenting part may cause it to become edematous. In a vertex presentation this is seen as *caput succedaneum,* or edema of the scalp. Figure 18-18 compares cephalhematoma and caput succedaneum. Note bleeding is *under* the periosteum in Figure 18-18, *B*.

Examination of the head may reveal the following warning signs:
- Widely spaced suture lines or abnormally large fontanelles
- Abnormally small fontanelles or suture lines that do not override or that have spaces
- Bulging fontanelles, a sign of increased intracranial pressure
- Depressed fontanelles, possibly associated with dehydration
- Large cephalhematoma, possibly associated with skull fracture, extreme molding, or intracranial bleeding
- Lacerations of the scalp with widely separated wound edges, which may need suturing
- Malformations of the head, face, or spine

Clinical Decision

Baby Ann has a cephalhematoma over the right side of her head and swollen soft scalp over the occiput. Describe the differences between cephalhematoma and caput succedaneum. What effect may cephalhematoma have on an infant's recovery?

- Abnormal head circumference (see general examination for warning signs)

Eyes

The examiner observes for symmetry and size of the eyes, color of the sclera and iris, and the presence of exudate or any other deviations from normal. The eyes should be equal in size and symmetrically placed. The angle of slant from inner to outer canthus is noted (Figure 18-19, *A*). A mongolian slant is upward from inner to outer canthus; the opposite is an antimongolian slant. The sclera may be white to blue-white; subconjunctival hemorrhage can result from the pressure on the infant's face and head during delivery. The iris varies with heredity from darker or lighter slate blue to brown. Speckling of the iris (**Brushfield's spots**), **epicanthal folds** (a vertical fold of skin covering the inner canthus), and a slant up or down from the inner canthus to the outer are associated with trisomy 21. Chemical conjunctivitis from eye prophylaxis may produce whitish exudate within the first 24 hours. Pressure during the birth may cause the eyelids to become

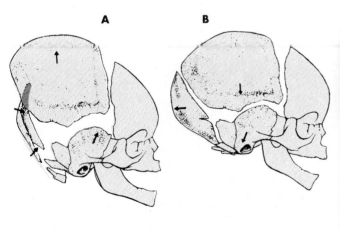

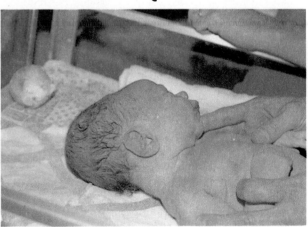

FIGURE 18-17 Molding during birth process causes overlapping and movement of cranial bones (**A**) and reexpansion of cranium on third day with return to normal positions (**B**). **C,** Molding of head evident in newborn. (**A** and **B** courtesy Mead Johnson. **C** courtesy Marjorie Pyle, RNC, *Lifecircle.*)

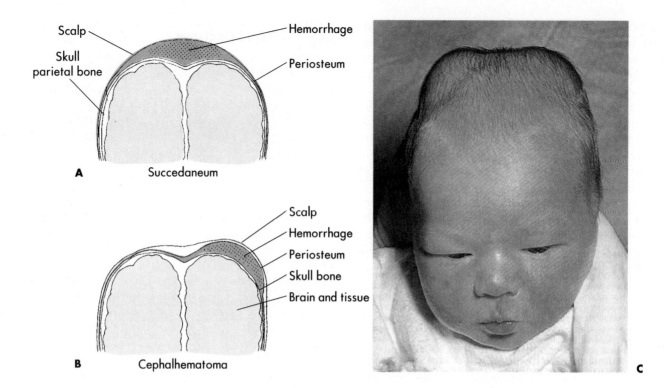

FIGURE 18-18 Note the differences between **A,** caput succedaneum, and **B,** cephalhematoma. **C,** Bilateral cephalhematoma. (C reprinted with permission of Harcourt-Brace Jovanovich Group [Australia]. From Beischer AA, MacKay EV, eds: *Obstetrics and the newborn,* ed 3, Philadelphia, 1993, WB Saunders.)

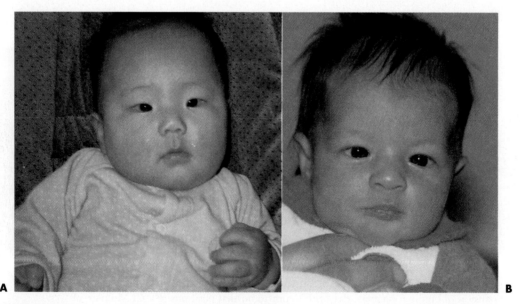

FIGURE 18-19 **A,** Epicanthal folds. **B,** Strabismus is normal in this week-old girl. (**A** courtesy S Ruhstaller; **B** courtesy R and B Silverman.)

edematous. The **sun-setting sign** (Figure 18-20, *A*) appears as a crescent of sclera over the iris and is caused by retraction of the upper lid; it is seen with hydrocephalus. When open, the lids should cover only the top part of the iris; drooping or ptosis is a sign of neuromuscular weakness. The examiner turns the infant's head from side to side and observes for **doll's eyes movement** (Figure 18-20, *B*); a lag in eye movement is normal in the newborn.

The examiner places the infant in the supine position and inspects the pupillary reflex by shining a light first into one eye and then the other. Pupillary reflexes appear at 30 weeks' gestational age and should be equal. The **red reflex,** a circular red area of light at the pupil, is noted. The red reflex should be equal and round. Inability to elicit this reflex indicates congenital cataract (opacity of the lens). The observation is commonly documented when checking PERRL (pupils equal, round, reactive to light).

Ocular movements are observed when the infant is alert. The examiner holds a light or red object 10 to 12 inches from the eyes and tries to get the infant to follow. The full-term infant should be able to follow a bright object or a face for 180 degrees horizontally and for 30 degrees vertically; however the eyes may not move smoothly and in unison because of immature muscular control. This is seen as crossing of the eyes, or **strabismus** (Figure 18-19, *B*). The infant should blink in response to bright light (optical blink reflex) but will show habituation to this response.

Newborn infants are relatively nearsighted and focus best on an object held at a distance of 10 to 12 inches.

The normal newborn shows interest in highly contrasting, brightly colored patterns. This is why the human face, with its sharply contrasting features, holds the neonate's attention.

The bright lights and hasty administration of eye prophylaxis in conventional delivery room settings are deterrents to neonatal vision. In spite of their normally decreased visual acuity, infants delivered in an environment where the lighting is dimmed will open their eyes and scan the area. When eye prophylaxis is delayed, the neonate will make eye-to-eye contact, an important part of early parent-infant interaction and bonding.

Ears

The placement of the ears is noted by using a straight edge and visualizing a line between the pinna and the inner canthus of the eye (Figure 18-21). The configuration, firmness, and degree of incurving of the pinna are observed. (This is an important part of gestational age assessment.) Examination of the canal and tympanic membrane (eardrum) soon after birth usually is not possible because vernix fills the canal. After vernix is absorbed, the membrane is visualized by pulling the ear lobe down and back. The membrane should appear light, pearly gray, and translucent. Often this examination is not included in the initial neonatal inspection.

Skin tags and preauricular sinuses may be innocuous or associated with renal malformations, and low-set or otherwise malformed ears are associated with chromosomal aberrations.

Hearing

Hearing may be impaired in the normal neonate if the external auditory canal is filled with amniotic fluid or vernix. This usually resolves within days.

The examiner observes the infant's startle reflex in response to loud noise and preference for high-pitched voices. The normal newborn will turn to the sound of

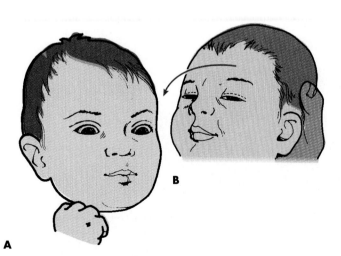

FIGURE 18-20 *A*, Sun-setting sign. *B*, Doll's eyes movement. (Courtesy Mead Johnson.)

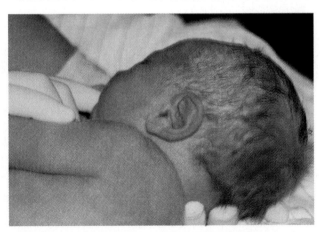

FIGURE 18-21 Ear placement. (Courtesy Marjorie Pyle, RNC, *Lifecircle*.)

the human voice and shows preference to the mother's voice. Refer to the Brazelton neonatal behavioral assessment (p. 468) for a description of the infant's ability to habituate to repetitive, noisy stimuli.

Warning signs for eye and ear problems follow:
- Exudate that is copious, greenish yellow, or persists or appears after 24 hours of age, possibly caused by an infectious process
- Jaundice of the sclera caused by hyperbilirubinemia
- Ptosis
- Sun-setting sign
- Brushfield's spots, epicanthal folds, and mongolian slant associated with Down syndrome
- Antimongolian slant associated with chromosomal abnormalities
- Cataract associated with congenital rubella
- Lack of optical blink reflex or failure to follow objects associated with blindness
- Short palpebral fissures associated with fetal alcohol syndrome
- Failure to respond to loud noise or human voice, or both
- Low-set or malformed ears

Nose

The examiner observes for gross abnormalities of the nose and face and for nasal patency by closing the infant's mouth and noting slight nasal flaring as the baby breathes. A soft catheter can be passed through both nares, but the previous method is less traumatic. Air should easily enter through the nose. A small amount of clear or white nasal discharge may stimulate the sneeze reflex, which is not a sign of illness. Copious nasal discharge may be a sign of congenital syphilis, and difficulty with nasal breathing may be associated with *choanal atresia* (blocked posterior nasal passages). Neonates are obligate nasal breathers—they will not breathe through the mouth if nasal passages are blocked. Therefore assessment of nasal patency is vital.

Mouth

While the infant is quiet, the lips and mouth are inspected for external defects and symmetry. There should be no obvious defects. Mucous membranes should be moist and pink. All movements of the mouth should be symmetric; asymmetric facial movement may be caused by facial nerve palsy (commonly associated with forceps delivery). The examiner places a gloved finger near the mouth to note rooting, then places the finger in the infant's mouth to test sucking, and runs the finger over the hard and soft palates (Figure 18-22, *A*) or uses a tongue blade to stimulate the gag reflex, which should be easily elicited. Sucking and rooting reflexes should be strong and coordinated with swallowing. Weak or absent root, suck, or swallow reflexes may be associated with neonatal depression caused by maternal medication or perinatal asphyxia.

When the infant cries, the examiner notes the size of the tongue and its coordination with the soft palate and uvula during movement and observes for the presence of natal teeth. Figure 18-22, *B*, shows an infant's mouth with thrush infection.

Neck

To properly visualize the anterior aspect of the normally short neonatal neck, the examiner extends it by placing one hand behind the neck and allowing the head to fall back slightly. The neck is inspected for skin tags, masses, and pits, and the posterior portion is observed for skin folds, the hairline, and the contour of the neck. The head should rotate freely during this process.

The examiner pulls the infant to a sitting position and looks for **head lag**, noting how well the infant can use the neck extensors and flexors to control the head in the upright position (Figure 18-23). This is the only time that the examiner does not support the infant's head.

The clavicles are palpated. Fractures may be sustained if a large baby has shoulder dystocia during delivery. The examiner may note a "crunchy" feeling (crepitus) or ac-

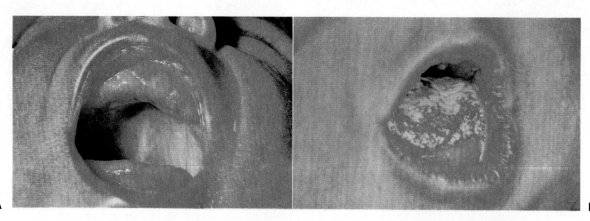

FIGURE 18-22 A, Normal mouth and palate. **B,** Mouth with thrush. (Courtesy Mead Johnson.)

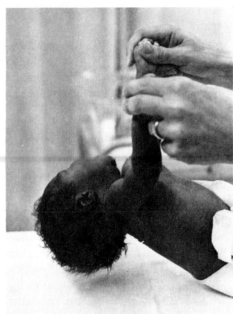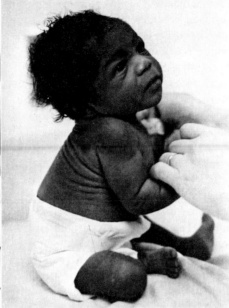

A **B**

FIGURE 18-23 **A,** Pulling to sit. **B,** Sitting. Note head lag. (Courtesy Mary Olsen Johnson.)

tually feel the two ends of the broken bone. The sternocleidomastoid muscle is palpated and any masses noted.

The following *warning signs require further investigation for nose, mouth, and neck problems:*

Nose
- Occluded nares
- Copious nasal discharge

Mouth
- Cleft lip or palate, or both
- Large or small mouth
- Thin upper lip and smooth philtrum (bow of lip)
- Weak or absent root, suck, swallow, or gag reflexes
- Poorly coordinated suck and swallow
- Asymmetric facial movement or appearance
- Large tongue
- Natal teeth or other masses

Neck
- Masses, pits, or skin tags
- Abnormal hair line
- Head lag
- Crepitus, poor arm movement

Test Yourself

- The _____ reflex is checked to document PERRL, which means pupils _____, _____, and _____.

- What do skin tags and sinuses near the ears signify?

- List the important steps in examination of nose and mouth.

Neuromuscular System
NORMAL TRANSITION

During intrauterine life the normally developing fetus exhibits voluntary and involuntary activities that increase in complexity and frequency with maturity. These prepare the infant for many behaviors vital for healthy extrauterine life. Chest wall movements encourage pulmonary development; rooting, sucking, and swallowing reflexes prepare for feeding; arm and leg movements keep limbs supple and promote symmetric muscular growth. Increasing muscle tone produces a posture of increasing flexion as pregnancy advances. This will help the newborn conserve body heat by exposing less body surface to the cooler environment, as well as keeping the hands positioned close to the mouth, encouraging rooting and sucking. Although reflexes such as the Moro and grasp must have had a positive survival value for our evolutionary ancestors, they now have no critical use.

The normal intrauterine environment provides only minimal variations in temperature, tactile sensation, light, and sound. Labor and delivery bring wider extremes. The infant is quickly subjected to the colder temperature, firmer touch, brighter light, and louder sound of the extrauterine world. These are functional because they provide the neonatal nervous system with necessary stimuli, as do rising carbon dioxide levels during the second stage of labor. Efforts can be made, however, for a gentler transition during the immediate neonatal period by shielding the newborn's eyes from harsh, direct lighting and by handling and speaking gently to the infant. A gentle delivery is especially important, a time when pressure from maternal structures and assisting hands or instruments can injure delicate nerves, bones, and connective tissue.

The close relationship of the neurologic and musculoskeletal systems, both functionally and anatomically, allows simultaneous assessment. Normal structure and behaviors, both voluntary and involuntary, are indicators of normal fetal development and future neonatal function.

ASSESSMENT

Assessment of fetal neuromuscular status begins during the observation of heart rate variability and accelerations with movement. These initial observations of the neonate's neurologic status are included in the Apgar score. The rest of the neurologic examination may be delayed for 24 hours to allow for recovery from birth and partial metabolism of any medications given to the mother. The examination is divided into three parts: general assessment; evaluation of motor function, developmental reflexes, and cranial nerve function; and behavioral assessment. This assessment is time consuming and tiring for the infant. It may not be completed in the setting; the demands in a busy unit may require an abbreviated examination.

General Assessment

Overall assessment should take place when the infant is quiet and neither too sleepy nor too hungry. The examiner should always remember to maintain warmth and especially to note the following:
1. Weight, height, and head and chest sizes (abnormal growth and development are associated with neurologic dysfunction)
2. Presence of any obvious congenital anomalies
3. Resting posture: position other than flexion (in a full-term infant) may be due to the effect of maternal medications, sepsis, or congenital neuromuscular disease
4. Tremors (repetitive vibratory motions); may be due to metabolic imbalance, neonatal drug withdrawal, or neurologic disorders
5. Abnormal eye movements or repetitive leg movements such as bicycling (leg movements in a cycling motion), tonic posturing, lip smacking, or rapid flexion-extension (clonic movements)
6. Level of responsiveness (see behavioral assessment)

Changes in neurologic status often are early markers for abnormalities of other systems; for example, lethargy is an important sign of sepsis and quality of cry a sign of some congenital syndromes.

Back. The back is inspected for anomalies by placing the infant in a prone position and observing; observe for birthmarks, hair distribution, dimples, or hair tufts anywhere along the spine (associated with spina bifida occulta). There should be no obvious defects. Mongolian spots and nevi may be seen (see assessment of the skin) (Figure 18-24).

The extremities are observed for symmetry of movement and size, posture at rest, fractures, lacerations, bruising, or deficiencies in function. No evidence of trauma should be noted. The full-term infant should lie in a position of flexion (normal intrauterine posture) at rest.

Extremities. An infant who has assumed the frank breech position in utero will lie with the hips flexed, with knees fully extended. These infants are at high risk for congenital dislocation of the hip. The following characteristics indicate dislocation (Figure 18-25).
1. There is limited abduction of the affected hip.
2. The femur will appear shortened on the affected side.
3. The placement of thigh creases (gluteal folds) is deeper on the affected side.

The examiner inspects for number of digits, normal formation of the hands and feet, and condition of the nails. There should be no deformities. Fingernails should not be stained with meconium and should reach the ends of the fingertips at term. The degree and pattern of sole and palmar creases are noted. At term, creases are found over the entire sole. A single crease in the palm, the **simian line,** is associated with Down syndrome (see Chapter 27). Moro reflex is elicited to evaluate whether there is any damage to the structure of the extremities and the function of the peripheral and central nervous systems (see Table 18-3). The Moro reflex should be brisk and complete bilaterally. The extremities should move symmetrically and return to the flexed position when movement ceases. Warning signs are listed at the end of this discussion.

The back is palpated by holding the infant under the chest and lifting horizontally, allowing the spine to flex. The examiner stimulates the trunk incurvation reflex by firmly running a fingertip along the back from shoulder to hip just lateral to the spine and then running the fingers over the entire spine from neck to sacrum. The examiner palpates for masses and absent vertebrae. Flexion and extension of the spine should be smooth and regular. Flexion should be elicited with the incurvation reflex.

Obvious defects may be a meningocele or meningomyelocele associated with hydrocephalus and deformities of the feet (see Chapter 27). **Ortolani's test** is performed during examination for the presence of congenital hip dislocation, with the infant placed in the supine position. The examiner places the middle fingers

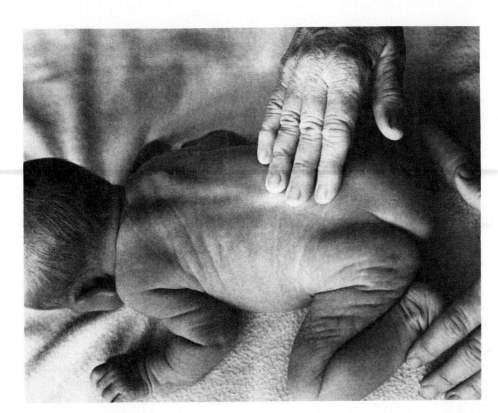

FIGURE 18-24 Inspection of back. (Courtesy John Young.)

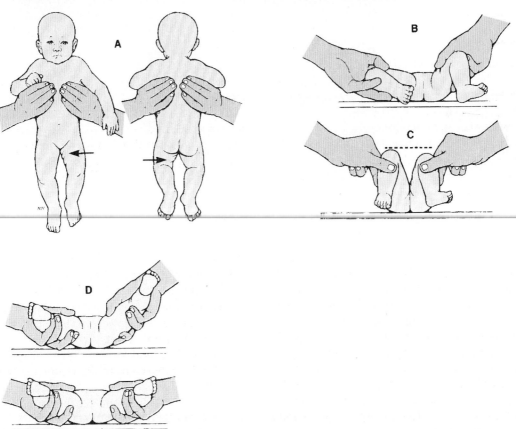

FIGURE 18-25 Signs of congenital dislocation of hip. **A,** Asymmetry of gluteal and thigh folds. **B,** Limited hip abduction, as seen in flexion. **C,** Apparent shortening of femur, as indicated by level of knees in flexion. **D,** Ortolani's click (if infant is younger than 4 weeks of age). (From Wong DL: *Whaley and Wong's essentials of pediatric nursing,* ed 4, St Louis, 1993, Mosby.)

TABLE 18-3 Motor Function

OBSERVATION	NORMAL RESPONSE	ABNORMAL RESPONSE	CAUSES
Resting posture	Flexion, even in sleep for first 2-3 wk	Hypotonia* ("frog leg posture")	Hypoxia, prematurity, metabolic disturbances (e.g., hypoglycemia, hypothyroidism, hypermagnesemia), Down syndrome
Tone	Normal tone: some head lag; flexion at elbow and knee becomes extension when pulled to sitting	Hypertonia: infant moves "as a block"; no head lag, no elbow or knee extension when pulled to sitting Hypotonia: excessive head lag	Hypoxia, intracranial bleeding, drug withdrawal
Symmetry†	No difference between two sides of body or upper and lower extremities	Tone increased or decreased from right to left or upper and lower parts of body	Hypoxia, intracranial bleeding, drug withdrawal, injuries to nerve plexus, fractures
Strength	Strong cry, spontaneous movements, resistance to painful or unnatural posture	Weak cry, lack of movement or response	Hypotonia, prematurity
Movement	Smooth when opening and closing hands, moving hand to mouth, kicking spontaneously	Seizure activity, tremors	Hypoxia, drug withdrawal
Fasciculations (fine tremors)	None noted	Fine tremors of fingers and toes at rest or during sleep, reduced spontaneous activity	Hypotonia
Spine Evidence of trauma to cervical area	Tonic neck reflex, symmetric Moro reflex, normal grasp	Lack of response unilaterally or bilaterally	Erb's palsy if unilateral, dislocation of cervical spine if bilateral, fractures
Lumbosacral disruption	Normal appearance and reflexes	Acute injury, bruising, mass in area, spinal shock, loss of knee and ankle reflexes	Congenital anomalies, traumatic breech delivery

*To demonstrate uncertain hypotonia note position of head as infant is placed back on bed from sitting posture. As vertex of head touches bed, infant with normal muscle tone will flex head so weight of head is on occiput. Hypotonic infant will not be able to flex head.
†Head should be held in midline to avoid stimulating tonic neck reflex during evaluation of symmetry.

on the outside of the femur (at the greater trochanter) and the thumb on the inside (at the lesser trochanter), flexing the infant's legs until the hips and knees are at right angles. The knees are abducted by pressing them toward the examining table. A click is heard and felt during this motion if the hip is dislocated (see Figure 18-25).

If the feet seem to be abnormally positioned, an attempt is made to manipulate them gently into a neutral or midline position. This should be easy to do if the malposition has resulted from pressure in utero rather than structural deformity.

The following are *warning signs for back and extremity problems:*

- Absence of limbs or digits, usually isolated deformities
- Deformities of digits, including fusion (syndactyly) and an extra digit (polydactyly), also usually isolated deformities
- Simian line associated with Down syndrome
- Lack of movement of limb, possibly from brachial nerve palsy caused by excessive traction and flexion of the neck during delivery (arm held adducted and internally rotated) or fracture
- Limited abduction and unequal femur length
- Asymmetric thigh creases or positive Ortolani's maneuver (clicks indicating congenital hip dislocation)

Motor Function

The infant's posture is observed for tone and movement on the basis of the head, back, and extremity examination results. Table 18-3 can be used as a guide.

Developmental Reflexes

Assessment of neonatal reflexes should be performed with expectations appropriate for the infant's gestational age. Table 18-4 reviews assessment of **developmental reflexes.**

Cranial Nerves

Observation of cranial nerve function is more detailed than other parts of the neurologic assessment; however, many parameters are assessed during other parts of the physical examination. For instance, as the examiner looks for forceps marks, the mouth can be observed for symmetric movement because the same excessive pressure that damaged the skin can cause facial nerve palsy. Pupillary response and eye movements indicate functioning of optic and oculomotor nerves. Rooting and sucking reflexes test the trigeminal and facial nerves. Startle response to a loud noise indicates the health of the eighth nerve.

These *neuromuscular warning signs* must be assessed with consideration of gestational age:

- Low birth weight, short height, and/or small head size
- Hypertonia or hypotonia
- Lethargy, irritability, abnormal cry
- Tremors
- Repetitive movements of the eyes or limbs
- Asymmetric development, movement, and/or strength
- Deformities of back or limbs
- Limited abduction and unequal femur length
- Asymmetric thigh creases or positive Ortolani's maneuver
- Poor or weak Moro reflex and grasp
- Absent or uncoordinated root, suck, and swallow
- Lack of self-quieting behaviors
- Failure to change behavioral states smoothly (see Brazelton assessment on p. 468)

Test Yourself

- What are the three parts of the neuromuscular examination? Why is Ortolani's test done?
- How can the rooting reflex be used to help the mother with breast-feeding?

TABLE 18-4 Developmental Reflexes

TECHNIQUE	NORMAL RESPONSE	ABNORMAL RESPONSE
MORO REFLEX Use your hand and forearm to support infant's head and back as you lift upper body off the surface and drop supporting hand to simulate falling (see photo). (This allows you to test response to sensation of falling. Using loud noise to elicit startle reflex tests response to sound.)	Abduction and extension of arms and at least fingers three to five occurs, followed by adduction and flexion of upper extremities (see photo). Infant may startle and cry. Disappears: 4 months.	Asymmetry means hemiparesis, fractured humerus or clavicle, or brachial plexus injury. Sluggish responses are seen in premature and ill infants.
TONIC NECK REFLEX (TNR) Position infant on back and turn head to side.	Same-sided arm and leg show extension and increased tone, whereas arm and leg on opposite side flex and show decreased tone ("fencing position"). Infant's response may vary. Disappears: around 4 months.	Infant who is unable to break this posture soon after it is elicited exhibits abnormal obligatory response.
STEPPING REFLEX Hold infant upright and place one foot in contact with firm surface (see photo).	Leg in contact with surface extends while other flexes. Infant then appears to take steps.	Hypertonic means both legs will be in extension. Hypotonic means infant will not extend legs.

Continued.

TABLE 18-4 **Developmental Reflexes—cont'd**

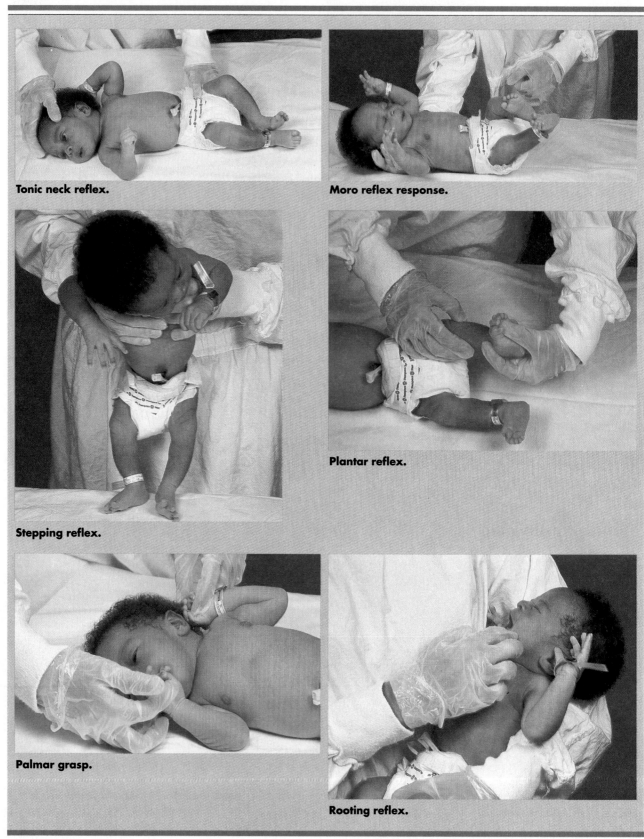

Tonic neck reflex.

Moro reflex response.

Stepping reflex.

Plantar reflex.

Palmar grasp.

Rooting reflex.

From Seidel HM et al, eds: Mosby's guide to physical examination, ed 2, St Louis, 1991, Mosby.

TABLE 18-4 Developmental Reflexes—cont'd

TECHNIQUE	NORMAL RESPONSE	ABNORMAL RESPONSE
BABINSKI'S REFLEX Stroke lateral aspect of infant's sole from heel to toe (see photo).	Dorsiflexion of great toe with extension of other toes occurs. Disappears: by 2 years.	Response may indicate neurologic dysfunction.
PLANTAR GRASP Press your finger to infant's sole just below toes (see photo).	Toes flex around your finger. Disappears: 10 months.	Absence of reflex is seen in infants with hypotonia or spinal cord or lumbosacral plexus injuries.
PALMAR GRASP Place object in palm of infant's hand.	Flexion of fingers with grasping of object occurs (see photo). This grasp is strong enough to allow infant to be lifted from bed (see traction response).	Lack of grasp seen in infants with hypotonia perinatal asphyxia.
TRACTION RESPONSE Place infant on back and firmly place one finger in each palm. After infant grasps your fingers, pull up.	Infant grasps your fingers and can be pulled to sitting position.	Lack of response indicates hypotonia.
ROOTING REFLEX When infant is awake, touch cheek (see photo).	Infant turns head and mouth toward stimulus. Disappears: 6 months.	Response may not be elicited in normal infants who have just been fed; it is weak in infants with facial nerve palsy or central nervous system depression.
SUCK REFLEX When infant is awake, place clean finger or nipple in mouth.	Infant begins to suck.	Weak or absent suck.
SWALLOW AND GAG REFLEX Observe infant swallowing during feeding.	Infant sucks and swallows fluid without distress. Coughs or gags appropriately.	Drooling, lack of swallow, and lack of coordination between suck and swallow.

Clinical Decision

What do you think of the following two findings? Is either a cause for concern? Why?
a. You note a full-term baby assumes a resting posture of extension and feels "floppy"._____
b. You note an asymmetric Moro reflex after an especially long second stage of labor._____

Brazelton Neonatal Behavioral Assessment Scale

Brazelton's research during the past two decades has changed the way health care personnel think about a newborn infant's capabilities. Previously, neonates were thought to be passive receivers of environmental stimuli. It is now known that the normal full-term infant can influence the amount of stimuli intake and the care givers' responses (Brazelton, 1984). Neonates can attend to their surroundings (Figure 18-26) or sleep or can remain agitated and distressed or use self-quieting activities for consolation. Normal infants differ in these

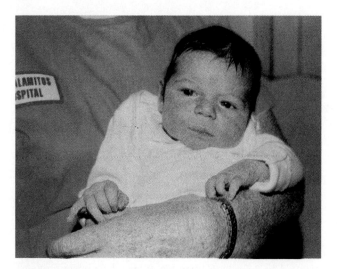

FIGURE 18-26 Quiet and alert. (Courtesy Marjorie Pyle, RNC, *Lifecircle*.)

abilities, but the normal full-term infant should make the transition between states smoothly. Use of the *Brazelton neonatal behavioral assessment scale (BNBAS)* as a research tool is limited to those who have completed an examiners' workshop training program. Nurses, however, can use items from this tool to assess the responses of infants and increase parental understanding of infant temperament and behavior patterns.

The Brazelton scale consists of 28 items in 7 categories (Box 18-5). Before the assessment is begun, the infant's state of consciousness is determined (Box 18-6). Recognition of their infant's state is especially important to parents because it can cue them to the appropriateness of their parenting behaviors. For example, it is not appropriate to attempt to play with an infant who is sleeping; to do so only encourages a sense of failure. However, the parent who recognizes the alert

---

BOX 18-5   Brazelton Neonatal Behavioral Assessment Scale

- *Habituation:* Infant's ability to decrease response to external stimuli (bright light, rattle, bell, and tactile stimulation to the foot)
- *Orientation:* Infant's ability to attend to, focus on, and interact with animate and inanimate stimuli (auditory and visual)
- *Motor performance:* Infant's ability to organize and control motor activity
- *Range of state:* State of consciousness during the entire examination period
- *Regulation of state:* Infant's self-quieting abilities
- *Autonomic regulation:* Skin color
- *Reflexes:* Primary neonatal reflexes

BOX 18-6   Neonatal States of Consciousness

SLEEP STATES
State I
- *Deep sleep:* Regular breathing, eyes closed with no movements, no spontaneous activity except startles

State II
- *Light sleep:* Irregular respirations, eyes closed with rapid eye movements, low activity level with sucking behaviors

AWAKE STATES
State III
- *Drowsy:* Variable activity level, eyes open or closed with lids fluttering, dazed expression

State IV
- *Alert:* Minimal motor activity, bright look with attention focused on source of stimulation, may appear dazed but easy to "break through" to infant

State V
- *Eyes open:* Much motor activity, thrusting movements of extremities, reacting to stimuli with increasing activity and/or startles

State VI
- *Crying:* High motor activity and intense crying, difficult to "break through" to infant
  Adapted from Brazelton TB: *Neonatal behavioral assessment scale,* ed 2, Philadelphia, 1984, JB Lippincott.

---

state and initiates play will more likely be rewarded by responses. Parents also can be made aware that their infant's hand-to-mouth activity is a self-quieting behavior (Figure 20-14), not a bad habit to be eliminated. Fostering this kind of awareness may help new parents to understand their newborn. (See Chapter 20 for further discussion.)

Gestational Age Assessment

The gestational age of the newborn infant is calculated in weeks from the last menstrual period (LMP) (see Chapter 7). Prenatally, fetal age can be assessed by various indirect means (e.g., ultrasonic determination of biparietal diameter and crown-rump length. After birth, physical examination leads to a more accurate assessment of maturity. It is important to determine the maturity of each infant because complications of the neonatal period vary greatly with maturity; premature and postmature infants have the most difficulty adapting to extrauterine life.

METHOD

Several attempts have been made to develop a system of gestational age assessment that is easy to perform, is replicable by many examiners, and has a high correlation with actual gestational age (Ballard et al, 1979; Dubowitz et al, 1970; Lubchenco, 1970). Physical characteristics may be assessed soon after birth, some of which may have been noted during an early assessment. Figure 18-27 can be used to note the special observations needed for gestational age assessment by circling the box on the tool that most closely represents the characteristic of each parameter. Then you will use the charts in Figure 18-28 to evaluate the size of the baby in relation to gestational age.

The examiner assesses the skin first by noting color, peeling and/or cracking, and visible blood vessels. The *skin* thickens with maturity, causing peeling and making the blood vessels less visible. The amount and distribu-

ESTIMATION OF GESTATIONAL AGE BY MATURITY RATING

Symbols: X - 1st Exam O - 2nd Exam

NEUROMUSCULAR MATURITY

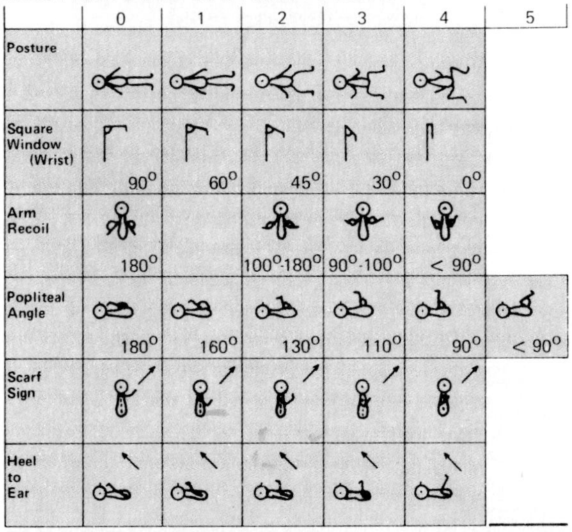

	0	1	2	3	4	5
Posture						
Square Window (Wrist)	90°	60°	45°	30°	0°	
Arm Recoil	180°		100°-180°	90°-100°	< 90°	
Popliteal Angle	180°	160°	130°	110°	90°	< 90°
Scarf Sign						
Heel to Ear						

PHYSICAL MATURITY

	0	1	2	3	4	5
SKIN	gelatinous red, transparent	smooth pink, visible veins	superficial peeling &/or rash, few veins	cracking pale area, rare veins	parchment, deep cracking, no vessels	leathery, cracked, wrinkled
LANUGO	none	abundant	thinning	bald areas	mostly bald	
PLANTAR CREASES	no crease	faint red marks	anterior transverse crease only	creases ant. 2/3	creases cover entire sole	
BREAST	barely percept.	flat areola, no bud	stippled areola, 1–2 mm bud	raised areola, 3–4 mm bud	full areola, 5–10 mm bud	
EAR	pinna flat, stays folded	sl. curved pinna, soft with slow recoil	well-curv. pinna, soft but ready recoil	formed & firm with instant recoil	thick cartilage, ear stiff	
GENITALS Male	scrotum empty, no rugae		testes descending, few rugae	testes down, good rugae	testes pendulous, deep rugae	
GENITALS Female	prominent clitoris & labia minora		majora & minora equally prominent	majora large, minora small	clitoris & minora completely covered	

Gestation by Dates ______ wks

Birth Date ______ Hour ______ am/pm

APGAR ______ 1 min ______ 5 min

MATURITY RATING

Score	Wks
5	26
10	28
15	30
20	32
25	34
30	36
35	38
40	40
45	42
50	44

SCORING SECTION

	1st Exam=X	2nd Exam=O
Estimating Gest Age by Maturity Rating	______ Weeks	______ Weeks
Time of Exam	Date ______ Hour ______ am/pm	Date ______ Hour ______ am/pm
Age at Exam	______ Hours	______ Hours
Signature of Examiner	______ M.D.	______ M.D.

FIGURE 18-27 Newborn maturity rating. Add points scored for neuromuscular maturity to those scored for physical maturity. Then circle score and corresponding gestational age. (Courtesy Mead Johnson.)

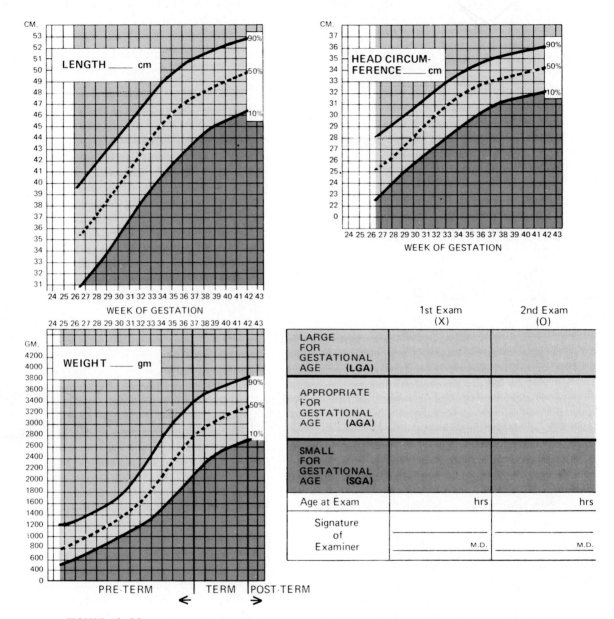

CLASSIFICATION OF NEWBORNS –
BASED ON MATURITY AND INTRAUTERINE GROWTH
Symbols: X - 1st Exam   O - 2nd Exam

FIGURE 18-28 Newborn classification. Plot gestational age against weight, height, and head circumference on appropriate graph. These should not be in widely divergent percentiles. If infant is AGA, weight will fall between 10th and 90th percentiles. Infant whose weight is below 10th percentile is SGA; infant whose weight is above 90th percentile is LGA. Problems associated with each are reviewed in Chapter 27. (Courtesy Mead Johnson.)

tion of *lanugo*, which appears early in gestation and disappears as pregnancy progresses, are observed. Next the *sole creases* are inspected (Figure 18-29); these increase in number and depth with gestational age. The *breast areolae* are palpated and their diameter measured. The areolae will be barely visible in the very immature infant and grow to 5 to 10 mm in diameter close to term. The *pinnae* of the infant's ears curve in with increasing gestational age (Figure 18-21). Carti-

lage formation also causes the pinnae to become stiffer and recoil after being folded in the more mature infant. Last, the *genitalia* are examined. In the male infant the testes descend through the inguinal canal as gestational age increases. As this occurs, the scrotum becomes larger with rugae (see Figure 18-12). In the female infant the labia majora grow to cover the clitoris and labia minora (see Figure 18-11). At the conclusion of physical assessment, the examiner totals the sum of the

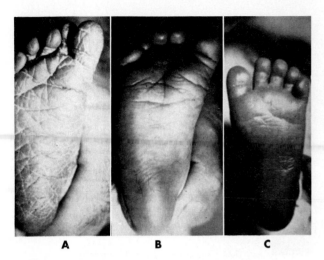

FIGURE 18-29 Plantar creases. Infant's sole becomes more creased with maturity. At 36 weeks there is only anterior transverse crease. By term, creases are found on entire sole. **A,** Postterm. **B,** Term. **C,** Preterm.

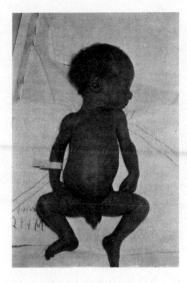

FIGURE 18-30 Neuromuscular maturity assessment posture for preterm infant. (For full-term posture, see Figure 19-7.) (Courtesy Kenneth Holt, MD.)

physical characteristics and records the number in the space provided (Figure 18-27).

Neuromuscular assessment should be postponed for 24 hours to allow the infant to recover from the stress of birth. First the infant's *resting posture* is observed (Figure 18-30). The preterm infant lies in a position of extension, which becomes gradually more flexed with maturity. Next the *angle of the square window* is determined by flexing the hand onto the forearm and noting the angle at which resistance is felt (see Figure 18-31). The angle decreases with increasing gestational age. The *degree of arm recoil* is assessed by first flexing and then extending the infant's arms for 5 seconds and then releasing them. The angle formed as the arms recoil also decreases with increasing gestational age. The *popliteal angle* is assessed by placing the infant on his or her back. The examiner extends one leg, taking care not to allow the buttocks to lift off the bed and noting the point at which resistance is met. The angle becomes more acute as gestation progresses. While the infant is on his or her back, the *scarf sign* is assessed by wrapping one arm across the baby's chest until resistance is met (Figure 18-32) and noting where the elbow lies in relation to the infant's midline. Finally, *heel-to-ear flexibility* is assessed by grasping the foot loosely, extending it toward the ear and letting go (allowing the back to rise up off the bed if necessary) and noting the point at which the foot slips out of grasp. The score for neuromuscular assessment is totaled as for the physical characteristics.

Add the two scores together and find the corresponding gestational age (Figure 18-27). After gestational age is determined, it is plotted against birth weight on the graph in Figure 18-28 and the infant is diagnosed as *small,* *appropriate,* or *large for gestational age* (*SGA,*

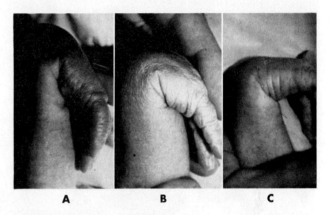

FIGURE 18-31 Square window. Flex the hand onto forearm and note the angle at which resistance is met. **A,** Postterm. **B,** Term. **C,** Preterm.

AGA, or LGA). Normally there is a positive relationship between gestational age and birth weight. This relationship, however, can be disturbed as a result of complications of pregnancy such as infection, diabetes, and hypertension. The weight of an infant who is AGA falls between the 10th and 90th percentile. SGA or LGA infants fall below and above these limits, respectively. The *interaction* of gestational age and birth weight greatly influences neonatal well-being (Figure 18-33). In addition, appropriateness of size and gestational age influences clinical decisions.

Assessment of neonatal health will not be complete for 24 hours, when all three areas of assessment (history, physical examination, and gestational age) are completed. Box 18-7 summarizes complete neonatal physical assessment. Every infant should be completely assessed soon after birth and then just before discharge. Assessments for skin color and cardiovascular and neuromuscular status are performed as necessary.

A   B

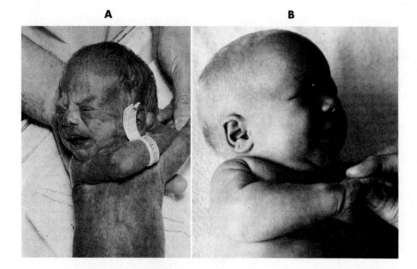

FIGURE 18-32 Scarf sign. Attempt to pull the arm across the upper chest until resistance is met. Note position of elbow in relation to midline. **A,** Preterm. **B,** Term. (**A** courtesy Kenneth Holt, MD; **B** courtesy John Young.)

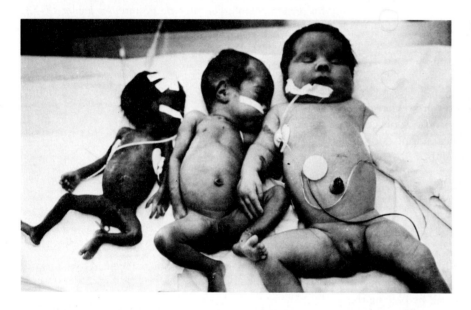

FIGURE 18-33 Three infants of same gestational age, weighing 600 g, 1400 g, and 2750 g, respectively, from left to right. (From Korones SB: *High-risk newborn infants: the basis for intensive nursing care,* ed 4, St Louis, 1986, Mosby.)

 Clinical Decision

Your assessment of baby boy R. reveals the following characteristics. Using gestational age assessment and Figures 18-29 to 18-32, determine the total score for this infant and the age in weeks. If baby R. weighed 2040 g at birth, is he SGA, AGA, or LGA? Plot weight against gestational age on the graph in Figure 18-28.

NEUROLOGIC CHARACTERISTICS
Posture: all extremities flexed
Square window: 30 degrees
Arm recoil: 90 degrees

Popliteal angle: 90 degrees
Scarf sign: elbow will not reach midline
Heel to ear: lower leg at right angle to trunk

PHYSICAL CHARACTERISTICS
Skin: cracking, pale, few veins
Lanugo: mostly gone
Sole creases: two thirds of sole
Breast: full areola, 5 mm bud
Ear: well formed and firm
Genitalia: good rugae, testes descended

BOX 18-7   Neonatal Physical Assessment

Date _____

Name of infant _____ Sex _____

Date and time of delivery _____ Age now_____

ADMISSION DATA

Time of admission _____

Placed in warmer? _____ Isolette _____ Servo temperature _____

Eye prophylaxis _____

Vitamin K _____ Time _____

Location _____

CORD BLOOD

Blood type and Rh _____

Direct Coombs' test _____

VDRL (serology) _____

INITIAL PHYSICAL EXAMINATION

Date _____ Time _____ Age of infant _____

FINDINGS

General

Vital signs: Temperature _____ Pulse _____ Respirations _____ BP _____

Weight _____ Height _____ Head circumference _____ Chest circumference _____

Color _____ Activity _____

State _____ Cry _____

Skin

Color _____ Lesions _____

Desquamation _____ Vernix caseosa _____

Hair distribution _____

Petechiae/ecchymosis/trauma _____

Nails (length) _____

Turgor (evidence of subcutaneous loss) _____

Other _____

Head

Circumference _____ Shape _____

Molding _____

Fontanelles/sutures (size, placement, fullness) _____

Birth trauma _____ Forceps marks _____

Caput succedaneum _____ Cephalhematoma _____

Facial symmetry _____ Other _____

Ears

Position _____ Size _____

Cartilage formation _____ Other _____

Eyes

Position (slant, hypertelorism) _____

Size _____ Iris _____

Sclerae _____ Drainage _____

Other _____

Continued.

BOX 18-7 Neonatal Physical Assessment—cont'd

Nose

Patency _____ Flaring _____
Nasolabial folds _____ Other _____

Throat and mouth

Lips (color, formation) _____ Symmetric facial movement _____
Palate _____ Gums/teeth _____
Tongue (midline, gag) _____ Secretions _____
Other _____

Neck

Webbing _____ Masses _____
Range of motion _____ Other _____

Chest

Circumference _____
Respiratory rate and quality (retractions/grunting) _____
Breath sounds _____
Thorax (symmetry of movement, anteroposterior diameter, bulging) _____
Breast tissue _____ Other _____

Cardiovascular

Color: cyanosis (location), pallor, plethora _____
Heart rate _____ Unusual rhythm/murmers _____
Location of PMI _____
Pulses: brachial _____ femoral _____
Capillary filling _____ Cyanosis/pallor/ruddiness _____
HCT (if done) _____ Other _____

Abdomen

Shape _____
Umbilical cord/vessels/color/size/drainage _____
Liver _____ Spleen _____
Kidneys _____ Anus (patency, location) _____
Other _____

Extremities and back

Spine _____
Upper extremities (digits, symmetry of size, movement, tone) _____
Lower extremities (digits, symmetry of size, movement, tone) _____
Gluteal and thigh creases _____ Ortolani's maneuver _____
Other _____

Genitalia

Female

Labia majora/minor/clitoris/vagina _____
Discharge _____ Edema/ecchymosis _____
Placement of urinary meatus and anus _____ Patency of anus _____
Other _____

Male

Penis (hypospadias or epispadias) _____
Scrotum _____ Testes _____
Patency and placement of anus _____
Other _____

BOX 18-7   Neonatal Physical Assessment—cont'd

Neurologic/behavioral

Reflexes

Moro _____	Tonic neck _____
Neck righting _____	Stepping _____
Babinski _____	Palmar grasp _____
Traction response _____	Plantar grasp _____
Rooting _____	Sucking _____
Swallowing _____	Other _____

Behavioral

State _____

Visual following _____	Auditory following _____
Consolableness _____	Hand-to-mouth activity _____

Tremors

Description (location, type) _____

Stimulus related _____

ASSESSMENT OF GESTATIONAL AGE

Via dates _____	Via ultrasound _____
Via examination: initial _____	After 24 hours _____

Classification:

Preterm   **Term**   **Postterm**

SGA
AGA
LGA

KEY POINTS

- The purposes of assessment are to identify those infants experiencing a difficult transition to extrauterine life and to aid in bonding between family and newborn; therefore at least one assessment in the presence of the family is advised. Each neonate should be assessed fully at birth and before discharge. If the infant is born at home or discharged early, assessment at 24 and 48 hours is recommended.
- Nurses caring for newborn infants should be proficient in neonatal assessment and necessary urgent interventions.
- Directions concerning communication of information obtained from assessment must be clear.

STUDY QUESTIONS

18-1 For the following statements, select an appropriate key term used in this chapter.
   a. Skin that is dry and peeling just after birth
   b. An unusual line crossing the center of the palm of the hand
   c. Enlarged breast tissue caused by maternal hormones in male or female infants at birth
   d. Formation of an exudate from the eye as a result of infection with gonorrhea
   e. Color of an infant who is anemic
   f. Color of an infant whose hematocrit value is over 65%

   g. Actions taken internally and externally to protect the infant from chilling

18-2 The infant's father is concerned because the baby's hands and feet are deep blue. How would you respond to his concern?
   a. The baby must have a low blood oxygen level. I'll get the oxygen right away!"
   b. Don't worry about that now; we'll ask the pediatrician about it later."
   c. "It's normal. Once the baby's peripheral circulation is established, her extremities will become pink."

d. "As long as she's moving, her color doesn't really matter."

18-3 Your assessment of baby boy R. reveals the following (refer to Figure 18-27, *A*). How would you score each characteristic? What is the infant's gestational age?

Neurologic characteristics

a. Posture: flexion of all four extremities
b. Square window: 30 degrees
c. Arm recoil: 90 to 100 degrees
d. Popliteal angle: 90 degrees
e. Scarf sign: elbow will not reach midline
f. Heel to ear: lower leg at right angle to trunk

Physical characteristics

g. Skin: cracking, pale areas with few veins
h. Lanugo: mostly gone
i. Plantar creases: cover two thirds of sole
j. Breast: full areola, with 5- to 10-mm bud
k. Ear: well formed and firm
l. Genitalia: good rugae, both testes in scrotum

18-4 Baby boy R. weighs 2040 g. He is:

a. LGA
b. SGA
c. AGA

18-5 Match the cardiac sounds with the appropriate events.

a. S_1 1. Systole
b. S_2 2. Diastole
c. S_1 to S_2 3. Closure of atrioventricular valves
d. S_2 to S_1 4. Closure of semilunar valves

18-6 Match the stage with the numbered manifestations.

a. First period of reactivity
b. First sleep
c. Second period of reactivity

1. Meconium passage
2. Labile vital signs
3. Active and alert
4. Onset of bowel sounds
5. Increased mucus secretions

18-7 When assessing the skin, you note that an 18-hour-old infant is jaundiced "from head to toe." Your conclusion is that:

a. This is a normal developmental event and not of concern.
b. There must be a maternal-infant blood incompatibility.
c. The jaundice must have begun in utero.
d. This is *not* normal and must be investigated.

18-8 After a forceps-assisted delivery, it is *most* important to assess for:

a. Facial nerve palsy
b. Umbilical hernia
c. Hepatosplenomegaly
d. Microcephaly

Answer Key

2 18-6 a. 2, 3, b. 4, c. 1, 5 18-7 d 18-8 a

18-3 a. 3, b. 3, c. 3, d. 4, e. 3, f. 3, g. 3, h. 4, i. 3, j. 4, k. 3, l. 3, gestational age 39 weeks 18-4 SGA 18-5 a. 3, b. 4, c. 1, d.

18-1 a. Desquamation b. Simian c. Gynecomastia d. Ophthalmia neonatorum e. Pallor f. Plethoric g. Thermoregulation. 18-2 c

REFERENCES

Ballard JL et al: A simplified score for assessment of fetal maturation or newly born infants, *J Pediatr* 95:769, 1979.

Brazelton TB: *Neonatal behavioral assessment scale,* ed 2, Philadelphia, 1984, JB Lippincott.

Dubowitz LMS et al: Clinical assessment of gestational age in the newborn infant, *J Pediatr* 77:1, 1970.

Hazle NR: Hydration in labor: is routine hydration necessary? *J Nurse Midwifery* 31:171, 1986.

Keppler AB: The use of intravenous fluids during labor, *Birth* 15(2):75, 1988.

Lubchenco LO: Assessment of gestational age and development at birth, *Pediatr Clin North Am* 17:125, 1970.

News, *Birth* 18:2, 1991.

 STUDENT RESOURCE SHELF

Seidel HM et al: *Mosby's guide to physical examination,* ed 2, St Louis, 1991, Mosby. This book provides an excellent general introduction to the skills needed for physical examination. It is extensively illustrated with interpretation of findings; however, the focus is not specifically on assessment of the newborn.

Scanlon JW et al: *A system of newborn physical examination,* Baltimore, 1979, University Park Press. This is the best manual for newborn physical assessment. It is comprehensive and will help the learner to interpret findings.

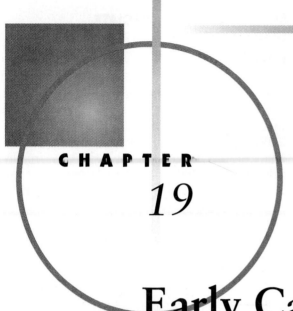

CHAPTER

19

Early Care of the Normal Newborn

KEY TERMS

Acrocyanosis
Apgar Score
Conduction
Convection
Desquamation
Evaporation
Grunting
Jaundice
Meconium
Ophthalmia
  Neonatorum
Pallor
Periodic Breathing
Plethora
Prepuce

Radiation
Rales
Smegma

Stridor
Thermoregulation

LEARNING OBJECTIVES

1. *Assess the infant's transition to extrauterine life on the basis of the Apgar score.*
2. *Recognize changes in reactivity and status during the first 24 hours of transition.*
3. *Describe supportive interventions to maintain temperature, circulation, respirations, and glucose levels.*
4. *Explain pros and cons regarding neonatal circumcision.*
5. *Describe components of feeding the newborn related to neurologic development, interactions between mother and infant, and problems in underfeeding or overfeeding.*
6. *Determine need for referrals on the basis of physical and psychosocial assessment.*
7. *Describe methods and parameters for evaluation of newborn health before discharge home.*
8. *Assess parental knowledge related to infant care before formulating a teaching plan.*

The nurse supports and assesses the normal newborn's body system adjustment in the transition period. In some birth settings it can be as long as 24 hours before a physician is required to examine a new baby. These first hours are crucial because multiple organ systems are making the transition from intrauterine to extrauterine functions. Nurses must be skilled enough to identify the baby who is having difficulty so that proper

therapy can be instituted. They also need to remember to protect themselves and their clients from communicable diseases by using universal precautions with barriers such as gloves until the normal newborn has the first bath.

Psychosocial support given during the early neonatal period coincides with the "maternal sensitive period" (Klaus and Kennell, 1982), during which infant-parent attachment begins. An environment that allows this process is vital in facilitating attachment. Families vary in their ability to recover from interruptions during this period. Although controversy continues regarding the importance of the maternal sensitive period, every attempt should be made to keep interruptions to a minimum. Assessment of infant-family interaction and parental knowledge regarding infant care must be performed before an individualized health education plan can be written.

Nursing Responsibilities for Care of the Newborn

Care given immediately after birth should be limited to measures necessary to support neonatal life, provide for identification of the neonate, and promote infant-parent attachment. All other interventions, such as eye prophylaxis, vitamin K administration, and extended physical examination should be postponed until the parents and infant have become acquainted.

The setting for the birth may vary, but materials needed for care during the immediate period do not. The following supplies are needed:
1. A radiant warmer with oxygen supply
2. Warmed blankets or towels
3. Materials for identification (footprint ink pad and sheet, name bands)
4. Suction apparatus: bulb syringe and wall suction with modified DeLee tray and catheters (size 8 and 10 French)
5. Stethoscope with neonatal bell and diaphragm
6. Plastic cord clamp (sterile)
7. Documentation forms

All materials may be placed on a cart or shelf for easy access but need not be visible. The radiant warmer should be turned on when a birth is imminent.

▶ ASSESSMENT OF IMMEDIATE TRANSITION

Apgar Score

In 1953 Virginia Apgar, an anesthesiologist, designed a tool for evaluating newborn infants. The **Apgar score** provides a quick assessment of an infant's immediate adjustment to birth, tells when an infant needs help, and indicates whether interventions have been successful. The score has limitations but is used in virtually all birth settings in this country. An assessment of five characteristics of adjustment is performed between 55 and 60 seconds after birth (the 1-minute score) and again at 5 minutes after birth. If problems continue, a 10-minute Apgar score is recorded as well (Table 19-1).

Low gestational age appears to invalidate the significance of Apgar scoring because prematurity affects the heart rate (higher), respiratory rate (more irregular), muscle tone (more flaccid), and reflex responses (less responsive). Nevertheless, the Apgar scoring method has led to significant changes in the ways newborns are supported in the crucial first few minutes. Five parameters are examined by an "independent" person, usually the nurse. Apgar scores should not be assigned by the person who delivers the infant because the score may be higher than warranted (Jepson et al, 1991). Scoring begins 55 seconds after birth, but one should not wait until 1 minute to begin assistance if it is obvious the baby is having a difficult first few seconds of transition. (See resuscitation methods in Chapter 28.)

Five parameters are examined and scored (Table 19-1) as follows:
1. *Heart rate:* Listen to the apical heart rate or palpate the pulsations of the umbilical cord. Do not count for a full minute; with experience you will know a dangerously slow heart rate almost instantly. Count 6 seconds and multiply by 10.

TABLE 19-1 Apgar Newborn Scoring System*

	SIGN	SCORE		
Acronym		0	1	2
A—Appearance	Heart rate	Not detectable	Below 100	Above 100
P—Pulse	Respiratory effort	Absent	Weak cry, hyperventilates	Good strong cry
G—Grimace	Muscle tone	Flaccid, limp	Some flexion of extremities	Well flexed
A—Attitude (tone)				
R—Respirations	Reflex irritability	No response	Grimace, some motion	Cough, sneeze, or cry
	Color	Blue, pale	Body, pink; extremities, blue (acrocyanosis)	Completely pink undertone

*If the child is not light skinned, alternative tests for color are applied, such as color of mucous membranes of mouth and conjunctiva, color of lips, palms, hands, and soles of feet.

2. *Respiratory effort:* You may count the respiratory rate by watching the infant's chest rise and fall, but it is best to assess air entry by auscultation. The normal neonate's irregular pattern of respiration may make it difficult to recognize weak, irregular respiratory effort. Observation for central cyanosis will help; the infant who has a pink tongue and mucous membranes has adequate oxygenation.

3. *Muscle tone:* Observe the position of the infant at rest. The full-term infant who is not distressed will be well flexed at the elbows and hips. Attempts to straighten the extremities will be met with some but not rigid resistance, and the extremity will recoil to its original flexion when released.

4. *Reflex irritability:* Observe the infant's reaction to suctioning or to stimulation of the sole of the foot. Either action should elicit a cry or at least a grimace. In practice the infant who has a heart rate over 100 beats/min, well-established respirations, good muscle tone, and pink or acrocyanotic color does not have to be stimulated to assess reflex irritability; any irritating stimuli such as drying with a towel will cause a cry, a grimace, or some motion. Assess the response to a catheter in the infant who is being resuscitated; crying, grimacing, and even pushing away tubes are signs of success.

5. *Color:* Observe the infant's peripheral (skin) and central (tongue and mucous membranes) color. Most infants are cyanotic for a short time after birth as drastic alterations in fetal circulation take place. The bluish color, termed **acrocyanosis,** may persist in the extremities. The face and trunk of the infant should show oxygenated color (pink undertone) after only a few respirations. Because brown-skinned babies may look "ashy" rather than cyanotic, the mucous membranes of the lips, mouth, and tongue are assessed for central cyanosis.

In the normal infant, the Apgar score often is 9 at 1 minute and 9 or 10 at 5 minutes (Figure 19-1). The lower the score the more acidotic the infant usually is; in addition, infants with lower scores have worsening cardiorespiratory function (see Asphyxia, Chapter 28). By 5 minutes of age, scores should improve markedly. A falling score or a 5-minute score below 7 indicates that neonatal intensive care must be instituted. (Refer to Chapter 28 for care.)

The 5-minute score is a better predictor of neurologic abnormality at 1 year, but the 1-minute score predicts survival more accurately (Jepson et al, 1991). The score's sensitivity is inadequate to predict acidosis because when the baby is in trouble, the adrenal hormones—*catecholamines*—may be elevated. These substances increase respiratory and heart rates and reflex responses in an effort to compensate for the acidosis. Thus it is apparent that, if catecholamines were elevated, the score result would improve. Yet the low *pH,* indicating metabolic acidosis, may be similar. (See Table 14-2 for a comparison of fetal acidity with the Apgar score.) In general, if the cord pH is over 7.24, the 1-minute score will be above 8. If the cord pH is 7.0 to 7.23, the score will be between 4 and 7. When pH is below 7.0, the infant is seriously acidotic, and the Apgar score will reflect a rating of 1 to 3 (Apgar et al, 1958).

▶ NURSING DIAGNOSES

Early nursing diagnoses that guide newborn care are as follows:

1. Ineffective thermoregulation related to limited ability to adjust to environmental temperature

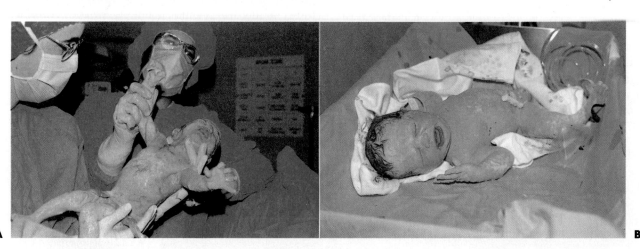

FIGURE 19-1 A, Note color and activity just after birth. **B,** Observe color of lips and mucous membranes on newborns rather than color of extremities. (Courtesy Marjorie Pyle, RNC, *Lifecircle.*)

2. Potential for aspiration or ineffective airway clearance related to early oropharyngeal mucus
3. Altered parenting related to attachment, preventing abduction
4. Risk of altered protection related to low production of immune factors; potential of low vitamin K resulting in increased bleeding rates
5. Altered nutrition: less than required related to delayed sucking, limited intake, or potential hypoglycemia

▶ EXPECTED OUTCOMES

1. Environmental temperature control methods to maintain infant core temperature
2. Respirations established; oxygenated color maintained
3. Protected from abduction or injury by parents and staff
4. Infection avoided as well as any untoward bleeding
5. Suck and swallow coordinated to enable adequate intake and avoid hypoglycemia, dehydration

▶ NURSING INTERVENTIONS

Maintenance of Respiration

Maintenance of a patent airway for respiration is a priority. As the infant's head is delivered, secretions are squeezed out of the mouth and nose by the pressure of the birth canal. The infant's airway may be occluded by respiratory secretions, mucus and blood from the maternal birth canal, or amniotic fluid mixed with meconium and vernix. To prevent aspiration the mouth and then the nose can be suctioned with a bulb syringe before the rest of the infant is delivered and the first breath is taken.

After the body is born, the infant is placed in a 15-degree, head-dependent, side-lying position to promote drainage of secretions. The infant is positioned either on the mother's abdomen or under a radiant warmer. Care is taken in positioning not to extend the infant's neck too far because overextension can cause compression of the soft trachea.

The oral airway is cleared first inasmuch as suctioning the nose stimulates a gasp that could cause aspiration of blood and mucus. In cases of infection (amnionitis), gastric aspirate is required as well. A sterile DeLee trap is used to suction the infant's stomach. At one time the strength of suction was controlled by the nurse using a plastic mouthpiece of the trap as a straw, but because of universal precautions against human immunodeficiency virus (HIV), the mouthpiece must be connected to low mechanical suction. Oversuction must be avoided. If the infant is breathing, has equal bilateral breath sounds, a heart rate in the normal range, and is pink to acrocyanotic, suctioning is stopped. The infant will complete airway clearance by coughing (Figure 19-2). This early suctioning is especially important in cases of suspected meconium aspiration or maternal serum hepatitis or HIV infection (MacDonald, 1990).

The following signs indicate that the airway has become clear:

- An irregular respiratory rate of 40 to 60 breaths/min with periods of apnea lasting less than 5 seconds
- Symmetric rise and fall of the chest and abdomen with each breath
- Absent or minimal nasal flaring, grunting, or retractions
- Pink mucous membranes and tongue (absence of central cyanosis)
- Spontaneous activity with good muscle tone—a reliable sign of adequate oxygenation

(See notes)

Maintenance of Circulation

A patent airway and adequate respiration are indicated by an apical heart rate of 110 to 160 beats/min easily heard on the left side of the chest near the nipple and absence of central cyanosis. Spontaneous activity with good muscle tone is a reliable sign of adequate oxygenation. Infants who cannot maintain *airway, breathing,* and *circulation (ABCs)* are at high risk and include those with low Apgar scores or other problems that interrupt this process.

Cord clamping. The cord stops pulsating as the first breaths reverse fetal circulation. Because it becomes

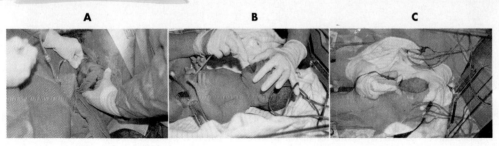

A   **B**   **C**

FIGURE 19-2 Suction equipment. **A,** Suctioning on the perineum with tubing attached to low suction at the wall. **B,** Suction of oropharynx with straight catheter. **C,** Suctioning with bulb syringe. (Courtesy Marjorie Pyle, RNC, *Lifecircle.*)

limp and a pulse cannot be felt through it, it does not need to be cut immediately. A reason for clamping and then cutting just after delivery is that it facilitates care in the warmer away from the mother. If, however, she is to hold the infant on her abdomen for a period of time, the cord may be clamped by the midwife and cut later. The possibility of transfusion of blood back into the placenta by gravity flow is another reason for clamping and cutting the cord just after delivery. For the same reason the baby should not be held for a long period below the perineum; this position could transfuse extra blood into the baby and cause a high hematocrit level (**plethora**) with associated jaundice (see Chapter 28).

Two metal hemostats are used to clamp the umbilical cord at delivery, and the cord is cut between them. The cord is examined for two arteries and one vein before the plastic clamp is applied. A sterile plastic or metal clamp is applied 2 cm from the skin. The clamp is not placed closer to the skin because if an intravenous infusion is needed for an ill infant, catheterization of the vessels in a cord that is too short is difficult.

(See notes)

Maintenance of Warmth

Thermoregulation is easily overlooked in the busy atmosphere of the birthing room. If the infant's core temperature is not maintained, the transition to extrauterine life can be compromised.

Four mechanisms cause heat loss. The first way in which an infant begins to lose heat is by **evaporation** of amniotic fluid and secretions. Drying with warmed towels or blankets not only removes these fluids but also provides tactile stimulation, which encourages continued respiration. Some units use large soft paper towels for first drying.

Heat loss by **conduction** to colder surfaces is controlled by placing the infant on the mother's abdomen or on a prewarmed bed and covering the baby with prewarmed blankets.

Heat loss by **radiation** to colder air masses is controlled by placing the infant under a radiant heat source or on the mother's abdomen. Because much body heat is lost through radiation from the head, covering the head with a warmed cap has been used (see Temperature Control).

Heat loss by **convection** is difficult to control because it necessitates limitation of air conditioning and other sources of air currents. There are thermal receptors on the face and body as well. The best way to control convective loss is to limit the number of persons attending the delivery and keep the environmental temperature as warm as possible.

Many nursing actions are available to prevent heat loss. The least heat loss occurs when the infant is dried promptly, the cord clamped, and the infant is placed in a warmed incubator. Because this procedure does not allow for bonding, other methods have developed. The use of an overhead radiant warmer is standard care in the birthing room and delivery room (Figure 19-3). Skin-to-skin maternal contact is also a way to warm the infant whose body is dry and head is covered. Greer (1988) compared use of an insulated bonnet, a stockinette cap, and no head covering in a birth setting where a radiant warmer was used. Her results showed that the stockinette cap was the least useful in maintaining heat, perhaps because the wet hair transmitted moisture to the cap, and evaporation continued. Mean rectal heat loss was between 0.65° F and 1.2° F in each case with use of the same radiant overhead warmer. Her conclusion was that when a radiant heater was used, a

— monitor temp q 1-2°

If all 4 mech. of heat loss have been v'd & infant cont. to loose heat – must check environmental factors

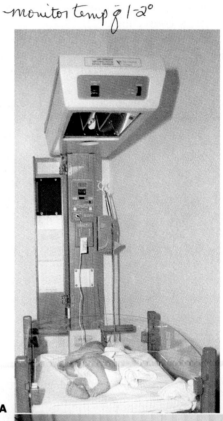

FIGURE 19-3 A, Overhead warmer. **B,** Birth weight obtained quickly to prevent chilling. Note large amount of vernix on infant. (Courtesy Marjorie Pyle, RNC, *Lifecircle*.)

stockinette cap should not be used. On the basis of this research, it may be wise not to use a stockinette cap until after the bath, when the hair is completely dry and the baby is in an open crib.

In our setting, babies were persistently cold under the overhead radiant warmer. It took some investigation to realize that the ceiling air-conditioning vent delivered cold air at an angle to disperse the warm air. We then used clear plastic food wrap placed over the sides and top to shield the baby's body until engineering services could adapt the vent flow.

Some suggestions for nursing care to prevent heat loss after birth include the following.

1. Birth rooms should be warmer than most customarily are. Doors should be shut and personnel limited to reduce convection.
2. Radiant warmer hoods may be placed above the baby and mother while the initial bonding period occurs; however, the mother may become too warm.
3. Infant should be dried well with warmed, large, soft paper towels and then cocoon-wrapped in one or two warmed baby blankets and placed by the mother's side or on her abdomen.
4. Head should be uncovered or an insulated bonnet applied if infant is under a radiant warmer. If a warmer is not used, an insulated bonnet or blanket loosely covering the scalp will reduce loss from evaporation and convection.
5. Oxygen should be administered by tube (not mask) held close to the baby's nose only for as long as needed. Oxygen is cold and will trigger the many receptors on the face.

Initiation of Infant-Parent Attachment

Assisting the new family in the acquaintance process is an important part of maternal-infant nursing care. The bonding process begins before birth (see Chapter 8). Ideally, the nurse facilitates the following measures to encourage further bonding:

1. Skin-to-skin and eye-to-eye contact
2. Privacy and comfort for both parents
3. Initial breast-feeding if desired

The first hour of life is an ideal time for initial infant-parent interaction because the infant is quiet and alert and may be eager to nurse or at least may make an attempt to nurse.

Skin-to-skin contact is promoted by encouraging the mother to hold the infant. In some settings the infant is

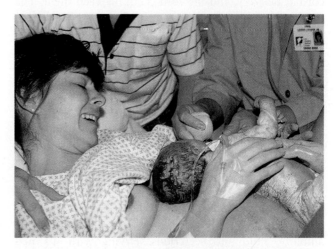

FIGURE 19-4 Skin-to-skin contact while suctioning is done allows the mother the opportunity to "claim" her baby. (Courtesy Marjorie Pyle, RNC, *Lifecircle*.)

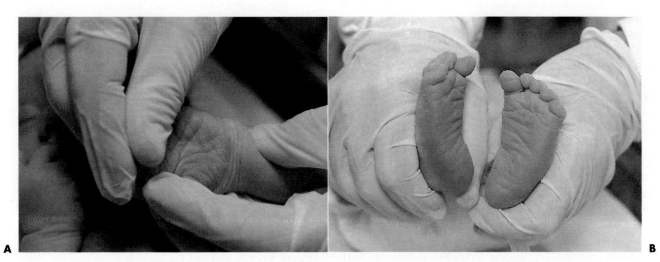

A   B

FIGURE 19-5 Check normal creases on hand (**A**) and sole (**B**) when doing footprints. (From Seidel HM et al: *Mosby's guide to physical examination*, ed 2, St Louis, 1991, Mosby.)

immediately placed on the mother's abdomen after birth. (An overhead radiant warmer should be used if there is concern about thermal environment.)

Infants who are breast-fed during the first hour of life are more likely to continue breast-feeding longer (Klaus and Kennell, 1982). During this period the nurse observes for signs of positive interaction, keeping in mind individual variations in behavior. This behavior includes hesitant touching that progresses to more confident touching, *en face* contact, expressions of approval, comparing baby with other family members, and calling the baby by name (Figure 19-4).

Identification

Identification (ID) of each newborn infant always takes place in the immediate neonatal period before the mother and infant are separated. Prints of the newborn's soles and the mother's right index finger are placed on the "footprint sheet" (Figure 19-5). This document also contains other information such as the date and time of birth, mother and infant's hospital numbers, and the infant's sex, race, weight, and length, as well as the signature of the person by whom it was completed (Figure 19-6).

Parents enjoy receiving a copy of this form. Hospitals may use only ID bands today because newborn footprints have not been as useful as expected in later identification. A set of name bands with preprinted matching identification numbers also is affixed to the infant's wrist or ankle and the mother's wrist. If mother and infant are separated at any time, the matching preprinted numbers are used to verify the infant's identity on discharge (Figure 19-7).

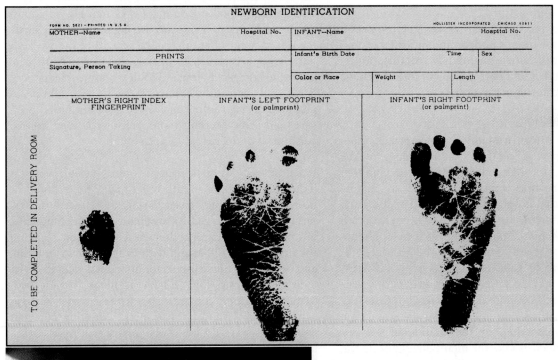

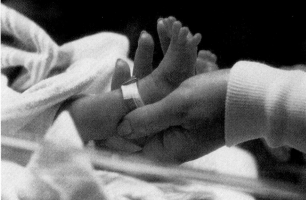

FIGURE 19-6 A, Identification process with footprint and mother's right index fingerprint. **B,** Hospital band on baby's ankle. (**B** courtesy St John's Mercy Medical Center, St Louis, Mo.)

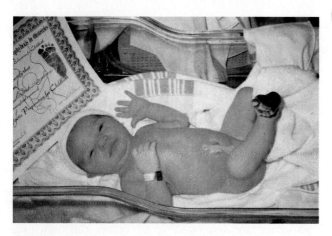

FIGURE 19-7 Footprinted and banded, this healthy newborn is ready to meet the world. Note hat for warmth. (Courtesy BL Silverman.)

These methods of identification are not foolproof, however; prints are often smudged and unreadable, and bands can fall off. When an infant's identification is questioned, blood and tissue typing or other genetic markers are used for confirmation.

Preventing Abduction

Infant abduction from hospitals has happened, especially where there is rooming-in. According to the National Center for Missing and Exploited Children (NCMEC), in the first 6 months of 1991 six infants were abducted from hospitals in the United States. Each year 12 to 18 infants are abducted. The typical case involves an "unknown," almost always female, abductor who impersonates a nurse, hospital employee, volunteer, or relative to gain access to a baby. NCMEC guidelines explain: "Because there is generally easier access to a patient's room than to the newborn nursery and a newborn infant spends increasingly more time with mother rather than in the traditional nursery setting, most abductors take the infant directly from the mother's arms" (News, *Birth,* 1992.)

Without frightening the mother, the nurse must provide specific precautions:

1. Do not leave the infant alone in the room.
2. Be alert for unidentified visitors—every hospital employee should wear an ID displayed on the uniform.
3. Check ID bands when the infant is returned to or brought from nursery.

Several hospitals have instituted bands with beeper alarms that are activated if the baby is illegally carried out of the maternity unit. These beepers are removed at the discharge hour in the mother's presence. If the mother is discharged before the baby, she keeps her ID bracelet and shows it when the infant is discharged.

Pulse and Blood Pressure

An infant with a pulse in the normal range (100 to 150 beats/min) with an underlying pink skin tone and mucous membranes should have sufficient oxygen, which the nurse usually can check at a glance. Cyanosis will develop if oxygen tension falls below 50 mm Hg pressure. (The normal range is above 70 to 80.) Cyanosis first appears around the mouth (circumoral) and then spreads to the face and trunk before appearing in extremities. A baby may turn "dusky," with a grayish undertone to the skin. Periods of apnea may occur in some seemingly normal newborns. If this occurs, the infant should be quickly stimulated to see if the color "pinks up." Oxygen and suction equipment are placed in each nursery but not in each mother's room.

Newborn blood pressure is taken initially in an upper and lower extremity to compare pressures, which should be equal. (See Table 18-1 for the normal range.) The average blood pressure is 68/41 mm Hg on admission to the nursery. Pressures are higher just after birth, then drop somewhat, and stabilize within the week. A baby who becomes pale during sleep or a baby with **pallor** may have a lower blood volume. Hematocrit levels will indicate anemia and low blood volume. A **plethoric** (ruddy) infant may have a higher blood pressure and may become more jaundiced than normal because of an increased blood volume.

Respirations. Nasal passages should be clear, which is indicated by lack of mouth breathing. There should be no respiratory effort, nasal flaring, or retractions. Respirations are observed by watching the diaphragmatic line between chest and abdomen. After the initial period the rate averages 30 to 60, with irregularities in rhythm and depth. The nurse listens for abnormal sounds. **Rales** indicate amniotic fluid still in the lungs. **Stridor** indicates inspiratory constriction of the larynx perhaps caused by too vigorous suctioning. **Grunting** indicates expiratory phase closure of the larynx that raises alveolar pressure, a classic sign of respiratory distress. **Periodic breathing** is a more irregular rate and rhythm accompanied by periods of apnea of 5 to 15 seconds. A baby with repeated episodes of periodic breathing should be followed up because of a related risk of sudden infant death syndrome (SIDS) (see Chapter 28).

Temperature. Monitoring of the infant's temperature continues, usually on a schedule of every 1 to 2 hours in the first 4 hours of life. Axillary or inguinal sites are preferable to rectal (Figure 19-8). Rectal temperatures measured only 2.5 cm into the rectum may not be an accurate core temperature, and deeper insertion increases the possibility of trauma to rectal mucosa and stimulation of the vagus nerve, which can cause bradycardia.

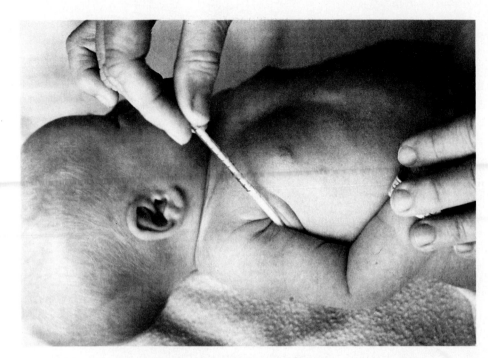

FIGURE 19-8 Taking axillary temperature. (Courtesy John Young.)

Located lateral to the femoral artery, the femoral inguinal site has many advantages over the rectal or axillary. There is no brown adipose tissue here as in the axillary site, the tissues come together more firmly, and the thermometer registers accurately within 5 minutes. In a recent series of studies, it has been shown that there is little difference between axillary and rectal temperature in the newborn. The mean differences range from 0.2° F by axillary and rectal sites and 0.8° F for inguinal and rectal sites. Axillary temperature took longer to reach maximum temperature (11 minutes) but rose only 0.1° F after 5 to 6 minutes (Bliss-Holtz, 1989). On the basis of these findings, a 5-minute limit for temperature taken in the axillary or inguinal site with a glass and mercury thermometer is adequate. The site should be noted and the fact acknowledged that inguinal temperatures average 0.2° F lower than axillary and 0.8° F lower than rectal. With an electronic thermometer the time of register is significantly shorter.

The infant usually is maintained under an overhead warmer until axillary temperature approaches 97.8° or 98.0° F. Then the first complete bath is given under the warmer. If the infant's temperature is higher, the nurse investigates dehydration first and then looks at the environmental temperature. Often, feeding the infant will bring the temperature down to the normal range. Signs of infection should be considered as well (review Chapter 18). A persistent low temperature should be investigated; one reason is hypoglycemia. In addition, environmental temperature and sources of convection should be checked.

Hypoglycemia and Early Feeding

In birthing rooms and in labor, delivery, and recovery rooms, the infant is put to the breast as soon as the mother is ready. Then, after about 1 hour the sleep phase begins, and the infant is fed again on awakening. Routines of feeding every 4 hours were adhered to when one or two nurses had a nursery population of 10 to 20 babies to feed. With rooming-in or LDRP the mother keeps a record of feeding times *on infant demand* and records intake and output (see Nutrition in this chapter). The system involves the parents immediately, promotes bonding, and allows staff members to assess for problems before early discharge.

Testing for hypoglycemia. Tests for whole blood glucose and calcium levels are performed on any infant who is small for gestational age (SGA) or large for gestational age (LGA), an infant of a diabetic mother (IDM), or an infant who was stressed during labor and delivery. Some of the signs of a hypoglycemic infant are hypothermia, tremors, high-pitched cry, cyanosis, and respiratory distress.   *a common problem*

Any baby who seems slow in transition in color, temperature, or neurologic state may be tested at the nurse's discretion. In this case testing follows a schedule of 30 to 60 minutes after birth, then every hour for 4 hours, and then every 4 hours for 24 hours. (For technique, see Figure 19-18.)

Infants with hypocalcemia exhibit signs similar to those seen with hypoglycemia. Blood levels are measured by means of a sample sent to the laboratory.

PROCEDURE 19-1   Eye Prophylaxis

- Within 1 hour of birth, wash infant's face with mild soap and water to remove maternal blood and body fluids and to reduce the risk of hepatitis B virus (HBV) and human immunodeficiency virus (HIV) transmission via mucous membrane.
- Dry the face.
- Place forefinger on ridge of eyebrow and thumb on cheekbone, and spread eyelid to expose subconjunctival sac.
- Place a *1 to 2 cm ribbon* of antibiotic into each conjunctival sac and gently close the eyelid. Wait for 1 minute, and wipe off excess ointment from the eyelid or 2 drops of silver nitrate 1% and flush eye with saline after 1 minute.

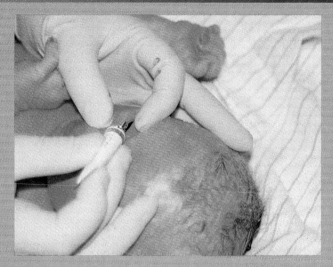

FIGURE 19-9 Eye prophylaxis. Instillation of 1 cm ophthalmic erythromycin ointment into subconjunctival sac for prevention of chlamydia and gonorrhea. Note that nurse is wearing gloves. (Courtesy Marjorie Pyle, RNC, *Lifecircle*.)

•   •   •

OPTIONAL ACTIVITY: Write a sample nursing note correctly documenting the performance of this procedure.

Hypoglycemia or hypocalcemia will delay an infant's discharge. Care is discussed in Chapter 28.

Test Yourself

- What is the schedule for testing a 10-lb newborn infant for hypoglycemia? Would you report a finding of 60 mg/dl?
- What additional information should you collect to evaluate an infant whose glucose capillary strip read below 45 mg/dl?

Eye Prophylaxis (Procedure 19-1)

Eye prophylaxis is mandated within 1 hour of birth in the United States to prevent **ophthalmia neonatorum.** The newborn may become infected with microorganisms during the descent through the vaginal canal at birth. Because 4 million women each year report symptoms of *Chlamydia trachomatis* and 2 million cases of gonorrhea are diagnosed each year (Hammerschlag et al, 1991), universal prophylaxis effective for both infections is now standard practice.

Test Yourself

- Why is erythromycin ointment recommended for newborn eye prophylaxis instead of silver nitrate?

Silver nitrate 1% is still used in some places, but antibiotic ointments are standard in the United States because these ointments are effective against both infections (Drug Profiles 19-1 and 19-2). Untreated infections and inadequately treated infections result in classic signs—swollen, bruised-looking eyelids with yellow exudate—that can result in corneal damage and blindness if left untreated (see Figure 25-2).

Before discharge, parents should be taught about the difference between the chemical conjunctivitis caused by treatment and inflammation from inadequately treated conjunctivitis. Chemical conjunctivitis causes some edema and inflammation that will subside within 48 hours. Inadequately treated conjunctivitis will progress with increasing amounts of exudate, and parents should contact a pediatrician for the baby to receive repeat treatment before complications occur.

Eye prophylaxis is delayed until after bonding has been initiated because the irritation can disrupt initial infant-parent eye contact. However, within 1 hour of birth the nurse should administer the medication. Improper technique is thought to be responsible for many cases of inadequately treated ophthalmia neonatorum.

Drug Profile 19-1

Silver nitrate 1%
Action

Disrupts cell membrane of susceptible organisms. Not effective against *Chlamydia* organisms.

Dosage

1 to 2 drops in each conjunctival sac—do not drop on cornea. Wait 1 minute and flush eye with normal saline then wipe each eyelid with cotton ball.

Side effects/adverse reactions

Periorbital edema. May stain skin. Chemical conjunctivitis occurs in 90% within first 48 hours.

Nursing considerations

Protect wax ampules from heat. Timing important—do within 1 hour of birth.
Wear gloves for procedure.

Drug Profile 19-2

Erythromycin ophthalmic ointment 0.5% (Ilotycin)
Available in single-dose tube

Tetracycline ophthalmic ointment 1%

Chlortetracycline ophthalmic ointment 1% (Achromycin ophthalmic 1%) Available in single-dose tube

Action

Bacteriostatic, bactericidal, inhibits protein synthesis. Must be used within 1 hour of birth. Effective against *Chlamydia* and gonorrhea.

Dosage

Instill 1 to 2 cm ribbon of ointment into subconjunctival sac. Wait 1 minute, then wipe excess off lid.

Side effects/adverse effects

Chemical conjunctivitis in about 20% lasting 24 to 48 hours.

Nursing considerations

Inadequate instillation may result in inflammation with organisms beginning about 3 days. Inform mother to observe and report. Be sure to wash maternal blood off face and eyes before manipulating eyelids. Wear gloves. Observe for hypersensitivity.

PROCEDURE 19-2   Vitamin K Injection

- The infant should be bathed before the skin is punctured to prevent tracking HBV or HIV into the tissues. An alternate choice is to use chlorhexidine (Hibiclens) solution for cleansing the site (Ross and Dickason, 1992). Alcohol is ineffective against these viruses unless it is allowed to dry on the skin for a full minute (MacDonald, 1990).
- Select site by measuring distance from trochanter to knee. Place in center with site in the midanterior portion of the thigh (vastus lateralis muscle).
- Prevent movement by pressing on knee with lower palm while grasping muscle with thumb and forefinger of other hand.
- The intramuscular (IM) injection is administered with a 1-ml syringe with a 25-gauge ⅝-inch needle (Figure 19-10). Observe for signs of bleeding from the site.

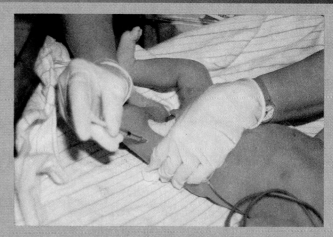

FIGURE 19-10 Vitamin K injection into midanterior lateral thigh. (Courtesy Marjorie Pyle, RNC, *Lifecircle*.)

• • •

OPTIONAL ACTIVITY: Write a sample nursing note correctly documenting the performance of this procedure.

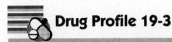

Drug Profile 19-3

Vitamin K (phytonadione)
(Aquamephyton, Konakion)

Action

Vitamin essential in the coagulation cycle

Dosage

Instill 0.5 to 1 mg by IM injection any time during the first 6 hours of life. Administer IM into the midanterior thigh (vastus lateralis muscle), using a tuberculin syringe and 25-gauge, ⅝-inch needle.

Adverse reactions

Sweating, flushing, erythema, pain, edema or hematoma at injection site

Nursing considerations

Observe for signs of oozing from cord or petechiae or postcircumcision bleeding.

Vitamin K

Hemorrhagic disease of the newborn (HDNB) is a result of a deficiency of prothrombin and other clotting factors. Vitamin K–dependent factors are low in the newborn. The vitamin is produced in the bowel by means of bacterial flora that are initially low in newborns and continue to be so in those infants being breast-fed. Infants who are breast-fed exclusively have different bacterial colonization (Faucher and Jackson, 1992).

A routine procedure is to administer 1 mg of vitamin K within 6 hours of birth (Drug Profile 19-3). Vitamin K may cross the placenta, and some have used it in mothers in the last week of pregnancy with expected preterm births. In the United States, however, parenteral vitamin K is used for newborns (Procedure 19-2). A number of countries give oral vitamin K_1, 1 mg, or vitamin K_2, 5 mg. Research comparing the two methods has not been definitive (Faucher and Jackson, 1992).

Hepatitis prophylaxis. The Centers for Disease Control (CDC) recommend hepatitis B vaccination (HBV) to begin for newborns within 48 hours of birth (CDC, 1991). Infants born to mothers with hepatitis B positivity are also given hepatitis B immunoglobulin (HBIG) within 12 hours of birth (see Chapter 25 and Table 19-5).

▶ EVALUATION

1. Did infant maintain a stable temperature in an open crib?

2. Was infant well acquainted and safe with parents?
3. Were all medications administered and lab tests completed?
4. Did infant get established with feedings?

Daily Care of the Neonate

Nursing responsibilities include preparing the parent for care of the newborn. With short hospital stays this instruction must include written material and video-taped programs. Whenever the nurse is with the client, some instruction should take place. When the baby is at the bedside, instruction is facilitated. At a minimum the mother should know bathing, cord care, circumcision and perineal care, and nutrition and elimination requirements, as well as infant behavior, characteristics, and signs of problems. There is much a new parent must learn; with the current early discharges much of this knowledge must be gained at home. The nurse, however, should maximize the limited time with the new parents to equip them with the knowledge and resources they will need to feel confident at home.

Universal precautions until 1st complete bath!

HYGIENE

The infant does not have protective skin flora at birth and is exposed to a variety of infectious agents. Abrasions from forceps or fetal scalp electrode, as well as the wound on the tip of the umbilical stump, can provide entry points for such agents. The newborn has passive immunity from the mother, but this immunity will not protect against all organisms. Acquired agents such as HIV may be transmitted to the infant or to medical staff personnel from the mother's blood and fluids on the baby's skin. Therefore all supplies used in care of newborns must be medically clean and not interchanged with other infants' supplies. Universal precautions require the use of gloves until the newborn has been bathed and for contact with blood such as occurs in drawing capillary samples.

Recommendations for skin care during the neonatal period have changed. Previously, dry care was advised; the infant was washed only as necessary for the first days to preserve the protective function of the vernix caseosa. However, the possible presence of HIV in maternal body fluids has led to the complete bathing of neonates soon after birth, with careful attention to stabilization of body temperature. Sponge baths are used thereafter to keep the cord dry until it is detached. At birth and after the cord falls off, infants may be immersed in water and usually express pleasure at being in water again.

First bath (Procedure 19-3)

The first bath has assumed new importance because of universal precautions. Because of rising numbers of

PROCEDURE 19-3   **First Bath**

Nurse protection: Waterproof gown and gloves.

- *Preparation:* Determine that axillary temperature is above 97.8° F (36.5° C). Under radiant warmer set at 36.5° C, place disposable pad under baby.
- *Equipment:* Plastic disposable bath basin, warm water (access to running water adjacent to warmer is helpful), gauze squares, disposable washcloth or sponge. (Some units save Hibiclens sponges with soft plastic brushes for the hair wash; others use small combs.) Two warm blankets, one for a towel, or use large, soft paper toweling.
- *Soap:* Ideal is Hibiclens diluted to 4% to 5%. Alternative choice is a mild soap that does not change skin pH.
- *Face:* Wash face with soap and water; infant will not open eyes. Rinse once. Lingering antiseptic may be beneficial. In some studies Hibiclens was not rinsed, with no untoward effect (Cowan et al, 1979).
- *Body:* With some small amount of friction, soap entire body, paying attention to creases where blood may linger.

- *Rinse:* You may immerse infant in warm water (some have suggested a small shower head) or liberally squeeze water from sponge onto infant. In any case, rinse water should be clean (do not put soapy cloth or sponge into the water). Lift infant out of water onto towel and dry thoroughly.
- *Wrap:* Wrap the body in a cocoon wrap.
- *Hair:* With sponge or gauze squares, soap hair, scrubbing firmly to remove all blood and mucus from hair. Rinse and dry hair as much as possible.
- *Rewarming:* Infant may remain under the radiant warmer for ½ to 1 hour—in this case, unwrap body and attach servomechanism temperature probe. Or infant, completely dressed, may be placed into a crib with a stockinette cap and double blanket. Temperature should be rechecked ½ to 1 hour after the bath. The skilled nurse can complete this bath in a very short period, protecting the infant from chilling.

• • •

OPTIONAL ACTIVITY: Write a sample nursing note correctly documenting the performance of this procedure.

women with HIV and HBV, use *baby universal precautions* to protect the baby as much as possible from the maternal virus that may be transmitted during the birth process (MacDonald, 1990).

Removing birth blood and fluids from the infant's skin is the first line of defense in the postbirth period. This should be done before eye medications (less than 1 hour) or parenteral medication (up to 6 hours) after birth. If the complete bath must be delayed because of unstable body temperature, then only the face is washed before eye medication is instilled. By 6 hours the temperature should have stabilized enough to wash the infant under an overhead radiant warmer.

Bathing at Home

Until the cord detaches, a sponge bath is given. The sequence is the same as the complete bath; hair washing

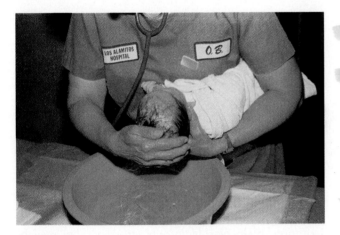

FIGURE 19-11 In daily care wash hair after bath to prevent heat loss from wet scalp. (Courtesy Marjorie Pyle, RNC, *Lifecircle*.)

is done last (Figure 19-11). Because parents tend to use too much soap, they should be instructed to use very little of a mild soap. The room in which the bath is given should be warm, without drafts. All bathing articles and the infant's change of clothes should be available before bathing begins. Parents should be shown how to safely handle the infant during the bath (Figure 19-12). The tub bath can be a time for sociability. Many parents find that the evening bath relaxes the baby before sleep. This routine carries through effectively for the older infant. The father may be more available to help, and this can be a special time for him and the infant.

Any safe receptacle may be used for a tub. If the kitchen sink is used, it first must be scrubbed. Place a soft towel on the bottom of the sink or use a "bath raft," a sponge pad to support the baby. Some parents use a commercially obtained tub, but its usefulness is brief because the baby grows so fast. Water must be tested for temperature and the infant protected against chilling. *✱ TEST c̄ Elbow NOT your hand*

CORD CARE

After the first bath the cord stump and clamp may be painted with a bacteriostatic agent such as alcohol or Triple Dye (a mix of brilliant green, proflavine, hemisulfate, and crystal violet), which colors the cord and adjacent skin dark purple. Daily care in the nursery involves application of Triple Dye or alcohol (protocol varies) and folding the diaper under the cord stump to prevent wetting from urine.

The plastic clamp is removed when the cord appears shriveled and drier, usually on the second day (Figure 19-13). In cases of early discharge the cord clamp may be kept on until the cord falls off; it does no harm. The

Nail trimming is contraindicated 1ˢᵗ few days of life. Nail separates from tips ā about a week. Then need to be trimmed c̄ blunt ended cuticle scissors

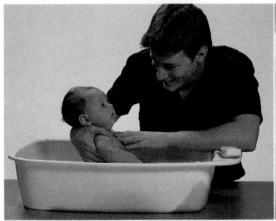
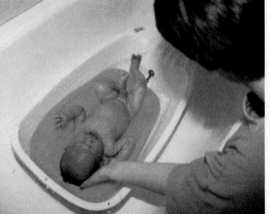

A   B

FIGURE 19-12 **A,** Bathing baby. **B,** Bathing using sponge mat for safety. (A courtesy Ross Laboratories, Columbus, Ohio; B courtesy M Schult.)

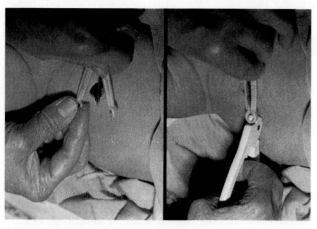

FIGURE 19-13 Plastic cord clamp is removed when cord is dry. (Courtesy Marjorie Pyle, RNC, *Lifecircle*.)

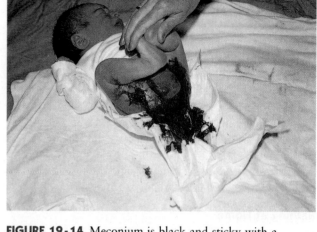

FIGURE 19-14 Meconium is black and sticky with a consistency like peanut butter. (Courtesy Marjorie Pyle, RNC, *Lifecircle*.)

mother should be told that there may be a small oozing site where the stump separated. She should be instructed to keep the stump clean and continue to swab alcohol over it after each diaper change. The cord usually will fall off after about 10 to 14 days. If it remains soft and red or begins to have a foul odor, the infant should be checked by the primary care provider. *Omphalitis* is an infection of the umbilical cord that begins with these color and odor changes, is potentially dangerous, and can lead to septicemia.

ELIMINATION

Meconium usually is passed within the first 24 hours and is characteristically dark greenish black (Figure 19-14). As feeding is established, meconium stools gradually are replaced by a stool that is light greenish brown (transitional stool). Gradual change in the color and consistency of the stool varies with the type of feeding (breast- or bottle-feeding). A breast-fed infant may pass four or more variable stools in 24 hours but also may have as little as one stool in 3 days. The stool may be looser and more pasty than that of bottle-fed infants and will reflect changes in the mother's diet. As long as stool is not hard and has a characteristic consistency and color, a variable pattern is acceptable.

Bottle-fed infants have stools that are firmer and stronger smelling. Constipation and diarrhea usually occur with other signs such as fever, vomiting, and anorexia.

Most infants void within the first 12 hours and will wet six to eight diapers a day. Actual urine output varies with intake. Parents should understand the connection between intake and output (i.e., that more concentrated urine means that the infant needs more fluids).

PERINEAL HYGIENE

Cloth or paper diapers may be used. Diaper changes should be done with each feeding and as necessary. The perineal area should be cleansed from front to back, using a wash cloth with plain water or a commercial cleansing wipe. A soap that removes normal skin flora should not be used. Although **smegma** may be gently washed off, it has a protective function and can remain. The use of plastic diaper covers that prevent air circulation should be avoided. If cloth diapers are used, "breathable covers" are satisfactory. To protect from irritation, plain petroleum jelly (from a tube) may be applied after the skin is dry. If a rash develops, a zinc oxide ointment is recommended.

CIRCUMCISION

Circumcision is a surgical procedure that involves separating and excising the prepuce from the glans penis; it allows exposure of the glans for easier cleaning. Circumcision has been practiced in many cultures throughout history, often as a coming-of-age ritual. Arabs, Jews, and many Christians base the practice of circumcision on religious principles. North and South American Indians, African groups, Australian aborigines, and many Pacific Islanders use circumcision as well (Gelbaum, 1992). Most families from the Orient and parts of Europe do not. The rates in Europe, England, and Scandinavia are about 1%. The current rate in the United States is about 50%; circumcision is the most commonly performed operation on males today (Gelbaum, 1992).

Issues

Opponents of routine neonatal circumcision note that they are advocates of choice; the newborn has no choice. They state that it is a human rights issue. According to the National Organization of Circumcision Information Resource Center, "There is perinatal encoding of the brain with violence, excruciating pain, interruption of maternal-infant bonding, betrayal of infant trust, and denial of the right to a sexually intact body by genitalia mutilation, as well as the right to individual religious freedom to choose" (Milos and Macris, 1992). Proponents cite religious beliefs, hygiene, and possible decreases in infection (Table 19-2).

How can the parents decide? For some the decision is made before birth. For others the decision is made for them, because of number of insurance companies and public hospitals have stopped paying for or doing newborn circumcisions, even by request, as a cost-cutting measure (Poland, 1990).

In 1989 the American Academy of Pediatrics changed its position and now supports routine circumcision because increased data suggested some medical benefits. Urologists have contributed data that indicate about 10% of males will require later circumcision for various reasons. In addition, uncircumcised males have developed penile cancer at rates two times that of circumcised males. Yet penile cancer is rare. Studies of urinary tract and sexually transmitted infection rates have shown conflicting results. A new report (Gelbaum, 1992) states that there is an increased incidence of HIV in the uncircumcised male, perhaps because the virus can linger behind the foreskin. Human papillomavirus has been implicated in increased rates of cervical cancer in the sexual partners of infected men who are uncircumcised.

Risks

Risks of the procedure are about 0.25% for any complication. Most are minor and result from lack of skill of the physician. Serious complications are rare and involve bleeding in unrecognized cases of hemophilia, infection, or surgical trauma (Gelbaum, 1992). Since 1948 there have been only three recorded circumcision-related deaths of newborns (AAP task force, 1989).

Contraindications

A sick, premature, or poorly adjusting infant should not be considered for circumcision. Boys with *hypospadias,* an opening of the meatus on the underside of the penis, may need the foreskin for future repair of the defect and should not be circumcised at birth. A boy with a very small penis also should not be circumcised.

Care

Parents who do not want their son to be circumcised need to know how to give penile care and teach their son penile self-care later. Knowledge of the development of the foreskin and glans helps this process. As the foreskin begins to develop, it grows from the base of the glans toward the tip. It is composed of inner and outer layers of skin, which adhere to the glans and protect the end of the penis. Small areas of separation begin to develop during the third trimester of pregnancy. Total separation of these layers is necessary before the foreskin can be completely retracted from the penis, usually by 3 to 4 years of age.

Parents are concerned about smegma, which is a harmless sterile material formed by the normal sloughing of the epithelial cells as the prepuce gradually

---

TABLE 19-2 Reasons to Proceed with or to Avoid Neonatal Circumcision

REASONS TO PERFORM NEONATAL CIRCUMCISION	REASONS NOT TO PERFORM NEONATAL CIRCUMCISION
HEALTH	
Penile cancer is more common if not done	Rates of penile cancer are extremely low
Cervical cancer is more common in female partners if men have human papilloma virus (HPV)	Conflicting evidence; admit some HPV involvement but advocate other ways to treat
Facilitates better hygiene	Removes natural protection of sensitive glans
May decrease urinary tract infections and balanitis	Minor infections are treatable
Procedure done early is less traumatic	Infants feel and remember pain; encode trauma, upset; breaks trust
RELIGION AND CULTURE	
Religious requirement or custom for Arabs, Jews, and many Christians	Should allow child to choose
Boy will develop sexual and cultural identity with father if he is circumcised	Some state it reduces sexual pleasure

Data from American Academy of Pediatrics task force, 1989; Gelbaum, 1992; Poland, 1990.

Cultural Aspects of Care

I remember the day of my son's briss. It was hot and sunny and 50 well-wishers were crammed into my small house. I chose to remain in the next room, and as I handed him over to my best friend, I thought of the meaning of this 5000-year-old ritual. I wished that it did not involve pain for my baby, but I embraced it as a physical, visual acceptance of the covenant and the beginning of Adam's life as a Jewish boy and man. Our family grew closer on that day, both to each other and to our heritage.

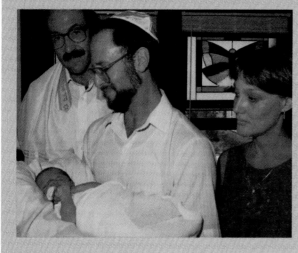

separates from the glans. The uncircumcised penis is cared for as is the rest of the body. Only the exposed surface should be cleaned until gradual separation of the foreskin from the glans is completed. The foreskin should not be forcibly retracted to cleanse the underlying surface. *Paraphimosis,* a condition in which the foreskin cannot be replaced, will cause pain and edema. Medical help must be sought.

The question of circumcision should be discussed with parents during the prenatal period. If this has not been done, the nurse will need to take the time to listen and provide information so they can make a decision. Parents who choose to have their son circumcised need to know about the procedure, which usually is performed in the hospital on the second day. With early discharge, circumcision may take place later.

For the Jewish male infant a ritual circumcision known as a *briss* occurs on the eighth day of life to celebrate the covenant between God and the Jewish people (see Cultural Aspects of Care). Women, including the baby's mother, have traditionally been banned from the room. In recent times, however, all adult family members and guests are included. There is special attention and love directed to the mother during this time.

The ceremony is performed by a *mohel,* a person trained in both the religious and surgical aspects of

briss. Some mohels require the bilirubin be no higher than 8 mg before they will perform the circumcision. If the infant is still in the hospital, the ceremony can be arranged there. The actual ceremony is quite short, with the principal honor being given to the *sondek* (godfather), who holds the infant during the procedure. The infant is swaddled in clean, white garments. Afterward the baby is placed in his father's arms and given sweet wine on clean gauze.

Methods

To prevent possible vomiting the infant is not fed for 1 hour before circumcision. His hunger may add to his discomfort and irritability. A molded plastic "circ board" is used to restrain him when the procedure is done in the hospital (Figure 19-15).

The plastibel method uses a plastic ring placed between the glans and prepuce and secured with a suture. The prepuce is then removed, and the plastibel remains in place until it falls off spontaneously, in about 10 days (Figure 19-16).

The Gomco method uses a bell-shaped apparatus that is fitted over the glans. A ring is then placed over the prepuce and tightened for 3 to 5 minutes. The prepuce is then excised. Gauze coated with petroleum jelly is wound around the penis. This gauze usually falls off within a day.

Although little attention has been paid to neonatal pain during any procedures, it is increasingly unacceptable to circumcise an infant without the use of anesthesia. Use of pacifiers and audiotapes of music and maternal heart beats during painful procedures has led to reduced crying but may not reduce pain during circumcisions and heel sticks. Marchette et al (1991) found significant elevations in heart rate and systolic blood pressure, with reductions in transcutaneous oxygen values, during the invasive steps of the procedure. These changes indicate pain response, and it seems

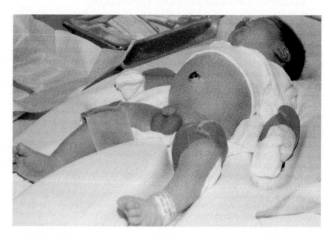

FIGURE 19-15 "Circ board" restrains infant during circumcision. (Courtesy Marjorie Pyle, RNC, *Lifecircle.*)

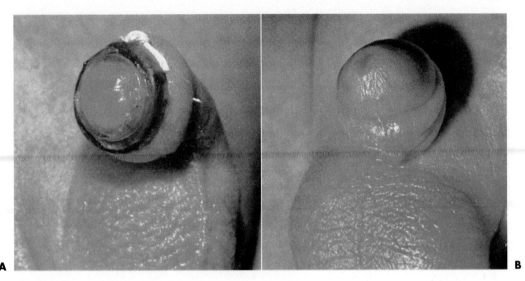

FIGURE 19-16   Circumcision using Hollister plastibel. **A,** Suture around rim of plastibel controls bleeding. **B,** Plastic rim and suture drop off in 7 to 10 days. (Courtesy Hollister, Inc, Chicago.)

BOX 19-1   Home Care of Circumcision

1. Keep area clean by using plain water *only* around area, not on sore area.
   - Vaseline gauze around penis may detach or be taken off within 12 to 24 hours. Use a big dab of Vaseline on a 4-inch sterile gauze square and place over penis to protect it against rubbing of the diaper.
   - If the plastibel method was used, expect the plastic ring to detach when the scab is dry. Use Vaseline as described previously.
2. The normal healing process will look like this:
   - Slightly swollen under the head of the penis, which should be quite pinkish red for several days. If head of penis is bluish, check amount of swelling and *call* healthcare provider.
   - There may be a watery pink-yellow oozing but no bright red bleeding.
   - A small blood clot may form underneath the head of the penis.
3. *Call* if any of the following happen:
   - Active bleeding: apply pressure with a sterile gauze for 5 minutes. If it does not stop, *call* us, and keep applying pressure.
   - Baby does not urinate after he is at home. If more than 12 to 18 hours, *call*, and check swelling of penis.
   - Infection will show redness and swelling after the first few days. Look for any pus or fever and *call*.
   - *Call* if baby is not eating or sleeping well.

important to use local anesthesia during circumcision (Mudge and Younger, 1989). Practitioners may use either a topical or local anesthetic to block pain impulses via the dorsal penile nerve. Even with the use of anesthesia, the infant may be irritable or lethargic for several hours after the procedure. Comfort measures include cuddling and offering feeding, which may be taken eagerly or rejected.

Aftercare

Circumcision care involves keeping the exposed glans covered with gauze squares on which sterile ointment has been placed. This protects the area from abrasion, excessive bleeding, and infection. Routine cleaning may begin after about 1 to 5 days with use of a soft cloth and omitting soap. Cleansing should be done with every diaper change, and diapers should be applied loosely. The care giver observes for early complications such as bleeding, infection, or difficulty voiding. Complications that may occur later include meatitis (inflammation of the meatus), adhesions of the remnants of the foreskin to the glans, or meatal stenosis caused by meatitis. See Box 19-1 for parental instructions.

Nutritional Needs

In the past the well neonate was not fed until 4 to 12 hours after birth to allow for adjustment to extrauterine life. Now, early feedings are standard for the well full-term infant for the following reasons.

1. During the first period of reactivity, the neonate is alert and eager to feed, making this an ideal time to start breast-feeding or bottle-feeding.

Teach Mom immed. how to use bulg syringe when taking infant in for 1st feeding

2. Early feedings stimulate early passage of meconium, which reduces enterohepatic circulation and later bilirubin elevations.

3. Early ingestion of colostrum coats the gastrointestinal tract with secretory IgE and other immune factors, which may offer protection against gastroenteritis.

4. The infant's gastrointestinal tract is also colonized with "friendly" organisms, allowing less opportunity for pathogens to proliferate.

5. Early feedings may lessen the chance of hypoglycemia because the act of feeding stimulates glucagon secretion and therefore glycolysis.

Feeding is a complex system that involves several components (Frappier, 1987). Examination of each of these is crucial in determining whether the neonate is feeding successfully.

NEUROLOGIC COMPONENT

Eating involves a chain of responses that are reflexive in nature. Recall that the **rooting reflex** is elicited by touching the cheek, which causes the infant to turn toward the stimulus. This survival maneuver allows the infant to seek food. Swallowing is an automatic mechanism that helps propel food into the stomach. The *gag reflex* protects the trachea by preventing aspiration. Coordination among sucking, swallowing, and breathing are necessary for successful feeding and should be present by about week 34 of gestation. All infants, whether breast- or bottle-fed, used to be offered a "test feeding" of sterile water to check suck, swallow, and gag reflexes. Now, water is not offered to breast-feeding infants before first feeds. Feeding also is part of the assessment for congenital anomalies. Infants with tracheoesophageal fistula and esophageal atresia will choke and become cyanotic when first fed.

Nurse should remain ē mom for 1st feeding.

NUTRITIONAL COMPONENT

Breast milk or formula provides the major source of calories during the first 6 months. The energy requirement for a healthy infant is 115 kcal/kg/day during this period. Fluid requirements vary with the age of the infant and range from 80 to 160 ml/kg/day (Table 19-3). The calories to fluid ratio of formula is the correct one to achieve needed fluid intake (20 kcal/30 ml). During the first day of life the infant will need 80 ml/kg/day. This increases to 100 to 110 ml/kg/day on the second and third days of life and to 150 ml/kg/day by the end of the first week. Adequate intake will ensure that the young infant gains about 30 g daily. It should be kept in mind that normal infants will lose up to 5% of birth weight initially because of the loss of extracellular fluid, primarily in the form of stool and urine.

TABLE 19-3 Recommended Dietary Allowances for Infants during the First Year of Life

	0–6 MO (0.0–0.5 YR)	6–12 MO (0.5–1.0 YR)
WEIGHT	6 kg (13 lb)	9 kg (20 lb)
HEIGHT	60 cm (24 in)	71 cm (28 in)
KILOCALORIES	kg × 115	kg × 108
PROTEIN, G	(kg × 2.2) 13	(kg × 2.0) 14
FAT-SOLUBLE VITAMINS		
Vitamin A, μ RE	375	375
Vitamin D, μg	7.5	10
Vitamin E, mg TE	3	4
WATER-SOLUBLE VITAMINS		
Ascorbic acid, mg	30	35
Folate, μg	25	35
Niacin, mg NE	5	6
Riboflavin, mg	0.4	0.5
Thiamin, mg	0.3	0.4
Vitamin B_6, mg	0.3	0.6
Vitamin B_{12}, μg	0.3	0.5
MINERALS		
Calcium, mg	400	600
Phosphorus, mg	300	500
Iodine, μg	40	50
Iron, mg	6	10
Magnesium, mg	40	60
Zinc, mg	5	5

Modified from *Recommended daily dietary allowances*, 10, Washington, DC, 1989, National Academy of Sciences. *RE*, Retinol equivalents; *TE*, α-tocopherol equivalents; *NE*, niacin equivalents.

Test Yourself

- Baby Jones weighed 3900 g at birth. On the basis of his weight, what are his 24-hour caloric needs _____ and fluid needs _____ ?

Weight gain. The average weight gain is 7 kg in the first year. Half of that, 3.5 kg, is gained in the first 4 months. After the first week, this means that the neonate will gain at a rate of 5 to 6 ounces per week, doubling the birth weight by 4 months. At about 5 months the rate of growth slows, and the baby becomes ready for the gradual introduction of other foods (Table 19-4).

Triples birth wt by 1st yr.

TABLE 19-4 Developmental Milestones and Suggested Infant Feeding Guidelines: Birth to Five Months

	0-2 WK	2 WKS-2 MO	2 MO	3 MO
Breast milk/formula				
Volume per feeding	2–3 oz	3–5 oz	5 oz	6–6.5 oz
Number of feedings (per day)	6–8	5–6	5–6	4–5
Average total	20 oz	28 oz	30 oz	32–34 oz
Recommended calories (115 kcal/kg)	403	483–598	598	656
Total calories	440	560	600	660–680

During the first 2 months of life, infants display the following oral and muscular development related to feeding; rooting, sucking, and swallowing. During the third month, the extrusion reflex diminishes and sucking becomes voluntary. Therefore, liquid is the appropriate food texture.

During months 4 and 5, the infant learns to put hands to mouth and develops a grasp. By the sixth month, chewing begins and the lips can be put more accurately to the rim of a cup. Food texture will continue to include liquids but baby soft foods can be added.

From Bronner YL, Paige DM: Current concepts in infant nutrition, *J Nurs Midwifery* 37 (suppl 2):475, 1992.

INTERACTIONAL COMPONENT

Satisfactory feeding not only affects the relationship between parent and infant; it depends on the quality of interaction between parent and infant. The parent should have the ability to focus attention on the baby during the feeding, read cues accurately, and respond to these appropriately.

Feeding meets several basic human needs. It satisfies the infant's craving for oral satisfaction and gives an infant a sense of security and love while providing parents with positive feedback about their ability to nurture a child. (See development of the senses in Chapter 20 for the great value feeding time has in infant development.)

These factors should be kept in mind in assessing the infant's ability to feed. The nurse observes the following:

1. Coordination of root, suck, and swallow reflexes
2. Quantity of intake sufficient for growth
3. Output in stool and urine is adequate
4. Skin turgor is elastic

Nursing Responsibilities

Nursing responsibilities in establishing feeding include evaluating the mother's knowledge within the very brief hospitalization period. Because extended families usually are not readily available to support the new mother, literature and resources for support become critical in most situations (see Chapter 17).

Breast-fed Infant

The breast-feeding infant is given a first try just after birth or during the first recovery hour if the condition is stable. The infant should again be breast-fed during the second period of reactivity. Advantages of this early feeding are seen in establishing early attachment; stimulation of maternal oxytocin secretion occurs as well. The infant should be fed on demand, that is, when crying from hunger. The intervals between feedings vary from 2 to 3 hours. At first, not all infants will demand feeding. Some infants may be sleepy. Variations always exist because of different methods of birth and analgesic and anesthetic use. For this reason close observation and output assessment are important. An infant may have to be coaxed the first few days.

Successful breast-feeding depends on the mother's desire and is influenced by her level of understanding and her support persons in the home (Figure 19-17; see also Chapter 17 for techniques and maternal support and see Box 19-2 for advantages of breast milk). Most mothers who are new at breast-feeding are concerned about adequate intake. Frequent feeding is the best way to establish lactation. Signs of satisfaction include a content baby after feeding who shows a weight gain of about 25 to 30 g/day in the first few months. There will be an average of six to eight wet diapers per day, with skin turgor elastic and soft or pasty stools. There may be frequent stools or stools every other day, depending on the maternal diet.

The mother who eats a balanced diet with adequate fluid intake will produce milk in adequate quantities for her infant's growth. If she does not drink enough fluids, the quantity of milk will be *reduced* while the quality stays stable. (See Maternal Nutrition, Chapter 17.)

Mothers often ask about offering water supplements. Initially water through a rubber nipple may result in "nipple confusion" because the sucking action is differ-

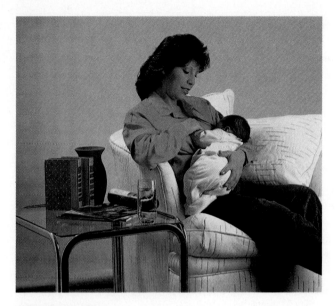

FIGURE 19-17 Breast-feeding. (Courtesy Ross Laboratories, Columbus, Ohio.)

ent. Later, especially in hot weather, water may be given between feedings but must be boiled and cooled and placed in a clean bottle.

Bottle-fed Infant

Bottle-feeding allows fathers and siblings to participate in feeding. Some mothers feel that they have more freedom when feeding responsibilities are shared. Infants usually require less frequent feeds because of the slower digestion of the larger milk curd. Demand feeding should be encouraged. Initially the infant may need to feed every 2 to 3 hours, but as the baby matures, feedings may be further apart.

Although many brands of formula are available, mothers tend to buy the brand that was given in the hospital. The formula companies provide free samples to hospitals for this reason (Novak, 1988). All formula companies in the United States must follow strict regulations and are attempting to make their products as similar to breast milk as possible. Parents should be told that cow's milk (whole or skim) is not to be added to the infant's diet until after 1 year of age. Cow's milk curd is not well digested unless the milk is boiled. Thus fresh whole milk is not advised. In addition, skim milk has a low fat content, and to gain sufficient calories would require too much fluid volume. Infant formulas are available in several forms, which influence the ease of preparation.

1. Powdered formula is mixed with boiled water in specific quantities to yield full-strength formula.
2. 13 ounces of concentrated formula when mixed with 13 ounces of boiled water yields 26 ounces of full-strength formula.

BOX 19-2   Advantages of Human Milk vs Cow's Milk

Contains adequate (not excessive) protein; has greater quantities of certain amino acids, including cystine and taurine
Contains more lactalbumin (produces easily digested curds) than casein (produces large, hard curds)
Contains more lactose, which in the gut stimulates growth of microorganisms, which synthesize some B vitamins and produce organic acids that may retard growth of harmful bacteria
Contains more monounsaturated fatty acids, which enhance absorption of fat and calcium
Contains adequate (not excessive) minerals with exception of fluoride (low in both)
Amounts of iron and zinc are low but more readily absorbed
Contains less calcium and phosphorus but a more favorable ratio of the minerals, which prevents excessive calcium excretion
Contains adequate amounts of vitamins A, B complex, and E; vitamin C content depends on maternal intake; vitamin D is low but more readily absorbed (vitamin C, D, and E are low in cow's milk, but K is higher)
Contains growth modulators that modify growth or maturation
Offers several immunologic benefits: contains various immunoglobulins (Ig), especially IgA; macrophages; granulocytes; T- and B-cell lymphocytes; and other factors that inhibit bacterial growth
Has laxative effect
Is economical, readily available, and sanitary
Has psychologic benefits of close bond between infant and mother during feeding

From Wong DL: *Whaley and Wong's essentials of pediatric nursing,* ed 4, St Louis, 1993, Mosby.

---

3. Ready-to-use formula in 32-ounce cans is convenient but expensive.
4. 4-ounce feeders like those used in the hospital are available but expensive.

Some health care professionals want parents to sterilize the bottles and nipples. Others believe that washing with hot, sudsy water and a hot-water rinse is enough. All agree that the water used to mix the formula should be boiled before using.

Addition of Solids

The most desirable diet for infants up to 6 months is breast milk. Bottle-feeding with commercially prepared formula is an acceptable substitute. The Academy of Pediatrics (Broussard, 1984) recommends that supplemental food not be introduced before 4 to 6 months.

Anticipatory guidance is required in explaining this because parents have cultural habits and backgrounds that will influence their choices of food. Parents need to know that there is a time of readiness for introduction of solids. The baby's weight, activity, and appetite are factors to consider in this decision. Signals of the infant's readiness include the following:

1. Has doubled birth weight
2. Demands breast feeding more than 8 to 10 times in a 24-hour period
3. Drinks more than a quart of formula per day
4. Often seems hungry

Parents need to know that adding solids does not initially increase the infant's nutrition; rather the infant is experimenting with the texture and taste of new foods and probably will not consume very much. Introducing new foods one at a time, at weekly intervals, allows for identification of allergies. Solids are introduced at the beginning of a meal when the child is hungriest and may be thinned with formula and fed by spoon. Solids should not be mixed in the bottle of formula. Sucking thickened liquid can cause choking and also will deprive the infant of learning spoon feeding. At first the infant may push the food away and appear dissatisfied. The *extrusion reflex,* the tongue thrusting of sucking, makes the infant appear to be "spitting out" the food. Feedings, although messy, should be enjoyable for both parents and child. Recommendations for the introduction of solid food are as follows:

1. From birth to 1 year, breast milk or formula is the food of choice. Whole, nonmodified cow's milk is introduced only after 1 year, which allows for maturation of the gastrointestinal tract.
2. Between the ages of 4 and 6 months, continue with breast milk or formula. Begin introducing solids in the following order: rice cereal (offered first because it is least allergenic and also supplies dietary iron), fruits, barley/oatmeal, and prepared vegetables and meats (with applesauce-like texture). Commercial baby foods free of added sugar and salt or home-blended food can be used.

Weaning

A baby can be successfully weaned when it can grasp with both hands, reach, and sit well. Babies often lose interest in breast-feeding after 7 to 8 months; others will continue longer. The mother who is breast-feeding can wean directly to a cup. A bottle-fed baby often will hold on to the night bottle until well into the second or even third year. The baby gets satisfaction from sucking, and it will do no harm if only a small amount of juice or milk is given. Diluting the drink with water may hasten the weaning. Parents should be cautioned *never* to allow an infant to fall asleep while drinking anything, even water, from a nursing bottle. This causes a pattern of tooth decay called "nursing bottle mouth," which can be severe enough to necessitate extraction of the affected teeth.

To begin weaning the baby, the mother should put a small amount of milk in a sturdy shallow cup. Training cups are available that have two handles, covers, spouts, and rounded bottoms to cope with the inevitable spills. Each baby differs in adjustment to drinking from a cup. The amount of milk consumed may decrease until the baby gets used to drinking from a cup. Water can be offered from a bottle to give the baby intake during transition.

Supplements

Parents often are concerned about vitamin and mineral supplements. Supplements of individual vitamins rarely are used for infants, however, with the exception of vitamin K at birth to prevent hemorrhagic disease of the newborn and vitamin E to prevent hemolytic anemia in premature infants. It is common for the pediatric health care provider to prescribe selected multivitamin preparations (Tri-Vi-Flor or Poly-Vi-Sol), but probably unnecessary. Full-term infants normally are born with iron supplies adequate for the first 4 months of life. Breast milk, although relatively deficient in iron, provides adequate supplies because the breast milk iron is more easily digested. Bottle-feeding with iron-supplemented formulas sometimes *increases* iron deficiency because the harder stool can cause microhemorrhages.

Fluoride supplements. Fluoride is incorporated in structures of the dental enamel that forms during the early months of life before teething occurs. Fluoride supplementation (prescribed if the local water supply is not fluorinated) can cause a 50% to 70% decrease in dental caries.

Discharge Planning
EVALUATION OF NEWBORN TRANSITION

A complete assessment includes review of the prenatal, intrapartal, and neonatal history. A complete physical examination should have been performed within the first 24 hours after delivery. Examining the infant in the parents' presence just before discharge gives them the opportunity to ask questions pertaining to the infant's status, as well as the opportunity for the examiner to observe early parent-infant interaction. Several deviations become evident in the first day, whereas others do not manifest until after several days. (See list of warning signs in Chapter 18.)

The physician will evaluate the newborn's condition and sign a discharge release. When mother and child are

Clinical Decision

Mrs. Jones wants to breast-feed exclusively but is afraid she won't have enough milk. Nutrition counseling should include which three principles?

She should be able to state that her infant is eating satisfactorily if which three events are occurring?

discharged early (less than 24 hours after delivery), it is necessary to perform another physical examination during a home visit and to have newborn follow-up at 1 or 2 weeks of life.

Predischarge testing and metabolic screening. Metabolic screening tests provide for early diagnosis and treatment of *inborn errors of metabolism (IEM),* which can prevent or lessen the severity of potential handicaps. In the United States, metabolic study programs use the filter paper spot technique. Capillary blood specimens from a heel stick are obtained (Figure 19-18). Blood samples are placed on the filter paper to fill and saturate each circle. The samples are analyzed for levels of enzymes, metabolites, and other substances. If these are not within normal limits, further testing takes place.

Phenylketonia (PKU) is an inherited autosomal recessive disorder caused by the absence of phenylalanine hydroxylase, an enzyme necessary for the conversion of the essential amino acid phenylalanine to tyrosine. Tyrosine is needed for the synthesis of hormones, skin, and hair pigment, and its absence leads to brain damage. This is why PKU is seen more frequently in fair-haired (or lightly pigmented) persons. Because maternal metabolism of fetal phenylalanine occurs in utero, clinical signs will not be seen immediately in the neonate. The screening test must be performed after the newborn has consumed enough milk that contains phenylalanine (either breast milk or formula) to produce levels high enough for detection. Newborns who are discharged early need to be *retested* by the primary care provider. Once the diagnosis is established, diet therapy that restricts phenylalanine intake is begun. During infancy, Lofenalac formula is recommended.

Primary congenital hypothyroidism is a defect in which the thyroid gland does not produce adequate thyroxine (T_4). If left untreated, severe brain damage may result. Clinical signs include hypotonia, widely spaced fontanelles, a large tongue that may cause feeding difficulties, and prolonged jaundice. Treatment consists of thyroid hormone replacement therapy.

Congenital galactosemia is a hereditary disorder of galactose metabolism. Signs that occur after the infant begins feeding include lethargy, hypotonia, and diarrhea. Treatment is elimination of galactose from the diet for 6 to 8 years. During infancy, lactose-free formulas such as Nutramigen or Prosobee are recommended.

Congenital lactose intolerance, a deficiency of the enzyme lactase (needed for the digestion of lactose), becomes evident in early infancy but is not life-threatening. Diagnosis is based on a history of diarrhea, abdominal pain, distention, and flatus after ingestion of milk containing lactose. Clinitest tablets are used to test the stool for malabsorbed sugar (reducing substances). Elimination of milk products and their gradual reintroduction while observing for return of symptoms is the easiest way to confirm the diagnosis. Treatment includes elimination of cow's milk products and substitution of a commercial formula such as Isomil and Prosobee. Dairy products that have been fermented such as yogurt can be consumed safely. Lactose-reduced milk (Lactaid) also may be used. At 1 year of age the child is observed for any digestive difficulties as milk products are slowly reintroduced. (See Chapter 27 for racial groups that carry genes for lactose intolerance.)

Other Rare Inborn Errors of Metabolism

There are a number of rare inborn errors. In general, if there is *failure to thrive, unusual stools,* or *difficulty digesting feedings,* the infant should be screened for an IEM. In many cases these metabolic problems can be treated with strict diet modifications.

Figure 19-18 indicates the usual genetic conditions included on the initial testing. Hemoglobinopathies such as sickle cell anemia and glucose-6-phosphate dehydrogenase deficiency are tested for as well. (These problems are discussed in Chapter 23.)

HIV Testing

The final blot on the test paper may be reserved for HIV maternal antibody testing. Currently a number of states perform *blind testing* of newborns, that is, without identification of the individual. Only the state and hospital are listed, and reports are sent back to notify these agencies of the rate of HIV-positive mothers in their units. Newborns of HIV-positive women will show the presence of maternal antibodies in their blood. No permit is obtained from the mother because there is no individual identification. (See Chapter 25 for the current status of the infant of an HIV-positive woman.)

Bilirubin. Hyperbilirubinemia occurs when the normal pathways of bilirubin metabolism and excretion are impeded. This may occur when the mother and infant blood types are incompatible (see Chapter 9). Cord blood is used to determine the infant's blood type and

go to → See pg 507

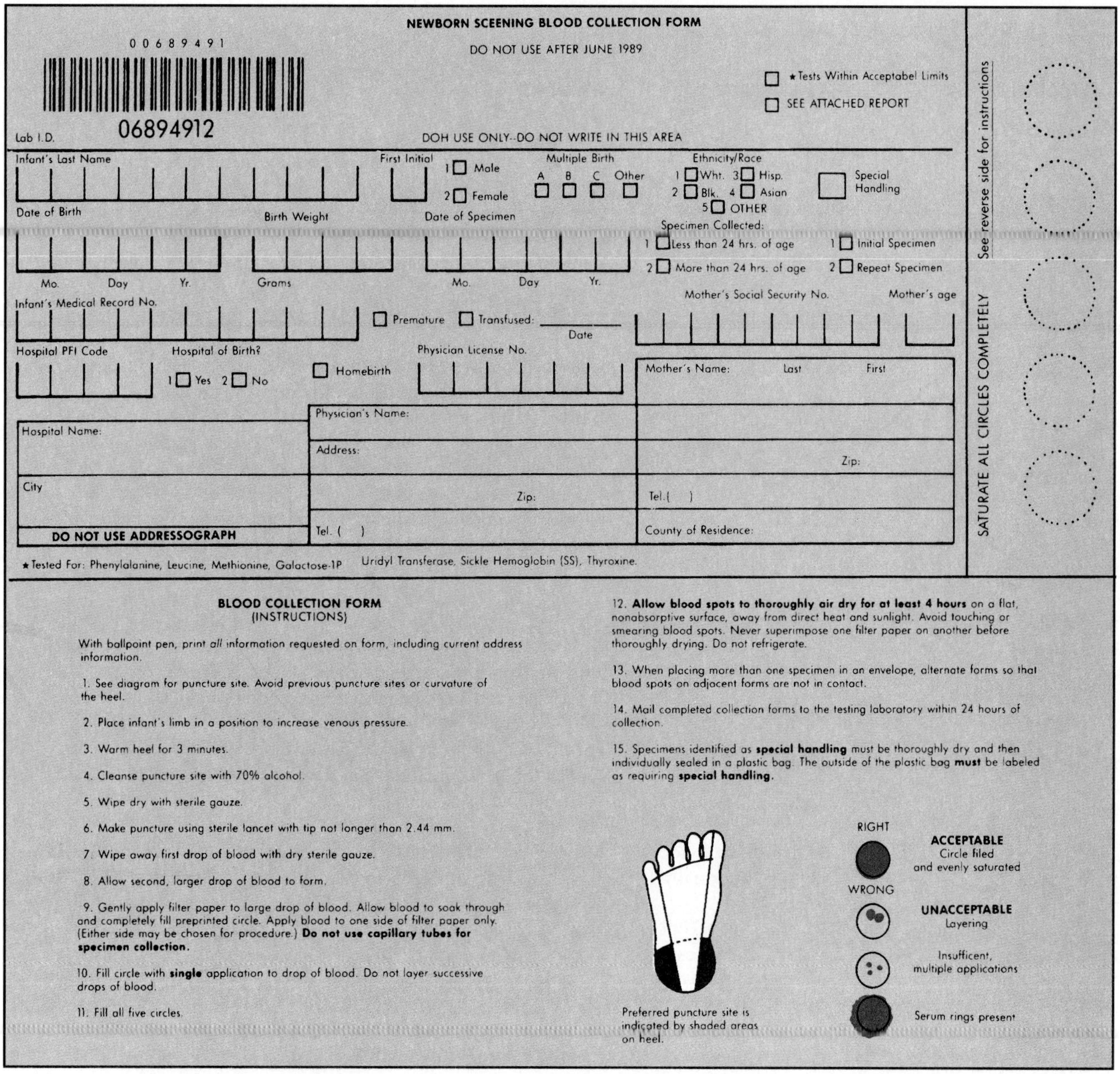

NEWBORN SCEENING BLOOD COLLECTION FORM

DO NOT USE AFTER JUNE 1989

0 0 6 8 9 4 9 1

Lab I.D. 06894912

★Tests Within Acceptabel Limits

SEE ATTACHED REPORT

DOH USE ONLY--DO NOT WRITE IN THIS AREA

Infant's Last Name | First Initial | 1 Male | 2 Female | Multiple Birth A B C Other | Ethnicity/Race 1 Wht. 3 Hisp. 2 Blk. 4 Asian 5 OTHER | Special Handling

Date of Birth (Mo. Day Yr.) | Birth Weight (Grams) | Date of Specimen (Mo. Day Yr.) | Specimen Collected: 1 Less than 24 hrs. of age 2 More than 24 hrs. of age | 1 Initial Specimen 2 Repeat Specimen

Infant's Medical Record No. | Premature | Transfused: ______ Date | Mother's Social Security No. | Mother's age

Hospital PFI Code | Hospital of Birth? 1 Yes 2 No | Homebirth | Physician License No. | Mother's Name: Last First

Hospital Name: | Physician's Name: | Address: | Zip:

City | Zip: | Tel.( )

DO NOT USE ADDRESSOGRAPH | Tel. ( ) | County of Residence:

★Tested For: Phenylalanine, Leucine, Methionine, Galactose-1P Uridyl Transferase, Sickle Hemoglobin (SS), Thyroxine.

See reverse side for instructions

SATURATE ALL CIRCLES COMPLETELY

A

BLOOD COLLECTION FORM (INSTRUCTIONS)

With ballpoint pen, print *all* information requested on form, including current address information.

1. See diagram for puncture site. Avoid previous puncture sites or curvature of the heel.
2. Place infant's limb in a position to increase venous pressure.
3. Warm heel for 3 minutes.
4. Cleanse puncture site with 70% alcohol.
5. Wipe dry with sterile gauze.
6. Make puncture using sterile lancet with tip not longer than 2.44 mm.
7. Wipe away first drop of blood with dry sterile gauze.
8. Allow second, larger drop of blood to form.
9. Gently apply filter paper to large drop of blood. Allow blood to soak through and completely fill preprinted circle. Apply blood to one side of filter paper only. (Either side may be chosen for procedure.) **Do not use capillary tubes for specimen collection.**
10. Fill circle with **single** application to drop of blood. Do not layer successive drops of blood.
11. Fill all five circles.
12. **Allow blood spots to thoroughly air dry for at least 4 hours** on a flat, nonabsorptive surface, away from direct heat and sunlight. Avoid touching or smearing blood spots. Never superimpose one filter paper on another before thoroughly drying. Do not refrigerate.
13. When placing more than one specimen in an envelope, alternate forms so that blood spots on adjacent forms are not in contact.
14. Mail completed collection forms to the testing laboratory within 24 hours of collection.
15. Specimens identified as **special handling** must be thoroughly dry and then individually sealed in a plastic bag. The outside of the plastic bag **must** be labeled as requiring **special handling.**

Preferred puncture site is indicated by shaded areas on heel.

RIGHT — **ACCEPTABLE** Circle filed and evenly saturated

WRONG — **UNACCEPTABLE** Layering; Insufficent, multiple applications; Serum rings present

B

FIGURE 19-18 A, Metabolic screening form. B, Blood collection form instructions. Note that circles must be completely saturated with blood to ensure identification of metabolic disorders. (Courtesy Newborn Screening Program, Wadsworth Center for Laboratories and Research, New York State Department of Health, Albany, N.Y.)

Rh factor, as well as the direct Coombs test (which detects antibodies on the neonatal erythrocytes). When an infant is found to be jaundiced (no matter what the reason), serum bilirubin levels are determined from a capillary heel stick sample. Various treatments are available (see Chapter 28). The infant's discharge will be delayed until this problem has resolved.

VDRL

The Venereal Disease Research Laboratory (VDRL) is a serologic screen for congenital syphilis. This has been mandated by law in the United States as one of the cord blood tests (see Chapter 25). As a cost-saving move, currently many hospitals save cord blood to examine only if the newly delivered woman's blood test result is positive. Table 19-5 summarizes common tests for newborns.

Early Discharge Teaching

Parenting is both a learned and an instinctive behavior. Even for those who are "natural parents," the first time

TABLE 19-5 Diagnostic Tests for Newborn Infants

LABORATORY TESTS	NORMAL RESULTS	COMMENTS
CORD BLOOD		
Blood type	A, B, AB, O	Potential for incompatibility, especially if infant is type A or B with a type O mother.
Rh factor	Negative or positive	Potential for incompatibility if mother is type Rh negative and infant is Rh positive.
Direct Coombs test	Negative	Detects sensitized red blood cells. Does not define blocking agent.
Bilirubin	1.0–1.8 mg/dl	Elevated level at birth indicates that fetal hemolysis is present.
Serology-antibody titers		
Syphilis	Negative	If mother has been treated during pregnancy, newborn titers may still be positive but should decrease by 3 months.
IgM	Negative	If present, indicates maternal infection during pregnancy with transfer of IgM antibodies to fetus. Specific antibody titers of mother and infant are compared to rule out infections such as TORCH (see Chapter 27).
IgG	Negative	Formed in infant in response to antigen and does not cross placenta. If found, indicates that infant responded to maternal infection.
HEEL-STICK CAPILLARY BLOOD		
Glucose	Range: 45–90 mg/dl	If Dextrostix below 45 mg/dl, take venous sample for lab analysis. Infants of diabetic mothers, infants <5½ lb, over > 8 lb, preterm, and stressed infants need additional testing.
Hematocrit	40%-65%	<40% anemia, >65% polycythemia.
Bilirubin	At 3–4 days normal elevation of 4–6 mg/dl	For infant with levels elevated above normal, expect q12h tests, extra oral fluids, infant may receive phototherapy if over 10-14 mg/dl.
Thyroid screening		
T_4 level	Less than 6 µg/dl at 3 days is abnormally low	Done on all infants at 2–3 days; especially important for those with wide-open suture lines and large fontanelles, thickened tongues.
TSH on suspected hypothyroid	TSH level >20 µU/dl at 3 days is diagnostic of hypothyroidism	Signs of thyroid deficiency develop by the first week.
IEM		
PKU	Blood levels of 4 mg or more by 48 hr indicate a problem	PKU needs to be repeated by pediatrician if infant discharged early, before adequate milk intake.
Histidinemia		Ferric chloride reaction will turn urine blue-green.
Glucose-6-phosphate dehydrogenase	Elevated indirect bilirubin if infant affected by maternal drug	Consult list of drugs causing hemolysis that may be excreted in breast milk and affect infant.
Sickle cell trait/ disease	Absent	Usually no initial problems. Watch for reduced oxygen tension.
MECONIUM		
Cystic fibrosis	No elevated albumin in meconium	Test strip changes to deep blue if positive. Sweat test done to measure sodium and chloride concentrations of collected sweat.

TABLE 19-5 Diagnostic Tests for Newborn Infants—cont'd

LABORATORY TESTS	NORMAL RESULTS	COMMENTS
PERIPHERAL CULTURES		
Cord, anorectal, ear canal, nasopharyngeal	Negative	Use varies. Done especially if mother had premature rupture of membranes or if nursery epidemic occurs.
Any lesion		
URINE		
Urinalysis	1.004–1.018 specific gravity	Urobilinogen associated with jaundice in infant.
Possible culture	Uric acid crystals; no protein or red blood cells	

TORCH, Toxoplasmosis, rubella, cytomegalovirus, and herpes simplex; *TSH,* thyroid-stimulating hormone.

caring for an infant is a time of turmoil and decreased confidence. The perinatal nurse will find that most couples need education to reduce knowledge deficits related to infant care. Taking the time to provide the family with more knowledge about their infant will increase their confidence and ability to care comfortably for their newborn. Box 19-3 includes common questions asked by new parents.

The best time for teaching varies with experience and prenatal preparation. The nurse must assess readiness to learn and the knowledge base and support systems available once the mother and infant are discharged.

OBJECTIVES FOR PARENT EDUCATION

1. Parents describe a positive support system and adequate housing.
2. Basic needs of the newborn infant are described.
3. Parents state signs of difficulty in nutritional intake and know how to seek help.
4. Parents evaluate home environment for hazards, infections, and temperature control and plan to childproof the home against accidents (including car seats).
5. Parents state recommendations for immunizations and schedule of visits.
6. Parents describe when to notify health care provider regarding alterations in infant status, and they consistently follow up as necessary.
7. Parents start the attachment-bonding process, giving indication that this will continue to develop.

Planning for bringing the newborn home begins well before birth as families gather the materials necessary for their baby's care, begin to educate themselves about parenthood, and anticipate life-style changes. Still, there is much to be done after the birth. Traditionally, new mothers and infants remained in the hospital for at least 3 days after birth, allowing time for assessment of parent needs and appropriate teaching. However, mothers and babies may now leave as soon as 12 hours after birth with home care follow-up.

Families who choose early discharge feel that the healthy new family is safer and more comfortable at home. They may be concerned about finances (see Box 1-1). It is vital that these families have a solid support system at home and that provisions are made for assessment of both mother and newborn on the third postpartum day. The mother is evaluated as described in Chapter 17. Neonatal adjustment is assessed in the same manner as described in Chapter 18, with special attention to the presence of cardiorespiratory difficulty or jaundice, and skin turgor.

Because of time constraints, teaching must be efficient and effective. Some suggestions are the following:

1. Begin classes in the prenatal period, reviewing infant care, growth, and development.
2. Perform predischarge infant assessments while the parents are present.
3. Give written information to reinforce verbal instructions.
4. Follow up with telephone contact from a nursery staff member or other designated provider.

EXTENDED STAY

Unfortunately, some families have to extend the hospital stay because of maternal or neonatal illness. Prematurity, sepsis, and congenital anomalies are the most common reasons for extended hospitalization of neonates. These conditions and their effects on family interaction are discussed in Chapter 28.

Assessment of parental needs is completed before the infant is discharged, and each plan is individualized according to the parent's knowledge base. Nursing interventions reflect common concerns parents express about infant care and safety. (See Nursing Care Plan.)

BOX 19-3   Common Questions Parents Ask Concerning Infant Care

HYGIENE

How often should a baby be bathed?
When can I give my baby a tub bath?
How do I care for the diaper area?
How do I care for his circumcision?

FEEDING

What is the best diet for a baby in the first year of life?

If breast-feeding:

What kind of diet should I follow while breast-feeding?
How long should I let my baby nurse? how often?
Should I offer my baby extra water?
Does my baby need extra formula?
How should I hold my baby when she nurses?
How do I burp my baby?
Should I let him use a pacifier?
When should I start offering solids?
When should I wean my baby?

If bottle-feeding:

What type of formula should I use?
How do I sterilize bottles, caps, and nipples?
How much should he feed? how often?
Should I offer her extra water?
How do I burp my baby?
Should I let him use a pacifier?
When should I start offering solids?

TEMPERATURE

How do I know if my baby is too hot or cold?
How should I dress my baby when going outdoors?
How warm or cool should I keep the house?
Is extra humidity necessary?

SAFETY

How do I choose a car seat, stroller, crib, or infant carrier?
How do I "childproof" my house?
I have a pet—is that safe for my baby?

SLEEP NEEDS

What are the normal patterns of sleep for a baby in the first year?
How can I help my baby go to sleep?
What do I do if my baby has colic?

HEALTH MAINTENANCE

When do I bring my baby back for a check-up?
When will my baby be immunized? Are there risks?
How will I know if my baby is sick?
How do I take my baby's temperature?
How can I keep my baby from getting sick?
When should I call my doctor or nurse practitioner?

 Clinical Decision

- *When cord blood reports return from the laboratory, you note the following: Blood type A+, Coombs test negative (mother is O+) Hemoglobin 20 g/dl, hematocrit 68%, VDRL negative Which finding is reportable?*
- *On the discharge day (day 3) the baby looks jaundiced. Why was the baby more likely to become jaundiced at this time?*

READINESS FOR DISCHARGE

Questions that may elicit evaluative data on parental and newborn readiness for discharge include the following:

1. Is the infant within normal parameters of vital signs, bilirubin, gestational age, and behavior?
2. Have feeding behaviors been established? Are there feeding problems that need referral? Do parents know whom to call if help is needed?
3. Have parents read handouts and asked questions? (Were handouts available in their primary language?)
4. Have all laboratory tests been performed? Does the parent know when to obtain results and when to see pediatrician or nurse clinician?
5. Do parents know the signs of illness and when to report problems?
6. Do parents indicate they have a car seat and understand safety guidelines?
7. Do parents indicate a support system, or do there seem to be problems with attachment, bonding, or support?

Referrals

If at any time before or during the discharge process a question arises about the abilities of the parents to care for the newborn, the family should be referred to an appropriate community agency. Usually this is done by the primary nurse with help from social services. Referral forms should be made out in advance so that early contact can be made with the family. (See Figure 19-19 for sample interagency referral.)

The women, infants, and children (WIC) program is a program of the federal government that provides pregnant and lactating women and their children with adequate nutrition. Essential foods are supplied to those who qualify. Referrals should be made prenatally or after birth.

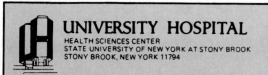

INTERAGENCY REFERRAL

Baby boy - white
MR# 014687
D.O.B. 5-29-94

Address: 28 Byrne Road West Islip, NY

Telephone: 516 - 927 - 4560   Unit: New born   Date of Discharge: 6-7-94

Family Names: Jessie - mother   Martha - grandmother

Directions to Home: Southern state to Sunrise Highway

Diagnosis: mother had no prenatal care
baby SGA

Information given to family re: Prognosis: good

Reasons for Referral:
• mother 14 years old, single, living with grandmother
• no prenatal care
• infant SGA   BW 4 pounds 8 ounces   Apgar 8¹ 9⁵
current weight 5 pounds 5 ounces

Review infant care to include:
• bathing
• feeding
• common problems in infancy

PROBLEMS	PLAN
① Knowledge deficit R/T lack of experience	A- review infant bath
	B- review infant safety
	C- review infant nutrition
② Altered nutrition: less than body requirements R/T birth history	A- weigh infant
	B- monitor feedings

Patient's discharge information sheet including medications, treatments, referrals and individualized care plan   □ is attached
□ will be sent upon discharge

	Name	Signature	Phone	Date
Nurse	S. Peterson	S. Peterson	444-0100	6-7-94
Social Worker	P. Callan	P. Callan		
Physician	C. Garber	C. Garber		

Additional referrals made to: WIC referral

Report to be sent back to: Head Nurse

Referral given to: Name Jody Mitchell   Telephone Number:

FIGURE 19-19 Interagency referral. Note use of nursing diagnosis in planning this referral to public health nurse. (Courtesy University Hospital at State University of New York at Stony Brook.)

NURSING CARE PLAN • Infant Discharge

CASE: Baby boy Jones was born at 41 weeks; weight 3900 g, Apgar score 9–9. He made a rapid adjustment in spite of a hematocrit of 68%. Jaundice of 7 mg/dl appeared at 3 days, but discharge with instructions was allowed. No circumcision was to be done at this time. Mary and Jed live near her parents, in a one-bedroom apartment. Mary was para 0000 with little experience of baby care but wants to breast-feed.

ASSESSMENT

1. Infant's date of birth, date of discharge
   Infant status, physical assessment, laboratory results
   Measurements, type of birth, recovery pattern
2. Infant response to breast-feeding
3. Parents' ages, experiences with infant care, mother's parity
4. Parents' knowledge of infant care and observed interaction with infant
5. Parents' realistic expectations and support systems
6. Knowledge of health maintenance measures, breast-feeding

NURSING DIAGNOSES

1. Health-seeking behaviors by parent
2. Altered nutrition: Less than body requirements related to initial breast-feeding and body weight
3. High risk for delayed metabolism of bilirubin related to hematocrit level and large breast-fed infant

EXPECTED OUTCOMES

1. Will attain adequate knowledge of home care of infant and demonstrate attachment behaviors with infant
2. Will establish breast-feeding and recognize infant satisfaction and weight gain
3. Will prevent adverse effects by bilirubin intervention
4. Will arrange a hazard-free home

NURSING INTERVENTIONS

1. *Hygiene:* Teach cord, skin, and diaper care.
   Safety: Teach position, handling, dressing for environment. Assess safety of home, baby care equipment, toys, use of infant seat in car.
   Interaction: Demonstrate baby behaviors; assess parental response. Teach infant needs for safety, security, and stimulation.
2. *Support:* Assess parent's support system. Refer to home care if necessary.
3. *Feeding:* Teach breast-feeding technique, difficulties. Provide referral telephone number. Encourage additional fluid with more frequent feedings until jaundice level decreases.
4. *Follow-up:* Give clinic appointments within 1 week for jaundice check. Teach signs of illness and whom to call. Refer to home health nurse for infant jaundice, breast-feeding follow-up.

EVALUATION

1. Do parents demonstrate basic care techniques? Are there positive attachment signs?
2. Does mother state signs of infant satisfaction with feeding? Does she use breast-feeding techniques adequately?
3. Do they describe when to seek referrals and clinic follow-up on bilirubin status, on any signs of illness, and for well-baby check?
4. Do parents state their plan to assess home for safety and use car seat?

The following families and infants must have referrals to social service and home care agencies:

1. Maternal problems
   a. Medical disorders
   b. 16 years old or younger at time of delivery
   c. Birth at less than 28 weeks' gestation
   d. Birth at home or en route to the hospital
   e. No prenatal care or came for less than four visits *F. Economically Disadvantaged ? ref. to WIC*
2. Infant problems
   a. Multiple gestation
   b. Weight less than 2001 g at birth
   c. Major congenital anomaly
   d. Inherited metabolic disease
   e. Discharged to home from the NICU

See Chapter 26 for a model of follow-up in home care of mother and infant.

The infant and mother are ready for discharge when the health care giver has completed the newborn physical assessment and necessary parental teaching, and the parents demonstrate an ability to care for their child (Figure 19-20). Instructions should be written and a

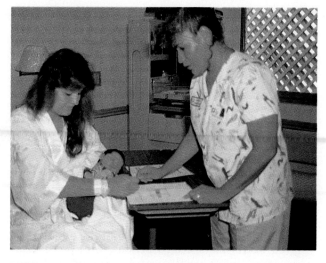

FIGURE 19-20 Before discharge, the mother examines the identification form and signs it. It is witnessed by the nurse. (Courtesy Marjorie Pyle, RNC, *Lifecircle*.)

copy given to the parents for future referral. See Box 19-4 for an example of a discharge summary sheet.

BOX 19-4 **Discharge Summary Sheet**

Name _____

Date of birth _____ Date of discharge _____

Birth weight _____ Weight at discharge _____ Length _____

Suggested diet _____

_____

Medications _____

Activity _____

_____

Community referral/resources _____

_____

_____

Poison control No. _____ Hospital No. _____

Private physician No. _____ Clinic No. _____

Return visit: Date _____ Time _____

               Place _____ Phone _____

Special instructions:

1. Continue applying alcohol to the cord with each diaper change.
2. Sponge bathe your baby every day until the cord falls off. Then a tub bath may be given when the cord is completely healed.
3. Buckle baby in infant seat with infant facing rear of car.

Other instructions:

_____

_____

_____

_____

A carbon copy is made so that parents can use this as a reference guide after discharge.

KEY POINTS

- Monitoring infant transition is critical and guided by Apgar scoring. Vital signs must be monitored frequently during the first 4 hours of life.
- The nurse's role in assessment of the newborn is based on knowledge of growth and development. The nurse is responsible for detecting variations from normal and reporting findings to the appropriate person.
- Protection from heat loss and infection are primary nursing responsibilities in the transitional period.
- Nurses have a major role in prevention of infant abduction from hospital settings.
- Routine medications in the newborn period must be given within the specified periods, with precautions to prevent infection.
- There is controversy about the value of circumcision. Nurses need to be prepared to discuss pros and cons of circumcision with parents.

- Education for care of the infant can be accomplished by demonstration, literature, and audiovisual materials. Teaching related to all aspects of newborn care should be covered before discharge.
- Documentation of client's levels of understanding should be included in nursing care plans and discharge notes.
- Nutritional needs begin soon after birth. When transition is troubled, the infant should be assessed for hypoglycemia.
- Some tests for metabolic screening may need repetition if the infant is discharged early.
- A referral for home care should be made whenever problems are identified in the immediate newborn period.

STUDY QUESTIONS

19-1 Match Key Terms to the following statements.
   a. A noisy breath on inspiration _Stridor_
   b. A sign of respiratory distress _grunting_
   c. Black, sticky first stools _meconium_
   d. White, cheesy material secreted at female and male genitalia _smegma_

19-2 Baby girl M. is delivered at term by normal spontaneous delivery (NSD) to a 28-year-old woman after an uneventful pregnancy, labor, and delivery. No maternal analgesia or anesthesia was used. She coughs several times, and you observe moderate amounts of white mucus expelled from her mouth and nose. You note that she is moving her arms and legs vigorously and that for the first minute she is pink but her hands and feet are blue. Select the points for each of the five items of the Apgar score at 1 minute.
   a. Heart rate 2; respirations 2; tone 2; reflexes 2; color 1, = 9
   b. Heart rate 0; respirations 2; tone 2; reflexes 0; color 0, = 4
   c. Heart rate 1; respirations 2; tone 2; reflexes 1; color 2, = 8
   d. Looks like 6 or 7.

19-3 At 5 minutes of age, the Apgar score is unchanged. What should you do?
   a. Chart the Apgar score, and continue to observe her.
   b. Start positive pressure ventilation with 80% oxygen via bag and mask.
   c. Move the baby from the warmer to footprint her and put on the identification band.
   d. Obtain another Apgar score.

19-4 Which mechanism of heat loss is prevented by the following methods of temperature control in the delivery area:
   a. Place the infant on warmed surfaces only _Conduction_
   b. Dry the infant thoroughly _Evaporation_
   c. Place the infant under a radiant warmer if the baby is not placed on the mother's abdomen _radiation_
   d. Minimize air-conditioning currents and movement of people _convection_

19-5 A pulse rate of 110/min in a deeply asleep term baby most probably indicates:
   a. A normal response for this phase of sleep.
   b. A heart problem to be evaluated.
   c. Bigeminal pulse deficit.
   d. Dehydration.

19-6 Baby R. is circumcised the morning of discharge. Which statement is inaccurate regarding immediate postcircumcision care?
   a. Check for bleeding from site for the first 12 hours.
   b. Clean penile area thoroughly with each diaper change.
   c. Use Vaseline as lubricant to prevent diaper irritation.
   d. Observe for and chart voiding before discharge.

2500g - 4000 g   3400g 7½#

19-7 Which of the following mothers should receive a referral for home care?
a. Primipara with a 4000 g full-term male infant and adequate support systems at home
b. Mother of twins with two siblings at home
c. Mother of 2400 g female infant who had elevated bilirubin level at 3 days of age and was discharged on the fourth day.
d. Diabetic mother of 3300 g full-term female infant.

Answer Key

19-1 a. Stridor, b. Grunting, c. Meconium, d. Smegma. 19-2 a 19-3 a 19-4 a. Conduction, b. Evaporation, c. Radiation, d. Convection. 19-5 a 19-6 b 19-7 b, c, d

REFERENCES

American Academy of Pediatrics, Committee on Fetus and Newborn: Use and abuse of Apgar score, *Pediatrics* 78:1148, 1986.

American Academy of Pediatrics: Report of the task force on circumcision, *Pediatrics* 84(4):388, 1989.

Apgar V et al: Evaluation of the newborn infant—second report, *JAMA* 168:1985, 1958.

Beachy P, Deacon J: Preventing neonatal kidnapping, *JOGNN* 20(1):12, 1992.

Birth News, *Birth* 19(1):45, 1992.

Bliss-Holtz J: Comparison of rectal, axillary and inguinal temperatures in full-term infants, *Nurs Res* 38(2):85, 1989.

Bronner YL, Paige DM: Current concepts in infant nutrition, *J Nurse Midwifery* 37(suppl 2):59s, 1992.

Broussard A: Anticipatory guidance: adding solids to an infant's diet, *JOGNN* 13(6):239, 1984.

Centers for Disease Control (CDC): Immunization Practice Advisory Committee: Hepatitis B virus: a comprehensive strategy for eliminating transmission in the US through universal childhood vaccination, *MMWR* 1-25, Nov 22, 1991.

Conrad PD et al: Safety of newborn discharge in less than 36 hours in an indigent population, *Am J Dis Child* 143(1):98, 1989.

Cowen J et al: Absorption of chlorhexidine from intact skin of newborn infants, *Arch Dis Child* 54:379, 1979.

Doherty LB et al: Detection of phenylketonuria in the very early newborn blood specimen, *Pediatrics* 87(2):240, 1991.

Faucher MA, Jackson G: Pharmaceutical preparations: a review of drugs commonly used during the neonatal period, *J Nurse Midwifery* 37(suppl 2):74S, 1992.

Frappier P et al: Nursing assessment of feeding problems, *J Pediatr Nurs* 2(1):37, 1987.

Gelbaum I: Circumcision, *J Nurse Midwifery* 37(suppl 2):97s, 1992.

Greenberg G.: *How to run a traditional Jewish household*, New York, 1983, Simon & Schuster.

Greer PS: Head coverings for newborns under radiant warmers, *JOGNN* 17(4):265, 1988.

Haddock B, Vincent P, Merrow D: Axillary and rectal temperatures of full-term neonates: are they different? *Neonat Network* 5(8):36, 1986.

Hammerschlag MR et al: Efficacy of neonatal ocular prophylaxis for the prevention of chlamydial and gonococcal conjunctivitis, *N Engl J Med* 320(12):769, 1991.

Herzog LW: Urinary tract infections and circumcision, *Am J Dis Child* 143(3):348, 1989.

Jepson Helen A et al: The Apgar score: evolution, limitations, and scoring guidelines, *Birth* 18(2):83, 1991.

Kemper D et al: Jaundice, terminating breast-feeding, and the vulnerable child, *Pediatrics* 84(5):773, 1989.

Klaus M, Kennell J: *Parent-infant bonding*, St Louis, 1982, Mosby.

Larsen GL et al: Postneonatal circumcision—population profile, *Pediatrics* 85(5):808, 1990.

Lemmer CM: Early discharge: outcomes of primiparas and their infants, *JOGNN* 16(4):230, 1987.

MacDonald M: Infection control considerations for management of the newborn in the delivery room, *Pediatr AIDS HIV Infect: Fetus to Adoles* 1(1):16, 1990.

Marchette L, Main R, Redick E: Pain reduction during neonatal circumcision, *Pediatr Nurs* 15:207, 1989.

Marchette L et al: Pain reduction interventions during neonatal circumcision, *Nurs Res* 40(4):241, 1991.

Marecki MA: Chlamydial trachomatis: a developing perinatal problem, *J Perinat Neonat Nurs* 1(4):1, 1988.

Milos MF, Macris D: Circumcision, *J Nurse Midwifery* 37(suppl 2):87s, 1992.

Mudge D, Younger J: The effects of topical lidocaine on infants' response to circumcision, *J Nurse Midwifery* 24:335, 1989.

Newborn screening for sickle cell disease and other hemoglobinopathies, *Pediatrics* 83(5; entire suppl), 1989.

Novak J: Formula for profit, *Common Cause* Mar/Apr, p 18, 1988.

O'Brien C et al: Effect of bathing with 4% chlorhexidine gluconate solution on neonatal bacterial colonization, *J Hosp Infect* 5(supple A):141, 1984.

O'Neill J et al: Percutaneous absorption potential of chlorhexidine in neonates, *Curr Ther Res* 31(3):485, 1982.

Osborn LM, Metcalf TJ: Hygienic care in uncircumcised infants, *Pediatrics* 67(3):365, 1981.

Poland RL: The question of routine neonatal circumcision, *N Engl J Med* 322(18):1312, 1990.

Ream S: Infant nutrition and supplements, *JOGNN* 14(5):371, 1985.

Ross T, Dickason EJ: Nursing alert: vertical transmission of HIV and HBV, *MCN* 17(4):192, 1992.

Schmidt B et al: Strengths and limitations of the Apgar score: a critical appraisal, *J Clin Epidemiol* 41(9):843, 1988.

Schoen EJ: The status of circumcision of newborns, *N Engl J Med* 322(18):1308, 1990.

Schoen EJ: The foreskin and urinary tract infections, *J Pediatr* 115(4):663, 1989.

Sutton MB et al: Baby bottoms and environmental conundrums—disposable diapers and the pediatrician, *Pediatrics* 88(2):386, 1991.

Tsang RC, Nichols BL, editors: *Nutrition during pregnancy*, St Louis, 1988, Mosby.

Valdes-Dapena M: Iatrogenic disease in the perinatal period, *Pediatr Clin North Am* 36(1):67, 1989.

Wiswell TE et al: *Staphylococcus aureus* colonization after neonatal circumcision in relation to device used, *J Pediatr* 119(2):302, 1991.

STUDENT RESOURCE SHELF

J Nurse Midwife 37(suppl 2), 1992. Entire issue devoted to infant care issues: infant nutrition, assessment, circumcision, and drug use.

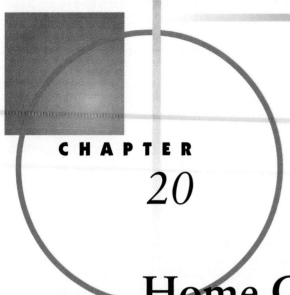

CHAPTER

20

Home Care of the Young Infant

LEARNING OBJECTIVES

1. *Identify the teaching topics for basic home care of the infant.*
2. *Describe immunizations needed during the first year.*
3. *Review safety measures necessary for the infant's environment.*
4. *Describe anticipatory guidance for parents on common problems during early infancy.*
5. *Determine the need for follow-up care and referral to various home care agencies.*
6. *Help the parent use the MABI scale and understand that there are various infant temperaments.*
7. *Discuss the infant cues to learning as well as the process of stimulation.*
8. *Compare normal growth and development milestones, while recognizing the unique qualities of a particular infant.*
9. *Describe how to assess initial attachment and demonstrate the infant's interaction activities to promote parent-infant bonding.*
10. *Know adoption and foster care guidelines.*

Coming home with a newborn infant is an experience requiring the total attention of the parents. Everything is new, and the infant's needs are largely unknown and somewhat frightening. Growing into the role of new parent will take approximately 1 to 3 months; being comfortable with reading the infant's cues to hunger, distress, boredom, or anger; and being able to satisfy the baby's needs. Small successes breed greater confidence, and confidence is what the new parents require.

Anyone assisting parents must remember not to "do it for them" but to enable them to do parenting tasks well. Anticipatory guidance about the growth and development of the infant's abilities and its needs can always emphasize the way parents will be able to recognize needs and manage care.

The nurse's role is guiding and teaching. When in the place of the visiting nurse in the home or in a neonatal follow-up setting, the nurse will be involved in assessment of the ways baby and parents are managing this transition. The nurse in the postpartum or nursery area usually may only provide immediate help and anticipatory guidance. The pages to follow introduce basic home care of the young infant.

Health Maintenance

Health maintenance is important because it allows the normal processes of growth and development to occur. In a positive setting, the infant is protected from the hazards of the environment. Social skills are encouraged as the infant gradually learns to regulate behavior. The infant whose physical and psychologic health is maintained is better prepared to live in an increasingly challenging world.

Nursing care includes teaching parents about hazards to the infant. A young infant is vulnerable to temperature extremes, environmental hazards, and choking.

SAFETY RESPONSIBILITIES

Temperature Control

Infants are frequently overheated and overdressed. When an infant is dressed in a shirt, diaper, and sleeper, the temperature of the room may be kept as low as 70° F which is comfortable for most adults. Add extra layers if the temperature drops further. Where houses are heated, avoid overheating and a dry atmosphere by placing a bowl of water near the source of heat or using a cold spray humidifier (must be cleaned daily). Parents should be cautioned against extremes in temperature and may need to monitor air conditioning. Care must be taken to keep the infant well hydrated, especially during spells of extreme heat and humidity, if no air conditioning is available.

Show parents how to dress the baby appropriately for the weather, using as many layers of clothing as they themselves need. Always *cover the head, hands, and feet* when going out in cold or windy weather. A hat is advisable during the summer months to protect the infant from the heat of the sun. (To prevent burning, use sun screen, even on brown-skinned infants when exposed to sunlight.)

Eliminating Hazards

Encourage parents to take a baby's eye view of the house to identify ways in which it is not safe. The Injury Prevention Program (Farmingham Safety Survey) sponsored by the American Academy of Pediatrics helps parents assess basic home items (Figure 20-1). This survey may be self-administered by parents, who will fill in the form while the health care professional reviews "at risk" answers. The survey should be used first at the 2-month health visit. Other similar surveys are available for parents of toddlers and preschoolers.

Pets. Pets may respond to infants with jealousy, regression, withdrawal, and hostility (Bahr, 1981). There are several guidelines to prepare the pet for the infant's arrival:

1. Discipline the pet not to enter the infant's room.
2. Never allow the pet to sleep in the empty crib.
3. Expose the pet to another newborn. Once the baby is brought home, allow the pet to smell the infant to establish identity.
4. Take time to play with the pet and give individual attention.
5. Keep the pet's immunizations current.

Auto safety. Automobile safety laws in most states require the use of a car restraint system for infants and children through 4 years of age. Many hospital policies require the use of a car seat before allowing the newborn infant to be discharged. Many civic groups sponsor a car seat lending program for a small deposit, which is reimbursed when the seat is returned. Usually the hospital provides management of the program so that seats are available and demonstrated before leaving the hospital. The nurse must educate and reinforce the importance of using a car seat.

Adults and infants who use a restraint system reduce their chances of serious injury or death during an accident. Holding an infant in one's lap is *unsafe* and underestimates the collision force that will propel the infant both in and out of the vehicle on impact (Krozy and McKolgan, 1985).

Seat restraints have the following purposes:

1. To help to absorb and dissipate the shock and minimize the impact.
2. To hold the infant in place during travel.
3. To regulate the infant's behavior, which allows parents to drive safely.

The two types of restraints available are the nonconvertible type, which is used for newborns and infants and faces toward the rear of the car in a reclined position, and the convertible type, which is intended for children through the toddler years. (This faces backward for infants and forward for older children.) All car seats must meet the following Federal Motor Vehicle Safety Standards criteria: (1) seats are tested for front end collision at 30 MPH, (2) harnesses must have buckles that require adult strength to open, and (3) the device must have directions clearly displayed. Safety depends on correct installation of the seat within the car.

Safety issues should be addressed before the baby is born. Parents should be asked:

1. How do you plan to take your baby home?
2. Do you know where to rent or buy a car seat?
3. Can you recognize a safe car seat?

FARMINGHAM SAFETY SURVEY
The First Year of Life

tipp
THE INJURY PREVENTION PROGRAM
SAFETY IS YOUR BEST PRESCRIPTION

Name _____   Date _____

Please X through one answer

1. Do you put the crib side up whenever you leave the baby unattended?	Always	Sometimes	Never
2. Do you use a crib, playpen, or portacrib made before 1976?	Yes	No	Don't know
3. Do you leave the baby unattended on tables or beds?	Frequently	Occasionally	Never
4. Do you leave the baby alone in the house?	Frequently	Occasionally	Never
5. Do you keep plastic wrappers, plastic bags, and balloons out of reach of your children?	Always	Sometimes	Never
6. Does your child play wth small objects such as beads or nuts?	Always	Sometimes	Never
7. Have any of your children ever had an accident requiring a visit to the doctor or hospital?	Yes	Don't remember _____ How many visits	No
8. Are any of your babysitters less than 13 years old?	Yes	No	Don't know
9. How frequently do you check the heating system in your house?	Never	At least once/ year	Every few years
10. Do you smoke in bed?	Frequently	Occasionally	Never
11. Do you have a plan for escape from the house in the event of a fire?	Yes	No	
12. Do you have working fire extinguishers in the house?	Yes	Don't know	No
13. Do you have smoke or fire detectors in the house?	Yes	No	
14. Do you watch for young children before handling hot liquids?	Always	Sometimes	Never
15. Do you ever use woodstoves, kerosene, or quartz heaters?	Yes	No	
16. Do you leave the baby alone in a tub of water?	Frequently	Occasionally	Never
17. Where do you seat your children in the car?	Front	Rear	Front or Rear
18. What type of car seat do you use when your child rides in a car?		_____ Indicate brand	None used
19. Does your child ride on your bicycle with you?	Always	Sometimes	Never

American Academy of Pediatrics

FIGURE 20-1 Farmingham Safety Survey. Note that the survey is for the first year of life. The injury Prevention Program has other surveys for use with growing children. (Courtesy American Academy of Pediatrics. Developed in part by the Division of Maternal and Child Health, DHHS.)

Giving this guidance before parents purchase a car seat is the responsibility of the health care provider (Figure 20-2). Never leave an infant unattended in a car seat. The intense heat or cold with the windows shut is potentially lethal; abduction is also a threat.

Accidents. Accidents are the leading cause of death to children in the United States, and 50% of all children will require medical attention for injuries sustained in an accident. The greatest dangers to the helpless baby are burns, drowning, suffocation, and falls. Parents are

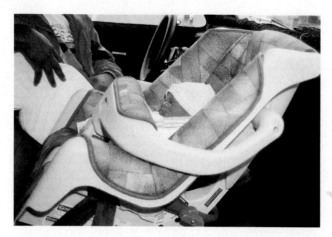

FIGURE 20-2 Position of car seat for a young infant. (Courtesy Marjorie Pyle, RNC, *Lifecircle*.)

responsible for maintenance of their child's environment but may not know how to provide one that is both safe and stimulating. Provide parents with these specific guidelines:

1. Check the temperature of hot water, regulate the water heater to less than 140° F. When you run the bath, turn on the cold water first and then add hot. Never leave the infant alone in the bath for any reason. Place the baby in the bath after the water is drawn and the faucets are turned off.
2. You must provide full supervision for an infant at all times. If you must leave the infant out of sight (parents do need to use the bathroom), the only

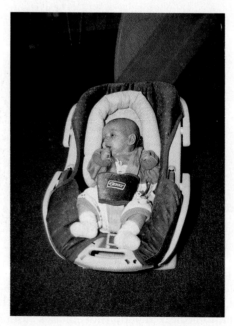

FIGURE 20-3 Infant seat placed on the floor for safety. (Courtesy Marjorie Pyle, RNC, *Lifecircle*.)

safe places for a small infant are the crib, playpen, or a sturdy infant seat with restraint buckled, placed on the floor (Figure 20-3).

3. Keep plastic bags, telephone cords, soft pillows, heavy blankets, small objects, and balloons away from the infant.
4. Keep pins and other sharp objects out of reach.
5. Keep infant away from the stove and other hot surfaces, such as wood stoves, fireplaces, and space heaters.

Furnishings and toys. There are so many new baby furnishings on the market, parents must be cautious. Standards are set by the United States Consumer Product Safety Commission for infant furnishings, and these should be used as a guide when making a purchase. Be aware that babies need both comfort and safety. Figure 20-4 illustrates safety features for cribs, strollers, and baby carriers. This guide is especially important for parents who receive or borrow used equipment.

Toy safety is an important hazard area. The first toys bought for an infant are often gifts not chosen by parents. The ability to select toys appropriate for age, interest, and play value is a skill (Box 20-1). The long-range usefulness of a toy lies in its play value, safety, and ability to capture the child's interest and imagination. Instructions should be read carefully until understood. Be aware that toys can be dangerous if they are not related to the age level of the child. Observe especially for any sharp edges and loosened parts. Finally, safe disposal is necessary if the toy is no longer usable.

Choking. Choking is the leading cause of accidental death in infants under 1 year of age (Effron, 1986). Prevention of choking includes teaching parents not to force-feed their infants and to check toys for small loose parts.

Every parent should know how to help a child (or adult) who is choking (Figure 20-5). The following standards for infants to 1 year of age are from the American Heart Association (Guidelines, 1992).

Airway obstructions usually occur in an infant while eating or playing. Before intervening, parents must determine that the airway is actually obstructed. The child's respirations will become increasingly difficult, coughing will be ineffective and have a high-pitched crowing quality, and the infant will become cyanotic or pale.

- Do *not* sweep mouth or pharynx with a finger.
- Supporting the head and neck with one hand, place the infant face downward, head lower than trunk over your forearm, supported on your thigh.
- Deliver four back blows forcefully between the shoulder blades with the heel of the hand (Figure 20-6, *A*).

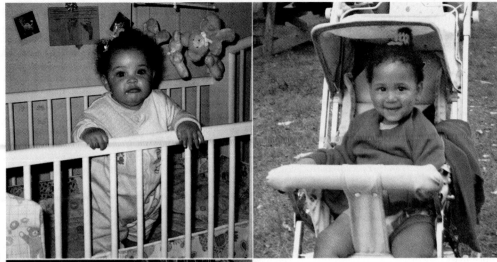

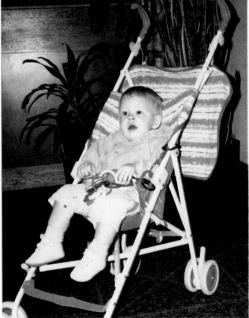

FIGURE 20-4 Safety features for cribs and strollers. **A,** Note the narrow crib slats to prevent injury. Sides need to be adjustable as the baby grows. **B,** This stroller is one that will adjust to a growing baby and saves money in the long run. **C,** A portable stroller is less expensive but not usable for as many months. The baby's back is always flexed in this stroller. (**A** and **B** courtesy Camille Bodden; **C** courtesy Marjorie Pyle, RNC, *Lifecircle.*)

BOX 20-1 Age-Appropriate Toys

NEWBORN TO 3 MONTHS

Toys should be visual, auditory, and tactile.
- Something to watch over crib: hanging mobile that is colorful with contrasting geometric designs and faces.
- Stuffed toys that are soft, small, cuddly, and washable.
- Bath toys such as sponges or squeeze toys.
- Music box.
- Safety mirror to see their own image.
- Soft and firm chewable "teethers."
- Crib gym with items to hold, push, and pull.

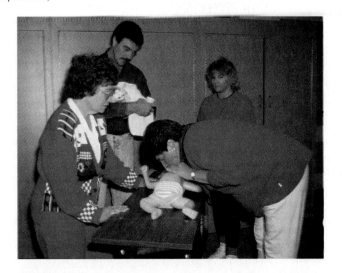

FIGURE 20-5 Parents learn mouth-to-mouth resuscitation in class. (Courtesy Marjorie Pyle, RNC, *Lifecircle.*)

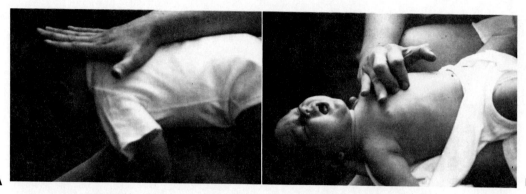

FIGURE 20-6 Modified Heimlich technique for choking infant. **A,** Four back blows with palm of hand between scapulae. **B,** Four chest thrusts by placing two fingers below nipple line and pressing down 1/2 inch. (Courtesy RO Roberson.)

- While supporting the head, sandwich the infant between your hands and turn him on his back, head lower than trunk.
- Deliver 4 chest thrusts in the midline, one finger-breadth below the nipple line in the same manner as external chest compressions (Figure 20-6, *B*).
- Open airway with head-tilt/chin-lift maneuver.
- If infant is not breathing, attempt one ventilation, and then turn over and repeat the the back blows and chest thrusts until the foreign body is expelled or the infant becomes unconscious.
- Once the infant does lose consciousness, CPR should be started (Procedure 20-1).

Test Yourself

A 2-month-old has inhaled a small object. Describe the necessary actions you would take.

PREVENTING ILLNESS

Communication must flow in both directions for illness prevention education to be effective. Assess parental knowledge by asking yourself what parents need to know. Addressing parental concerns first will alleviate their anxiety. Parents are especially anxious when a newborn seems ill.

Warning signs of illness in a newborn should be taught to the new parents. Call the primary health care provider* when:

- The eyes, umbilical cord, or circumcision site is red or swollen.
- The baby appears lethargic or sleeps a lot.
- The baby does not cry normally.

---

*This list may be given to parents on discharge from hospital or by home health nurse.

- The baby is not eating well or vomits feedings.
- The baby does not move all extremities well.
- The baby's skin seems yellow, even in sunlight.
- The baby's stools are watery and frequent.
- The baby has a stuffy nose and seems to have difficulty breathing (breathing very rapidly, more than 60 times a minute).
- You notice anything unusual or have a vague, uneasy feeling that all is not well.

Immunizations

All children should be immunized against what were once common childhood infectious diseases. These diseases took a terrible toll in the days before immunizations became safe and standardized. It is a tragedy that in many underdeveloped countries, as well as in some populations within the United States, children who have not been immunized may die or be damaged by these preventable diseases. Cost should not be a deterrent—free immunizations are available at Department of Health Clinics; immigration status is not questioned.

Infants must weigh at least 10 pounds and be 2 months old to be immunized. Table 20-1 lists immunizations and guidelines for administration. However, be aware that schedules may vary with each health care provider. You must know the actions, adverse effects, contraindications, and implications for the vaccines you administer. Many of the vaccines are made from live-attenuated viruses. Thus, there is a low risk that multiplication of the virus may cause a reaction. There are problems with universal vaccination. The benefit-risk ratio should be considered for any infant with allergic or medical problems. Vaccination may be delayed. There are rare cases of allergic reaction to DPT with protracted crying, shock, or seizures. Rubella vaccine is associated in rare cases with acute arthritis. Immunization is postponed if the child has an acute, infectious febrile illness, since any reactions to the vaccine could be confused with disease symptoms. Children with

Observe color; tap, or gently shake shoulders.

Yell for help; if alone, perform CPR for 1 min before calling for help again.

Turn infant to back, supporting head and neck.

Place on firm, flat surface.

Clear airway, prn (see text).

Tilt head back gently to "sniffing" or neutral position; use head-tilt/chin-lift maneuver (Fig. 20-7, *A*).

Do not hyperextend neck.

Assess for evidence of breathing:

Observe for chest movement.

Listen for exhaled air, and feel for exhaled air flow.

Breathe for infant (Fig. 20-7, *B*):

Take a breath.

Open mouth wide and place over mouth and nose of infant to create seal.

NOTE: Repeat the word *ho* as you gently puff volume of air *in your* cheeks into infant. *Do not* force air.

Infant's chest should rise slightly with each puff; keep fingers on chest wall to sense air entry.

Give two slow breaths (1 to 1.5 sec/breath), pausing to inhale between breaths.

Check pulse of brachial artery (Fig. 20-7, *C*) while maintaining head tilt.

If pulse is present, initiate rescue breathing. Continue until spontaneous breathing resumes at rate of every 3 sec or 20 times/min.

If pulse is not present, initiate chest compressions and coordinate with breathing.

Chest compressions:

Maintain head tilt. With other hand, position fingers for chest compressions.

Place index finger of hand farthest from infant's head just under imaginary line drawn between nipples (Fig. 20-7, *D*). Move index finger to a position one finger-breadth below this intersection.

Using 2 or 3 fingers, compress sternum to depth of ½ or ¾ inch.

Release pressure without moving fingers from the position.

Repeat at a rate of at least 100 times/min; 5 compressions in 3 sec or less.

Perform 20 cycles of 5 compressions and 1 ventilation. (If possible, compressions are accompanied by positive-pressure ventilation at a rate of 40 to 60/min.) After cycles, check the brachial pulse to determine presence of pulse.

Discontinue compressions if spontaneous heart rate reaches or exceeds 80 beats/min.

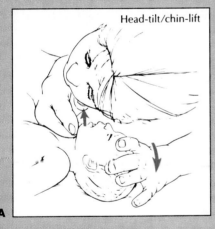
Head-tilt/chin-lift

A

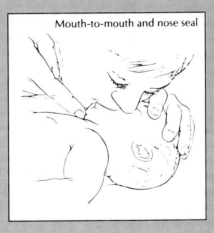
Mouth-to-mouth and nose seal

B

FIGURE 20-7 A-D, Procedures for cardiopulmonary resuscitation. (From Guidelines for Cardiopulmonary Resuscitation [CPR] and Emergency Cardiac Care [ECC]): *JAMA* 286[16]:2171, 1992.)

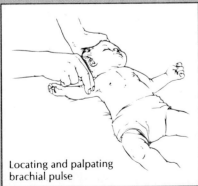
Locating and palpating brachial pulse

C

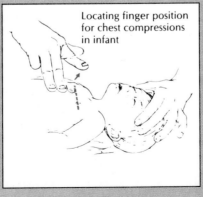
Locating finger position for chest compressions in infant

D

OPTIONAL ACTIVITY: Write a sample nursing note correctly documenting the performance of this procedure

TABLE 20-1 Immunization Recommendations During Infancy

TYPE	TIMING	POSSIBLE SIDE EFFECTS
Diphtheria		
Inactivated toxin called **toxoid**	2, 4, 6, and 18 months, then at 4 to 6 years	Erythema, induration, tenderness, mild to moderate fever, vomiting, malaise
Pertussis		
Killed vaccine	Begin at 2 months, same schedule for diphtheria, not administered over 6 years of age	See above side effects and central nervous system effects: local swelling, excessive tiredness, rare convulsions, encephalopathy
Tetanus		
Killed vaccine	Begin at 2 months, repeated at 8-week intervals for 3 doses	Fever, local soreness, swelling
Measles		
(Rubeola, 10-day measles) Live-attenuated virus	Administered usually at 15 months alone or with measles, mumps, and rubella (MMR)	Rash, fever about 10 days after immunization
Tuberculosis		
Limited immunity: BCG (Bacillus Calmette-Guérin vaccine); screening with tine test	If high risk, testing to be done every year starting at 12 months; if low risk, testing should be done at 12-15 months; should precede or be given simultaneously with measles vaccine because measles can give a false positive TB test	False negative can be produced if child exposed to childhood diseases within 4 weeks of TB testing. False positive reports if child has received BCG vaccine
Mumps		
Live-attenuated virus	Administered at 15 months with MMR	Mild fever 7 to 14 days after vaccine
Rubella		
(German measles, 3-day measles) Live-attenuated virus preparation	Administered at 15 months with MMR	Rash, joint pain, lymphadenopathy
Polio		
Live-attenuated virus (TOPV), containing three different viruses; use killed vaccine (IPV and Salk) for immunocompromised patients	TOPV (trivalent oral polio vaccine) administered at 2, 4, and 18 months and again between 4 to 6 years	No reaction; not administered to infant with HIV
HbCV		
(*Haemophilus influenza* type B conjugate vaccine) anti-*Haemophilus influenzae* serum	12-24 months, begin at 1 to 3 months if infant in day-care	Slight fever
Hepatitis B Vaccine		
For infants of hepatitis B negative women	Within 48 hours of birth or some start at 1-2 months; second dose 1 month later; third dose before age 18 months	Pain at IM site Possible fever
Infants of women who are hepatitis B positive plus	Within 12 hours of birth, then second and third dose as above	Report all adverse immunization effects to VAERS 1-800-822-7967
Hepatitis B Immunoglobulin	Within 12 hours of birth	

Modified from American Academy of Pediatrics: *Report of Committee on Infectious Diseases,* ed 22, Elk Grove, IL, 1991, The Academy.

malignancies (such as leukemia or lymphoma) who are receiving corticosteroids or radiation therapy or who have altered immune systems (HIV positive) should not be immunized with attenuated live virus. Rapid multiplication of the virus in these children can cause severe illness. Recently, with some publicized reactions to the pertussis vaccine, parents have been hesitant to have their infants receive DPT. It is true that many more children die or suffer damage from pertussis (or whooping cough) than from the vaccine. However, a neurologic history should be obtained before the administration of the pertussis vaccine because of certain adverse neurologic reactions. If there is any history of neurologic disorders, the vaccine should be omitted from the immunization regimen. Some parents are delaying their child's immunizations until school entrance or refusing to immunize them at all. As a result, there is an increase in the incidence of preventable diseases.

> **Test Yourself**
>
> Which infants should not receive immunizations on the regular schedule?

Common Illnesses

Fever. Fever causes anxiety for parents. Parents need to know that fever is a normal response to a viral or bacterial infection. Fever is a rectal temperature above 100.4° F (38° C) or an axillary temperature above 99° F (37.2° C). During the day, normal body temperature rises and peaks between 6 and 10 PM, then drops to its lowest between 2 and 4 AM. Febrile patterns follow the same cycle. Many infants will "spike" high fevers with an illness. Spontaneous visual and motor behaviors are more reliable indicators of the severity of illness than fever. However, fever should not be ignored. The primary health care provider should be notified if:

1. The infant appears dehydrated.
2. The fever is greater than 99° F.
3. The infant is irritable, difficult to awaken, has difficulty breathing, or holds his head and neck stiffly.

Interventions for treating a fever are as follows:

1. Monitor axillary temperature at least twice a day (morning and night) to account for diurnal variations. Hold the baby securely so the thermometer remains in place for at least 3 minutes. An inguinal temperature may also be taken (see Chapter 19).
2. Monitor temperature more often during the first day of illness and if the infant feels warm, is irritable, shivers, or is flushed.

3. Reduce the infant's activity to conserve energy.
4. Dress baby lightly.
5. Increase fluid intake.
6. Sponge bathe with tepid water if the temperature is greater than 103° F, and recheck the temperature after the bath.
7. Parents should be aware of the appropriate dosage of acetaminophen for their infant's age and weight; if not sure, call the health care provider. (Never give aspirin, because it is associated with **Reye's syndrome,** a severe neurologic disorder.)

Common colds. Common colds usually include cough, nasal congestion, and possibly anorexia and fever. Colds are viral illnesses and have no cure; thus, all treatment is for symptomatic relief. To prevent colds, keep the infant out of crowds and away from visitors who are sick. This may be difficult for the working mother, especially if she uses a day-care facility. The following interventions help ease the discomfort of the infant with a cold:

1. Use a cool mist vaporizer to increase the moisture to the infant's mucous membranes. Clean vaporizer daily.
2. Show parents how to use a bulb syringe to relieve nasal congestion especially before feeding and sleeping.
3. Increase intake of water.
4. Contact the primary health care provider for advice about medications that may ease symptoms.

If the baby looks sick, has a fever over 38.5° C (101° F), has a bad cough or a congested chest, is refusing liquids, or is pulling at his ears, then the problem may be more serious than a simple cold. Infants with these symptoms should be examined.

Vomiting and diarrhea. *Vomiting* should be distinguished from spitting up. Spitting up or regurgitation is expelling a small amount of liquid when the infant burps or is handled actively after feeding. Vomiting is not always associated with these activities; the amount of fluid expelled is also greater. It can be caused by factors such as overeating, food allergies, pyloric stenosis, or gastroenteritis, or it can be indicative of emotional problems. Diarrhea is an increase in the fluidity, frequency, and volume of stool and can be caused by some foods, excessive sugar intake, infections, allergies, or overintake of fluids. Dehydration is a serious complication of both diarrhea and vomiting. Assessment of the infant with these problems should include the following:

1. A description of the onset, duration, frequency, and color
2. Consistency and amount of the diarrhea and/or vomitus

3. Approximate oral intake within last 24 hours
4. Signs of dehydration—weight loss, sunken fontanelle, dry eyes and mucous membranes, decrease in number of wet diapers

Interventions will include the following:

1. Stop all milk intake.
2. Encourage clear fluids in small amounts.
3. The younger infant must be seen by the health care provider and then may be given an electrolyte formula such as Pedialyte, Vivonex, or sometimes Gatorade for 24 hours and then slowly restarted on breast-feeding or formula.
4. Refer any infant to the health care provider if there is:
   a. Vomiting and fever or bulging fontanelle
   b. Prolonged or persistent vomiting with dehydration
   c. Blood or bile in the vomitus
   d. Vomiting with abdominal distention, localized tenderness or pain, or palpable abdominal mass
   e. Vomiting with visible peristalsis or projectile vomiting, sunken fontanelle
   f. Vomiting and a history or suspicion of ingestion of a drug or poison

Constipation. A constipated baby has hard, dry, infrequent stools. This often begins when the baby is switched from formula or breast milk to cow's milk. Great effort is required to pass the stool, producing anal irritation, fistulas, and pain. Other causes of constipation include insufficient sugar in the formula, low fluid intake, starvation, prolonged vomiting spells, intestinal constriction, chronic disease, fissures, and severe diaper rash. Constipation can also be a sign of Hirschsprung's disease or hypothyroidism. Some older infants can withhold stool and will when there is pain. Early toilet training can cause psychologic problems with the same result. Constipation should be discussed with the primary care provider who may advise changes in diet. Infants should not be given laxatives or enemas. Sometimes a small amount of Karo syrup mixed into formula or water is effective.

Skin Problems

The epidermis and the immune system of the infant are immature, which increases susceptibility to irritation and infection. The addition of any irritating agent may cause the skin to become inflamed and lose its protective quality. There are many types of skin lesions, some of which are treated with prescription medication. Parents need to know how to relieve symptoms to increase an infant's comfort.

First look for and eliminate environmental factors that could cause irritation such as laundry soaps, laundry detergent, and wool clothing. Symptomatic relief can be achieved by a tepid bath or applying cool lotions to relieve the symptoms of itching, rubbing, and chafing. Apply cornstarch to areas that are not weeping wounds, taking care not to scatter powder. Do not use baby powder or scented talcs.

Cradle cap is seborrheic dermatitis, resulting in yellowish oily scales on the scalp. Seborrhea of the face is frequently seen as well. Rub a small amount of baby or mineral oil into the scalp before shampooing. After softening, a fine-tooth comb is used to remove the loose scales. Stubborn cases may require the use of an anti-dandruff shampoo and application of 0.5% hydrocortisone cream to the face. Do not attempt to remove all scales after the first treatment. It is safer to try several applications over a few days than try to loosen all the scales at once.

Diaper rash is diaper dermatitis, resulting in reddened, excoriated skin. Washing routines for cloth diapers should be reviewed. Changing detergents or fabric softeners may be all that is needed. Cloth diapers should be double rinsed in a solution of sodium borate (Borax). Some infants do not tolerate the use of plastic waterproof pants or paper diapers with plastic covers. A change in diet may add a new element in the stool or urine, which irritates the skin. Whatever the cause of the rash, the diaper area should be washed with water at each diaper change and exposed to air. A thick coat of ointment containing zinc oxide (Desitin) can be applied.

Candida albicans, monilia, can invade the infant's diaper area or mouth. This type of diaper rash has defined scalloped edges and a wet, oozing look. Lesions that seem like curdled milk will appear in the mouth. Feeding the baby plain water before examining the mouth can differentiate between milk residue and a monilial infection. Nystatin is the treatment of choice and can be obtained only by prescription.

Some infants develop *heat rash* (miliaria rubra) when they are too warm. Face, neck, trunk, and diaper areas are the first to break out with reddened papules. Cooling the infant with a tepid bath or changing to lighter clothing will improve the rash. In winter, turning down the thermostat might eliminate the problem. Cornstarch can be used sparingly in the creases around the neck and axilla.

Newborn Sleep Cycles

Infants have unique cycles of sleep and wakefulness. Some babies sleep through any noise, while others wake and cry more frequently. By 10 days of age the infant should be more tuned to the parents' sleep and wake cycles and begin to establish a consistent pattern of sleep. During the first few weeks of life, infants may sleep up to 5 hours at any time and awaken for feeding and social time. However, some infants spend a considerable block of time awake. Until 2 to 3 months of age, the infant will require about 18 to 20 hours of sleep daily. By 4 months of age, 95% of all infants sleep through the night (about 8 hours). During growth spurts the child may awaken for a feeding once a night. By 1 year of age, about 12 hours of sleep plus two nap times are needed. Routines should be set to establish good sleeping habits, although the age at which parents can anticipate an uninterrupted night's sleep varies.

Sleep disturbance. Problems occur when the infant does not accommodate the family's schedule. This often leaves the parents distressed, uncertain, and exhausted. Anticipatory guidance during the early infant period includes advising parents that, starting early in infancy, children need to be taught acceptance of bedtimes and nap times and that there is a special time and their own special place for sleeping. Young infants should sleep near but not with parents until they are 2 to 3 months old. Always leave the door open if the infant is in another room. In many ethnic groups, the "family bed" is used by some or all family members.

1. When an infant is not synchronized with day and night schedules, keep him awake rather than encouraging extra sleep during the day.
2. When an infant is a trained night feeder, make night feeding brief and boring. Do not use solids at bedtime because extra calories do not encourage sleep. Give the last feeding at 10 to 11 PM and not in the bed. *Do not prop the bottle* or let babies suck on bottles while falling asleep. This leads to "bottle mouth," tooth decay, and to inner-ear infection. Use a pacifier or an alternative if this is acceptable to parents.
3. When an infant is a trained night crier, it is often because the parent reinforces this behavior with extra attention. Soothe the infant as quickly as possible and leave the room. Place the infant in bed before he is asleep, so the last waking memory is of the crib and comfort toy or blanket and not the parent. Avoid changing diapers at night.
4. When an infant is a fearful night crier and suffers from separation anxiety (at about 6 months), give the infant a security object. Leave the door open and a nightlight on in the room.

Although infants appear to sleep longer on the abdomen, new studies on sudden infant death syndrome (SIDS) suggest that small babies should not be placed on the abdomen to sleep (Graves, 1992). Later when the SIDS risk is over (6 to 8 months), the infant may assume any position. Most infants, in fact, have a preferred sleep position after they are able to turn themselves.

Crying, fussiness, and colic. An infant's cry is his only means of communication, as well as a method of releasing tension. There are differences between cries of hunger, discomfort, boredom, and fatigue. Parents may become discouraged if their actions do not influence the infant's crying. The infant who cries inconsolably is a real challenge to both parents and health care providers. It must be determined that no functional or organic disorder exists that is causing the infant distress. A complete nursing history includes inquiring about maternal drug intake, both legal and illegal. Infants of mothers who use cocaine or crack are extremely irritable and may be inconsolable. The breast-fed infant may be receiving stimulating substances such as caffeine via breast milk.

Most newborns cry for about 2 hours out of every 24. Some do it all at once, others cry intermittently. Infants who cry for sustained periods during the first 3 months may have **colic**. These crying episodes are more likely to occur during the evening and late night as the baby is influenced by the fatigue, tension, and busyness of the parent at the end of the day. The pattern varies, but babies may cry for 4 or more hours without letting up. They appear very distressed after feeding, draw their legs up to the abdomen, and scream. The anxiety level, perhaps even the hostility of the parent, adds to the problem of quieting the colicky baby.

Instruct parents to hold the infant, use gentle motion, touch, and soothing words. Motion helps soothe. Parents can try placing the infant in a front-pack carrier that allows free movement of the parent's hands, take the infant for a ride in the car, play music, or use an infant swing. Encourage parents not to overfeed their crying infant as a way of inducing sleep. Allow at least 2 to 2½ hours between feeds. A pacifier may be used. Most important, urge the parents to seek help from friends and relatives, because they will need "time out."

Brazelton discovered early in his practice (1976) that half of his morning calls were about crying infants. He suggested many of the previous activities, which would work at first and then quickly failed. He found that as parents became worn out, the babies cried even more. Brazelton asked the parents to keep charts on crying, with the following results:

1. Total crying usually did not amount to more than 2 hours per day.
2. The more frantic the maneuvers a parent instituted, the more the baby cried.
3. If parents allowed a certain amount of crying and only periodically attempted to soothe the infant, the crying settled down to 2 hours each day.
4. The crying began to decrease by 7 weeks and by 10 weeks was just about gone.
5. By 12 weeks, the time of day formerly used for crying became the infant's most sociable period.

Armed with this information, Brazelton decided there is no easy solution to crying. It seems to be a channel for the baby's energies, a time to let off steam, or an exercise period. He now encourages parents to try various methods of quieting the baby and not to get excited if they do not work. If they are able to relax, they do not add to the infant's tension.

There are a certain group of infants who respond to outside stimuli with unusual amounts of crying and motor activity. They cry longer than 2 hours per day and are difficult to quiet. If the parents of these irritable infants do not remain calm, the babies can end up crying for as much as 12 hours a day. Follow-up studies on some of these overractive infants show that they often grow up to be extremely intelligent—which may be of some encouragement to distraught parents.

In 1970, an organization called Mothers Anonymous (now Parents Anonymous) was formed. Although called by different names in different locations (e.g., Parental Stress Hotline, COPE, CALM), it is a helpful resource for parents who have crying babies.

Parents' fatigue and frustration levels are often related to subsequent abuse of the infant. An irrational idea emerges that the baby deliberately is crying to irritate the parent. Interventions are important *before* this irrational idea becomes fixed. Unfortunately, in families where abuse is seen, often there is not a support network of people who are knowledgeable about growth and development. Often there is a repeated cycle of abuse (see Chapter 26).

Significance of Growth and Development

The first few months of life establish the groundwork for the ability to love and trust. Because the infant may sleep for a majority of the day, parents often regard the baby as unresponsive and believe he is not learning from them and the environment. In reality, the new infant is responding intensely, especially to the emotional tone of the care givers.

The extent to which the infant interacts with the environment has only begun to be appreciated. Informing parents of the newborn's visual, auditory, and cognitive abilities helps them to begin appropriate stimulation for intellectual, social, and emotional growth. They may also learn to prevent adverse stimulation.

Much has been realized about the vital importance of growth and development. The nurse who is able to assess the baby's progress may be able to identify delays in development and suggest interventions. Often, early intervention can overcome a developmental lag. A number of studies have found that the appropriate stimulation may allow premature infants to catch up. Studies show also that there are significant differences between infants whose mothers use appropriate stimulation and understand infant cues and those whose mothers do not (Mahler, Pine, and Berman, 1975). Because the goal is healthy development, these studies may guide your interaction with parents of new infants (Figure 20-8).

MATURATION

Biophysical maturation may be assessed by examining the infant's ability to control gross and fine motor movements, as well as the responses to sound, color, and light. Cognitive growth is assessed by observing the infant's curiosity and interest in the environment. The infant who reaches monthly milestones in a timely manner shows the ability to manipulate and interact with the environment.

The infant is observed for motor tone, social interaction, growth, and sleep patterns. If these are within the normal ranges, the infant is thought to be developing well.

Verbal growth is assessed by observing the infant's attempts at vocalization, his quality of voice, and communication with parents and others. For instance, in-

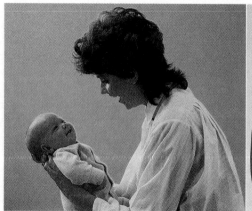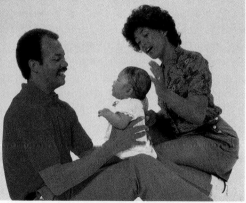

FIGURE 20-8 **A,** Social smile. **B,** Sitting up. (Courtesy Ross Laboratories, Columbus, Ohio.)

fants with hearing deficits often do not vocalize early. Healthier infants show increasing depth of comprehension and ability to communicate in verbal and nonverbal ways. This interaction reveals information about the infant's social and affective growth.

FIRST TASK: DEVELOPMENT OF TRUST

Each infant acts as if he is the center of the world. Infants are preoccupied with their own needs and believe that in some way, the outside world is connected to their inner world. It is as if the infant believes that there is a magical connection to the mother; this is the first understanding of relationship.

Positive, comforting early experiences, with **repetition, continuity, and routine** of the parenting experience, are the infant's building blocks for developing an internal framework that will allow use of the flood of perceptions. With *continuity* and *repetition,* perceptions are organized into the earliest memories. Because of the routine and physical gratification involved with feeding, its significance is great, and it is organized into memories of satisfaction and pleasure. These significant memories then make feeding even more important. Sensations in the infant's mouth and stomach while feeding are of such intense gratification that they become the unconscious essence of satisfaction throughout the infant's life.

The child is stimulated and gratified through feeding, cuddling, and simple play. The child responds and begins to subtly "understand" the personal warmth the mother transmits through her body and tender gestures. The infant directs growing amounts of attention toward the outer world through gratification of his needs.

Without parents who gratify and stimulate, the infant concentrates only on unmet inner needs, particularly the demands of hunger and touching. Left for long periods without personal contact or left to cry when food or other forms of attention are needed, the infant learns not to expect satisfaction of these needs (i.e., learns to *mistrust*). As a result, the baby may develop primarily in a self-involved way and exclude the outside world.

Thus, "spoiling" is not an issue in this early period. Rather, parents will want to meet the infant's needs in as comforting a way as possible. When parents understand the importance of their actions on future development, most are eager to do the correct things.

Perception of Feeling

While developing a relationship with the mother, the infant is learning the way the mother feels toward him. Later, as the ability to perceive and remember develops, the infant will remember particular things about their relationship but initially will only reflect and remember the mother's feeling tone. If a child has an adequate mother who can provide the necessary emotional atmosphere, the early impressions are of warmth, tenderness, comfort, and the satisfying milk that the mother gives. If the child has an inadequate mother who is unable to provide a healthy emotional tone, the early impressions are of isolation, frustration, coldness, and, as a result, "undesirable" milk. Even food can be given in such a way as to make it seem bitter.

Even at a very early stage, unhealthy mothering can greatly affect the child's development because the feelings at this stage are carried the rest of the child's life. Because basic feelings are so essential to personality makeup, adults who have not had a satisfying infancy may have the mark of infancy always with them. Some children continue to act in babyish ways until they reach adolescence. In adolescence, they rebel or overreact and may become destructive in their desire to be independent. As adults, they can be dependent and cling to friends, their spouses, or parents. This is one example of why it is necessary for infants to have relationships. The healthier the person is to whom they relate, the healthier their development will be.

DEVELOPMENT OF THE SENSES

The sensory system parallels other systems in that it is initially uncontrolled and unrefined and requires physical maturation and experience to develop. Thus, although the infant receives sensory input readily, the ability to interpret this input accompanies maturation.

Touch and Motion Perception

Perceptions of motion and touch are perhaps the most important to the new infant. Although tactile sensation has not been studied in depth, research has shown that the fetus in utero responds to manipulation of the mother's abdomen by squirming away. Research showed that a fetus stroked around the lips moved toward the stimulus. After birth, skin conveys sensations from patting, stroking, cuddling, carrying, and diapering. Touch creates quiet states and decreases tension. For instance, an infant will move around in a crib against the crib wall before relaxing and falling asleep. Infants wrapped snugly tend to sleep more soundly and be less fretful.

Response to stroking and the rooting reflex is increased over the first 5 days of life. Skin-to-skin stroking is most soothing for an adult, and many parents are now stroking infants lightly and perhaps misleadingly use the term *infant massage.* Infant stroking is a widely used relaxation therapy in other countries (e.g., in India where a baby is rubbed with oil several times a day). Strokes should move from central to distal and from head to toe. When stroking the head, move from the forehead to the occiput.

Stroking is used with premature infants because it promotes more regular respirations and reduces periods of apnea (Field, 1988). All children and most adults respond with satisfaction to hugging and loving touching. (When a child does not respond positively, question further into early tactile experiences.)

Vestibular sensitivity reflects body posture, balance, and the sense of falling. The canals of the inner ear are functional at birth but must develop further afterward. Vestibular sense is integrated with visual perception slowly; the baby is unaware of heights from just visual perception. Even up to 3 years, children will climb and jump with no real idea of how far they are above a surface.

The awareness of motion is already acute at birth, having been present in utero. Infants respond with pleasure to rocking rhythmic motion and to tactile sensations of warmth, closeness, and snugness (see Cultural Aspects of Care). An infant's consolability often relates to body position, e.g., an infant becomes more alert and quiet when held upright. Infants enjoy being rocked, riding in cars or strollers, or swinging. One of the signs of neglect is a child rocking himself, moving rhythmically and restlessly in the crib.

Recognizing the value of body contact gained from observation of cultures that use infant carriers, many American parents are now using such carriers for young infants. The infants sleep well and seem to find pleasure in being close to their parents in this way (Figure 20-9).

Hearing

At around 6 months of gestation, the fetus begins to move in rhythm with maternal speech. Response to music while in utero has been noted; babies are soothed by quiet music and become more active with noisy music.

Clinical Decision

Andy was born at 37 weeks but weighed 6 pounds, so he was sent home after a 2-day recovery in the hospital. Mary decided to bottle feed him. At first, his sucking was irregular; he would often pause to rest. Mary felt he "wasn't hungry" and tended to remove the bottle before he was satisfied. "Oh, you're done?" she'd say. "Well, time to go to sleep." She would put Andy down and leave the room. Within 10 minutes, he was crying again. This frustrating pattern developed early in the first month. Using the baseline data about feeling tone and feeding satisfaction, what interventions might help Mary and her baby develop better continuity?

I played rhythmic music and stroked my abdomen in the same rhythm as well as talking often to the fetus. After the baby was born, I continued this activity. My baby does seem to demonstrate an alert responsiveness to music and rhythm in his early infant months.

At birth the auditory canal is shorter in the baby than for the adult, and higher tones are tolerated more easily than those of lower frequency (resonance). The closer the infant is to the sound, the easier it will be to discriminate it. Little reaction occurs below the level of normal speaking voices (50 to 60 decibels). Infants tend to like sounds around the range of the human voice and are sensitive to rhythmic and continuous sound. Infants

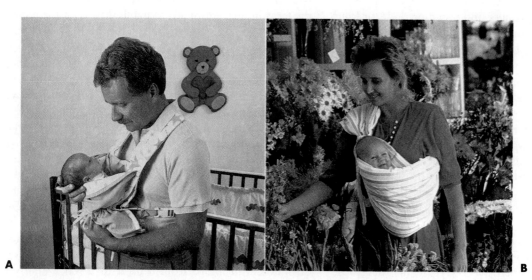

FIGURE 20-9 A, Father with Snugli carrier. **B,** Mother with sling carrier. (**A** courtesy Ross Laboratories, Columbus, Ohio; **B** courtesy Marjorie Pyle, RNC, *Lifecircle*.)

Cultural Aspects of Care

The mothering pattern of the Kikuyu tribe of central Kenya stands out as strikingly different from many American styles. Infants are almost never put down, either to sleep or for any other reason. They are continuously carried, usually tied on their mothers' backs and therefore are rarely deprived of physical contact with their mothers.

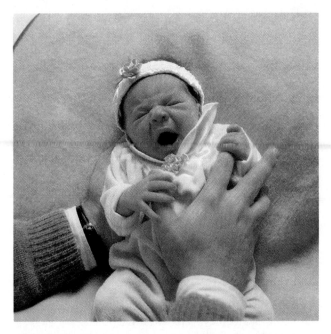

FIGURE 20-10 Infant grimace may mean many things. (Courtesy Marjorie Pyle, RNC, *Lifecircle*.)

like to listen to sentences uttered with exaggerated variation in pitch.

Hearing responses in infancy:

4 to 5 weeks. Occasional turning of eyes in direction of sound origin

4 months. Consistent turning of head toward site of sound; widening of eyes; quiet, listening attitude (audiovisual link important)

6 months. Turning toward sound; recognizing it below eye level first, then above eye level

Groundwork for verbal ability begins to be developed long before words appear. Many observers feel that infants whose mothers often talk to them tend to begin speaking earlier than infants who are not exposed to such sounds (Table 20-2). The ability to listen and discriminate among sounds is an important task to be undertaken in the second half of the first year.

Smelling and Tasting

The sensation of smell is demonstrated by placing an alcohol swab under the infant's nose, eliciting a startle reflex and a turn away from the smell. Facial expressions of rejection are similar to adult expressions (Figure 20-10). The infant quickly becomes more sensitive to smell, and by the fifth day a less potent smell elicits the same response. By the end of the first week, the infant can distinguish between the mother and a stranger by smell. The most noted study was done by McFarlane (1975) with infants at 6, 8, and 10 days of age. When presented a breast pad, these infants showed a stable preference for the breast pad used by their own mother.

Most recent research has shown that the infant can discriminate tastes. Infants especially savor fluid that has been sweetened. The infant sucks harder and consumes more sweet fluid. When a sour and bitter taste is presented, facial expressions of rejection are similar to those of children and adults (Haith, 1986).

Seeing

The visual ability of the fetus at 16 weeks has been demonstrated by a startle reflex when strong light was shone on the mother's abdomen. All neurologic development for visual perception is functional before birth, but a number of studies indicate that the visual system goes through marked growth and development during the first 6 months (Box 20-2). At birth, the infant's skill is an important factor in parent-infant attachment because it allows the infant to find, concentrate on, and prefer the human face to all other stimuli. Eyes can fixate on one object for a specific time and are especially attracted to contrasting patterns. The best focal point at first is approximately 10 to 12 inches away; this is the distance between faces when the infant is being held in the traditional feeding position. The infant can coordinate both eyes to move together and track a moving object for a short arc. The eyes can be oriented to an area

TABLE 20-2 Normal Speech and Language Development

AGE	SPEECH
1 month	Throaty sounds
2 months	Vowel sounds ("eh"), coos
3 months	Babbles, initial vowels
4 months	Guttural sounds ("ah," "goo") and consonants
6 months	Vocalizes to toys
	Imitates sounds

BOX 20-2   Early Visual Awareness

Newborn

Can perceive changes in light intensity and movement

Protective blinking; ability to follow bright object to midline if 6 to 8 inches from eyes; doll's eye phenomenon may be present (see Chapter 17)

5 to 6 weeks

Ability to fix gaze on an object if 12 to 24 inches in distance and patterned (interesting)

6 to 8 weeks

Ability to follow objects well established if still kept close to eyes

3 to 5 months

Visual and tactile links rapidly developing (see-touch-grasp); begins to inspect hands; focusing distance increasing

Data from Holt K: *Developmental pediatrics,* London, 1977, Butterworths.

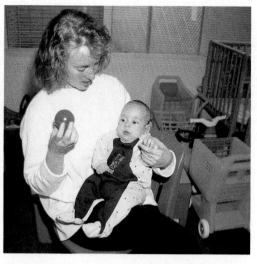

FIGURE 20-11 Quiet alert state following red ball. (Courtesy Marjorie Pyle, RNC, *Lifecircle.*)

INFANT TEMPERAMENT

Differences in children puzzle parents. One child will be easy to raise, the next difficult. Parents will point out how different a child is from themselves and search for **claiming cues**—is he like my own father or my brother? Does she react like this because of some way I am treating her?

Today it is fairly clear that **temperament** is distinctly identifiable early in infancy. Chess and Thomas (1985) said that temperament is "the general nature or characteristic mood of the individual determining the general way a person behaves." When parents need help in understanding their infant, the *Infant Temperament Questionnaire (ITQ)* (Carey and McDevitt, 1978) may

to find an object (Figure 20-11). Changes in looking occur by about 2 months. Babies then detect changes in structure in pictures (e.g., smiley faces with a frown or a box with a piece missing) indicating that perhaps structure is being recognized (Haith, 1986). Infants appear to enjoy primary colors, black and white contrasts, and colored mobiles that move (Figure 20-12).

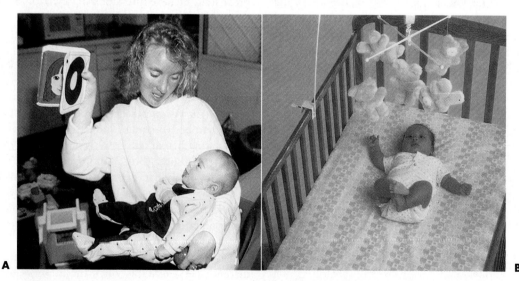

FIGURE 20-12 A, Presenting black and white diagrams for infant interest. **B,** Crib mobiles keep baby interested. (**A** courtesy Marjorie Pyle, RNC, *Lifecircle;* B courtesy Ross Laboratories, Columbus, Ohio.)

be used to assess parents' perception of their infant between 4 and 8 months of age. Today, there are many questionnaires based on this ITQ. The ITQ assumes that temperament is a stable characteristic. When scored, the behaviors are clustered into one of the following groups: (1) easy, (2) slow to warm, (3) difficult, (4) intermediate high difficulty, and (5) intermediate low difficulty. The ITQ appears to be a useful tool in acquainting the parents with their infant. Because there are more than 90 questions, Box 20-3 shows only a sample of the questions that may be asked for each of nine categories.

1. The *easy child* is characterized by a positive rhythmic mood, with a low to moderate intensity of reaction. The child is adaptable and predictable as long as expectations are consistent. Consistent parenting helps the child to compare home with the real world. The child will adapt to any practice or ritual, so parents must take care concerning things to which the child is exposed.

2. The *slow-to-warm-up* child is less active, responds with tentative withdrawal and slower adaptability, lower intensity, and a mildly negative mood. The child gradually adapts to new situations as long as the parent is patient, relaxed, and does not force the child into strict rules. The parents must identify acceptable behaviors. Repetition and routines are needed for successful daily experiences.

3. The *difficult child* is unpredictable, intense, and tends to withdraw in situations and have a negative mood. The parents must help the child with clear limits, which requires a patient and positive set of parental behaviors. Often parents must be reassured that their own parenting skills are not at fault. The child will need gradual and repeated negative and positive reinforcement. Rules should be simple and few. Plan specific outlets for this energetic child.

4. The *intermediate child* is one that is a mix of these three sets of characteristics and may be of intermediate high difficulty or intermediate low difficulty.

BOX 20-3 Sample Items by Category from the Revised ITQ*

Activity

The infant moves about much (kicks, grabs, squirms) during diapering and dressing.

The infant plays actively with parents—much movement of arms, legs, body.

Rhythmicity

The infant wants and takes milk feedings at about the same times (within 1 hour) from day to day.

The infant's bowel movements come at different times day to day (over 1 hour's difference).

Approach/withdrawal

The infant accepts right away any change in place or position of feeding or person giving it.

For the first few minutes in a new place or situation (new store or home), the infant is fretful.

Adaptability

The infant objects to being bathed in a different place or by a different person, even after two or three tries (after 3 months).

The infant accepts regular procedures (hair brushing, face washing) any time without protest.

Intensity

The infant reacts strongly to foods, whether positively (smacks lips, laughs, squeals) or negatively (cries).

The infant reacts mildly to meeting familiar people (quiet smiles or no response).

Mood

The infant is pleasant (smiles, laughs) when first arriving in unfamiliar places (friend's house, store).

Persistence

The infant amuses self for half an hour or more in crib or playpen (looking at mobile, playing with toy).

The infant watches other children playing for under a minute and then looks elsewhere.

Distractibility

The infant stops play and watches when someone walks by.

The infant continues to cry in spite of several minutes of soothing.

Threshold

The infant reacts even to a gentle touch (startle, wriggle, laugh, cry).

The infant reacts to a disliked food even if it is mixed with a preferred one.

*The mother rates each of the following items on a scale of 1 to 6; *1* almost never; 6 almost always. Rev 1977 by WB Carey and SC McDevitt. The entire instrument is available for $10. Send to WB Carey, MD, 319 West Front Street, Media, PA 19063.

Infants show distinct individuality in temperament in the first weeks of life. Responsiveness to stimulation is directly related to infant temperament. For instance, Korner (1990) has shown a significant relationship between neonatal activity and responses with later activity levels and temperament between ages 4 and 8 years. The infant's and his parents' temperaments determine the **goodness-of-fit** or how well the infant integrates into the family (see Chapter 2). If the infant easily meets the parents' expectations, the transition is easy.

Infant Stimulation Programs

It is now accepted and written into regulations that early stimulation be provided for high-risk infants. The parents of normal newborns have concern about how much and how soon their infants should receive extra stimulation. This question never arose in the past; in extended families infants were always with some family member, and practices of child rearing were very different. Today, the infant may be with a baby-sitter, in day-care, or have only a single parent with whom to interact. There are activities parents may do to stimulate an infant, but there must be a balance. Anxious, usually well-educated parents may misguidedly never give their infant a chance to build a routine or to relax because they insist on presenting multiple stimuli. On the other hand, as Horowitz (1990) indicates, it may be the parent's inability to *modulate infant state* (i.e., to console or calm a tired, crying infant) which predicts the future possibility of child abuse. The person who cannot deal with a crying infant may in frustration hit or hurt the infant. A more subtle abuse may be psychosocial, not allowing the infant or child to develop in a way that fits their unique temperament.

Therefore, nursing interventions can focus on teaching parents what to look for in infant state and responses and then how to console so as to alter the tension shown in an upset, crying state. Use the *Funke-Irby Mother Infant Assessment* for early assessment of mother-infant interaction. Just as a low Apgar score demands attention, a low FIMI score indicates the need for prompt intervention (Table 20-3).

The goals for parent learning of infant cues have been spelled out in a number of early intervention programs. These goals include (Rauh et al, 1990):

1. Assisting the parent to focus on the infant's ways of responding by pointing out positive infant cues and the best interaction periods.
2. Encouraging the parent to recognize signs of fatigue, exhaustion, overload, and hunger in the infant.
3. Teaching parents when to stimulate, when to comfort, when to decrease stimulation, and how to encourage sleep.

4. Teaching parents the progression of growth and development so they can enjoy and note the infant's rapid progress.

Most of the work in infant stimulation studies has been done with preterm infants, but findings can be useful for parents of normal full-term infants.

Cues to Infant Responses

The kinds of visual cues the baby gives are related to time, attention, and gaze. In the early weeks, a newborn cannot maintain looking or gazing for more than a short period. As eye muscle control improves, the baby will scan and focus, if interested, looking at an object for longer periods. By 2 months, **gaze aversion** signals that a baby needs a break from interaction. Adults respond in similar ways.

Brazelton (1978) made it clear that the infant has a drive to learn, seeks external satisfaction, and only "turns off" attention when it is too much, too fast, or when fatigue sets in.

Infants learn best in the quiet alert state. If a baby becomes hyperalert, wide-eyed, almost staring during extended stimulation, he may be *overstimulated* and unable to break away. Encourage the parent to break eye contact to allow the baby to quiet down. Persistent stimulation (often by siblings) may cause the infant to turn away. Sometimes the palm becomes outstretched, and the arms stiffen. Stiffening and pulling away indicate that the baby wants a change. Body language is the baby's way to communicate.

On the other hand, early positive signs of enjoyment are lip pursing or sucking, leaning toward an object, or cuddling into the person holding the infant. Breathing and pulse become slower when the infant is interested (Haith, 1986). Families can learn to read their infant's messages easily after these messages are pointed out (Figure 20-13).

Self-consolation is observed when you are doing the **Brazelton Neonatal Assessment Scale.** You can point out these cues to infant responses and encourage the mother to become aware of her infant's responses. For instance, the baby shows pleasure or tension by nonnutritive sucking; infants need at least 120 minutes of sucking each day. If an infant takes formula or breast milk rapidly, a pacifier may supplement sucking time, or

Self-Discovery

Think about the temperaments expressed in your siblings and parents. Are there clashes in temperament? How does your family work these out?

TABLE 20-3   FIMI: Funke-Irbe Mother-Infant Interactional Assessment*†

COLUMN I	COLUMN II	COLUMN III	COLUMN IV
FEEDING			
Force-feeds baby. Disrupts feeding pattern of baby. Stops feeding before baby's need is met. Withdraws and then offers repeatedly.	Feeds baby only after several minutes of crying.	Wakes baby for scheduled feeding. Hurries baby while feeding. Displays neutral affect during feeding. Occupies time more with observer than with baby once feeding has begun.	Maintains eye contact with baby. Feeds baby immediately on demand. Spends most of time looking at baby. Responds to baby's behavior by changing own behavior (that is, withdraws nipple when baby spits out milk on side of mouth).
MOVING AND HOLDING			
Restrains or controls baby's movements.	Changes baby's position only after baby has cried for 3 to 4 minutes. Does not change baby's position; is unaware of baby's need for positional comfort.	Displays inconsistent awareness of baby's need for positional comfort; at times changes baby's position to meet baby's needs and other times does not. Enfolds baby in arms with some rigidness.	Rocks baby gently. Enfolds baby close to body. Changes baby's position gently. Responds to baby's need for positional comfort.
CLEANING AND DIAPERING			
Wipes baby compulsively, disruptively. Cleans roughly. Displays verbal or facial displeasure at and rejection of cleaning activity. Does not respond to baby's need for cleaning or change of clothing.	Delays cleaning 4 to 5 minutes when baby is in need of cleaning. Changes baby's diapers only after baby fusses for 3 to 4 minutes.	Delays cleaning slightly, 1 to 2 minutes, when baby is in need of cleaning. Does not interact during cleaning activities; is task-oriented.	Responds immediately to baby's need for cleaning. Keeps baby well groomed.
TOUCHING			
Touches baby roughly. Does not touch baby.	Touches baby only after 3 to 4 minutes of baby's demands.	Touches baby infrequently, only 3 to 4 times during specific activity. Displays protective touching only.	Kisses. Fingers. Strokes. Gently pats.
NONVERBAL AND VERBAL COMMUNICATION			
Commands baby. Voices negative criticism. Angrily voices disapproval. Displays angry facial expression. Makes no eye contact. Refers to baby as "it."	Speaks to baby but withholds affect. Makes eye contact only 3 to 4 times. Is inconsistently pleasant and harsh in voice.	Refers to baby as "he" or "she." Speaks to baby casually. Displays inconsistent eye contact.	Calls baby by name. Speaks with affection. Empathizes. Maintains eye contact. Uses a warm vocal tone.

*For characteristics of interaction observed during early acquaintance and attachment periods.
†This assessment is one of many tools and is useful as you learn to really "look" at the interaction.
Column I, poor adaptation; column IV, positive attachment.
From Funke J, Irbe MI: An instrument to assess the quality of maternity behavior, *JOGNN* 7(5):19, 1978.

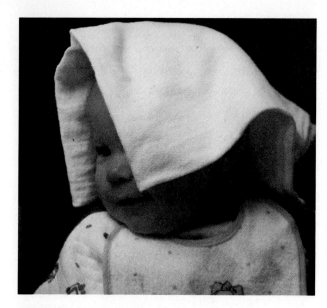

FIGURE 20-13 Teach parents how to play games with baby. (Courtesy Eric Schult.)

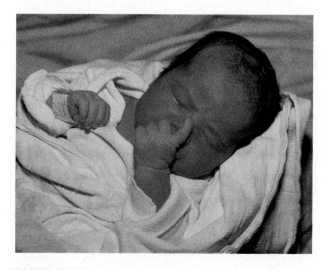

FIGURE 20-14 Hand-to-mouth consolation. (Courtesy Marjorie Pyle, RNC, *Lifecircle*.)

the infant may quickly find a finger or thumb (Figure 20-14). Use of a pacifier is often a very important self-quieting tool for the baby. You can help parents to feel more accepting toward this behavior by using parallel examples in adults' self-consoling behaviors such as chewing gum or eating when upset. Sucking needs to be done in an emotionally positive atmosphere. As a result propping a bottle should be avoided because it denies the gratification of interaction.

The **Mother's Assessment of the Behavior of Her Infant** (MABI) scale may be used to assist the mother of a baby to become aware of her infant's patterns (Field et al, 1978). The scale is keyed to the Brazelton Assess-

ment Scale. It was found that the use of the MABI scale with lower socioeconomic status teenage mothers of premature infants was useful and appeared to be significant in their increased interaction with their infants. They suggest that early use of the Brazelton scale at the bedside and the MABI may be a cost-effective way of affecting mother-infant interaction and contribute to better learning in infants (Box 20-4).

PARENTAL INTERVENTIONS FOR STIMULATION

The following activities are some of the many suggestions a care giver may use to help parents understand and promote early infant learning:

1. Explain the normal development of the senses and the relation of sleep states to responses. Babies respond best in the quiet alert state.
2. Assess the abilities of each infant before demonstrating how a baby responds. There is much variation in a newborn and infant response. Use the differences to introduce the topic of the uniqueness of each child.
3. Place the infant in a position that will promote eye-to-eye contact. Use mobiles over the infant's seat or crib.
   a. Make mobiles out of cardboard with colors of dark and light contrast and medium intensity.
   b. Use black and white contrast in stripes and checkerboards, as well as for smiley faces.
   c. Make the mobile light enough to respond to air movement.
   d. Place the mobile low enough so the older baby can touch it, preferably with the feet.
   e. Add auditory stimulation when possible.
4. Use soft, rhythmic sounds (singing, music boxes) but regulate the loudness (decibels). Talk in a higher tone with variations in pitch.
5. Promote tactile stimulation by encouraging skin-to-skin contact. Provide toys that have different textures. Use a soft crib bumper.
   a. Learn baby stroking techniques.
   b. Carry the baby in soft body carrier on front of parent; backpacks are appropriate only for older infants.
6. A baby learns through exploration and play so creative play should be fostered. Several books on games to play with babies are available for parents. These games were often passed on in extended families but may have been forgotten in a generation of nuclear families.

Parental Cues

Some early cues to parental responses have been identified by Kodadek (1986). **Claiming cues** are observed in

BOX 20-4   Questionnaire for Mothers Modified from the Neonatal Behavioral Assessment Scale

Directions to the mother: Because a mother knows her baby better than anyone else, we would like you to give us your impressions of your baby by circling your answer to these questions. To answer these questions, you might want to watch your baby for a while and try playing some of the games with him or her. For example, to answer question No. 9, we ask you to shake a rattle to the side of your baby's face to see if he turns to look at the rattle. We have discovered that newborn babies can do lots of interesting things that you will probably discover in your baby too.

1. (Predominant state) When you play with your baby he or she is often:
   □ Sleepy (1–2, 2–3)
   □ Alert (3–4, 4–5)
   □ Upset (5–6)
2. (Descriptive paragraph) How would you describe your baby?
   □ Fairly attractive (1)
   □ Quite attractive (2)
   □ Very attractive (3)
3. (Descriptive paragraph) How much do you have to stimulate your baby to get her to look at you?
   □ Not very much (1)
   □ A fair amount (2)
   □ A lot (3)
4. (Descriptive paragraph) When your baby is upset, what does he do to quiet himself?
   □ Brings his hand to his mouth (1)
   □ Sucks with nothing in his mouth (2)
   □ Looks at you (3)
5. (#9) Try talking to your baby holding your face about 1 foot away from his or her face and then slowly move your face to one side and then to the other as you continue talking. When you do this, your baby:
   □ Doesn't look at you (1–2)
   □ Becomes quiet and looks at you (3–4)
   □ Follows your face to each side with his or her head and eyes (5–7)
   □ Follows your face with his or her head and eyes, up and down and to each side (8–9)
6. (#7) Now try the same thing, only move your face without talking. When you do this, your baby:
   □ Doesn't look at you (1–2)
   □ Becomes quiet (3–4
   □ Follows your face with his or her head and eyes (5–7)
   □ Follows your face with his or her head and eyes, up and down and to each side (8–9)
7. (#8) Try talking to your baby from one side of his or her head and then from the other. When you do this, he or she:
   □ Has no reaction or blinks (1–2)
   □ Becomes quiet (3–4)
   □ Turns his or her eyes and head to your voice once or twice (5–7)
   □ Turns his or her eyes and head to your voice more than twice (8–9)

8. (#5) Now try holding a colorful toy or some shiny object in front of your baby's face and then move it slowly to each side of his or her head and then up and down in front of the face. When you do this, he or she:
   □ Doesn't look at the toy (1–2)
   □ Becomes quiet and looks at toy (3–4)
   □ Follows the toy you are moving with his or her head and eyes (5–7)
   □ Follows the toy you are moving with his or her head and eyes, up and down and to each side (8–9)
9. (#6) Try shaking a rattle on one side of your baby's head and then on the other side. When you do this, he or she:
   □ Has no reaction or blinks (1–2)
   □ Becomes quiet (3–4)
   □ Turns his or her eyes and head to the rattle once or twice (5–7)
   □ Turns his or her eyes and head to the rattle more than twice (8–9)
10. (#10) When you did the above things with your baby, he or she usually:
   □ Paid little attention to you or the toy (1–2)
   □ Had short periods of watching you or the toy (3–4)
   □ Watched you or the toy for a fairly long time (5–7)
   □ Paid attention most of the time (8–9)
11. (#11) How does your baby feel when you handle or hold him or her?
   □ Limp like a rag doll (1–2)
   □ Limp some of the time (3–4)
   □ Relaxed but firm (5–6)
   □ Very tense (7–9)
12. (#12) When your baby moves his or her arms, the movements are:
   □ Jerky most of the time (1–2)
   □ Jerky some of the time (3–4)
   □ Smooth some of the time (5–7)
   □ Smooth most of the time (8–9)
13. (#14) When you pick up your baby and hold him or her in a rocking position, he or she:
   □ Often swings his or her arms and kicks his or her legs and squirms (1–2)
   □ Is like a sack of meal in your arms (3–4)
   □ Relaxes and nestles his or her head in the crook of your arms (5–7)
   □ Moves his or her face toward you and reaches his or her hands out to grab your clothing (8–9)

Continued.

BOX 20-4   Questionnaire for Mothers, Modified from the Neonatal Behavioral Assessment Scale—cont'd

14. (#16) When your baby is crying very hard:
□ Nothing seems to quiet him or her (1)
□ Only a pacifier will quiet him or her (2)
□ Holding and rocking will quiet him or her (3–6)
□ Talking to him or her and holding your hand on the stomach quiets him or her (7–9)

15. (#17) How would you describe your baby most of the time?
□ Very sleepy (1–2)
□ Awake a lot of the time and quiet (3–4)
□ Crying occasionally but easily quieted (5–7)
□ Crying a lot and difficult to quiet (8–9)

16. (#19) Please circle those activities that upset your baby:
□ Changing diaper (1–2)
□ Undressing or dressing (3–4)
□ Putting him or her back in her bassinet (5–7)
□ Lying him or her on the stomach (8–9)

17. (#20) How active is your baby?
□ Not very active (1–2)
□ Somewhat active (3–4)
□ Quite active (5–6)
□ Very active (7–9)

18. (#21) How often does your baby tremble when he or she is warmly dressed?
□ Not very often (1–2)
□ Occasionally (3–4)
□ Fairly often (5–6)
□ Very often (7–9)

19. (#23) How would you describe your baby's color changes?
□ Rarely changes color (1–2)
□ Changes to blue around the mouth when uncovered and red when crying but only for a minute (3–4)
□ Changes color when uncovered or crying but changes back to his or her natural color when covered up or comfortable (5–6)

□ Seems to get blue or red very often but will get his or her natural color back after you've been holding her for a while (7–9)

20. (#24) How are your baby's mood swings—how often do they occur and how quickly do they change?
□ Sleeps most of the time and hardly ever cries (1–2)
□ Is quiet much of the time (3–4)
□ Goes back and forth from being quiet to crying fairly often (5–6)
□ Often changes from being sleepy or quiet to crying and then back again—changes mood often and very quickly (7–9)

21. (#25) When your baby is crying, how successful is he or she at self-quieting activities:
□ Cannot quiet self (1–2)
□ Makes several attempts to quiet self but is usually unsuccessful (3–4)
□ Has many brief successes at quieting self (5–6)
□ Often quiets self for long periods (7–9)

22. (#26) How would you describe your baby's hand-to-mouth activity?
□ Makes no attempt to bring hands to his or her mouth (1–2)
□ Often brings hands next to his or her mouth (3–5)
□ Sometimes puts fist or fingers in his or her mouth (6–7)
□ Sometimes sucks on fist or fingers for as long as 15 seconds at a time (8–9)

23. (#27) How many times has your baby looked like she or he was smiling at you?

Modified from Field T: University of Miami Medical Center, Mailman Center for Child Development, Miami, FL 33152. By permission of the author and *Infant Behavior and Development* 1:156, 1978.
*Note how questions parallel Brazelton items and scoring. The numbers of the Brazelton items that correspond to the MABI items have been written before the questions. The corresponding Brazelton rating is in parentheses after each MABI rating.

the immediate postnatal period, when the parents begin to explore and touch the infant with fingertips. Parents will describe characteristics that the infant shares with other family members, as well as remark on unique features. (This initial reaction is important, even if the baby is stillborn.)

Degree of consolidation cues are observed during the first 2 months, when the parent talks to the infant in endearing terms and infant response is observed. Parents are still uncertain and often seek guidance and

reassurance that they are perceiving their infants' responses correctly.

Growth in parental role cues are observed as parents adjust to their infant. These cues are seen after the second month as parents become comfortable with infant care. The box indicates clues to difficulty in parent-infant interaction. More data must be collected before conclusions are made. Early intervention through tools and time with the parent will usually bring long-term positive changes.

Clinical Decision

Andy's father did not know what to "say to a baby." He was a serious businessman who had had no prior experience with infants. He stated that he "felt silly" talking with an infant who could not respond. How could he be encouraged to vocalize with his infant?

Attachment after Birth

Achievement of the motherhood self-image is built on attachment to the fantasy baby. After birth the parents must reconcile this image with the real infant. In addition to the physical separation of birth, there is a psychologic process of separating from the unity and oneness of pregnancy and forming a new relationship with the child in the outside world (Rubin, 1977). Many factors can influence how well this attachment proceeds, including maternal parity, previous parenting experiences, parental attitudes to the infant, socioeconomic status, and the condition of the mother and infant. A stable parent-child bond is the result of a bonding process that takes place during *acquaintance, attachment,* and *bond formation.*

ACQUAINTANCE

During pregnancy, an infant's health can be inferred only from secondary sources such as fetal monitors or ultrasound. After delivery, however, the mother can observe her newborn directly and is hungry for affirmation from those around her. This is demonstrated when she asks if the baby is all right, even before she looks at it.

There is a strong urge for visual, then tactile, observations. The visual contact helps her to psychologically relocate her baby as existing outside of herself. If the baby is healthy, she touches it, beginning with a light fingertip inquiry, tracing contours, counting fingers and toes, and feeling the texture of hair and skin, moving toward the center of the body. This process of **acquaintance** will be repeated over and over in the early days until her discoveries are confirmed and stabilized for recognition (Rubin, 1984).

With her discoveries, each facet of the newborn's appearance or behavior will be bound into the self and family system by the process of claiming. This is one of the early tasks of parenthood. You often observe new parents claiming that features "look like" his or hers (or grandmother's or another family member's). This linking is a way of claiming the newborn and incorporating it into the family system.

At the same time, the new mother is examining the "fit" of this new relationship. As she examines her baby's body with her fingertips (Figure 20-15), she looks for cues from the infant. Fingertip touch causes the newborn to turn toward the touch and to contract the muscle tissues around it. The infant finds his mother's touch pleasurable. When his lips are touched, he produces a "kiss" or "smile," or when his palm is stroked, he grasps his mother's finger. Sometimes, the touch is not as pleasurable to the infant; when his mother strokes his brow, he may grimace, thus causing the mother to withdraw and resume exploration elsewhere. Through the repeated experience of "reading" the baby's cues, the new mother gains a sense of predictability and competence in her mothering ability.

ATTACHMENT

After recognizing and claiming the infant as her own, the mother begins to form bonds with her infant; these bonds will assure her commitment to its care.

Studies have shown that a predictable group of reciprocal interactions takes place with each encounter to foster and reinforce **attachment.** Each interaction between the mother and her newborn elicits a response in the other that is satisfying to both. For example, the baby cries, triggering the mother to soothe and comfort

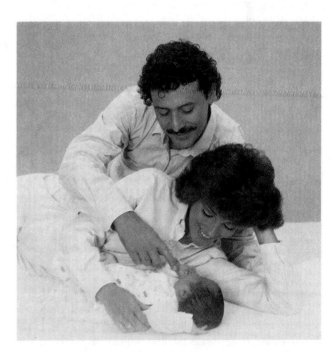

FIGURE 20-15 Fingertip exploration. (Courtesy Marjorie Pyle, RNC, *Lifecircle.*)

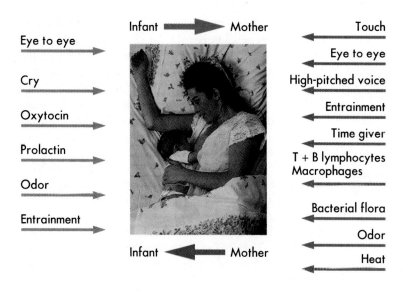

Infant ➡ Mother

Eye to eye ➡
Cry ➡
Oxytocin ➡
Prolactin ➡
Odor ➡
Entrainment ➡

⬅ Touch
⬅ Eye to eye
⬅ High-pitched voice
⬅ Entrainment
⬅ Time giver
⬅ T + B lymphocytes Macrophages
⬅ Bacterial flora
⬅ Odor
⬅ Heat

Infant ⬅ Mother

FIGURE 20-16 Mother-to-infant and infant-to-mother interactions can occur simultaneously in first days of life. (Modified from Klaus MH, Kennell JH: *Parent-infant bonding*, ed 2, St Louis, 1982, Mosby. Photo courtesy Ross Laboratories, Columbus, Ohio.)

(satisfying to the baby); the baby becomes quiet (satisfying to the mother and enhancing her self-esteem and confidence in her mothering skills) (Figure 20-16).

Touch

By touch, the new mother gains knowledge of her infant's responses and a kinesthetic sense of his texture, temperature, moisture, and contours. Descriptive terms denoting her pleasure in this action include "silky-smooth" and "downy soft." Maternal touch helps the baby to define his body boundaries and will contribute to his sense of self as worthwhile in the months to come. The mother will touch the infant first with her fingertips and then progress to massage with palm contact. The mother will position the infant in the en face position for eye-to-eye contact, which helps to establish the infant's identity and provide positive feedback to the parents; this is called *reciprocal interaction*.

Eye Contact

For new mothers, the need for the baby to open its eyes is nearly universal. Comments like "Open your eyes and then I'll know that you're real" are common. Babies held upright in the face-to-face (*en face*) position attempt to focus on the eyes of the holder. This contact strongly evokes parental feeling (Figure 20-17).

Pitch of the Voice

Everyone who has ever engaged in "baby talk" knows that people raise their voices when talking to babies, even when they do not know that babies prefer sounds in the higher range. Babies are more responsive to and comfortable with high-pitched voices, enhancing the probability that the speaker will continue to speak in this range. Because of vibrations in the inner ear, the

baby may cry when approached by a person with a deep, loud voice.

Cry

Crying brings an immediate reaction from the care giver to soothe or look for the cause of distress. The ability to interpret the cry and comfort the baby will enhance the parent's self-esteem. The inability to comfort leads to feelings of failure. Thus, it is difficult for parents to care for an infant with colic or withdrawal from drugs.

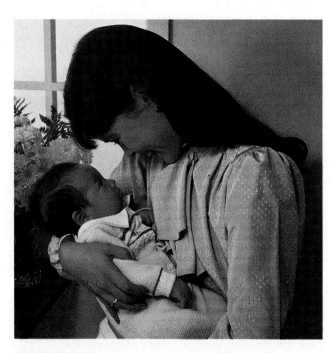

FIGURE 20-17 Mother-infant gazing. (Courtesy Ross Laboratories, Columbus, Ohio.)

Entrainment

Entrainment is the synchronization of the baby's movement to the patterns and rhythms of the mother's speech. When there is a change in the speech pattern such as a pause or accented syllable, subtle changes in the baby's behavior are noted.

Odor

The olfactory sense also helps the process of identification and attachment. Studies have indicated that by about 5 days of age, breast-fed infants can discriminate the breast pads of their own mother from those of others. Many mothers report that each of their babies had its own scent.

Heat

The mother once provided heat for her baby by wrapping and placing him close against her body. This aspect of bonding is less important in our culture because of central heat.

Time-giver

The rhythm of the mother's speech is only a part of entrainment. The intricate pattern of response of the fetus to its mother's sleep-wake cycle and hormonal patterns are thrown out of equilibrium by birth. As a result, the mother becomes a "time giver" for the infant after he is born; in other words, she causes the formation of **rhythmic neonatal functions** (Klaus and Kennell, 1982). An example of this is the frequency with which the mother holds the infant in the alert state (which reinforces the infant). In this state, he is awake and ready to respond to her cues (which is reinforcing to the mother). The mother's steady routine of holding the baby when she wants him awake and of quieting when she wishes him to sleep helps to establish predictable sleeping and waking patterns.

Hormonal Stimulation

The infant's breast-feeding or stimulation of the breast by licking or touch induces the release of the maternal hormones oxytocin and prolactin.

BONDING

Attachment that leads to the maternal-infant bond depends on the infant's responsiveness. This response reinforces the mother and encourages her to continue interaction. The result is a stable bond between the infant and parents that will endure and not be extinguished in spite of separations. Bond formation is an outgrowth of reciprocal attachment stimulus-response and affectional ties to form a coordinated, constructive social relationship. You can only infer that bonding is progressing satisfactorily through observation of attachment behavior (i.e., behaviors that serve to maintain contact and demonstrate affection toward the baby). Examples of this behavior include kissing, fondling and cuddling, and holding in the *en face* position to maintain eye contact (Figure 20-18). See Box 20-5 for clues to difficulty in parent-infant bonding.

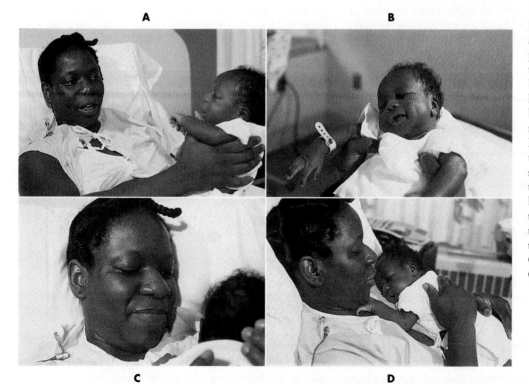

FIGURE 20-18 **A,** Early acquaintance process proceeding well. **B,** First the mother holds the baby away to look at her. **C,** Then the mother brings her baby close, noticing details. **D,** Finally, she cuddles her up close. The nurse should wait and allow the natural sequence of bonding to occur rather than urging the mother to immediately cuddle the baby. (Courtesy Concept Media, Irvine, Calif.)

BOX 20-5 Clues to Difficulty in Parent-Infant Bonding

- The nurse will be alerted to potential problems in parent-child bonding if:
  - ° The mother is young or immature.
  - ° The mother must struggle against a nonsupportive or isolated environment.
  - ° The mother is beset by stress-causing situations (e.g., poor environmental conditions, serious illness in the family, severe disappointment, rapid and repeated pregnancies) and the arrival of the new infant.
  - ° The mother was separated from her infant for a prolonged period after birth (e.g., prematurity, maternal illness).
- The nurse will strongly suspect that there is a problem in parent–child bonding if:
  - ° The parent expresses inappropriate feelings (e.g., anger, frustration, helplessness) in response to infant's crying.
  - ° The parent fails to express anything about the infant that she or he likes (i.e., the parent has not found in the infant a physical or psychologic attribute valued in self).
  - ° The parent expresses unresolved feelings over a "dream" child (e.g., disappointment over sex of infant).
  - ° The parent expresses mostly negative feelings about the infant (e.g., disgust over messy diapers or a perception that the infant is too demanding).
  - ° The parent expresses expectations of infant far beyond the baby's developmental potentials.
  - ° The parent fails to exhibit close, gentle, physical contact with the infant (e.g., holds infant away from body, plays roughly, or avoids eye contact and the en face position).

Separation from Birth Mother

Many infants do not become a part of the families into which they were born. These infants are placed in adoptive or foster homes. The reasons for the parents' inability to care for the child are as widespread and varied as the situations and personalities of the people themselves. Some parents recognize that, because of their circumstances, they can not care for a baby or raise a child, at least at this point in their lives. Other parents, because of social pressures, drug addiction, or mental illness, give up or abandon children or have the child removed from the home by protective agencies. There are many other reasons that children are given up temporarily or completely.

For parents to recognize that they are unable to care for a child requires great maturity and courage. Such an individual needs understanding and support.

Clinical Decision

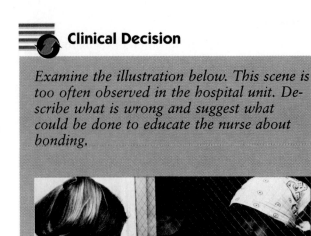

Examine the illustration below. This scene is too often observed in the hospital unit. Describe what is wrong and suggest what could be done to educate the nurse about bonding.

Infants who go into adoptive or foster home placement frequently remain in the hospital nursery longer than other infants. The staff should plan to supply the missing personal attention, warmth, and comfort that an enthusiastic and loving parent would normally provide. Although all their physical needs may be met, these infants have great need for psychologic stimulation from tender and playful handling. Studies have shown that infants in institutions without personal contact, given adequate food and comfortable but unstimulating surroundings are retarded in their physical and psychologic development, and in extreme cases may even die (Bowlby, 1965).

Nurses who establish some type of relationship with an infant risk feelings of attachment to the child. Nurses who have become attached to an infant left for several weeks in the hospital have suffered feelings of separation, loss, and grief when the infant was taken away. Although these feelings are painful, they are normal signs of separation and prove that the infant has had a relationship that will help to approximate a normal experience.

ADOPTION

Adoption is the legal process by which the state gives full responsibility for the child to suitable parents, with the child becoming an actual legal member of the family. Adoption requires that the child's biologic mother voluntarily give up her legal rights to the child or that a court terminate her rights, usually on the basis of abandonment. After a period of placement, usually 1 year, the adoption is legally finalized in the courts, and in most states a new birth certificate is issued showing the adoptive parents as the only parents. At this point, there should be complete protection against removal of the child from home because of claims to the child made by another party.

There have been challenges, and the legal scene is changing. Focus is now on the needs and rights of the child to be in a home that provides the best chance for optimum growth and development. Challenges based on cross-cultural considerations are being made.

After the child is adopted, the adoptive parents are entirely responsible for the child's life. Adoption assures the child of having continuing family relationships throughout life. These relationships can begin as soon as the infant leaves the hospital, sometimes 1 or 2 weeks after birth.

FOSTER CARE

Other babies leave the hospital's nursery for foster homes. If the biologic mother chooses not to give up her rights to the child and remains at least somewhat interested in the child so abandonment cannot be proved (even though the biologic mother may be unable to care for the child herself), the child is placed in a foster home. Often, foster care is used for children who could be adopted but for whom adoptive homes are difficult to find because the children are older, are of a minority race, or have medical problems.

Foster care in theory is temporary placement with the goal of stabilizing the biologic parent or finding adoptive parents. The child is placed with a family that is given major responsibility for the child's care. Legal responsibility for the child is assigned to a state agency or a state-licensed private agency. Foster homes are usually administered directly through these agencies. Foster parents are paid a monthly rate through the agency or the child's expenses plus medical and other expenses. A social worker is assigned to each home to give professional assistance. The social worker works with the biologic parent toward resolution of the uncertainty of the child's status by proving abandonment, voluntary surrender of the rights to the child, or return of the child to the biologic mother. Unfortunately, there are a number of problems today related to an overwhelming number of placements (often related to drug-using parents) and a shortage of supervising personnel.

LEGAL ISSUES

The distinction, then, between a child who can be placed for adoption and a child who is placed in a foster home for extended care is usually a legal one. The child must be free for adoption, which means that there is no parental claim to the child. Biologic parents may voluntarily surrender their rights to the child by signing affidavits stating that this is their wish. Biologic parents can also be sued in court and have their rights to children severed. The judicial systems of many states have in the past favored the *blood bond* over the *psychologic bond* that the child has to the family with whom he lives, but this appears to be changing. Complete abandonment of the child by biologic parents is one reason the courts usually sever parental rights.

If the biologic parental rights remain intact while the child lives with a foster family, many psychologically damaging conflicts can cause problems for the child. The foster parents find it difficult to commit themselves totally to the child because of the possibility that he will be removed from their home to be returned to biologic parents. The child does not understand the situation and is confused by having two sets of parents (one set of which the child knows as his or her "real" parents but who in fact are hardly known); later the child is in conflict because he does not know where his identity and allegiance really lie. Finally, the biologic parents are also frequently in conflict over the situation, torn between guilt over not being able to care for their child and their sense of inadequacy for being unable to do so. Unresolved grief may continue over an extended period (Haberkern, 1988).

The foster care situation is difficult from the foster parents' viewpoint because legal uncertainties make them insecure in their feelings of love for their foster children. Many foster parents who commit themselves fully to children placed in their care suffer agonizing loss when the child is removed from their home, especially if the child is being returned to biologic parents whom the foster parents feel remain "unfit."

Even for the child who remains in the foster home, deep emotional conflicts can arise around matters such as visits from the biologic parents. Foster parents must be unusually strong to be able to reach out to the child and explain the very mixed feelings involved in this situation. An ideal arrangement is to have foster parents and biologic parents all working together for eventual return to the biologic parents. But this is not always feasible.

The trend in the legislative and judicial systems is to give the children and foster parents more rights. Children, even infants, are being assigned their own lawyers to protect their rights and to guarantee that the best possible living situation is available to them in terms of their psychologic and physical development. Every state has its own laws concerning foster care, but as an example of progressive legislation, New York has given foster parents who have had a child in their home for 2 or more years the right to a hearing before removal of the child from the home. This is a step protecting the *psychologic bonds,* the delicate, fragile feelings of relationship, between the foster child and parents. Foster care needs to be restructured legally to guarantee that the psychologic parents of the foster child will have the fullest possible opportunity to develop normal family relationships and—most important—that the child will have an opportunity to feel that he is a secure and wanted member of a family.

Many states also now have subsidized adoption for foster parents who cannot afford to adopt a child who has been their foster child. Subsidized adoption means that the state will continue to provide foster care payments to such a family. Such payments are usually subject to an annual review of the parents' income.

Compared with other forms of child care, foster care is the best way devised by our society of taking care of the child who cannot be brought up by the biologic parents. In a foster home, a child relates to a complete family and can form close relationships on an individual basis. Even in the present legal situation, it is possible for a child to enter a foster home immediately after birth and to remain as a member of the family throughout childhood and adolescence, although this usually does not happen. The infant who enters a foster home will be able to relate to a parent with whom he can form the comforting, satisfying, and stimulating relationship that every baby needs to be able to go on to more mature levels of psychologic development.

KEY POINTS

- Settings vary widely; nurses often do not have opportunity to evaluate their teaching interventions, but parental knowledge of basics that allow the normal infant to do well consist of the following:
    1. Parents describe a positive support system and adequate housing.
    2. Basic needs of the newborn infant are described.
    3. Parents describe signs of difficulty in nutritional intake and know how to seek help.
    4. Parents evaluate home environment for hazards, infections, and temperature control, and then will child-proof the home against accidents.
    5. Parents describe recommendations for immunizations.
    6. Parents describe when to notify health care providers regarding alterations in infant status and consistently follow up.
    7. Parents initiate the attachment bonding process, giving indication that this will continue to develop.

STUDY QUESTIONS

20-1 Match Key Terms to the following statements:
  a. The parents find that their new infant integrates well into the family. *Goodness of Fit*
  b. A child who responds with tentative withdrawal and slower adaptability. *Slow to warmup*
  c. The general nature or characteristic mood of the individual. *Temprament*
  d. For an infant, sucking a thumb is a way of *Self consolation*
  e. The infant cue of looking away when fatigued. *gaze aversion*
  f. Condition that can result from allowing an infant to fall asleep while nursing from a bottle. *Bottle mouth*
  g. Sustained periods of crying during the first 3 months. *Colic*

20-2 Which of the following behaviors is not present in a normal newborn infant by 1 week of age?
  a. The infant will be able to recognize the parents by sight.
  b. Habituation is used to block out stimuli.
  c. Loud noise will produce a startle response.
  d. The infant will distinguish between his mother and another by smell.

20-3 Parents question the nurse about newborn crying. The most helpful answer would be:
  a. "Infants cry to express frustration with their parents."
  b. "Crying only indicates a need for attention."
  c. "Newborns cry to release tension or ask for help."
  d. "This is their way of communicating with bigger people."

20-4 Mary M asks about whether her baby can "see." Choose the most appropriate answer the nurse could give.
  a. "Babies can follow a red ball or light like adults can."
  b. "Eye muscles are weak, so they cannot gaze more than a few minutes."
  c. "Babies focus on objects about 4 to 10 inches away, such as your face."
  d. "At first they probably see only black and white objects."

20-5 You note during a home visit that the mother has not provided toys for a new infant. She states that she can't afford fancy toys. Which intervention would be inappropriate for the nurse to do?

a. Help the mother make several visually interesting safe toys from household objects.

b. Agree with the mother that new babies do not need expensive toys.

c. Encourage the mother to find sources of used, safe toys.

d. Recognize she may be unable to provide other necessary items of care.

Answer Key

20 1 a. Goodness of fit, b. Slow to warm up, c. Temperament, d. Self-consolation, e. Gaze aversion, f. Bottle mouth,
g. Colic, 20-2 a 20-3 c 20-4 c 20-5 b

REFERENCES

American Academy of Pediatrics: *Report of Committee on Infectious Diseases,* ed 22, Elk Grove, IL, 1991, The Academy.

Anderson C: Enhancing reciprocity between mother and neonate, *Nurs Res* 30(2):89, 1981.

Anderson C: Integration of the Brazelton Neonatal Behavioral Assessment Scale into routine nursing care, *Issues Compr Pediatr Nurs* 9:341, 1986.

Bahr J: Canine and feline rivalry, *Pediatr Nurs* 1(4):18, 1981.

Betelheim B: *A good enough parent: a book on child-rearing,* New York, 1987, Alfred Knopf, Inc.

Bowlby J: *Child care and the growth of love,* Baltimore, 1965, Penguin Books.

Brazelton TB: The remarkable talents of the newborn, *Birth Family J* 5:187, Winter 1978.

Brazelton TB: *Doctor and child,* Boston, 1976, Delacourt Press.

Carey WB and McDevitt SC: Revision of the infant temperament questionnaire, *Pediatrics* 61(5):735, 1978.

Chess S, Thomas A: Temperament differences: a critical concept in child health care, *Pediatr Nurs* 21(2):167, 1985.

Choi E, Hamilton R: The effects of culture on mother-infant interaction, *J Obstet Gynecol Neonatal Nurs* 15(3):256, 1986.

Dean P, Morgan P, Towhe J: Making baby's acquaintance: a unique attachment strategy, *MCN* 7:37, 1982.

Donaher-Wagner BM, Braun DH: Infant cardiopulmonary resuscitation for expectant and new parents, *MCN* 17(1):27, 1992.

Effron D: *Cardiopulmonary resuscitation: CPR,* ed 3, Washington, DC, 1986, American Heart Association.

Field TM et al: The mother's assessment of the behavior of her infant, *Infant Behav Develop* 1:156, 1978.

Field TM et al: Tactile/kinesthetic stimulation effects on preterm neonates, *Pediatrics* 77(5):654, 1988.

Fuller BF: Acoustic discrimination of three types of infant cries, *Nurs Res* 40(3):156, 1991.

Funke J, Irbe MI: An instrument to assess the quality of maternity behavior, *JOGNN* 7(5):19, 1978.

Graves BW: Differential diagnosis of respiratory distress, *J Nurs Midwifery* 37(2):275, 1992.

Greenberg M, Morris N: Engrossment: the newborn's impact on the father, *Am J Orthopsychiatry* 44:520, 1974.

Haith M: Sensory and perceptual processes in early infancy, *J Pediatr* 109(1):158, 1986.

Haberkern RC: Adoption: new tasks for the pediatrician, *Pediatr Rev* 10(5):155, 1988.

Horowitz FD: Targeting infant stimulation efforts, *Clin Perinatol* 17(1):185, 1990.

Keefe MR: The irritable infant syndrome: theoretical perspectives and practice implications, *Adv Nurs Sci* 10:70, 1988.

Klaus M, Kennell J: *Parent-infant bonding,* St Louis, 1982, Mosby.

Kodadek MP: Parenting the newborn, NAACOG Update Series 5(10), 1986.

Korner, AF: Infant stimulation: issues of theory and research, *Clin Perinatol* 17(1):176, 1990.

Krozy R, McColgan J: Auto safety: pregnancy and the newborn, *JOGNN* 14(10):11, 1985.

Mahler M, Pine F, Berman A: *The psychological birth of the human infant,* New York, 1975, Basic Books.

McFarlane A: Olfaction in the development of social preferences in the human neonate. In Parent-infant interactions, *Ciba Found Symp* 33:103, 1975.

Rauh VA et al: The mother-infant transaction program, *Clin Perinatol* 17(1):91, 1990.

Rubin RA: Binding-in in the postpartum period, *Matern Child Nurs J* 6(2):67, 1977.

Rubin R: *Maternal identity and the maternal experience,* New York, 1984, Springer.

Schmitt B: The prevention of sleep problems and colic, *Pediatr Clin North Am* 33(4):763, 1986.

Sherwen LN et al: Common concerns of adoptive mothers, *Pediatr Nurs* 10:127, 1984.

Widmayer AM, Field TM: Effects of Brazelton demonstrations for mothers on the development of preterm infants, *Pediatrics* 67(5):711, 1981.

STUDENT RESOURCE SHELF

Broussard AB, Rich SK: Incorporating infant stimulation concepts into prenatal classes, *JOGNN* 19(5):381, 1990. Practical application of infant stimulation for nurses who are involved in teaching parents.

Lipsitt L: Learning in infancy: cognitive development in babies. *J Pediatr* 109(1):172, 1986.

Nugent JK: *Using the NBAS with infants and their families,* New York, 1985, March of Dimes Birth Defects Foundation.

Whitehouse H: How infants achieve self-organization and self-confidence: implications for health care professionals and parents, *Matern Child Nurs Currents* 34(5):1, 1987.

PARENT RESOURCES

Klaus MH, Klaus RH: *The amazing newborn,* Reading, MA, 1985, Addison-Wesley.

Ludington-Hoe SM: *How to have a smarter baby,* New York, 1985, Rawson Associates.

Ludington-Hoe S: Parents guide to infant stimulation, Los Angeles, Infant Stimulation Education Association. Also available for health care providers are samples of toys and recommendations for stimulation principles to hospital units. Write to Infant Stimulation Education Association, % Dr. Ludington-Hoe,

UCLA, Center for Health Sciences, Factor 5–90024, Los Angeles, CA 90024.

The sensational baby, Boston, Polymorph Films (film). Wallin C: Infant stimulation for parents, Washington, DC, 1982, ISEA Publications.

Thomas E: *Born dancing,* New York, 1988, Harper & Row.

Whitehouse H: *You and your baby,* Columbus, Ohio, 1987, Ross Laboratories. Free publication that talks about month-to-month ways parents can communicate with their infant to understand each other better while encouraging baby's development.

Five

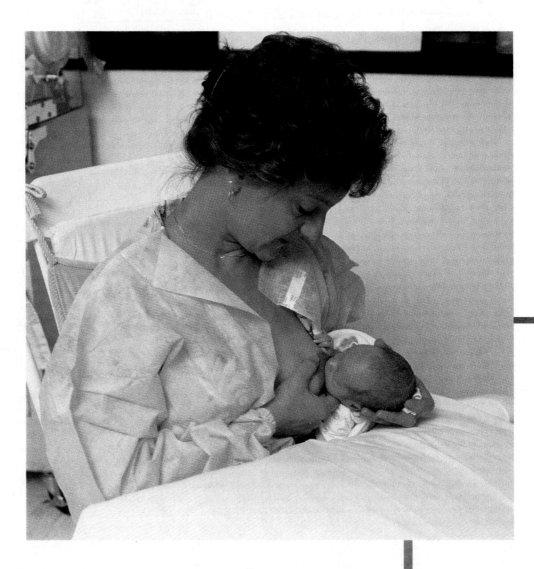

PREGNANCY AT RISK

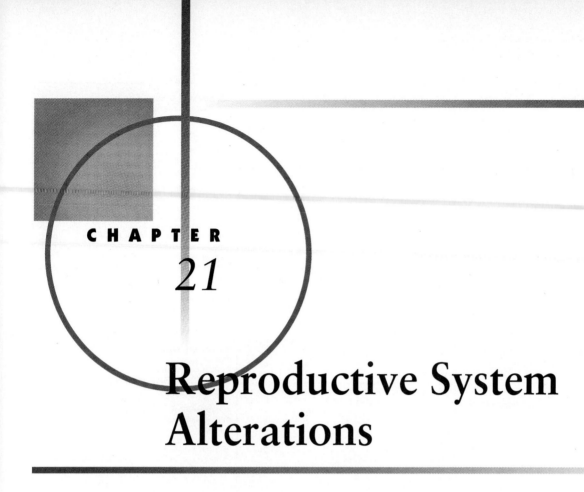

Reproductive System Alterations

KEY TERMS

Abruptio Placentae
Diovular Twins
Ectopic Pregnancy
Hemorrhage
Hydatidiform Mole
Hypovolemia
Induced Abortion
Intrauterine Fetal
Death (IUFD)
Laceration
Monovular Twins
Oligohydramnios
Placenta Accreta
Placenta Previa
Polyhydramnios
Preterm Birth

Spontaneous
Abortion
Tocolytics

Trophoblastic
Disease
Uterine Atony

LEARNING OBJECTIVES

1. *Apply the steps of the nursing process to planning care for a woman with complications of the reproductive system.*
2. *Plan preterm prevention strategies for a client in a selected life situation.*
3. *Correlate the changes of multiple pregnancy with the increased pregnancy discomforts and risks.*
4. *Describe current rules and regulations that affect elective abortion.*
5. *Summarize methods of psychosocial support for a woman when pregnancy is interrupted by spontaneous or elective abortion and by fetal death.*
6. *Associate reproductive anatomy with causes of bleeding during pregnancy and the birth process.*
7. *Compare and contrast signs and symptoms for each life-threatening cause of obstetric hemorrhage, and relate to intervention choices.*

The complications of pregnancy that cause high risk for the woman and infant are presented in the second half of this text. Approximately 85% of all pregnancies that progress to the birth date are normal and without problems. When problems do occur, extreme anxiety and fear for the safety of the woman and her infant often occur. Figure 21-1 illustrates the varied "things that can go wrong." These complications are documented in the new maternal and infant health portion of the birth certificate. Throughout these chapters it should be kept in mind that preventive care is the goal of all maternal and newborn interventions.

The reproductive system is complex and, if disturbed, can place a woman at risk for loss of her fetus

38a. MEDICAL RISK FACTORS FOR THIS PREGNANCY
(Check all that apply)

Anemia (Hct. <30/Hgb. <10) .... 01 □
Cardiac disease .... 02 □
Acute or chronic lung disease .... 03 □
Diabetes .... 04 □
Genital herpes .... 05 □
Hydramnios/Oligohydramnios .... 06 □
Hemoglobinopathy .... 07 □
Hypertension, chronic .... 08 □
Hypertension, pregnancy-associated .... 09 □
Eclampsia .... 10 □
Incompetent cervix .... 11 □
Previous infant 4000+ grams .... 12 □
Previous preterm or small-for-gestational-age
  infant .... 13 □
Renal disease .... 14 □
Rh sensitization .... 15 □
Uterine bleeding .... 16 □
None .... 00 □
Other _____ 17 □
(Specify)

38b. OTHER RISK FACTORS FOR THIS PREGNANCY
(Complete all items)

Tobacco use during pregnancy .... Yes □ No □
  Average number cigarettes per day _____
Alcohol use during pregnancy .... Yes □ No □
  Average number drinks per week _____
Weight gained during pregnancy _____ lbs.

39. OBSTETRIC PROCEDURES
(Check all that apply)

Amniocentesis .... 01 □
Electronic fetal monitoring .... 02 □
Induction of labor .... 03 □
Stimulation of labor .... 04 □
Tocolysis .... 05 □
Ultrasound .... 06 □
None .... 00 □
Other _____ 07 □
(Specify)

40. COMPLICATIONS OF LABOR AND/OR DELIVERY
(Check all that apply)

Febrile (>100°F. or 38°C.) .... 01 □
Meconium, moderate/heavy .... 02 □
Premature rupture of membrane (>12 hours) . 03 □
Abruptio placenta .... 04 □
Placenta previa .... 05 □
Other excessive bleeding .... 06 □
Seizures during labor .... 07 □
Precipitous labor (<3 hours) .... 08 □
Prolonged labor (>20 hours) .... 09 □
Dysfunctional labor .... 10 □
Breech/Malpresentation .... 11 □
Cephalopelvic disproportion .... 12 □
Cord prolapse .... 13 □
Anesthetic complications .... 14 □
Fetal distress .... 15 □
None .... 00 □
Other _____ 16 □
(Specify)

41. METHOD OF DELIVERY *(Check all that apply)*

Vaginal .... 01 □
Vaginal birth after previous C-section .... 02 □
Primary C-section .... 03 □
Repeat C-section .... 04 □
Forceps .... 05 □
Vacuum .... 06 □

42. ABNORMAL CONDITIONS OF THE NEWBORN
(Check all that apply)

Anemia (Hct. <39/Hgb. < 13) .... 01 □
Birth injury .... 02 □
Fetal alcohol syndrome .... 03 □
Hyaline membrane disease/RDS .... 04 □
Meconium aspiration syndrome .... 05 □
Assisted ventilation <30 min .... 06 □
Assisted ventilation ≥ 30 min .... 07 □
Seizures .... 08 □
None .... 00 □
Other _____ 09 □
(Specify)

43. CONGENITAL ANOMALIES OF CHILD
(Check all that apply)

Anencephalus .... 01 □
Spina bifida/Meningocele .... 02 □
Hydrocephalus .... 03 □
Microcephalus .... 04 □
Other central nervous system anomalies
  (Specify) _____ 05 □
Heart malformations .... 06 □
Other circulatory/respiratory anomalies
  (Specify) _____ 07 □
Rectal atresia/stenosis .... 08 □
Tracheo-esophageal fistula/Esophageal atresia ... 09 □
Omphalocele/Gastroschisis .... 10 □
Other gastrointestinal anomalies
  (Specify) _____ 11 □
Malformed genitalia .... 12 □
Renal agenesis .... 13 □
Other urogenital anomalies
  (Specify) _____ 14 □
Cleft lip/palate .... 15 □
Polydactyly/Syndactyly/Adactyly .... 16 □
Club foot .... 17 □
Diaphragmatic hernia .... 18 □
Other musculoskeletal/integumental anomalies
  (Specify) _____ 19 □
Down's syndrome .... 20 □
Other chromosomal anomalies
  (Specify) _____ 21 □
None .... 00 □
Other _____ 22 □
(Specify)

FIGURE 21-1 New maternal and infant health items from the 1989 revision of the U.S. Standard Certificate of Live Birth.

or potentially her own life. In this chapter the focus is on reproductive problems related to preterm labor and multiple pregnancy. Abnormal functions such as polyhydramnios or oligohydramnios, hydatidiform mole, and ectopic implantation have underlying pathologic conditions. Loss of the pregnancy before viability (abortion) or after viability (intrauterine fetal death) result in common interventions. Abnormal placental function underlies major bleeding problems during the perinatal period.

Preterm Birth

Preterm birth is a leading cause of perinatal morbidity and mortality throughout the world. The less mature the infant the higher the risk of problems from immaturity of body systems. Prematurity accounts for 6% to 10% of all newborn deaths and is related to 60% to 75% of all neonatal morbidity in the United States (Graber, 1992). An emphasis on reducing the U.S. rate has not been as successful as programs in other developed countries because of the fragmentation of health care here. In fact, in spite of many early intervention programs, the rate has risen from 8.9% in 1980 to 10.2% in 1988 (*MMWR*, 1992). In addition, the current rate of premature births of 18.9% for African-American mothers contrasts with the rate of 8.8% for white mothers.

The causes of preterm birth are related to nutrition, poverty, drug use, maternal chronic disease, multiple births, and predominantly infection (see Table 21-1). To reduce the incidence of prematurity a number of factors must be considered, including high-risk socioeconomic or physical situations that require improved preventive interventions. Home monitoring of preterm labor coupled with nursing management and support is a growing and necessary field. Every nurse needs to know the sequence of preterm labor and recommended interventions.

The diagnosis of preterm labor usually is made when the following criteria are present (Beringer and Niebyl, 1990):

- Gestational age of 20 to 37 weeks
- Uterine contractions of four in 20 minutes or eight or more in 60 minutes and ruptured membranes *or*
- Intact membranes with clinical effacement of 50% or more and dilation of more than 2 cm

TABLE 21-1 Preterm Labor Risk Factors

FACTOR	SCORE	FACTOR	SCORE
SOCIAL HISTORY		**HISTORY OF MEDICAL PROBLEMS–CONT'D**	
Maternal age			
Under 17	4	Uterine anomaly	5
Over 40	2	Insulin-dependent diabetes	2
Single	2	**HISTORY OF PRETERM LABORS**	
Maternal education		Prior premature rupture of membrane	No. × 10
Grades 9-11	1		
Under grade 8	2	Prior preterm birth	No. × 10
		Prior full-term birth	No. × 10
Weight above/below standard			
Prepregnancy <45.5 kg	3	**PROBLEMS WITH PRESENT PREGNANCY**	
Weight gain by 22 wk >3.3 kg	2		
Weight loss by 22 wk >2.3 kg	3	Vaginal infection	3
		Bacteriuria	2
Height <152 cm	3	Fibroids	3
No. preschool children at home	Use actual number	Engagement >32 wk	3
Loss of pregnancy	1 (if two or more)	Bleeding after 12 wk	4
No. of first-trimester abortions	Use actual number	Cervical length <1 cm	4
No. second-trimester abortions	Use actual number	Dilation of internal os	4
		Uterus irritable	4
Last birth within the year	1	Placenta previa	5
Work outside the home	1	Oligohydramnios	5
Heavy work	3	Multiple pregnancy	10
Long commute	3	Cervical surgery	2
		Abdominal surgery	1
Smoking, drug use		Illness with fever	3
More than 11 cigarettes a day	2	Protein in urine >1+	2
Any cocaine use	4	Hypertension	2
Heavy use	10		
HISTORY OF MEDICAL PROBLEMS			
Pyelonephritis	4		
Cone biopsy	5		

Modified from Herron MA, Dulock HL: *Preterm labor,* series 2: *Prenatal care,* module 5, ed 2, White Plains, NY, 1987, The March of Dimes Birth Defects Foundation, 1987, p. 31, with permission of the copyright holders and the authors.

RISK

More than 40 factors (Table 21-1) have been identified as placing women at increased risk for preterm birth. In general, those who have preterm birth fall into one of the following categories: (1) almost one third of preterm births are related to maternal medical complications such as pregnancy-induced hypertension (PIH), cardiac disease (see Chapter 22), and complications such as placenta previa and cervical incompetence; (2) another one third result from rupture of membranes (ROM) before term, causing labor; and (3) among one third of women, labor begins with no apparent reason. These last two probably have an underlying cause of infection.

Women who give birth prematurely more frequently have amniotic fluid infection and postpartum endometritis, and neonatal pneumonia develops more frequently in their infants (Daikoku et al, 1982). A study that took into account the duration of labor and ROM showed histologic evidence of inflammation among 53% of placental membranes from preterm births, compared with 16% of membranes from full-term births (Hillier, 1988).

The microorganisms associated with increased risk of preterm birth include *Neisseria gonorrhoeae, Gardnerella vaginalis, Chlamydia trachomatis, Mycoplasma hominis, Ureaplasma urealyticum, Trichomonas vaginalis,* group B streptococcus, and aerobic and anaerobic microorganisms found in organisms that cause *bacterial vaginosis* (BV). Microbial colonization and resultant inflammation cause disruption of the decidua and membranes and a release of prostaglandins. Some vaginal flora also produce enzymes that increase the concentration of *arachidonic acid* (a precursor of prostaglandins). Microorganisms and host white blood cells produce a variety of *proteolytic enzymes,* substances that break down protein (McGregor, 1988). In addition, microorganisms may break down the mucous plug and facilitate the entrance of vaginal and cervical bacteria into the uterus.

Lactobacillus organisms normally present in the vagina have a protective effect against preterm labor. Preventive strategies are being studied. Use of metronidazole and intravaginal clindamycin seem the most promising but are not yet approved for use during pregnancy (McDonald et al, 1992).

SIGNS: CONTRACTION PATTERNS

Beginning after weeks 20 to 28, normal uterine activity includes low-intensity contractions of less than 15 mm Hg pressure, which very gradually increase in frequency and intensity until term when there should be fewer than four per hour by the external tocotransducer (the woman may not sense these mild contractions). Normal diurnal activity occurs with two periods of more frequent contractions and two *quiet periods* between 4 and 11 AM and 2 and 10 PM. This *diurnal* (twice a day) pattern is absent when preterm uterine activity is irritable (Figure 21-2).

Preterm uterine irritability may begin as early as 24 weeks. These low-amplitude, high-frequency (LAHF) waves are an early warning sign. This hyperactivity is evidenced as erratic but frequent mild, wavelike contractions. The rate increases before 28 weeks to more than 8 to 10 per hour, and the intensity may exceed 15 mm Hg (Figure 21-3).

Without intervention, contractions will become organized and more intense, resulting in premature birth (Eganhouse and Burnside, 1992).

Through home monitoring it has been shown that there is a *sudden increase* in numbers of contractions per hour in the 24-hour period before overt signs of preterm labor. If women can learn to detect this increased activity, they can receive intervention *before* excessive cervical dilation occurs.

In preterm labor, membranes may rupture without subsequent organized labor contractions, or contractions may begin without membrane rupture. Some women can recognize contractions; others talk of "feeling something change." Because the *subtle signs of preterm labor* may be missed, these signs should be taught to every pregnant woman and reinforced frequently for anyone at risk (Box 21-1).

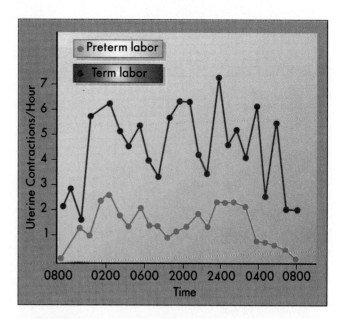

FIGURE 21-2 Comparison of contraction rates in 24 hours in normal pregnancies (*red*) and those with uterine irritability (*blue*). (Modified from Schwenzor TH, Schumann R, Halberstadt F: The importance of 24 hour cardiotocographic monitoring during tocolytic therapy. In Jung H, Lambert G, eds: *Beta-mimetic drugs in obstetrics and perinatology,* New York, 1982, Thieme-Stratton, p. 60.)

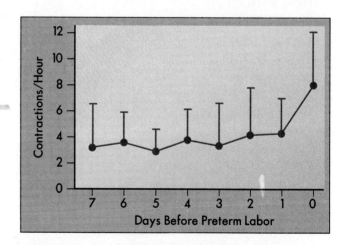

FIGURE 21-3 Frequency of contractions during the last 7 days before preterm labor. (From Katz M, Newman RB, Gill PJ: Assessment of uterine activity in ambulatory patients at high risk of preterm labor and delivery, *Am J Obstet Gynecol* 154:44, 1986. Used by permission.)

CLINICAL MANAGEMENT

A number of approaches have been attempted to standardize early detection of the potential for preterm labor. Women in the risk categories are observed more frequently, and most are instructed in self-monitoring of contractions. Recently, researchers have found that the *mammary stimulation test (MST)* (see Chapter 11) has been a predictor of approximately 85% of cases of

BOX 21-1 Subtle Signs of Preterm Labor

Menstrual-like abdominal aching or thigh cramps

Rhythmic dull backache or pelvic ache

Heavy feeling in the pelvis

Increased vaginal discharge—more mucus: watery or blood-tinged

Intermittent uterine cramping, more than four per 20 minutes, or eight per hour, often not sensed as painful

Intestinal cramping with or without diarrhea

preterm labor. Eden and Sokol (1992) found that the MST, performed between 24 and 32 weeks of gestation for women with risk factors, could identify most of those who actually experienced preterm labor. In addition, 95% of those who had full-term births were identified by the presence of a negative response to the MST (Box 21-2).

The MST for this purpose is brief (20 minutes) and inexpensive, and it can be conducted in the clinic or office. A Doppler fetal heart monitor and tocotransducer are attached to the woman's abdomen. Baseline uterine activity is observed for 10 minutes. If uterine activity is present, it is evaluated for preterm labor characteristics and the test is *not* initiated. If uterine activity is *not present*, the woman lightly stimulates one nipple through her clothing for 2 minutes, followed by a rest period of 2 minutes. The monitor record is observed for contraction activity. If there is no uterine response, the nipple is stimulated once more for 2 minutes, with a 2-minute rest period. Absence of uterine contractions after stimulation indicates a negative test response almost ensuring that the woman will

BOX 21-2 Mammary Stimulation Test Criteria

Positive test

Any spontaneous uterine contraction(s) > 40 seconds before initiation of nipple stimulation

Any uterine contraction(s) of > 40 seconds by the completion of two stimulation cycles (8 minutes from the onset of stimulation)

Negative test

Absence of uterine activity (contraction[s] that last for > 40 seconds before or during stimulation)

From Eden RD et al: The mammary stimulation test—a predictor of preterm delivery? *Am J Obstet Gynecol* 164:1409, 1991; with permission.

proceed to full term. Those with uterine contractions are considered at risk for preterm labor and should be followed up with home monitoring and other interventions.

If the woman has been under care, understands her situation, and reports findings or if the home monitor transmits increased uterine activity, she is observed in the labor unit while a decision is made about her status. Remember, the earlier she comes for diagnosis, the more likely it is that interventions will be effective.

Uterine cramping is monitored externally. A careful speculum examination is performed to assess cervical dilation and to note the presence of bulging membranes and amniotic fluid in the vagina. A positive Nitrazine test result will show a more alkaline pH if membranes are leaking. Often preterm labor is not experienced as painful. Therefore, to assess cervical effacement a careful digital examination follows the speculum examination. Thereafter vaginal examinations are kept to a minimum.

Assessment for preterm labor includes evaluating risk factors and subtle signs. If a woman is sent home after evaluation, careful documentation of the assessment is crucial to prevent risk of liability later should she deliver unexpectedly and blame the personnel for sending her home.

The woman always is monitored for at least 1 hour in the labor area until a decision is made regarding potential outcome. Treatment consists of intravenous (IV) hydration with 500 ml in 1 hour (Beringer and Niebyl, 1990). A more rapid fluid intake is not advised in the event tocolytic agents are to be used because fluid retention with pulmonary edema may occur. During this hour the woman maintains a side-lying position and is monitored. The goal is to relax the uterine muscle with these interventions. If contractions stop, she may remain in the area for a few more hours but may assume a sitting position. If contractions do not improve and the cervix is less than 3 to 4 cm dilated, tocolytic therapy will be instituted.

dehydra is a prim. cause for preterm labor.

Tocolytic Agents

Tocolytics belong to a class of drugs that inhibit contractions by affecting smooth muscle action. Analyses of tocolytic effectiveness show that these drugs will

 Clinical Decision

Mary is being monitored before an MST. What should you say to her if after 20 minutes you assess the strip and see mild contractions every 5 to 6 minutes?

delay labor at least 24 to 48 hours and sometimes up to several weeks, but there are many failures. In cases of possible infection, the addition of antibiotic therapy has improved effectiveness ratings (McGregor, 1988). The cervix must not be too far effaced or dilated. If the cervix is more than 3 or 4 cm dilated, with intense contractions, ruptured membranes, or if the woman has a medical contraindication, labor will be allowed to progress (Table 21-2).

A number of drugs are in trial and require informed consent for their use. The only tocolytic drug approved by the Food & Drug Administration (FDA) for this purpose is *ritodrine* (Yutopar), but it is used less often because of unpleasant side effects related to its beta-mimetic activity. *Terbutaline* (Brethine) is commonly used. A drug used for asthma to relax bronchioles, it has fewer side effects than does ritodrine although it is in the same category. These beta-mimetics have a group of actions illustrated in Figure 21-4. *Nefedipine*, a calcium channel blocker used for hypertension, has been found useful because it relaxes smooth muscle. The most frequently used agent is *magnesium sulfate*. Effective as a neuromuscular blocking agent in cases of hypertension during pregnancy, it also relaxes smooth muscle by affecting the flow of calcium out of the muscle cell. Magnesium sulfate is a familiar drug in labor and birth and has fewer side effects than do other tocolytic agents (Figure 21-5). Finally, certain antiprostaglandins have been used; currently *indomethacin* is in frequent use. Table 21-2 shows benefits and risks of these therapies.

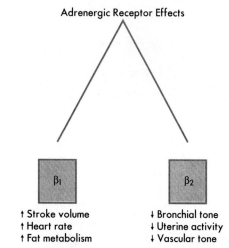

FIGURE 21-4 Adrenergic receptor effects. (α, Stimulation; β, inhibition.) β_1 and β_2 receptor effects often overlap. Search is for drug that has more specific β_2 effects.

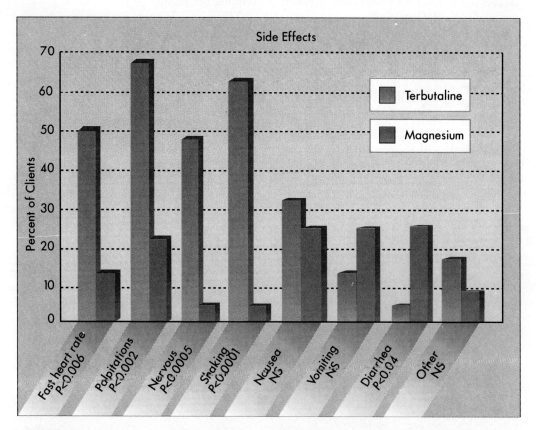

FIGURE 21-5 Percentage of patients reporting side effects with oral terbutaline and oral magnesium oxide. (Redrawn from Ridgeway LE et al: A prospective randomized comparison of oral terbutaline and magnesium oxide for the maintenance of tocolysis, *Am J Obstet Gynecol* 163:879, 1990.)

TABLE 21-2 Tocolytic Drugs

DRUG/DOSE/ROUTE	MATERNAL/FETAL EFFECTS	MONITORING
BETA-ADRENERGIC AGONISTS *Ritodrine (Yutopar)* *Dosage:* IV bolus 0.25 mg, then mix 150 mg/500 ml IV solution to run at 20 ml/hr. Increments of 10 ml/hr q10 min to a maximum of 350 µg (70 ml/hr) until contractions cease. Continue for 24 hr, then phase in PO dose of 5-10 mg q2-4 hr. Stabilize before sending home on PO doses. *Action:* β-adrenergic receptor stimulant; T½, 6-9 min at first, then 2-3 hr. Tolerance develops quickly. *Contraindications:* Hypovolemia, bleeding, hypertension, thyroid dysfunction, cardiac disease of any kind, diabetes, migraines, significant chronic fetal distress, infection. *Terbutaline (Brethine)* *Dosage:* 0.25-0.5 mg SC q1-4 hr until contractions stop. Then 5 mg PO or SC q4 hr for 48 hr. Maintenance dose is 5 mg q6 hr. May be delivered by terbutaline pump, SC. *Action:* Acts on β₂-receptor in smooth muscle of uterus, bronchi, t½, 3.7 hr. Also used with fetal distress to reduce hypertonic contractions and increase placental blood flow. *Contraindications:* Not used for diabetes, cardiac, asthma, severe PIH, thyroid conditions. Risk of pulmonary edema with IV fluid related to colloid osmotic pressure (COP), especially with betamethasone use. **MAGNESIUM** *Magnesium sulfate* *Dosage:* Loading dose, 4 g of 10% solution (40 ml) over 20 min, then 1 to 3 g/hr until contractions stop. Then PO with 500 mg tab: q4 hr for 24 hr. Many physicians use magnesium sulfate after terbutaline or ritodrine in lower doses with good effect.	*Maternal* Effects are dose-related, and dose is titrated by woman's response; screen ECG before starting dose. *CV:* tachycardia, premature ventricular contractions, chest pain, increased systolic or decreased diastolic pressure; *CNS:* tremors, headache, malaise, anxiousness, weakness; *GI:* nausea, vomiting, bloated feeling, diarrhea, constipation; *metabolic:* hyperglycemia, hypokalemia, metabolic acidosis; *other:* erythema, sweating, chills, hyperventilation. *Fetal* Only with severe maternal effects: tachycardia, acidosis, hypoxia. Check newborn for these effects and paralytic ileus, hypotension, and hypoglycemia at birth. *Maternal* *CV:* increases systolic, decreases diastolic pressures related to peripheral vascular resistance; increases heart rate CO, SV; pounding heart, flushing, palpitations; *CNS:* tremors, nervousness, headache; *GI:* nausea, vomiting, *metabolic:* glucose metabolism altered, hypokalemia, ketonuria. *Fetal* Tachycardia; monitor glucose, heart rate. *Maternal* *CV:* hypotension, circulatory collapse; *CNS:* depressed deep tendon reflexes, depressed respirations, muscle weakness, paralytic ileus, confusion; *other:* sweating, flushing, hypothermia, oliguria.	Vital signs: BP q5 min until stable then q15 min during IV route, then q4 hr until stable. Pulse, respirations every hour. Notify physician if pulse is over 100. Auscultate chest for rales and rhonchi. Daily weight. Urine for ketones. Blood for electrolytes, glucose. Give antiemetic, ice chips at first. Maintain quiet, restful environment with side-lying or Fowler's position. Reassure for anxiety. Teach to self-monitor contractions and fetal movements at home. Often use home monitoring. Discontinue drug 6 hr before birth. Screen baseline glucose status; follow urinary ketones and serum glucose levels during treatment, as well as electrolytes and serial hematocrit values. Screen baseline ECG; follow maternal-fetal vital signs closely; strict I&O Fetal heart tone and contractions. If unsuccessful, discontinue infusion 2 hr before expected delivery of infant. Discontinue solutions if any adverse effects occur. Antidote is calcium gluconate. Excreted unchanged in urine. Observe I & O. Check respiratory rate >14/min; check reflexes.

Continued.

TABLE 21-2 Tocolytic Drugs—cont'd

DRUG/DOSE/ROUTE	MATERNAL/FETAL EFFECTS	MONITORING
Action: Blocks myoneural junction, thus affecting contraction intensity. Short t½; difficult to obtain therapeutic level of 4.5 mg/dl. Toxic level may occur if renal function poor. *Contraindications:* Renal impairment, hypotension, myocardial damage.	*Newborn* Hypermagnesemia, lethargy, hypotonia, possible magnesium toxicity and neuromuscular and respiratory depression.	Fetal heart tones and contractions. Maternal vital signs. Bed rest in left lateral position. Obtain laboratory data: electrolyte levels. Monitor blood status.
CALCIUM CHANNEL BLOCKERS *Nifedipine (Adalat Procardia)* *Dosage:* Sublingual for quick onset using gelatin capsule. Then PO 20 mg four times a day (qid), chew and swallow with water. Reduce dosage after 3 days to two times a day (bid) for 5 days *Action:* Inhibits calcium flow in muscle tissue, relaxes smooth muscle; suppresses prostaglandin- and oxytocin-induced contractions; extra benefit if woman has hypertension. t½, 2-3 hr. *Contraindications:* Hypersensitivity. increases effects of β-blockers; with other β-blockers, may cause cardiac failure, hypotension. Caution: not FDA approved.	*Maternal* CV: palpitations, hypotension, peripheral edema; CNS: headache, weakness, dizziness, transient facial flushing, disturbed sleep; *EENT:* nasal congestion, dyspnea, cough, wheezing, blurred vision; *GI:* nausea, heartburn, diarrhea, abdominal cramps; *other:* muscle cramps, joint pain, fever, chills. *Fetal* Tachycardia.	
ANTIPROSTAGLANDINS *Indomethacin* *Dose:* Rectal suppository 50-100 mg, then 25 mg PO q6h until contractions cease. Or 50 mg PO, then 25 mg PO q4h 24 hr. Observe contractions and repeat for another 24 hr if recur. Sometimes used with ritodrine. Usually not used after 35 weeks to avoid potential of ductus arteriosus closure. *Action:* Prostaglardin inhibition. t½, 2-3 hr. Transferred across placenta. Neonatal t½, 11-15 hr and longer if very immature. *Contraindications:* Woman with any bleeding potential or peptic ulcer (because of slight anticoagulant effect).	*Maternal* Few effects, no change in heart rate or BP; nausea, heartburn, and vomiting occur; rare postpartum hemorrhage *Fetal* Potential of premature closure of ductus arteriosus—used for this purpose in neonate. Oligohydramnios—inhibits production of amniotic fluid. Used as therapy for these women.	*Monitoring:* In small doses few side effects. Observe contraction patterns for dizziness, drowsiness. Avoid alcohol, salicylates. Observe for change in bleeding pattern postpartum.

PO, By mouth; *t ½,* half-life; *CV,* cardiovascular; *CNS,* central nervous system; *GI,* gastrointestinal; *BP,* blood pressure; *SC,* subcutaneous; *CO,* cardiac output; *SV,* stroke volume; *qid,* four times daily; *bid,* twice a day; *ECG,* electrocardiogram; *FDA,* Food and Drug Administration; *EENT,* eyes, ears, nose, and throat; *I & O,* intake and output.

Drug Profile 21-1

Betamethasone (Celestone)

Action

Used in pregnant women to stimulate maturity of fetal lungs in cases of preterm labor. Steroid action with onset 10 minutes with IM route, duration 1⅛ days.

Dosage/route

12 mg IM 24 to 48 hours before preterm delivery. Repeat once 12 to 24 hours after first injection. Inject deep into large-muscle mass with 21-gauge needle. Avoid deltoid.

Side/adverse effects

Contraindicated for woman taking phenytoin or indomethacin.

When birth is inevitable, the woman is given *betamethasone* intramuscularly to stimulate production of surfactant. For the greatest effect, one or two doses 12 hours apart must precede birth by 24 to 48 hours (Drug Profile 21-1).

Nursing Responsibilities
▶ ASSESSMENT

A collaborative effort is required to determine if preterm labor is indeed present or advancing (see Clinical Management). All the assessment activities are carried out by the nurse, physician, or midwife.

▶ NURSING DIAGNOSES

Preterm labor may require extended bed rest at home or in the hospital. In addition, women in preterm labor may have the following nursing diagnoses:

- Sleep pattern disturbance related to frequency of medication, contractions, or monitoring
- Anxiety related to outcome as well as side effects of medication
- Self-esteem disturbance related to feeling she may have caused preterm labor to begin
- High risk for infection if membranes have been leaking

▶ EXPECTED OUTCOMES

The following are examples of expected outcomes that may apply to preterm labor clients:

- Obtains adequate sleep and rest using side-lying position

- Maintains adequate fluid intake
- Copes with limitations on life-style as a result of medication or bed rest
- Understands and complies with self-monitoring and medication regimen
- Labor and infection inhibited because of treatments

▶ NURSING INTERVENTIONS

Nursing interventions are crucial in effective prevention programs. A pattern of care that is producing positive results includes the following (Eganhouse and Burnside, 1992):

- Instruction on early signs and preventive care for all pregnant clients (Box 21-3)
- Identification of those at risk for preterm labor
- Instruction on self-monitoring of contractions twice a day from weeks 20 to 36 for women at high risk
- A 24-hour "hot line" to a nurse in the labor unit, clinic, or prevention program
- Staff education so that uniform responses are made to clients' telephone calls
- Frequently scheduled visits to evaluate clients at high risk
- Telephone contact with high-risk clients between visits
- Home uterine monitoring for a selected number who have had one episode of preterm labor
- Home care visits for those needing medication and monitoring at home

Women need instruction regarding premature labor signs, and each pregnant woman should be given an illustrated handout that teaches self-monitoring of contractions. If she develops symptoms of preterm labor, she is instructed to do the following:

- Empty her bladder
- Drink 3 to 4 cups of juice and water
- Palpate for contractions and record times
- Rest in a side-lying position for 30 minutes, then gradually resume activity if contractions diminish
- Notify health care provider if symptoms persist

Care during Tocolytic Therapy

Once tocolysis has been chosen, care will depend on the agent. Table 21-2 lists doses, side effects, and monitoring requirements. Beta-mimetic agents and magnesium sulfate demand closer initial monitoring than do calcium channel blockers or antiprostaglandins because of cardiovascular and renal effects. Ritodrine and magnesium sulfate are begun with an IV bolus dose and then are titrated to the woman's responses. Once contractions have stopped, oral doses may be started but always overlapping the IV doses. Drug and electrolyte levels must be followed during this period. Each woman should have written instructions for medication times,

BOX 21-3   Home Instructions for Prevention of Preterm Labor

Rest periods

Lie down on your left side for an hour twice a day. The physician may prescribe more rest if needed.

Fluid intake

Make sure to drink 8 to 10 cups of fluid each day. If you are having increased contractions, drink 3 to 4 cups within the first hour.

Strenuous activity

Do not perform any strenuous activity, including jogging, running, tennis, long walks, heavy lifting, or frequent trips up and down stairs. Do not do heavy cleaning, scrubbing floors, changing curtains, or moving furniture. Discuss long trips by car with your physician or midwife.

Employment

You may have to decrease, stop, or modify your work pattern.

Sexual activity

You may have to limit or stop vaginal intercourse depending on the cause of preterm labor. If after vaginal intercourse, you have a marked increase in contractions, report this to the physician.

Breast preparation

Avoid breast massage, and nipple stimulation, or preparation for breast-feeding until 2 weeks before your due date.

Childbirth classes

Attend childbirth education class unless your physician or midwife has prescribed bed rest. Avoid the physical exercises, but practice breathing techniques.

Stress reduction

Discuss stressful or anxiety-producing situations with your support person, physician, or midwife. Seek appropriate helpers.

Modified from Johnson FF: *MCN* 14(3):158, 1989.

with side effects noted and directions for notification of her primary care person.

Terbutaline is begun by subcutaneous (SC) injections every half hour until contractions cease and then is given orally. Because these three medications have short half-lives, dosage interval is frequent and the drug may have to be taken during the night.

It is important for a woman going home on an oral tocolytic regimen to have regular nursing checks, as well as 24-hour telephone contact with a knowledgeable staff member. She needs reassurance that everyone is doing whatever is possible to keep the pregnancy intact for as long as possible.

Home Therapy by Terbutaline Pump

In addition to the oral route, SC terbutaline infusion by portable pump is available for home use. Figure 21-6, which illustrates the pump size, can be programed to deliver small volumes of medication or bolus doses if contractions should reappear (Gill, Smith, McGregor, 1989). *more prem. contract Evening/late afternoon*

Candidates for this technique include women who have multiple pregnancies, prior episodes of preterm labor, previously delivered preterm infants, and those with risk factors known to increase the incidence of preterm labor, including a positive MST result. The in-home monitor consists of a tocotransducer, which the woman is instructed to use twice a day for 1 hour and at any time unusual contractions occur. The data are stored in the monitor and sent by a telephone modem to the health care provider (physician or perinatal clinical nurse specialist) for daily analysis. Uterine activity is compared with the client's usual pattern and a standard baseline of no more than three to six mild contractions per hour. If she is taking tocolytics at home, drug therapy will be adjusted and she will be asked to return to the hospital for adjustment of the dose and more complete evaluation.

Problems connected with in-home monitoring are cost and the ability of the woman to comply with the testing schedule. Women most in need of in-home monitoring often are those who are most affected by these factors; thus in-home monitoring currently is not used by all who may need it.

Knowledge deficits may exist about the cause of preterm labor or about self-monitoring. Careful instruction about signs and symptoms and the reasons for the

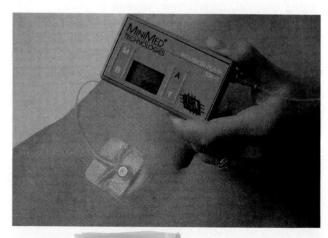

FIGURE 21-6 Terbutaline pump. (Courtesy Minimed Technologies.)

Clinical Decision

Lisa is receiving IV magnesium sulfate, 2 g/hr, because of preterm labor. She complains of a heavy feeling in her limbs and of feeling too warm. What assessments must be done, and what would you expect to find? (See Table 21-2 and Drug Profile 22-1.)

drug interventions will help the woman to cooperate with clinical management. She especially needs to understand the effects of tocolytic drugs. Symptoms such as palpitations and nervousness may be alarming unless understood as part of the drug effect. Any misinformation about fetal well-being or potential outcome should be corrected.

The woman often feels *powerless,* and it helps to encourage decision making in other aspects of her life. Family coping and support during this time are important. Financial concerns related to prolonged hospitalization need to be discussed with the social worker.

When preterm birth becomes likely, maternal transport to a tertiary center may be indicated if a local supportive service or neonatal intensive care unit (NICU) is unavailable. Distance from home will intensify feelings of loneliness and depression. Interventions to help the woman remain hopeful and interested in her environment are important. Primary nursing can be an important factor in the continued support for this client. If the infant is premature, anxiety over outcome is a crucial factor. (The support for parents of a premature infant is outlined in Chapter 28.)

Test Yourself

• Why is early detection of an irritable uterus important?
• List the early warning signs of preterm labor.

▶ EVALUATION

The following questions may be asked to evaluate expected outcomes for preterm labor care.
• Were sleep and rest patterns maintained satisfactorily?
• Did the woman cope adequately with changes in life-style?
• Did her increased understanding of the preterm labor process prevent loss of self-esteem?
• Was infection controlled?
• Was labor delayed long enough to benefit the baby?

Multiple Pregnancy

A multiple pregnancy carries a higher risk of perinatal morbidity and mortality because preterm birth occurs much more frequently, compared with single births. Perinatal mortality for twins is 3 to 11 times higher than for single infants (Hollenbach & Hickok, 1990). The greater the number of fetuses, the higher the rate of premature birth and poor survival. Therefore medical intervention is aimed at achieving the best possible outcome by maintaining the pregnancy as long as possible. The goal of treatment is to maintain a healthy pregnancy to at least 34 weeks' gestation. Bed rest in the last weeks, accompanied by administration of tocolytic agents, may be used to prevent premature labor.

TYPES

Monovular twins (monozygous) are the result of a single fertilized ovum that has divided into two before implantation. This process of "twoing," or twinning, *but before implantation* may occur from 2 to 7 days after fertilization. The time of division affects whether the fetuses have separate amnions and chorions, but there always is a single

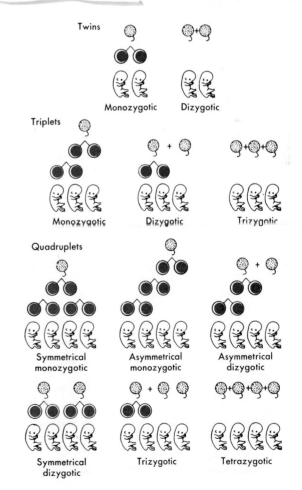

FIGURE 21-7 Possible embryologic origin of multiple pregnancies. (From Hafez ESE: *J Reprod Med* 12:88, 1974.)

placenta when separation has occurred early; later separation may result in two placentas (Figure 21-7). Placentas must be saved for complete examination. Each of the blastocysts develops into an individual with similar intelligence, physical characteristics, and sex.

Monovular, or identical, twins are interesting to study from psychosocial and biologic aspects because both individuals have the same genetic make-up. Incidence is 3 to 4 per 1000 worldwide, a fairly steady rate in every area.

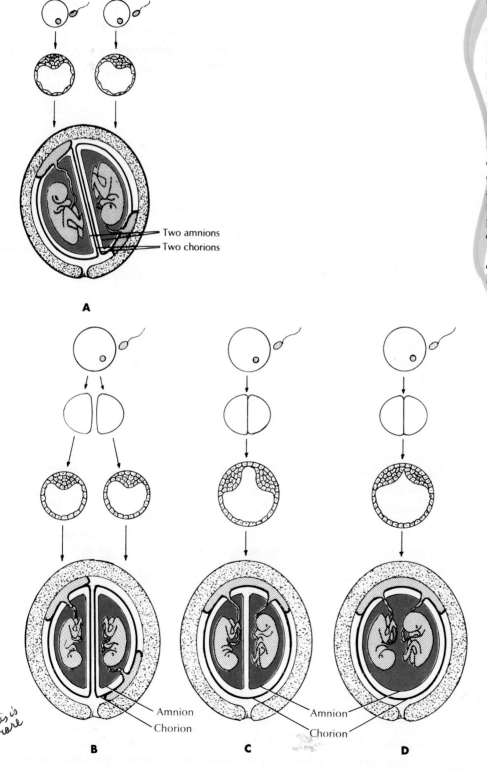

Two amnions
Two chorions

A

Amnion
Chorion

Amnion

Chorion

this is rare

B   C   D

FIGURE 21-8 **A,** Formation of dizygotic twins; fertilization of two ova, two implantations, two placentas, two chorions, and two amnions. **B-D,** Formation of monozygotic twins. **B,** One fertilization: blastomeres separate, resulting in two implantations, two placentas, and two sets of membranes. **C,** One blastomere with two inner cell masses, one fused placenta, one chorion, and separate amnions. **D,** Later separation of inner cell masses, with fused placenta and single amnion and chorion. (From Whaley LF: *Understanding inherited disorders,* St Louis, 1974, Mosby.)

Diovular twins, or fraternal twins, stem from two ova released at the same time, either from one ovary or one from each ovary. The placentas may fuse together or develop separately (Figure 21-8). Even if the placentas fuse, each has an individual chorion and amnion. Fraternal twins (dizygous) may look so much alike that they may be thought identical, or they may be as different in size, coloring, personality, and ability as other brothers and sisters in a family. The incidence of diovular or dizygotic twins varies with racial groups. The rate is highest, 1:25 to 1:50, in those of African descent. The rate is 1:100 in white women and 1:150 in Japanese women. There is a family tendency, passed through the maternal line, to release more than one ovum at a time.

Triplets and quadruplets may be diovular or monovular, but single-ovum pregnancies are less frequent. There may be mixed groups, with a set of monovular infants and one or two diovular infants.

Quintuplets and sextuplets are rarely the product of single-ovum pregnancies. In most cases, two or three distinct placentas or masses of two or three have fused together. These pregnancies most often are linked to drugs that cause hyperovulation. Ovulation stimulants have increased the incidence (see Chapter 6). A few physicians advocate selective abortion of one or more of the embryos to improve the outcome for the remaining ones.

Conjoined twins are caused by the failure of the fertilized ovum to separate completely. If the embryonic disk divides after 13½ days, it will remain united at one or more connections. The thorax, abdomen, and umbilical cord are common fusion sites. Sometimes surgery is possible when all organs are fully formed and function independently (Reed, Clariceaux, Bain, 1989).

Tests for Twin Type

Blood factors are identical in monovular twins, as are chemical substances such as haptoglobins and gamma globulins.

Footprints and fingerprints are nearly the same. "Ear prints," however, can assist in identifying identical twins because ear formations are distinctive from birth onward. Often an identical twin appears to be a mirror image of the other (e.g., the whorl of hair on the crown of the head is on the opposite side). Skin grafts from one identical twin always will be accepted by the other twin (Figure 21-9).

Placental structure is studied for relationships of the chorion and amnion. The examiner searches for one or two chorionic membranes. (Monochorionic membrane means a monovular twinning.) In the United States approximately 28% of twins are monozygous, and 72% are dizygous.

Twins may differ considerably in weight. Especially in fraternal girl-boy pairs, girls often weigh less than the

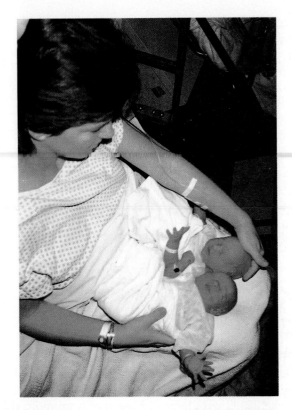

FIGURE 21-9 New twins meet their mother. (Courtesy James Suddath.)

boy at birth. Sometimes one infant has dominated because of better placement of its placenta. The small infant is called the *discordant twin* and may have severe intrauterine growth retardation (IUGR) and postnatal problems.

SIGNS

Twins often came as a surprise in the past when confirmation depended only on palpation and auscultation of fetal heartbeat. Today, diagnosis occurs by ultrasonographic examination at 8 to 10 weeks (see Figure 11-1). Occasionally, if more than two fetuses are present, diagnosis may be complicated by overlapping outlines. At times, there is one more baby than predicted.

Although most multiple pregnancies follow a normal course, delivery comes early. The length of gestation from the onset of the last menses to birth is about 22 days less than in a single birth, averaging 37 weeks. Pregnancy proceeds normally during the first trimester, when the embryos are small, with the exception that blood volume increases to a higher level. The only early problem noted by some is increased nausea and vomiting, which may indicate increased levels of human chorionic gonadotropin (hCG). Because of these increased levels of placental hormones, the mother may experience more frequent

Clinical Decision

Jenny visits the clinic at 16 weeks. She has had nausea, fatigue, and urinary frequency longer in this pregnancy than the last one. In addition, she is worried about her rapid weight gain. All the signs of pregnancy are present, and physical examination shows that her fundus is 2 cm below the umbilicus.
- *Is this finding appropriate for estimated gestational age?*
- *What anticipatory guidance should she receive if twin gestation is diagnosed?*

hot flashes and sweating. The major physiologic problems are caused by pressure of the overlarge uterus on the surrounding organs, anemia, and fatigue.

Pressure Effects

The uterus causes pressure on the ureters, bladder, intestines, vena cava, and renal vasculature, and later on the diaphragm. Increased pressure from more than one fetus may lead to varicose veins of the rectal, saphenous, or vulvar veins. In addition, many women experience marked dependent edema in the lower portion of their legs (see Figure 22-2). Constipation and digestive problems may be accentuated during the second and third trimesters. Pressure on the ureters may favor urinary stasis and infection. Pressure effects in each case are relieved by the side-lying position when the mother rests. Finally, during the day she may have to wear a maternity corset to provide some support for the abdomen.

CLINICAL MANAGEMENT

Anemia/Nutrition

Maternal anemia may be prevented by a diet rich in iron and the addition of supplemental iron and folic acid. The iron requirement is increased for a multiple pregnancy; iron needs are 60 to 80 mg/day. In addition to the normal (2000 to 2800 calories) requirements of pregnancy, there is an additional 300 calories per fetus for multiple-gestation pregnancies. The woman usually can tolerate only small meals because of increased pressure on the stomach.

Rest and Activity

Rest for the woman carrying more than one fetus is the most important factor in preventing preterm delivery. Toward the end of the third trimester, she may use the semi-Fowler's position for sleep. The chance of develop-

ing PIH is more common in multiple gestations, but the reasons for this increased incidence are unknown. A regimen of bed rest should help to diminish the incidence of hypertension, edema, and albuminuria.

Test Yourself

- List the expected maternal discomforts from pressure effects during a twin pregnancy.
- What are the modifications of diet for a woman with multiple pregnancy?

Early Monitoring

Because of the higher incidence of preterm labor, a multiple pregnancy is monitored early and often. Home uterine monitoring may be prescribed. Contraction monitoring for preterm irritability is important because the overdistended uterus may begin significant contractions sooner than expected. During nonstress testing (NST) each twin's heartbeat is located. Fetal heart reactivity of 15 beats/min and 15 seconds' duration is more valid a measurement *after* 32 weeks. The younger fetus tends to have a heart rate above 150, is less reactive, and has a lower beat-to-beat variability. The biophysical profile will be used to clarify fetal condition. It can differentiate the sleeping from the sick fetus (Eganhouse, 1992).

Unfortunately, contraction monitors commonly in use in labor units may not pick up preterm labor well, especially contractions before 26 weeks. In one large study, after 27 weeks only 78% of contractions that were indicated by the more sensitive home monitors were picked up by monitors in the labor unit (Hess et al, 1990). Home monitors correlate well with internal pressure catheters.

During labor, fetal monitors with dual capability are desirable. A spiral electrode may have to be placed on the first infant and an external ultrasound transducer for the second infant. Or both may be monitored externally by means of the newer technology: the monitor strip of one machine shows two fetal heart rates, and two tracings are provided by which to read the rates (Figure 21-10). Heart rates are never identical. If they appear to be, the transducer should be adjusted because one fetus is being recorded on both transducers. Monitoring of the fetal heart rates should continue during the birth process because there is up to a 30-minute delay in the birth of the second twin. A longer delay may necessitate a cesarean delivery for the second twin.

Presenting baby is labeled "A", all others consecutive B, C, D

Altered Labor Process

With therapy the mother may approach nearer to term than has been customary in the past. She is observed

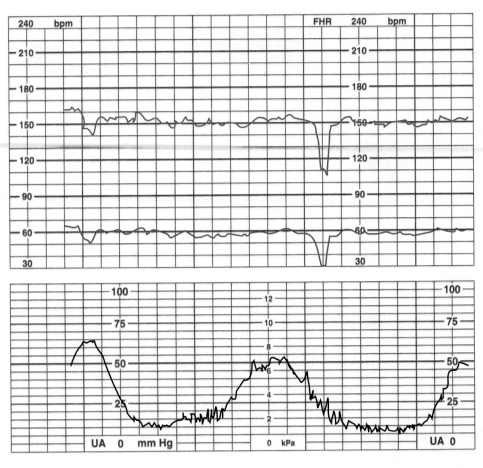

FIGURE 21-10 The first twin is accidentally monitored by both spiral electrode and cardiotransducer. Monitor paper with separate scales shows identical fetal heart rate tracings, but heart beats are never identical. (Redrawn from Eganhouse DJ: Fetal monitoring of twins, *JOGNN* 21[1]:17, 1992.)

carefully, and the condition of the cervix checked each week. She is instructed to notify the physician when contractions begin regularly. Usually considerable dilation and effacement of the cervix have already taken place during prelabor; thus it appears that the active phase of labor is shortened.

Uterine overdistension with resultant ineffective contractions is a problem during labor. Abnormal presentations of one fetus may cause special hazards to the second. The first infant may have a vertex presentation, but the second often is in a transverse or breech position, with the attendant problems of difficult delivery and possible prolapse of the cord. When regional anesthesia is used, the risk of hemorrhage after birth is slightly higher. Cesarean birth under regional anesthesia is planned when there is any question of fetal positions. General anesthesia is not used because the infants would be exposed too long a time and become depressed.

Preparation for a multiple delivery requires a multidisciplinary approach. Neonatologists, anesthesiologist,

obstetrician, and nurses must coordinate activities. Resuscitation equipment for several infants must be available, and if necessary, the premature infant nursery must be ready to receive the infants. Each cord is tagged at the maternal side, and each infant is identified in order of birth. After delivery the placentas are examined to aid in the diagnosis of zygosity.

High Risk for Hemorrhage

Because of the enlarged placental site, the internal os may be completely or partially covered. The warning signs of bleeding before labor should be noted carefully. During delivery a lower uterine or a cervical tear is not uncommon. After delivery the woman may have postpartum hemorrhage because of uterine atony and the large placental site.

Recovery and Planning Home Care

Parents who expect the arrival of more than one infant have time to prepare psychologically and financially to receive them. The birth of more than one infant often rallies the whole family to help. Extended hospitalization for preterm infants may be costly, however. Every possible referral to supportive agencies may be needed.

Because multiple births occur more often in women who have had children, it is important to prepare older siblings for the babies (Figure 21-11). Most parents find that it makes no difference whether the infants are fraternal or identical in the first year. One infant may be behind the other in developmental tasks, however, and the parents may suffer undue anxiety. The nurse can assist in helping the parent recognize the uniqueness of each infant.

Test Yourself

• Which complications of labor and delivery are more possible with a multiple pregnancy?

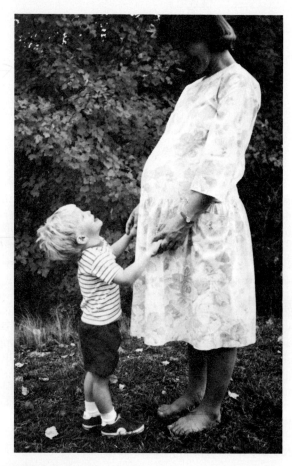

FIGURE 21-11 Siblings need special attention when twins are coming to "take up the space."

Ectopic Placement

An **ectopic pregnancy** is "out of place." In these cases the placenta usually implants in the fallopian tube (95% to 98%) but rarely may develop on the ovary or be attached to the broad ligament and intestine. Cell growth proceeds at the same phenomenal rate of speed whether the blastocyst implants in the fallopian tube, ovary, cervix, interstitial area of the fundus, or in the peritoneal areas (Figure 21-12). The rapidly developing embryo and placental tissue usually begin to show specific pressure effects by 10 weeks of gestation, and by 12 weeks, all overt signs are evident. As the placenta and embryo grow in the abnormal location, blood vessels proliferate, and when the pressure is too intense, the tube will rupture.

RISK

Ectopic implantation occurs in an average of 1 in 200 pregnancies in the general population. The number is considerably higher for women of low socioeconomic status, however, and is associated with general lack of prenatal care. The rate in inner-city areas of the United States is 1 in 80 to 1 in 120, whereas in areas of higher income the rate may be as low as 1 in 500 (Ellerbrock et al, 1987). Since 1982, ectopic pregnancy has become the second leading cause of maternal mortality in the United States. Two thirds of the deaths are related to misdiagnosis or delayed diagnosis. With prompt medical intervention and earlier diagnosis, the death rate should be drastically reduced.

The following conditions contribute to the development of an ectopic pregnancy:

1. Adhesions in the fallopian tubes from pelvic infections (salpingitis), especially from sexually transmitted diseases. The incidence is slightly increased in those who use intrauterine devices (IUDs) and in those who have had infections after previous pregnancies.

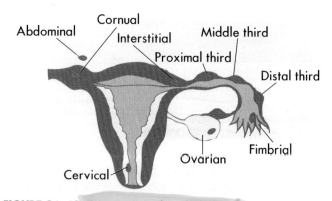

FIGURE 21-12 Ectopic sites of implantation. (From Breen JL: A 21-year survey of 654 ectopic pregnancies, *Am J Obstet Gynecol* 106:1004, 1970.)

2. Scars with adhesions from prior pelvic surgery.
3. Low levels of estrogen and progesterone, causing a delay in transport of the fertilized ovum.
4. Ovum migrating to the opposite tube, implanting when ready.
5. Presence of uterine benign muscle tumors (fibroids).

The incidence with future pregnancies is increased when the contributing conditions still are present or when one tube has been damaged and removed.

SIGNS

All signs of early pregnancy are present: amenorrhea, breast tenderness, nausea, and hCG levels are usually lower than in normal pregnancy (<25 mg IU/L), which indicates the presence of chorionic tissue. This usually occurs when a woman is confirming pregnancy and before she seeks prenatal care. Signs and symptoms may be confusing and may lead her to delay seeking a diagnosis (Table 21-3).

Before rupture, signs are related to increasing pressure or hidden bleeding. Pressure in the tube increases fairly rapidly, and by 10 weeks the woman will feel pelvic discomfort, beginning with dull aching and cramping and increasing to sharp stabbing pain in the lower portion of the abdomen. She may have referred shoulder pain (Figure 21-13) because blood in the peritoneal cavity causes irritation to the phrenic nerve, or pain may be referred to other parts of the body. If the

TABLE 21-3   Signs and Symptoms of Tubal Implantation*

SIGNS AND SYMPTOMS	COMMENTS
BLEEDING	
Painless, periodic vaginal spotting may resemble a light menstrual period.	Client may not notify physician. Bleeding may be caused by breakdown of decidual tissue after death of embryo in tube.
Hidden bleeding into peritoneum ("slow leak") causes symptoms of lower abdominal pressure (dark unclotted blood collects in cul-de-sac).	Hidden bleeding is caused by slow separation of placenta.
Sudden massive bleeding associated with rupture of tubal site causes woman to go into hypovolemic shock.	Bleeding usually is preceded by pain.
ANEMIA	
Fatigue and pale mucous membranes (out of proportion to observed blood loss) occur.	Hemoglobin and hematocrit levels fall slowly, especially with hidden slow bleeding.
ABDOMINAL PAIN	
Feeling of fullness in lower part of abdomen or backache and mild abdominal aching occur.	Three to five weeks after the woman misses the first period, symptoms begin, gradually increasing in intensity. (See Figure 21-12 for sites.)
Pain may be referred and occur at time of usual menstrual period.	
Pain may be excruciating during vaginal examination when cervix is moved.	Vaginal examination often brings first clue.
Intense, "tearing" pain may occur at time of rupture of tube.	Pain may still masquerade as appendicitis (See Figure 21-13).
SYNCOPE	
Light-headedness and fainting have been observed in 35% to 50% of ectopic pregnancies. It is called the *bathroom sign* because fainting often occurs while straining to defecate.	Bathroom sign is a response to feeling of fullness and pressure in rectal area. Cause is pressure of growing embryo or collection of blood in cul-de-sac or pressure on nerves of the perineal area.
EARLY SYMPTOMS OF PREGNANCY	
There will be breast tenderness, nausea for about 50%, a positive pregnancy test result, and uterus enlarged to about an 8-week size.	As long as corpus luteum is functioning, effects of pregnancy hormones will be experienced.

*Early diagnosis and intervention will prevent more serious signs.

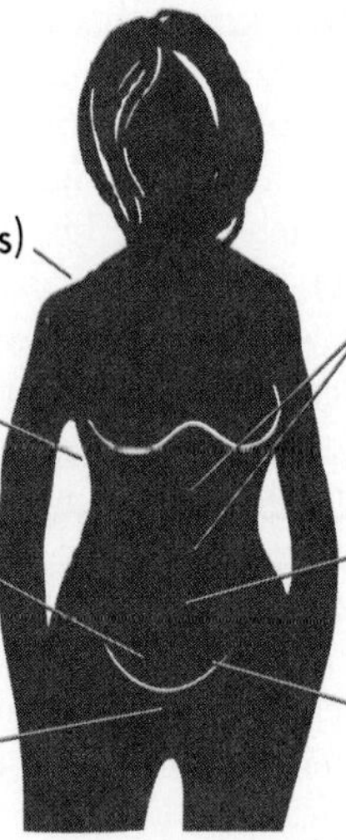

FIGURE 21-13 Sites of referred pain from ectopic pregnancies. (From Breen JL: A 21-year survey of 654 ectopic pregnancies, *Am J Obstet Gynecol* 106:1004, 1970.)

ectopic pregnancy ruptures, an episode of severe pain occurs, and the woman may show rapid signs of hypovolemic shock from blood loss into the peritoneum.

Depending on the site, bleeding may be visible or internal and begins as a slow leak. Blood may collect in the peritoneal cavity in the cul-de-sac behind the vagina and anterior to the rectum. The woman feels pressure and the need to defecate; the "bathroom sign" includes feeling faint when pressing down to evacuate the bowels. An abdominal examination elicits pain over the tube or ovary from pressure and chronic bleeding. The abdomen may be rigid and tender. During vaginal examination, if the cervix is moved, severe pain may occur. If there has been extensive bleeding, Cullen's sign shows a bluish tinge to the umbilicus.

> **Test Yourself**
> - Which early signs of pregnancy are missing when there is an ectopic pregnancy?

CLINICAL MANAGEMENT

The clinical problem is confirmed by the following tests:
1. Pelvic examination for masses and cervical signs of pregnancy
2. Ultrasound to verify placement of gestational sac in an unruptured tubal or intraabdominal pregnancy; transvaginal sonography is most accurate
3. Culdoscopy or culdocentesis to extract old blood from the cul-de-sac or to view the site with fiberoptic light

Laboratory tests reveal low hemoglobin and rising leukocyte counts. The red blood cell count is low, and the sedimentation rate is elevated. The serum hCG level, which is followed every 48 hours if there is any question, is lower than in normal pregnancy. One study reports a 95% predictive diagnostic success with ultrasound and hCG levels. If used early enough, these tests may reduce the chance of rupture (Stock, 1991).

Medical treatment is to remove the ectopic pregnancy, stop the bleeding, and when possible repair the tubal damage. A tuboplasty may be performed to save the tube, or the tube may have to be removed because scar tissue here would raise the risk of a future ectopic pregnancy. *Methotrexate,* a folic acid antagonist that inhibits cell division, has been used as an adjunct to surgery (Ichinoe et al, 1987).

When a woman desires to have a future pregnancy, the tube is not removed; instead newer conservative treatments are performed by laparoscopy. Depending on the gestational size and tubal damage, one of the following techniques is used:
- Salpingotomy (incision and closure of the tube)
- Salpingostomy (incision and evacuation of the tubal contents)
- Segmental resection of the tube

ADVERSE RESULTS

When conservative treatment is used, adverse effects can include a persistent ectopic pregnancy, that is, a failure to disrupt placental growth. hCG levels remain elevated and pain persists; 5% require a second surgical procedure or instillation of methotrexate (Stock, 1991). There is no guarantee of future fertility, and tuboplasty has led to occasions for lawsuits. Documentation is critical, and often, as evidence, photographs are taken of the tubal damage and the repair technique.

If rupture occurs, the peritoneal blood provides an ideal medium for the growth of bacteria. Therefore prophylactic antibiotics are ordered. The risk of paralytic ileus is increased because of abdominal surgery and irritation to the bowel.

On the woman's admission, vital signs and blood loss are observed and recorded frequently. If emergency surgery is required, preparation may be done in the emergency or operating room. A urine sample is obtained, perhaps from the Foley catheter inserted before surgery. The blood must be typed and cross-matched. IV fluids through a large-bore catheter are continued throughout this initial period.

After return from the recovery room, the woman will have nothing by mouth until bowel sounds are heard. Paralytic ileus is a possibility because of the proximity of the bowel. Ambulation is encouraged to promote movement of flatus, and bowel sounds are monitored.

Recovery depends on the degree of blood loss and the complexity of the surgery. Because of the significant blood loss the client is observed for signs and symptoms of infection and anemia. She also is given prophylactic antibiotics during recovery. All Rh-negative women receive RhD immunoglobulin to prevent sensitization.

The nurse initiates discussion of recovery and future pregnancies and teaches the use of contraception and the method most suitable for at least three menstrual cycles. The woman is encouraged to allow time for recovery. Finally, she should know the signs of ectopic implantation because there is a greater risk of recurrence if one tube has been removed.

Abnormal Placental Tissue: Molar Pregnancy

In fairly rare instances the placental chorionic villi undergo abnormal degenerative changes in which the trophoblastic epithelium proliferates to form grapelike cysts (Figure 21-14). These cysts eventually completely fill the uterus. Only a calcified embryo may be left. This change is termed **hydatidiform mole** or molar pregnancy. It also may be called **trophoblastic disease**. The complete mole has only the paternal chromosome present and thus is called an "empty ovum." In this case there is no embryonic tissue or membrane, only swollen, cystic villi. Because chorionic tissue is proliferating, large amounts of hCG are produced. Without treatment, choriocarcinoma of the endometrium will develop in about 20% to 50% of the cases.

A partial mole has some normally formed villi. There is only focal hyperplasia of tissue and a calcified or macerated embryo with chromosomal changes. hCG

titers are lower with a partial mole, and the levels return to normal more quickly after removal. A partial mole is less often malignant.

RISK

This abnormal condition occurs in 1 in 1200 to 1500 conceptions. Some other parts of the world, particularly Southeast Asia, India, and Mexico, report an incidence as high as 1 in 200. A relationship may exist between low protein intake or low socioeconomic status and its occurrence. The cause is unknown; however, contributing factors may include malnutrition, chromosomal abnormalities, and hormonal imbalance. It has been seen more frequently after use of clomiphene to induce ovulation. The chance of having a repeat molar pregnancy is 2% to 3% greater, especially if the woman is older than 40 years (Mehta and Young, 1988).

SIGNS

This clinical problem is determined by an abnormally rapidly growing uterus and signs of threatened abor-

Clinical Decision

Ann is in emergency admission with abdominal pain and suspected ectopic pregnancy of 10 weeks' gestation. What is the first care priority? List questions you could ask during assessment.

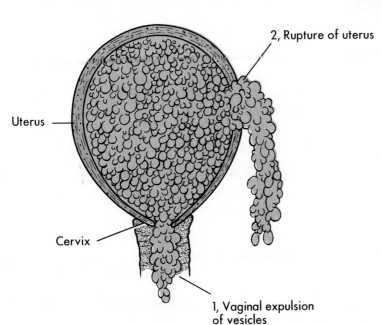

2, Rupture of uterus

Uterus

Cervix

1, Vaginal expulsion of vesicles

FIGURE 21-14 Uterine rupture with hydatidiform mole. *1,* Evacuation of mole through cervix. *2,* Rupture of uterus and spillage of mole into peritoneal cavity (rare). (From Bobak I: *Maternity and gynecologic care: the nurse and the family,* ed 5, 1993, Mosby.)

tion. Bright red or brownish vaginal bleeding may occur by the sixteenth week, with vaginal discharge of clear vesicles. Symptoms of hypertension may be present before 24 weeks. Nausea and vomiting may be much more severe than normal.

Laboratory tests reveal hCG levels completely out of the normal range, and levels may be 1 to 2 million IU, compared with hCG levels of under 300,000 IU in normal pregnancy. hCG levels may be normally elevated in multiple gestation; unlike usual pregnancies, however, these levels remain elevated after day 100 of pregnancy. Other values show reduced hematocrit and lower estriol, pregnanediol, and 17-ketosteroid levels. Because of elevated triiodothyronine (T_3) and thyroxine (T_4) levels, maternal pulse may be faster (Berkowitz and Goldstein, 1984), and sweating and intolerance to heat may be increased.

The problem is confirmed by use of ultrasound, which reveals the absence of fetal or skeletal growth. Multiple diffuse echoes are seen.

Prompt & compliant TX is critical.

CLINICAL MANAGEMENT

Medical treatment is to remove the molar tissue by dilation and curettage (D&C), depending on the length of gestation. If diagnosis is made in the second trimester, a hysterotomy must be performed to empty the uterus. The woman's desire for future pregnancy is an important factor in the choice of treatment. The woman's condition must be closely assessed for at least a year. Some physicians recommend a prophylactic course of methotrexate, although this management is controversial. One year without malignancy and with normal hCG titers is considered hopeful.

If choriocarcinoma occurs, hCG titers remain elevated 3 to 4 months after pregnancy termination. Chemotherapy is then carried out. The results from therapy can be excellent. In contrast, if the woman is untreated and metastases occur to the lungs, liver, and brain, death may result within a few months. Some women developed metastases, unaware of the life-threatening complications, because they did not have medical help after having a spontaneous abortion of a molar pregnancy.

Depending on the degree of development of the mole, bleeding, or other adverse signs, the woman will be scheduled for immediate evacuation of the uterus by D&C. The client is prepared for surgery while blood loss is monitored and, if necessary, replaced. The nurse should assess anxiety level and determine the level of understanding regarding the diagnosis and immediate treatment.

After surgery it is important that the woman become knowledgeable about self-care in the follow-up period. She must not skip weekly laboratory evaluations. The

year of waiting will be difficult, similar to a cancer client's wait to know if treatment has been effective. The woman's fears for herself may be well founded, depending on the outcome of the treatment; therefore she should not be reassured lightly.

Because recurrence is possible, the woman should be instructed about early signs, including vaginal bleeding, hypertension, aggravated nausea, and rapid uterine enlargement. She should be determined to wait at least a year before trying pregnancy again. This means that selection and use of an effective method of delaying pregnancy are important.

Because the variation in uterine growth is so strange and the prognosis so variable, the woman may suffer from lack of self-esteem, as well as fear for herself. She may ask, "Why me?" The nurse can be a supportive contact person for her during follow-up care in the clinic and if chemotherapy is advised. The woman's future may be determined by her decision and ability to comply with diagnostic testing and treatment.

Outcomes

The outcomes of treatment can be summarized as follows (Mehta and Young, 1988):

1. About 80% of moles are benign and have 100% cure rate with prompt treatment.
2. About 16% become malignant but are nonmetastatic, and most are cured with prompt treatment.
3. About 4% become malignant and metastasize. If there are no liver or brain metastases, there is hope that they may be cured.
4. In the worst case, if there have been previous chemotherapy and metastases, the prognosis is poor.

Continuity of care, teaching, and support needed when a molar pregnancy is confirmed may be a very significant nursing role. The woman's involvement in her care and, consequently, the outcomes may be largely determined by successful nursing interventions. Continuity of nursing care, particularly with primary nursing, is most desirable in this rare but potentially life-threatening disease.

Abnormal Amniotic Fluid Volume

Polyhydramnios and **oligohydramnios** exist when the normal volumes of amniotic fluid are not maintained. These volumes average as follows:

1. 16 weeks—200 ml
2. 34 to 35 weeks—980 ml
3. 40 weeks—800 ml
4. 42 weeks—540 ml and decreasing 150 ml/wk thereafter

Fluid volume is maintained by means of various mechanisms that change in ratio as pregnancy progresses:

alveolar secretions from the lungs transfer across fetal skin and membranes of the sac and umbilical cord. After 20 weeks, fetal urine is added to the volume of fluid, increasing from 5 to 50 ml/24 hr at 38 weeks. Fetal swallowing removes fluid at a rate of 15 to 20 ml/hr at term; because fluid is reabsorbed across membranes, the balance should be precise. Even a small variation either way will lead to too much or too little fluid.

OLIGOHYDRAMNIOS

A long list of congenital anomalies will produce oligohydramnios, especially defects in renal and gastrointestinal systems. In cases in which urine is not excreted or swallowing is affected, imbalance occurs quickly. Maternal hypertension, vasoconstriction, and IUGR will affect volume. Premature rupture of membranes (PROM) is always considered, and vaginal pH must be tested for alkalinity (See Preterm Labor). If ultrasound examination reveals a cramped fetal position and few pockets of fluid (<1 to 2 cm), or if the biophysical profile shows poor fetal breathing expansion, a diagnosis of oligohydramnios is made. Amniotic fluid is necessary for lung development. If diminished fluid volume occurs, lungs may be poorly functioning. Severe oligohydramnios that occurs early may be life threatening because the fetus cannot move freely or exercise the lungs with fetal breathing. *Pulmonary hypoplasia* may be lethal in the fetus. Furthermore, diminished fluid occurs normally with increasing gestational age, and it is expected that the postmature infant may have fetal distress from compression of the cord related to diminished fluid. (See Chapter 14 for the intervention of *amnioinfusion* during labor.) Finally, certain drugs such as the prostaglandin inhibitors indomethacin and ibuprofen have been shown to diminish fluid (Beringer and Niebyl, 1990).

As labor approaches, if oligohydramnios is acute or related to earlier rupture of membranes that did not result in preterm labor, maternal blood volume is increased by a rapid infusion of 1000 ml lactated Ringer's solution. If it is chronic, evaluation for congenital defects takes place. In any case, if the pockets of fluid are less than 2 cm, a cesarean section is planned because it is believed that the fetus cannot withstand the pressures of labor (see Chapter 14).

POLYHYDRAMNIOS/HYDRAMNIOS

The production of an abnormally large amount of amniotic fluid can precipitate premature labor and the uterus may resemble a multiple gestation. Hydramnios is more common in multiple pregnancies and pregnancies in which renal or gastrointestinal anomalies occur in the infant. If even a 1 or 2 ml imbalance occurs, the buildup of pressure can be quite dramatic. The uterus enlarges more rapidly than normal in the second half of pregnancy, and the pressure symptoms felt by the mother may be quite severe. An amniocentesis may be one way of relieving pressure, but a definite risk is connected to repeated tapping of the amniotic sac. As a further complication, when membranes rupture before or during labor, the risk of a prolapsed cord is much greater.

Pregnancy Loss

A pregnancy may be terminated by **spontaneous abortion** (in lay terms, a miscarriage) or by **induced abortion** for elective or therapeutic medical reasons. Abortions are further divided into early abortions, which take place before the sixteenth week of gestation, and late abortions, which occur between the sixteenth and twentieth weeks of gestation. To be classed as an abortion or *previable*, the fetus must weigh less than 500 g and have a crown-rump (CR) length of less than 16.5 cm. The *age of viability* is considered to be the beginning of the twentieth week, although very few of the 20- to 25-week-old infants are able to survive, even with intensive support. These infants are counted as potentially viable for vital statistics. *prior to 20 wks previable*
p̄ 20wks — fetal death .

SPONTANEOUS ABORTION

There are several types of spontaneous, involuntary abortion. The following descriptions are based on the woman's presenting signs and are listed in order of severity:

Threatened—Slight bleeding with mild uterine cramping and backache. The cervix is closed.

Inevitable—Moderate to severe bleeding with uterine cramping similar to labor contractions. The os is dilating.

Incomplete—Heavy bleeding with severe uterine cramping, with some tissue already partially out of uterus in the vagina.

Complete—Products of conception are totally passed. There remains slight bleeding with mild to moderate uterine cramping.

Missed—Slight bleeding with no uterine cramping, closed os. Embryo or fetus dies but is retained. Pregnancy growth ceases.

Habitual—Any of the above repeated in three consecutive pregnancies, usually after 16 weeks.

Risk

It is estimated that 15% of all conceptions are lost spontaneously, many so early that the woman is hardly aware of it. More than half of these spontaneous abortions are caused by fetoplacental defects, such as genetic defects or implantation abnormalities. Other causes are maternal problems such as poor nutrition or low hormone levels, severe diabetes, infections, uterine structure (e.g., fibroids or incompetent cervix), and rarely, severe trauma such as an automobile accident or abuse. Some evidence indicates that emotional shock results in abortion through an elevation in maternal epinephrine, which then leads to vasoconstriction and necrosis of the decidua basalis.

Signs

Cramping or spotting that leads to frank bleeding is the major sign of spontaneous abortion. Membranes may rupture at this time. The clinical problem is confirmed by history, pelvic examination, and ultrasound to determine the presence of a gestational sac as early as 6 weeks. Laboratory values may show a decrease in hemoglobin (less than 10.5 g/dl) with bleeding and an increase in white blood cell count if infection is present; hCG levels are not helpful because they may not decrease for 2 weeks. Serial ultrasound examination may document lack of fetal growth if there is a question about missed abortion.

A spontaneous abortion may become septic, with signs of fever, odorous bleeding, and a tender uterus. The later in the gestation the abortion occurs, the more bleeding there may be.

Clinical Management

Treatment of threatened abortion consists of limiting activities for 24 to 48 hours and observing the result. Controlled studies have failed to prove that bed rest, progesterone, or sedatives have any effect on the outcome of a threatened abortion (Grimes, 1984). Some centers are treating the woman with corticosteroids and low doses of acetylsalicylic acid (ASA) as an antiprostaglandin. If the bleeding can be stopped, it will do so within 48 hours. The woman may be asked to avoid stress, intercourse, fatigue, and extended activity until the pregnancy seems to be progressing satisfactorily. It is important to realize that a spontaneous abortion often occurs because something is not going well with the fetus. Thus a woman who has a rocky beginning may in fact have a fetus with a structural or genetic defect, or a hormonal support may be deficient.

INEVITABLE ABORTION

A threatened abortion may reverse itself or progress to an *inevitable* abortion. After cervical dilation is established and progressing, no therapy works. The products of conception will be expelled *completely* or *incompletely.*

Complete abortion occurs when all the parts of the conceptus pass out of the uterus. This may happen in the home, and the woman reports a delayed menses with much heavier flow at the next menses, or tissue is passed as large clots. The recovery period is one of normal involution, and most women do not need therapy. In cases in which an inevitable abortion has been completed at home and the products of conception not seen by the health care provider, the woman may be observed, undergo blood tests, and receive follow-up care in a clinic or private office within 2 days.

Incomplete abortion is accompanied by heavy bleeding as fragments of the conceptus are expelled. Bleeding does not stop, and most women seek medical help. The nurse should be aware that sometimes an incomplete abortion is the result of an incompetent abortion performed by a nonlicensed person. If the woman is seen by a physician or midwife, the products of conception should be examined for completeness and sent for pathologic examination. If the products are completely expelled, the woman receives oxytocin and prophylactic antibiotics and is observed for 1 day.

When the abortion is incomplete, the client is anesthetized for an obligatory D&C. Oxytocin and antibiotics are given postoperatively. Depending on the client's condition, she may then be discharged.

Missed abortion is diagnosed when the uterus fails to grow, and the signs of pregnancy begin to diminish. Although a fetal heartbeat may have been obtained at a prenatal visit, ultrasound examination will confirm the absence of fetal movement and heartbeat. Because placental function may continue for some weeks after fetal death, tests such as that for hCG may be misleading. Fibrinogen levels are checked; levels below 150 mg/dl are significant. Retention of a dead fetus is physically and psychologically harmful; thus evacuation is planned as soon as possible. After the procedure a woman is observed for clotting problems and normal signs of recovery.

Habitual abortion may be caused by genetic, structural, immunologic, or hormonal problems. The search for cause may take time. Most commonly, for many possible reasons, the cervix loses its muscular integrity and begins dilation in the second trimester.

INDUCED ABORTION

The U.S. Supreme Court in 1973 *(Roe v. Wade)* ruled that elective abortions could follow these guidelines: (1) during the first 12 weeks, the state could not bar a woman from obtaining an abortion by a licensed physician, (2) between 12 and 20 weeks the state could regulate the performance of an abortion to protect the woman's health, and (3) after 20 weeks the state could regulate and prohibit abortion except those deemed necessary to protect the woman's health or life. The state may impose safeguards for the fetus. Most state laws have "conscience clauses" that allow a physician, nurse, or other hospital personnel to refuse without fear of reprisal to assist in abortion if it conflicts with their ethical or religious principles.

Abortion is an issue of intense debate in the United States. The trends in rules and regulations are following the Supreme Court decisions of 1986, 1989, 1990, and 1991. There will be yet more challenges to *Roe v. Wade* (1973) as individual states and groups of citizens seek through legal recourse to change the way abortions are allowed or restricted. Challenges have resulted in many states passing laws that restrict the *times* (only first trimester), the *reasons* (only life/health of the mother, rape, incest, or fetal anomaly), and the *notification* or permission requirements before an abortion. Finally, the issues of who may counsel women, who may do an abortion, and who pays the bill are subjects of a bitter battle, the result of which is to limit accessibility for indigent women who would have to continue the pregnancy, whereas more affluent women will have access to services. Thus the balance between those who can and those who cannot obtain abortions remains proportionately the same as before 1973, although abortion is not now illegal in any state (Harrison and Naylor, 1991). The nurse will want to update knowledge of any change in this controversial choice, especially for individual states. (See Chapter 30 for legal issues arising from or surrounding elective abortion.)

Induced abortion may be chosen for many reasons:
1. Inability to care for or support a child
2. Desire not to be pregnant
3. Interference with current or long-range life goals
4. Rape or incest
5. Emotional problems and/or mental incompetence

Medically advised abortion may be for maternal disorders such as heart disease, cancer, sickle cell disease, neurologic disorders, or psychiatric disorders. Fetal disorders such as those discovered by amniocentesis include chromosome disorders, severe structural defects, and gene defects (see Chapter 27).

Risk

Approximately 1.6 million abortions are performed in the United States each year, a rate that has continued at almost the same level since 1981. Compared with the maternal mortality risk of 9 per 100,000 live births, the mortality rate for induced abortion is 0.5 per 100,000 (Harrison and Naylor, 1991). The proportion of second-trimester abortions has declined since 1973. Personal reasons that cause the delay until the second trimester are less amenable to public health intervention (Grimes, 1984). The development of dilation and evacuation procedure for later, safer abortions has reduced the frequency of transabdominal methods. Efforts continue to find safer abortifacients. Rulings on Ru 486 may change all these statistics in the future (see Chapter 5).

Follow-up care on the effects of repeated abortions on fertility and birth complications also is important. Hemorrhage is the most common problem after abortion, contributing to the maternal mortality rate of 0.5 per 100,000.

Asherman's syndrome. With repeated and frequent abortions, a condition known as *Asherman's syndrome* may exist. Although this syndrome may be caused by other problems such as hormonal imbalance, repeated surgery by D&C will affect the endometrium. In Asherman's syndrome the endometrium does not build up an adequate lining during the proliferative period of the cycle because of *adhesions*, usually from infections. No shedding or menstruation occurs, and occasionally the inner uterine tissue may adhere. (In some cases, an IUD may be used to separate the uterine tissue while hormones are used to build up the endometrium [Klein, 1987].)

Clinical Management

Pregnancy is confirmed by a positive pregnancy test result and a pelvic examination to estimate gestational size. If size is questioned, ultrasound may be used. A low-lying placenta and fibroids, which would affect the safety of the procedure, also may be identified by ultrasound. Laboratory tests are performed to determine Rh factor, blood type, and hemoglobin and hematocrit levels. A health history is taken to assess special needs and risks. Counseling is offered to determine knowledge of alternative options and to ensure that abortion is the woman's choice.

Methods. *Dilation and evacuation (D&E)* is the method of choice for an early termination of pregnancy of 7 to 8 weeks' gestation. The cervix must be dilated enough to allow the passage of instruments. Dilation is the most difficult part of the procedure because it must proceed slowly and may be met with considerable resistance, especially in the nullipara. (See Figure 21-15 for method.)

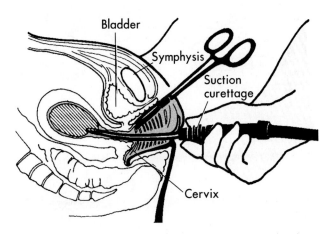

FIGURE 21-15 Technique of suction evacuation of uterus.

Dilation and curettage (D&C) may be performed toward the end of the first trimester. Instead of a suction device, a spoon-shaped instrument is used to scrape the lining out of the uterus. Dilation of the cervix is achieved as in a suction evacuation. A D&C usually is not performed after the first trimester because the uterine lining becomes thinner and could be penetrated (Figure 21-16).

Transabdominal prostaglandin F_2 (PGF_2) may be used to induce labor. An amniocentesis needle is inserted through the abdominal wall into amniotic fluid and 20 to 40 mg PGF_2 is inserted. Labor begins within 1 to 2 hours or up to 24 hours later. Labor contractions follow the usual pattern of mild to increasingly strong intensity until the fetus is delivered, usually when the cervix is 4 to 5 cm dilated. The placental tissue must be checked to see if it is intact. Side effects may be nausea and vomiting, and appropriate medication is administered.

Transabdominal instillation is performed by inserting an amniocentesis needle and withdrawing 200 ml of amniotic fluid and replacing it with 20% saline or a urea solution. Contractions begin within 8 to 12 hours and may last 48 hours before the fetus is delivered. To shorten the waiting period, oxytocin infusion may be used. Side effects may be significant, especially if saline is inadvertently drawn into the maternal circulation. For this reason, saline abortions are performed less frequently today.

The use of *prostaglandin E_2 (PGE_2)* is the most convenient method, with the fewest side effects (see Drug Profile 15-1 for use to induce labor). For an

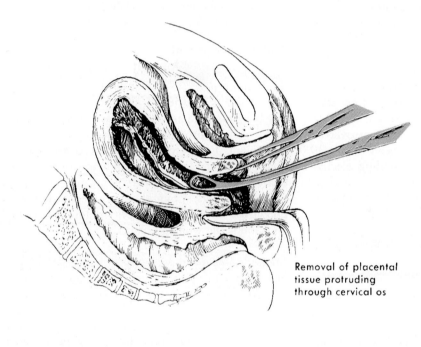

FIGURE 21-16 Use of ring forceps to remove placental tissue. (From Willson JR: *Management of obstetric difficulties*, ed 6, St Louis, 1961, Mosby.)

Removal of placental tissue protruding through cervical os

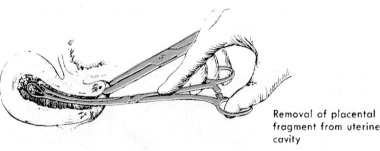

Removal of placental fragment from uterine cavity

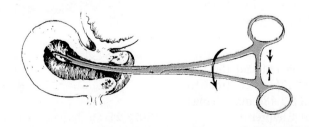

abortifacient to work, the cervix must become dilated. To speed this process, laminarin, dried seaweed that absorbs water, has been used, but recently Lamicel (hydrogenous cervical dilator) has replaced laminarin (Mueller, 1991). This rod is inserted 10 to 24 hours before induction, the substance swells three to four times its original size, and painless cervical dilation takes place. The Lamicel is removed and a 20 mg PGE$_2$ suppository is inserted into the posterior vaginal canal and repeated every 3 to 5 hours until delivery. Birth of the fetus should take place within 24 hours. Oxytocin may be used to shorten the time for a more advanced pregnancy (see Intrauterine Fetal Death).

INTRAUTERINE FETAL DEATH

After the age of viability a fetus that dies in the uterus or during the process of birth is an **intrauterine fetal death** (IUFD). *Stillbirth* is another term used to define the status of a fetus that does not breathe, exhibit a heartbeat, or show pulsation of the umbilical cord or movement of voluntary muscles at birth. Fifty percent of the perinatal mortality rate is related to IUFD. The causes are numerous. Maternal conditions that result in loss of placental functioning, including abruptio placentae, severe hypertension, or an aging placenta, lead to fetal hypoxia and acidosis. Chronic maternal conditions such as severe Rh sensitization, sickle cell disease, or diabetes mellitus may make an intrauterine environment incompatible with life. Unusual events such as trauma or uterine rupture may lead to death. Fetal conditions include genetic conditions not supportive of life, IUGR, prolapse of the cord, nuchal cord, true knot in the cord, chronic fetal distress that worsens during labor, and, finally, many unknown reasons.

Clinical Management

The only warning signs are changes in fetal movement patterns (see Chapter 11). Once fetal death has been diagnosed before labor begins, treatment involves waiting up to 2 weeks for spontaneous labor to begin. Coagulation problems such as disseminated intravascular coagulation (DIC) may develop if a dead fetus is retained longer. Laboratory evaluation of coagulation levels help to monitor early changes that lead to DIC. If labor does not occur naturally, it will be stimulated with oxytocin infusion or vaginal prostaglandin insertion. If the placenta is still functioning, progesterone inhibits oxytocin, and several attempts may be needed to deliver the fetus. Physicians are hesitant to subject the woman to surgery for a nonviable infant.

Nursing Responsibilities

Few nurses using this text will work with women seeking induced abortion in the first trimester because most are seen in specialized clinics. All nurses, however, need to examine their own positions on these issues. Often, too, a nurse's counsel is informally sought in the community. In addition, nursing organizations and individual nurses may lobby for whichever position best provides women's health (see Chapter 4).

Elective Abortion Approaches

When the woman is debating whether to have an abortion, the nurse gives her information about the procedure. If she decides to proceed with the pregnancy, she should be informed about available resources. The woman should have a supportive environment while she deals with the issues and results of her decision. Many young women in their teens have not had an opportunity to develop their own values and to differentiate themselves from other people. This may be the first time that some have had to make a decision about their own bodies.

Choice of attitudes. Nurses must develop an understanding of their own attitudes toward pregnancy termination so they can effectively approach a woman seeking abortion. The confusion resulting from ambivalent feelings or incompletely understood ideas interferes with a therapeutic approach to such clients.

Burchell (1979) has identified five possible positions on abortion and effectively discusses professional questions, attitudes, and approaches to it. He notes that legal changes do not usually affect deeply held attitudes, which he describes as follows.

1. The first position allows no indication for abortion. Carried to its extreme, an ectopic pregnancy could not be removed, nor could a client with pelvic cancer be treated until the baby was born.
2. The second position holds that no direct abortion is accepted, but if necessary, an indirect abortion secondary to a life-saving procedure may be performed. It appears that most persons against elective abortion hold this position.
3. The third position allows medical indications to govern whether an abortion is necessary. This

 Self-Discovery

Consider the five positions discussed in light of your own ethical, moral, religious convictions. For an imaginary early pregnancy in your current life situation, can you identify your position? How would you counsel another person? What considerations would you want to know about in the situation?

position promoted therapeutic abortions. The indications, however, became so vague that restrictions were almost negligible if the client could afford to obtain different medical opinions. The physician became the one who governed the choice of instituting an abortion.

4. The fourth position supports direct abortion based on the judgment of the physician and client. The reasons may be social, economic, or medical, but it is a fairly joint decision. The physician, however, may refuse to perform the procedure.

5. The fifth position allows the client to be the sole deciding agent (i.e., abortion on request, based on the woman's judgment alone). This last position has no restrictions, and although she may be counseled otherwise, the woman has the responsibility of the final decision.

Most people in the United States agree that abortion should not be used as a method of contraception. Therefore professional nurses involved in health education can help a woman to prevent future conception when pregnancy is unwelcome. Nurses who have gained a degree of empathy with a woman going through an unwanted pregnancy can begin to comprehend the aspects of her choice. Making a decision oneself is far different from making it for someone else.

Abortion in the Second Trimester

Today a woman seeking second-trimester abortion has a set of psychosocial problems with which to cope. In some cases this decision is based on a fetal anomaly established after many tests, which included a waiting period for results. For others, denial of the pregnancy or financial considerations caused the delay. In any case these women need nursing assessment, support, and guidance.

▶ ASSESSMENT

The nurse establishes communication to elicit the woman's reasons for waiting for the procedure and completes required tests and assessments, depending on the week of pregnancy and the situation. The client usually is in the labor area for this procedure (see also IFUD therapy).

▶ NURSING DIAGNOSES

The following diagnoses may apply to those with spontaneous abortions or with induced abortions.

- Ineffective individual coping or dysfunctional grieving related to unresolved feelings about loss of pregnancy or choosing elective abortion
- Spiritual distress related to conflicts in choices or reasons for loss

- Knowledge deficit related to methods, outcomes, or use of family planning in recovery period
- High risk for infection, depending on procedure
- Potential for injury related to Rh-negativity and isoimmunization possibility

▶ EXPECTED OUTCOMES

- Verbalizes to at least one person her feelings about pregnancy termination
- Seeks spiritual help as needed
- Describes what method of preventing pregnancy she will use during recovery
- Methods prevent injury from infection or hemorrhage
- Experiences grieving that is not dysfunctional

▶ NURSING INTERVENTIONS

Recovery Care for Early Abortion

After an elective abortion the woman is taught to look for symptoms of infection such as a change in vaginal discharge, uterine cramping, nausea, vomiting, or chills. She should call the clinic or physician if these signs occur. An oxytocic agent and an antibiotic will be prescribed. After a gestation of 59 days, all Rh-negative, Coombs' negative women will receive gamma globulin to prevent isoimmunization. The nurse explores with the woman the reasons she became pregnant, counsels and teaches her about contraceptive methods that may be more acceptable to her, and, finally, acknowledges the client's statements about the pregnancy in relation to her religious beliefs. She may wish to have the conceptus baptized, for instance. It may be important for her to talk with a chaplain or clergyperson.

The prevailing mood for a woman who has chosen to terminate an early pregnancy is relief. A period of grieving may still follow, and the nurse can prepare the woman for such an event. The importance of good counseling cannot be overemphasized. It is critical to prevent long-term adverse effects of the abortion process. The goal is to prevent *recidivism,* or repeated elective abortions (Mueller, 1991).

Second-Trimester Care

Care at the bedside involves monitoring and treating the side effects of PGE_2 administration, which are nausea, vomiting, and diarrhea. Scopolamine, promethazine (Phenergan), diphenoxylate (Lomotil), and acetaminophen (Tylenol) may be used. For more severe pain of contractions, maternal comfort can be achieved with adequate doses of morphine or meperidine (Demerol) because fetal depression need not be considered. In some cases of IUFD an epidural anesthetic is offered.

The woman must go through the process of labor, although often with a shortened second stage because of the size of the fetus. (See also support techniques of labor care.) Especially in cases of IUFD or an anomalous fetus, the behavior of the health care team during labor and birth and during recovery sets the tone and model for a woman's grieving. Avoidance, lack of empathy, and inability to initiate discussions retard a woman's grief work (see Chapter 29). Therefore it is the nurse's responsibility to initiate discussion and to show empathy but not to give false reassurance. Time to explore the woman's feelings and responses is required. For instance, autopsy may be desired and useful to gain information about causes. The physician introduces the topic of autopsy with the rationale that at least the woman and her family will know there was no evident contributing cause. It may be helpful in the grieving process to know there are no known avoidable reasons for death. The woman should be encouraged to express her feelings and fears to reduce anxiety about the autopsy. The nurse may suggest clergy support and baptism, depending on the woman's beliefs.

Recovery follows a usual pattern, with lochia and lactation. To suppress lactation, bromocriptine may be given (see Drug Profile 17-1). The standard postpartum recovery instructions are given. It should be emphasized to a family member that if the woman has had previous unresolved losses and shows symptoms of extended denial or anger or delayed grieving, she may need to be referred to a counselor.

Test Yourself

- Describe interventions for threatened abortion.
- Compare and contrast the use of PGE$_2$ for induction and second-trimester abortion in terms of dosage, timing, and precautions.

▶ **EVALUATION**

Depending on the reason for pregnancy loss, its conclusion may bring great relief or great sadness. The nurse refers to data and expected outcomes while asking evaluative questions such as the following:

- Was there a supportive milieu for her?
- Is there support for her in the home situation?
- Does she talk of managing care in the recovery period? Is she aware of family planning method to use?
- Was pregnancy terminated without infection or hemorrhage?
- Does she know self-care for involution?
- Has she received Rh D immunoglobulin, if indicated?

Hemorrhage in Obstetrics

During pregnancy the blood supply to the uterus increases enormously to provide for placental circulation. The myometrium is supplied mainly from the uterine and ovarian arteries, and as these arteries enter the uterine muscle, they coil and loop to allow for the stretching of the growing uterus (Figure 21-17). Their pathways into the myometrium at every level of the uterus from cervix to fundus allow the uterine muscle to act as an elastic web to control blood flow by constricting vessels that pass through it as the uterus contracts and by allowing normal flow as the uterus relaxes. For hemostasis the myometrium must function to close off blood vessels.

This unusual action of the uterus does not provide hemostasis in cases such as low implantation or ectopic pregnancy in which the placental blood supply is not under the control of uterine contraction.

When the placenta is correctly implanted in the body of the uterus, bleeding may occur because of separation of part of the placenta. Until delivery and uterine contraction, hemorrhage may be rapid. Remember that 500 ml/min circulate through the placenta in the last part of pregnancy. Without hemostasis, this amount can be lost from the placenta during each minute. Uncontrolled, the result is hypovolemic shock.

Hemorrhage is rapid loss of blood of more than 1% of body weight, or 10% of blood volume. This is calculated as follows: 1 ml of blood is equivalent to 1 g of body weight. In a woman weighing 50 kg (110 pounds) or 50,000 g, 1% of body weight is 500 g or 500 ml. Blood loss of more than 500 ml can cause inadequate tissue perfusion, deprivation of glucose and oxygen in tissue, and build-up of waste products. Most healthy persons tolerate loss of 500 ml with replacement of oral fluids (e.g., when donating a pint of blood).

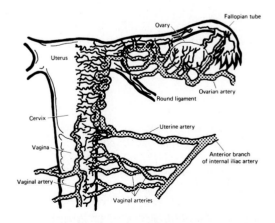

FIGURE 21-17 Blood supply to uterus. Note how vessels enter at every level.

Hypovolemic shock begins if bleeding progresses to 1.5 to 2 L. Fortunately, normal pregnant women are protected against **hypovolemia** by the excess plasma and red blood cells already present by 14 weeks. With the exception of very small women and those who bleed steadily during the antepartum period or those with severe preeclampsia with its reduced blood volume, signs of hypovolemia do not become clearly evident until 30% to 35% of volume is lost. By then, tachycardia and recognizable signs may be present, but the shock is *more advanced* than it would appear (Foster, 1984). Body responses are initiated to maintain tissue perfusion; intricate processes for hemostasis and reflex vasoconstriction begin.

General treatment follows these guidelines:
1. Replacement of fluid to restore adequate blood volume
2. Repair or removal of causes of bleeding
3. Support of body systems during treatment

A summary of medical and nursing assessment and support is outlined in Table 21-4. Hemorrhage affects 7% to 8% of pregnancies. Of these 1% are related to placental location, 1.5% to placental separation, and the rest to all other causes during birth and recovery. Today with careful monitoring, morbidity and mortality may be reduced to a very low rate (Hyashi and Castillo, 1986; see also Chapter 23).

TABLE 21-4 Hypovolemic Shock

PHYSIOLOGIC CHANGES	CLIENT SYMPTOMS	INTERVENTIONS
CARDIAC AND CIRCULATORY STATUS		
Decreased venous pressure, cardiac output, pulse pressure, arterial pressure	Client feels weak, anxious, dizzy and may feel rapid heartbeat.	Record vital signs; if necessary, take apical pulse. Support blood volume with plasma expanders, whole blood, Ringer's lactate solution. Military antishock trousers (MAST) may be used.
Peripheral vasoconstriction: to protect vital organs, adrenal medulla is stimulated to produce catecholamines, adding to vasoconstriction	Client feels cold; peripheral tissues are pale. Nails blanch slowly; client feels restless, anxious, fearful.	Keep client warm; check skin color, turgor, mucous membrane moisture, temperature. Reassure client. Record expressed statements, observations.
RESPIRATORY STATUS		
Tachypnea Respiratory center stimulated by hypoxia	Client complains of "air hunger," shortness of breath.	Note rate, rhythm, depth of respirations. Administer oxygen by mask. Place client in side-lying position or in left-lateral tilt with legs at 45-degree angle to hips.
GASTROINTESTINAL STATUS		
Fluid shift from interstitial tissues and intestinal tract to vascular compartment (takes several hours)	Sensation of thirst increases.	Drop in Hct observed after shift. Draw blood for serial hemoglobin and Hct determinations. Allow nothing by mouth if returning to operating room or delivery room for correction of bleeding.
Decreased parasympathetic activity plus reduced gastrointestinal motility, secretions	Nausea may occur.	Nasogastric tube may be inserted.
RENAL STATUS		
Conservation of fluids and salts stimulated by vasoconstriction of renal arterioles (needs 70 mm Hg pressure to effectively filtrate blood)	Client may have no sensation of need to void.	Observe closely for oliguria (lower limit of normal 30 ml/hr). Record hourly output and specific gravity from Foley catheter.

PLACENTA PREVIA

Placenta previa occurs when the placenta is attached in the lower uterine segment rather than in the body of the uterus. Because a thinner decidual layer is located here, the placenta develops over a larger surface and may cover the internal os *completely, partially,* or *marginally* or may be *low-lying*. The types of previa are categorized by the amount of placental tissue over the os (Figure 21-18).

Toward the last part of pregnancy the cervix slowly effaces. With this movement, it *pulls away* from the poorly situated placenta and bleeding begins. The earlier the bleeding begins, the more serious the type of previa. The cause may be unknown, but predisposing factors include uterine scarring from prior surgery such as uterine curettage or cesarean delivery, multiple gestation with a large placental site, infection with endometritis, and a previous episode of low implantation. Women with problems of infertility and older multiparas account for many of the cases (Rose and Chapman, 1988).

Risk

Lower uterine attachment occurs in 0.5% (1 in 200) of pregnancies and is a significant cause of perinatal mortality. Because blood is lost over an extended period, the fetus may be affected by maternal anemia and intrauterine hypoxia. Prematurity is a problem because early delivery may be necessary if bleeding becomes excessive. Because of effective treatment in the last decade, maternal mortality is very low.

Signs

There may have been spotting in the first trimester. The classic sign by 28 weeks, however, is intermittent, painless vaginal bleeding. Bright red bleeding may begin slowly as spotting or may come in intermittent gushes. Continuous bleeding is less common. Bleeding is not related to activity level, and the uterus is relaxed and nontender. Placental location prevents movement of the fetus into the pelvic canal, and its position may be transverse, oblique, or breech.

Clinical Management

The clinical problem is confirmed by ultrasound to view placental position. If ultrasound examination is performed too early, the results may be misleading because the lower uterine segment develops further in the last part of pregnancy. Thus the placenta may appear to "move up on the wall" (Hyashi and Castillo, 1986). If bleeding is significant, the woman must be hospitalized and placed on a regimen of complete bed rest. Laboratory tests are ordered every 12 hours for hemoglobin and hematocrit levels. Blood will be typed and matched; two units will be kept on call. If Rh negative, the woman will be given gamma globulin to prevent sensitization. Fetal heart rate and activity will be monitored at regular intervals.

The amount of bleeding and the woman's response will be weighed against the age of the fetus. When the risk to either seems greater than the risk associated with birth, the baby will be delivered. The result of this waiting and watching is increased anxiety.

There is a chance of dislodging more of the placenta if a vigorous pelvic examination is performed. Therefore, after the first speculum examination, no vaginal examinations are done. If the cervix is even partially dilated, the placental tissue may be visualized at the cervical os. Ultrasonography has allowed precise diagnosis.

After diagnosis is made of the degree of placental growth over the os, fetal age is determined. A recommendation for continuing the pregnancy and for the type of birth is made (Table 21-5).

Bleeding may not begin until the time of labor with grades 1 (low-lying) and 2 (marginal), and the cause may be confused with premature separation of the

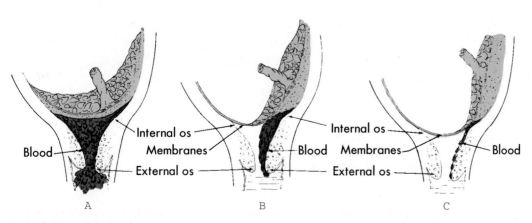

FIGURE 21-18 Types of placenta previa. **A,** Total, or complete, placenta previa. **B,** Partial placenta previa. **C,** Low implantation. (From Bobak IM: *Maternity and gynecologic care: the nurse and the family,* ed 5, 1993, Mosby.)

TABLE 21-5 Management Strategies for Placenta Previa

GRADES 1 AND 2*	GRADES 3 AND 4†
AMOUNT OF BLEEDING	
Later bleeding in gestation	Early bleeding, often by 28 to 30 weeks
MANAGEMENT	
Bed rest with bathroom privileges at home	Complete bed rest in hospital
Frequent monitoring of fetal heart rate and movements	NST and amniocentesis
	Maintenance of pregnancy to 35 weeks and deliver by 35 weeks of age
Vaginal birth possible	Cesarean delivery always

*Low-lying and marginal.
†Partial and complete.

placenta. Vaginal delivery may be possible if the head is well down in the birth canal; the head may act as a pressure tourniquet in this case. If the placenta *partially* (grade 3) or *completely* (grade 4) covers the os, bleeding begins earlier and a cesarean delivery always will be required. Eighty percent of women with placenta previa require operative delivery. Surgery must be performed with care, especially if the placenta is lying over the anterior part of the lower uterine wall, because it is possible to cut blood vessels and cause more bleeding.

After delivery the placenta must be examined carefully. Fragments may adhere to the placental site, leading to infection. Hemorrhage may occur because the lower uterine segment does not have the same muscle strength in contraction to shut off the bleeding.

PREMATURE PLACENTAL SEPARATION

Premature separation of the normally implanted placenta is known as **abruptio placentae.** Separation occurs in many degrees (Box 21-4) and occurs after 20 to 24 weeks, often at labor. Severity is classified by grades 0 to 3, or as mild, moderate, or severe, depending on the location and amount of bleeding (Figure 21-19). Separation may be (1) partial, with separation occurring in the center of the placenta so that no bleeding is observable, (2) marginal, at the edge of the placenta, with bleeding seen at the vagina, or (3) complete, with bleeding trapped in the uterus or visible at the vagina. Differentiating types of placental separation is difficult, and it often may be confused with placenta previa. Differences between the conditions are listed in Table 21-6. The cause varies, but any condition that contributes to vascular changes at the placental level contributes to separation. In some cases the vessels may necrose, and infarcts (dead tissue) occur, which may split

BOX 21-4 Degrees of Abruptio Placentae

Mild
Grade 0
No external bleeding or less than 250 ml
Placenta showing infarcted areas of less than one sixth of placenta

Moderate
Grade 1
Retroplacental or vaginal bleeding of less than 1000 ml, separation of less than one half of placenta, cramping and mild abdominal aching to more severe pain, fetal heart tone present but may show irregularities

Severe
Grade 2
Up to two thirds of placenta separated; uterus du bois (woodlike), uterine tenderness, rigidity, severe pain, Couvelaire uterus: bruising of uterine muscle; fetal heart tones usually absent or showing severe distress

Grade 3
Entire separation; maternal shock, fetal death; severe pain; disseminated intravascular coagulation DIC

from the decidua. If the infarct is thought of as a stroke in the placental vessels, it is easier to relate the possible precursors; hypertension is present in 50% of the cases, and multiparas older than 35 years are more commonly affected (Beischer and MacKay, 1993). In addition, severe diabetes and renal disease with vascular changes are associated with separation. Chronic smoking also

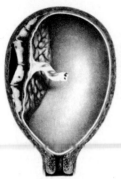 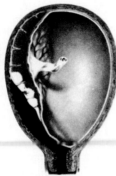 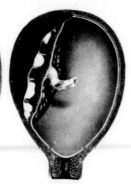

Partial separation (concealed hemorrhage) Partial separation (apparent hemorrhage) Complete separation (concealed hemorrhage)

FIGURE 21-19 Abruptio placentae. Premature separation of normally implanted placenta. (Courtesy Ross Laboratories, Columbus, Ohio.)

TABLE 21-6 Comparison of Placenta Previa and Abruptio Placentae

PLACENTA PREVIA	ABRUPTIO PLACENTAE
No underlying chronic disease	Associated with hypertension, diabetes, and kidney diseases
Warning signs of spotting hemorrhage always externally visible	Usually no warning signs
No pain	Hemorrhage may be internal or externally visible
Occurs rarely during labor but is unrelated to labor	Pain may be present in varying degrees
Fetal heart tones and movement usually present and unaffected	Usually occurs in labor
	Fetal heart tones reflecting uteroplacental insufficiency
Placenta in lower uterine segment	Placental attachment in normal locations
Soft uterus	Uterus tender to woodlike

contributes to vascular changes. Mechanical factors may be responsible in some cases, including trauma from automobile accidents (see Chapter 23). Sudden release of a large amount of amniotic fluid or rapid descent of an infant with an unusually short cord pulling part of the placenta away may contribute. In many clients, however, there is no clear cause (Box 21-5).

Risk

Between 0.5% and 1.5% of all pregnancies have premature separation of some grade; most are minor. However, separation accounts for more than 15% of perinatal deaths. If separation begins at home and if there is a delay in obtaining assistance, maternal mortality is about 6% when complete separation occurs. The rate has increased significantly between 1974 and 1987 (Saftlas, 1991). Much of the increase is attributed to crack and cocaine use. Although perinatal mortality has decreased, the rate still is 20% to 40%.

Signs

Signs of separation often occur as labor begins (Box 21-6). If the woman is at home, the first sign may be

BOX 21-5 Factors Underlying Abruptio Placentae

Chronic hypertension/preeclampsia
Sudden uterine decompression (trauma, accidents)
Malnutrition
Smoking
Cocaine and crack use
Vena caval compression, short cord
Fibroids
Premature rupture of membranes
Severe diabetes/renal disease
Multiple gestation

vaginal bleeding. Fetal movements may become hyperactive and then cease. If membranes break, meconium staining may be observed. Pain may occur; persistent escalating pain indicates concealed bleeding with an enlarging clot.

When blood loss is significant, signs of shock will be present. If the woman is in labor in a hospital setting, the monitor strip will show uteroplacental insufficiency

---

BOX 21-6   **Early Signs of Abruption**

- Vaginal bleeding
- Uterine tenderness or severe pain
- Back pain
- Fetal distress—late decelerations decreased variability
- Change in contractions:
  —Rising baseline tonus
  —Hypertonic, frequent

(UPI), with baseline changes and reduced variability. Tonus will rise, and contraction patterns will change. In addition, if bleeding is concealed, erratic hypertonic contractions, uterine tension, and severe pain will be present. There may be bruising of the uterine muscles (Couvelaire uterus), with poor hemostasis after birth. Fetal condition deteriorates rapidly, and emergency surgical intervention is instituted.

Laboratory tests show a decrease in complete blood cell count values, and coagulation factors may change. In case of severe abruptio placentae, 10% to 30% develop DIC (see Chapter 23).

Clinical Management

Treatment is determined by the amount of separation and blood loss compared with fetal age and status. For grade 0 (mild) with concealed or overt blood loss of less than 250 ml, conservative treatment of bed rest, sedatives, and close observation is continued until the fetus is 37 weeks of age. In cases of moderate blood loss, when 250 to 1000 ml have been lost but less than one half of the placenta is affected, cesarean delivery will be performed after stabilization of maternal and fetal perfusion. Severe cases that affect more than one half the placenta often result in fetal death in utero. The woman has a rigid abdomen and pain, and her condition is serious. If she is in shock, her condition must be stabilized enough to undergo anesthesia. This condition may cause an intermingling of maternal and fetal blood; therefore Rh-negative women receive RhD immunoglobulin.

UTERINE RUPTURE

Rupture is uncommon but usually related to separation of a prior uterine scar. Sudden and unexpected, it is a major concern with vaginal birth after cesarean (VBAC). When the placenta invades the endometrium where the scar is located, it is more likely to invade into the myometrium (**placenta accreta**) or be associated with rupture.

Risk

Uterine rupture results in serious maternal morbidity and mortality. Depending on where it occurs—at home or in the delivery unit—the blood loss will be significant, usually concealed, and into the peritoneum. Depending on placement of the placenta, the perinatal mortality ranges from 8% to 56%, depending on geographic location (Phelan, 1991). *Hysterectomy*, removal of the uterus, or repair of the rupture must be chosen. If repair is possible, the woman is not allowed to labor in a subsequent pregnancy but is scheduled for cesarean birth when fetal lungs show maturity, about week 36.

Signs

Signs of uterine rupture include a change in station of the presenting part during labor, with the fetal body rising up in the abdomen, or a change in contour of the abdomen. Abnormal fetal tracings signal distress. About 18% of women have pain that may be confused with abruptio placentae. With upper or miduterine rupture, there may be tearing pain, collapse, and shock. The fetus usually dies.

Ultrasound evaluation may quickly establish the presence of blood in the peritoneum and a shift in fetal position. Maternal signs of hypovolemia rapidly progress, and emergency cesarean must be carried out as soon as possible.

With rupture of the lower uterine segment, which is less vascular, signs may be less dramatic. Fetal distress, with aching or pain in the lower abdomen, will be evident. Labor contractions change or cease at the same time. In these less dramatic cases, the tear in the lower uterine wall may be seen only after birth, when exploration of the cause of bleeding occurs.

Hemorrhage Related to Birth Method

Common factors that raise the risk for hemorrhage include a history of previous hemorrhage, often for unknown reasons, such as the higher risk for Asian and Hispanic women. Underlying medical problems related to hypertension/preeclampsia, reduced platelets (see

 Clinical Decision

Sally B. comes to the unit with moderate vaginal bleeding at 36 weeks' gestation. Immediate physical assessment includes fetal heart tones and activity, visualization of type and volume of blood on pad or at vagina, and which other actions?

Chapter 22), anemias, and infection place the woman at risk. Bleeding happens more often with a nullipara than a multipara unless she has had four or more births, a *grand multipara*. Finally, any woman with a long labor and a prolonged second stage is at risk for bleeding. Fatigue of the muscle from these causes, as well as overstretching of the uterine muscles related to multiple pregnancy, increases risk (Table 21-7).

RISKS WITH VAGINAL BIRTH

Vaginal birth adds risks related to forceps or vacuum extraction, prolonged third stage, mediolateral or midline episiotomy, and lacerations of the birth canal. Bleeding averages 500 ml at birth, including the first few hours of recovery (Combs, Murphy, and Laros, 1990).

RISKS WITH CESAREAN BIRTH

The main cause is general anesthesia, which quickly exerts a vasodilating effect. Bleeding with cesarean birth averages 900 to 1100 ml and may total much more as risk factors are added. A classic surgical incision adds to blood loss as well. Any woman having an emergency section is at high risk because of factors leading to surgery—preeclampsia, uterine dystocia, second-stage arrest, and amnionitis. Therefore staff members must always be prepared for additional blood loss. Lowe (1991) estimates that 7% to 8% of women will exceed the average blood loss for vaginal and cesarean birth.

Hemorrhage After Birth

There may be hemorrhage as a result of uterine atony, trauma, or subinvolution with infection. Hemorrhage is described as *early or primary* in the first 24 hours or as *late* or *secondary* if heavy bleeding with clot formation occurs after 24 hours and up to 2 weeks. Causes may be factors that inhibit uterine contractions, trauma, or infection and subinvolution.

The placental site is a raw wound with numerous blood vessels that spill blood if ineffective uterine contractions are evident. If the uterus stays firmly contracted, its condition is good and blood loss follows the normal pattern. If reduced tone begins again after initial contraction, the newly formed clots on the surface of the placental site will be loosened, and fresh bleeding will begin.

UTERINE ATONY

Uterine atony is the most frequent cause of early bleeding. Reasons for poor contractility of the muscle are numerous (Box 21-7). Common reasons are a long, exhausting labor or uterine inertia with excessive oxytocin stimulation. Foremost is the effect of a distended bladder on the uterus. The bladder and the anterior lower portion of the uterus are attached by fascia. When the bladder becomes distended, the uterus must be pulled up with it and thus is unable to maintain contraction. With the fundal check, the uterus is found to be soft and located to the right side, at or above the

---

TABLE 21-7 Risk Factors for Hemorrhage

VAGINAL BIRTH	CESAREAN BIRTH
CAUSES IN DESCENDING ORDER OF OCCURRENCE*	
• Prolonged third stage Placenta accreta in some degree, manual extraction of placenta, which reflects **uterine atony**	General anesthesia Amnionitis
• Preeclampsia: low platelets and blood volume, and effects of magnesium sulfate	Preeclampsia
• Mediolateral episiotomy	
• Previous postpartum hemorrhage	Protracted active labor
• Twins or more than two fetuses	Prolonged second stage
• Prolonged second stage	
• Soft tissue lacerations	
• Oxytocin-augmented labor	
• Asian or Hispanic ethnicity	Being Asian or Hispanic
• Forceps/vacuum extraction	Classic uterine incision
• Midline episiotomy	
• Nulliparity (not multiparity unless >4)	

Data from Combs CA, Murphy EL, Laros RK Jr: Factors associated with hemorrhage, *Obstet Gynecol Surv* 46:362, 1991.
*For women who bled during labor or birth and whose hematocrit dropped 10 points or more from admission or who received a transfusion.

BOX 21-7   Risk Factors for Uterine Atony

- Multiparity
- Overdistended uterus, twins, polyhydramnios
- Placenta previa or abruptio placentae
- Fibroids causing asymmetric contraction
- Long, exhausting labor
- Prolonged second stage
- Oxytocin stimulation during labor
- General fatigue, anemia, and preeclampsia
- Distension of bladder
- Too vigorous massage of fundus

umbilicus. Signs may not be evident until fundal pressure is applied and clots are expressed.

A rare cause of bleeding is *placenta accreta,* an anomaly in which the placental trophoblastic tissue entered the myometrium when the placenta was formed. When placental separation after the birth is expected, parts adhere to the wall and prevent uterine contracture. This may be an emergency, and in some cases requires a hysterectomy to save the life of the woman.

LACERATIONS

Lacerations of the birth canal may occur with large infants, when breech or other dystocias are present or when forceps are used. The vagina and cervix are inspected after the birth to detect tears that need to be sutured. *Continuous bright red bleeding with a contracted uterus* indicates a laceration in the birth passage. The laceration may be in the lower uterine segment, and bleeding then is retroperitoneal and unobserved until signs of hypovolemia begin. Periurethral lacerations may accompany the birth of a large infant. Perineal lacerations are evident to the physician or midwife and may occur especially with precipitous or uncontrolled final moments of the descent phase of birth. See Box 15-4 for the description of each type of laceration.

HEMATOMA

A hematoma is a collection of blood within tissue. During birth certain vessels may be torn, with bleeding into tissues of the upper part of the vagina, around the perineum, or into the labia. Blood loss usually is underestimated and hidden. Pain often out of proportion to the size of the hematoma occurs. In most cases the hematoma is visible as a swelling within the vagina, at the labia, or in the rectal area. The pain may be severe and felt in the entire perirectal area. The woman may

have fever, chills, and thigh pain, and on occasion, if left undiscovered, leg edema. Treatment is to excise and evacuate the hematoma. Sometimes a pressure gauze pack is inserted for 12 hours. Then the incision is sutured and antibiotics are given. An ice compress applied intermittently is an important early treatment of a perineal hematoma.

SUBINVOLUTION

Hemorrhage may occur later as a result of poor involution of the uterus related to infection, or retained placental fragments or membranes. The woman should be given instructions regarding the expected changes in lochia. When bright red bleeding or clotting begins again, she should contact the physician at once because the amount may vary from a normal menstrual flow to volumes that precipitate shock.

Clinical Management

Treatment of inadequate uterine contraction is to strengthen muscle tone with oxytocic agents (see Chapter 15). Oxytocin, 10 U, may be given in a slow, diluted IV bolus in addition to IV fluids containing 20 U. Remember that oxytocin is an antidiuretic and delays diuresis if more than the usual dosage is administered. PGF_2 has been used as a direct injection into uterine muscle. If oxytocics do not cause muscle contraction, bimanual compression of the uterus may be instituted. Wearing a sterile glove, the physician compresses the cervix with the right fist while grasping the fundus and exerting downward pressure. This pressure should be released for 1 minute in every 5.

The *bladder* is the first area that must be checked if bleeding develops in the recovery area. There is a standing order for straight catheterization to keep the bladder empty.

Severe bleeding from rupture, lower uterine lacerations, and cervical or perineal lacerations must be repaired on the delivery table.

Management of Hemorrhage

The management of hemorrhage in obstetrics is a complex subject, and a summary of steps that are taken in collaborative care among physician, nurse, and anesthesiologist follows (Lowe, 1990; Zahn & Yeomans, 1991).

1. *Estimate the actual blood loss,* relate it to the prehemorrhage blood volume, and make a comparison. (Remember that small women and those with severe preeclampsia have lower than average volumes). Guessing by observing the blood is not accurate, as indicated by the saying, "One half of what the doctor estimates. . . ." When blood is on the floor or in the pads or

sheets, the only *accurate* way is to weigh pads, sheets, or sponges or to measure collected blood or clots. (A saturated perineal pad contains about 30 to 40 ml). In the emergency situation, no one can stop to do this, but later it may be useful.

2. *Find the source of the bleeding and correct the cause.* This complex and possibly time-consuming task is the physician's primary responsibility. The anesthesiologist and nurse assist in supporting the woman while this process proceeds. Laboratory determinations are required for clotting time, platelet counts, prothrombin time (PT), partial thromboplastin time (PTT), and thrombin time, which are important to direct the blood replacement and to detect DIC, which can lead to massive hemorrhage (see Chapter 23).

3. *Support blood volume and body functions until hemorrhage ceases and functions normalize.* Remember that the pregnant woman is protected by the 40% to 50% volume increase that occurred early in pregnancy. Therefore, before signs of hypovolemic shock occur, she must have lost at least 30% of her blood volume. Remember also that vital signs do not change at first because of the compensatory mechanisms of vasoconstriction and fluid shift to the central circulation. Often the only initial signs in the woman are pallor, cold wet skin, and oliguria, all related to vasoconstriction. There may be expressions of anxiety, restlessness, and "air hunger"—feeling short of breath. Fetal tachycardia may occur or late decelerations may be observed on the strip chart. Whether or not overt blood is observed, these early warnings of hypovolemia should always be assessed.

It is important to correct hypovolemia, if possible, before the signs of shock appear. This potential risk underlies the sometimes large amounts of IV fluids administered during a cesarean operation. Protecting the blood pressure will allow oxygen pressures to remain high enough for maternal and fetal tissues. If hypovolemia progresses to the second stage of blood loss, after about 30% to 35% of the volume is lost, preload will fall, cardiac output falls, pulse rises, and blood pressure (reflecting afterload) will drop, sometimes dramatically. Tissues become hypoxic. Uncorrected this leads to metabolic acidosis with damage to tissues, platelet consumption, and vasodilation reversing the protective vasoconstriction. Blood may pool in the peripheral circulation, causing further hypoxemia.

VOLUME EXPANSION

Blood volume is supported in several ways:

1. *Crystalloids* useful in expanding volume are normal saline (0.9%) and lactated Ringer's solution. The ratio is two to three times the estimated blood loss. Too great a volume of these fluids without albumin will

Clinical Decision

The client in labor says that she does not feel well. She is chilly, feels breathless, and is pale. You see no vaginal bleeding. List the assessment steps and early interventions you can do while notifying the physician.

lower the colloid osmotic pressure (COP) that regulates movement of fluid across body membranes. A lowered COP contributes to accumulation of interstitial fluid and pulmonary edema. Units of *albumin,* either 5% or 25%, may be given in these cases. (After cesarean birth significant edema sometimes may be noted, especially in the lower extremities, when all else appears normal. The nurse can check the volume of fluids received in the operative period as part of the assessment of this situation).

2. *Packed red blood cells (PRBC)* may be given to increase oxygen delivery. Later the hematocrit level will be checked; women do best if it is maintained above 28% (Lowe, 1990).

3. If bleeding continues and the clotting system appears to be affected, *platelets* are given to maintain counts above 80,000 /mm^3. *Cryoprecipitate* contains clotting factors and fibrinogen, and *fresh frozen plasma* contains clotting factors and albumin.

Unless the hematocrit level falls drastically, whole blood is avoided because of the slight risk of serum-induced viral infections. (See Box 21-8 for alternate choice of autologous transfusion.)

IV access must be maintained with a large-bore catheter (16 to 17 gauge). A second IV line will be started, and occasionally a *blood pump* attachment will be used to push in the fluids at a faster rate. Remember, if bleeding is arterial or from many sites around the placenta, the blood loss may be very rapid. (During pregnancy, 500 to 600 ml of blood circulates through the placenta per minute.)

After the first emergency stage of intervention is over and the client stabilized, a Foley catheter, if not already

BOX 21-8 Autologous Transfusion

The second trimester is an appropriate time for the woman who anticipates operative delivery to donate her own blood, which can be stored and used if needed. Blood volume is quickly replaced in this period. Such an arrangement eliminates the small risk accompanying blood transfusions (Kruskall, Leonard, and Klapholz, 1987).

in place, will be inserted and output evaluated by means of a bag with hourly volume markings. Infusions should maintain an output of 30 to 50 ml/hr and a hematocrit level of more than 30% (Zahn and Yeomans, 1991). If volume is difficult to correct, a central venous line may be placed using the neck (external jugular) or antecubital fossa (brachial) route, because fluid overload and pulmonary edema are significant possibilities. Central access must be carefully considered when there is a clotting deficiency inasmuch as localized bleeding can be dangerous.

Oxygen by mask or nasal cannula should be started at the first indication and the woman kept warm. Often overrapid infusion of room temperature IV fluid causes extreme chilling and a fall in core temperature. A *blood warmer* attachment may be used to avoid this problem.

Reversing blood loss during birth takes a coordinated team effort and is an obstetric emergency. Today, with the current technology and a competent team the woman almost always will survive the ordeal and recover well.

Nursing Responsibilities

The potential for antepartal bleeding must be considered in all care. Placental perfusion may diminish and fetal distress occur, so monitoring of the fetus always accompanies a risk of bleeding. Placenta previa may seem to subside, but at any time may recur with painless, silent bleeding. Women with risk factors for hemorrhage need closer monitoring of vital signs and intake and output. Documentation is critical since events may transpire so quickly.

▶ ASSESSMENT

The nurse ascertains risk factors in the woman's history, compares current vital signs and laboratory reports with the last prenatal visit, and assesses for signs and symptoms of blood loss. The highest priority for care in placenta previa stems from the potential for bleeding. On admission, if there is heavy bleeding, status is monitored frequently with assessment of amount on pads by visual comparison with a standard chart or by weighing the pads. Vital signs are monitored every hour with bleeding and every 4 hours when it subsides. Clients with a diagnosis of placenta previa that is more severe than grade 2 may not leave the hospital. Exceptions may be made if the woman lives nearby and has home help, easy transportation, and understands her self-care regimen completely. Bleeding related to abruption or rupture is a crisis, and assessment is a collaborative event in the labor area.

▶ NURSING DIAGNOSES

Nursing diagnoses that apply to the type and time of occurrence of bleeding in pregnancy are selected:

1. High risk for fluid volume deficit: active, related to loss of body fluid
2. Altered maternal or fetal tissue perfusion related to maternal anemia or hypovolemia
3. High risk for infection related to anemia, surgical procedures, and blood loss
4. Pain related to uterine rupture, placental abruption, surgical or traumatic events
5. Severe anxiety and fear for self and infant
6. High risk for altered parenting; delayed attachment with a potentially ill, preterm infant
7. Knowledge deficit related to multiple rapid tests and interventions

▶ EXPECTED OUTCOMES

Some outcomes that may be selected for clients with placenta previa, abruption, and birth-related bleeding are as follows:

1. Improvement or maintenance of blood volume and tissue perfusion, as evidenced by hematocrit level and normal fetal heart rate, maternal vital signs, and urine output
2. Management of pain, with relief
3. Expresses feelings about self and fetal risk; seeks support
4. States understanding of purpose of interventions and treatments
5. Speaks of fetus/newborn with hope and plans

▶ NURSING INTERVENTIONS

For *placenta previa*, the regimen is prolonged bed rest of 5 to 10 weeks. Even though bleeding is not aggravated by activity, bed rest appears to lessen the potential for it. However, all the body changes that accompany bed rest, including reduced muscle tone, constipation, fatigue, and calcium loss, become a problem. Therefore the woman must work toward maintaining normal body functions.

Fluid and food intake are encouraged. Because iron tablets are constipating, iron-bearing foods and roughage are included. No enemas are to be given. The woman is advised to change positions; sitting up in a chair may be as restful as lying in bed. The activity of walking to the bathroom is decided with the physician, depending on the grade of previa. To prevent calcium loss, the woman stands to bear weight several times a day. Isometric exercises and simple upper body and lower leg exercises must be done several times daily to retain muscle mass.

For an active person who feels well, bed rest is very distressing. She needs a full understanding of the care plan to gain her compliance. The plan should be clear so that those involved in her care do not insist on different regimens. A primary nurse should follow the woman's progress and initiate discussion about coping and family needs. The nurse refers the woman to social service and discusses plans with the family early in the hospitalization. An extended stay is very costly before birth and later for the premature infant. Because most families do not have adequate financial coverage, anxiety about financial matters will be a real factor.

The nurse ensures that the woman has a relationship with several staff members so she does not feel isolated; works to provide diversion, including books, handwork, and TV; and checks often on her mental state. Depression often occurs during prolonged bed rest.

After birth, the nurse carefully observes for hemorrhage from the larger placental site where muscles do not constrict as completely as in the fundus.

Mild placental separation is treated like placenta previa; there is bed rest and watchful waiting. Depending on the degree of separation, fetal age and well-being, and the woman's status, she may be sent home or kept under observation.

Conservative treatment of moderate separation includes watchful monitoring, analgesics, and evaluation of the degree of abruption by ultrasound examination. If the baby is mature enough, cesarean delivery is planned.

Severe separation is always an emergency; the client goes to surgery from the emergency or labor room. Until the placenta is removed, there is no hemostasis.

Remember the general high-risk diagnoses even during an emergency. The plan of treatment must be fully explained to the client and her partner. The nurse works with them to modify their escalating level of anxiety. When the woman has recovered, she should be encouraged to review what has happened so that she may understand and recover equilibrium. The nurse should enlist the family's support, keeping them informed. Because this problem may be a real threat to the woman's self-esteem, she should be encouraged to express her beliefs about why this has happened. When she is in early grieving, observe for signs that she has support from significant others.

For *postbirth hemorrhage* the initial nursing role includes monitoring and detection of developing problems. Remember, signs of shock, evidenced by an increase in pulse and a decrease in blood pressure, are *late results* of hemorrhage. In an emergency, the nurse supports blood volume by increasing flow rates of infusing fluids or by beginning an infusion with a large-bore intracatheter. Oxytocic agents are administered as ordered. The woman may be placed in a position that allows elevation of knees and lower legs to 45 degrees, or MAST may be applied (see Table 21-1). Hemorrhage may be rapid, and a team approach is essential.

If bleeding is local and the source is determined, initial application of an *ice pack* to the perineum may be effective. Most commonly, the condition can be corrected in the delivery area, and the client returns to the recovery area with blood volume restored. Hematocrit and hemoglobin levels may be low, but transfusions are used only if necessary. Laboratory values are monitored at least every 12 hours during recovery.

The hemorrhaging woman will be very anxious and requires explanations of the management and expected outcomes. It is always important to explain the rationale for treatment and give her as much information as she desires about the techniques being used to stop the bleeding.

The woman is at special risk for infection and usually is given prophylactic antibiotics. She should be taught the signs of lingering infection and subinvolution.

▶ EVALUATION

Questions similar to the following may be asked to form an evaluation of outcomes of care for a woman with bleeding from the reproductive tract.

1. Did the woman realize why treatments and interventions were performed?
2. Did both mother and infant receive adequate perfusion during the bleeding episode?
3. Was fluid volume monitored, with output in the normal range?
4. Did supportive staff and family members assist her in coping with anxiety?
5. Does she understand the signs of infection or changes in lochia in the recovery period?
6. Are referrals needed for home care or assistance?

NURSING CARE PLAN • Birth-Related Hemorrhage

CASE: Joan B, para 2012, had an extended second stage after a long first stage of labor. Membranes had been ruptured 16 hours before birth, and rectal temperature was 100°F. Because of lack of descent, a cesarean delivery occurred. During surgery, blood loss was 3000 ml. She received 2 U of PRBC and 6000 ml of crystalloids during surgery. She has now been transferred to the recovery area.

ASSESSMENT

1. Current IV fluids, rate, and replacement orders
   - Output per Foley catheter compared with amount of intake and oxytocin dosage
   - Status of vaginal or wound drainage, abdominal dressing
   - Vital signs, chest sounds, color of mucous membranes and nail beds
   - Level of consciousness and pain sensation
2. Laboratory assessments of CBC, PT, PTT, and platelets
3. Joan's knowledge of why and what happened

NURSING DIAGNOSES

1. High risk for fluid volume imbalance related to loss of body fluid and rapid replacement of crystalloids
2. High risk for infection related to blood loss, extended ROM, and surgical procedure
3. Pain related to fatigue, surgical procedure, and potential inflammation of tissues
4. Anxiety for self and infant related to complicated labor, potential newborn infection

EXPECTED OUTCOMES

1. Balanced fluid status is evidenced by hematocrit level above 28%, urine output of 30 to 50 ml/hr or more
2. Risk of infection avoided by antibiotics and adequate fluids after birth
3. Pain is managed, with relief
4. States understanding of reasons for cesarean. Speaks of newborn with hope and anticipation of going home.

NURSING INTERVENTIONS

1. Maintain warmth with extra blankets. Place all infusions on IV pumps.
   - Maintain pulse oximetry to assess oxygenation.
   - Monitor blood pressure, pulse, respiration. Evaluate lung sounds. Position in semi-Fowler's.
2. Advocate for reduced oxytocin dose to prevent antidiuretic action. Hourly output is compared with intake until active diuresis occurs.
3. Observe for signs of infection. Administer antibiotics. Monitor temperature, pulse, and respiration (TPR). Follow laboratory reports.
4. Depending on anesthetic, monitor postepidural narcotic responses or need for analgesic. Administer before severe pain returns. Assess if pain seems more severe than usual.
5. Include partner in discussion of progress. Orient family to reasons for surgery, responses to hemorrhage. Update frequently. Assure woman when signs of recovery are apparent. Inform her of newborn status.

EVALUATION

1. Did diuresis begin and hematocrit level remain above 28%? Did bleeding follow normal recovery patterns?
2. Was infection avoided/counteracted?
3. Did fatigue levels diminish? Was pain managed?
4. Did she demonstrate interest in the events through which she just passed? Does she recognize need for surgical interventions? Has she seen and begun attachment to infant?

KEY POINTS

- Approximately 85% of all pregnancies are completed normally without problems, but complications of the reproductive system may be life threatening for mother or fetus.
- Preterm labor remains a leading cause of morbidity and neonatal mortality. Every nurse should be knowledgeable about signs and symptoms and recommended interventions.
- Some risk factors for preterm labor are amenable to prevention, especially smoking, infection, stress, and drug abuse.
- Multiple gestation places extra stress on the woman from pressure effects, nutritional demands, and labor complications. Early monitoring is mandatory.
- Signs of ectopic implantation are confusing. Early diagnosis and intervention prevent morbidity. The embryo is lost and fertility may be altered.
- The age of viability is the dividing point in pregnancy loss. Early abortions have many serious implications.

- Second-trimester abortions present significantly greater maternal risk.
- There is a choice of attitude toward elective abortion, and nurses have the responsibility of becoming self-aware and cognizant of state rules and regulations.
- Hemorrhage in obstetrics is a risk because of the greater vascular supply to tissues during pregnancy.
- Pregnant women are protected against effects of moderate blood loss, but when hemorrhage exceeds 30% to 35% of blood volume, sudden signs of severe shock will occur.
- Risk factors for hemorrhage can be estimated, which facilitates the implementation of preventive watchful care.
- Nursing monitoring during labor and recovery will identify early warnings of hemorrhage.
- Care is collaborative when hemorrhage occurs. Documentation is essential because events transpire rapidly.

STUDY QUESTIONS

21-1 Provide the appropriate Key Term for each of the following statements:
   a. Abnormal site for implantation of the embryo *Ectopic*
   b. Too much amniotic fluid *polyhydramnios*
   c. Lack of maternal chromosomes results in an "empty ovum" *Hydatiform mole*
   d. A precursor of uterine cancer *Trophoblastic disease*
   e. Untreated result of an irritable uterus *preterm birth*
   f. Two embryos from one fertilized ovum *monovular*
   g. Agents to inhibit uterine contractions *tocolytic*

21-2 Jenny is pregnant with twins. She complains of being warm and sweating at 28 weeks. To further evaluate these findings you should first ask her about:
   a. Her weight gain pattern
   b. Her usual activity and rest pattern
   c. Any allergies or changes in environment
   d. Signs of infection

21-3 During the last trimester of a twin gestation, it would be most important to teach self-monitoring of which of the following?
   a. Fatigue levels and interrupted sleep patterns
   b. Patterns of edema in lower extremities
   c. Heartburn and inability to take full meals
   d. Changes in mild contraction patterns

21-4 After two warnings of impending labor, Sue calls to say that she is having abdominal aching, diarrhea, and increased watery vaginal mucus. Which instructions should be given over the phone?
   a. "Drink several glasses of water, void, and rest on your left side for 30 minutes."
   b. "Take an acetaminophen tablet and a glass of water. Try to sleep."
   c. "Come in to see us in the labor unit as soon as you can, and drink two glasses of water as you get ready."
   d. "Rest in a side-lying position and call again in an hour, because you tend to have these feelings off and on."

21-5 A woman would be at risk for premature labor if her history includes the following:
   a. Is working full time at a mildly active job
   b. Has gained 40 pounds by week 35 of gestation
   c. Was treated for a bladder infection and is now reinfected
   d. Is a vegetarian having difficulty getting enough iron in her diet

21-6 A woman in her first trimester of pregnancy calls, wondering if she is miscarrying. During a telephone assessment, which question is not pertinent?
   a. "What is the amount of bleeding and uterine cramping?"

b. "Do you know the time fetal movements stopped?"

c. "Was a pregnancy test done, and when?"

d. "Do you know the exact length of pregnancy?"

21-7 Nursing assessment of a woman admitted for an inevitable abortion at 18 weeks includes which of the following:

a. Determination of fetal heart sounds or movement

b. Evaluation of bleeding and frequent vital signs

c. Evaluation of character of the contractions

d. Measurement of height of fundus and time since membranes ruptured

21-8 Anna was admitted at 6 AM because of a painless bleeding episode during the night. She is 26 weeks pregnant and is frightened. Before the physician arrives to examine her, how can you help to limit her complication?

a. Perform a pelvic examination to determine bleeding site; place in Trendelenburg position.

b. Reassure her that this pregnancy may turn out normally, and explain admission process.

c. Maintain bed rest and monitor vital signs and bleeding.

d. Encourage bed rest, urge oral fluids, and ask companion to stay.

Answer Key

21-1 a. Ectopic pregnancy, b. Polyhydramnios, c. Hydatidiform mole, d. Trophoblastic disease, e. Preterm birth, f. Monovular twins, g. Tocolytics 21-2 a 21-3 d 21-4 c 21-5 c 21-6 b 21-7 b 21-8 c

REFERENCES

Beischer NA, MacKay EV, editors: *Obstetrics and the newborn*, ed 2, Philadelphia, 1986, WB Saunders.

Beringer RE, Niebyl JR: The safety and efficacy of tocolytic agents for the treatment of preterm labor, *Obstet Gynecol Rev* 45(7):415, 1990.

Berkowitz RS, Goldstein DP: Complications of molar pregnancy, *Contemp Obstet Gynecol*, 24:57, 1984.

Burchell RC: Professional perspectives on abortion, *JOGNN* 3(6):25, 1979.

Combs CA, Murphy EL, Laros RK Jr: Factors associated with hemorrhage, *Obstet Gynecol Surv* 46:362, 1991.

Daikoku NH et al: Premature rupture of membranes and spontaneous preterm labor, and maternal endometritis risk, *Obstet Gynecol* 59:13, 1982.

Eden RD, Sokol RJ: Predicting prematurity: the mammary stimulation test, *Clin Perinatol* 19(2):219, 1992.

Eden RD, Eaganhouse, Burnside et al: The mammary stimulation test—a predictor of preterm delivery? *Am J Obstet Gynecol* 164:1409, 1991.

Eganhouse DJ: Fetal monitoring of twin gestation, *JOGNN* 21(1):17, 1992.

Eganhouse DJ, Burnside SM: Nursing assessment and responsibilities in monitoring the preterm pregnancy, *JOGNN* 21(5):355, 1992.

Ellerbrock et al: Ectopic pregnancy mortality in the US 1979-82 (No SS-2), *MMWR* 36:13, 1987.

Foster CA: The pregnant trauma patient, *Nursing 84* 11:58, 1984.

Gill P, Smith M, McGregor C: Terbutaline by pump to prevent recurrent preterm labor, *MCN* 14(3):163, 1989.

Gill SA, editor: Twin pregnancy, *Clin Perinatol* 15(1):162, 1988.

Golan A et al: Incompetence of the uterine cervix, *Obstet Gyncol Rev* 44(2):96, 1989.

Graber EA: Prematurity 1992, *Obstet Gynecol Surv* 47(8):521, 1992.

Grimes DA: Second trimester abortion in U.S., *Fam Plann Perspect* 16(6):365, 1984.

Harrison LK, Naylor KL: The laws that affect abortion in the United States and their impact on women's health, *Nurs Pract* 16(12):53, 1991.

Herron MA, Dulock HL: Preterm labor (series 2, module 5), White Plains, NY, 1987, March of Dimes Foundation.

Hess RD et al: Correlation of uterine activity using the Term Guard monitor versus standard external tocodynamometry compared with intrauterine pressure catheters, *Obstet Gynecol* 76: 52S, 1990.

Hillier SL et al: A case-controlled study of chorioamnionitis in prematurity, *N Engl J Med* 319:972, 1988.

Hollenbach KA, Hickok K: Epidemiology and diagnosis of twin gestation, *Clin Obstet Gynecol* 33:3, 1990.

Hyashi RA, Castillo MS: Bleeding in pregnancy. In Krueppef RA, Drukker JE, editors: High risk pregnancy, Philadelphia, 1986, WB Saunders.

Ichinoe K et al: Nonsurgical therapy to preserve oviduct functioning in patients with tubal pregnancy, *Am J Obstet Gynecol* 156:2, 1987.

Johnson FF: Assessment and education to prevent preterm labor, *MCN* 14(3):157, 1989.

Jones JM, Sbarra AJ, Cetrulo CL: Antepartum management of twin gestation, *Clin Obstet Gynecol* 33:32, 1990.

Katz M, Goodyear K, Creasy RK: Early signs and symptoms of preterm labor, *Br J Obstet Gynaecol* 162:1150, 1990.

Kim Klein SM: Asherman's syndrome. In Speroff L, Simpson JL, Sciarra JJ, editors: *Gynecology and obstetrics*, vol 5, Philadelphia, 1987, Harper & Row.

Krohn MA et al: Vaginal *Bacterioides* species are associated with an increased rate of preterm delivery amoung women in preterm labor, *J Infect Dis* 164:988, 1991.

Kruskall MS, Leonard S, Klapholz H: Autologous blood donation during pregnancy: analysis of safety and blood use, *Obstet Gynecol* 70(6):938, 1987.

Lowe TW: Hypovolemia during hemorrhage, *Clin Obstet Gynecol* 33(3):454, 1990.

McDonald HM et al: Prenatal microbiologic risk factors associated with preterm birth, *Br J Obstet Gynaecol* 99:190, 1992.

McGregor JA: Prevention of preterm birth: new initiatives based on microbial:host interactions, *Obstet Gynecol Surv* 42(1):1, 1988.

Mehta I, Young ID: Recurrence risks of common complications of pregnancy: a review, *Obstet Gynecol Surv* 42(4):218, 1987.

Morbidity and Mortality Weekly Report, 1992.

Mueller L: Second-trimester termination of pregnancy: nursing care, *JOGNN* 20(4):284, 1991.

Phelan JP et al: Vaginal birth after cesarean, *Am J Obstet Gynecol* 157:1510, 1987.

Prepert JF, Donnenfeld AE: Oligohydramnios: a review, *Obstet Gynecol Rev* 46(6):325, 1991.

Rose GL, Chapman MG: Aetiological factors in placenta previa, *Br J Obstet Gynaecol* 93:586, 1988.

Sala DJ, Moise KJ: The treatment of preterm labor using a portable subcutaneous terbutaline pump, *JOGNN* 19(2):108, 1990.

Saftlas AF et al: National trends in the incidence of abruptio placentae, 1979-1987, *Obstet Gynecol* 78(6):1081, 1991.

Stock A: Ectopic pregnancy, *Clin Obstet Gynecol* 33(3):448, 1991.

Zahn CM, Yeomans ER: Postpartum hemorrhage: placenta accreta, uterine inversion and puerperal hematomas, *Clin Obstet Gynecol* 33(3):422, 1991.

 STUDENT RESOURCE SHELF

Eganhouse DJ, Burnside SM: Nursing assessment and responsibilities in monitoring preterm labor, *JOGNN* 21(5):355, 1992. Clear discussion of the importance of nursing interventions during preterm labor.

Harrison LK, Naylor KL: The laws that affect abortion in the United States and their impact on women's health, *Nurs Pract* 16(12):53, 1991. Review of Supreme Court rulings since 1973 with analysis of how they affect women's choices.

Nolan TE, Gallup DG: Massive transfusion: a current review, *Obstet Gynecol Surv* 46(5):289, 1991. Concise review of uses of blood components when massive hemorrhage occurs. Clarifies tests and reasons for using different blood fractions.

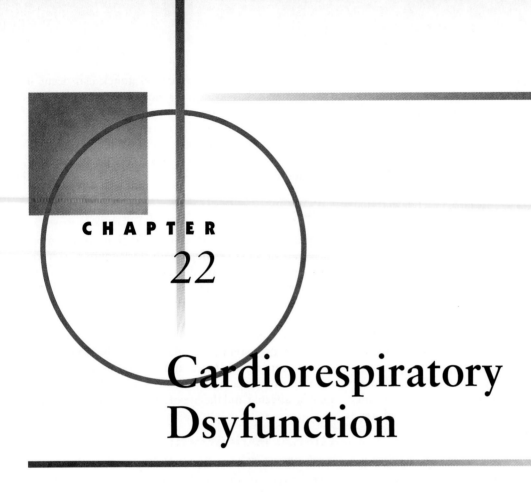

CHAPTER

22

Cardiorespiratory Dsyfunction

KEY TERMS

Adult Respiratory
  Distress Syndrome
  (ARDS)
Aggregation
Amnesia
Antiphospholipid
  Syndrome (APS)
Asthma
Colloid Osmotic
  Pressure
  (COP)
Congenital Heart
  Disease (CHD)
Eclampsia
Embolism
Epigastric Pain
Gestational
  Hypertension
Hemoconcentration

Obstetric Pulmonary
  Embolism
Papilledema
Photosensitivity
Preeclampsia
Pregnancy-Induced
    Hypertension (PIH)

Rheumatic Heart
  Disease (RHD)
Scotoma
Thrombocytopenia
Thrombophlebitis

LEARNING OBJECTIVES

1. *Apply steps of the nursing process to planning care for a woman with cardiorespiratory complications.*
2. *Describe self-care for the asthmatic client during pregnancy.*
3. *State strategies for preventing progression of pregnancy-induced hypertension.*
4. *Contrast normal hemodynamic changes of pregnancy with alterations caused by severe preeclampsia and pulmonary edema.*
5. *Compare events of embolic disorders with normal increases in clotting activity during pregnancy.*
6. *Describe the various subtle signs of antiphospholipid syndrome and lupus erythematosus.*
7. *Identify preventive health care instructions for a woman with pregnancy-induced hypertension, thromboembolic problems, and cardiac dysfunction.*

Various physical conditions have specific implications for the pregnant woman and her fetus and newborn. Expert nursing care requires knowledge of these conditions and their implications, as well as the techniques for assessment and intervention.

Cardiovascular problems can complicate pregnancy and delivery. Respiratory problems also place the pregnant woman at risk. The most common of these disorders is asthma.

The normal cardiorespiratory changes of pregnancy are quite distinct and would be considered abnormal in a nonpregnant adult. Each change has a purpose, and each affects the symptoms experienced by the pregnant woman. Understanding cardiorespiratory problems in pregnancy requires a knowledge of these normal changes. The changes in cardiac stroke volume and output, blood volume, and body water, as well as the effects of pregnancy hormones on blood vessels and the kidney, are reviewed in Chapter 9.

Asthma

Bronchial **asthma** is a complex chronic problem that includes airway hyperresponsiveness and obstruction. When airflow through the bronchioles and smaller bronchi is obstructed, the obstruction results in bronchospasm, edema and inflammation of the mucous membrane, and excessive mucus production. It also causes wheezing and rhonchi. Major precipitants are inhaled allergens such as pollens, dust, feathers, animal hair, and certain foods. Other precipitants include chemical irritants, emotional stress, exercise, steroid withdrawal, inhaler abuse, and bronchoconstrictive drugs.

Some pregnant women describe an improvement in their breathing, especially during the first trimester. Improvement probably is related to the increase in adrenal steroid hormones, cortisol and prednisolone, and to the higher levels of histaminase associated with pregnancy. Other women complain of attacks during the second and third trimesters, perhaps caused by emotional stress, weight gain, the pressure of the uterus against the diaphragm, or in some cases, pregnancy-induced hypertension.

RISK

In women of childbearing ages, 2% have asthma, and 0.1% have acute attacks during pregnancy, especially in the third trimester. Although it is not common for a woman to have an episode at the time of labor, very often after a cesarean delivery and during recovery, episodes will occur. An asthmatic woman is likely to repeat the same pattern of exacerbation with each pregnancy. The major risk to the woman is the development of *status asthmaticus,* a sustained period of reduced gas exchange. The risk to the fetus is related to the effects of medications and the hypoxia that may result from severe attacks.

Treatment now includes antiinflammatory therapy so that the bronchi may heal. Without this respite, chronic irreversible hypertrophy and other changes occur, which lead to disability and death even in young persons. In fact, the death rate has risen in the last 10 years, believed to be related solely to excessive use of bronchodilators (Gift, 1991).

Women may reduce their regular medication, fearing its effect on the fetus, and thus precipitate asthma symptoms. A severe or even fatal attack can occur if the woman takes aspirin or nonsteroidal antiinflammatory drugs and certain prostaglandins. If asthma is poorly controlled during pregnancy, intrauterine growth retardation (IUGR) and low birth weight will occur, as well as a higher risk of preterm birth or perinatal mortality.

SIGNS

Dyspnea with prolonged expiratory phase is accompanied by a productive cough with thick sputum, respiratory sounds, respiratory distress, and increased anxiety. Asthmatic wheezing must be differentiated from bronchitis, emphysema, congestive heart failure, and pulmonary embolism.

A sustained increase in respiratory distress may result in status asthmaticus. Blood gases become altered and indicate an advanced and dangerous stage of pulmonary obstruction. In these cases, fetal oxygenation may be affected and the life of the mother is in jeopardy.

CLINICAL MANAGEMENT

A chest x-ray film is a standard diagnostic tool that may reveal hyperinflation of the lungs. Pulmonary function tests are performed to evaluate the degree of obstruction. The usual findings are decreased vital capacity, increased residual volume, and decreased peak expiratory flow rates (PEFR). To determine the presence of pulmonary infection, a white blood cell count and sputum analysis are performed.

For all acute episodes, parenteral or inhalant epinephrine, bronchodilators, and corticosteroids are given. Supportive therapy includes oxygen, hydration, and chest physiotherapy. Drugs such as theophylline must be used with caution and the fetal condition monitored.

During labor, epidural anesthesia will be chosen. Because of respiratory compromise, narcotics and anesthesia that may depress respirations are to be avoided. Oxygen levels are monitored by pulse oximeter (SaO_2) during labor. Fetal responses are continuously monitored during this high-risk labor, and the infant is monitored for residual drug effects.

Interventions between episodes are important. During these periods the client must be evaluated for history of allergen contact, which may be treated by desensitization. Respiratory tract infections should be avoided, and if they occur, they must be aggressively treated.

Nursing Responsibilities

Asthma is a chronic problem, and the client brings a history of episodes, good or poor management and compliance, and her own responses to the disease. The nurse must include these factors in assessment and planning.

ASSESSMENT

Early detection of bronchospasm can be discovered by the client's self-monitoring of PEFR and comparing it with her best efforts. In addition, clients should record events that precipitate attacks so that they may be prevented if possible. Assessment includes vital signs, noting the timing and dosage of medications in relation to precipitating events. The woman's compliance and her understanding of the stresses of pregnancy need to be assessed and her knowledge of self-care and medication dosage.

NURSING DIAGNOSES

1. Ineffective airway clearance related to increased secretions in tracheobronchial tree
2. Impaired gas exchange related to chronic tissue hypoxia from inflammation of bronchial mucosa, severe bronchospasm, and copious secretions
3. Potential altered fetal tissue perfusion related to chronic oxygen deficit
4. Potential altered fetal growth and development
5. Anxiety related to lack of sleep as a result of stress of dyspnea or perceived threat to fetus
6. Knowledge deficits about self-care, medications
7. Potential noncompliance

EXPECTED OUTCOMES

1. Complies with medication regimen
2. Recognizes factors that precipitate attacks; able to maintain control of her environment, preventing contact with allergens
3. Works on reduction of stressors that may precipitate attacks
4. Asthmatic episodes quickly controlled

NURSING INTERVENTIONS

Although asthma is a chronic health problem, the nurse should not assume that the client is fully knowledgeable. Some women who have lived with asthma since childhood may have a very thorough knowledge of the disease and required medications. Others may be unaware of self-care requisites or may not follow recommendations. For instance, steam or mist inhalation helps clear mucus from the airway. The small home vaporizer used for this purpose must be cleaned carefully and frequently to avoid bacterial growth in the water; yet a number of clients do not do this task. The client and her family also should maintain a comfortable home temperature with a humidity of about 30%.

A number of young asthmatic persons are stressed by their disease and do not accept the rigorous self-care requirements. These young women may omit medica-

tion, expose themselves to stress or allergens, or overuse bronchodilators.

She should be provided with complete written information about medications that are taken at home, use of home therapy such as hand-held nebulizers, and signs and symptoms that require immediate medical care. In addition, she should be cautioned to avoid exposure to individuals with infections, especially upper respiratory tract infections. Further, the nurse validates the understanding of the cause, treatment, and impact of this disease on her present pregnancy and makes every attempt to capitalize on her present assets and incorporate them into a comprehensive health plan.

Self-care should be promoted in every way because she must manage her condition at home. The nurse can negotiate schedules, help her with analysis of potential stress areas, and engage her in achieving the best prenatal health status for the sake of the developing infant. Because there is a psychosocial component to asthma, it is wise for the plan of care to include only one or two nurses in primary care (Geiger-Bronsky, 1992). *need Rest p̄ an attack*

EVALUATION

1. Has the woman analyzed sources of stress in her home?
2. Has she identified and avoided allergens?
3. Does she describe her treatment plan correctly?
4. How rapidly did an asthma attack subside? What intervention was required?
5. Did the infant show deleterious effects from hypoxia or medications?

Hypertensive Disorders of Pregnancy

Approximately 23 million persons in the United States have hypertension, and many of them are not under treatment. Because an adult woman may seek health care for the first time when she becomes pregnant, it is important to recognize initial signs of chronic hypertension, renal disease causing hypertension, or **pregnancy-induced hypertension (PIH)**. Diagnosis may be difficult. Indeed, many women have been treated for PIH only to

Clinical Decision

Randi tells you that when she gets an asthmatic attack, she puffs on her bronchodilator inhaler like a "house afire." What do you need to know before teaching her correct use?

BOX 22-1   Classification of Hypertensive States

Pregnancy-induced hypertension (PIH)

Gestational hypertension:

Without edema or proteinuria: resolves within 6 weeks after birth

Preeclampsia:

With edema and proteinuria:
— Mild preeclampsia
— Severe preeclampsia/eclampsia

Eclampsia Seizures Coma

HELLP syndrome

Hypertension with hemolysis, elevated liver enzymes, and low platelet count

Preexisting hypertension, chronic

Occurs before 20 weeks and persists 6 weeks after birth
— With renal disease
— Without renal disease

find later that the signs really indicated a preexisting condition. This happens because an existing elevation in blood pressure (BP) may be masked by the normal BP decrease in the first half of pregnancy. It is important to be alert to symptoms, because untreated disease will progress in severity, will cause cardiovascular damage, and may result in fetal morbidity and mortality. Classification of hypertensive states is shown in Box 22-1.

GESTATIONAL HYPERTENSION

Transient or **gestational hypertension** occurs only in pregnancy. It develops because the woman has a predisposition to hypertension; under the cardiovascular stress of pregnancy, she has overt signs of a condition that may develop later in life. BP rises during pregnancy, but neither edema nor proteinuria develops. After the baby is born, the mother's BP returns to the baseline level. For this woman, treatment is symptomatic, with adequate rest and controlled diet that includes extra fluids. Medication usually is not needed. BP levels are monitored carefully. There should be no adverse effect on the infant.

PREECLAMPSIA

The Greek word, *eklampnis,* meaning "shining forth, or sudden development," refers to the sudden onset of the characteristic convulsion that divides **preeclampsia** from **eclampsia.** The term *toxemia of pregnancy,* as well as preeclamptic toxemia (PET), is still used in some areas. This type of hypertension has an insidious onset.

Preeclampsia is detected after the twentieth week of gestation when hypertension is accompanied by edema or proteinuria, or both. In the early phase, there is gradually developing vasoconstriction, sodium retention, and edema with increased plasma volume. If uncorrected, a late phase develops in which there is further sodium and water retention accompanied by hypertension, proteinuria, and a *reduced* plasma volume or **hemoconcentration.** Without treatment eclampsia may develop with convulsions and coma.

Although the earliest trigger for preeclampsia is unknown, recent studies have pinpointed prostaglandin *imbalance* as a primary factor. *Prostacyclin* (PGI_2) is a vasodilator and potent inhibitor of platelet aggregation (clumping, often causing thrombosis). Prostacyclin is produced in the vascular epithelium and should be present in higher amounts during pregnancy than in a nonpregnant state. *Thromboxane* A_2 (TXA_2), which is a powerful vasoconstrictor that stimulates platelet aggregation, is an important prostaglandin in the normal processes of hemostasis. What is not known is the exact cause of this imbalance. It is thought that a defect in placental development is involved wherein the muscular walls of the placental vessels *do not vasodilate normally* to accommodate the normal rapid increase in blood volume. This may be seen by Doppler flow–velocity waveforms in the uteroplacental circulation or the umbilical cord (see Chapter 11). *Lack of vasodilation* occurs, which may be detected early in the second trimester, before 18 weeks, long before any evident signs appear. The fragile blood vessel walls are injured by the increased blood flow. Platelets and fibrin are deposited and begin intrinsic processes that will inhibit normal prostacyclin. Secretion of TXA_2 occurs in increasing ratios and fosters vasoconstriction (Figure 22-1).

This theory can explain the vasoconstriction in placental vessels that leads to IUGR and abruptio placentae and to a higher risk of fetal death during the pregnancies of hypertensive women. Over time, placental perfusion diminishes and peripheral vasoconstriction increases, reducing perfusion to other vital organs.

The normal cardiovascular adjustments of pregnancy are altered in the following ways.

- Systolic and diastolic pressures rise above 30/15 mm Hg over baseline; mean arterial pressure (MAP) rises above 100 mm Hg.
- Systemic vascular resistance is increased, including pulmonary vascular resistance.
- Cardiac output is *lower* than normal.
- Blood volume becomes *lower* than normal as disease progresses.
- Hematocrit values are elevated.
- Platelet counts may fall below 150,000/mm³.
- Colloid osmotic pressure is lowered, contributing to generalized edema and potentially to pulmonary edema.

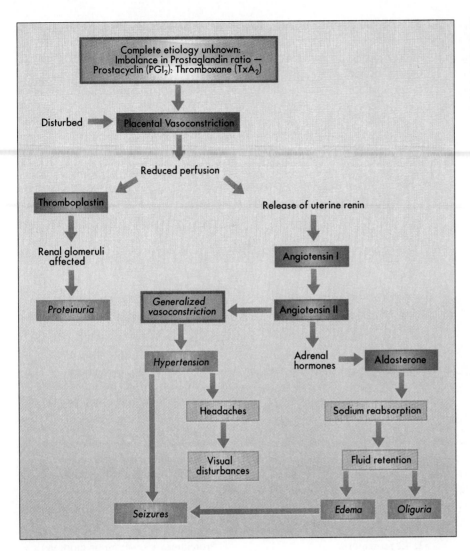

FIGURE 22-1 Cycle of responses in pregnancy-induced hypertension. (Data from Walsh SW: Preeclampsia: an imbalance in placental prostacyclin and thromboxane production, *Am J Obstet Gynecol* 150:335, 1985.)

Risk

Preeclampsia is most likely to develop during pregnancy in those women who already have hypertension or diabetes and those who have other complications of pregnancy such as multiple pregnancy, hydramnios, or hydatidiform mole. Primigravidas are susceptible, especially those younger than the age of 14 or older than 35. The association of preeclampsia with poverty and protein malnutrition is recognized but not really explained. Although black women have a two to three times higher prevalence of chronic hypertension than do white women, the incidence of preeclampsia is similar between populations of black and white women (Chesley, 1985).

The reported incidence of *all* hypertensive disorders of pregnancy is 20% to 30%. For PIH only the incidence is 6% to 7% of all pregnancies. The risk for preeclampsia superimposed on preexisting hypertension is 15% for those women with chronic hypertension.

Because recognition and treatment of early preeclampsia have improved, incidence of eclampsia has dropped during the last 20 years. Most perinatal deaths are from IUGR, intracranial hemorrhage, or prematurity.

Eclampsia still occurs in women who do not receive prenatal care and in chronically hypertensive women with superimposed PIH. It is a leading cause of maternal and fetal death worldwide.

Signs

Hypertension. Hypertension is a lasting elevation of BP to 140/90 or above or a change of 30 systolic and 15 diastolic points above a previously normal baseline reading, or MAP above 100 mm Hg in an adult and above 85 mm Hg in an adolescent. Technically, this elevation must be observed at two readings at least 6 hours apart. Readings should be taken several times at each prenatal visit. The trend of the readings is observed. For example, a woman who normally has a BP of 100/70 would demonstrate potential preeclamptic hypertension if her pressure increased to 130/80 or 130/85. *A diastolic pressure of 80 in a young woman should always be investigated.* The diastolic pressure is

Take in sitting position

more significant because it reflects the cardiac resting phase (Table 22-1).

The third-trimester BP reading must be compared with the baseline (a prepregnancy or first-trimester reading) to recognize pathologic significance in a third-trimester elevation. A baseline reading is a pressure obtained in the first trimester, if possible; otherwise the earliest clinic visit pressure is used. After 14 to 18 weeks, remember that the normal drop in diastolic (10 to 20 mm Hg) and systolic (0 to 5 mm Hg) may not be

TABLE 22-1 Signs and Symptoms of Preeclampsia and Eclampsia

MILD	MODERATE	SEVERE
WEIGHT GAIN: EDEMA		
More than 1-2 lb/wk	More than 1-2 lb/wk	Excessive weight gain; usually face puffy, rings hard to get off
No visible edema	Some edema above waist in abdomen, fingers, face, and extremities	
HYPERTENSION		
30/15 rise over baseline reading	Diastolic, 90 or above; 140/90 or above MAP >100	Systolic, 160 or above; diastolic, 110 or above; with preexisting hypertension, which may be very high
Diastolic 80-90 depending on baseline	Complains of headaches, lethargy, fatigue	Complaints of lasting frontal headache unrelieved by analgesics; cerebral and visual disturbances, ringing in ears, fainting episodes
Feels some lethargy, fatigue	Client appears alert and functions normally unless heavily sedated	Possible grand mal convulsion in sleep
		May experience amnesia up to 48 hours before convulsion
		Epigastric girdling pain, result of edema/hemorrhage in liver capsule (HELLP)
URINE: QUALITY/QUANTITY		
No proteinuria or just a trace	+1, +2 proteinuria	Proteinuria +3, +4; 5g or more in 24-hr specimen
Not much change	Scanty concentrated urine	Oliguria: 800 ml or less in 24 hr progressing to severe oliguria (400 ml), sometimes anuria
BLOOD CHANGES		
Some increase in plasma volume		Hct elevated because of hemoconcentration; plasma volume lowered; platelets lowered <100,000/mm^3
Hct lower		
Uric acid 26 mg/dl	Rising level	Uric acid above 6 mg/dl, BUN↑
FUNDAL CHANGES IN EYE		
Some retinal arteriolar spasm	More extensive spasm can be seen	Edema: papilledema, ischemia of retina
INFANT		
If delivered at this time, usually no problem	Usually no major problems if delivered at this phase; may be small for dates	Infants may be malnourished or small for dates because of placental changes
		Precipitate delivery may occur; infant anoxic, stillborn; premature separation of placenta may occur

evident in a client with preeclampsia. Remember also by the third trimester BP usually returns to normal prepregnant levels in a woman free of PIH.

Edema is NOT always assoc c Hypertension

Edema. The difference between *dependent edema* and *generalized edema* is important. In the last trimester, most pregnant women have pedal edema, especially toward evening. This dependent edema is so named because its development is caused by elevated femoral venous pressure, mechanical obstruction produced by the enlarging uterus, and the effects of gravity when the woman is in the upright position. Resting in bed in a lateral recumbent position relieves the collection of fluid in the interstitial spaces and causes diuresis to occur.

In PIH, edema is associated not only with these mechanical factors but also with salt retention and vasoconstriction. Intravascular fluid may move into both the intracellular and interstitial spaces, may be seen in the face, hands, and abdomen, and is unrelated to body position. The developing poor renal function results in a decreased serum albumin level. As the plasma **colloid osmotic pressure (COP)** decreases, more fluid moves into the intracellular spaces including the brain, liver, and kidneys. This kind of edema is *generalized edema.*

Because of the reduced flow to the kidneys, serum levels of blood urea nitrogen (BUN), uric acid, and creatinine become elevated. Sodium conservation is triggered, and urine output is decreased. Sodium retention increases the woman's sensitivity to angiotensin II (see Figure 22-1).

During healthy pregnancy the glomerular filtration rate in each kidney increases 50%, from about 55 ml/min to 75 ml/min. If sodium were not reabsorbed by the kidneys, the woman would soon be suffering from hyponatremia. For many years, retained sodium was considered the major cause of preeclampsia and women were put on rigid low-sodium diets. Now this regimen is considered to be *hazardous* to the mother (Chesley, 1985). A low-salt diet actually stimulates renin-angiotensin II output, whereas a less restricted salt diet and bed rest inhibit renin output.

Excessive weight gain (more than 2 pounds per week) indicates early generalized edema and is the *earliest* observed sign during the antepartum period. Often in severe states the woman gains 5 or more pounds in a week. *Pitting edema* is a sign of increasing generalized edema and can be demonstrated during assessment of the lower legs (Figure 22-2). When the examiner presses on the client's ankle or pretibial area for 15 seconds, pitting edema is present if the finger pad leaves an indentation in the tissue. Assessment of the degree of edema is summarized in Box 22-2.

Seemingly unrelated, a late sign in preeclampsia is **epigastric pain,** which is a result of severe edema of the

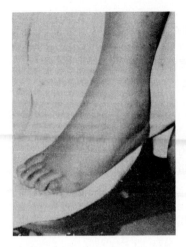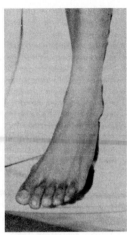

FIGURE 22-2 Pedal edema. Note pitting edema.

BOX 22-2   Assessment of Edema

- Minimal edema of lower extremities: +1
- Marked edema of lower extremities: +2
- Edema of lower extremities, face, and hands: +3
- Generalized massive edema, including the abdomen and face: +4

---

liver capsule. Because epigastric pain may be confused with symptoms of gastric illness, careful assessment is necessary.

Reason for routine Ua @ prenatal visits + to ↓ Ketones

Proteinuria. Renal involvement is produced by vasoconstriction and edema of the endothelial cells so that glomeruli look enlarged and bloodless. A lesion develops called *glomerular capillary endotheliosis.* Fibrin is deposited, and the function of the glomeruli is affected.

Renal ischemia and proteinuria of varying amounts correlate with the severity of renal involvement. Thus, spilling of protein of 1+ or more (>300 mg/L in 24 hours) is considered a sign of renal abnormality and a reason to begin treatment. Complete renal recovery occurs in most cases, with resolution of preeclampsia.

Proteinuria is often first recognized by the nurse from results of a glucose enzymatic test strip. A clean-voided midstream specimen must be obtained to eliminate secretions from the vagina that could distort findings. (All pregnant women have leukorrhea and should use clean-voided midstream urine for laboratory tests.) The degree of proteinuria is more accurately determined by a 24-hour urine collection. A level of 3 to 5 g/L in 24 hours is considered very serious.

Oliguria. Dark concentrated urine results from water and sodium retention with reduced renal output. Nor-

BOX 22-3   Deep Tendon Reflex Assessment Scale

- No response (abnormal): 0
- Diminished response (low normal): +1
- Average response (normal): +2
- Brisker than average response but not abnormal: +3
- Hyperactive (jerky or clonic) response: +4

mal urine output of 30 to 50 ml/hr is reduced and may lead to *oliguria* (<800 ml/24 hours) or to *anuria,* lack of urine production.

Other signs. Thrombocytopenia (<150,000/mm^3) occurs in 30% to 50% of women with moderate to severe preeclampsia. (See the HELLP syndrome for further discussion.)

Hyperreflexia develops as the brain becomes more irritable because of vasoconstriction and edema. Reflexes become increasingly hyperactive (see Box 22-3). Deep tendon reflexes are assessed regularly during therapy. Hyperactive (jerky or clonic) responses of +4 indicate the potential for a seizure (Box 22-3).

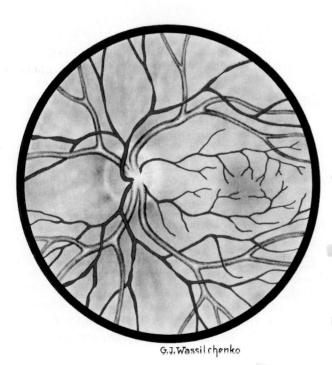

FIGURE 22-3 Funduscopic evidence of severe pregnancy-induced hypertension: arteriospasm, edema, hemorrhages, arteriovenous nicking, and exudates. (From Bobak IM: *Maternity and gynecologic care: the nurse and the family,* ed 5, St Louis, 1993, Mosby.)

Amnesia occurs in the few hours before a seizure. The woman may appear vague and confused and will have no memory of recent events.

Scotomas are visual changes related to retinoarterial spasm and edema of the optic disk that may include temporary loss of vision in one part of the eye (Figure 22-3). Spots, rings, or blurred vision accompanied by headache aggravated by bright lights also are signals of severe vasoconstriction in the eyegrounds. Partial lower retinal detachment may occur in 10% of cases of eclampsia and 1% of preeclampsia (Seidman, Seer, Ben-Rafael, 1991). It resolves spontaneously in most cases, within 2 weeks of the birth.

Blindness is a rare symptom of eclampsia, caused either by thrombosis or detachment of the retina or by cortical involvement with hypodense areas in the occipital lobes. This event also is reversible as vasospasm and edema diminish with treatment. A scan by computed tomography (CT) can be diagnostic.

SEVERE PREECLAMPSIA

If a woman's BP continues to rise in spite of treatment, severe preeclampsia will occur when one or more of the following criteria appear (Dekker and Sibai, 1991):

1. Systolic BP of 160 mm Hg or a diastolic BP of 110 mm Hg on two occasions at least 6 hours apart when the client has maintained bed rest
2. Proteinuria level of at least 5 g/24 hr, or +3 or +4 by semiquantitative analysis with Tes-Tape or Clinistix
3. Cerebral or visual disturbances, or epigastric pain
4. Late pulmonary edema or cyanosis

Abruptio placentae, disseminated intravascular coagulation (DIC), thrombocytopenia, pulmonary edema, congestive heart failure, cerebral hemorrhage, liver necrosis, or renal failure may develop in a woman with severe preeclampsia.

ECLAMPSIA

Severe preeclampsia becomes *eclampsia* when grand mal seizures or coma occurs. Warning signs are amnesia, epigastric pain, hyperreflexia, or clonus before a convulsion. Convulsions may occur during sleep, and contrary to some types of seizures, they are not specifically triggered by light or noise. The eclamptic convulsion is an acute emergency that can result in hypoxia, acidosis, cerebral hemorrhage, or physical injury. It can occur at any time after 20 weeks' gestation, before labor, during labor and birth, or within 14 days after birth. Late-onset seizures are those beginning after 48 hours until 14 days after birth. HELLP syndrome is associated with 30% to 50% of late-onset cases.

Eclamptic convulsions often begin with facial twitching. During the *tonic phase,* the client arches her back and muscles contract and stiffen. Her jaw closes tightly, sometimes injuring her tongue. Thoracic muscles contract tightly, and breathing stops temporarily. After 15 to 20 seconds, the *clonic phase* begins, during which the client thrashes about; muscles alternately contract and relax. Cyanosis, sometimes apnea, continues through this phase, and incontinence of urine or feces may occur. A coma usually follows, which if not treated might lead to another convulsion.

Hypoxia and acidosis may be present in both woman and fetus for several hours after a seizure. Measures are taken to control BP, seizures, and hypoxia. Delivery should be postponed if possible until seizures are controlled and she is responsive. Recovery begins with onset of diuresis of greater than 100 ml/hr for more than 2 hours, but there remains a risk of seizure in those with elevated blood pressures; thus therapy must be continued.

Risk

The overall incidence between 1978 and 1986 in the United States was 0.056% of all births, which is approximately 1:2000 births (Saftlas et al, 1990). Those with early antepartal eclampsia before 28 weeks have the highest risk of maternal and fetal morbidity and mortality. Women with chronic hypertension overlaid with preeclampsia fall more often into this category. If the seizure begins while the woman is in the hospital, chances are better for the woman and infant than if seizures begin at home.

HELLP SYNDROME

An unusual variation of PIH occurs with little warning and often no "regular signs." Blood pressures will appear to be near normal, no edema may be noted, but proteinuria may be present and epigastric pain has occurred in 90%. A woman may seek help from an internist or emergency department for this symptom. Because the diagnosis may be missed until a seizure occurs, it is important to look carefully at platelet counts and at liver enzyme levels, which may rise very high (Figure 22-4).

HELLP stands for hemolysis, elevated liver enzymes, and low platelet count. This syndrome, which was described only in 1982, occurs in every geographic area. Laboratory results will show diagnostic levels of low platelets—less than 150,000/mm³ and classic ratios of lactic dehydrogenase (LDH) levels higher than aspartate aminotransferase (AST, formerly SGOT) levels, which are higher than alanine aminotransferase (ALT, formerly SGPT) levels. A blood smear on a slide will show fractured, broken red blood cells (RBC) that have been torn by forceful passage through tightly constricted vessels. These are called *schistocytes* or *burr cells,* and once fractured are removed from the system, causing a lowered hemoglobin and hematocrit level and possibly an elevated serum bilirubin value (Table 22-2). The resultant condition is *microhemolytic anemia.*

Risk

This variation of PIH occurs anytime after 28 weeks but more often after birth, usually within 72 to 96 hours

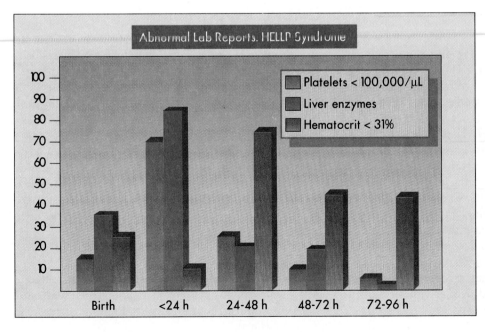

FIGURE 22-4 Liver enzyme levels. Percentage of clients with HELLP whose postpartum laboratory reports showed abnormal findings. Abnormalities tend to peak before 72 hours after birth—usually LDH > peak AST > ALT. (Data from Catanzarite V: HELLP syndrome and its complications, *Contemp Obstet Gynecol* 36[12]:13, 1991.)

TABLE 22-2   Comparison of Laboratory Values: Pregnancy-Induced Hypertension, HELLP, and Disseminated Intravascular Coagulation (Third Trimester)

VALUE	NORMAL	PIH (SEVERE)	HELLP	DIC
Hb	11.5-13	Same	<11 g/dl	Hemolysis
Hct	32%-40%	Elevated	<32%	
Burr cell (schistocyte)	Absent	Possibly some	Possibly some	Present
PT (sec)	10.2-13.8	Slightly shorter	Same as PIH	Prolonged
PTT (sec)	40-60	Slightly shorter	Same as PIH	Prolonged
Platelets (1000/mm^3)	200,000-400,000	<150,000	As low as 30,000	<150,000
Fibrinogen (mg/dl)	300-600	Same	Elevated	Decreased
Clotting time (min)	6-12	Same	Same	Varies
FSP	Absent	Absent	Usually absent	Always present
Creatinine	0.4-1.3	Higher	Higher	Unchanged
BUN	<11	>BUN	>BUN	Unchanged
Uric acid	<6 mg/dl	>6	>6	Unchanged
LDH (IU/dl)	Slight increase over nonpregnancy levels: 84-220	Same	>500	Unchanged
Proteinuria	Negative	2+-4+	1+-4+	Negative
Serum albumin	Down by 15%	Decreased		

Hb, Hemoglobin; *Hct,* hematocrit; *PT,* prothrombin time; *PTT,* partial thromboplastin time; *FSP,* fibrin split products; *BUN,* blood urea nitrogen; *LDH,* lactic dehydrogenase.

(Catanzarite, 1991). Until clear signs of improvement occur, the woman is at risk for adult respiratory distress syndrome (ARDS), seizures, liver hematoma, hepatic failure, renal failure, and death. Acute fatty liver of pregnancy may be confused with this syndrome. HELLP is managed in the same way as PIH.

Signs

Often edema of the extremities does not occur, and the first presenting sign is right upper quadrant pain. Thus the client may be seen by an internist for suspected hepatitis or gallbladder problems. Most also have diastolic pressures above 90 mm Hg and more than 2+ proteinuria (Catanzarite, 1991). The differential diagnosis of HELLP depends on recognizing this as a variation of PIH. Laboratory studies will clarify diagnosis. Liver enzymes are greatly elevated in the classic ratios of LDH > AST > ALT. Platelet levels may be lower than 50,000/mm^3 (class I) or below 100,000/mm^3 (class II). Platelets will be transfused if levels fall below 20,000/mm^3 because of the danger of hemorrhage from many sites (see DIC, Chapter 23). Hematocrit levels follow the microhemolytic process. Extreme hemoconcentration may occur, with fluid shifts out of the vascular compartment, and confuse the outlook. These clients are very ill and may have sudden seizures, or with PIH treatment they may recover within 4 to 5 days. Until platelet counts and liver enzymes return to normal, danger is present.

 Clinical Decision

Mrs. J. is 21 years old, para 0000, and 35 weeks pregnant. What should be the content of your instruction about warning signs of preeclampsia and the HELLP syndrome?

CHRONIC HYPERTENSION

The second group of hypertensive clients have preexisting *chronic hypertension.* Hypertension always is a secondary sign of a primary problem. Chronic hypertension exists when BP is 140/90 before pregnancy or is 140/90 before the twentieth week of gestation and persists more than 6 weeks after the birth. In this case, hypertension is not associated with pregnancy but may be aggravated by it. If a woman has had untreated or poorly controlled chronic hypertension for several years, she may show signs of hypertensive vascular disease. Vascular changes such as arteriosclerosis, retinal hemorrhage, or renal disease may be present. Pregnancy is stressful for these women.

Risk

Women with preexisting hypertension are considered at risk for superimposed PIH and are monitored with close supervision throughout pregnancy. Extreme increases in systolic pressure may occur; thus the risk of cerebral vascular accident (CVA) is increased.

Signs

When a woman with hypertension does not seek early prenatal care, differential diagnosis is obtained by several tests. An ophthalmologic examination reveals vascular sclerosis, hemorrhage, or **papilledema** (engorgement and swelling of the optic disk). Plasma urea nitrogen levels over 20 mg/dl and creatinine levels of more than 1 mg/dl indicate a chronic underlying problem. BP may soar above 160 systolic, and a CVA can occur. Placental injury leads to infarcts, with resulting poor circulation to the infant. Growth-retarded infants result. Finally, the damaged placenta may separate prematurely. During pregnancy a woman with chronic hypertension continues her usual antihypertensive medication unless it has an adverse effect on the fetus. Each newborn infant must be evaluated for drug effects.

Multiple nursing problems may arise in the care of a woman with hypertension. Assessment often reveals alterations in many body systems, as well as knowledge and self-care deficits. Problems with compliance also must be explored.

PIH SUPERIMPOSED ON CHRONIC HYPERTENSION

Some form of preeclampsia develops in about 25% of women with hypertension. Those with moderate to severe hypertension before pregnancy are in the most danger. These women fall into a very high risk category of the hypertensive states. The disease develops in pregnancy and moves to a crisis more rapidly than in other women. Severe renal failure, abruptio placentae, and more stillbirths are found in this group. In women who already have hypertension, preeclampsia tends to recur in about 30% to 40% with each subsequent pregnancy. In addition to a rise in systolic and diastolic BP over the usual reading, any of the classic signs of headache, fatigue, generalized edema, oliguria, and proteinuria indicate the onset of PIH. Hospitalization is the only safe way to care for these women.

Clinical Management of PIH

If a woman has hypertension but no renal involvement during pregnancy, her uric acid level remains in the normal range, below 4 mg/dl. The opposite phenomenon occurs in PIH. Because functions are decreased, uric acid, urea, and creatinine blood levels are increased, but levels in the urine are decreased. A serum uric acid level above 4.5 mg/dl is diagnostic of PIH, and a level above 5.5 mg/dl indicates severe PIH. Serum levels of creatinine and BUN also are elevated because of the decreased glomerular filtration rate. Management

depends on the diagnosis of chronic hypertension or PIH. If chronic hypertension exists, the woman will remain on her medication as long as there is no adverse fetal effect (Box 22-4).

Recently two new therapies have been recommended for PIH. Increased *calcium* supplement during pregnancy has been used to inhibit preterm birth. Increased calcium also is recommended for preeclampsia, although the woman with PIH excretes less calcium. In one study a level less than 195 mg/24 hr was predictive for PIH (Sanches-Ramos et al, 1991). The rationale is that calcium supplementation, which may reduce vascular as well as uterine muscle tone, may be therapeutic for both hypertension and preterm labor (Villar and Repke, 1990). Low zinc levels also have been linked with the development of PIH.

Low-dose *aspirin* has been used since the mid-1980s for cardiovascular and thrombotic disease because of its antiprostaglandin effect, reducing platelet aggregation and inactivating TXA_2. This effect may be seen in larger doses (1 to 2 g/24 hr), which also may actively inhibit the clotting mechanism.

As early as 1979 Crandon and Isherwood showed that women who took aspirin more than once every 2 weeks had significantly fewer cases of PIH. Only recently have low doses (60 to 100 mg daily) been used therapeutically for PIH, and results are exciting. A dosage as low as 0.45 mg/kg for 7 days will inhibit platelet TXA_2 production without significantly chang-

---

BOX 22-4 Antihypertensive Drugs in Pregnancy

Central sympatholytic agents
Methyldopa—Mild hypertension, side effects occur

β-Adrenergic receptor-blocking agents
Oxprenolol—May use with prazosin, hydralazine
Atenolol—Safe, but may slow fetal heart
Pindolol—Does not slow fetal heart
Propranolol—May slow fetal growth

α-Adrenergic receptor-blocking agents
Prazosin

α- and β-Adrenergic receptor-blocking agents
Labetalol—Safe; can be used IV in severe cases

Peripheral vasodilators
Hydralazine—Titrate dose, not over 250 mg qd
Nifedipine—In severe crises and with β-blockers

Data from Lubbe (1990) and Burke (1989).

mg is CNS & urinary depressant & respirators

ing prostacyclin production. Women had been warned against using regular doses of aspirin because of potential fetal and maternal bleeding and prolonged gestation and labor (Dekker and Sibai, 1993). Because of lingering doubts on the part of some practitioners, several large studies are in progress, and widespread therapy for PIH will not be approved until the results are in. Because its effectiveness is so singular, however, many physicians are using low doses with the woman's informed consent. Perhaps in the near future, we will not see severe preeclampsia/eclampsia in anyone who seeks prenatal care!

Anticonvulsants. The treatment of choice for prevention of eclamptic convulsions is *magnesium sulfate.* The magnesium ion provides a neuromuscular blockade at the myoneural junction by reducing acetylcholine release. Its parasympathetic effects on the vessel walls and on the flow of intracellular calcium cause peripheral vasodilation. Although the effect on the BP level is small, there is some reduction in smooth muscle tone, which increases blood flow to the placenta and in the brain. Because the frequency and intensity of labor contractions are decreased, it is used also as an agent to stop premature labor (see Chapter 21).

Magnesium sulfate inhibits muscle function. Thus toxic doses result in hypotonia, loss of deep tendon reflexes, respiratory failure, and cardiac arrest. Regulation of magnesium levels must be exact and is best achieved by monitoring serum levels. Dosage is planned to maintain a level between 4 and 7 mEq/dL. Normal serum levels are 1.5 to 2.0 mEq/dL (1.5 to 2.8 mg/dl or 0.75 to 1.2 mmol/L). Serum magnesium levels are drawn before the dose is ordered and reordered. Magnesium illustrates the small *window of effective concentration* (see Chapter 16) and the ease with which toxic levels may be reached. At regular intervals the three following standard observations are made and documented:

1. Determination of the presence of knee-jerk response. Deep tendon reflexes are lost if magnesium levels rise above 10 mEq/dl (Box 22-5).
2. Respiratory rate must remain above 14 breaths/min.

BOX 22-5   Magnesium Levels

Normal: 1.8-2.5 mEq/dl
Therapeutic: 4.0-8.0 mEq/dl
Hyporeflexia: 10.0-12.0 mEq/dl
Respiratory distress: >12.0 mEq/dl
Cardiac arrest: >15.0 mEq/dl

Calcium gluconate 1-3 g IV over 2-3 min as a bolus for **antidote**

---

3. Urine output should exceed 30 ml/hr through an indwelling catheter. The magnesium ion is excreted by the kidneys; oliguria would lead to a cumulative effect, causing magnesium toxicity. If assessment reveals any abnormal findings, doses are reduced while further evaluation is sought.

Administration. The usual route is by continuous intravenous infusion (Drug Profile 22-1). First a loading dose of 3 to 4 g in 200 to 250 ml D₅W is given over 15 to 20 minutes. Then by pump, 1 to 2 g/hr is continuously infused. The drug should be continued for at least 24 hours after birth.

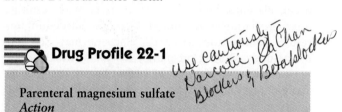

🔬 Drug Profile 22-1

Use cautiously Narcotic, Ca Chan Blockers & Betablockers

Parenteral magnesium sulfate
Action

Blocks release of acetylcholine at neuromuscular junction, thus decreasing neuromuscular irritability, including vasomotor and uterine irritability. Causes slight peripheral vasodilation, reduces edema in the brain, and increases perfusion to brain and placenta. Not used in kidney impairment because it is excreted unchanged from kidney. Cumulative doses may occur if output too low.

Dosage/route

IV by infusion pump: Loading dose 3-4 g in 250 D₅W over 15 to 20 min. Maintenance dose: To keep in therapeutic range of 4-7 mg/dl, must be 1.5 to 3 g/hr, regulated by titrating with client's responses of reflexes, output, respirations, and magnesium levels.

Antidote

Calcium gluconate 10%; keep syringe and ampule at bedside.

Side effects/adverse effects

Sweating, warmth, flushing, heavy feeling in limbs. May become lethargic and confused, with depressed reflexes and respirations.
Fetal effects: Decreased beat-to-beat variability, potential for tachycardia. Monitor newborn for magnesium levels, hypotonia, hyporeflexia.

Precautions

More difficult to obtain therapeutic levels in preterm labor than in PIH because kidney involvement in PIH delays excretion. Monitor for respiratory rate under 12-14/min, urine output under 30 ml/hr, and depressed reflexes, as well as neurologic check q4h. Assess for changes of headache, visual disturbances, epigastric pain. Continue seizure precautions for PIH. Monitor contractions and fetal heart tone in both preterm labor and PIH.

Intramuscular (IM) injections into the gluteus medius of a 50% solution are rarely ordered because they are painful. Sometimes 1 ml of 1% procaine is added to the solution if the client has no allergies. With the IM route there is a lag of 90 to 120 minutes before plasma levels are effective. This drug must be administered by Z-track injection using a sufficiently long needle to place the solution well into the body of the muscle. A subcutaneous injection would cause edema and pain and possibly result in an abscess. The loading dose is 5 g (50% solution) in the right and left dorsogluteal areas and then 3 to 5 g every 4 hours depending on client response.

Effect on fetus and newborn. The fetus is affected in direct proportion to the maternal serum levels because magnesium crosses the placenta. Loss of beat-to-beat variability may mimic fetal distress. Cord blood levels will reflect magnesium levels of the mother. Thus if the woman had been on continuous infusion before the infant was born, the newborn may demonstrate adverse signs of hypotonia, lethargy, and low Apgar scores related to reflexes and respirations. Magnesium is slowly excreted, unchanged, and the newborn should recover with supportive care.

When a seizure is imminent, *phenytoin* is being used with more frequency. The recommended dosage is 1 g by IV infusion, over 1 hour, diluted to give 10 to 12 µg/ml, and then one dose of 500 mg PO 10 hours later. The only side effects are transient burning at the IV site, mild euphoria, dizziness, nystagmus, and a mild decrease in BP (Miles et al, 1990).

Antihypertensives. Opinions differ on the use of antihypertensives for the treatment of preeclampsia, because the mechanism of action must not affect fetal perfusion. The usual approach is to delay their introduction unless the diastolic pressure rises above 100 mm Hg. Hydralazine then may be started first by IV push or infusion but titrated to BP response.

Hydralazine (Apresoline). Hydralazine is safe in pregnancy because it acts directly to relax arteriolar smooth muscle. A decrease in peripheral resistance brings about a reflex increase in cardiac output and better perfusion of the placenta. To maintain adequate blood flow to the placenta the diastolic pressure should not drop below 90 to 100 mm Hg when it has been elevated above this level. The fetal heart is monitored frequently during test doses and IV administration of hydralazine. *Continuous Fetal Monitoring & Maternal*

Although the drug has no direct action on the heart, *EKG monit.* reflex tachycardia, increased stroke volumes and cardiac output occur. Side effects include flushing, headache, dizziness, and cardiac irregularities. Doses should not exceed 200 mg/day. Because the drug must be titrated with BP responses, IV use always includes fetal and maternal continuous monitoring. After the BP is stabilized, the woman's condition may be controlled with oral doses. To block the reflex tachycardia, methyldopa (Aldomet) may be chosen as an adrenergic-blocking drug. In severe cases, if the diastolic pressure exceeds 110 mm Hg, IV methyldopa may be given, alternating with hydralazine. (See Box 22-4 for other antihypertensive agents.)

Propranolol sometimes is given (40 mg every 6 hr). Propranolol, however, crosses the placenta, causing fetal bradycardia.

Nursing Responsibilities

Chronic hypertension often is related to life stress, obesity, smoking, and poor nutrition. All prenatal assessment and instructions focus on preventing complications. Because hypertension is a frequent problem, all women need assistance to manage stress responses, nutrition, and contributing factors. Many nursing diagnoses and interventions for preeclampsia are valid for hypertensive crises of eclampsia and extreme high blood pressure (Burke, 1989). Nursing diagnoses focused on safety always involve the crisis related to convulsions and the aftermath of hypoxia or bleeding.

▶ ASSESSMENT

Admission BP is compared with the earliest available baseline pressure, and the MAP elevation is calculated; a MAP rise higher than 10 to 15 points is very serious. The BP is taken with the woman in a side-lying position, and the upper portion of the arm is used. Note from which arm the reading was taken and assess for signs of fetal distress by fetal monitor. On admission run a 10-minute strip for assessment of fetal status (see Chapters 11 and 14). Physical assessment will detect edema, proteinuria, and deep tendon reflex status. Query the client regarding visual changes, headache, fatigue, and apprehension. Note the woman's level of consciousness and her recall of past events and also query family members about changes noted in the last few days.

Often the woman with preeclampsia manifests several of the overt signs. More subtle changes established only by laboratory evaluations may be detected in cases of chronic renal disease, HELLP, and lupus erythematosus–induced hypertension. When a hypertensive crisis occurs, the entire health team works rapidly together to manage the life-threatening aspects of illness.

▶ NURSING DIAGNOSES

Nursing diagnoses will change in terms of the status of the condition:

1. Knowledge deficit regarding preventive care, stress reduction, nutrition, and smoking factors

2. Altered tissue perfusion related to generalized vasospasm; potential reduced fetal perfusion related to placental damage
3. Altered fluid volume in vascular compartment related to shift to interstitial tissue, renal involvement
4. High risk for injury caused by seizures, acidosis, hypoxia, and potential for thrombosis

▶ EXPECTED OUTCOMES

1. Injury does not occur.
2. Perfusion to woman and fetus is maintained.
3. Adequate oxygenation and airway clearance are maintained.
4. Woman and family know reason for interventions.

▶ NURSING INTERVENTION

Good prenatal care involves assessment to detect early signs of developing hypertensive problems. The nurse should telephone any client who skips an appointment and question her regarding signs of PIH. A home visit should be promptly scheduled if a client does not return to a clinic after showing signs of preeclampsia.

During each visit the client is weighed, and the reading is compared with previous measurements. Nutrition assessment may determine if the client's weight is related to intake or edema. It is difficult to gain more than 2 pounds a week through nutrition alone. Screening includes a urine test for glucose and protein, a BP reading, and an assessment of edema. The following *warning signals,* which are noted as part of the assessment process at each prenatal visit, should be taught to every client:

1. Visual disturbances (blurred vision or spots before her eyes)
2. Dizziness
3. Persistent headache unrelieved by mild analgesic
4. Edema in her face, hands, or legs on arising from sleep
5. Changes in urine color, consistency, and volume

The woman should understand the importance of following rest, diet, and fluid instructions. Cigarette smoking must be strongly discouraged because it promotes vasoconstriction. Conservative management involves bed rest on the woman's left or right side, increased oral fluids to 2500 or 3000 ml/day, and a high protein diet of 80 to 100 g/day. Following these instructions and making frequent prenatal visits may prevent the woman's condition from progressing to the more severe phases. If her condition does not resolve and PIH signs continue or worsen, hospitalization will be necessary.

Test Yourself
- Distinguish between the types of pregnancy-induced hypertension in relation to signs, onset, and adverse effects.
- Compare preeclampsia with chronic hypertension.

Care for Severe Pregnancy-Induced Hypertension

Levels of consciousness should be regularly assessed because the client can slip into a coma without a convulsion. A rapidly rising BP, decreasing urinary output, and increasing amounts of albumin in the urine are alarming signs of deterioration. Vital signs should be assessed by monitors and the MAP requires careful watching by this means. If no monitor is available, check BP every 15 minutes and temperature, pulse, and respirations every hour. BP measurements should be taken in the same arm, noting which arm. If in the dependent position there will be a higher reading. Uterine contractions and fetal heart rate are observed for late decelerations, changes in baseline variability, and other signs of distress.

Protection from hazards is important because the woman might have a convulsion even while she appears to be asleep. Her physical safety is protected by padding the sides of the bed or using pillows to prevent her from hitting her legs or arms on the side rails. With a seizure the chance of biting the tongue is real. If there is an opportunity, an airway should be inserted.

If the woman is not already in the left lateral position when the convulsion occurs, she should be positioned promptly to promote circulation to the placenta and to provide for drainage of mucus. On occasion the airway must be suctioned to clear away mucus. Oxygen is begun by mask or cannula, if not already in place.

The woman's status is continually assessed for circulatory or renal failure and signs of cerebral hemorrhage. She also is observed for signs of abruptio placentae, as evidenced by uterine rigidity, decreased fetal heart rate, and, at times, vaginal bleeding. The possibility of DIC exists (for discussion see Chapter 23). *Labor may begin during a convulsion.* In these cases it usually progresses rapidly to a precipitate delivery, often with excessive bleeding.

Intake and output recording takes place on an hourly basis. A Foley catheter must be in place with a urimeter bag. Protein levels are checked every hour as well. All infusions are by pump, usually for a *total* of 125 ml/hr. This means that to avoid overload, antibiotics, antihypertensive solutions, and mainline IV fluids are added together for the total. Sometimes a *bolus* of IV fluid is given to try to reverse the reduced blood volume. Precautions must be followed carefully, and the BP, pulse, respiratory rate, and chest sounds assessed frequently in case of pulmonary edema. Some units use **central venous pressure (CVP)** measurements that reflect pressures on the right side of the heart (*preload*) (see Figure 22-9). In serious cases the use of a triple pulmonary artery catheter (PAC) or quadruple lumen line (Swan-Ganz catheter) is recommended to continuously measure CVP and **pulmonary artery (PA)** pressures. **Pulmonary capillary wedge pressures (PCWP)** and **cardiac output (CO)** may be measured as well to ascertain how hard the heart is working. Systolic BP indicates the *afterload* (see Table 22-4; Kirshon and Cotton, 1987). Because the client requires intensive care, a one-to-one nursing ratio is mandatory.

Every client will receive magnesium sulfate by IV pump. With that infusion, hourly assessments of reflexes, respirations, and output give an indication of whether the serum concentration is in the therapeutic range. Only magnesium levels will indicate the exact range and these are drawn every 6 hours, but reports may be delayed. The physician is notified of adverse responses (see Drug Profile 22-1), and calcium gluconate 10% should be placed at the bedside for use as an antidote. Potassium depletion also is checked. Magnesium sulfate will be continued for 24 to 48 hours to ensure that convulsions do not occur. Of course, in the postdelivery period, ergot medications (ergotamine, methylergonovine [Methergine]) are contraindicated because they act as vasoconstrictors.

The family will be very anxious about the client. The woman with seizures will not remember events from before the convulsion to several hours after. Her family will be frightened and will need careful explanation of what is happening.

The time of birth will depend on the woman's condition and the presence of fetal distress. Recovery may be very rapid, with the BP returning to moderate levels within 48 hours. The mother is cared for in the labor recovery area until she is out of danger. Severely affected clients are not out of danger until they have given birth and diuresis begins (>100 ml/hr), showing that the edema and vasoconstriction in the brain and kidney have improved (see Nursing Care Plan).

▶ EVALUATION

1. Was perfusion maintained in mother and fetus?
2. Was safety maintained?
3. Did client progress without excessive bleeding?
4. Were family members and client kept informed of progress and clinical management decisions?

 Clinical Decision

Ms. Jones is hospitalized for severe pre-eclampsia. Magnesium sulfate is begun. Four hours after the loading dose, her assessment shows the following: tendon reflexes +2, BP 150/100, fetal heart rate 144, respirations 10/min, urine output 40 ml in the last 2 hours. Choose the appropriate action(s).

Thromboembolic Disease
ANTIPHOSPHOLIPID SYNDROME

Only 40 years ago autoimmune antibodies were first described. Of increasing interest in maternity care, antiphospholipid (APS)—with its partner, *lupus erythematosus*—is assigned a role in recurrent spontaneous abortion, IUGR, and severe PIH. This is an immune response gone awry. Antibodies should be formed against "nonself" foreign proteins by means of B and T lymphocytes. When activated, B cells produce an antibody substance that will bind to a specific antigen to form an **immune complex**. This complex is then eliminated from the body by means of a substance called **complement** (Figure 22-5). In this syndrome, immune complexes, after interacting with complement proteins, are *not* eliminated but are deposited in body tissue where they trigger antibody production against

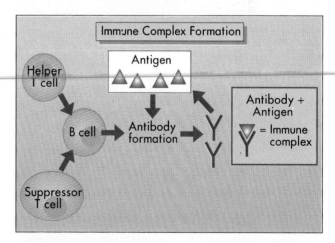

FIGURE 22-5 The immune system is composed of white blood cells. Four principal classes are involved: phagocytes (including macrophages), natural killer cells, and two kinds of lymphocytes, B cells and T cells. T cells include helper T cells and suppressor T cells. Three different kinds of cells mount attacks against the antigen-studded foreign cell in the center of the diagram. (Modified from Hadi HA and Treadwell EL: *Obstet Gynecol Surv* 45: 117, 1990.)

NURSING CARE PLAN • **Pregnancy-Induced Hypertension**

CASE: Karen, age 16, single, para 0000, first visited the clinic at 24 weeks' gestation. BP 120/76, weight 115 pounds. She was counseled on nutrition and warning signs and asked to return in 2 weeks. The next visit was at 32 weeks; she stated that she skipped coming because of headaches and feeling tired and "blue." Now weight gain is 17 pounds in last 8 weeks, BP 138/94, 2+ edema, 2+ proteinuria. Social History: Family support is moderate, with no support from father of child. She seems unimpressed with diagnosis and is resistant to being admitted to labor area for intensive monitoring and treatment.

ASSESSMENT

1. Adolescent, single, primigravida with unknown onset of hypertension. MAP is 108.
2. Weight gain of more than 2 pounds/week.
3. Complains of headaches, fatigue, down mood.
4. Verbalizes no need for assistance; appears frightened of hospitalization.
5. Demonstrates lack of knowledge of condition, implications.

NURSING DIAGNOSES

1. Fluid volume excess: edema related to sodium and water retention
2. Potential for injury related to seizure activity, hypoxia, fetal distress
3. Fear related to potential for injury to self and fetus and to unknown hospitalization events
4. Knowledge deficit related to signs, interventions for PIH, self-care
5. Potential noncompliance with therapies related to developmental age, anxiety

EXPECTED OUTCOMES

1. Weight gain will return to normal pace and control of BP by therapy.
2. No injury results from central nervous system involvement.
3. Verbalizes fears to primary nurse or physician regarding complications and treatments.
4. States signs and symptoms that indicate need for interventions.
5. Actively participates in decisions about treatments and follows therapy guidelines.

NURSING INTERVENTIONS

1. Monitor daily weight, vital signs, and fetal responses q4h. Monitor intake and output. Assess location and intensity of edema. Monitor urine for proteinuria q4h. Maintain bed rest in side-lying position.
2. Monitor for neurologic changes, and assess level of consciousness q4-8h. Administer magnesium sulfate as ordered, and monitor magnesium levels by respirations, output, and reflexes. Institute seizure precautions as per order.
3. Acknowledge validity of Karen's feelings. Assign a primary nurse to establish rapport. Provide emotional support. Involve family members in increasing support.
4. Provide Karen with accurate information about treatments and procedures. Involve her in measurement activities to gain a measure of control over events.
5. Discuss with Karen and family the decisions that must be made; give choices where possible. Arrange for counseling if necessary or requested.

EVALUATION

1. Did weight return to normal sequences? Did vital signs return to normal ranges?
2. Were neurologic changes, including seizures, experienced?
3. Did Karen verbalize feelings of fear for herself and infant? Did supplying support and information help reduce fears?
4. Did she state acceptance of therapies necessary to control PIH?
5. Did she actively participate in care?

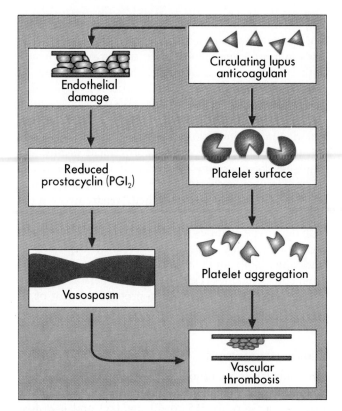

FIGURE 22-6 Two major pathways whereby lupus anticoagulant produces its thrombotic effect in vivo. (From Hadi HA, Treadwell EL: *Obstet Gynecol Surv* 45:117, 1990.)

the cells in the tissue. These *antinuclear antibodies* are against "self" proteins. Figure 22-6 illustrates how one type of autoimmune antibodies will attack platelets and stimulate formation of thrombi in the vessels, as well as upset the prostacyclin-TXA_2 ratio, which, as discussed, underlies PIH. (This does not mean that everyone with PIH has these antibodies but that those who have them and become pregnant most probably will have PIH.)

Box 22-6 lists different antibodies formed in this syndrome. It is confusing that some have one type and not others, whereas in more severe cases a person may demonstrate each type of antibody. The exact trigger is unknown but may be viral, with a genetic tendency as an underlying cause.

Persons with this syndrome experience varied health problems triggered by microthrombi and thus seek different health care specialists. Today a number of mysterious syndromes are believed to be associated with thrombosis, including Addison's disease, thromboembolic disorders, certain cerebral infarcts (strokes), and multiple microinfarcts that change mental status. In addition, pathologic conditions that lead to cardiomyopathy, valve obstruction, renal artery occlusion, and lupus erythematosus are antibody-antigen triggered (Asherson and Cervera, 1992). The client will be diag-

---

BOX 22-6 Tests for Lupus and Autoimmune Antibodies

1. Follow C3 and C4 levels (complement)
2. Follow PT and PTT times, blood cell levels
3. Antibody levels
- *Antinuclear antibody (ANA)* against person's own cells.
- *Lupus anticoagulant antibody (LA).* Causes thrombosis first and, when platelets are consumed, may cause bleeding. Releases TXA_2 from platelets, stimulating vasoconstriction and increased BP. May be activated by drugs such as chlorpromazine and procainamide. Gives false VDRL result.
- *Anticardiolipin antibody (ACL).* IgG, IgM, and IgA may cross placenta to affect fetus, depending on maternal level. High risk of deep venous thrombosis, arterial thrombosis with cerebral infarct, transient ischemic attack, and placental thrombosis. High risk of fetal loss.
- *Sicca syndrome: SS-A antibody.* Causes congenital heart block with fetal heart rate less than 90/min, and/or *SS-B antibody* sometimes results in neonatal lupus with rash when infant is exposed to ultraviolet rays.

Antiphospholipid syndrome

Presence of one or two of above without clear diagnosis of lupus

Modified from Hadi HA, Treadwell EL: Lupus anticoagulant and anticardiolipin antibodies in pregnancy: a review, *Obstet Gynecol Surv* 45:117, 1990.

---

nosed as having **antiphospholipid syndrome (APS)** if any one of the antibodies in the listing in Box 22-6 is present or if there is repeated fetal loss or thrombotic disease. Clinical management is discussed in the section that follows.

LUPUS ERYTHEMATOSUS

Lupus erythematosus (LE) usually is diagnosed by a rheumatologist because the most common presenting sign is *migrating arthritis*. Before the autoimmune theory was clarified, a person may have sought many sources for help, each treating only the presenting symptom. Usually damage was well advanced, and kidney failure was a common cause of death.

Pregnancy does not appear to worsen LE (Hadi and Treadwell, 1990), but if a woman becomes pregnant soon after or before an episode or already has significant renal damage and hypertension, placental damage can lead to spontaneous abortion. A flare during pregnancy is dangerous to mother and fetus. Ideally a pregnancy should be started only when the woman is in clear remission. There seems to be special risk in the postpartum period, perhaps related to the hormonal changes taking place. Nurses should be alert to the potential danger to any known lupus client or anyone with APS.

Risk

The incidence occurs in a ratio of ten women to one man, which is believed to relate to female hormonal patterns. LE occurs in 1:700 women between 15 and 64 years of age but is seen in African-American women in a ratio of 1:250. In past decades, life expectancy after diagnosis was 5 years. The outcome now depends on early diagnosis and treatment and is much more hopeful. The fetal outcome is less hopeful, and loss of the pregnancy occurs in about 30% in the first trimester and 20% in the second trimester (Out, Derksen, and Christiaens, 1989). The newborn is at risk for temporary neonatal lupus if the mother's serum contains any SS-B antibodies. **Photosensitivity** will cause a rash in the newborn, or the infant may have congenital heart block. Because these are maternal antibodies, the effect may gradually diminish; the infant *does not* continue to have a lupus syndrome.

Signs

Early signs are insidious and may contribute to a diagnosis of APS. These are malaise, joint aching, low-grade fever, hypertension, and a thrombotic event.

In pregnancy this may easily be confused with PIH. There may be new onset of migraines (see Chapter 23) and *amaurosis fugax,* which is a temporary "white out" with loss of vision in one eye, thought to be due to platelet clumping in the retinal arteries. Reynaud's disease also has been linked (Table 22-3).

There are flares and resolutions. Antibodies are found in increasing amounts (titers), and antibody titers are followed to show when improvement begins. Because of the migrating character of the symptoms, a client does not know what will occur next. Depending on where thrombi are deposited, renal involvement with signs of damage may be evident. Skin flare-ups include a typical lupus "butterfly" rash over the face, chest, and hands, that is triggered by exposure to ultraviolet light: sunlight, fluorescents, or even the light from copy machines (Figure 22-7). All persons with LE must use a sunscreen with a sun protection factor of 15 to 30 whenever they are exposed to these sources of light.

Clinical Management

Antibody levels are followed, along with renal tests and BP checks. Treatment includes a combination of low-dose corticosteroids (15 to 40 mg/day) and low-dose aspirin (75 to 80 mg/day) as an anti-TXA$_2$ agent. If an acute episode with rising antibody titers occurs, hospitalization is required, with higher doses of IV cortisone and heparin infusion. In very severe cases, human

TABLE 22-3 Criteria for Lupus Erythematosus*

SIGN	DESCRIPTION	CLIENTS WITH SIGN (%)
Malar rash (butterfly)	Erythema patches on face/hands	50
Discoid rash	Plaques, spread easily	Less often
Photosensitivity	Rash after UV exposure	25
Oral and nasal ulcers	Painless; on hard or soft palate, nasal septum	Less often
Arthritis/arthralgia	Symmetric morning stiffness; swelling in joints	90
History of pleuritis/pericarditis	Pleurisy, pleural effusion with URI	50-90
Proteinuria/renal signs	2-3+ with sediment, RBC, casts, and creatinine >1.6 mg	50
Psychosis, seizures	Grand mal, organic brain syndrome, CNS problems, microinfarcts	Rare, but especially after birth
Hematologic disorder	Thrombocytopenia, leukopenia, hemolytic anemia	Less often
Immunologic changes	Positive LE factor, VDRL; anti-DNA antibodies	20-30
Antinuclear antibodies	Abnormal titer	100

Modified from Revised criteria for classification of systemic lupus erythematosus and from Hadi HA, Treadwell EL: *Obstet Gynecol Surv* 45:117, 1990.
UV, Ultraviolet; *URI,* upper respiratory infection; *RBC,* red blood cell; *CNS,* central nervous system.
*Diagnosis of LE if 4 of 11 signs are present.

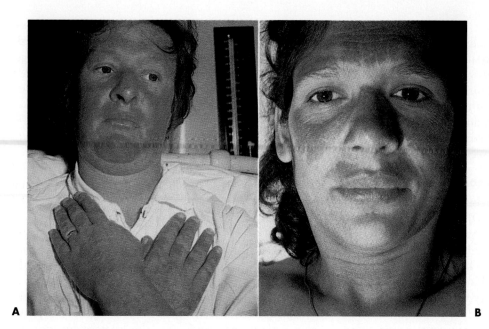

FIGURE 22-7 Comparison between lupus rash (**A**) and melasma (**B**). Note that lupus rash is much more reddened than normal melasma and is on face and chest. (Used with permission of Harcourt Brace Jovanovich Group [Australia] from Beischer NA, MacKay EV: *Obstetrics and the newborn,* ed 3, Sydney, 1993, WB Saunders.)

A   **B**

immunoglobulin may be transfused to reduce antibody levels, or *plasmapheresis* (plasma exchange transfusion) may be selected to quickly lower levels of antibodies. Immunosuppressive drugs such as azathroprine (Imuran) and cyclophosphamide (Cytoxan) have been used. Blood counts must be monitored closely.

Nursing Responsibilities

The woman with LE who wishes to be or is pregnant is vulnerable to fetal loss and usually understands the grave nature of her disease. Symptoms include fatigue and depression. If she is taking steroids, there may be changes in mood and fluid retention. She also may worry about the effect of medications on the fetus. The nurse can reassure her that without these drugs the effects of LE might be damaging but rarely do the doses she must take affect fetal growth and development. Because fatigue and depression are included in her symptoms, the family should be involved in observing the woman's mood and looking for signs of advancing depression or behavior changes.

Dental care may be required. Often there is a lack of saliva and increased caries, bleeding gums, oral ulcers, and candidal infection. The woman should be referred for evaluation and preventive care and taught precautions and care for exposure to ultraviolet rays.

The nurse must assess when confronted with confusing symptoms and remember the potential for exacerbation in the postpartum period. There have been rare cases of women who went through pregnancy with hypertension, gave birth safely, but then suddenly became less responsive and had seizures. The first thought is eclampsia, especially if albuminuria accompanies kidney involvement. But LE should be considered as well, because a form of cerebral lupus occurs in the postpartum period that results from multiple microinfarcts in the brain, beginning with restlessness, confusion, and vague personality changes, and leads to coma and death (Sala and Lentz, 1986).

I was assigned to Carmen, a young single mother who was frightened by the birth. She was thought to be somewhat "slow" mentally, which seemed the cause of her lack of understanding of self-care. She was flushed and frightened during labor. A rash was noted on her neck, chest, and face. I took her to the shower. She needed help undressing, and during the shower she moved her bowels. I got her back to bed and called for help with assessment. Vital signs were normal, but her mental state was bizarre. She wouldn't look at the baby and kept moving her head back and forth in the bed. She became progressively unresponsive over the next hour while being examined by a number of persons. She was taken to the ICU where after extensive work-up her diagnosis was LE with cerebral involvement. She died 2 weeks later.

The client requires education about her drugs. Because steroids may mask infection, she needs particularly to avoid sources of infection. The nurse should discuss with her her desire to breast-feed, checking dosage with drug tables; steroid doses under 30 mg/day are thought to be acceptable. The infant should be followed up for growth ratios when the lactating mother is on a daily medication regimen. She will benefit by referral to one of the support groups for persons with LE. Certainly, if there is any disability, she will need referrals for home care follow-up.

THROMBOPHLEBITIS

Although **thrombophlebitis** (clot formation, with inflammation, in the venous system) may occur during pregnancy, it is primarily a recovery problem because of physiologic factors. Increased thrombocytosis (increased circulating platelets), increased thromboplastin release, and an increase in some blood clotting factors contribute to the development of a thrombus in the venous system. A client with APS may have recurrent episodes.

Superficial Vein Thrombophlebitis

Superficial vein thrombophlebitis (SVT), one of the thromboembolic diseases (TED), is seen most often in saphenous veins. Women who have preexisting varicose veins or prior episodes are at higher risk (see Chapter 9). Other predisposing factors are obesity, high parity, advanced maternal age, and previous heart disease. In addition, bed rest with immobility associated with surgery, anesthesia, or complications can result in thromboembolic disease. Estrogens once were used to suppress lactation but rarely are used now because of an association with an increased incidence of emboli.

SVT is accompanied by moderate to severe inflammation, causing pain and swelling over the site. Sometimes there is a low-grade fever and an elevated pulse.

Deep Vein Thrombus

The onset of deep vein thrombus (DVT) varies; a few cases begin during the antepartum period, but most begin within 72 hours of birth, with some occurring as late as 22 days after birth. A related cause is antiphospholipid antibodies (see discussion of LE). When a thrombus forms in the deep veins of the leg, the swollen leg becomes cyanotic or may be pale. Reflex arteriolar spasm causes severe pain. The location of the pain depends on the vein involved: in the popliteal and lateral tibial areas, in the low calf and foot, in the inguinal area, or even in the pelvic veins.

Risk. SVT occurs in approximately 1.5:1000 women who have vaginal births and has been reported in slightly higher levels after cesarean birth. Early ambulation has reduced the incidence. Deeper vein embolus has a much lower incidence but is very serious when it occurs.

DVT carries a risk of pulmonary embolism. In addition, Bergquist et al (1990) found that a postphlebotic syndrome could persist in 3.4% of her clients. This included intermittent swelling of the extremity, pain, cramping, and in some cases later ulceration of the lower leg. *Osteoporosis* may occur with prolonged heparin therapy. Whenever possible, an oral anticoagulant (warfarin [Coumadin]) is substituted after birth (Cosico et al, 1993).

Clinical management. A physical examination usually cannot pinpoint the trouble, and Doppler ultrasound, contrast venography, or a computerized tomography (CT) scan may be used. Anticoagulants rarely are used for SVT. The clot is fixed and small, and there is little danger of an embolus to the heart or lungs. Management of DVT includes all the treatment used for SVT plus anticoagulants, antibiotics, and venous compression when the leg improves. A heparin loading dose of 100 U/kg is followed by 15 to 20 U/kg/hr until there is a stable *activated partial thromboplastin time (aPTT)* of approximately 1.5 to 2.0 times the control. After a week of IV heparin therapy, subcutaneous therapy twice a day is begun (Drug Profile). Sometimes low molecular weight heparin (with a longer half-life (t½) is used as a single daily injection (Hull et al, 1992).

In rare critical cases of threatened pulmonary embolism, surgical treatment may be indicated; the client may undergo an embolectomy, or a screening tent may be placed in the vena cava to prevent passage of emboli to the lungs. Clotting and thromboplastin times are tested at regular intervals. Analgesics usually are needed. However, aspirin and agents that alter platelet function are contraindicated. Phenylbutazone and other antiinflammatory agents should not be given during the first trimester because of embryotoxicity. These agents also pass into breast milk and are not used for lactating mothers.

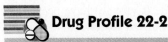

Drug Profile 22-2

Heparin sodium
Action

Inhibits clotting sequence. Acts at multiple sites. Does not dissolve existing clots. Because large molecule does not cross placenta, it may be used up to 4 hours before birth inasmuch as t½ is rapid. Lower molecular weight type has a longer t½ and can be used as a daily dose.

Dose/route

SC, never IM. 5000 U q12h or as an IV infusion continuously over 24 hours. Titrated to aPTT levels and clotting time, which are measured regularly. Protamine sulfate is antagonist, given over 20- to 30-minute intervals if bleeding occurs.

Side effects/adverse effects

Thrombocytopenia, hemorrhage with oozing from mucous membranes, ecchymosis. Hypersensitivity with fever, urticaria. IV site may become locally irritated and SC site ecchymotic. Sometimes rash, diarrhea. Long-term use (5 to 6 months) may lead to osteoporosis.

Precautions

Rotate SC sites carefully. Do not aspirate or use site with less than one half inch fatty tissue. Mother may breast-feed. Observe for signs of oozing or hemorrhage. Note laboratory reports.

Nursing Responsibilities

Supportive interventions for SVT include bed rest until pain and swelling subside. Legs are elevated to reduce edema and to shunt blood into the deep veins. Moist heat is applied to dilate the veins and improve circulation. Analgesics are given for inflammation and pain. Anticoagulants rarely are necessary.

Because varicose veins are so commonly associated with SVT, as soon as the swelling decreases, the client is measured for pressure-gradient elastic stockings and encouraged to ambulate. To be effective, these stockings must be applied before she sits or stands. Until her custom-fitted stockings arrive, elastic bandaging is used. The woman must learn how to put on the stockings or how to bandage her legs. In addition, she must avoid prolonged standing or sitting with crossed legs.

The same treatment for SVT is used with DVT, plus anticoagulant and antibiotic therapy. The client may be anxious about moving because she fears loosening the clot. The nurse helps her to comply with the regimen of bed rest until pain and swelling have disappeared.

The client needs to learn self-injection with heparin if she is going home on this therapy regimen. Encourage self-injection during the hospital stay, helping her maintain some control, and teaching her to observe for any signs of bleeding tendency that might develop with prolonged therapy.

Because of prolonged bed rest with DVT, active and passive range of motion exercises are important to enhance venous flow. The extended period of bed rest will be difficult to adjust to and may markedly upset family life. Social service personnel should be involved in arrangements if there are children at home.

AMNIOTIC FLUID EMBOLISM

In very rare instances, amniotic fluid is drawn into the woman's venous circulation (Figure 22-8). The fluid contains debris such as meconium, vernix, and lanugo, which along with other abnormal substances in the fluid triggers cardiogenic shock. Amniotic fluid embolism (AFE) occurs after an intense, tumultuous labor, a hypertonic oxytocin stimulation of labor, or uterine or abdominal trauma. It also has occurred in the postpartum period as late as 48 hours after birth (Clark, 1990).

AFE cannot be predicted or prevented; it constitutes a medical emergency in which every member of the health team must work rapidly to sustain the life of the mother and fetus. *AFE occurs usually during labor*

Risk

AFE is rare (1 in 37,000 births), with a high maternal mortality rate of 85% (Duff, 1984). It is a leading cause of maternal death in many countries, including the United States (Franks et al, 1990).

Signs

In an otherwise healthy woman, AFE manifests by sudden dyspnea with a bluish gray pallor, coughing

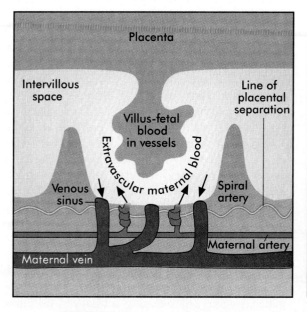
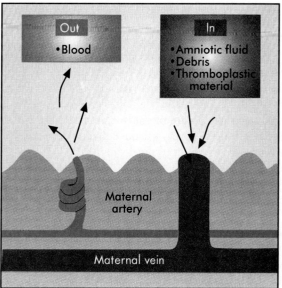

FIGURE 22-8 Amniotic fluid embolism. The placental circulation may suck amniotic fluid into the venous flow.

with frothy pink sputum, and hypotension. Respiratory collapse and cor pulmonale occur as fluid substances infiltrate the lung circulation. Signs of shock appear, preceded by chills, diaphoresis, and extreme anxiety. There may be seizures. Uterine atony occurs, leading to hemorrhage. Disseminated intravascular coagulation may complicate treatment of hemorrhage, and adult respiratory distress syndrome with pulmonary edema may occur. Fetal distress is clearly evident, and fetal death may occur.

Clinical Management

Cardiopulmonary life support must be started at once by means of oxygen and support of blood volume. A PAC line is monitored to prevent fluid overload. Depending on the incident in relation to birth, a cesarean may be performed to save the infant. Only with skilled, prompt intervention is there a chance to save the woman's life.

OBSTETRIC PULMONARY EMBOLISM

In some instances a clot breaks off from the deep femoral or pelvic vein thrombosis and travels to the heart and then to the pulmonary artery, causing a pulmonary **embolism**. Respiratory signs may be sudden, and the syndrome progresses rapidly. Sometimes this occurs after the client has returned home; either the thrombus develops late or is undiscovered before she is discharged.

Risk

A client at risk for embolus has a prior history of thrombophlebitis and varicose veins, cardiac disease, and obesity, is an older multipara, or has been placed on lengthy bed rest because of complications. Of women with DVT in the femoral or iliac veins 10% to 15% will have a pulmonary episode (Beischer and MacKay, 1993). Pulmonary embolism was the leading cause of maternal mortality before early ambulation. In many countries, emboli still are a major cause of maternal death. Today in the United States pulmonary embolism is the most common medical cause of maternal mortality (Communicable Disease Center, 1991). The client may complain of sharp stabbing pain in her chest that mimics a heart attack. She may make statements that she "is going to die."

Signs

Classic signs are as follows:

- Tachypnea
- Dyspnea
- Pleuritic pain
- Apprehension
- Cough/hemoptysis
- Diaphoresis
- Fever
- Râles

Signs such as sudden shortness of breath, cyanosis, and hemoptysis may be accompanied by a sense of pressure in the bowel or rectum. Collapse may occur within seconds or minutes if a large blood vessel is blocked. If smaller vessels are blocked, lung tissue is deprived of blood and dies (infarct). In this case, signs are tachycardia, tachypnea, and cough with blood-tinged sputum.

Clinical Management

If a pulmonary embolism is suspected, clinical therapy should begin immediately. Electrocardiogram, x-ray films, and laboratory tests are not always accurate and take valuable time. Pulmonary arteriography and ventilation-perfusion scan (V/Q scan) are diagnostic. Death could occur if treatment is postponed to collect diagnostic data. Strict bed rest in high Fowler's position should be maintained and nasal oxygen administered. A heparin infusion, pain medication, and sedation are begun. Fibrolytic therapy, such as streptokinase, may be attempted to lyse a large clot. An embolectomy may be necessary for this critical condition.

PULMONARY EDEMA

A number of factors predispose the woman to the high risk of *pulmonary edema* when complications of pregnancy occur. First, the physiologic changes of pregnancy include hemodilution because of physiologic hypervolemia, lowered serum albumin with a lower colloid osmotic pressure (COP), and renal changes. These normal variations may be exaggerated by hemorrhage when infusion of crystalloid fluids is given rapidly. Tocolytic therapy with ritodrine or terbutaline has resulted in pulmonary edema. Excessive duration and amount of oxytocin infusion have been implicated in water retention because of an antidiuretic action. When corticosteroids are used (for asthma, preterm labor), permeability of the lung tissue is affected and the risk increases. Other factors are severe anemia (see Chapter 23), hypokalemia with magnesium sulfate infusion, preeclampsia, chronic cocaine use, and severe cardiac and renal disease. Sepsis may precipitate pulmonary edema from noncardiogenic reasons related to increased permeability of the lung tissue to fluids.

Acute lung injury—*adult respiratory distress syndrome (ARDS)* is characterized by *noncardiogenic* pulmonary edema and is a major cause of morbidity and mortality in obstetrics today. ARDS is precipitated by indirect injury to the lungs related to shock, sepsis, and disseminated intravascular coagulation (Chapter 23), and may result from trauma. In these cases normal blood flow through the lungs is reduced for some reason and platelets aggregate, releasing substances, including histamine, serotonin, and bradykinin, that damage alveolar membranes (Shailor, Roach, and Weisnor, 1992).

TABLE 22-4   Alterations in Normal Pregnancy Hemodynamics

NORMAL VALUES*	ALTERATIONS
CENTRAL VENOUS PRESSURE	
1-7 mm Hg (responds slowly to changes)	Low = Severe volume depletion
POSITIVE AIRWAY PRESSURE	
Pulmonary artery systolic: 18-30 mm Hg indicates right afterload	Low = Volume depletion, decreased right preload
Pulmonary artery diastolic: 6-10 mm Hg (similar to PCWP)	High = Fluid overload
PULMONARY CAPILLARY WEDGE PRESSURE	
Intermittent: 6-10 mm Hg	Low = Decreased left preload
	High = Increased left preload
Cardiac output 6-7 L/min	Low = Volume depletion
	High = Volume excess
ARTERIAL BP	
Measures left afterload	

*Measured by PAC.

Fluid leaks into the lungs, lung volume decreases, and hypoxia develops. A vicious cycle develops rapidly as lung damage impairs surfactant supply and gas exchange. The same process is reflected in the preterm infant (see Chapter 28), and providing oxygen by mask does not correct the worsening hypoxia and respiratory distress. Even with tachypnea, oxygen levels fall. Metabolic acidosis worsens.

ARDS in one survey was found in preeclampsia, HELLP syndrome, acute fatty liver of pregnancy, amnionitis, bacterial sepsis, pyelonephritis, status epilepticus, and after aspiration and trauma from motor vehicle accidents (Catanzarite et al, 1991).

Signs

Signs of pulmonary edema are as follows:
- Hypoxia, cyanosis
- Tachypnea
- Tachycardia
- Pulmonary infiltration: crackling sounds, wheezing
- Increased BP, depending on precipitating factor
- Cool, moist skin
- Restlessness, confusion
- Fetal distress

Clinical Management of Adult Respiratory Distress Syndrome

ARDS must be managed with intubation and ventilator-regulated oxygenation, positioning, antibiotics, and fluid volume regulation monitored with a PAC. In spite of treatment the result often is fatal for the fetus and mother.

Management of Pulmonary Edema

Early diagnosis of the susceptible client will prevent iatrogenic causes such as fluid overload. PAC monitoring greatly assists management in certain cases (Table 22-4 and Figure 22-8). Oxygen must be delivered by means of intermittent positive pressure. If the cause is fluid imbalance, it must be corrected, either by modifying the IV infusion or by diuretics. Furosemide commonly is used. A Foley catheter must be in place for hourly urine output measurements. The causative factors are corrected: vasodilators for vasospasm, antibiotics for infection, and albumin or hetastarch to raise low COP. Morphine sulfate is given to diminish anxiety and for its benefit as a vasodilator, thus reducing preload temporarily. The client is placed on vital sign monitors, and IV pumps control infusions. If the woman is in labor, epidural anesthesia may help to reduce preload by vasodilation of the circulation in the lower extremities. Rapid reversal of symptoms of pulmonary edema occurs with correct interventions. If the woman's condition deteriorates, ARDS and multiorgan failure must be suspected.

Cardiac Disease during Pregnancy

Every pregnancy affects the cardiovascular system. The increased blood volume especially may be a problem for a woman with cardiac compromise, because of the peak volume at 28 to 32 weeks of gestation. A woman with a healthy heart can tolerate the stress of pregnancy, but when heart function has been affected by heart disease, pregnancy can be complicated.

CLASSIFICATION OF DISABILITY

An important determinant is the degree of disability caused by the heart disease. The following New York Heart Association functional classification of heart disease is accepted as a standard guide:

Class I   No symptoms of cardiac insufficiency on exertion (uncompromised)
No limitations on physical activity

Class II   Symptoms felt on ordinary exertion (slightly compromised)
A slight limitation of physical activity

Class III   Symptoms felt even during limited activity (moderately compromised)

Class IV   Symptoms occurring during any physical activity, even at rest (severely compromised)

The three major types of heart disease encountered in pregnant women are rheumatic heart disease, congenital heart anomalies, and heart changes resulting from hypertension.

Risk

It is estimated that some form of heart disease occurs in 1% to 2% of pregnant women (Danforth and Scott, 1987). Spontaneous abortion and premature labor are more prevalent in these women than in other childbearing women. Respiratory acidosis in severe cases may cause fetal distress if the baby is prematurely born. Some newborns appear growth-retarded, probably as a result of low oxygen pressure in women who have severe cardiac disease. Finally, the incidence of myocardial infarction during pregnancy is 1 in 10,000 (Kirkland, 1991; Lamb, 1987).

Test Yourself

Match the description of the management of heart disease in a pregnant woman with the classification of heart disease determined by the New York Heart Association.

a. Bed rest is necessary for most of the day. Client is hospitalized for final weeks of pregnancy; cardiac symptoms occur during and after labor.

b. Stress should be limited; additional periods of rest are recommended after meals and at night. Vaginal delivery is planned with use of oxygen and monitoring.

c. Cardiac signs and symptoms occur at rest.

1. Class I
2. Class II
3. Class III

RHEUMATIC HEART DISEASE

Rheumatic heart disease (RHD) is the most common cause of heart disease encountered in childbearing women. RHD previously accounted for 60% to 80% of all heart disease during pregnancy, but its incidence has decreased in the past 20 years, probably because of improved childhood treatment. Studies, however, report a resurgence of RHD in some parts of the country (Veasey, 1987); therefore it remains an important health problem.

RHD must be considered when a pregnant woman complains of chest or joint pains or if she has an unexplained fever or dyspnea and orthopnea, which can be signs of congestive heart failure. RHD often causes mitral stenosis, which restricts cardiac output, causing fatigue, the most common symptom. As blood flow to the left atrium becomes obstructed, pressures then become elevated in the left atrium, pulmonary veins, and pulmonary capillaries. The left atrium becomes distended, which results in pulmonary congestion, causing symptoms of dyspnea and orthopnea, usually by the twentieth week. Pulmonary artery pressures increase, causing failure of the right side of the heart. If atrial fibrillation ensues, the normal changes of cardiac output, slight tachycardia, and normal fluid retention of pregnancy contribute toward deterioration in the woman's functional status. The risk of thrombus formation increases. Management of thrombotic problems is discussed earlier in this chapter.

Clinical management of **mitral stenosis** in a pregnant woman involves antibiotic therapy, because this condition is believed to be caused exclusively by previous RHD. If despite antibiotic therapy her pulmonary congestion does not improve, on rare occasion mitral commissurotomy may be performed. Valve replacement also can be performed during pregnancy, but fetal loss may be as high as 35%.

Mitral regurgitation may be caused by RHD, as well as by previous endocarditis or, rarely, by structural factors. The client complains of fatigue related to a decrease in blood flow from the left ventricle. It usually is a much less severe condition than that resulting from mitral stenosis. Some clients with mitral regurgitation remain symptom free for years, even during pregnancy. Prophylaxis against streptococcal endocarditis is indicated. Surgery is unnecessary.

Aortic regurgitation occurs as a result of RHD, endocarditis, rheumatic arthritis, systemic lupus erythematosis, or Marfan's syndrome. Because of aortic valve incompetence, some of the left ventricle output flows back into the left ventricle during diastole. The left ventricle dilates in an effort to compensate. The left ventricle pressure causes pulmonary congestion. With rest, this condition sometimes is tolerated during pregnancy. If pulmonary congestion occurs, bed rest, diuretics, and digitalis, as well as antibiotic prophylaxis, are recommended.

CONGENITAL HEART DISEASE

The number of women with **congenital heart disease** (**CHD**) recently has increased because of better survival as a result of treatment during early childhood. Women with successfully repaired childhood defects will have little or no problem. The degree to which the woman's condition is compromised depends on the defect. Some women have left-to-right shunts because of an atrial septal defect or a patent ductus arteriosus. Some women are unaware of defects until they reach adulthood or become pregnant. These defects often are tolerated by the well-monitored pregnant woman, unless pulmonary hypertension develops.

Right-to-left shunts carry a higher risk of mortality. They usually occur from tetralogy of Fallot, which is a combination of an atrial septal defect, ventral septal defect, and patent ductus arteriosus. Certain degrees of cyanosis and clubbing develop in these clients, and chest x-ray films reveal right ventricular hypertrophy. If pulmonary hypertension occurs, there is a 50% mortality rate.

Any woman with congenital heart disease who shows cyanosis or clubbing of the fingers must be counseled about the risks of pregnancy for herself and her fetus.

DISSECTING ANEURYSM OF THE AORTA

Aortic aneurysm is a rare but dangerous occurrence in childbearing women. It sometimes is associated with Marfan's syndrome, an autosomal dominant inherited disorder of the connective tissue.

Necrosis and tearing occur in the aortic wall, possibly resulting from the increased blood volume and a general softening of collagen during pregnancy. Because of the characteristic locations of these tears, it is thought that they are caused by the systolic force. Aortic branches can become occluded, and the aortic valve can become detached. The fetus is at risk because the placenta does not receive sufficient blood flow (see Roth, Riley, and Cohen, 1992, for a case example).

Medical management of dissecting aortic aneurysm requires medications (e.g., propranolol) that decrease blood pressure and the force of myocardial contractions. Cardiopulmonary bypass is required for surgical correction.

HEART DISEASE RELATED TO HYPERTENSION

Women with chronic hypertension may exhibit heart disease. Recently many women have postponed child-bearing until their later years. Some of these women have stressful careers, live fast-paced lives, and have poor health habits. These women should be promptly screened for hypertension and cardiovascular problems (Burke, 1989).

Clinical Management

The woman is interviewed carefully for subjective symptoms of cardiac insufficiency. In addition, the functional classification of her heart condition is evaluated, including the following:

1. Shortness of breath or fatigue during her usual activities of daily living (ADL)
2. Frequent coughing, with or without hemoptysis
3. Feelings of "palpitations" or recognized arrhythmias

Physical examination reveals objective symptoms, such as generalized edema, rales at the lung bases, and cardiac arrhythmias such as murmurs. The clinical diagnosis of heart disease requires a complete physical examination, x-ray films to determine cardiac enlargement, electrocardiogram (ECG), and examination by ultrasound or echocardiogram.

The woman might be asked to keep several appointments per week, especially between 28 and 32 weeks of gestation, when her blood volume is highest. She will be reevaluated for functional classification, based on her disability at that time. Sometimes, if cardiac status is deteriorating, she must be hospitalized for stabilization during the third trimester.

Labor Precautions

Monitoring during labor of clients with class III or IV disability includes central hemodynamic monitoring (Figure 22-9) and electrocardiographic continuous readings. Pain must be managed to reduce stress and heart rate. Low-dose morphine (2 to 3 mg) and low-dose bupivacaine (0.25%) via epidural catheter has been found useful to manage pain (see Chapter 16). Delivery is accomplished as smoothly as possible; vaginal birth without intense pushing or Valsalva's maneuver is important. *Cardiac stress from surgical delivery is equal to or greater than that from vaginal delivery;* therefore operative delivery is done only for obstetric reasons.

Nursing Responsibilities
▶ ASSESSMENT

Care focuses on assessment, education, and monitoring of compliance, often with restrictive activity levels and medication routines. The woman must be a full partner in care decisions.

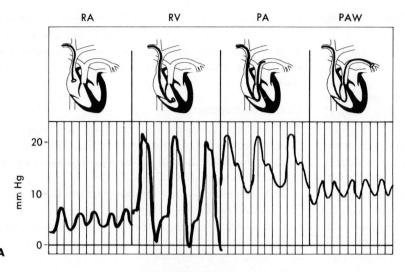

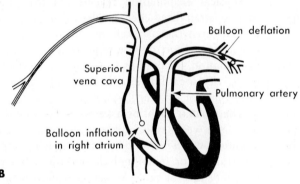

FIGURE 22-9 A, Flow-directed, balloon-tipped catheter locations with corresponding pressure tracings. **B,** Flow-directed, balloon-tipped catheter showing inflation of balloon in the right atrium and consequent "floating" of the catheter through the right ventricle and out to a distal pulmonary artery branch. The balloon is deflated, advanced slightly, and reinflated slightly to obtain a pulmonary artery wedge pressure. (From Schroeder JS, Daily EK: Hemodynamic monitoring [slide series], Tarpon Springs, Fla, 1976, Tampa Tracings.)

▶ NURSING DIAGNOSES

1. Decreased cardiac output related to cardiac disease hemodynamics plus changes induced by pregnancy
2. Activity intolerance related to decreased perfusion of vital organs
3. High risk for fluid volume deficit related to daily use of diuretics
4. High risk for fluid volume excess related to infusions during labor or anesthesia
5. Altered comfort related to anxiety, contractions, and central hemodynamic monitoring during labor
6. Potential for infection or phlebitis related to method of birth, susceptibility to valvular disease, thromboembolism
7. Altered parenting related to fatigue, activity restrictions

▶ EXPECTED OUTCOMES

1. Tissue perfusion is maintained.
2. Fetal growth and development are within normal limits.
3. Woman remains free of infection or thromboembolism.
4. She monitors medications, effects, and cardiac symptoms and reports promptly.

5. She finds ways to cope with stress of pregnancy, rests as advised.
6. She finds balance between activity limitation and parenting activities.

▶ NURSING INTERVENTIONS

The primary nursing problems are alteration in cardiac output and activity intolerance. Activities and interventions are directed toward helping the woman to minimize the stress of her pregnancy, as well as to preserve her cardiac function.

Interventions include frequent assessment of vital signs, subjective symptoms, and activity tolerance. An appropriate activity level will be evaluated and established by the physician and supported by the nurse. The woman will be counseled about her activity limitation and her needs for sleep and rest periods to improve cardiac reserve. Knowledge deficits about medications and nutritional demands of pregnancy must be explored and the woman's positive self-care behaviors reinforced.

At this time the woman and her family want to begin planning for childbirth, and they will have many concerns. Anxiety and ineffective coping are common during the third trimester. The nurse must offer emotional support during such a high-risk pregnancy.

Labor and delivery can be stressful for the woman and fetus. The management of the birth depends on the recent functional classification of the woman's disability and the response of woman and fetus to labor stress.

The main goals are to reduce maternal exertion and promote cardiac reserve. Promote relaxation throughout labor while monitoring maternal vital signs, fetal heart rate, and labor progress. Continuously monitor maternal cardiac status. Position the woman on her left side in Semi-Folwer's position to promote cardiac emptying and placental perfusion. Give oxygen by mask because laboring women usually breathe by mouth. Diuretics, digitalis, and analgesics must be accessible if needed. IV fluids must be carefully monitored to *prevent fluid overload.*

The second stage of labor is especially stressful. The woman who is allowed to push is instructed to *prevent the Valsalva maneuver* by using shorter open-glottis pushes. She must not become short of oxygen by holding her breath. The woman is encouraged to relax between pushes. She should be allowed to follow her own instinctive desires to push rather than being forced to bear down with each contraction (Cosner and de-Jong, 1993). After expulsion of the placenta, even with blood loss during delivery, additional blood volume may strain the woman's cardiac reserves. Extravascular fluid now moves into her bloodstream, and blood flow through the heart is greatly increased for approximately 1 week. Continuous cardiac and postpartum monitoring and laboratory tests are used to assess the maternal condition for at least 48 hours.

Because there is a potential for infection, prophylactic antibiotics are administered during labor and throughout the postpartum time. The woman should be in a private room if possible. She must be protected until clinical evaluation reveals that she is free from bacterial endocarditis.

Bed rest is crucial for women with classes II, III, and IV disability until cardiac function is stabilized and they can tolerate increased activity and progressive ambula-

tion. This activity limitation poses other problems. Constipation is a particularly serious problem for the woman with cardiac disease because she should not strain during bowel movements. She should receive high-fiber food, adequate fluid intake, and prescribed stool softeners to draw water into the stool. A self-care deficit exists, and total or partial care is necessary, depending on her status.

The nurse will need to work on the alteration in parenting roles related to the separation of the newborn from its mother. If the mother is fatigued, the infant should be kept at the mother's bedside while a nurse or family member provides infant care and feeding. Touching and eye contact are important for establishing an emotional bond between mother and infant, without causing a weak mother to exert herself or lift her baby.

Although women with class I or II disability usually can breast-feed without any problem, antibiotics or other medications must be evaluated for potential effects on the newborn. Usually, because lactation presents increased requirements for rest and nutrition, class III and IV cardiac clients do not breast-feed.

Discharge requires careful nursing assessment and planning. The mother needs to balance her requirements for rest and her energy potential with her parenting responsibilities. Together, the nurse and woman must evaluate her self-care capability. The available home support for mother and baby must be evaluated. Appropriate home referrals must be initiated promptly.

▶ EVALUATION

1. Was the newborn's growth normal?
2. Did infection or thromboembolism occur?
3. Did monitoring detect problems that were quickly corrected?
4. Is the woman knowledgeable regarding self- and infant care?
5. Have referrals or home care been processed?

KEY POINTS

- Inadequate or noncompliant care for asthma may lead to irreversible hypertrophy, disability, and death.
- Management of asthma depends primarily on the client's recognition of early changes in her peak expiratory flow rate (PEFR) and instituting corrective medication before events escalate.
- Diagnosis of pregnancy-induced hypertension (PIH) is difficult because of the prevalence of undiscovered chronic hypertension and the antiphospholipid syndrome.
- Platelet counts have assumed a new importance in PIH and HELLP syndrome. Levels below 100,000/mm^3 are

considered signals of serious risk of bleeding and a pathologic condition.
- Prevention of eclampsia is necessary because of the potential of death and cerebral damage associated with vasoconstriction, edema, and seizures. Seizures may occur at any time.
- Lupus erythematosus is diagnosed more commonly than in the past, and pregnancy loss, thromboembolism, and hypertension often are related to autoimmune antibody formation.
- Preventive care for superficial vein thrombosis (SVT) and deep vein thrombosis (DVT), types of throm-

boembolic disease, must be begun before pregnancy in susceptible women. Pregnancy alters the clotting mechanisms, which increases risk in these cases.

- Amniotic fluid embolism and pulmonary embolism are critical events for which intense collaborative care is required to prevent maternal or fetal mortality.
- Pulmonary edema may occur with an abnormally low colloid osmotic pressure (COP) or a fluid over-

load, both of which may occur in crisis situations unless there is very careful monitoring of fluids and hemodynamic status.

- The pregnancy outcome of a client with cardiac disability depends primarily on her functional cardiac status. Special care and monitoring are required during the third trimester, labor, and recovery periods.

STUDY QUESTIONS

22-1 Select a Key Term in this chapter to fit each of the following statements.

   a. When the hematocrit level is elevated and blood volume lowered there is _Hemoconcentratio_

   b. The result of infection in heart muscle or valves is _RHD_

   c. The single sign of hypertension accompanying pregnancy occurs in the condition called _gestational hypertension_

   d. The condition of sudden dyspnea, cyanosis, and hemoptysis after birth could be caused by _Obstetric Pulmonary Embolism_ [Amniotic Fluid Embolism]

   e. A rash forms on the face, chest, or arms when a person is exposed to ultraviolet rays _Photosensitiy_

   f. Resulting from PIH, a defect of vision in one or both eyes is _Scotoma_

   g. Change in permeability of tissue barriers is a result of lowered _Colloid Osmotic Pressure_

   h. Lowered platelet counts result in a condition called _Thrombocytopenia_

22-2 Janice Smith, 33 and para 2010, is admitted to the antepartum unit because of signs of preeclampsia. During the nursing history interview, which statement by her increases the risk of serious hypertension?

   a. Previous history of several spontaneous abortions

   b. Maternal grandmother died of cerebrovascular accident

   c. Client has had borderline hypertension for 3 years

   d. Client did not begin prenatal care until 6 weeks before admission

22-3 Which of the following would indicate that preeclampsia had progressed to eclampsia?

   a. Headaches persisting in spite of analgesia

   b. Oliguria of 400 ml/24 hours

   c. Vasospasm seen in the fundus of the eye

   d. Amnesia leading to coma

22-4 Which of the following statements by a postpartum client complaining of pain would be most alarming?

   a. "It's a chest pain that comes and goes."

   b. "It's a sharp chest pain when I burp."

   c. "It's a sharp chest pain, and I can't get my breath."

   d. "It's a catching pain when I breathe deeply."

22-5 Physical examination, ECG, and chest x-ray examination reveal mitral stenosis. Ms. York is classified as having class II cardiac disease. She asks you what is meant by class II. Your best response is:

   a. "You are able to carry on with your regular activities."

   b. "You must really limit most of your activity to prevent symptoms."

   c. "You must follow strict bed rest orders. It is stressful for you to have any physical activity."

   d. "No increase in activity is good for you. Your symptoms occur if you rush at all."

22-6 Ms. York is reevaluated at 28 weeks of gestation. The physician tells her that she may perform ADL and light activity. She asks you, "May I continue my waitress job?" The best immediate response is:

   a. "I don't know. Ask the doctor."

   b. "Your job sounds tiring. Would you consider asking your manager for a sedentary job, perhaps as a cashier, sitting down?"

   c. "You can continue your job until you feel too dyspneic, fatigued, or uncomfortable."

22-7 The primary antepartum nursing goal for Ms. York is:

   a. To preserve her cardiac reserve function.

   b. To have successful antibiotic prophylaxis.

   c. Adequate rest when she feels short of breath or has palpitations.

   d. To have family understand her condition and help with her care.

REFERENCES

Asherson RA, Cervera R: The antiphosphiolipid syndrome: a syndrome in evolution, *Ann Rheum Dis* 51:147, 1992.

Austin M, Davis PA: Valvular disease in pregnancy, *J Perinat Neonatal Nurs* 5(2):13, 1991.

Beischer NA, MacKay EV, eds: *Obstetrics and the newborn*, ed 3, Philadelphia, 1993, WB Saunders.

Bergquist A et al: Late symptoms after pregnancy-related deep vein thrombosis, *Br J Obstet Gynaecol* 97:338, 1990.

Burke ME: Hypertensive crisis and the perinatal period, *J Perinat Neonatal Nurs* (5):33, 1989.

Catanzarite V: HELLP syndrome and its complications, *Contemp Obstet Gynecol* 36(12):13, 1991.

Chesley LC: Hypertensive disorders in pregnancy, *J Nurse Midwifery* 30(2):99, 1985.

Clark SL: New concepts of amniotic fluid embolism: a review, *Obstet Gynecol Surv* 45(6):360, 1990.

Communicable Disease Center: *MMWR* 40 (ss-1):1, 1991.

Cosico JN et al: Indications, management and patient education for anticoagulant therapy during pregnancy, *MCN* 17(3):130, 1993.

Cosner KR, deJong E: Physiologic second-stage labor, *MCN* 18(1):38, 1993.

Crandon AJ, Isherwood DM: Effect of aspirin on incidence of preeclampsia, *Lancet* 1:1356, 1979.

Danforth D, Scott J, eds: *Obstetrics and gynecology*, ed 5, New York, 1987, JB Lippincott.

Dekker GA, Sibai BM: Early detection of preeclampsia, *Am J Obstet Gynecol* 165:160, 1991.

Dekker GA, Sibai BM: Low dose aspirin in the prevention of preeclampsia and fetal growth retardation: rationale, mechanisms and clinical trials, *Am J Obstet Gynecol* 168(1):224, 1993.

Duff P: The dangers of amniotic fluid embolism, *Contemp Obstet Gynecol* 24:127, 1984.

Eganhouse DJ, Burnside SM: Nursing assessment and responsibilities in monitoring preterm labor, *JOGGN* 21(5):335, 1992.

Expert Panel Report: Guidelines for the diagnosis and management of asthma, *Pediatr Asthma, Allergy Immunol* 5:2, 1991.

Gant N, Worley R: *Hypertension in pregnancy: concepts and management*, New York, 1980, Appleton-Century-Crofts.

Geiger-Bronsky MJ: Asthma and pregnancy: opportunities for enhancing outcomes, *J Perinat Neonatal Nurs* 6(2):35, 1992.

Gift AG: Psychologic and physiologic aspects of acute dyspnea in asthmatics, *Nurs Res* 40(4):196, 1991.

Hadi HA, Treadwell EL: Lupus anticoagulant and anticardiolipin antibodies in pregnancy: a review, *Obstet Gynecol Surv* 45:117, 1990.

Hull RD et al: Subcutaneous low–molecular weight heparin compared with continuous intravenous heparin in the treatment of proximal-vein thrombosis, *N Engl J Med* 326:975, 1992.

Kirkland CJ: Myocardial infarction during pregnancy, *J Perinat Neonatal Nurs* 5(2):38, 1991.

Kirshon B, Cotton DB: Invasive hemodynamic monitoring in the obstetric patient, *Clin Obstet Gynecol* 30(3):579, 1987.

Lamb M: Myocardial infarction during pregnancy: a team challenge, *Heart Lung* 16(6):658, 1987.

Lubbe WF: Treatment of hypertension in pregnancy, *J Cardiovasc Pharmacol* 16(suppl 7):S110, 1990.

McParland P, Pearce JM, Chamberlain GVP: Doppler ultrasound and aspirin in recognition and prevention of pregnancy-induced hypertension, *Lancet* 335:1552, 1990.

Miles JF et al: Postpartum eclampsia: recurring perinatal dilemma, *Obstet Gynecol* 76(3) Pt I:329, 1990.

New York Heart Association: *Nomenclature and criteria for diagnoses and diseases of the heart and blood vessels*, ed 5, New York, 1955, The Association.

Out HJ, Derksen RH, Christiaens GC: Systemic lupus erythematosus and pregnancy, *Obstet Gynecol Surv* 44(8):585, 1989.

Poole JH: Getting perspective on the HELLP syndrome, *MCN* 13(6):432, 1988.

Porter KB et al: Finapres: a noninvasive device to monitor blood pressure, *Obstet Gynecol* 78(3):431, 1991.

Roth CK, Riley B, Cohen SM: Intrapartum care of a woman with aortic aneurysms, *JOGNN* 21(4):316, 1992.

Sabai BM et al: Low-dose aspirin in pregnancy, *Obstet Gynecol* 74:551, 1989.

Saftlas AF et al: Epidemology of preeclampsia and eclampsia in the United States, 1979-1986, *Am J Obstet Gynecol* 163:460, 1990.

Sala J, Lentz JR: Pregnant women with systemic lupus erythematosus, *MCN* 11(6): 382, 1986.

Sanches-Ramos et al: Urinary calcium as an early marker for preeclampsia, *Obstet Gynecol* 77(5):685, 1991.

Seidman DS, Seir DM, Ben-Rafael Z: Renal and ocular manifestations of hypertensive disease of pregnancy, *Obstet Gynecol Surv* 46(2):71, 1991.

Shailor TL, Roach D, Weisnor D: Challenging diagnosis: management of the obstetric patient with adult respiratory distress syndrome, *J Perinat Neonatal Nurs* 6(2):25, 1992.

Sharts-Engle NC: Aspirin for prevention of pregnancy-induced hypertension, *MCN* 17(3):169, 1993.

Tso E et al: Late postpartum eclampsia, *Ann Emerg Med* 16:907, 1987.

Veasey L: Resurgence of acute rheumatic fever in the intermountain area of the U.S., *N Engl J Med* 316:421, 1987.

Witry AW: Pulmonary embolus in pregnancy, *J Perinat Neonatal Nurs* 6(2):1, 1992.

Witry AW: Pulmonary edema in pregnancy, *JOGNN* 21(3):177, 1992.

STUDENT RESOURCE SHELF

Anderson B: An overview of drug therapy for chronic adult asthma, *Nurs Pract* 16(12):39, 1991. Asthma control includes balancing a variety of medications, which is reviewed clearly in this article.

Arnone B: Amniotic fluid embolism: a case report, *J Nurse Midwifery* 42(2):92, 1989. Pulmonary embolism occurs rarely but needs crisis interventions, learned best through studying cases like these.

Harvey M: Critical care for the maternity patient, *MCN* 17(6):296, 1992. Emphasizes the collaborative role in high-risk care and presents several cases for illustration.

Legun LA: Systemic lupus erythematosus during pregnancy, *JOGNN* 19(4):304, 1990. Lupus assumes a new importance in triggering other embolic events as seen in this review of the current information.

Roth CK, Riley B, Cohen SM: Intrapartum care of a woman with aortic aneurysm, *JOGNN* 21(4):310, 1992. One example of well-planned care for a high-risk cardiac client during labor and delivery.

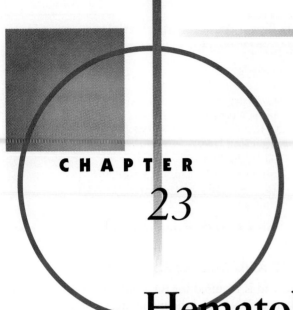

Hematologic, Immunologic, and Neurologic Problems

LEARNING OBJECTIVES

1. *Analyze diets for iron- and folic acid–bearing foods.*
2. *Describe effects of hemoglobinopathies on pregnancy.*
3. *Correlate effects of low platelet levels with assessment findings.*
4. *Describe the necessary adaptations in cardiopulmonary resuscitation for pregnant women.*
5. *Discuss the cause of fetal distress after blunt trauma.*
6. *Formulate questions that encourage clients to discover their own strengths in self-care and planning for infant care.*
7. *Plan care that supports independence in self-care for women with epilepsy, multiple sclerosis, or spinal cord injury.*

Anemia

The major function of red blood cells is to transport oxygen to the tissues. When the number of red blood cells is deficient, tissues do not receive enough oxygen and *anemia* results. Inadequate blood production to maintain a normal hemoglobin level may result from a variety of causes. Most prominent among them are lack of "building blocks" for blood cells such as iron, folic acid, and vitamin B_{12}. Hormonal stimulation for erythrocyte production also may be inadequate, and the bone marrow structure or the hematopoietic (blood-producing) stem cells in the marrow may be damaged. When tissues do not receive enough oxygen, the body attempts to compensate by increasing cardiac output and respirations.

IRON DEFICIENCY ANEMIA

Iron deficiency anemia which is the most common type of anemia in pregnancy, is 10 times more common than other anemias (Beischer and MacKay, 1993). Iron is essential for oxygen transport and is incorporated into hemoglobin. Iron deficiency is strongly suggested when hemoglobin concentrations are below 11.5 g/dl and the hematocrit (Hct) value is less than 32%.

Risk

Iron deficiency anemia can develop because of inadequate dietary intake, alcohol abuse, increased need for iron as a result of pregnancy, excessive blood loss at birth, and closely spaced pregnancies (Figure 23-1). After pregnancy, heavy menstrual flow may affect some women, and certain women may become anemic during menopause. Populations at greatest risk for iron deficiency anemia are women, minorities, low-income groups, infants younger than the age of 2, and elderly persons (Dudek, 1987).

Signs

A major symptom of anemia is activity intolerance. The woman may complain of weakness or fatigue when performing normal activities. In addition, she might have sensory-perceptual alterations such as dizziness and light-headedness. She may appear paler than usual.

The presence of iron deficiency anemia is established when the Hct value—a measure of the size, capacity, and number of red blood cells in ratio to plasma—is less than 32% and the hemoglobin (the oxygen-carrying pigment of red blood cells) is less than 11.5 g/dl. See Box 23-1 for a list of tests used to determine iron deficiency anemia.

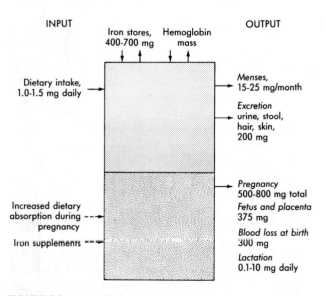

FIGURE 23-1 Iron balance in nonpregnant women compared with iron demands of pregnancy.

BOX 23-1   Tests for Iron Deficiency Anemia

- Hemoglobin
- Hematocrit (Hct)
- Mean corpuscular volume (MCV)
- Mean corpuscular hemoglobin concentration (MCHC)
- Serum iron levels
- Transferrin levels
- Serum protein/albumin 3.5 g/dl
- Red blood cell count
- Serum folic acid

FOLIC ACID DEFICIENCY

Folic acid is required for the synthesis of deoxyribonucleic acid (DNA) and the maintenance of normal levels of mature red blood cells. Folic acid deficiency results in macrocytic or megaloblastic anemia, which is characterized by large immature red blood cells. Pregnant women are especially susceptible to this condition because of the increasing demand for this vitamin by the trophoblast, the rapidly developing fetus, and the expanding maternal red cell mass. The normal nonpregnant daily requirement is increased sixfold or sevenfold during pregnancy.

Depletion of folates results from an inadequate dietary intake of foods such as green, leafy vegetables, organ meats, milk, and eggs and impaired absorption or altered metabolism related to alcohol abuse. Other causes include parasitic infections and ingestion of anticonvulsant drugs such as diphenylhydantoin and certain antibiotics that impair the absorption and use of folates. Serum folate levels of less than 3.2 ng/ml indicate folic acid deficiency (Dudek, 1987).

Risk

Folate deficiency is common in all parts of the world and is the second most frequent cause of anemia during pregnancy in the United States. It occurs in approximately 15% to 20% of clients who are anemic during pregnancy (Danforth and Scott, 1987).

THALASSEMIA

Thalassemia has a distinctly different mechanism and effect from iron-deficiency anemia. Thalassemia is characterized by anemia caused by *decreased or defective production* of red blood cells. This health deviation is widespread; it is genetically determined and found commonly in 4% to 6% of persons of southern Italian, Greek, or Cypriot origin and in other Mediterranean countries, as well as in persons from Asia (Figure 23-2). Immigration patterns have made this type of anemia

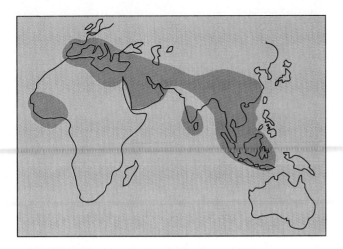

FIGURE 23-2 Areas where thalassemia is most often found. (Courtesy National Foundation March of Dimes, White Plains, N.Y.)

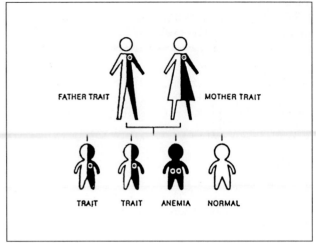

FIGURE 23-3 Genetic inheritance risk for sickle cell anemia. (Courtesy National Foundation March of Dimes, White Plains, N.Y.)

a concern in the United States and Canada (Chui, Wong, and Scriver, 1991). Any woman from these areas of the world should be tested if anemia is discovered.

The varying severity of anemia is related directly to the degree of defect in either of the alpha chains of the hemoglobin molecule or in the beta chains (see Chapter 27).

Risks

Those with defects in both beta chains of the hemoglobin molecule have *thalassemia major,* a serious chronic disease (Cooley's anemia, Mediterranean anemia). Affected children depend on transfusions and have enlargement of the spleen and liver with decreased resistance to infection and bone changes. Very few of these persons ever live beyond adolescence or become pregnant.

Effects of defects in one of the alpha chains of the hemoglobin molecule vary widely, with increasingly severe degrees of anemia. When both alpha pairs are dysfunctional, the fetus does not survive. Because the course of pregnancy with any of the two heterozygous forms is variable, therapy must be individualized.

If only one of the beta chains is affected, the person is heterozygous for beta thalassemia. *Thalassemia minor* is mild, and signs vary widely. Some persons are completely free of symptoms; others have episodes of severe anemia. This heterozygous form may be combined with sickle cell trait (Figure 23-3) and also may occur in 2% of African-Americans (Mayberry et al, 1990). There are other variations such as thalassemia intermedia (mild Cooley's anemia) and thalassemia minima (similar to showing a trait but without symptoms).

Signs

Fewer red cells are produced, and cells have a shorter life span. As a result hemoglobin values may range from 5 to 9 g/dl, and Hct values may range from 15% to 30%.

Bilirubin levels may be elevated as well, reflecting red blood cell destruction. Laboratory tests to establish mean cell volume (MCV) and mean corpuscular hemoglobin (MCH) can detect abnormal erythrocyte populations. These tests identify anemias as normocytic, microcytic, or macrocytic. Normal MCV range is 82 to 98 μm^3, and the MCH is 27 to 31 pg. Values below these suggest thalassemia. There may be during pregnancy several anemic episodes plus increased pregnancy-induced hypertension (PIH) and hemorrhage.

GLUCOSE-6-PHOSPHATE DEHYDROGENASE

Glucose-6-phosphate dehydrogenase (G6PD) deficiency is an *enzyme disorder* (enzymopathic condition) that shortens the survival time of red blood cells. The deficiency is carried on the female sex chromosome and therefore is expressed more often in male offspring (see Chapter 27). When drugs such as nitrofurantoin or primaquine are taken, red blood cells disintegrate, and hematuria occurs (Box 23-2). Stressors such as infection, fever, or pregnancy also may precipitate a hemolytic crisis as hemoglobin values drop rapidly.

Risks

The major maternal risk is increased susceptibility to infection. The fetus is at risk for development of decreased neonatal iron stores, neonatal jaundice, intrauterine growth retardation, and death. In the United States, G6PD can be seen in certain people with a history of immigration from areas shown in Figure 23-2. G6PD is also prevalent in southern Europe and northern Africa in much the same pattern as thalassemia. Another variation of G6PD is found in high rates in certain Jewish populations as well.

BOX 23-2　Some Drugs Causing Hemolytic Reaction in Clients with G6PD

Nitrofurans
- Furaltadone (Altafur)
- Furazolidone
- Nitrofurantoin
- Nitrofurazone

Antimalarials
- Pamaquine
- Pentaquine
- Primaquine phosphate
- Quinacrine
- Hydrochloride
- Quinidine
- Quinine
- Quinocide

Antipyretics and analgesics
Acetanilide
Acetophenetidin
Acetylsalicylic acid
Aminopyrine
Antipyrine
Para-aminosalicylic acid

Sulfonamides
- Salicylsulfapyridine
- Sulfanilimide
- Sulfapyridine
- Sulfisoxazole (Gantrisin)

Others
- Chloramphenicol
- Chloroquine hydrochloride
- Fava beans
- Methylene blue
- Nalidixic acid
- Naphthalene (moth balls, moth spray)
- Probenecid
- Tolbutamide
- Vitamin K (water soluble)

From Buckley K and Kulb N: *Handbook of maternal-newborn nursing*, New York, © 1983, John Wiley & Sons.

Signs

After insult with a stressor such as a food or chemical, rapid hemolysis of red blood cells takes place; the client suddenly becomes very anemic. Hemolytic jaundice develops as the bilirubin level rises because of the increased rate of red blood cell destruction.

Clinical Management

Treatment of *iron deficiency anemia* during pregnancy consists of increasing dietary intake and absorption of iron by means of a daily iron supplement. Without supplementation and an improvement in dietary iron intake, more severe iron deficiency anemia and decreased neonatal iron stores can develop. On rare occasions, parenteral iron (Imferon) is administered intravenously or intramuscularly when response to oral iron is poor.

Treatment of *folic acid deficiency* consists of oral supplementation of 1 mg/day during pregnancy and lactation. The dosage may be increased in pregnant women with alcohol dependency and in those with chronic infections, hemolytic anemia, or anticonvulsant therapy.

Diagnosis of *G6PD* is made by the methemoglobin reduction test. Withdrawal of the offending drug, plus folic acid and iron supplementation, nutrition counseling, and drug education, are vital components of care.

Nursing Responsibilities

When a primary health need is information, the nurse and client should collaborate to develop a plan of care. The woman should be instructed to take iron preparations between meals with a citrus fruit to enhance its absorption. She should avoid ingestion of iron with substances such as tea, coffee, milk, and antacids because such substances inhibit iron absorption. In addition, the nurse identifies foods rich in iron and folic acid and emphasizes the importance of their daily inclusion in the diet. The woman is encouraged to take the prescribed medication. When appropriate, she is given information about the interaction of folic acid with alcohol, antibiotics, chronic infections, and anticonvulsants. Untoward effects such as constipation and gastric irritation should be reviewed, and the client should report these symptoms to her health care provider.

Test Yourself
- Which iron-bearing foods would you recommend to a vegetarian?
- Which substances inhibit iron absorption?
- Which substances interact negatively with folic acid?

Care for Clients with G6PD

During the prenatal history of women of African, Mediterranean, Asian, or Middle Eastern descent, the nurse asks about any episodes of jaundice of unknown origin; notes whether the woman has been anemic, and asks if she has ever been tested for G6PD. In addition, the client is assessed for signs of anemia.

The nurse asks for the names of prescription and over-the-counter medications that the woman is taking or has taken in the past. In addition, stress the importance of avoiding infections and getting prompt medical attention if they occur. Review a written list of medications that induce hemolytic anemia, including name, purpose, and potential side effects. Identify for the client the problems she will encounter using over-the-counter analgesics such as compounds that contain aspirin or sulfa drugs that may be inadvertently prescribed. Emphasize the importance of medical follow-up care. In addition, instruct her to inform any new health care provider about her diagnosis. Finally, all newborn infants are now screened for this enzymopathic condition, and the mother should be informed if her infant has G6PD.

Test Yourself

- If a worried neighbor tells you that her 8-year-old son has suddenly become very pale and tired, what assessment questions should you ask?

Care for Clients with Thalassemia

Nursing diagnoses and outcomes of care for thalassemia clients are similar to those for sickle cell disease.

Sickle Cell Disease

More than 1000 possible genetic abnormalities affect the production, structure, and function of hemoglobin. The most common of these are found in clients with sickle cell disease (hemoglobin SS), sickle cell trait (Hb AS), sickle C disease (Hb CC), or a combination of sickle cell with sickle C disease (Hb SC). These **hemoglobinopathic conditions** are inherited equally by males and females. In the healthy population, approximately 97% of adult hemoglobin is composed of Hb A; the rest is Hb A_2 and Hb F (Table 23-1). In contrast, the person

with sickle cell anemia has primarily Hb S. Sickle cells have a half-life of 5 to 20 days compared with 120 days for a normal red blood cell. Thus bilirubin levels are higher, and immature cells are present in larger quantities.

SICKLE CELL TRAIT

Approximately 9% of African-Americans have the sickle cell trait (Hb AS) and are carriers of the affected gene. These persons have about 35% to 40% Hb S but are symptom-free. Symptoms rarely occur in this relatively benign condition, and pregnancy is not associated with any adverse maternal or fetal effects. Pregnant clients with Hb AS, however, have a twofold increase in genitourinary infections and should have regular urine cultures during pregnancy (Danforth and Scott, 1987).

SICKLE CELL ANEMIA

Persons with sickle cell disease primarily have Hb S instead of Hb A. At low oxygen tensions, red blood cells containing Hb S assume a sickle shape and the form of a rigid, semisolid gel. Intravascular sickling results in stasis of blood flow, accelerated erythrocyte destruction, and increased blood viscosity, which causes the cells to flow poorly through the vessels. This "sludging" results in stasis of blood tissue hypoxia, ischemia, and microinfarcts in the affected organs, especially the kidney, spleen, bones, lungs, and gastrointestinal tract (Figure 23-4). These events probably cause the pain that accompanies sickle cell crisis (Ouimette, 1986).

HEMOGLOBIN C DISEASE

Hemoglobin C disease is a less common hemoglobinopathic condition occurring in 2% of African-Americans (Beischer and MacKay, 1993). Clients with the combination Hb SC disease have mild symptoms. Health problems may not be noticed until a hemolytic crisis occurs during pregnancy. Although pregnant women with Hb CC have less morbidity than do women with Hb SS, an increased incidence of early spontaneous abortion and PIH occurs. Prenatal care should be the same as that provided to clients with Hb SS.

Test Yourself

- If Mr. Smith has the sickle trait and Mrs. Smith is free of any genetic inheritance, what is the inheritance risk for their child? (See Figure 27-9 if you need assistance.)

TABLE 23-1 Hemoglobin Types

TYPE	NORMAL (%)	SICKLE CELL ANEMIA (%)	TRAIT (%)
Hb A (adult)	95	0	60
Hb A_2	2–3	2–3	2–3
Hb F	<1	<2	<1
Hb S	<1	80–90	35–40

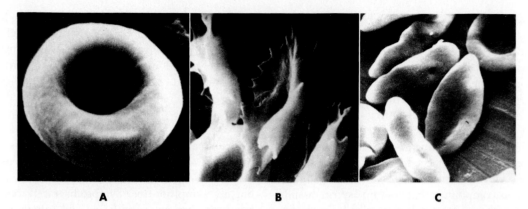

A   **B**   **C**

FIGURE 23-4 Process of sickling and unsickling of red cells. **A,** Stereoscan electron micrograph of normally oxygenated red cell showing classic biconcave disk with central cavity and slight surface irregularity. **B,** Deoxygenated cells take on typical holly-leaf sickle shape. If reoxygenated, cells unsickle. Process may progress to irreversible state. **C,** In oxygenated state, irreversibly sickled cells have characteristic oval or cigar shape with smooth membrane. If deoxygenated and then reoxygenated, cells return to this shape. (From Lessin, Jensen, and Klug: Sickling damages red-cell membrane, *Medical World News,* Jan 26, 1973.)

Risk

The sickle mutation is found in populations of Africa, the Middle East, and Asia (Figure 23-5). Consequently, the gene is most commonly found among descendants of people who originated in these areas. In the United States the incidence of *sickle cell anemia* is highest among African-Americans. However, testing of all newborns shows about a 0.3% rate of the trait (see Chapter 19).

The impact of the disease on future offspring is a major concern. The child conceived by two parents with sickle cell trait will have a 50% chance of carrying the trait and a 25% risk of having sickle cell anemia. The same risk accompanies sickle C trait (see Figure 23-3).

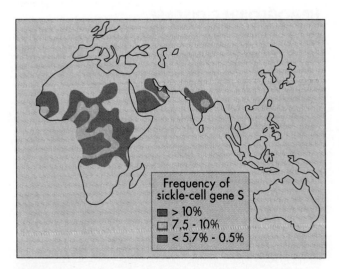

FIGURE 23-5 Areas where sickle cell S and C disease is seen in greatest numbers. (From Kan YW: *Hemoglobin Abnormalities,* New York, 1982, Academic Press.)

Severe sickle cell disease with anemia hinders fertility. If a woman does conceive, many potential complications exist: the potential for a crisis, infection, and anemia. If the woman must have frequent blood transfusions, there is a small risk of hepatitis, human immunodeficiency virus (HIV), and febrile reactions (Ouimette, 1986).

The risks of a poor pregnancy outcome are greater in this population. Spontaneous abortion and intrauterine death because of impaired blood flow to the placenta and inadequate oxygenation of the fetus are more frequent (Ship-Horowitz, 1983). The incidence of premature and low-birth-weight infants also is higher.

Signs

The manifestation of sickle hemoglobin may range from serious disease to an absence of symptoms. The diagnosis of sickle hemoglobinopathies is made by screening with hemoglobin electrophoresis.

Painful vasoocclusive episodes involving multiple organs are the clinical hallmark of sickle cell anemia. The most common sites are the extremities, joints, and abdomen. Sickle cell anemia can affect every organ system. Osteomyelitis caused by *Salmonella* organisms is common. Sickling may occur in the renal medulla, resulting in papillary necrosis. Because of chronic hemolysis and decreased red blood cell survival, clients often have jaundice. In addition, the increased cardiac work imposed by chronic anemia can cause left ventricular hypertrophy, cardiomegaly, and congestive heart failure.

Clinical Management

The care of the pregnant woman with sickle cell anemia requires collaboration among health team members and a thorough understanding of the effect of sickle cell anemia on the woman, developing fetus, and support system. Because of vulnerability to infections, especially of the genitourinary tract, urine cultures should be performed frequently. Any infection should be treated immediately because a hemolytic crisis may be precipitated.

As soon as pregnancy is confirmed, a folic acid supplement of 1 mg/day and promotion of good dietary habits are begun. Although hemoglobin and Hct levels are decreased, iron supplements are not routinely given. If, however, serum iron levels (which should be checked monthly) become low, the client may be advised to take daily iron supplementation. Additional oral fluids maintain hydration and are a major self-care intervention to prevent the precipitation of a crisis.

Some perinatal centers give *prophylactic* transfusions to pregnant women with sickle cell anemia. Transfusions usually begin after 28 weeks. The benefit seems to be a reduction in crises but no better fetal outcome (Koshy et al, 1988). About 50% will require transfusions. The goal of transfusions is to maintain the percentage of hemoglobin A above 20% at all times and the Hct value above 25%. A new technology is being tried; recombinant erythropoietin is a genetically engineered substance to stimulate formation of red blood cells.

During labor, the client should be in the left lateral recumbent position and receive supplemental oxygen. Adequate hydration should be maintained. Unless complications occur, vaginal delivery is preferable to a cesarean birth. Conduction anesthesia is recommended.

Nursing Responsibilities
▶ ASSESSMENT

A nursing assessment of the client's knowledge of self-care practices and support systems is required. Stress, exertion, and dehydration can increase sickling and precipitate a crisis. Explore with the client coping mechanisms she has used in stressful situations. Maladaptive behaviors should be evaluated and alternatives suggested.

▶ NURSING DIAGNOSES

1. Altered renal tissue perfusion related to decreased circulation secondary to hemolytic destruction
2. Altered peripheral and cardiopulmonary tissue perfusion related to decreased circulation secondary to inflammatory process and occlusion of blood vessels
3. Acute pain related to hemolysis in joints
4. Knowledge deficit regarding factors that can precipitate hemolytic crisis and preventive self-care practices

▶ EXPECTED OUTCOMES

Depending on the severity of the sickle cell disease the following outcomes could be chosen.
1. Fluid intake and elimination will be balanced.
2. She inquires about and assesses her life situation for factors that precipitate hemolytic crisis.
3. She complies with measures that help prevent crises.

▶ NURSING INTERVENTIONS

Help the client meet her self-care needs through validation of information, counseling, promotion of self-care, physical care, referral, and collaboration with other health care professionals (see Nursing Care Plan). To assess the client and to enhance her ability to care for herself, the nurse must know potential risks and complications and interventions that may improve perinatal outcome.

Nutritional counseling helps the woman identify foods high in folic acid and iron. Emphasize daily intake of folic acid with vitamin C. If iron supplements also are prescribed, discuss information about self-administration and side effects. In addition, it is essential that she drink adequate fluid; eight glasses a day is recommended.

Infection is a major hazard. Explain how to prevent infection by avoiding sick people and crowds. Clean-catch urines will be collected once each month to monitor for urinary tract infections.

▶ EVALUATION

1. Did urinary infection or anemia occur?
2. Has she complied with recommended treatment?
3. Was the infant full term, of average gestational age, and neurologically normal?
4. Did hemoglobin and hematocrit remain normal?

Disseminated Intravascular Coagulation

Normal pregnancy causes an increase in coagulation factors, especially fibrinogen. The coagulation system involves both factors that assist in blood clotting and those that affect breakdown, or lysis, of a clot. **Disseminated intravascular coagulation (DIC)** is a condition in which the coagulation sequence is activated in a clinically inappropriate manner and leads to a series of events that may result in hemorrhage or thrombosis, or both (Figure 23-6). If clotting factors have been used and yet are being broken down before adequate hemostasis is obtained, the woman first has multiple small clots and then massive hemorrhage because the clotting

NURSING CARE PLAN · Sickle Cell Disease during Pregnancy

CASE: Naome E. is a 23-year-old African-American woman with sickle cell anemia. She is in her first trimester of pregnancy. Physical examination reveals a short female who appears to be underweight. Vital signs are within normal limits. Laboratory studies reveal a borderline normal erythrocyte count, low hemoglobin and Hct values (9.4 g/dl and 28%, respectively), and an iron level of 125 mg/dl. The results of a hemoglobin electrophoresis were Hb F 20%, Hb A2 3%, Hb S 77%, and Hb A 0%. A peripheral blood smear reveals sickled forms of red blood cells, a positive sickle test result, and a blood type of 0+.

ASSESSMENT

1. Lack of knowledge of hemolytic crisis during pregnancy
2. Verbalizes fear for self and fetus
3. Inadequate dietary and fluid intake; weight gain less than expected
4. Compare urine values, blood values with norms

NURSING DIAGNOSES

1. Knowledge deficit about factors in pregnancy that precipitate hemolytic crisis
2. Anxiety related to health of developing fetus
3. Alteration in nutrition: less than body requirements
4. Potential for infection related to lowered resistance

EXPECTED OUTCOMES

1. States the factors that precipitate hemolytic crisis; identifies measures that prevent episodes
2. Gains at least 25 pounds during pregnancy; selects a balanced diet that includes foods rich in folic acid, iron
3. Uses methods to help to decrease risks of infection
4. Experiences uneventful pregnancy and birth

NURSING INTERVENTIONS

1. Provide written and verbal information about the health deviation. Discuss effective self-care measures. Provide information about community resources. Review factors that precipitate sickle cell crisis.
2. Assist client in identifying ways to decrease anxiety. Help client to focus on positive coping behaviors that reduce anxiety.
3. Consult with nutritionist regarding dietary requirements. Perform nutritional assessment at each antepartum visit. Review sources and reinforce importance of folic acid, iron.
4. Identify ways to prevent infection. Review sources of infection and preventive care. Monitor urine during each visit.

EVALUATION

1. Can she state causes, signs, and symptoms of sickle cell disease and use of measures to promote health and prevent hemolytic crisis?
2. Has she identified community resources?
3. Is her weight gain in the range of at least 25 pounds during pregnancy? Did she report taking folate supplements daily and eating diet high in folic acid?
4. Were urine specimens free of pathogens?
5. Did Hbg and Hct levels remain in the normal range?

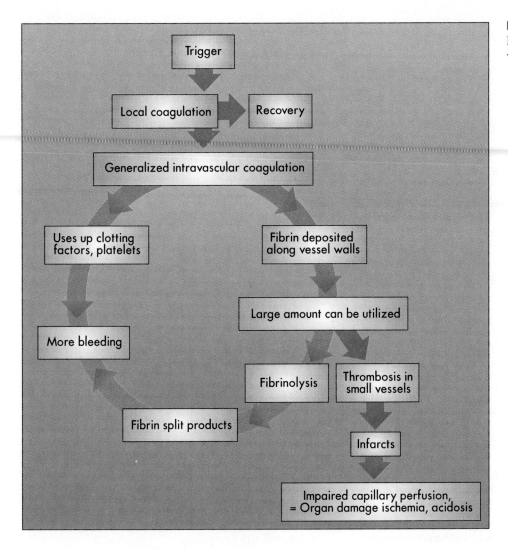

FIGURE 23-6 Mechanisms of DIC can escalate into a vicious cycle.

process is overwhelmed. Other terms sometimes used to describe various aspects of this condition include *consumptive coagulopathy* and *defibrination syndrome.*

TRIGGERS

Disseminated Intravascular coagulation

The coagulation sequence always is triggered by prior problems such as exchange of incompatible red blood cells, amniotic fluid into the maternal circulation, or possible low fibrin levels after severe hemorrhage from the uterus (Letsky, 1987).

Low-grade DIC may be seen in moderate preeclampsia, intrauterine fetal death (IUFD), or intrauterine infection. More severe effects may occur with severe abruptio placentae or severe preeclampsia, HELLP syndrome, amniotic fluid embolism, hydatidiform mole, sepsis, or prolonged shock from any cause (Letsky, 1987).

DIC, which always results from another trigger, has the following characteristics.

- Signs vary widely.
- Condition may remain chronic or low grade.
- It may escalate suddenly.

- If priorities are followed, the client's own liver will clear fibrin split products and platelets will be formed.

SIGNS

DIC may first be identified when a tube of blood fails to clot or *oozing* occurs at a venipuncture site or *bruising* occurs after a blood pressure cuff has been used. There may be petechiae, ecchymosis, and purpura. Bleeding from the gastrointestinal tract and into urine also occurs (Box 23-3).

CLINICAL MANAGEMENT

Because the major effect of DIC in pregnancy is uncontrolled bleeding, the site of hemorrhage must be assessed for possible repair. On occasion a hysterectomy is required. The following priorities must be followed in severe cases.

- Correct trigger cause if possible.
- Maintain central blood volume.

BOX 23-3 Key Signs of Disseminated Intravascular Coagulation

- Oozing at venipuncture site; mucous membranes of mouth, nose
- Hematoma enlarging or wound drainage increasing
- Bruising from BP cuff
- Hematuria or oliguria, or both, related to renal infarcts
- Pain at site of organ infarcts
- Adult respiratory distress syndrome (ARDS) from thrombosis in lung capillaries
- Acute fatty liver of pregnancy (AFLP) with liver failure

- Replace deficiencies (see Chapter 21).
- Support body system functions.

Laboratory evaluation may reveal fractured (broken) red blood cells called *Burr's cells* or schistocytes, elevated fibrin split product (FSP), increased partial thromboplastin time (PTT) and prothrombin time (PT), and decreased fibrinogen levels. (See Table 22-2, which presents variations found in PIH and HELLP syndrome, for comparison.)

If blood coagulability is questioned, the following screening tests are performed: bleeding time, clotting time, PT (factors II, V, VII, X), and PTT (all factors except VII and XIII). Although DIC of a clinically significant degree is uncommon, self-limiting episodes may occur. These episodes usually clear up spontaneously within a few hours and do not initiate the cycle described. In situations in which the state is transient or can be dealt with (delivery of infant, removal of placenta), treatment may not be indicated or required.

Clinical Decision

Mary M. has had a long labor with amnionitis and finally a cesarean delivery. She returns to the recovery room with a Foley catheter in place, O₂ by nasal catheter, and IV fluids with oxytocin. On her admission, urine was clear. An hour later you note hematuria and in checking her skin under the BP cuff, you find bruising. Including further assessment, what actions should you now take?

Immune Disorders: Platelet Dysfunction

The significance of platelets has increased because of the similarities in findings of low platelets in severe preeclampsia, HELLP syndrome, and systemic lupus erythematosus (SLE). **Thrombocytopenia,** low platelet counts, may be the first sign of SLE and HELLP. Levels are followed carefully and are directly related to the severity of these syndromes.

Thrombocytopenia may occur in severe folate deficiencies or because of idiosyncratic responses to medications, sepsis, or excessive alcohol intake. Of special concern is an immunologic disorder that causes **idiopathic (immune) thrombocytopenic purpura (ITP).** This disorder is more common in women than in men (3:1), in which circulating antiplatelet antibodies, immunoglobulin G (IgG), accelerate the destruction of platelets because of changes in the platelet surface (Giacoia and Azubuike, 1991). The result is a much higher risk of hemorrhage and hematoma formation if levels are below $50,000/mm^3$. (For this reason, anesthesiologists will not use the epidural route if platelet counts are low.)

A second type is called *thrombotic thrombocytopenic purpura* (TTP), which is a severe form that results in thrombosis in capillaries and organ damage. Five indicators occur (Watson, Katz, and Bowes, 1990):

- Thrombocytopenia below $50,000/mm^3$
- Microangiopathic anemia
- Renal abnormalities
- Fever
- Neurologic symptoms

The usual corticosteroid management has poor results in TTP.

FETAL RISK

The IgG antibody may cross the placenta to affect fetal platelets and cause bleeding. The major risk is trauma-induced intracranial bleeding during birth. Consequently it has become the practice in known cases to analyze fetal scalp capillary blood for platelets early in labor. If the count is below $50,000/mm^3$ a cesarean usually will be the method of birth to avoid trauma to the fetal head. Fetal thrombocytopenia usually clears in the neonatal period, but steroid treatment may be required.

Signs

In addition to low platelets, there may be prolonged bleeding times and petechiae and purpura on the skin and mucous membranes. Any client who has abnormal bleeding from wounds, petechiae, or bruising, similar to those signs of DIC, needs to be evaluated for ITP.

Clinical Management

In chronic ITP, steroids are used to keep platelet levels up. Corticosteroids in the range of 60 to 80 mg/day for 1 to 2 weeks are given; then the dose is tapered to a maintenance level. Although not performed during pregnancy, a splenectomy may be used to control platelet levels. The spleen functions to remove platelets and is believed to contribute to platelet antibody formation (Giacoia and Azubuike, 1991).

Intravenous immunoglobulin (IV IgG) is now a standard of care in these cases. High-dose IV IgG has been useful in several immune disorders and is very effective in management of ITP. During the last weeks of pregnancy, infusion of 0.4 g/kg/day for 3 days has raised platelet counts into the normal range, thus protecting the mother against hemorrhage during labor and birth. Fetal response may be reduced by already transferred antiplatelet antibodies. IV IgG also is used in Rh-negative women who have been immunized and in SLE to reduce antibody levels.

Plasmapheresis is an expensive therapy in which the client's blood is withdrawn and cells (RBC, WBC, and platelets) are spun out and resuspended in a new solution. This solution is replaced into the circulation. By removing a portion of the person's plasma, adverse substances such as antibodies are removed, so that plasmapheresis is a type of *exchange transfusion*. One or two exchanges of 3 L each often results in rapid improvement (Watson, Katz, and Bowes, 1990).

Trauma during Pregnancy

The incidence of trauma varies. Minor trauma may be treated in the physician's office. Major trauma is treated in the emergency department. Because two lives are at stake, the following questions take priority.

- Does the injury affect the pregnancy?
- Does being pregnant worsen the effect of the injury?

Remember that the physiologic changes of pregnancy must be considered in trauma treatment. Significant cardiovascular changes that influence care are as follows.

- A higher preload of 40% to 50% greater blood volume is present.
- Before signs of shock will be evident, 30% to 35% of blood volume must be lost.
- Physiologic alkalemia (higher than normal pH) occurs.
- Physiologic anemia (lower Hct and Hb levels) is present.
- Placental circulation is completely dependent on maternal blood pressure.

In cases of hypovolemia, shunting of blood to vital organs takes place. The *uterus is not a vital organ in this process*, and blood may be shunted to maintain maternal blood pressure; yet the placental flow is poor. Thus fetal monitoring often shows signs of distress *before* any changes in maternal signs. Therefore maternal blood pressure must be protected to avoid fetal hypoxia.

TYPES OF INJURY

Falls

Falls tend to be caused by a pregnant woman losing balance as a result of the shift in weight or because of orthostatic hypotension. Education for prevention is important (see Chapter 9).

Burns

Burns receive standard burn therapy. Major trauma from fire or electrical burns requires emergency care. If more than one third of the body is affected, the pregnancy will be threatened (Deitch et al, 1989). First-trimester abortion is common. In later pregnancy, preterm labor is frequent. Severe burns require hemodynamic monitoring while fluid balance is regulated. Topical preparations with iodine should be avoided (Sherer and Schenker, 1989).

Electric Shock

Electric shock usually passes through the hand and then through the fetus on the way to the feet and ground. It has resulted in fetal death (Leiberman et al, 1986), intrauterine growth retardation (IUGR), and oligohydramnios. If electric shock occurs, the woman should be monitored closely for fetal movements. Nonstress test (NST) and amniotic fluid volume measurements may be ordered at regular intervals.

Motor Vehicle Accidents

Motor vehicle accidents are the leading cause of accidental injury during pregnancy. How seat belts are used is the primary determinant of the severity of injury (see Chapter 9). Three-point shoulder and lap belts are mandatory, and the lap belt should be located below the abdominal bulge. Correct use of three-point belts has reduced injury to the mother, especially from ejection. The fetus is not so fortunate because the sudden deceleration is powerful enough to throw the fetus against the uterine wall and cause a shearing force to separate the placenta. Normally, amniotic fluid cushions the fetus in the early months, but by the third trimester the baby is larger and there is less fluid. The fetus itself may be injured by blunt trauma; broken bones, skull fracture, and intracranial hemorrhage have been reported.

In a study of 441 pregnant trauma patients, Crosby and Costello (1971) defined a list of observations that holds true today.

1. Internal injuries often are associated with hidden intraperitoneal bleeding and hypovolemic shock.
2. Placental abruption and shock are major causes of fetal death.
3. The most common cause of fetal death is maternal death.
4. Maternal death is most often from head injuries sustained during ejection from an automobile.
5. Pelvic fractures are extremely hazardous for mother and infant and almost always are associated with placental separation.
6. Pelvic fractures carry a high risk of concealed retroperitoneal bleeding. The bladder and urethra may be torn by the fractured bone.

Gunshot and Stab Wounds

Gunshot and stab wounds that penetrate the abdomen may injure the fetus more severely than the pregnant woman if the angle is directly into the uterine tissue. If the wound is in the upper or lateral abdomen, the woman's vital organs may be lacerated. The puncture wound often must be evaluated by peritoneal lavage before the decision for laparotomy is made. If there is a return of red blood cells, leukocytes, or gastrointestinal contents an exploratory laparotomy is performed.

Physical Abuse

Physical abuse may include blows to the pregnant woman's abdomen. The skin surfaces may be bruised, but blunt trauma may have injured underlying tissues more severely (see Chapter 26).

CLINICAL MANAGEMENT

Cardiopulmonary Resuscitation

The need for cardiopulmonary resuscitation (CPR) always includes initial assessment by evaluating airway, breathing, and circulation (ABCs). Bleeding is controlled and broken bones immobilized. The CPR variations for pregnant women recommended by the American Heart Association include steps found in Box 23-4. (See Troiano [1989] for detailed instruction.)

Supporting Perfusion

Supporting blood volume and pressure using a large-bore IV line and a central venous pressure (CVP) line is necessary because pregnancy volumes are critical to support fetal perfusion. Military antishock trousers (MAST) may be used on the lower extremities but *not* over the abdomen (Sherer and Schenker, 1989). Oxygen at 8 to 10 L/min by mask is started. An indwelling Foley catheter is necessary to monitor output and note hematuria. A nasogastric tube decompresses the stomach and prevents aspiration.

BOX 23-4   Principles of Basic Life Support during Pregnancy

Airway
- Determine unresponsiveness.
- Call for help.
- Position patient on firm flat surface.
- *Displace uterus laterally* either manually or with wedge.
- Open the airway with head-tilt and chin-lift or jaw-thrust maneuver.

Breathing
- Look, listen, and feel for air movement.
- If breathing is absent, deliver two slow breaths.

Circulation
- Feel for presence of carotid pulse.
- If pulse is absent, begin external chest compressions at a rate of 80 to 100 per minute.
- Alternate 15 chest compressions with two slow breaths.
- Reassess patient after four complete cycles.
- If breathing and pulse are absent, continue CPR.

Two-rescuer CPR
- Same as above, except five compressions are followed by a pause to allow delivery of one slow breath.

The intubated patient
- Same as for two-rescuer CPR, except compressions and ventilations asynchronous.
- Perform compressions at a rate of 80 to 100 per minute.
- Perform ventilations independently at a rate of 12 to 15 per minute.

Modified from American Heart Association: *Textbook of advanced cardiac life support*, Dallas, Tex, 1987, The Association.

Assessing Fetal Condition

As soon as the woman's condition is initially stabilized, the fetal condition must be monitored. Ultrasonography is used if abdominal wounds prevent placing a belt. Monitoring should continue during any procedure.

Test Yourself
- Why does the fetal heart rate show distress signs before the woman's signs of shock become evident?

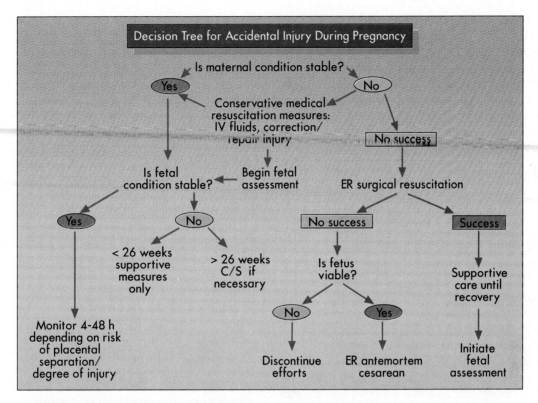

FIGURE 23-7 Decision tree for accidental injury during pregnancy. If resuscitation of woman is successful, the fetal assessment sequence is followed. (Modified from Sherer DM, Schenker JG: Accidental injury during pregnancy, *Obstet Gynecol Surv* 44[5]:330, 1989.)

Every trauma client should have fetal and contraction monitoring for at least 4 hours in mild cases and continuously until stabilized in more severe cases. Placental separation may be indicated by late decelerations, rising baseline, and falling beat-to-beat variability.

Preventing Isoimmunization

Often fetomaternal transfusion occurs as placental tissue or the uterus is injured. The fetus may be bleeding. The Kleihauer-Betke test for fetal cells in the maternal circulation may be used to follow the levels. If a woman is Rh-negative, she must receive the correct dose of $Rh_o(D)$ immune globulin.

Perimortem Cesarean Section

In situations in which the woman is brain dead, is dying from fatal head or chest injuries, or has just died, it may be possible to rescue the fetus through a cesarean delivery performed in the emergency department. Choices must be made quickly and, of course, with informed consent of the next of kin. Sometimes rapid surgery relieves the woman's body of the uterine pressure and her condition improves. The following criteria are recommended in these cases (Sherer and Schenker, 1989):

1. Fetal age more than 28 weeks
2. Surgery less than 15 minutes after maternal clinical death
3. Continuous resuscitation, ventilation, and cardiac massage before and during the procedure
4. Intensive neonatal care

Sherer and Schenker also recommend a decision tree (Figure 23-7). All health care staff members need to be aware of procedures in these difficult cases.

Nursing Responsibilities

The trauma client will be seen first in the emergency room (ER) for evaluation. If any blunt trauma has occurred but is not life threatening, she will be transferred to labor and delivery for fetal and contraction monitoring. Amniocentesis may be used to identify red blood cells in the fluid, as well as to determine fetal lung maturity. Monitoring will continue until signs indicate good fetal activity and beat-to-beat variability, without abnormal decelerations. The woman will be instructed in counting fetal movements and asked to return on a regular basis for monitoring. Preventive education concerning preterm labor is included because of the risk of continuing problems.

If major trauma occurs, the maternity nurse works in collaboration with the emergency department team, providing monitoring expertise and assessment of the pregnancy complications. When the client is transferred to the intensive care unit (ICU) after stabilization, the nurses there may utilize the maternity nurse's expertise for consultation (Johnson and Oakley, 1990).

Neurologic Disorders during Pregnancy
EPILEPSY

Neurologic disorders form a diverse group of health deviations in pregnancy. They range from annoying conditions (headache) to life-threatening conditions (intracranial hemorrhage). Epilepsy is the most common major neurologic disorder that complicates pregnancy (Gabbe, Kneibyl, and Simpson, 1986). Epilepsy is characterized by recurrent seizures that are the symptoms of abnormal electrical discharges in the brain. There are a wide variety of seizures that cause problems in motor, sensory, or conscious function, depending on their type. Seizures commonly are classified into two groups: **partial seizures,** which are localized or originate in a specific part of the brain, and **generalized seizures,** which involve the entire brain simultaneously. In pregnant women, generalized tonic-clonic (grand mal) or similar convulsive seizures are of greatest concern because of potential harm to the fetus.

Most epilepsy is **idiopathic** (no clearly determined cause), but some cases are due to conditions such as congenital anomalies, head injuries, intracranial tumors, meningitis, hypoxia, toxin exposure, hypoglycemia, uremia, hypoparathyroidism, and excessive hydration. In persons with a lowered threshold for seizures, a seizure may be precipitated by bright lights, fatigue, stress, and excessive use of or withdrawal from drug or alcohol abuse.

> **Test Yourself**
> • Name two factors that the client herself can control to decrease the likelihood of seizures.

Risk

Seizures tend to increase during pregnancy in more than one third of epileptic women (Conley and Olshansky, 1987). Seizure frequency tends to increase mostly at the beginning or end of pregnancy and is thought to be related to low levels of **antiepileptic drug (AED),** noncompliance, and possibly maternal sleep deprivation. The normal physiologic alterations of pregnancy can lower the concentration of AEDs in the blood. Nausea and vomiting, decreased gastric motility, increased plasma volume, fetal and placental growth and development, and an increased extracellular fluid may change the distribution of anticonvulsants and thus lower the serum levels (see Chapter 16).

Noncompliance in taking AEDs as prescribed may be related to the mother's concern about teratogenic effects. Psychologic stress, physical fatigue, and anemia also may contribute to a lowered seizure threshold.

Not all seizures carry the same threat to the fetus. Generalized convulsive seizures carry the highest risk because of the potential for hypoxia and acidosis. Emergency cesarean delivery may be necessary if the fetus is severely affected by the seizure. **Status epilepticus,** a series of seizures with little or no recovery in between, is rare during pregnancy but carries a high mortality risk for fetus and mother. Seizures that cause an alteration in consciousness (such as complex partial seizures) may not affect fetal oxygenation but can increase the risk for accidental injury. Simple partial seizures are not believed to pose a risk to the fetus unless they progress to generalized seizures.

> **Test Yourself**
> • Which physiologic changes of pregnancy might lower the AED levels during pregnancy and thus precipitate a seizure if dosage is not adjusted?

All AEDs have substantial *teratogenic risks.* In addition, valproic acid has been linked to the higher rate of neural tube defects. Phenytoin has been more frequently associated with fetal malformations than are other AEDs, but this may be due to its widespread use. Other drugs used to treat seizures include *carbamazepine, phenobarbital, primidone, ethosuximide,* and benzodiazepine derivatives such as *clonazepam.* AEDs have been associated with depressed folate levels, which can result in anemia, as well as being a possible factor in fetal defects. Long-term use of phenytoin can lower vitamin D levels in the mother. All AEDs depress vitamin K–dependent clotting factors, which can result in fetal and neonatal hemorrhage. The *teratogenic risks* of these drugs appear to be dose-dependent, so use of the lowest dosage that controls seizures adequately is the therapeutic goal. Because teratogenic risks also increase when more than one AED is used, monotherapy is preferred during pregnancy.

Clinical Management

As indicated, a variety of problems can cause seizures. Consequently, testing is extensive but varies according to individual history and circumstances. Laboratory tests usually include awake and asleep electroencephalogram (EEG), skull x-ray films, and computed tomography (CT) or magnetic resonance imaging (MRI) scan of the brain to detect skull injury or lesions. Radiation risk from CT scans is minimal when the client is properly shielded. An MRI involves no radiation, and no harmful effects on the fetus have been established. If metabolic problems are the suspected cause of seizures, serum electrolyte, calcium, magnesium, and glucose levels are obtained. Ultrasonic scanning should be done at 18 weeks' gestation to evaluate the fetus for possible anomalies. Echocardiography, serial ultrasound studies, and amniocentesis also are performed to evaluate the status of the fetus.

Seizures are treated with the AEDs recommended for the seizure type that the person is experiencing. If seizure control is not achieved with one drug, others may be added until better control is achieved.

Treatment of known underlying causes is instituted. Counseling or psychotherapy is recommended when the client has poor coping abilities or low self-esteem related to the disorder.

When possible, the woman should be counseled before conception. If pregnancy is desired, daily vitamin supplements and folic acid are begun before conception. Attempts are then made to gradually withdraw the anticonvulsant and substitute less potentially teratogenic drugs. During this process, anticonvulsant drug levels should be monitored weekly until the woman is stable. Once medication doses keep the client within a therapeutic range, she can then be advised to conceive. If, however, seizures recur, maintenance drugs are reinstated.

In some cases, discontinuation of AED therapy may be possible if the client has been seizure-free for a long period of time. This is a complex decision that needs to be made after thorough evaluation with the client's physician.

Supplements. Mothers taking AEDs may be given vitamin K supplements in the last month of pregnancy, and neonates can be given vitamin K to prevent hemorrhage. Folic acid usually is prescribed. Women who are taking phenytoin should take supplementary vitamin D throughout pregnancy.

Labor and recovery. Later, depending on dosage, anticonvulsant drugs are given during labor even if fluids are withheld. In addition, drug levels are monitored frequently during the postpartum period, and the client is carefully observed for warning signs of seizures.

Effect on newborn. AEDs may produce neonatal depression, which is characterized by sedation, hypotonia,

and poor breathing or sucking. The symptoms appear at birth and disappear within 2 to 8 days. Withdrawal symptoms develop in some newborns, including excessive crying, disturbed sleep, hyperactivity, tremors, myoclonic jerks, hypertonia, hyperreflexia, hyperventilation, hyperphagia, vomiting, sneezing, and yawning. Breast-feeding is not totally contraindicated for women with epilepsy, depending on the specific drug. Many AEDs are excreted in breast milk, which can be a concern. Sedative AEDs such as phenobarbital have been associated with feeding difficulties in the infant. If a mother decides to breast-feed, she should discuss her decision with her physician and observe the suggestions about timing doses in relation to feeding times (see Chapter 16), as well as observe the infant for any unusual symptoms.

Nursing Responsibilities
▶ ASSESSMENT

Assessment of status always should include the frequency and type of seizures that have occurred. The characteristics of a seizure, such as eye movement, changes in consciousness and body movement, and the **postictal** state (after seizure), are all important observations. The client may be able to provide this information. If alteration in consciousness occurred, it must come from observers. The nurse also can explore with the client if there were any precipitating factors before the seizure, such as stress, fatigue, or alcohol ingestion.

Assessment of AED compliance is crucial. Open-ended, nonthreatening questions such as, "How are you taking your medications? Is it hard to remember them? Do you have any concerns about your medications?" may elicit more information than accusing a person of failing to take medication. It also is important to assess the client for any signs of drug toxicity and to determine if she knows what those signs are and how to report them to the physician.

The client should be assessed for her knowledge about what to do if she has a seizure. Does she have a plan formulated with her physician about steps to take if she has a seizure while pregnant? Are her family, friends, and co-workers aware of what to do if a seizure occurs? During pregnancy it is particularly important that the woman with epilepsy has a clear understanding of her prevention and treatment plan, including factors she can control such as stress or fatigue.

▶ NURSING DIAGNOSES

Although epileptic states vary widely in degrees of severity, the following diagnoses may apply:

- Health-seeking behaviors related to information about plan of treatment and precautions during pregnancy
- High risk for noncompliance for medication related to anxiety over effect on fetus
- High risk for injury to client or fetus related to seizure activity during pregnancy or birth

▶ EXPECTED OUTCOMES

Samples of outcomes for the pregnant woman with epilepsy are as follows:

- Verbalizes plan discussed with physician regarding self-care during pregnancy
- Lists precautions concerning triggers to seizure activity
- States dose, timing, and potential side effects of prescribed medication
- Informs family and relevant others about signs of seizure onset and methods of assistance to maintain safety
- Both client and family able to state plan for follow-up care should a seizure occur

▶ NURSING INTERVENTIONS

Monitoring Medications

The nurse must help the client understand the risks and benefits of her AEDs during pregnancy. Pregnant women with epilepsy often decrease the dosage on their own for fear of harming the fetus. They need to understand that changing dosages may harm themselves and the fetus even more. Plans for testing AED levels, dietary supplements, and follow-up evaluation need to be coordinated with the neurologist and obstetrician so that holistic care is given.

Ensure that the client is familiar with signs and symptoms of toxicity:

- Ataxia
- Blurred vision or diplopia
- Nausea (may be confused with pregnancy changes)
- Lethargy or other symptoms of the specific AED

Discuss the woman's plans to minimize stress and lack of sleep, and assess how pregnancy is affecting her diet and vitamin intake. Check the early nausea of pregnancy to see if she is tolerating her doses. Encourage her to express fears related to fetal outcome. Additional counseling may be needed if anxiety is overwhelming. Referrals to local epilepsy support groups have been helpful.

After the birth AED dosage may be continued at the same level initially, but blood levels must be checked within a few weeks. Be sure she is made aware of signs of withdrawal in the infant and when to report to the physician. If the infant has neonatal depression related to AEDs but the condition is borderline and continued hospitalization is not required, the mother may need help in knowing how to encourage feeding. For the parents whose infant has a congenital defect, special support and information will be needed.

▶ EVALUATION

- Did she remain seizure-free?
- Were medication and testing regimens followed?
- Did she verbalize and implement plans to minimize impact on pregnancy and life-style?
- Did the family positively and knowledgeably support her?

HEADACHE

Almost 30% of women in the United States suffer from headaches that may continue to be a problem during pregnancy. There are a variety of types of headache with varying or unknown causes. Generally, they may be classified as *vascular,* such as migraine, cluster, or hypertensive headaches, *muscle contraction* tension headaches, or *traction and inflammatory* headaches related to mass lesions, cranial hemorrhage, strokes, temporomandibular joint disease, and various other diseases of the ears, eyes, nose, throat, and teeth.

Signs

Migraines have a wide variety of frequency, duration, and intensity. They usually start on one side of the head and may be accompanied by anorexia and then nausea and vomiting. In classic migraine a visual, sensory, or motor aura precedes the headache. Because there seems to be a relationship between steroid hormone levels and migraines, menses and pregnancy often affect migraine status. In pregnancy a complete cessation of migraine or a decrease in frequency often occurs. This usually begins in the third or fourth month and does not seem to be related to emotional status. It is possible, however, for migraines to continue and even become aggravated during pregnancy.

Muscle contraction headaches are characterized by a sensation of pressure or aching that usually is bilateral and may cover the head like a tight cap. There is a sustained contraction of muscles around the scalp, and no aura precedes the pain, which may last for a few hours or as long as several months. There are many theories about the causes of these headaches, including vascular and muscular factors, as well as psychologic factors.

Traction and inflammatory headaches are infrequent but can indicate serious problems. They may be caused by inflammation or displacement of cranial structures and are characterized by an ache that be-

BOX 23-5 Assessment Questions for Headaches

- Is there a history of similar headaches?
- If so, have you been seen by a physician?
- Describe the onset; was there a prodrome or aura?
- Where is the pain located?
- How would you describe the character and duration of the pain?
- Are there associated symptoms such as photophobia, nausea, vomiting, or neurologic symptoms? Did you lose vision in part or all of an eye even temporarily?
- Can you pinpoint any aggravating factors?
- Can you describe any relieving factors you have tried?

comes continuous and progressively worse. Coughing or straining precipitates or aggravates the pain. Symptoms of neurologic impairment may appear. Intracranial tumors may grow rapidly during pregnancy because of fluid shifts or hormonal stimulation and can cause this type of headache. Intracranial hemorrhage is characterized by severe explosive headache that requires immediate interventions to avoid death. In pregnancy, most strokes occur during the puerperium.

Although this type of headache can have severe, life-threatening causes, it also can be characteristic of more benign disorders of the head and neck so that assessment is needed before any hasty conclusions are drawn. Information to assess origin and significance of the headache is noted in Box 23-5. A headache of acute onset with no previous history and with progressive symptoms is more cause for concern than a characteristic headache in a person who has a history of migraines or muscle contraction headaches that may have been thoroughly evaluated. During pregnancy, increases in frequency or severity of any headaches are signs that need further evaluation.

Test Yourself

Match the headache type with its typical characteristic:

- Migraine
- Muscle contraction
- Traction/inflammatory

- Coughing makes pain worse
- Feels like a tight cap over head
- Often preceded by an aura

Clinical Management

A complete history and physical examination are performed, and laboratory tests such as complete blood count (CBC), sedimentation rate, blood glucose, urinalysis, and electrocardiogram (ECG) may be ordered to rule out systemic causes. Depending on the headache profile, other procedures may be ordered, such as EEG, thermographic examination, x-ray studies of the skull, spine, and paranasal sinuses, a CT scan, MRI, and a lumbar puncture.

Migraines and muscle contraction headaches usually are treated primarily with drugs, but during pregnancy it is preferable to use nonpharmacologic interventions. Biofeedback and relaxation techniques are effective for both migraine and muscle contraction headaches. For migraine sufferers, comfort measure such as the use of ice packs for at least 12 minutes and rest in a dark quiet room can be helpful. Some migraines have trigger factors that can be minimized; examples are fatigue, heat, and fasting for more than 5 hours during the day or 13 hours at night. Some may find that certain chemicals trigger migraines; these include tyramine, phenylthylamine, nitrites, and monosodium glutamate (MSG). Offending foods include red wine, chocolate, aged cheese, caffeine, alcohol, hot dogs, and some Chinese foods.

In addition, psychologic interventions such as expressing emotions, adjustment of work patterns, or modification of other stress factors may be useful. Physical interventions such as a cervical collar or dental treatment may help if muscle contraction headaches are caused by a poor alignment.

When the woman is not pregnant, muscle contraction headaches commonly are treated with acetaminophen, acetylsalicylic acid (ASA), diazepam, and amitriptyline. Except for diazepam and ASA, these are used during the first trimester with minimal risk for the fetus (Khurana, 1992). Of the commonly used migraine drugs, *ergotamine* is avoided because of its oxytocic potential. Meperidine and acetaminophen may be used to treat acute attacks during pregnancy. Propranolol and amitryptyline sometimes are used despite some risk of growth retardation with propranolol. The use of multiple drugs is discouraged, and prophylactic drugs usually are discontinued 2 weeks before delivery. As with any drugs used during pregnancy, a woman should have a clear understanding of the benefit to risk ratio before taking the drug.

Nursing Responsibilities

A nurse may be the first health care provider contacted regarding a headache. Take a thorough history to ascertain if further evaluation is needed. Certainly the pregnant client should be referred to her physician for the acute development of a progressively severe headache, especially if there has been no history or work-up in the past. An increase in frequency and severity of any headache should be evaluated. Even if the headache is benign, the client will need reassurance and education about alternative measures to pharmacotherapy. If drugs have been the only therapy in the past, it may be a daunting prospect to face a headache without such intervention. The client may need to explore ways to reduce stress or identify triggers once she realizes that such factors may contribute to headache. Pregnancy can become an opportunity for the woman to assume more initiative in preventing and treating her headaches without dependence on drugs. If medication is necessary to achieve adequate relief, describe the risk and appropriate doses. In any case the primary goals are to support the client and assist her in obtaining adequate pain relief while minimizing risk to the fetus.

PERIPHERAL NERVOUS SYSTEM DISORDERS

Two common peripheral nervous system disorders that can occur in pregnancy are carpal tunnel syndrome and Bell's palsy (Table 23-2). These conditions are basically benign but can cause a good deal of discomfort, inconvenience, and even debilitation. Because the initial symptoms may be alarming to the client, prompt diagnosis is helpful. She will need supportive symptomatic care as she waits for her symptoms to resolve (Felsenthal, 1992).

MULTIPLE SCLEROSIS

Multiple sclerosis (MS) is characterized by episodic inflammation and demyelination in the brain, optic nerves, and spinal cord. A wide range of symptoms may result, depending on the specific areas affected. Motor and visual impairment are common. Urinary problems and spasticity can occur and some clients with MS have impairment of cognitive or emotional functions. The client usually has periods of exacerbation and remission that occur in unpredictable patterns, with a gradual decline in overall neurologic function. In rare cases there is a progressive form that has no remissions and results in death in a few months. The general course of the disease, however, can be quite long, with an average duration of more than 30 years.

 Clinical Decision

Choose questions to ask Debra, 3 months pregnant, who calls to say, "I have a terrible headache! What should I do?"

TABLE 23-2 Bell's Palsy and Carpal Tunnel Syndrome

CHARACTERISTIC	EFFECT
BELL'S PALSY	
• Unilateral seventh cranial nerve facial weakness	Facial weakness/paralysis of one side of forehead and lower portion of face
• Occurs in third trimester or within 2 weeks of birth	Client may be concerned she has had a stroke; thus prompt diagnosis is helpful
• Cause unclear; may be related to edema, hormonal changes in pregnancy, or a virus	Treatment usually is symptomatic, with eye patch, artificial tears, facial massage, and exercises as needed; if lesion is severe, corticosteriods may be used Generally resolves in 3-12 weeks
CARPAL TUNNEL SYNDROME	
• Compression of median nerve at the wrist	Burning or numbness in fingers that may arouse client at night and may be relieved by shaking the hands
• More often in dominant hand	Weak lifting and grasping ability
• Onset is usually between months 4 and 9 of pregnancy	Splinting the wrist may help; other treatments are nonsteroidal antiinflammatory drugs or local steroid injections
• *Possible* causes: edema, relaxation of the transverse carpal ligament	Most cases resolve spontaneously and gradually by 3 months postpartum; surgery may be used in the few cases that do not resolve

The onset of MS is most common between the ages of 20 and 35, and women are twice as likely to be affected as men. The etiology of MS is unknown, but recent theories suggest that some environmental factor, possibly a viral infection, triggers an autoimmune attack on the central nervous system myelin in a person with a genetic susceptibility. Because treatment is limited and often ineffective and the course of the disease so unpredictable, the psychologic challenge of coping with MS is tremendous. The individual's degree of disability does not necessarily determine the psychosocial problems a person with MS may have. Physical limitations are one factor, but other factors such as social support, how she perceives her condition, and her relationship with care givers and health care providers seem to contribute also. Sometimes a person with minor physical limitations may experience severe psychosocial problems and a person with pronounced physical limitations may be able to adjust surprisingly well.

Risk: Pregnancy and Multiple Sclerosis

MS does not affect a woman's fertility and has little impact on the course and outcome of a pregnancy. Pregnancy does not cause MS; in fact the onset of MS is less likely during a pregnancy. The condition of most women with MS stabilizes or improves during pregnancy, particularly during the second and third trimesters. This effect is thought to be due to the physiologic **immune suppression** that occurs during pregnancy. At this time research does not show that pregnancy has any worsening effect on the overall course of MS, but *after* birth there is a high risk of a relapse or exacerbation in the first 3 to 6 months. This factor is important to consider in planning child care and postpartum work schedules. Although a susceptibility to MS is inherited, the risk of transmitting it to the infant is not present.

Clinical Management

No treatment exists that is effective in the long-term course of MS. Acute exacerbations may be treated with high-dose corticosteroids or adrenocorticotropic hormone (ACTH) in an attempt to shorten the duration of the event. These treatments may or may not have any effect. Treatment with immunosuppressive drugs is being tried, but with unclear results. Physical therapy and orthotic devices can help maximize physical abilities. The person with MS also is often advised to obtain adequate rest and avoid excessive exposure to sunlight and heat, factors that may cause exacerbations. Spasticity and bladder dysfunction or infections may be treated with various medications. Psychosocial support and counseling often are important components of adequate care for the person with MS.

A primary factor to consider in the discussion with her health care provider about the impact of MS on her

decision to have children will be the effect on her ability to perform self-care and to care for her child. Other factors influencing this ability will be the economic situation, social support, and her own adaptation to the disease. A discussion of MS treatment during pregnancy also is appropriate. Prednisone and ACTH should be avoided if possible, especially in the first trimester. Low doses of prednisone for short periods of time may be used later on. Because the use of immunosuppressive drugs has been associated with some fetal malformations, a careful consideration of the *benefit-risk ratio* is necessary. Avoidance of anemia is important. Persons with MS tend to have more urinary tract infections and may need prophylaxis with nitrofurantoin or ampicillin.

Labor and delivery are managed routinely. The rate of exhaustion may be higher, resulting in use of forceps more often. Because of a possible link with relapse, spinal anesthesia is avoided; epidural is believed to be safer (Goldstein and Stern, 1992). If the woman is being treated with more than 10 or 20 mg prednisone, she must receive steroid coverage during labor and delivery, usually in the form of intramuscularly or intravenously administered hydrocortisone.

Breast-feeding is not contraindicated in women with MS. It does not seem to cause or prevent exacerbations. Often, however, the woman is advised to avoid exhaustion, which might mean that night feedings of milk pumped during waking hours be given by someone else. If the mother is being treated with drugs, she should discuss the advisability of breast-feeding because of potential adverse effects on the baby.

Test Yourself

- What self-care advice is needed for pregnant women with MS?
- Which types of infections most frequently affect women with MS?
- When as a result of pregnancy does risk of MS exacerbation occur?

Nursing Responsibilities

It may be helpful to explore with the woman her strengths and limitations. She may be facing hostility and emphasis on her disability from other people who disagree with the couple's decision to have a child. An honest exploration of her physical, emotional, and cognitive status is more likely to occur in an accepting environment. Her need for education or consultation can be assessed through questions such as the following.

1. Have her questions about MS and pregnancy/parenthood been answered adequately?
2. Does she have realistic plans for self-care during pregnancy and for child care?
3. Does she have an active support system, and what is the reaction of significant others to the pregnancy?
4. Is she aware of resources in her community such as MS support groups and other disabled mothers who can serve as emotional and informational resources?

The time to resolve these questions is before the pregnancy. The nurse's role is to help the client make an informed decision and maximize her potential for self-care and parenting. The way to help a woman consider the decision more thoroughly is by being aware of the questions MS raises for the woman contemplating pregnancy, some of which are listed in Box 23-6. Although education about medical considerations and drug information and access to articles, books, and community resources are important the decision to have a child is up to the woman with MS, not the medical establishment.

The client herself may provide an education for the nurse, because she is considering the situation on a personal level. In the hospital setting it is important to accommodate and assist her when needed but not to take over unnecessarily. The client herself usually is the best person to consult about what is needed because she knows her own abilities. The postpartum nurse will need carefully to assess the woman's comfort level in managing child care and to arrange appropriate referrals if needed—for example, with a social worker or for occupational therapy. The nurse should remember that some anxiety about caring for the newborn is entirely normal. Encouragement with appropriate humor and a spirit of innovation can go a long way in facing parenthood with a chronic disease.

SPINAL CORD INJURY

The most common causes of spinal cord injury in women are motor vehicle accidents, followed by falls, acts of violence, and sports-related injuries (Goldstein and Stern, 1992). Some women who have been injured decide to become pregnant, whereas others are injured during the pregnancy. In the latter case, the care and needs of the woman are multiplied as she adjusts to her injury, as well as to its impact on her pregnancy. The challenges faced by a pregnant woman with a spinal cord injury vary, depending on the level of her injury and disability. In addition to the cord level of the lesion, the degree of disability depends on whether the lesion is complete or incomplete, which establishes if some motor or sensory function is left below the level of injury. Paraplegia usually is not a contraindication to vaginal delivery as long as the injury did not include pelvic fractures or occur before puberty, both of which could cause insufficient pelvic diameters. In any case the woman herself is likely to be the most accurate source for information on her abilities and limitations.

BOX 23-6   Issues to Consider in Multiple Sclerosis and Pregnancy

Decision to become pregnant

Will my MS symptoms get worse with pregnancy?
Can I do anything to lessen the chance of postpartum relapse?
Will my overall disability be worse as a result of pregnancy?
Will my baby inherit MS?

MS and pregnancy

How will MS affect the medical management of my pregnancy?
Will termination of pregnancy affect my MS?
How can MS affect labor and delivery?
What drugs are safe during pregnancy and breast-feeding?
Should my MS treatments be changed?

MS and postpartum issues

What assistance will I need to adequately care for my infant?
What adaptations of home and equipment will be needed?
What contingency plans do I have for exacerbations?
How much can I rely on my support systems?
How can I maximize rest?
What community resources and written material are available to provide additional support and information?

 Clinical Decision

Maggie, who has had MS for 3 years, is admitted to the postpartum unit after the birth of her first child. If she had a normal vaginal birth, how can you determine what her needs will be? List potential nursing diagnoses for her and a plan of self-care education.

Risk

It is uncommon to encounter a pregnant woman with a spinal cord injury, but as rescue and treatment modes improve, more victims of trauma are surviving. There are approximately 10,000 spinal cord injuries in the United States every year, and one fifth of those injured are women. Because many are young women, fertility is unimpaired and a desire for a family may coexist with varying degrees of motor impairment. Chief problems to be managed are urinary tract infections, autonomic dysreflexia, and decubitus ulcers.

Clinical Management

Urinary tract infections are common problems for women with spinal cord injuries, especially because of the use of catheters for bladder management. Because the likelihood of urinary tract infection increases during pregnancy as a result of hormonal changes, frequent urine cultures and sometimes prophylactic antibiotics are used to manage infection. As pregnancy advances, increasing difficulty with self-catheterization and with incontinence may occur. Some women may choose to use an indwelling catheter for a period of time.

Autonomic dysreflexia. A number of stimuli, including labor contractions, may cause muscle spasms related to **autonomic dysreflexia.** This adverse effect occurs most often in persons with lesions at T6 or higher. Noxious stimuli that cause hyperreflexia include the following:

- Distension, contraction, or manipulation of cervix, rectum, bladder, uterus
- Excessive deep breathing
- Cold water, cold weather

Hyperreflexia is a response of the sympathetic nervous system to noxious sensory stimuli from the skin, a distended bladder, an impacted bowel, a pelvic examination, or labor. Urinary tract infections, pressure ulcers, tight clothing, monitor straps, and even breast-feeding have caused autonomic dysreflexia. Symptoms include a severe pounding headache related to hypertension, profuse sweating, blotching of the skin or flushing and piloerection (erect hairs on skin) above the level of cord lesion, and tachycardia or sometimes bradycardia. The symptoms may be confused with PIH, but the hypertension is transient and episodic; for instance, it may occur during the contraction and subside during the rest period. In severe cases hypertension can result in loss of consciousness, seizures, intracranial bleeding, and death.

Prevention of autonomic dysreflexia is important. Careful attention to bladder and bowel management and maintenance of skin integrity can eliminate the most common prelabor causes. Other preventive measures include the following:

- A semisitting position for a speculum or digital vaginal examination
- Use of an indwelling catheter to avoid bladder distension during labor
- Anesthetic ointments for pelvic examinations or catheter manipulation

If an episode does occur, the woman should be put in a sitting position and any constrictive clothing loosened. Then the primary cause needs to be found and treated; often a distended bladder is the cause. The hypertension is managed pharmacologically during an acute episode or in some cases with epidural analgesia such as meperidine (Baraka, 1985). Epidural anesthesia is favored for the labor and birth.

Labor. Unrecognized labor can be a problem in paraplegia. In women with spinal cord injury, labor usually is painless if the injury is above T10 (Nygaard, Bartscht, and Cole, 1991). A gush of amniotic fluid may be confused with incontinence. The first symptoms of labor that some women perceive may be those of autonomic dysreflexia. Others feel back discomfort, nausea, or abdominal spasms. A woman may be taught to feel for a hardening of the uterine muscle. There have been instances of a paraplegic woman delivering an infant at home alone because of little warning of active labor. For this reason some physicians advise admitting paraplegic women at 36 to 37 weeks' gestation, or even earlier if they have any indication of early effacement. Others may advocate periodic home uterine monitoring to help detect the onset of contractions. During the labor process, extra help may be needed for spasms. Frequent positioning will be very important, including soft restraints and propping legs with pillows. A birthing chair may be helpful in adding gravity to the pushing effort, as well as helping to prevent autonomic dysreflexia.

Nursing Responsibilities

Persons with disabilities often encounter reactions from others that include treating them as if they are lacking in intelligence or to be pitied or admired for "courage"; if they are ill or dependent, conversation may be directed toward a relative or friend rather than to the person herself. A nurse may have common misconceptions—that paraplegic women always need cesarean births, that disabled persons will not be able to parent adequately, or that paraplegic and quadriplegic women will have no pain during labor. A woman with a history of spinal cord injury may be asked to retell "how it happened" to each new nurse that works with her.

Collaboratively develop a plan of care that meets the woman's individual needs. Determine how advancing pregnancy changes her ADL level. Remember these clients have worked intensely in rehabilitation to become independent in self-care, and this independence must be protected.

ASSESSMENT

Speak frankly and directly to the woman herself, asking her what assistance is needed before assuming she needs help or leaving her alone in a difficult situation. Assessment includes finding out her abilities and how her care can be facilitated by asking questions such as "What do you find inconvenient in our setup?" or "How can I help?" Nurses have an obligation to become informed about each type of disability when their clients include women with spinal cord injury. Collect data to prepare for a discharge plan.

NURSING DIAGNOSES

A number of diagnoses may apply, depending on the level of injury and the accompanying problems, some of which are listed:

1. Alteration in urinary pattern: incontinence secondary to impaired voluntary control
2. High risk for urinary tract infection related to changes of pregnancy, weight, difficulty with self-catheterization
3. High risk for impaired skin integrity secondary to immobility, edema, incontinence, and impaired vascular tone
4. High risk for injury related to altered center of gravity, orthostatic hypotension
5. Alteration in self concept secondary to altered ability for self-care, isolation in managing pregnancy and parenting

EXPECTED OUTCOMES

1. Maintains bladder management program.
2. Maintains nutrition and fluid intake to prevent constipation and urinary tract infection.
3. Woman uses methods to prevent edema and skin breakdown.
4. Exhibits self-confidence in independence of care, seeks support as needed.
5. Identifies early signs of labor.

NURSING INTERVENTIONS

As weight and size increase with pregnancy, the woman may begin to find her limited mobility further impaired. Transfer may be difficult, for example, even to the point of needing assistance with toileting or driving. An increase in disability, even though temporary, can be traumatic and can feel like regression. Avoiding excessive weight gain and maximizing upper body-

strengthening exercises may be helpful. Medical staff members will need to be alert about providing adequate help for transfer to the examination table and toilet during later pregnancy.

Women who spend long hours in a wheelchair may already have orthostatic edema, which can be compounded by pregnancy. Elevating the feet above hip level at regular intervals, wearing elastic support hose, and range of motion exercises can help decrease edema. Prevention or treatment of anemia, careful attention to position changes, padding chairs, and daily skin inspection are helpful in preventing skin breakdown. Explain the changes of pregnancy that may affect her established patterns of care, and remind her that constipation can be a major problem for pregnant women, as it may already be for her. Instruct her about the expected urinary changes.

The woman will need a modified version of the warning signs of pregnancy for impending labor. Teach her to look for the signs that can be noticed, such as the mucous plug extrusion, and abdominal contractions that may be palpated and are progressively regular and frequent. Both the woman and her family should be reminded that autonomic dysreflexia—about which she already will be familiar, may be an early sign of labor.

A birth plan should have been devised before labor so that early in labor, special needs and concerns are discussed with the woman and solutions found (Figure 23-8). Many paraplegic women have felt they had to keep track of their own special needs because no one was prepared for them. During labor someone should keep careful track of repositioning (every 30 to 60 minutes) to prevent skin pressure. Bladder management usually is handled by an indwelling Foley catheter or by periodic straight catheterization (remember to use anesthetic ointment). Fetal monitoring usually is instituted, but the straps must not be too tight. Internal fetal electrocardiogram or use of a soft stretchable band to hold both tocotransducer and ultrasonic transducer is helpful. Because varying reports indicate that at least half of all paraplegic cases will experience hyperreflexia during labor, the entire staff should be acquainted with the event and planned therapy.

Adequate help for transfers should be arranged, and a physical therapist may be consulted. The use of a birth chair or bed will be helpful in adding gravity to the process, but long periods in one position should be avoided to prevent skin breakdown.

After delivery, mobilization is important to avoid deep vein thrombosis and preserve skin integrity. The assistance of a physical therapist may be appropriate. Bladder management must be carefully followed to avoid new problems with infection. Because lochial flow and sanitary pads may cause skin irritation, commercial disposable diapers and frequent perineal care are advisable.

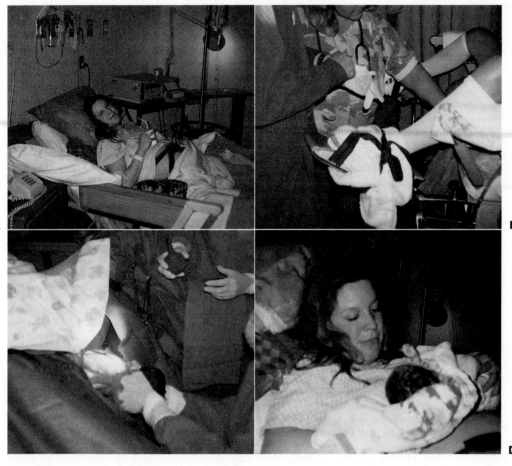

FIGURE 23-8 Birth sequence of woman with spinal cord injury. **A,** Padding with many pillows makes labor positions more comfortable. **B,** Legs are tied onto the leg holders, and knees are padded against pressure of the birthing bed's side rails. **C** and **D,** First look at her baby.

In the recovery period the woman will be fatigued, and the nursing care plan should include extra assistance for self-care. The disability should not distract from common needs for adjustment and learning that any new mother has. Rehearsing infant care in the hospital, including baths and hygienic care, is important. Discuss her planning for home care, including how the infant will be placed in a car seat. Referring her to other resources such as other mothers with disabilities, occupational therapy, and appropriate literature may help with practical ideas. (See Figure 23-9 for a crib adaptation.)

▶ EVALUATION

1. Is she able to verbalize a positive response to the experience? Did she feel her independence was honored?
2. Did planning take place for increased self-care needs and modification of the home for infant care?
3. Was hyperreflexia avoided or managed without risk to mother and infant?
4. Is she free of bladder infection and pressure sores?

I found out that I was pregnant 7 weeks into the pregnancy. I was extremely excited. My spinal cord injury is at T12 so I have full use and feeling in my arms and torso but no feeling in my legs. I began wondering who I could turn to for advice and realized I would have to blaze my own path, network as best I could, and read what little had been published.

My pregnancy was marked by a series of hard-to-treat urinary tract infections. Life became scientific—tracking intervals between catheterizations, increasing fluid intake to flush the kidneys, and analyzing methods of cleaning catheters for reuse since it is cost-prohibitive to use a new one every time. One way I could tell a UTI was raging was when voiding began and was frequent until the infection was under control. I had to have extra supplies (adult superabsorbent diapers) on hand for "accidents." My greatest fear was that the antibiotic I needed to take would adversely affect the baby. I was assured by my specialist that the risks were small and would be greater if no action were taken. I had to wear clothes and underwear with an access for catheterization when away from home, since it became more difficult to remove clothing. I did self-catheterization all during pregnancy with no problems except that I had to watch my balance and recline more fully in the chair to do it.

One piece of advice I would give nurses is not to assume or make decisions for a person with a disability.

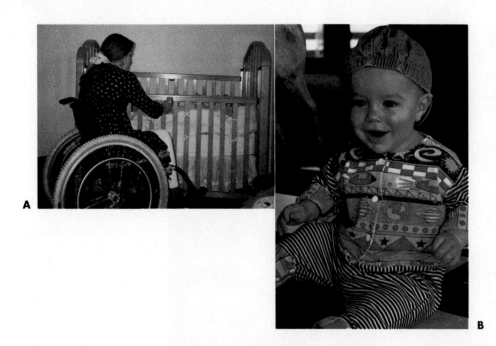

FIGURE 23-9 A, Wheelchair adaptations for a new mother with spinal cord injury. **B,** It is difficult to lift a heavy boy in and out of cribs and car seats, but he is worth it.

Sometimes, too, nurses seemed to be intimidated by leg spasms and didn't know what to do—just ask. If my leg is spasming, it helps if a person holds my leg and bends it at the knee, which usually stops the spasm.

Lower back pain was crippling from time to time, as my weight increased and the center of gravity shifted. The best remedy was a visit out of the chair, lying on a heating pad. If I could not leave the chair, I put my chest on my lap to stretch out the spasm.

Things went smoothly until the seventh month when the excess weight I had gained began to limit my already limited mobility. Transfers from chair to bed and to toilet, and from chair to car, became more strenuous and risky. I was unable to go up even slight uphill slopes like curb cuts. I had to choose carefully for the flattest route anywhere. I gained so much weight, I almost got too big for the wheelchair. Looking back, I would try to limit weight gain since it affected my mobility so greatly.

The worst problem of the last month was edema in my feet. I did elevate my feet at night and wore TED hose. The edema never traveled much past the midcalf, which worried me, since I had previously had deep vein thrombosis in my upper thigh. Exercise such as stretching also might have helped, especially with a partner to assist.

I went to the hospital several times with Braxton Hicks because they seemed so strong, but real labor was more painful. We timed the contractions from 12 midnight to 7 AM until they were close and more regular, then went to the hospital. I had a lot of stomach and back pain and asked for pain relief. They gave me intrathecal morphine, which relieved the pain; I was alert and the labor went well. I did have side effects of itching and a severe headache for 3 days afterward. I wanted my legs secured so that if I had spasms they would not get in the way. A birthing chair was available, but it was not offered until late in the labor and I did not want to transfer then. I was aware of when the contractions began and ended and when the baby's head reached the perineal area, and I was able to push. They did use suction to get the baby's head out. I had a healthy baby boy. The doctor gave me local anesthetic for my episiotomy even though I didn't need it—he couldn't stand doing it without! I felt great all through the labor but was completely exhausted after birth.

Fatigue was one of my biggest problems postpartum. The combination of fatigue, having lots of discharge, and needing to catheterize made perineal care incredibly difficult. Many nurses asked me how my injury happened, when questions about what was happening with me currently would have been more helpful. I didn't get a shower until the second day when someone thought to get a shower chair from another floor. Once I got home, child care seemed overwhelming. Role playing with someone at the hospital might have been helpful. Bathing the baby was difficult because sinks are too high. I couldn't walk or rock the baby to comfort him. So a battery-operated swing really helped. It was difficult to get my baby into his car seat safely while supporting his head. A friend devised a sling to help with this. Disability is often costly, so people don't usually have a lot of extra money for equipment. A crib with a hand-operated gate rather than foot-controlled, as well as a good seamstress, were helpful. A nearby college engineering department sometimes helps with adapting equipment as a student project.

Finally, my advice to nurses is to talk directly to a person with a disability. Feel free to admit, "I don't know—tell me what I can do," as many nurses did with me. Try to think in advance about what special needs may come up and how to address them. An increase in disability, even if temporary, can be frustrating and scary—you can help by being sensitive to needs for assistance and independence.

KEY POINTS

- Anemia underlies many chronic health problems and during pregnancy is intensified by physiologic demands for iron.
- Anemia related to genetic causes is a widespread problem, made worse by poor nutrition in many parts of the world.
- Because of its prevalence in the United States there is universal newborn testing for the sickle trait.
- Disseminated intravascular coagulation (DIC) may be at a low level in preeclampsia or may escalate suddenly in a variety of pregnancy complications.
- Rapid diagnosis of DIC and intervention are critical to stop hemorrhage and save the woman's life.
- Platelets have assumed new importance for several problems: pregnancy-induced hypertension, HELLP, systemic lupus erythematosus, and idiopathic thrombocytopenia show blood platelet disorders of varying severity.
- After blunt trauma the fetal status should be assessed for at least 4 hours because abruptio plancentae is the most common result.
- The Rh status must be assessed after trauma because fetomaternal transfusion is common.
- CPR must be modified for the pregnant woman by ensuring that the vena caval syndrome is avoided.

- Perimortem cesarean delivery may save the life of the fetus.
- The importance of maintaining independence in self-care cannot be overemphasized when pregnant women have chronic disease or disabilities.
- Epilepsy is caused by abnormal electrical discharges in the brain and has many trigger events.
- Generalized convulsive seizures such as tonic-clonic have the greatest potential for harmful impact on the fetus.
- Changes in levels of antiepilepsy drugs during pregnancy may be due to physiologic changes or to noncompliance with medication regimen: all these drugs carry some teratogenic risk.
- The physiologic immune suppression of pregnancy appears to stabilize or improve multiple sclerosis temporarily, but relapses are common in the postpartum period.
- Women with spinal cord injury are fertile, and many retain some sexual feeling; therefore pregnancies can be expected.
- The chief problems to anticipate in spinal cord injury are preterm labor, autonomic dysreflexia, and need for operative assistance.

STUDY QUESTIONS

23-1 Fill in the blanks with a Key Term in this chapter.
   a. AEDs may depress _Folate_ levels and can result in anemia.
   b. After a seizure a person may be difficult to arouse in the _____ state. _Postictal_
   c. When seizures happen continuously: _____. _Status Elepticus_
   d. Bleeding from mucous membranes occurs in _____. _DIC disseminate intravascular coagulation_
   e. A person with spinal cord injury may have _Autonomic dysreflexia_ when noxious stimuli occur.
   f. A condition of lowered platelet levels is _____. _Thrombocytopenia_

23-2 Note if the statement is true or false:
   _F_ a. Pregnancy causes MS to worsen in its overall course.
   _T_ b. AEDs should be given during labor even if fluids are being withheld.

_F_ c. Paraplegic and quadraplegic women have no pain during labor.
_T_ d. High fluid intake is protective for a client with sickle cell disease.

23-3 What nursing interventions are *not used* when autonomic dysreflexia occurs?
   a. Loosen tight clothing.
   b. Move woman to a sitting or high Fowler's position.
   c. Turn woman onto left side, and prop with pillows.
   d. Empty the bladder, if full.

23-4 Which intervention is unique for a pregnant woman receiving CPR?
   a. Slightly elevate the legs to increase central circulation.
   b. Use a ratio of chest compression to breaths of 10 to 1.

Anti Epileptic Drugs

c. Listen for fetal heart rate before using extraordinary methods.

d. Position so that vena caval compression does not occur.

23-5 Mrs. Sapolous comes to the clinic with anemia indicated by an Hb level of 9.4 and Hct value of 28%. You should obtain information from her regarding use or ingestion of:
   a. Acetaminophen
   b. Naphthalene moth balls
   c. Kidney beans
   d. Okra

23-6 Folic acid, 1 mg daily, is prescribed. Its effectiveness will be enhanced if a person takes it with:

a. Skim milk
b. Orange juice
c. Cranberry juice cocktail
d. 8 ounces of water

23-7 You emphasize that a client with sickle cell disease can decrease the precipitation of crisis by:
   a. Using meditation as an effective stress management technique
   b. Taking prophylactic antibiotics to avoid infection
   c. Drinking at least eight glasses of water daily
   d. Eating a variety of foods high in iron

Answer Key

23-1 a. Folate, b. Postictal, c. Status epilepticus, d. DIC, e. Autonomic dysreflexia, f. Thrombocytopenia, 23-2 a. False, b. True, c. False, d. True, 23-3 c 23-4 d 23-5 b 23-6 b 23-7 d

REFERENCES

Baraka: Epidural meperidine for control of autonomic hyperreflexia in a paraplegic patient, *Anaesthesia* 62:688, 1985.

Beischer NA, MacKay EV: *Obstetrics and the newborn,* ed 2, Philadelphia, 1993, WB Saunders.

Birk K et al: The clinical course of multiple sclerosis during pregnancy and the puerperium, *Arch Neurol* 47:738, 1990.

Carty EM, Conic TA, Hall C: Comprehensive health promotion for the pregnant woman who is disabled: role of the nurse midwife, *J Nurse Midwifery* 35(3):133, 1990.

Chui DHK, Wong SC, Scriver CR: The thalassemias and health care in Canada: a place for genetics in medicine, *Can Med Assoc J* 144(1):21, 1991.

Conley NH, Olshansky E: Current controversies in pregnancy and epilepsy: a unique challenge to nursing, *JOGNN* 16(5):321, 1987.

Crosby WM, Costello J: Safety of lap-belt restraint for pregnant victims of automobile collisions, *N Engl J Med* 284:632, 1971.

Daddario JB: Trauma in pregnancy, *J Perinat Neonatal Nurs* 3(2):14, 1989.

Danforth D, Scott J, eds: *Obstetrics and gynecology,* ed 5, New York, 1987, JB Lippincott.

Davis RK, Maslow AS: Multiple sclerosis in pregnancy: a review, *Obstet Gynecol Surv* 47:190, 1992.

Deitch EA et al: Management of burns in pregnant women, *Am J Obstet Gynecol* 161(1):1, 1989.

Dudek S: *Nutrition handbook for nursing practice,* New York, 1987, JB Lippincott Co.

Felsenthal G: Peripheral nervous system disorders and pregnancy. In Goldstein PJ, Stein BJ, eds: *Neurological disorders of pregnancy,* Mt Kisco, NY, 1992, Future Publishing.

France-Dawson M: Sickle cell disease: implications for nursing care, *J Adv Nurs* 11:729, 1986.

Gabbe S, Niebyl J, Simpson J, eds: *Obstetrics: normal and problem pregnancies,* New York, 1987, Churchill Livingstone.

Giacoia GP, Azubuike K: Autoimmune diseases in pregnancy: their effect on the fetus and newborn, *Obstet Gynecol Surv* 46(11):723, 1991.

Goldstein PJ, Stern BJ, eds: *Neurological disorders of pregnancy,* Mt Kisco, NY, 1992, Future Publishing.

Harvey M: OB critical care: beyond high-risk pregnancy, *MCN* 17(6):296, 1992.

Hughes SJ et al: Management of the pregnant woman with spinal cord injuries, *Br J Obstet Gynaecol* 948:513, 1991.

Johnson JD, Oakley LE: Managing minor trauma during pregnancy, *JOGNN* 20(5):379, 1990.

Khurana R: Headache. In Goldstein PJ and Stern BJ, eds: *Neurological disorders of pregnancy,* Mt Kisco, NY, 1992, Future Publishing.

Koshy M et al: Prophylactic red-cell transfusions in pregnant patients with sickle cell disease, *N Eng J Med* 319:1447, 1988.

Leiberman JR et al: Electrical accidents during pregnancy, *Obstet Gynecol* 67:861, 1986.

Letsky EA: Disseminated intravascular coagulation. In Morgan B, ed: *Problems in obstetric anesthesia,* New York, 1987, John Wiley & Sons.

Mayberry MC et al: Pregnancy complicated by hemoglobin CC and C-thalassemia disease, *Obstet Gynecol* 76(2):324, 1990.

McManus KJ: Effects on the fetus and newborn of medications commonly used during pregnancy, *J Perinat Neonatal Nurs* 3:73, 1990.

Meadow, R: Anticonvulsants in pregnancy, *Arch Dis Child* 66:62, 1991.

Nygaard I, Bartscht KD, Cole S: Sexuality and reproduction in spinal cord injured women, *Obstet Gynecol Surv* 46(10):727, 1991.

Ouimette J: *Perinatal nursing care of the high risk mother and infant,* Boston, 1986, Jones & Bartlett.

Pearlman MD, Tintinalli JE, Lorenz RP: Blunt trauma during pregnancy, *N Engl J Med* 323:1609, 1990.

Shailor TL, Roach D, Weisnor D: Adult respiratory distress syndrome, *J Perinat Neonatal Nurs* 6(2):25, 1992.

Sherer DM, Schenker JG: Accidental injury during pregnancy, *Obstet Gynecol Surv* 44(5):330, 1989.

Ship-Horowitz T: Nursing care of the sickle cell anemic patient in labor, *JOGNN* 11(6):381, 1983.

Smith CIE, Hammarstrom SL: Intravenous immunoglobulin in pregnancy, *Obstet Gynecol* 66(suppl):39, 1985.

Troiano NH: Cardiopulmonary resuscitation of the pregnant woman, *J Perinat Neonatal Nurs* 3(5):1, 1989.

Warner MB, Rageth CJ, Zack GA: Pregnancy and autonomic hyperreflexia in patients with spinal cord injury, *Paraplegia* 25:482, 1987.

Watson WJ, Katz VL, Bowes WA: Plasmapheresis during pregnancy, *Obstet Gynecol* 76(3 Pt I):451, 1990.

Willens JS, Copel LC: Performing CPR on adults, *Nursing '89* 1:34, 1989.

Wineman, NM: Adaptation to multiple sclerosis: the role of social support, functional disability, and perceived uncertainty, *Nurs Res* 39:294, 1990.

STUDENT RESOURCE SHELF

Campion JM: *The baby challenge: a handbook on pregnancy for women with a physical disability,* New York, 1990, Tavistock/Routledge. An exploration of issues from deciding to have a child to delivery and beyond, including chapters on specific disabilities and one for health professionals.

Johnson JD, Oakley LE: Managing minor trauma during pregnancy, *JOGNN* 20(5):379, 1991. Discussion of nursing responsibilities with a detailed care plan for the injured woman.

Kopula B: Mothers with impaired mobility speak out, *MCN* 14:115, 1989. Seven mothers with disabilities discuss obstacles they faced in becoming parents; includes a detailed annotated bibliography of literature for parents with disabilities.

McEwan CE et al: Comprehensive health promotion for the pregnant woman who is disabled, *J Nurse Midwifery* 35:133, 1990. Considerations for health professionals working with disabled women during pregnancy, labor, and postpartum, with specific discussion of rheumatoid arthritis, spinal cord injury, and hearing and vision impairment.

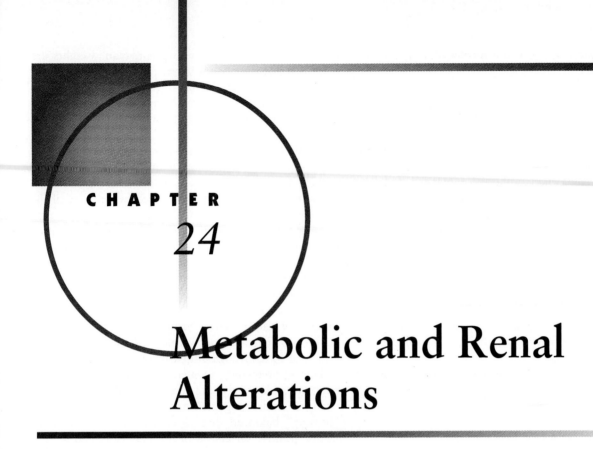

CHAPTER
24

Metabolic and Renal Alterations

KEY TERMS

Acute Cystitis (AC)
Acute Urethral
  Syndrome
Asymptomatic
  Bacteriuria (ASB)
Diabetes Mellitus
  (DM)
Euglycemia
Gestational Diabetes
  Mellitus (GDM)
Glucagon
Hyperglycemia
Hypoglycemia
Hyperthyroidism
Hypothyroidism
Infant of a Diabetic
  Mother (IDM)

Insulin Dependent
  Diabetic Mellitus (IDDM)
Macrosomia
Pyelonephritis

LEARNING OBJECTIVES

1. *Describe the effects of each metabolic disorder on the pregnancy, as well as the effect of pregnancy on the disorder.*
2. *Compare various types of urinary tract infections.*
3. *Summarize nutritional teaching specifically for conditions of overweight, hyperthyroidism, and insulin dysfunction.*
4. *Compare variations in nursing interventions for hyperthyroidism and hypothyroidism.*
5. *Discuss common methods for monitoring blood glucose during pregnancy, and describe two methods of insulin administration.*
6. *Prepare a teaching plan for the possible difficulties in diabetic control during pregnancy, labor, and immediately after birth.*
7. *Discuss at least two considerations in planning pregnancy for a woman who has had a kidney transplant.*

Nutritional Problems During Pregnancy

Pregnancy may be considered a laboratory examination of the working order of the female body, testing every organ system and part. Obviously the metabolic system receives its share; it is subject to 40 weeks of stress that often reveals some fascinating reactions and responses. Many of these have appeared predictably enough that health care givers act as alert investigators to discover the first indication that any of these distinctive conditions has appeared and warrants further scrutiny and/or treatment.

OBESITY

The most common metabolic disorder in this country is **obesity.** An estimated 15% of adults are overweight, with women outnumbering men. Simple gain is present when body weight exceeds the recommended amount by 10%; *obesity* is the term used when weight is 20% or more above ideal before pregnancy.

Risk

Invariably, among pregnant women there will be some who are obese, whose bodies are taxed by two simultaneous stresses, pregnancy and overweight. Obese women are at higher risk for the following:

1. Chronic hypertension
2. Latent diabetes with large-for-gestational-age infants
3. Uterine dysfunction because of oversized fetus
4. Abnormal presentations and cesarean birth
5. Increased anesthetic and operative risk; and in the recovery period, thromboembolism and febrile morbidity (Friedman and Kim, 1985)

Large birth weight infants tend to be taller and heavier throughout childhood and are at increased risk for obesity in adult life (Binkin, 1988). Women with similar weight gains who are thinner before pregnancy tend to have smaller babies than obese women.

Excessive weight gain during pregnancy is associated with increased birth weight of infants and its consequences, that is, risk of fetopelvic disproportion, risk of cesarean delivery, birth trauma, asphyxia, and mortality. Excessive weight gain can also place women at a greater risk of obesity and its health-related problems such as hypertension and diabetes in the future.

Nursing Responsibilities

The nurse must participate with the entire health care team to ensure clients have the best possible outcome of pregnancy. Use the period of pregnancy to teach diet related healthy behaviors that will influence the health of the woman postpartum and her child. Identify problem areas that impact on the client's ability to maintain expected weight gains as her pregnancy advances. Discuss poor or excessive weight gains on a nonjudgmental basis and support appropriate changes in the client's diet. Issues that are related to excess weight for height should be addressed postpartum, not during pregnancy.

The best indicator for appropriate weight gain during pregnancy is based on the maternal prepregnancy weight (see Chapter 10). Women's weight should always be measured at each health care visit, even if the woman is in her second or third trimester at the time of the first encounter. Although prepregnant weights are helpful in assessing gain patterns, women do not always contact a member of the health care team until they are well into their first trimester or may tell you unrealistic prepregnant weights. At that time, the rate of weight gain can be used as a marker of acceptable gains over time. When abnormal gains in weight are noted, a discussion with the pregnant woman should be planned to help work with her to establish possible causes to explain the gain in weight, followed by a review of the findings with the health care team.

Severe dietary restrictions should never be attempted during pregnancy. This practice can lead to catabolism (breakdown) of fat stores and formation of ketones. Protein restriction, especially during the first trimester, can negatively affect fetal brain cell multiplication and lead to irreversible damage. Dieting and fasting during pregnancy lead to ketone formation and hypoglycemia, conditions that are poorly tolerated by the fetus, and may lead to neurologic impairment.

During pregnancy, women are very receptive to nutritional guidance and are accepting of dietary behavior changes. Addressing concerns of a pregnant woman's "healthy" balanced diet vs empty calories may have lasting positive effects on health behaviors and dietary practices in the future. Pregnant women may find that an increase in the insoluble fiber content of their diets (wheat bran) will help relieve the common problem of constipation. Nurses should use any situation or "teachable moment" made available to them to promote preventive health patterns to their clients.

It is always best to discuss the changes women experience including weight gain goals before pregnancy, but, if unable to do this, a review of dietary intake and food preferences are useful tools to use in establishing expected weight gain during pregnancy.

MATERNAL PHENYLKETONURIA (PKU)

Almost all protein sources contain the amino acid phenylalanine which should be metabolized to tyrosine. The biochemical defect in PKU is a deficiency of the liver enzyme *phenylalanine 4-hydroxylase* needed to metabolize phenylalanine. Excessive accumulation of this amino acid and its abnormal metabolites, phenylpyruvic acid and phenylacetic acid, leads to progressive and irreversible brain damage. This inborn error of metabolism (IEM) is genetically inherited in a recessive pattern; two parents may carry the trait and have a homozygous infant (see Chapter 27). There are severe and milder forms. The rate of occurrence is 1:16,000 births and the risk is higher for people from northern European heritage. Since 1967 all newborns in the United States and Canada have been screened for PKU and a diagnosed infant has been treated with a phenylalanine-free diet. Unfortunately, until the late

1970s it was thought that one "grew out of" this problem. Today, studies show that a modified diet should be continued, and especially just before and during pregnancy there should be a return to a strict diet.

Maternal PKU has arisen as a threat as a generation of young women who were treated are now entering their childbearing years. Some may not know about the PKU effect on a fetus, and screening is important.

Risk

The harmful effects of poorly regulated maternal PKU have a teratogenic result; an increased incidence of intrauterine growth retardation, microcephaly, mental retardation and a greater risk of heart defects. If the maternal phenylalanine concentration can be kept below 150 μmol/L (<2.0 mg/dl) during pregnancy, there is a better outcome (Acosta and Wright, 1992).

Signs

In the infant there is decreased pigmentation—fair skinned, blond infants often seen with eczema, hypertonicity, irritability and sometimes with seizures. Untreated, severe mental retardation develops.

In the adult, additional signs are a distinct "mousey" or "barnlike" odor, rashes, seizures or poor coordination (Acosta and Wright, 1992). For instance, it might be possible for a retarded woman to have a diagnosis of epilepsy, and be an undiagnosed PKU client. So screening is important and is done as for the newborn infant.

Clinical Management

The data achieved so far by the National Maternal PKU Collaborative Study, which began in 1984, has shown that control of maternal blood phenylalanine levels before pregnancy improves pregnancy outcome. More than 3000 women of childbearing age have been successfully treated. Strict dietary treatment of the young infant with PKU has resulted in the child being able to achieve the average intellectual abilities appropriate in his family.

The foundation of treatment is removal from the diet of all protein containing phenylalanine. Since this is an essential amino acid, a balanced diet is gained by a protein modified supplement taken especially just prior to and during pregnancy to keep the blood levels between 60 and 180 μmol/L (Smith et al, 1990). This medical nutrition is expensive. Supplements for a year cost $4,500. Women, Infants and Children (WIC), insurance company funds, and the Collaborative Study are sources from which to obtain this supplement. The rest of the diet is made up of low-protein cereals, fruits, fats, and vegetables. Iron and zinc levels are monitored. Blood phenylalanine and tyrosine levels are monitored every 2 to 4 weeks during early pregnancy and may be done every week in later pregnancy.

Nursing Responsibilities

Every woman should be asked if she was on special diet in childhood. Any woman should be tested if she has an infant who is mentally retarded or has microcephaly. Nutrition counseling and follow-up are critical. The nurse and nutritionist will work as a team in care of this client.

Thyroid Problems

Circulating iodine from food or iodized salt is synthesized by the thyroid gland into two thyroid hormones: triiodothyronine (T_3) or thyroxine (T_4), controlled by thyroid-releasing factor from the hypothalamus and TSH from the pituitary. Balance is maintained by a feedback mechanism, which increases or decreases the amount of each for healthy functioning.

Normal pregnancy mimics a slightly hyperthyroid state; there is an increase in basal metabolic rate, cardiac output, heat intolerance, emotional liability, and amenorrhea. The thyroid hormone increases the production of intracellular proteins and energy which results in increased consumption of carbohydrates, fats and oxygen, and increased heat production as the BMR is increased (Figure 24-1).

During pregnancy, maternal thyroid function is normal. The serum thyroxine T_4 levels increase during the first trimester due to an increased binding capacity of thyroid binding globulins (TBG) secondary to the elevated estrogen level. These effects will last for one to three months after birth.

Fetal thyroid activity usually starts around 2 months gestation; by the end of the first trimester the fetal pituitary begins secretion of TSH. Apparently, T_4, T_3, and TSH do not cross the placenta in any significant amount.

HYPERTHYROID STATES

Graves' disease is an autoimmune disorder that occurs in genetically susceptible individuals. Characterized by exacerbations and remissions, the peak incidence occurs during the reproductive years (Pederson, 1989). When a woman with Graves' disease becomes pregnant, there are two patients, the fetus and the woman herself. The woman may be evaluated relatively quickly, but the fetus is at risk of an abnormal growth environment and viability is in jeopardy. Fetal loss is common, with some infants stillborn or prematurely born.

Risk

Some newborns are born with autoimmune disease, or with a goiter, exopthalamos and a hypermetabolic state. In most cases, infants have a transient disorder lasting less than 5 months and completely treatable.

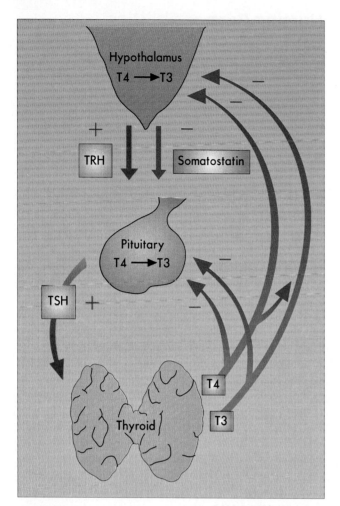

FIGURE 24-1 Diagram of hypothalamic-pituitary-thyroid axis showing the feedback cycle. (From Martin JB, Reichlin S: *Clinical endocrinology*, ed 2, Philadelphia, 1985, FA Davis.)

Signs

Characteristics of hyperthyroidism are listed in Table 24-1. Greatly elevated levels of T_4 and T_3 are found. Diagnostic studies with radioactive iodine (RAI) are not recommended during pregnancy since RAI crosses the placenta and would affect the fetal thyroid.

Clinical Management

Pregnant women with Graves' disease require medication to control their symptoms. The goal is to achieve acceptable hormone levels for pregnancy to prevent fetal difficulty. Propylthiouracil (PTU) is the drug of choice for women with hyperthyroidism since it crosses the placenta more slowly and blocks synthesis of T_4 and conversion of T_4 to T_3 in peripheral tissues.

In most cases, thyroid hormone levels are stabilized within 4 weeks. If medical management cannot control hyperthyroidism, surgical management with a subtotal thyroidectomy may be considered only during the sec-

ond trimester. The baby after birth should be closely observed for signs and symptoms of imbalance.

Nursing Responsibilities
▶ ASSESSMENT

Review the signs of hyperthyroid states and include observations for these signs in physical assessment and history taking.

▶ NURSING DIAGNOSES

Based on the presenting symptomatology and the woman's history of thyroid problems the following diagnoses may be chosen.
1. Activity intolerance related to fatigue, weight loss, hyperthermia, and insomnia.
2. Altered nutrition, less than body requirements related to increased metabolic rate resulting in poor weight gain.
3. Knowledge deficit about effect of hyperthyroidism on fetus; new medications.
4. Self-concept or body image disturbance related to goiter and exophthalmos.

▶ EXPECTED OUTCOMES

1. General feelings of health return as noted by temperature stability, sleep patterns and muscle strength.
2. Resumes normal weight progression and appetite.
3. Is able to discuss feelings about self and body image.
4. Is aware of treatment plan and medication requirements.

▶ NURSING INTERVENTION

During the actual hyperthyroid state, the woman will have increased dietary needs. Guidance as to the appropriate food choice for a well-balanced intake (with suggestions for snacks and extra fluid intake to compensate for increased perspiration, urination, and metabolism) is a real contribution by the nurse counselor. Some women are afflicted with diarrhea. Question the client about foods that particularly cause diarrhea for her (highly seasoned and fibrous foods frequently speed peristalsis).

Daily weights should be charted by the client. Instruct her to weigh at the same time every morning, after voiding and before breakfast.

The environment needs to be made comfortable for her. Since initially, there will be restlessness, anxiety, insomnia and diaphoresis, the nurse should try to create a stress-free environment by limiting visitors to those the woman chooses, reducing noise, dimming lights, and changing linens as needed. Until the treatment plan takes

TABLE 24-1 **Signs and Symptoms of Thyroid Imbalances**

HYPERTHYROIDISM	HYPOTHYROIDISM
• Nervousness • Hyperactivity • Diaphoresis • Skin texture warm, velvety, soft, damp • Hair silky • Hypersensitivity to heat • Weakness • Fatigue	• Lethargy • Dry skin, thick at knees and elbows • Hair is coarse • Cold intolerance • Weakness • Mental impairment (slowed cognitive ability, poor memory, forgetfulness, depressed affect)
• Palpitation • Tachycardia • Dyspnea • Angina • Increased appetite • Weight loss • Absence of forehead wrinkling on upward gaze • Nail loose or detached from bed	• Chest pain • Dyspnea • Anorexia • Weight gain • Facial edema (especially periorbital) • Pale skin; coarse, dry, cold with a yellow tinge (normal sclerae)
• Diarrhea • Eye symptoms (burning, tearing, diplopia, lid lag, prominent eyes [exophthalmia], stare, eyelid tremors when closed) • Hyperreflexia • Goiter	• Constipation • Thinned lateral aspect of eyebrows • Sluggish return of reflexes • Thyroid shows diffuse enlargement or is not palpable • Heavy, prolonged menses, infertility
• Decreased or absent menses • Susceptibility to infection	• Deafness (in third of population)

effect, these measures will make the initial period tolerable. Work together with the client to achieve these goals.

Because of nutritional imbalance, intake and output are important. Vital signs will reflect recovery with a decreased pulse rate and temperature. Remember to repeat and reinforce information. When a person is under physiologic stress, ability to retain information is decreased.

In implementing all teaching, including medication information, the following points are helpful:

1. Because the hyperthyroid client may be anxious, go slowly with instruction, repeating as necessary and having her repeat for verification of understanding. Personalize instructions and write out directions.
2. Teach names and dosages of drugs, and specify exact hours for taking each one.
3. Be sure the woman knows she must continue medication as long as the physician considers it necessary. She will soon feel better, but she must not stop medication prematurely. Often PTU is withdrawn by the physician several weeks before delivery because 30% of gravidas will have returned to a normal thyroid state (Ouimette, 1986).

4. Granulocytosis is a rare but serious side effect with PTU. Medication should be stopped promptly with appearance of fever or sore throat, and the health provider contacted immediately.
5. Breastfeeding is not contraindicated if PTU therapy must continue after birth.

If an eye condition leads to dryness and discomfort, soothing drops will be ordered, to be administered by either client or nurse. The client is included in every step of care, with the nurse giving rational explanation to all questions and providing information to alleviate anxiety or fear.

▶ EVALUATION

The following questions may be asked:

1. Did she participate in and state satisfaction with environmental comfort?
2. Can she state how signs began and current level of responses to therapy?
3. Does she relate the plan of care and precautions on medications for home therapy?
4. Has she discussed with the team the implications of thyroid imbalance on the fetus?

HYPOTHYROIDISM

Low T_4 levels frequently prevent conception, so hypothyroidism is rare in pregnant women. If it occurs, it is usually secondary to a known disorder such as Hashimoto's disease or to, prior thyroid gland ablation by RAI or surgery. Any of these disorders may have been diagnosed prior to pregnancy and thyroid replacement hormone given orally to normalize balance. Because of the demands of pregnancy, thyroid replacement may be inadequate.

Every system of the body is affected by a low thyroxin level (see Table 24-1). Primary hypothyroidism is caused by inability to produce or release thyroid hormones due to irradiation, surgical removal of tissue or defects in synthesis because of antithyroid drugs or iodine deficiency. This leads to increased secretion of TSH from the pituitary gland without a corresponding release of T_3 and T_4 from the thyroid. Secondary and tertiary hypothyroidism is a result of deficiency in TSH and TRH production and release. Hypothyroid states are more commonly found in Caucasians.

Risk

A decreased rate of conception is common. When adequate replacement of the hormone is taken, pregnancy outcome appears good. Sensitivity to anesthetic agents is a real problem in uncorrected hypothyroidism and places the woman at increased risk for complications.

Clinical Management

Thyroid hormone replacement taken daily achieves normal levels. Symptoms fade gradually and pregnant women may need higher doses than when nonpregnant. Blood levels should be monitored closely by the obstetrician and endocrinologist.

Nursing Responsibilities

The woman should understand that a balanced state is achieved slowly. Comfort needs should be seriously addressed. For example, these needs include extra clothing if cold intolerant, small frequent meals and extra fluids, and fiber in the diet to counteract constipation. Skin will be dry and itchy and hair dry, so skin and hair care needs to be adapted. As serum thyroid levels stabilize, symptoms should disappear. The importance of continuing daily medication must be stressed even though signs have resolved. If there are children at home, reinforce safety concerning medications. An intake of thyroid replacement tablets (L-thyroxin, Synthroid) by children can lead to acute hyperthyroidism and all its consequences.

Diabetes Mellitus

Diabetes mellitus, from the Greek *diabetes* (siphon) and the Latin *mellitus* (honey-sweet), is the inability to metabolize glucose properly. It is a chronic systemic disease, manifesting metabolic and vascular changes affecting virtually every organ in the body. The basic defect is an absolute or relative lack of insulin, which leads to alterations of carbohydrate protein, and fat metabolism. The attendant vascular changes include thickening of basement membranes, microaneurysms, peripheral vascular disease, early and widespread atherosclerosis. Transient and permanent neuropathies commonly develop.

There are several types of DM. *Type I: Insulin-dependent diabetes mellitus* (IDDM) (previously juvenile or ketosis-prone diabetes). IDDM can occur at any age and thus is no longer labeled "juvenile." This person is dependent on insulin for life; without daily injections ketoacidosis will develop.

Recently, IDDM has been shown to be linked to the HLA region of chromosome 6, which also has immunologic functions (Reece, Hagay, and Hobbins, 1991).

According to Lipman (1988), diabetes mellitus type I is inherited recessively, with 75% of the population free of diabetes, 20% not diabetic but able to transmit the gene, and 5% who are diabetic, although not necessarily symptomatic and who can and do transfer the disease to offspring. Although not specifically race-related, the incidence of diabetes type I is somewhat higher in Caucasian Americans than in African-Americans. Widely distributed geographically, the greatest prevalence occurs in northern Europe; it decreases in the Mediterranean region and still further in eastern Asia (Lipman, 1988). (See Table 24-2 for a summary of each type of diabetes.)

TABLE 24-2 Characteristics Associated with Glucose Intolerance

DIAGNOSES ASSOCIATED WITH GLUCOSE INTOLERANCE	CHARACTERISTICS
DIABETES MELLITUS (DM) *Type I Insulin Dependent (IDDM)* Insulin deficient	• Prone to produce ketone • Due to islet cell destruction • Associated with specific HLA types • Common in young, occurs at any age
Type II Non-insulin dependent (NIDDM) Insulin resistant	• Does not produce ketones • Common in adults • Associated with increased BMR (overweight) • Seen in families as autosomal dominant recessive trait
DM associated with conditions or syndromes	• Hyperglycemia due to pancreatic disease • Drug or chemically induced DM • Insulin-receptor disorders • Certain genetic syndromes
IMPAIRED GLUCOSE TOLERANCE (IGT) (Secondary diabetes)	• Abnormal glucose levels but less than those noted in overt DM • Can improve, remain static, or progress to overt DM
GESTATIONAL DIABETES MELLITUS (GDM)	• Glucose intolerance occurring during pregnancy

Modified from *Diabetes Care* 15(2):4, 1992.

Type II: non-insulin dependent diabetes mellitus (NIDDM). In the past type II was called *adult* or *maturity-onset diabetes mellitus* and has been further subgrouped into insulin-requiring and non-insulin–requiring. NIDDM is thought to be a problem of peripheral insulin resistance rather than insulin deficiency. Type II clients are usually middle-aged and overweight at onset. Type II is found more commonly in African-Americans and is also associated with hypertension.

Type II diabetes is usually controlled by diet, but women may need insulin when stressed or pregnant (Douglas, 1990). The key difference is that they may require insulin to prevent hypoglycemia but are not insulin dependent to sustain life.

Other types (secondary diabetes) include diseases causing carbohydrate intolerance such as pancreatic disease, hormonally and chemically induced diabetes, insulin receptor abnormalities, and certain genetic syndromes.

In *impaired glucose tolerance (IGT)* serum glucose levels are higher than normal, but are not in themselves diagnostic for diabetes mellitus.

Gestational diabetes mellitus (GDM) is an alteration in carbohydrate intolerance initially noted during pregnancy. It occurs in about 3% of pregnant women and the symptoms and abnormalities in glucose tolerance disappear after delivery. The symptoms of hyperglycemia are usually mild but the risks of this hyperglycemia to the fetus can be serious as in other types of DM. The diagnosis of GDM applies whether or not insulin is

BOX 24-1 White's Classification

For diabetes during pregnancy, the following classification is specific and may be still used (White, 1978):
1. Class A: Slightly abnormal glucose tolerance test. Dietary control sufficient; no insulin required
2. Class B: Onset after age 20; duration less than 10 years; no vascular disease
3. Class C: Onset between ages 10 and 20; duration 10 to 19 years; minimal or no vascular disease (that is, arteriosclerosis or calcification of the leg vessels only)
4. Class D: Onset before 10 years, duration more than 20 years; vascular disease demonstrated by retinitis, transitory albuminuria, or transitory hypertension
5. Class F: Kidney involvement
6. Class H: Heart involvement
7. Class R: Pathologic changes in the retina, including preretinal hemorrhages and evidence of new blood vessels or scars
8. Class T: Pregnant after renal transplant
Classification may change during the course of pregnancy and may be different in subsequent pregnancies.

included in the treatment plan or if the hyperglycemia persists after delivery. Physicians will also use pregnancy classifications in Box 24-1.

PREGNANCY UNMASKS DM

In normal pregnancies, the maternal plasma glucose level fluctuates between 60 mg/dl and 120 mg/dl. The glucose balance is affected by changes in estrogen and progesterone levels leading to B-cell hyperplasia (enlarged insulin secreting cells in the pancreas). Since peripheral utilization of glucose is increased during pregnancy this in turn leads to lower glucose levels. Maternal glucose crosses the placenta but maternal insulin does not. In pregnancies complicated by diabetes, maternal hyperglycemia leads to fetal hyperglycemia. Fetal hyperglycemia in turn stimulates the fetal pancreas β-cells to produce increased insulin. The increased insulin produces β-cell hyperplasia and fetal hyperinsulinemia. (See Chapter 28 for treatment of the **infant of a diabetic mother [IDM].**)

Hypoglycemia in ♀ is Øusually TX during preg. unless other Sx occur Ø

RISK

Women with IDDM who have vasculopathy or unstable diabetes are at the greatest risk for complications and death during pregnancy. Benign diabetic retinopathy may worsen during pregnancy but usually regresses following birth. The same cannot be said of women with untreated proliferative retinopathy prior to pregnancy, since worsening of the condition and possibly vision loss may occur.

Fetal Risk for IDM

There is increasing evidence that the degree of control for an IDDM woman prior to conception greatly affects the fetal outcome. Metabolic control seems to reduce the risk of perinatal mortality to that similar to the general population (Coustan, 1988). Studies find that poor maternal glucose control underlies the incidence of congenital malformations in IDM (Box 24-2).

The morbidity and mortality factors for IDM are macrosomia or IUGR, intrauterine death, delayed pulmonary maturation with respiratory distress syndrome. At any age, the IDM is 5 to 6 times more likely to develop respiratory distress syndrome. Why does this happen? Insulin is an important growth factor during fetal development, and hyperinsulinism results in excessive fetal growth or **macrosomia** (Figure 24-2) and delays pulmonary maturation of surfactant. On the other hand, if the woman is a severe diabetic with poor control, the fetus may be IUGR and have mental deficiency or die from prolonged exposure to ketonemia. What about successful completion of the pregnancy? After 36 weeks, fetal mortality appears to increase in women with DM. For this reason, frequent NST and BPS are done and delivery is scheduled by induction soon after 37 weeks.

Risk for GDM Infants

Women who have fasting and postprandial glucose elevations are at higher risk for intrauterine or neonatal

BOX 24-2 Congenital Malformations in Infants of Diabetic Mothers

Cardiovascular
- Transposition great vessels
- Ventral septal defect
- Atrial septal defect
- Hypoplastic left ventricle

Skeletal
- Cordal regression syndrome
- Spina bifida

Gastrointestinal
- Tracheoesophageal fistula
- Bowel atresia
- Imperforate anus

Central Nervous System
- Meningomyelocele
- Anencephaly
- Encephalocele
- Microcephaly

Genitourinary
- Absent kidneys
- Polycystic kidneys

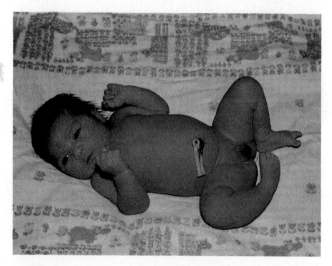

FIGURE 24-2 Large for gestational age, macrosomic infant of a diabetic mother (IDM). (Courtesy Marjory Pyle, RNC, *Lifecircle*.)

mortality. Well-controlled glucose levels in maternal GDM leads to less risk. Approximately 25% of infants of GDM mothers have a characteristic triad of problems, such as hypoglycemia, hypocalcemia and hyperbilirubinemia during recovery (see Chapter 28). They also may

not @risk for congeni malformation

have cardiomyopathy, polycythemia, and small left-colon syndrome.

SIGNS

The symptoms of uncontrolled or new onset diabetes include excessive thirst, hunger, and weight loss (Box 24-3). There may be blurred vision and possibly recurrent, hard to resolve infections. DM can develop rapidly and lead to hospitalization for acute symptoms. It can also develop slowly, with symptoms appearing gradually so as not to be initially noticed. GDM women have no overt signs although hypertension and overweight may be present.

Pregnant women with IDDM are at increased risk for development of diabetic ketoacidosis (DKA). The presence of an infection with increased insulin requirements is the most common cause. Infection precipitates a rise in plasma glucose levels. If not addressed quickly by increasing the insulin doses there may be formation of plasma ketones. The pregnant woman will then experience diuresis, dehydration and hyperosmolality. When malaise, drowsiness and hyperventilation are noted, a severe illness requiring hospitalization is present and an endocrinologist as well as a perinatologist will be needed to treat the mother and fetus. Fluid replacement, stabilization of serum electrolytes and correction of acidosis are part of the treatment plan for this medical emergency.

CLINICAL MANAGEMENT

The American Diabetes Association (ADA) Position Statement on GDM (1990) states that all pregnant

---

BOX 24-3   Signs and Symptoms of Overt Diabetes

• Polyuria (excess urination)
• Polydipsia (excess thirst and fluid intake)
• Polyphagia (excess hunger and food intake)
• Neuritis (pain in the fingers and toes)
• Skin disturbances (for example, pruritus [itching] and slow healing)
• Weight loss
• Weakness, fatigue, drowsiness

BOX 24-4   Classification of Diabetes Mellitus

Diabetes mellitus

• Random plasma glucose level ≥200 mg/dl with symptoms of diabetes
• Fasting plasma glucose level ≥140 mg/dl on two occasions
• 2 oral glucose tolerance tests with the 2 hour sample ≥200 mg/dl and one other value ≥200 mg/dl after 75 g of glucose

Gestational diabetes mellitus

• Two or more plasma glucose levels equal to or greater than those noted below, following a 100 g oral glucose intake

fasting	105 mg/dl
1 hour postglucose load	190 mg/dl
2 hour postglucose load	165 mg/dl
3 hour postglucose load	145 mg/dl

Modified from American Diabetes Association, 1992.

---

women should be screened for glucose intolerance between 24 and 28 weeks of pregnancy. Any woman with a history of glucose intolerance would be tested in the first trimester. Box 24-4 lists diagnostic criteria, and Figure 24-3 lists decisions based on testing results.

First a glucose challenge of 50 grams is given, and 1 hour later, blood is drawn for glucose levels. If levels are over 140 mg/dl the woman is tested with a larger dose in the glucose tolerance test (GTT). Three days before a GTT, the client should be put on a diet of 150 grams of carbohydrate per day, fasting after midnight on the day of the test and having taken no caffeine or nicotine.

A history of elevated glucose may be seen by two laboratory tests. Hemoglobin A_{1c} (HbA_{1c}) is a measure used to estimate blood glucose levels over the previous 4 to 6 weeks, in effect, a lie detector. It is an irreversible bond of glucose to a fraction of hemoglobin protein. Since the lifecycle of a red blood cell is 120 days, an elevated HbA_{1c} indicates significant past hyperglycemia. This test will be used throughout the pregnancy to monitor levels. Levels greater than normal reflect poor control of blood glucose. The following outcomes have been documented by long term studies (Barss, 1989).

Excellent control < 6.9% = outcome has shown
                              no infant malformation
Good control < 7 to 8.5% = outcome has
                              shown 5% malformations
Poor control > 8.6% = outcome has shown
                              22% malformations

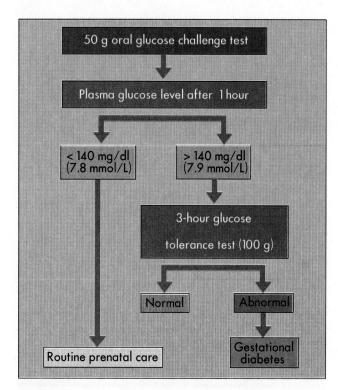

FIGURE 24-3 Screening plan for all pregnant women. (From American Diabetes Association Council on Diabetes in Pregnancy.)

There may be false results with anemia (low) and renal failure, stress and steroids (high). The second measure is the use of fructosamine glycosylated albumin which indicates the average serum glucose for the last 1 to 3 weeks since the lifespan of albumin is 28 to 40 days. High fructosamine glycosylated albumin has been seen in women with large babies.

The goals of treatment for diabetes are to (1) maintain metabolic control of glucose levels (Box 24-5) and (2) prevent acute and chronic complications.

The pregnant woman with DM should work together with members of the diabetes health care team, including obstetrician, specialist in diabetes, certified diabetes nurse educator, and a nutritionist; as labor approaches, a perinatologist joins the team. All should agree that she is in good control as she plans to conceive. Because she will need extra care, she and her

---

BOX 24-5   Good Control of Glucose Levels

	Type I	Type II
Fasting	< 120mg/dl	< 140 mg/dl
Postprandial	< 180 mg/dl	< 200 mg/dl

Modified from the American Diabetes Association, 1988.

---

partner should understand the cost of pregnancy in money and time spent in being monitored, at home or in the hospital.

Since oral hypoglycemic agents are known to cross the placenta, use is avoided during pregnancy due to adverse effects on fetal development. Yet, a woman with DM type II may seek care in the first trimester while still taking oral agents. Risks associated with oral agents will need to be discussed with the client.

The four major areas to be addressed in management are blood glucose monitoring, insulin, nutrition, and exercise.

Blood Glucose Monitoring

Today glucose monitoring in the home is essential for pregnant DM women. Blood glucometers requiring only one drop of blood from a finger stick sample are easy to use, give rapid results and are small and portable. Measurements should be taken on a schedule as seen in Box 24-4. Ideally, levels should be checked before meals, two hours postprandial, at bedtime and around 2 to 3 AM when there is increased risk of nocturnal hypoglycemia. In reality, it is very difficult for the woman to be so precise. She needs a number of incentives and much encouragement to inflict needle sticks so many times a day. The nurse works with her to encourage compliance. Keeping a chart is an incentive, especially when she brings it to clinic each visit. Women soon learn their own patterns and can then omit one or two testing times because they understand their daily fluctuations. Teach her that blood is taken only from the side of a finger, using all ten fingers in a rotation so that there is time to heal (see Procedure 24-1). When she is in the hospital, encourage her to continue doing her own checks since she causes herself less pain and can be more consistent. In this way she keeps a measure of independence in the hospital setting. She should also monitor the first morning specimen for ketones each day to see if blood glucose exceeds 150 mg/dl.

Insulin

Most pregnant woman have a general lowering of plasma glucose levels during the first trimester related to estrogen action. Therefore IDDM clients are at greater risk of hypoglycemia. The woman will need to know how to adjust insulin levels in response to glucose testing. With metabolic changes in the second and third trimesters, insulin requirements are increased as much as two to three times. She is not becoming worse; this physiologic effect will return to normal after birth.

However, greater need for insulin means administering divided doses and often 3 to 4 injections each day. Again, these are procedures which are time consuming and require attention. Thus, the woman may begin to feel that she is sick and can become fearful or noncom-

PROCEDURE 24-1   Glucose Screening

Capillary blood sugar

- Wash hands in warm water (warmth promotes circulation).
- Choose a finger, and, using spring-driven lancet, stick the finger on the side or outer edge (least painful sites).
- Drop hand to side, below heart. (Perhaps "milk" the finger, using other hand, gently squeezing finger from hand to fingertip.) Be sure there is enough blood to cover both pads on plastic glucose-oxidase impregnated strips for testing capillary blood glucose.
- Put drop of blood on strip as instructed by health team, following timing and wiping away excess blood as directed by method.
- Read visually or on reflectance meter and record.
- Repeat on recommended schedule (Figure 24-4)

Urine for glucose and ketones

- Empty bladder completely (the "long specimen").
- Using a clean container, 30 minutes later void again and collect specimen (the "short specimen").
- Test "short specimen" for glucose and ketones.
- Repeat in morning each day (or as otherwise instructed).

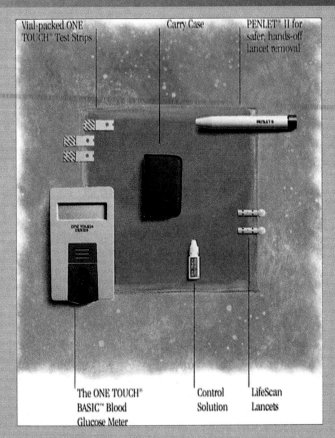

FIGURE 24-4 One Touch glucose testing equipment. (Courtesy Life Scan, Milpitas, Calif.)

•   •   •

OPTIONAL ACTIVITY: Write a sample nursing note correctly documenting the performance of this procedure.

pliant. Nursing intervention is extremely important during these weeks to keep her focused on the goal of having a healthy baby.

A number of changes have been made in recommendations for insulin administration, not all of which have been put into practice correctly on hospital units (See annotated reference from Diabetes Care, 1990). In the following, note how the concern to protect tissue integrity *overrides* certain routine habits of injection.

- Human insulin should be used during pregnancy because of a more rapid onset and shorter duration of action. Human insulin triggers fewer antibodies and is recommended for women beginning insulin, such as for GDM or NIDDM mothers placed on insulin. A pregnant woman already using another type or brand of insulin should remain on that brand, even in the hospital. *Do not change brands* without careful supervision since there are different levels of action.
- Insulin only requires refrigeration for long term storage. The currently opened vial should be kept at room temperature for up to 30 days. It has been found that refrigerated, cold insulin irritates the tissue more than that at room temperature.
- NPH and regular insulin may be premixed into the same syringe without any change in stability. At home, these may be mixed in the morning and given at the specified intervals throughout the day.
- At home, insulin needles and syringes may be reused until the needle is dull. This is true as long as the needle is recapped immediately after use. Do not wipe needle with alcohol which removes the silicone covering that prevents trauma during injection.
- Insulin should be given at a 90 degree angle without aspiration or massage of the site. It is not necessary to cleanse the skin with alcohol, since alcohol tracked down with the needle irritates the tissue. If alcohol is used, be sure the skin is dry before injection.
- Different sites as well as exercise following insulin administration will affect the rate of absorption. In a crisis, if not IV, the IM route has the fastest absorption rate.
- Sites should be used for a week, with *rotation within the site.* This allows an area to completely heal in 3 to 4 weeks before again being used.
- Whenever possible insulin should be self-injected by the client, even in hospital or in labor. Always ask her to inject and only do for her at her request.

Insulin pump. In certain cases, a woman may not be able to achieve a balanced glucose level, **euglycemia,** with the standard administration regimen. The continuous subcutaneous insulin infusion (CSII) pump is often a life-saver for these women. The CSII pump has a small syringe that holds a 2 day supply of insulin. A thin catheter attaches to the insulin syringe in the pump. The end of the catheter has a small subcutaneous needle that is placed in recommended sites. The pump is programmed to deliver a basal rate of insulin in units per hour. The pump user programs the desired bolus of insulin prior to meals and snacks. Multiple BG measurements are needed to ensure that the basal rates and dose of insulin are appropriate. Because of requiring precise control, the use of a CSII pump can only be an option to a select group of compliant pregnant women with DM. Cost is also a factor in availability for use.

Nutrition

The nutritional recommendations are similar to those of the American Heart Association. The proportions change slightly. Total calories are calculated to achieve desired body weight and the weight gain needed during pregnancy. The distribution of calories is recommended by the ADA (1990) as follows:

Carbohydrates   55%–60% with most in form of complex carbohydrates

Fats   < 30%

Protein   0.8g/kg body weight, unless renal disease is present

The average daily intake should be between 2000 and 2500 kcal. A gravida should be encouraged to increase the amount of fiber to at least 30 g/day to assist in glycemic control, relieve constipation, and to satisfy the appetite.

Fiber. Fiber is an important part of the diet. Addition of certain forms of dietary fiber to the diet of diabetics significantly decreases postprandial hyperglycemia. The American Diabetes Association suggests a fiber intake as high as 20 to 30 g/1000 calories. This amount would be derived from complex, unrefined carbohydrates and from a generous amount of vegetables, salads, and fresh fruits.

The absorption rate of glucose into the blood has led to labeling carbohydrates as "slowly" and "rapidly absorbed." The slowly absorbed carbohydrates (complex, high in fiber) are preferred above the rapidly absorbed carbohydrates (simple sugars and disaccharides).

Since pregnancy is a dynamic state, frequent adjustments to the diet are made as gestation advances. Attention is focused on food preferences and life-style to increase the woman's ability to maintain appropriate intake. A daily planned pattern of three meals and three to four snacks is essential whether or not nausea is present (Table 24-3). Since nocturnal hypoglycemia is common in IDDM women, emphasis is placed on the importance of the bedtime snack. If the woman is in the

TABLE 24-3 Sample Menu and Distribution of Food with Insulin*

TIME	MENU
MORNING MEAL†	
Split between 7:30 AM and 10 AM;	2 slices low-fat cheese or $\frac{1}{2}$ cup cottage cheese
7 AM glucose test and insulin—regular and long acting	2 slices wheat or rye bread or 1 cup oatmeal
	2 tsp margarine or butter
	1 cup skim milk
	1 fresh fruit
NOON MEAL	
Split between 12:30 PM and 3 PM;	3 oz of fish, poultry or meat (trim fat)
Noon glucose test	1 serving mixed salad
	2 slices wheat or rye bread or 1 cup rice
	2 tsp of margarine or mayonnaise
	1 cup skim milk or plain low-fat yogurt
	1 fresh fruit
EVENING MEAL	
Split between 5:30 PM and 8 PM;	4 oz fish, poultry, or meat (trim fat)
5 PM glucose test and regular insulin	$\frac{1}{2}$ to 1 cup cooked vegetables
	1 serving mixed salad
	1 cup corn or lima beans
	2 tsp margarine or oil
	1 cup skim milk or buttermilk
BEDTIME SNACK	
10:30 PM;	$\frac{1}{2}$ cup cottage cheese, 2 slices low-fat cheese, or 2 tsp of
some clients need to be tested at night.	peanut butter
	1 slice wheat or rye bread
	1 fresh fruit

Available from the American Dietetic Association (216 West Jackson Boulevard, Chicago, Illinois 60606), the "diabetic exchange list" can be used as a guide to high-fiber foods.
*2000 Calories.
†Reduce carbohydrates in morning meal. Distribute food from each list between the meal and the snack after the meal.

hospital, she should participate in meal and snack planning, for often the usual snacks provided are inadequate for her.

Obese pregnant women with NIDDM present a problem regarding diet and glucose levels. Since NIDDM is usually symptom free, they may not be as motivated to make lifestyle changes early in pregnancy. Remember, this type of DM is related to insulin-resistance, making glucose regulation difficult. Insulin will often be initiated, so the woman must learn all the self-care factors. Under no condition should any weight loss be considered during pregnancy.

Women with GDM should follow the same general nutrition guidelines as seen in Table 24-3. Dietary modification is the first step in control of hyperglycemia. In general, attempts are made to maintain blood glucose between 60 mg/dl and 120 mg/dl. Although she may not need insulin, she should divide food intake into three meals and three snacks and maintain the ratio of fats, protein and complex carbohydrates.

Exercise

Pregnant women with DM should only begin exercise programs after discussing the frequency, intensity and duration of the exercise with the diabetes care team. Hopefully, a woman with IDDM has already been using a personal exercise program. Exercise lowers blood glucose levels and decreases cardiovascular risk factors such as high blood pressure and hyperlipidemia. It also affects fuel utilization and insulin sensitivity in Type II diabetes. Thus it lowers insulin requirements. There are risks involved in exercise; hypoglycemia is a possibility as well as ketoacidosis if exercise is done when blood glucose levels are over 250 mg/dl. The benefits of exercise can be obtained through scheduled sessions lasting 20 to 45 minutes, 3 days a week.

INTRAPARTUM MANAGEMENT

Infants of DM women are usually delivered just before or at term. Acceptable results of weekly and then biweekly nonstress testing and of an L/S ratio of >2.0 from amniotic fluid are positive indicators of fetal well-being and pulmonary maturity. Sonography should aid the obstetrician in identifying the infant who may require a cesarean birth because of macrosomia.

Regardless of what a fetal maturity test may show, early delivery is required when PIH, repeated ketoacidosis, increasing polyhydramnios, advancing maternal retinopathy, or preexisting renal disease with hypertension or albuminuria occurs.

Intrapartum management requires attention to glucose levels, glucose infusion rates, and insulin dosage. Bedside BG testing during labor is mandatory on a schedule of q 2 h in early labor and q 1 h in late labor and immediate recovery. Labor is equivalent to moderate exercise so less insulin is needed for control. An IDDM patient will usually have an IV of 1000 ml D_5LR with 10 U regular insulin, to run at 100 ml/hr. This rate provides 1 U per hour. An additional bolus may be given as needed.

If the plan is for cesarean birth (and the nationwide cesarean delivery rate in diabetes varies from 55% to 85% [Pritchard et al, 1986]), it should be done very early in the morning with no glucose or insulin administered until after delivery if blood sugar is 80 to 120 mg/dl. A neonatologist must be present at the delivery.

POSTPARTUM MANAGEMENT

Blood glucose management following birth can be difficult due to endocrine and metabolic changes. At separation of the placenta with removal of insulin antagonists (hPL, estrogen, and progesterone) and a reduction in plasma cortisol, there is a reduced need for insulin. After the second day, hPL is gone, and insulin shock is possible if usual doses of insulin are continued. During the first 24 hours, no long-acting insulin is given; monitoring blood glucose every 4 hours will determine the need for additional cover insulin. The prepregnancy amount is usually ordered by the 2nd morning after birth.

Breast-feeding is not contraindicated, but an increase in the diet of 500 to 600 calories per day is required (Vaughn, 1986), with insulin dosage recalculated accordingly. Hypoglycemia decreases milk supply and inhibits the let down reflex. If ketonuria is present and persists, breast-feeding must be discontinued. For contraception, barrier methods are preferable. Oral contraception may change insulin requirements as a result of altered carbohydrate metabolism. Many diabetic women eventually choose tubal ligation.

The majority of cases of gestational diabetes revert to normoglycemia after birth. Nonetheless, it is important after delivery to reassess women with an abnormal glucose tolerance to determine whether it returns to normal. The test is best repeated 6 weeks after birth. The woman should be warned that there is a 90% chance that diabetes will recur in each subsequent pregnancy and if she remains overweight, there is a greater chance of developing diabetes later in life. All these factors make pregnancy an ideal time for teaching nutrition and self-care.

Nursing Responsibilities
▶ ASSESSMENT

Never assume a pregnant woman with known diabetes is fully knowledgeable about her survival needs. Glucose monitoring, insulin administration and adjustment, meal planning and timing, nutritional balance, preventive health habits, and management of acute imbalance of glucose all should be reviewed. Although it may not be a first exposure, follow through on assessment carefully. You may find that she is much more aware of her own needs than you are, but you may also find areas of ignorance that are surprising. Many women will be diagnosed for the first time as type II or as GDM and will need the complete range of teaching. Use the Diabetes Knowledge Screen in the initial assessment (Box 24-6).

▶ NURSING DIAGNOSES

Depending on data collection, you may choose nursing diagnoses similar to the following for a pregnant woman identified as a diabetic.

 Clinical Decision

Debra, an insulin-dependent diabetic, is scheduled for induction at 8 AM. She is anxious about the preparation for labor. Give rationale why each of these plans would be helpful or harmful.
- *Give her nothing by mouth after midnight with a fasting blood sugar drawn before transfer to the labor area.*
- *Give both insulin and glucose by intravenous pump during labor.*
- *Provide a special early breakfast.*
- *Begin intravenous therapy with D_5W, 1000 ml before the onset of labor.*

BOX 24-6   Diabetes in Pregnancy Knowledge Screen

Below are questions about diabetes during pregnancy. Answering these questions will help us determine your current knowledge about diabetes during pregnancy and enable us to provide the best care possible during your pregnancy. Many questions have more than one answer, therefore circle "I don't know" rather than guessing. By answering to the best of your knowledge, we will be able to counsel you most effectively about diabetes during your pregnancy.

1. Which of the following feelings may result from a reaction? (Circle all that might happen, not just those that have happened to you)
   A. Difficulty thinking
   B. Blurred vision
   C. Nervousness or shaky
   D. Numbness
   E. Sweating
   F. I don't know

2. What should you do if you have a reaction? (Circle all that apply)
   A. Walk it off
   B. Sit down and rest
   C. Eat crackers or cheese
   D. Drink milk
   E. I don't know

3. Glycosylated hemoglobin levels are drawn about once per month during pregnancy. Why are these levels taken?
   A. They measure previous blood sugar control
   B. They measure the amount of iron in your blood
   C. They measure how helpful your diet is in controlling your blood sugar
   D. I don't know

4. When planning vigorous exercise (e.g., swimming, playing tennis), what changes should you make in your daily diabetes routine? (Circle all that apply)
   A. Decrease insulin
   B. Carefully time when to do your exercising
   C. Increase amount of carbohydrates (e.g., bread, fruits) you eat
   D. Increase the amount of protein (e.g., meat, cheese) you eat
   E. I don't know

5. On days when you are sick, what steps should you take to control your diabetes?
   A. Increase the amount of water or other fluids
   B. Stop your insulin
   C. Call your doctor
   D. I don't know

6. The normal range for blood sugar during pregnancy is:
   A. 40–150 mg/dl
   B. 60–120 mg/dl
   C. 100–200 mg/dl
   D. I don't know

7. A specific meal plan has been devised for you by the dietitian. Which of the following statements about your meal plan are correct. (Circle all that apply)
   A. You should eat everything on your meal plan
   B. You can reduce the amount of food you eat if you're not hungry
   C. You should control the amount of food you eat all the time
   D. You can eat your meals any time during the day as long as you eat everything on your plan
   E. I don't know

8. Bedtime snacks are an important part of your meal plan because they help you avoid having reactions overnight. (Circle one)
   True or False

9. Margarine is mainly:
   A. Protein
   B. Carbohydrate
   C. Fat
   D. Mineral and vitamin
   E. I don't know

10. Rice is mainly:
    A. Protein
    B. Carbohydrate
    C. Fat
    D. Mineral and vitamin
    E. I don't know

11. If you don't feel like having the egg on your diet for breakfast, you can: (Circle two)
    A. Have extra toast
    B. Substitute one small chop
    C. Have an ounce of cheese instead
    D. Skip the egg, and don't eat anything else
    E. I don't know

12. If you have problems controlling your blood sugar during pregnancy, what are some of the possible effects on your baby after birth? (Circle all that apply)
    A. Could be born with low blood sugar (hypoglycemia)
    B. Could be a large baby making delivery more difficult
    C. Could have breathing problems after birth
    D. I don't know

13. What does glucagon do?
    A. It helps the liver release more sugar into the blood
    B. It makes the liver stop releasing sugar into the blood
    C. It helps the pancreas release more insulin
    D. It stops the pancreas from releasing insulin
    E. I don't know

14. After using glucagon, it's most important to:
    A. Drink plenty of fluids
    B. Get plenty of rest

Spirito A et al: Screening measure to assess knowledge of diabetes in pregnancy, *Diabetic Care* 13(7):712, 1990.

1. Anxiety over implications of diagnosis, risks for self and fetus, testing and cost of pregnancy.
2. Health-seeking behaviors related to need to manage diabetic self-care.
3. High risk for maternal or fetal injury related to glucose imbalance.
4. High risk for noncompliance related to restrictions in diet, frequent glucose measurements, lifestyle changes.
5. Increased potential for infection due to hyperglycemic state.

▶ EXPECTED OUTCOMES

All of the outcomes center on the woman learning self-monitoring and self-care so well that she can manage "day-to-day operations."
1. Discusses the plan of care to determine fetal status and outcome.
2. Verbalizes her understanding of how the pregnancy changes DM control.
3. Demonstrates dietary control, insulin self medication and glucose regulation.
4. Maintains blood glucose within advised range as seen by HbA_{1c} tests.
5. Persists with skin care, infection prevention, and exercise requirements.

▶ NURSING INTERVENTIONS

The nurse plays an important role in care and in counseling a pregnant DM woman. She may be eager to learn or angry and resistant because of the diagnosis. It is essential that she soon learn how to manage her situation and she may need hospitalization during this learning interval, for regulation is difficult in the first trimester. She will need frequent prenatal visits and supervision by a diabetologist and nutritionist. Reinforce the idea that the health care team also desires a stable pregnancy and healthy baby. Assist her to understand the ways hyperglycemia or hypoglycemia may injure her or her fetus. Without raising severe anxiety, assist her to understand the daily need for euglycemia. Remember, with good control, fetal defects and intrauterine deaths are practically at the same levels as for nondiabetic pregnancies.

She should be made aware of potential signs of complications of infection, hypertension and vascular disease. She should keep a record of insulin intake, glucose monitoring, and dietary schedules and amounts, noting her own ups and downs. She brings this record with her at each visit. Weight gain should follow the normal pattern, based on BMR. With the nutritionist counseling, her cultural and ethnic patterns will be considered. The nurse can reinforce nutritional choices she has planned.

Urinary ketones should be monitored daily by dipstick since ketonuria is common in the third trimester. Any pregnant woman is more likely to spill ketones because calories from glucose and amino acids are diverted to the fetus, leading to increased breakdown of maternal fats. Significant ketonuria can alert the woman to the possibility of DKA, which carries an increased risk of fetal death.

Education is the key to a successful pregnancy. She needs to learn all signs of hyperglycemia and ketosis, and how to use emergency sugars for hypoglycemia when out of the home. At home or in the hospital, the first line of defense for hypoglycemia is a *glass of milk* because protein sustains a glucose level for a longer period. If the blood glucose level has dropped below 50 mg/dl and she is becoming confused, a rapid simple sugar such as orange juice can be offered. In very labile situations, **glucagon** may be administered IM by a nurse or a family member who has been instructed. And finally IV glucose may be administered, usually by the physician. Venous and capillary blood sugars should be tested 30 min to 1 hr after such administration. Remember, *capillary levels are slightly below venous blood levels.*

The following areas must be part of the teaching plan for the newly pregnant diabetic:
1. The importance of early prenatal care and of keeping all appointments.
2. The role of the diet for good nutrition and diabetic control. Meals must be eaten on time and never skipped. Keeping a diet diary is a useful tool for reviewing or learning meal planning, calorie counting, and food values.
3. Testing capillary blood sugar and urine for ketones.
4. Recognizing the signs and symptoms of hypoglycemia and hyperglycemia and understanding why she may be more labile. Friends and colleagues should be told of her diabetes. She should wear identification as a diabetic.
5. Carry fast-acting carbohydrate for emergency use and use milk as first choice when hypoglycemic.
6. Importance of reporting any infections or illness to the physician.
7. Importance of care of teeth, skin, feet, personal hygiene.
8. Exercise and rest.
   Exercise after a meal, not when blood sugar may be low. Do not administer insulin into an extremity that will be used immediately in exercise and monitor blood glucose to determine its variations with exercise.
9. Method of administration of insulin, if needed. Familiarity with type or types of insulin to be used. Protocol for sites of injection, rotation of sites, and skin inspection; technique for preparing materials and injection skills.

NURSING CARE PLAN • Diabetes during Pregnancy

CASE: Denise, Para 2002, was a type II diabetic managed on diet alone until this pregnancy. She is 130% of baseline weight. She earns a small weekly income and is a single parent living with her two active sons at her mother's home. At her eighth week visit, she was placed on insulin because of a high Hb A_{1c}. She was counseled regarding risk of defects, and she needs extensive support and teaching about using insulin. She is begin medicated for bacteriuria.

ASSESSMENT DATA

1. Prior knowledge of diabetes and self-care with nutrition, exercise.
2. Makes inaccurate choices in diet plan.
3. New to insulin; has used only urine dipstick for checking glucose.
4. Bacteriuria now being treated.
5. Life situation indicates need for extensive support during this pregnancy.

NURSING DIAGNOSES

1. Knowledge deficit regarding meaning of diagnosis, testing, and management throughout pregnancy.
2. High risk for noncompliance related to lack of adequate support systems, anxiety, and need to work full time.
3. High risk for fetal or maternal injury related to hyperglycemia.
4. High risk for infection related to glycosuria, inadequate knowledge of preventive measures.
5. Altered individual coping related to increased risk of diagnosis, stress of pregnancy, lack of resources.

EXPECTED OUTCOMES

1. Maintains euglycemia at 60-120 mg/dl as seen by periodic Hb A_{1c} testing.
2. Keeps accurate records of glucose tests and dietary intake.
3. Masters insulin requirements and methods.
4. Identifies self-care requirements during pregnancy; prevention of infection, increased exercise, good skin care.
5. Participates in planning care, keeps clinic appointments and follows through on referrals for additional assistance.

NURSING INTERVENTIONS

1. Engage Denise in reviewing what she knows and in identifying areas needing improved monitoring. Review learning needs for this pregnancy as well.
2. Determine her understanding of warning signs of hypoglycemia or hyperglycemia and which interventions to use. Acertain if she knows when to call physician or nurses for questions.
3. Review customary diet and help plan modifications.
4. Ensure her understanding of relationships between calories, fiber, exercise, and insulin balance.
5. Instruct in record keeping, Dextrostix procedure.
6. Demonstrate and then determine ability to select, measure, draw, and administer insulin injection.
7. Refer for assistance in obtaining supplies, glucometer, test stips, lancets, syringes, and insulin. Refer to social services and WIC program.
8. Review self-care needs for skin, infection prevention, adequate sleep and rest, and social support. Discuss ways she handles single parenting and full-time work. Set up home care liaison if possible.
9. Refer for identified coping problems. Reinforce positive behaviors. Assign contact person for her in office or clinic setting. Give telephone number.

EVALUATION

1. Is there appropriate weight gain for gestational age?
2. Had Denise maintained euglycemia? Did she manage diet modifications, glucose testing, and insulin accurately?
3. Did infection or other signs of complications occur?
4. Has she managed her social environment satisfactorily with referrals and support?

10. In last trimester how to monitor and record level of fetal movements three times a day for 1 hour; report any changes.
11. Reasons for referral to other health professionals (visiting nurse, Diabetes Association, homemaker, dietitian or nutritionist, social worker, other physicians, childbirth educator).

▶ EVALUATION

1. Did she demonstrate understanding and compliance with plan of care in maintaining diabetic diet and following insulin requirements?
2. By maintaining adequate glucose balance, did client avoid injury to self and infant?

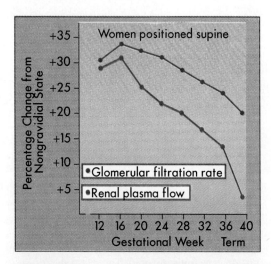

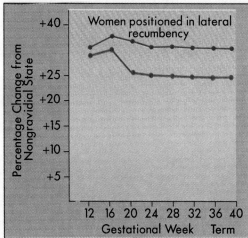

FIGURE 24-5 Renal hemodynamics in pregnancy. Differences in glomerular filtration rate and renal plasma flow in supine and lateral positions. Increases occur early in pregnancy and are sustained to term if women maintain lateral recumbency position. (From Lindheimer M, Katz A: *Contemp Obstet Gynecol* 3[1]:49, 1974.)

3. Were abnormal symptoms reported promptly and appropriately?
4. Did family coping mechanisms appear positive?

Renal Alterations During Pregnancy

Renal plasma flow and glomerular filtration rates increase greatly during pregnancy. Beginning in the first trimester and increasing until just after delivery, this increase is partly due to the increased cardiac output and decreased vascular resistance (Figure 24-5).

INFECTION

Women seem to be at a greater risk than men for developing urinary tract infections (UTIs), probably due to anatomic factors as well as personal hygiene and sexual practice. The progression of enteric bacteria into the bladder is thought to occur by bowel flora (bacteria) colonizing in the perineum, vaginal vestibule, urethra, and bladder. The proximity of the anus, vagina, and urethra aids this process. Therefore routine hygiene factors after toileting and sexual intercourse are important to reinforce during pregnancy (Box 24-7).

Asymptomatic Bacteriuria (ASB)

The definition of this condition is made by the presence of more than 100,000 organisms/mm^3 in urine, without symptoms of fever, dysuria, urinary frequency, or flank pain. A great deal of research has been directed toward urinary tract infection because of a link with preterm labor, but ASB does not in itself appear to be causative. However, ASB may develop into acute cystitis (AC) and then a positive link with preterm labor becomes present.

Acute Cystitis

In about 1% of pregnant women, signs of bladder infection become evident. Symptoms include the classic signs of urgency, frequency, dysuria, and pyuria. Suprapubic tenderness is present but fever and flank pain are absent. There may be a strong unpleasant odor to the

---

BOX 24-7   Perineal Hygiene

* Wipe front to back after each bowel movement with a fresh tissue
* Cleanse the urethral area with a fresh tissue
* Adequate fluid intake
* No douching
* Warm water perineal flush recommended

urine and blood on the toilet tissues. Urine cultures test positive for the same organisms as in ASB.

Approximately 30% of these women with acute symptoms may have sterile urine cultures. In this case, they are considered to have **acute urethral syndrome,** a condition most commonly associated with *Chylamydia trachomatis* infection (see Chapter 25), and require treatment for that condition.

Acute Pyelonephritis

Women with cystitis may progress to develop acute pyelonephritis. Acute **pyelonephritis** is the most common, nonobstetric cause for hospitalization during pregnancy.

Risk. The risk of maternal and fetal morbidity from pyelonephritis is significant. Up to 10% of pregnant women with pyelonephritis have bacteremia (positive blood cultures). Recurrent pyelonephritis, chronic renal disease, septicemia, septic shock, and adult respiratory distress syndrome are potential complications of pyelonephritis (Cunningham, Lucas, and Hankins, 1987). In addition, the fetus is at risk from preterm labor and birth and potential teratogenic effects of maternal fever and antibiotic therapy (McGrady, Daling, and Peterson, 1985).

The presence of asymptomatic bacteriuria is the most common risk factor for acute pyelonephritis during pregnancy. Other risk factors for pyelonephritis are the same as for ASB (that is, lower socio-economic status, increasing age, parity, sickle cell trait, and chronic medical illness).

Signs. The clinical diagnosis of pyelonephritis is based on subjective complaints of chills, fever, back pain, dysuria, urgency, frequency, nausea, vomiting, and physical findings of temperature greater than 101° F, costovertebral angle tenderness, and laboratory findings of pyuria and bacteriuria. During the early clinical course, the client may be afebrile but still complain of these symptoms.

Clinical management. Since almost one half of the pregnant women with ASB will develop an acute infection if left untreated, most obstetricians believe that treatment is warranted (Davison et al, 1989). Women should have urine recultured within 3 to 4 days after the antibiotic course is completed and regularly throughout the rest of the pregnancy. Remember, pregnant women need a midstream, clean voided specimen or a straight catheterized specimen to avoid mixing urine with vaginal mucus. The woman should be taught to complete the course of antibiotics, which sometimes causes nausea. For ASB and cystitis, treatment is recommended for 10 to 14 days with nitrofurantoins, gantrisin, or ampicillin. Sulfonamide antibiotics like gantrisin are avoided in the third trimester of pregnancy because of the

association between their use and newborn hyperbilirubinemia.

Some authorities recommend that women with recurrent ASB during pregnancy should be given antimicrobial suppression by low doses of antimicrobials daily for the remainder of the pregnancy.

Pregnant women with pyelonephritis require hospitalization and close monitoring of maternal status, intravenous hydration, and antibiotic therapy. Choice of antibiotics includes broad spectrum antibiotics or those that provide coverage for the microorganisms most often found. Combinations of ampicillin or a cephalosporin with an aminoglycoside are usually initiated. This combination therapy is recommended because microorganisms resistant to ampicillin and cephalosporins are increasingly recovered from women with pyelonephritis. The high incidence of bacteremia and potential for endotoxin sepsis warrants the use of broad spectrum antimicrobial agents. Ampicillin is indicated because a small portion of pyelonephritis is associated with group B streptococcus and enterococcus. Intravenous antibiotics are generally continued until the client is afebrile at least 24 hours and able to tolerate oral medication. The majority of clients are usually afebrile within 48 hours of treatment onset. If the client continues to be febrile, a repeat urine culture for antimicrobial sensitivities is performed to evaluate for the presence of microorganism resistance. Frequently, a change or addition of antibiotics is then made. After discontinuation of intravenous antibiotics, the client continues oral antibiotics for 10 to 14 days on an outpatient basis.

CHRONIC RENAL PROBLEMS

Among the background renal conditions that may be complicated by pregnancy are chronic glomerulonephritis, nephrotic syndrome, polycystic kidney, class F diabetes, solitary kidney, and kidney transplant. Significant proteinuria will invariably accompany these conditions, leading the physician to investigate. Normally BP falls during early pregnancy. An elevation and serum urea may be the earliest signs of a developing renal problem. The most common causes of acute renal failure are abruptio placentae and eclampsia.

Chronic Glomerulonephritis

Ranging in severity from tolerable impairment of kidney function to severe disability, *chronic glomerulonephritis* was once incompatible with pregnancy. Now it is considered manageable in a cooperative client. Usually a sequel to a severe systemic disease, most notably streptococcal glomerulonephritis, chronic glomerulonephritis results in proteinuria and/or persistent urinary sediment. Because streptococcal infections are now treated aggressively, this condition is becoming less prevalent. In pregnancy, it produces palpitation, visual disturbances, headaches, fatigue, dizziness, nausea, vomiting, edema, hypertension, and eventually some degree of cardiovascular disease and renal insufficiency. Anemia is usually severe enough to require transfusion. After pregnancy, the mother's condition returns to the state present at conception.

Nephrotic Syndrome

If *nephrotic syndrome* appears during pregnancy, the findings may indicate preeclampsia, edema, massive protein in the urine, low blood protein, and lipemia, with or without hypertension. Renal biopsy is required for definitive diagnosis. Usually the kidney functions enough to allow the pregnancy to continue; interruption is indicated by severe malfunction, hypertension, or uremia. Thromboembolism (caused by an elevated fibrinogen or depressed antithrombin level) and infection as a consequence of low gamma globulin level must also be anticipated. Depending on the cause, recovery may take place or the disease may progress to renal failure and death. Pregnancy seems to have no serious effect on the course of the disease.

Solitary Kidney or Kidney Transplant

In the past a woman would have one kidney because of congenital anomaly or trauma, but modern medicine has introduced kidney transplant. The following criteria are applied in not discouraging a woman with a renal transplant from becoming pregnant (Pritchard, 1986):

1. Good general health
2. No elevation in BP for 2 years after treatment
3. No evidence of graft reaction
4. No persisting proteinuria

If for any reason a cesarean birth is needed, a midline incision is preferable because it minimizes danger to the transplanted kidney if it is pelvically located.

When only one kidney is present, it will enlarge to compensate for the extra demands of pregnancy. Pregnancy does not seem to cause any other special problems. The duration of the solitary kidney condition, the present ability of that kidney to function, and the cause of the condition must be taken into account.

Following renal transplantation, renal and endocrine functions return to normal quickly. Over 90% of pregnancies that continue past the first trimester end successfully (Davison, 1987), although only 1 in 50 women of childbearing age postrenal transplant become pregnant. Careful consideration is needed by a couple in which the woman has had a renal transplant. Most centers advise that the women be 2 years posttransplant before considering becoming pregnant.

Risk. Katz et al (1980) reported that women with renal disease who became pregnant did not have the natural course of their disease affected, but that during pregnancy clinical signs worsened. In all series of pregnant women with chronic renal disease, fetal mortality increased; Ferris (1980) found a 7% fetal mortality if maternal blood pressure was normal and a 45% mortality if the mother was hypertensive.

Fertility is decreased as renal function decreases. If a woman with renal disease becomes pregnant before speaking with her physicians, the question of whether the pregnancy should continue must be answered.

Clinical management. All women with chronic renal disease should have a counseling session with her gynecologist and nephrologist before considering a pregnancy. Complete renal function studies including creatinine clearance with protein excretion should be obtained before conception so that studies taken during pregnancy can be compared to the prepregnant state. There is an increased incidence of renal infections in these women and frequent urine cultures are followed for infection. Ultrasound studies assist in the evaluation of fetal growth during the pregnancy. Hypertensive women should have antepartum fetal monitoring and be delivered when fetal pulmonary maturity is acceptable. The development of preeclampsia may lead to the need for an emergency preterm delivery.

Clients with chronic renal disease should be followed more closely than other pregnant women. Their needs include evaluation of the following:

1. *Renal function.* To monitor status of renal function frequently (monthly), urine collections should be followed assessing both creatinine clearance and protein excretion. If deterioration is noted, further studies need to be planned.
2. *Blood pressure.* Most of the risks of hypertension are secondary to superimposed preeclampsia. High blood pressure is treated more aggressively during pregnancy to preserve renal function.
3. *Fetal growth and development.* Measurements of fetal well-being are important, since there is an association between renal disease and intrauterine growth retardation. Fetal growth and development are important markers should an emergency delivery be necessary.

Provided that no infection or hypertension intervenes, pregnancy progresses to term. If renal function deteriorates at any stage of gestation, reversible causes, such as urinary tract infections, subtle dehydration, and electrolyte imbalance, should be sought. Failure to find such a reversible cause is grounds for recommending termination of the pregnancy. For *glomerulonephritis* generally, therapy includes administration of antihypertensive agents and, with cardiac insufficiency, digitalis and perhaps diuretics. When modification of customary prenatal diet is indicated, it should be undertaken with the principles of good nutrition. Diet prescription in kidney disease is generally high in protein, allowing for fetal growth and maternal needs. Sodium may be restricted. Consideration should be given to avoid dehydration, electrolyte imbalance, and anemia.

Preeclampsia necessitates hospitalization. *Azotemia* (nitrogen in the blood), *hyperkalemia* (high potassium content in the blood), and continuing BP rise indicate the need to interrupt the pregnancy. *Nephrotic syndrome* is treated according to symptoms and the other conditions accompanying it. Bed rest in the lateral recumbent position; a high-protein, restricted-sodium diet; and diuretics are commonly ordered. Steroids are contraindicated during the first 2 months of gestation. Infections must be vigorously treated.

Nursing Responsibilities

All pregnant women should be screened for asymptomatic bacteriuria at specific times during their pregnancy at prenatal visits. Waiting for acute symptoms to develop may have serious consequences to the mother and fetus. Women with high risk for UTIs should provide clean-catch urine samples for culture. Women at high risk include those with history of UTIs, sickle cell trait, or renal stones.

Pregnant women with AC are usually uncomfortable and they need to be reassured that the symptoms will lessen within 48 hours. As in the treatment of all infec-

tions, the woman must understand the importance of following the dosing schedule and the completion of the entire course of treatment in order to prevent relapse, recurrence, or worsening or traveling of this infection. Increased fluid intake is usually recommended to ensure hydration and to help flush the urinary system.

The nurse's role in working with pregnant women with chronic renal disease is to help identify gaps in the client's knowledge base that may affect completion of successful pregnancy. Nutrition knowledge and dietary changes such as appropriate protein intake and sodium requirements need to be addressed throughout pregnancy. Proper technique and timing of urine collections should be reviewed. Home care referrals should be made as appropriate to women whose activities have been restricted. Emotional and social support systems should be developed to aid in the woman's adherence to the treatment plan.

She may require interpretation and teaching about all the drugs she may be given (for example, digitalis, diuretics, antihypertensives, steroids, antibiotics) whether she is going to take them at home or receive them as an inpatient. If bed rest has been prescribed, she will need to explore her emotional response to this order and discover activities that can keep her from boredom. The side-lying position is critical for her (see Figure 24-5). If the baby has a problem, the nurse can provide support and information and help during the grief process.

(KEY) POINTS

- Metabolic changes accompanying pregnancy may complicate preexisting disease or unmask potential problems in glucose or thyroid balance.
- Assessment during prenatal care always includes measurements for glucose levels, weight gain, and the presence of infection.
- Self-monitoring is the key to good control of diabetes and overweight.
- After diagnosis of glucose imbalance, an intensive educational program is required so that the woman can manage her daily care.

- Nutrition is the key to control in PKU and diabetes.
- Clients need a good knowledge of prescribed medications because of the frequency of adverse effects.
- Pregnancy alters insulin effects requiring increased doses as gestation progresses.
- After birth, insulin needs drop swiftly and overdose is a risk. Careful intrapartal monitoring is required.
- The team approach is unusually important in metabolic and renal problems during pregnancy.

STUDY QUESTIONS

24-1. Use the Key Terms for this chapter to complete the following statements.
   a. A test that gives evidence of hyperglycemia within the prior 6 weeks is ___Hgb A₁c___
   b. When hyperglycemia is unmasked by the metabolic changes of the second and third trimesters, it is called ___gestat. diab-___
   c. A hormone of pregnancy that acts as a direct insulin antagonist is ___HPL___.

   d. The definition for ___obesity___ is to be more than 20% over the normal weight for height.
   e. A balanced normal amount of glucose in the blood is ___Euglycemia___
   f. When signs of frequency, dysuria and urgency occur infection is causing ___cystitis___

24-2. Which of the following are true regarding the effect of pregnancy on insulin and carbohydrate metabolism?

F a. The fasting blood sugar is higher in pregnancy.

F b. Estrogen and progesterone reduce insulin production.

F c. As pregnancy progresses, maternal insulin requirements are lower.

T d. HPL is an insulin antagonist.

24-3. If a diabetic woman shows signs of insulin overdose because she did not adjust her insulin dosage, which change in her normal pattern has probably occurred?

   a. She added extra simple sugars in her diet.

   (b.) She has had nausea, vomiting, and loss of appetite for a week.

   c. It rained all week so she omitted exercise.

   d. She had additional intake of high sodium in restaurant dinner.

24-4. Birth several weeks before the due date may be induced for diabetic women to:

   a. Prevent hypoglycemia in the fetus

   b. Reduce the chances of neonatal respiratory difficulty

   c. Provide an easier labor and birth because babies tend to be larger

   (d.) Avoid the chance of unexpected intrauterine fetal death

24-5. When a woman has a urine laboratory report of 100,000 colonies/mm³ with no other symptoms, you would understand the diagnosis to be:

   a. Urethritis

   (b.) Asymptomatic bacteriuria

   c. Cystitis

   d. Pyelonephritis

24-6. When a woman in her second trimester begins to experience urinary frequency and dysuria, she should

   (a.) Drink more fluids.

   (b.) Call her health care provider for advice.

   c. Try resting and call her health care provider if the symptoms do not pass.

   d. Realize that these are expected sensations during advance pregnancy.

Answer Key.

24-1 a. HbA₁c, b. Gestational (GDM), c. HPL, d. Obesity, e. Euglycemia, f. Cystitis 24-2 d 24-3 b 24-4 d 24-5 b 24-6 a and b

REFERENCES

Acosta PB, Wright L: Nurses' role in preventing birth defects in offspring of women with phenylketonuria, *JOGNN* 21(4):270, 1992.

ADA Position Statement: Office guide to diagnosis and classification of diabetes mellitus and other categories of glucose intolerance, *Diabetes Care* 13(1)Suppl 1:3, 1990.

ADA Position Statement: Gestational diabetes mellitus, *Diabetes Care* 13(1)Suppl 1:5, 1990.

Barss V: Diabetes and pregnancy, *Med Clin North Am* 73:685, 1989.

Binkin NJ et al: Birth weight and childhood growth, *Pediatrics* 82:828, 1988.

Blackburn ST, Loper DL: *Maternal, fetal, and neonatal physiology,* Philadelphia, 1992, Saunders.

Coustan DR: Pregnancy in diabetic women, *N Engl J Med* 319(25):1663, 1988.

Cunningham FG, Lucas MJ, Hankins GDV: Pulmonary injury complication of antepartum pyelonephritis, *Am J Obstet Gynecol* 156:797, 1987.

Czoizel AE, Dudas I: Prevention of the first occurrence of neural tube defects by periconceptional vitamin supplementation, *N Engl J Med* 327(26):1832, 1992.

Davis LE, Leven KJ, Cunningham FG: Hypothyroidism complicating pregnancy, *Obstet Gynecol* 72(1):108, 1988.

Davison JM, Lindheimer MD: Pregnancy and the kidney: an update. In *1985 Yearbook of obstetrics and gynecology,* Chicago, 1985, Year-Book Publishers.

Davison JM, Lindheimer MD: Renal disorders. In Creasy R, Resnick R, eds: *Maternal-fetal medicine: principles and practice,* ed 2, Philadelphia, 1989, Saunders.

Douglas JG: Hypertension and diabetes in Blacks, *Diabetes Care* 13(11)Suppl 4: 1191, 1990.

Friedman CI, Kim MH: Obesity and its effect on reproductive function, *Clin Obstet Gynecol* 28(3):645, 1985.

Gabbe SG: Gestational diabetes mellitus, *N Engl J Med* 315:1025, 1986.

Guthrie R: Maternal PKU–a continuing problem, *Am J Public Health* 78(7):771, 1988.

Herbert V: Folate and neural tube defects, *Nutrition Today* 27(66):30, 1992.

Insulin administration, *Diabetes Care* 13 (Suppl 1):28, 1990.

Katz AI et al: Pregnancy in women with kidney disease, *Kidney Int* 28:192, 1980.

Kracic B: Antepartal management of Graves' disease, *JOGNN* 15(8):214, 1986.

Lipman T: What causes diabetes? *MCN* 18(1):40, 1988.

McGrady GA, Daling JR and Peterson DR: Maternal urinary tract infections and adverse fetal outcomes, *Am J Epidemiol* 121(3):377, 1985.

National Academy of Sciences, Committee on Nutritional Status During Pregnancy and Lactation: *Nutrition during pregnancy, Part 1: Weight gain,* Washington, DC, 1990, National Academy Press.

Pritchard JA et al: Metabolic conditions in pregnancy. In *Williams' Obstetrics,* ed 17, East Norwalk, Conn, 1986, Appleton-Century-Crofts.

Reece EA et al: Assessment of carbohydrate tolerance in pregnancy, *Obstet Gynecol Surv* 46(1):1, 1991.

Reece EA, Hagay Z, Hobbins JC: Insulin-dependent diabetes mellitus and immunogenetics: maternal and fetal considerations, *Obstet Gynecol Surv* 46 (5):255, 1991.

Smith JE: Pregnancy complicated by thyroid disease, *J Nurse Midwifery* 35(3):143, 1990.

Smith JE: Pregnancy complicated by thyroid disease, *J Nurse Midwifery* 35(3):143, 1990.

Spirito A et al: Screening measure to assess knowledge of diabetes in pregnancy, *Diabetes Care* 11(7):712, 1990.

Thompson GN et al: Pregnancy in phenylketonuria: dietary treatment aimed at normalizing maternal plasma phenylalanine, *Arch Dis Child* 66:1346, 1991.

White P: Classification of obstetrical diabetes, *Am J Obstet Gynecol* 130:228, 1978.

STUDENT RESOURCE SHELF

Acosta PB, Wright L: Nurses' role in preventing birth defects in offspring of women with phenylketonuria, *JOGNN* 21(4):270, 1992. Describes diagnosis and treatment of varying degrees of PKU. Precautions for the woman while pregnant will often ensure a healthy outcome.

ADA: Insulin Administration, *Diabetes Care* 13(1), suppl 1, S28, 1990. Nursing practice must keep up with the new recommenda-tions. Each student should read this article and then compare with practices in the hospital setting.

ADA Position Statement: Nutritional recommendations and prin-ciples for individuals with diabetes mellitus, *Diabetes Care* 13(1), suppl 1:18, 1990. A clear description of the current recommenda-tions for each type of diabetes.

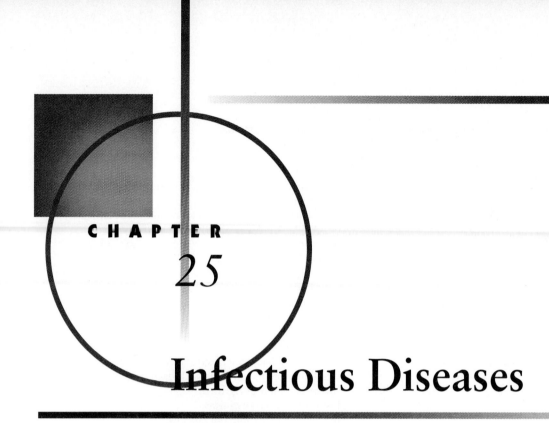

CHAPTER 25

Infectious Diseases

KEY TERMS

Active Immunity
Ascending Infection
Chancre
Cofactor
Friable Cervix
Horizontal
  Transmission
Host Defense
  Mechanisms
Humoral Response
Hyperimmune
  Globulin
Latent Period
Macrophages
Opportunistic
  Infection

Passive Immunity
Pathogen
Primary Infection
Reinfection

T4 Lymphocytes
Universal Precautions
Vaccination
Vertical Transmission

LEARNING OBJECTIVES

1. Describe briefly the maternal immunologic adaptations during pregnancy.
2. Describe vertical and horizontal transmission of organisms.
3. Enumerate all methods of transmission of sexually related diseases.
4. Recognize errors in preventive care for the mother at risk for infection during labor, birth, or recovery.
5. List methods to prevent transmission of infections acquired through blood and body fluids.
6. Describe the subtle signs of infection in the woman, fetus, or newborn.
7. Choose appropriate nursing diagnoses for women with perinatal infections.
8. Locate and describe isolation requirements for each perinatal infection.

Pregnant women may acquire any infectious disease. Infectious diseases during pregnancy are of special concern because they may occur more frequently or more severely in pregnant women, they may threaten the well-being of the fetus or newborn with little or no physiologic effect on the mother, or the fetus and mother may be seriously affected. In addition, infections may occur as a result of events related to the pregnancy and birth experience.

Infectious diseases are caused by a wide variety of microorganisms, including bacteria, viruses, fungi, rickettsiae, protozoa, and parasites. Any microorganism may cause disease under the appropriate circumstances. For infection to develop, transmission of the microorganism must occur and then entry gained to the body. The immune status of the woman governs whether the **pathogen** is to survive, reproduce, and cause damage.

667

TABLE 25-1 Host Defense Mechanisms

NONSPECIFIC AND SPECIFIC HOST DEFENSE MECHANISMS	MECHANISMS OF PROTECTION
NONSPECIFIC	
Physical barriers	
Epithelial surfaces	Cell turnover and sloughing remove adherent microorganisms.
Unidirectional flow of fluid within organs or on mucosal surfaces	Unidirectional flow washes microorganisms away.
Mucociliary system	Cilia on mucous membranes trap microorganisms and carry them out of the body.
Cervical mucus	Mucus blocks cervical opening and helps to prevent ascent of microorganisms into uterine cavity.
Amniochorion	This structure aids in prevention of ascent of microorganisms into uterine cavity.
Biochemical mechanisms	
Secretory products in mucosal surface fluids	Lysozyme is a bactericidal substance. Lactoferrin, an iron-binding protein, competes with bacteria for iron, which bacteria require for growth.
Variation in pH	This inhibits microorganisms.
Unsaturated fatty acids	This inhibits many microorganisms.
Amniotic fluid—antibacterial system	This inhibits growth of microorganisms.
MICROORGANISM COLONIZATION	
Colonization mechanism	Colonization of epithelial and mucosal surfaces with non-pathogenic bacteria helps to inhibit growth of pathogenic bacteria. This likely occurs by production of antibacterial substances, competition for host receptors, and alteration of microenvironment.
Inflammatory response	Microorganism invasion of tissue leads to dilation of blood vessels (redness). It also causes capillary permeability (edema) and migration of neutrophils and macrophages to area.
Neutrophils, monocytes, and macrophages	These phagocytize (ingest) and destroy microorganisms.
Complement	This responds to certain microorganisms' surface structures or antigen-antibody complexes. It promotes chemotaxis, opsonization, and microorganism lysis.
SPECIFIC RESPONSES	
Secretory IgA and other immunoglobulins in mucosal surface fluids	These inhibit attachment of bacteria and viruses to cell surfaces.
Immune response	
Humoral immune response	This causes production of specific antibodies to microorganisms by B-cell lymphocytes. Antibodies and complement coat microorganisms to enhance phagocytosis (ingestion by leukocytes).
Cell-mediated immune response	Sensitized lymphocytes release factors that stimulate macrophages to migrate to area and enhance phagocytosis; sensitized lymphocytes stimulate multiplication of other T-cell and B-cell lymphocytes, which destroy and produce antibody to the microorganisms, respectively. As infection is contained, biologically active substances released in this response stimulate T-cell lymphocytes to halt response. Memory T-cells and B-cell lymphocytes remain in circulation.

Initiatives to combat infection are directed toward each of these steps in the pathogenic process.

Host Defense Mechanisms

All organisms have evolved a variety of mechanisms by which they protect themselves from hostile agents in their environment. These mechanisms may be inborn or acquired, nonspecific or specific. *Nonspecific protective mechanisms* are numerous and frequently taken for granted. Examples include the intact skin and mucous membranes, ciliated epithelial cells of the respiratory tract, secretions that bathe mucous membrane surfaces, and "normal flora," microorganisms that colonize our body surfaces but do not cause disease. The **nonspecific host defense mechanisms** generally are not altered during pregnancy.

Specific **host defense mechanisms** remain responsive to invading microorganisms during pregnancy and at the same time allow the fetus to develop and thrive. Reasons the fetus is not rejected as a foreign tissue are not understood. Complex alterations within the cell-mediated immune system appear to occur primarily locally in the uterus and are regulated in part by placental and sex steroid hormones. The specific host defense mechanisms—humoral and cell-mediated immune responses—are depressed during pregnancy. This depression and other changes allow the fetus to survive while the woman's immune system can still respond to microorganisms. However, these immunologic changes may in fact *impair* the pregnant individual's response to some infections. Table 25-1 lists examples of mechanisms by which human beings resist microbial infections.

Vaginal microbiology is complex. The normal flora of the vagina undergoes a shift in the type of microorganisms that predominate during pregnancy. A wide variety of microorganisms *colonize* the vagina, including mainly nonpathogenic *Lactobacillus* species and more potentially pathogenic aerobic and anaerobic bacteria. As gestation progresses, vaginal *Lactobacillus* species increase in number, and anaerobic bacteria decrease in number. This shift in vaginal flora prepares a benign microbial environment for birth. As an additional protection, amniotic fluid contains substances that inhibit the growth of many pathogenic bacteria, and the maternal serum leukocyte count increases. Finally, increased numbers of neutrophils are found in the cervix and uterine decidua during labor (Figure 25-1).

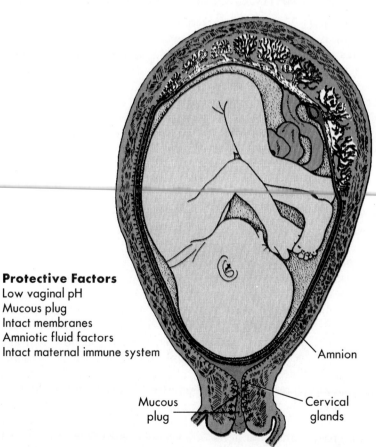

Contributing Factors
Higher amniotic fluid pH
Loss of mucous plug
Ruptured membranes
Cervical dilation
Vaginal exams
Artificially ruptured membranes
Fetal pH sampling
FECG electrode
Intrauterine pressure monitor
Lacerations
Operative delivery

Protective Factors
Low vaginal pH
Mucous plug
Intact membranes
Amniotic fluid factors
Intact maternal immune system

Amnion

Mucous plug

Cervical glands

FIGURE 25-1 Ascending infection during labor. (Modified from Corliss CE: *Patten's human embryology,* ed 4, New York, 1976, McGraw-Hill.)

EXTRA RISK DURING LABOR

The processes of labor challenge the host defense systems. Loss of the cervical mucous plug, cervical dilation, and rupture of the fetal membranes allow microorganisms of the vagina to ascend to the uterus and fetus. The pH of amniotic fluid is considerably more basic than that of the normal vagina; a high pH favors the growth of the potentially more pathogenic anaerobic bacteria.

Obstetric practice may disrupt the natural defenses. Practices such as amniocentesis, cervical examinations, artificial rupture of membranes (AROM), intrauterine monitoring, fetal blood sampling, and fetal operative procedures may introduce bacteria into the amniotic fluid. General anesthesia and cesarean birth also are associated with increased risk of postpartum infection.

IMMUNIZATION DURING PREGNANCY

When a foreign substance enters the body, there is a series of complex interactions—the immune response (Table 25-1). This response occurs when microorganisms invade the body from the environment or are purposefully induced through immunization.

Active Immunity

Active vaccination is the most effective means of disease prevention. **Active immunity** occurs when an individual produces antibodies in response to a specific infectious agent. Active immunity may be induced by administration of the following:

- Bacterial extracellular toxin (exotoxin) that has been altered to retain antigenicity without toxicity (called *toxoids*), for example, tetanus-diphtheria toxoid
- Whole organisms or portions of killed bacteria or virus administered to induce immunity, for example, typhoid
- Attenuated live virus vaccines created by repeated inoculation of the virus through animals or tissue culture until it loses its virulence, for example, rubella, measles, and mumps

Vaccinations should be given *before conception.* Only after evaluation of the woman's risk of exposure, susceptibility to the disease, gestational age, and type of vaccine will any vaccine be given during pregnancy because *live attenuated vaccines* generally cause a *subclinical* or mild illness, as well as transplacental passage and possible fetal infection. Women who are inadvertently immunized with **live virus vaccines** within 3 months before or after conception should be reported to the Centers for Disease Control (CDC) in Atlanta, Georgia, so their infants may be followed up closely for potential adverse effects. *Killed virus or bacteria* preparations probably are safe for use in pregnancy.

Passive Immunity

To prevent illness, **passive immunity** is achieved by administration of antibody that is derived from human or animal sources. Immunity is immediate *but transient.* Immune serum globulin may be given to provide nonspecific immunity, or a specific **hyperimmune globulin** may be given to provide postexposure immunity against specific infections such as varicella-zoster and hepatitis. Appendix 4 lists immunization recommendations for the most commonly encountered infectious agents for which vaccinations are available.

Test Yourself

- List one difference among the following immunizing agents:
  —Toxoids
  —Attenuated live virus
  —Killed bacteria
- Which type is not recommended during pregnancy, and why?

ANTIMICROBIAL USE DURING PREGNANCY

More than one third of all pregnant women will receive some form of antimicrobial treatment during pregnancy. Antibiotics should be used with discretion because toxic side effects and development of resistant bacterial strains may result.

Antibiotics may be given in full therapeutic doses for infection or prophylactically for a shorter duration to reduce the risk of infection. No antibiotic is approved by the Food and Drug Administration (FDA) for use during pregnancy, largely because of the lack of research on safety for pregnant women and fetuses. Such research is unlikely to occur because of ethical reasons. However, long-time use of some antibiotics during pregnancy provides enough information to use them with confidence.

Antibiotic *pharmacokinetics* are altered by the physiologic changes of pregnancy. Antibiotics must be distributed over a larger area within the body; thus the overall concentration of circulating antibiotic will be *reduced* if usual adult dosages are given. Blood volume, maternal cardiac output, renal blood flow, and glomerular filtration are increased, and plasma albumin is decreased. These physiologic changes facilitate increased renal clearance of the drugs. Increased rate of hepatic breakdown may further interfere with obtaining effective serum antibiotic levels. Overall, circulating antibiotic levels are thought to be from 10% to 50% *lower* during pregnancy than among nonpregnant women (Chow and Jewesson, 1985). In addition, placental transport of antimicrobial agents generally increases as gestation progresses because of progressive thinning of the placental membrane. Commonly used antibiotics and special considerations during pregnancy and lactation are listed in Appendix 4.

ISOLATION PROCEDURES

Isolation procedures are implemented to prevent transmission of the microorganism or disease. Basic medical-surgical isolation procedures also apply to obstetric clients with infectious diseases. Guidelines for whether mother and infant are isolated are listed in boxes that accompany each description of infection. These guidelines are based on recommendations by Abrams and Wexler (1983), the American College of Obstetricians and Gynecologists (ACOG), and CDC (Ginsberg, 1991). The purpose of isolation procedures and precautions is to prevent the transmission of disease. The rationales for these procedures are explained in Box 25-1.

Universal precautions required for the human immunodeficiency virus (HIV) and hepatitis B virus (HBV), discussed in Chapter 13, include blood and body fluid precautions. Universal precautions are intended to *supplement, not eliminate,* other types of isolation precautions. Each infection listed in this chapter identifies

---

BOX 25-1   Isolation Procedures and Precautions

Respiratory isolation

Reduces risk of transmission of organisms by droplets dispersed into the environment from the upper respiratory tract or lungs

Enteric precautions

Avoids contact with feces or objects contaminated with feces

Wound precautions

Avoids contact with contaminated wounds or secretions from contaminated wounds

Blood precautions

Avoids contact with blood or objects contaminated with blood

Body fluids

Usually added to blood precautions, ensuring prevention against contact with additional body fluids—urine, sweat, saliva, and tears

---

TABLE 25-2 Health Care Workers* Acquiring HIV through the Work Setting

Percutaneous route	28
Mucocutaneous route	4
Other route	1
TOTAL	33

*From HIV/AIDS Surveillance Report: *CDC and prevention,* Atlanta, Feb. 1993. Nurses and laboratory technicians totaled 24 of the 33 cases.

those fluids that contain infectious material. For instance, the rate of transmission of HIV through tears and saliva seems very low. The nursing responsibility for precautions is primary: first, to arrange for correct protective clothing and devices and for disposal and second, to follow the precautions and insist that others do so as well. Finally, every health care worker should monitor her or his own hand-washing practice and the practice of co-workers.

RISKS TO HEALTH CARE WORKERS

Compliance with universal precautions has often been uneven in labor and delivery units, perhaps because of an attitude of denial of risk or being rushed. In addition, in areas of the country in which prevalence of HIV, HBV, and herpes simplex virus (HSV) are lower, the level of intensive infection control may not be considered necessary. Noncompliance is found both in nursing and medical personnel, especially in starting intravenous (IV) infusions, in hand washing, in eye or hair protection, and in double gloving (Morrison et al, 1991). Several studies recommend *double gloving* for surgical procedures because of the frequency of needle punctures (Ginsberg, 1991). Current statistics indicate that nurses and laboratory technicians have a high rate of seroconversion (changing antibody response) after contact (see Table 25-2 for figures released in 1993).

Community-Acquired Infections

Community-acquired infections are acquired by an individual from the environment. These infections may be spread or acquired by a wide variety of mechanisms, including direct person-to-person contact, hand-to-mouth contact, or sexual contact, by carriage through air (coughing, talking), water, soil, foods, or contaminated fomites, or by infected animals and insect bites. Assessment of an individual's potential susceptibility for a community-acquired infection is obtained through interview, observation, review of records, physical examination, and laboratory testing. Knowledge of the incidence of infections in the community, their mode of transmission, potential risks, signs and symptoms, preventive strategies, treatments, and follow-up care will aid the nurse in asking directed questions, making observations, reviewing records, and obtaining physical findings and laboratory data so that actual and potential problems or needs may be identified. Nursing care plans may then be developed to address these problems.

Sexually Transmitted Diseases

Sexually transmitted diseases (STDs) are specific infections or syndromes transmitted primarily during sexual contact. They may be caused by bacteria, viruses, protozoa, fungal agents, or ectoparasites. More than 20 different diseases are recognized as sexually transmitted. Although STDs traditionally were considered to most commonly afflict men, it is especially young women and their unborn or newly born infants who suffer the most severe symptoms and complications. A wide variety of STDs have been associated with serious complications during pregnancy, including spontaneous abortion, preterm birth, intrauterine growth retardation (IUGR), stillbirth, neonatal death, congenital infection, and postpartum endometritis. As a group, STDs constitute a major, largely *preventable health threat* to women and infants. Public health initiatives for STD prevention have been directed at the primary areas of health education, disease detection, optimal treatment, partner tracing, and research. Health care providers and the public at large should apply this information more effectively.

CHLAMYDIA

least severe STD to affect infant, partners must also be Tx

Today, infection with the bacteria *Chlamydia trachomatis* is a widespread STD in the United States; an estimated 4 million persons are affected annually. The infection has not been a reportable disease; therefore the actual incidence is difficult to determine. Generally, among pregnant women, 8% to 12% have positive cervical chlamydia cultures (CDC, 1985). Groups at risk for other STDs also are at increased risk for contracting chlamydial infection. Women at high risk include those who are young (less than 24 years), single, or poor or who are using an oral contraceptive method or nonbarrier contraceptive method; who have contact with a man with nongonococcal urethritis; and who have histories of new partners in the preceding few months or multiple sexual partners (Handsfield et al, 1986).

The organisms invade and reproduce inside the cells that line the cervix, endometrium, fallopian tubes, and urethra, among other tissues. Different types of *C. trachomatis* are associated with three major groups of infections, including lymphogranuloma venereum, trachoma, and oculogenital infections. Lymphogranuloma venereum (LGV) is an STD that begins with a painless genital ulcer and progresses to lymphadenopathy, systemic symptoms, fever, myalgia, and progressive tissue destruction. LGV is extremely rare in the United States and is more common among tropical countries, including South America, the West Indies, East and West Africa, and Southeast Asia. Trachoma, caused by other types of *C. trachomatis*, is the leading cause of blindness worldwide but is rare in the United States.

Risk

C. trachomatis infection in the United States causes a variety of clinical conditions, including cervicitis, endometritis, irregular menses, acute salpingitis, urethritis, bartholinitis, Fitz-Hugh–Curtis syndrome (perihepatitis), and possibly infertility. Pelvic inflammatory disease (PID) may lead to infertility and ectopic pregnancy. Women with chlamydia infections have two to three times the risk of ectopic pregnancy (Pearlman and McNeeley, 1992). During pregnancy, cervical chlamydial infection has been associated with premature labor, premature rupture of membranes (PROM), and preterm birth.

Neonatal risk. If chlamydiae are present at the time of vaginal birth, 50% to 60% of infants become infected. Chlamydial conjunctivitis develops within the first week of life among 20% to 50% of exposed infants, and pneumonia will develop in 10% to 20% of exposed infants within the first 3 months of life (Schacter et al, 1986).

Signs

Women with cervical chlamydial infection frequently are symptom free or may have nonspecific symptoms such as increased discharge. On pelvic examination the presence of a mucopurulent cervical discharge and **friable cervix** (bleeding when cervix is touched) indicates chlamydial infection. With endometritis signs are evident at about 2 days after vaginal delivery.

Neonatal signs. Conjunctivitis consists of edema of eyelids, conjunctival redness, and mucopurulent discharge. Untreated, the cornea may become scarred (Figure 25-2). *C. trachomatis* pneumonia occurs within 2 to 3 months of birth. Signs are afebrile cough and tachypnea, malaise, cyanosis, and poor weight gain. Diffuse bacterial infiltrates appear on the chest x-ray film.

Clinical Management

Because evidence of chlamydial infection often is not apparent by clinical examination, laboratory methods such as cell culture, antigen detection, or the enzyme-

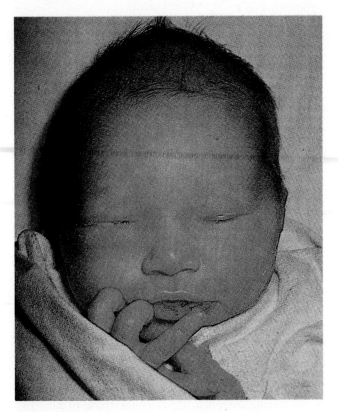

FIGURE 25-2 *Chlamydia trachomatis* eye infection. Note puffy, bruised-looking eyelid. (Used with permission of Harcourt, Brace, Jovanovich Group [Australia]. From Beischer NA, MacKay EV: *Obstetrics and the newborn,* ed 3, Sydney, 1993, Saunders.)

linked immunosorbent assay (ELISA) are required to identify infection. The partner usually will be infected and also should be treated. Condoms must be used during treatment to prevent reinfection although sexual intercourse should be avoided during treatment. Recommendations for treatment during pregnancy are shown in Box 25-2.

In addition to primary prevention strategies, screening for chlamydial cervical infection of all pregnant women at their first prenatal visit has been recommended. Additional screening at 36 weeks for high-risk women is recommended.

Posttreatment *test-of-cure* cultures generally are not required because antibiotic resistance has not been identified.

Neonatal treatment. The best prevention is maternal treatment in the last trimester. Topical prophylaxis with the mandated erythromycin ointment does not treat other sites of infection. Once *conjunctivitis* is diagnosed, the treatment in Box 25-3 is recommended.

Nursing Responsibilities

The woman should be instructed to insist on use of a condom during therapy and to encourage the partner to go for treatment. If he does not, condom prophylaxis should be continued during pregnancy. The woman should be informed about signs of recurrence: increased vaginal mucus, abdominal aching, and preterm labor. She needs to be taught that chlamydial infection leads to PID, ectopic pregnancy, and spontaneous abortion. After birth, she should be instructed to look for signs of infection in herself and in her infant. When the infant is diagnosed with chlamydial infection, the parents should be referred for examination, treatment, and counseling. Box 25-4 lists isolation precautions.

GONORRHEA

Gonorrhea is the most commonly reported communicable disease in the United States. Up to 3 million cases

---

BOX 25-2   Pharmacologic Treatment of Chlamydial Infection during Pregnancy

One of the following is used:
   Erythromycin base 500 mg q6h for 7 days
   Sulfisoxazole 500 mg q6h for 7 days
   Amoxicillin 500 mg q8h for 7 days
   Clindamycin 300 mg q6h for 7 days

BOX 25-3   Pharmacologic Treatment of Neonatal Chlamydial Infection

Erythromycin 50 mg/kg/day in 4 doses for 7-14 days

For pneumonia
Erythromycin 50 mg/kg/day in 4 doses for 14-21 days

BOX 25-4   Isolation Precautions: Chlamydial

Infected mother and infant
No isolation
Careful hand washing: prevent contact with vaginal fluids

Breast-feeding
Permissible if antibiotic therapy permits

of gonorrhea are thought to occur annually in the United States, and up to 7% of pregnant women are infected with gonorrhea. The bacteria *Neisseria gonorrhoeae* lives preferentially in the types of cells that line the cervix, endometrium, fallopian tubes, and urethra.

Gonorrhea may cause uncomplicated genitourinary tract infection (urethritis and cervicitis) and upper genital tract infections such as endometritis and PID. Urethritis, epididymitis, and prostatitis occur in men. Gonorrhea may cause Fitz-Hugh–Curtis syndrome (inflammation of the liver), disseminated gonorrhea with associated arthritis, and rarely, endocarditis or meningitis. Disseminated gonorrhea appears to be more frequent among pregnant women than nonpregnant women, but the reason for this is unknown.

Risk

Neonatal gonococcal ophthalmia, ophthalmia neonatorum, is a serious complication of gonorrhea infection during pregnancy. Newborns acquire the infection during passage through the infected cervix. Untreated gonorrhea during pregnancy also has been associated with increased risk of PROM, preterm birth, chorioamnionitis, neonatal sepsis, and puerperal sepsis.

Signs

Nonpregnant women with gonorrhea may be symptom free, or they may have dysuria, urinary frequency, increased vaginal discharge, or abnormal uterine bleeding, whereas pregnant women most commonly have no symptoms.

Neonatal signs. In the newborn, purulent conjunctivitis occurs usually within 4 days of birth and, without treatment, may progress rapidly to corneal ulcerations and, ultimately, blindness. In a review of neonatal gonococcal infection, Desenclos et al (1992) found 81% of cases had ophthalmia neonatorum, 6% had genital infection, 3% showed infection in gastric or respiratory aspirates, and 1% had skin infection, scalp abscesses, or ear infection.

Clinical Management

Gonorrhea is detected by recovery of the bacteria *N. gonorrhoeae* by culture. The medium is inoculated with discharge from the endocervix, urethra, rectum, or pharynx with a cotton swab. Appropriate handling of the culture is essential for obtaining accurate results. First the media must be at room temperature before inoculation; colder temperatures kill the gonococcus. Then, after inoculation, the culture must be placed in a carbon dioxide atmosphere to ensure bacterial survival.

Most gonococcal strains are sensitive to penicillins and are eradicated by single-dose therapy of ampicillin 3.5 g or amoxicillin 3.0 g orally followed by probenicid 1.0 g by mouth. Probenicid inhibits renal excretion of

---

BOX 25-5   Pharmacologic Treatment of Gonorrhea

Ceftriaxone 250 mg IM
For women who cannot take ceftriaxone:
    Spectinomycin 2 g IM
When type of gonorrhea is not resistant to penicillin:
    Amoxicillin 3 g PO, with 1 g probenecid

---

penicillins and usually increases plasma levels of these antibiotics. Because of penicillin resistance, the current CDC recommendations for treatment of gonorrhea are shown in Box 25-5 (CDC, 1989). Compliance with treatment is achieved because only one dose is needed. Nonetheless, a follow-up culture is needed to test the cure. The *reinfection* rate is estimated to be 5% to 8% (Cavenee et al, 1993).

Strategies to prevent gonorrhea infection involve methods of personal prevention (See Table 25-14). Secondary prevention includes screening all pregnant women for gonococcal infection early in pregnancy and again during the third trimester for those of high-risk populations. Women with positive cultures are reported to the state health department to ensure treatment and counseling of sexual contacts. Isolation precautions are listed in Box 25-6.

HERPES SIMPLEX VIRUS

Herpes simplex virus (HSV) is a member of the herpesvirus group, which includes varicella-zoster virus, cytomegalovirus, and Epstein-Barr virus. Herpesviruses are composed of DNA material enclosed in a protein coat and surrounded by a lipid envelope. Herpesvirus infection occurs by attachment of the viral particle to the susceptible cell membrane, penetration into the cell, and subsequent release of the viral DNA into the cell cytoplasm. Viral DNA is transported to and incorporated into the cell nucleus. The cell then begins to produce viral proteins and to replicate viral DNA.

BOX 25-6   Isolation Precautions: Gonorrhea

Maternal and infant isolation
Careful hand washing. Avoid genital contact until initiation of therapy.

Breast-feeding
Permitted if antibiotic regimen safe for breast-feeding.

These viruses are formed within the nucleus and then transported through the cell to the extracellular fluid.

Transmission of HSV infection occurs by direct contact of the virus onto susceptible mucosal tissues (oropharynx, labia, cervix, vagina, conjunctiva) or onto broken skin. (Spread by fomites or aerosol is unlikely because *HSV does not survive drying and room temperature.*) Historically, herpes lesions "above the waist" were attributed to HSV type 1, and genital herpes was attributed to HSV type 2. For reasons that are incompletely understood but likely involve changes in sexual practices, the number of persons with genital HSV-1 infection or oral HSV-2 infection have increased. The distinction between HSV-1 and HSV-2 genital infections is of little value because both virus types may cause significant neonatal illness.

Risk

It is estimated that 20 million people in the United States have genital HSV (ACOG, 1988). Transmission to the infant occurs during passage through the infected birth canal or by ascending infection after rupture of membranes. Rarely has transplacental infection been noted. Transmission through close contact with an infected mother, relative, or health care provider may occur if simple precautions are not followed (Table 25-3).

Although the clinical course of the infection during pregnancy does not appear to be different from that of nonpregnant women, without treatment, approximately 50% of HSV-infected newborns die. An additional 50% of the survivors experience significant neurologic or ocular damage.

Primary HSV infection poses the greatest risk to the pregnancy. Primary HSV infection has been associated with increased risk of spontaneous abortion, low birth weight, and preterm delivery. The rate of transmission is approximately 50% if the infection is a primary one (ACOG, 1988). Recurrent HSV disease has not been associated with adverse outcome other than neonatal infection, with a transmission rate of 5%.

Signs

After inoculation with HSV, the infected person may have symptoms or may be symptom free, or asymptomatic. In either case, during primary (initial) HSV infection the virus ascends along peripheral sensory nerves, enters sensory or autonomic nerve root ganglia, and establishes latent infection (Figure 25-3). Nonspecific stimuli, including fever, sunlight, and stress, have been associated with stimulating recurrences of oral HSV-1. Such trigger mechanisms have not been characterized for HSV-2 infection. Persons reporting their first episode of genital herpes generally have milder symptoms if they have serologic evidence (antibodies) of either HSV-1 or HSV-2 infection.

Symptomatic *primary genital HSV* infection often is accompanied by prolonged systemic and local symptoms. Fever, headache, malaise, and myalgias are common and may persist for the first 3 to 4 days after lesions develop. Local symptoms include severe pain, itching, dysuria, vaginal or urethral discharge, and tender inguinal lymph nodes. Typical lesions appear as papules and progress to vesicles, which rupture and ulcerate. Lesions may spread over the genital area. Ulcerated lesions of primary herpes may persist for 4 to 15 days, before healing. HSV cervicitis occurs among 70% to 90% of women with primary HSV infection. In some cases symptoms occur, with increased and abnormal vaginal discharge and mucopurulent cervicitis.

Signs and symptoms of *recurrent genital HSV* are localized to the genital region and generally are less severe than in primary HSV. Lesions may last 4 to 10 days. Up to 50% of persons with recurrent HSV infection may note warning symptoms, including local tingling, itching, or shooting pains in buttock, legs, or hips. Frequency of recurrences differ, and in some persons, severity of individual recurrent episodes vary. HSV infection may involve solely the cervix, without external genital or extragenital lesions being noted. Viral shedding from the cervix may occur, without symptoms, at any time during the course of HSV

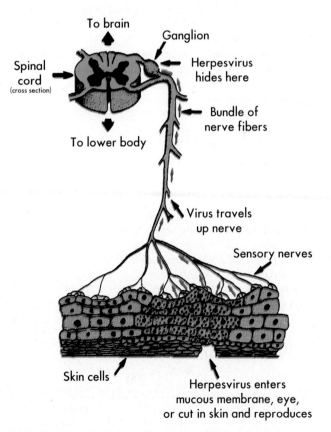

FIGURE 25-3 Path of the herpesvirus. The virus ascends to hide in the nerve ganglion. (Courtesy National Foundation March of Dimes, White Plains, N.Y.)

TABLE 25-3 Guidelines for Prevention of Perinatal Transmission of Herpes Simplex Virus

RECOMMENDATION	RATIONALE
PRENATAL	

Carefully question all pregnant women about:
  History of HSV infection
  Sores or lesions that recur in the same places
  Sexual contact (past or present) with a partner with history of HSV infection or sores that recur in same location
  Prior affected infant
	Identifies women with history of HSV infection, history that suggests HSV infection, or risk for acquiring infection. Allows for education about signs and symptoms of infection and guidelines for prevention of transmission (interpersonal and perinatal).

Obtain culture of any possible herpetic lesion during pregnancy if diagnosis not documented.	Confirms diagnosis of HSV.
INTRAPARTUM	
If no lesions are visible or no prodrome is occurring during labor, vaginal delivery is allowed.	Risk of perinatal transmission is small.
To ensure absence of virus at time of vaginal delivery, women with active lesions close to term and before labor or rupture of membranes have had cultures obtained every 3 to 5 days until one is negative. (Recent data show this is unnecessary.)	
Internal fetal cardiac monitoring, if indicated to adequately assess fetal well-being, is not contraindicated in women with history of HSV and no lesion or symptoms.	Fetal scalp electrodes only rarely have been associated with neonatal infection.
Culture of mother (cervix, vulva) or newborn (mouth, umbilicus, rectum) may be obtained at time of delivery.	May aid the pediatrician in determining need for newborn therapy. This protocol, however, may not prove beneficial because 70% of neonatal infections occur in women with no history of HSV.
Women in labor at term or with ruptured membranes at term who have visible lesions should have cesarean delivery (regardless of the duration of ruptured membranes).	Cesarean delivery will reduce the risk of neonatal herpes infection.
Women with PROM and active lesions should be managed individually and the risk of prematurity weighed against the risks of HSV.	Little information is available to provide universal recommendations.
POSTPARTUM	

Infant does not need to be isolated from mother.
  Avoid direct contact with lesions. Avoid kissing infant if oral-labial lesion present.
  Wash hands carefully before handling infant. Do not place child in parent's bed.
	Risk of transmission is low with careful hygiene precautions.

Breast-feeding is not contraindicated unless visible lesions are present on the breast.	Risk of transmission is low with avoidance of direct contact with lesions and careful hand washing.
Infected health care providers should not be prohibited from caring for these clients as long as direct contact with lesions is avoided and scrupulous hand washing is followed.	Risk of transmission from health care workers is low.
Private room is not required.	HSV infection is transmitted by direct contact with secretions from open lesions, not by fomites or casual contact.

Data from ACOG: Perinatal herpes simplex virus infection, *ACOG Technical Bulletin* 122, Nov 1988; Gibbs RS et al: Management of genital herpes infection in pregnancy, *Obstet Gynecol* 71(5):779, 1988 (editorial).

infection. Cervical viral shedding is detected among 70% to 90% of women during primary infection and among 15% to 30% of women with recurrent vulvar lesions. Up to 5% of women excrete the virus between recurrent episodes. Latex condoms may provide some protection.

Clinical Management

Diagnosis of HSV infection is made by a history of tingling, itching, or painful lesions on the genital area, thigh, or buttock, which appear as blisters that burst, ulcerate, then crust over, and heal. These lesions tend to recur periodically in the same location. Confirmation of HSV infection is best made by recovery of HSV from a viral culture of vesicle fluid. The ELISA test is in use but not as widely available.

Currently HSV infection is *incurable*. Acyclovir antiviral therapy shows promise in lessening the severity of primary illness and preventing recurrences among nonpregnant women. No teratogenic effects have been demonstrated in work with laboratory animals, but its use in human beings has been limited. At this time it is not recommended for use during pregnancy except in life-threatening, disseminated infection.

Recommendations for women with recurrent disease have been revised (ACOG, 1988). It has been determined that 60% of infants with neonatal HSV infection are born to women with no history of HSV and no lesions at the time of delivery. Current recommendations for prenatal screening, method of delivery, and postpartum care are outlined in Table 25-3. These recommendations will likely be modified further as HSV infection is further researched.

Nursing Responsibilities

Pregnant women should be carefully questioned regarding a history of genital or oral HSV, sores that seem to come and go in the same general place, or sexual contact with a current or past partner with a history of HSV infection or recurrent sores in the genital region, thigh, or buttock, or previous infant with HSV infection. Women who have no history of HSV or no history of possible contact with HSV should be counseled in ways to reduce their risk of acquiring HSV during pregnancy, as appropriate. Women who experience true primary infection during pregnancy will require considerable emotional support and information about HSV infection. See Box 25-7 for isolation precautions.

Palliative measures such as application of cool tea or milk compresses or use of warm-to-cool sitz baths may relieve lesion discomfort. Urination into bath water may avoid catheterization among women who have severe dysuria. Analgesic medications also may be required. Women should be counseled about their somewhat increased risk for pregnancy complications, in-

---

BOX 25-7 Isolation Precautions: Herpes Simplex

Active genital lesions at birth: see Table 25-3
History but no active lesions
  Careful hand washing, gloves for perineal care or lochia contact
Oral herpes lesions:
  No general isolation. Mother wears mask and prevents baby's contact with oral secretions until lesion healed.

---

cluding spontaneous abortion, preterm birth, and IUGR. Strategies for preventing perinatal HSV transmission should be carefully discussed.

HUMAN PAPILLOMAVIRUS

More than 50 types of HPV have been identified by laboratory techniques. These distinct viruses are numbered sequentially. Different skin manifestations are associated with different viral types, although mixed infections are common. Genital warts are the most common sign. Certain viral types are more commonly found in the female genital tract. There seems to be a direct role for HPV in lower genital tract cancer. Whether HPV virus acts alone or as a **cofactor** remains to be understood. It has been determined that heavy cigarette smoking among women with HPV infection increases their risk for cervical cancer (Hellberg et al, 1988). Chlamydia and herpesvirus may have a synergistic effect. Considerable research is directed toward understanding HPV infection, diagnosis, and treatment.

Risk

The overall rate is thought to be as high as 20% in pregnant women. During pregnancy, papillary lesions of HPV infection may increase in size and number. Decrease in cell-mediated immunity and growth factors present during pregnancy may be responsible. Lesions may become more vascular and friable during pregnancy, and, in a few cases, extreme growth on vulva and vagina may be noted.

HPV transmission to the infant occurs. Perinatal transmission occurs during passage through the contaminated birth canal, although ascent from the cervix and vagina into the uterus, transplacental passage, and postnatal transmission also are possible means for infection (Wood, 1991).

Signs

Diagnosis of clinical HPV infection is made by identification of the characteristic appearance of lesions. Cervical and vaginal HPV infections often are asymptomatic and are detected by cytologic identification of squamous cell changes on Papanicolaou's (Pap) smear or by colposcopy. Condyloma acuminatum may be noticed on external genital tissue from mons to the anorectal region. The lesions are most common on moist areas and may occur in the vagina or on the cervix. They may appear as soft, pink, white, or tan, cauliflower-like (papillary) masses and may be single or multiple or the size of a small pin, or they may cover several centimeters in area. The papules also may look like skin warts or be flat.

Clinical Management

Recommendations for follow-up care and treatment of HPV infection are likely to change in the next few years as more is learned about HPV pathogenesis. Pap smears on a regular basis are necessary. Treatment of HPV infection during pregnancy is controversial and problematic. Specific antiviral therapy is not available, and frequent recurrences are noted with existing therapy. Topical podophyllin has been a frequent treatment among nonpregnant women but is contraindicated during pregnancy because of increased potential for maternal and fetal toxicity. Excision of lesions with laser, electrocautery, sharp excision, or Cavitron ultrasonic suction aspiration are used only for very large lesions. Interferon has been used for persistent disease but not during pregnancy.

Recently, podofilex 0.5% solution has been found effective and practical. It is not yet approved in pregnancy and therefore must be used with caution, perhaps not in the first trimester, and with informed consent. Treatment consists of topical application by the woman herself, twice a day for 3 days (Figure 25-4). After a 4-day rest the cycle is repeated for 2 or 3 more weeks. No systemic effects have been reported (Patsner, 1991). Local effects diminish over the 3 weeks but are uncomfortable. These are pain, burning, stinging, itching, edema and some sloughing of skin, with odor (Baker et al, 1990).

HUMAN IMMUNODEFICIENCY VIRUS

HIV is an RNA retrovirus that establishes a chronic infection; it has a long latency period before causing progressive immunodeficiency. The virus, first isolated in 1983, has been shown to have caused human infection as early as 1958 in isolated areas of central Africa. During the 1970s and 1980s the virus spread extensively in Africa, the United States, and Western Europe. There is rapid spread also in Asia at this time. Recognition of the lethal nature of this virus and its epidemic spread was followed by extensive investigation, much of which continues. The reader should seek the most current references to learn about HIV infection.

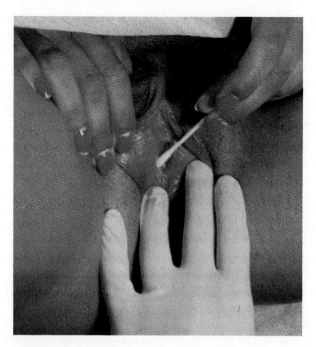

FIGURE 25-4 Client-applied topical application of podofilex for HPV warts. (Courtesy Patsner B: A patient-applied topical solution for genital warts, *Contemp OB/GYN* 36:12, 27, 1991.)

HIV attaches to and invades selected host cells. Viral RNA is translated by enzymes into DNA; this DNA can insert the viral code into the host cell genome (or genetic code). This code for viral DNA will be reproduced each time the cell divides. The code may remain silent (latent), instruct the host cells to begin to produce additional virus, or cause the cell to be destroyed. Antibodies to the viral coat proteins are produced, and all parts of the immune response are activated during HIV infection; yet these responses are unable to protect the host from infection. HIV appears to replicate only in certain white blood cell types, including cells of the central nervous system, intestinal tract, and possibly bone marrow.

HIV is unique among human viruses in that it infects and destroys **helper T lymphocytes** and **macrophages,** cells that are integral to the body's defense system. Helper T lymphocytes are a special class of thymus-derived lymphocytes that circulate in the blood and are programed to recognize the wide variety of foreign antigens to which the body is exposed. Individual T cells are programed to recognize different antigens. When a helper T cell recognizes its special antigen on a macrophage surface, the cell and antigen bind together and the T cell is activated. Activated helper T cells release biologically active substances that stimulate production of additional specific helper T cells, killer T cells, and B cells. The immune response is initiated. Activation of HIV-infected helper T cells causes rapid proliferation of the virus, which destroys the host T cell. Thus the immune response is disrupted. Destruction of helper T cells also is thought to be caused by other, as yet undefined, mechanisms. Viral replication appears to occur more slowly among other cell types and interferes with function rather than causes cell death.

Risk

High-risk groups include homosexual and bisexual men, IV drug users who share needles, transfusion recipients before 1985, and sexual partners of these persons. HIV infection continues to occur most frequently among homosexual and bisexual men; however, the incidence of heterosexual transmission is increasing.

HIV may be transmitted by sexual penetration between men, between women and men, and between women. Nonsexual transmission may occur by inoculation with contaminated blood, blood products, and possibly other selected bodily fluids. Inoculation with large numbers of virus during transfusion of contaminated blood or blood products almost universally causes HIV infection in the recipient. However, among individuals who received inadvertent needle sticks, which would involve much lower numbers of virus, transmission is infrequent; currently 0.5% among health workers after needle stick or other contamination (see Table 25-2). HIV has been detected in other body fluids, including saliva, tears, amniotic fluid, cerebrospinal fluid (CSF), synovial fluid, and peritoneal fluid; however, evidence of transmission by contamination with these fluids has not been detected because the viral load is lower in these fluids. Intact skin appears to be an effective barrier to HIV acquisition. Transmission of HIV to close household contacts of persons infected with HIV has not been demonstrated.

Pregnancy is associated with a modest suppression of cell-mediated immunity or a decrease in helper T cells. This, with HIV reduction of helper T cells, may increase the woman's susceptibility to opportunistic infections. Most women with HIV infection are of reproductive age and therefore also risk transmitting HIV perinatally.

Vertical transmission from mother to infant may occur transplacentally, during the intrapartum period from contamination with vaginal secretions and blood, or during breast-feeding.

Fetal and newborn risk. HIV infection is transmitted to approximately 30% of exposed infants. All infants of HIV-positive women show maternal antibodies at birth (Box 25-8), but 70% will show seroconversion to negative before 2 years of age because there is no viral infection in their systems. Infants who do have HIV infection appear to develop end-stage disease or AIDS after a much shorter incubation period (less than 1 year) than do adults (Figure 25-5).

Currently it is believed that HIV is transmitted to the fetus if the maternal viral load is high, such as occurs at the beginning of the infection and if the T4 cell count is low, such as toward the period when AIDS symptoms appear. In addition, it is now clear that *at the time of birth the baby may be inoculated with a virus load by contact with maternal blood and vaginal fluids.* This

---

BOX 25-8 Perinatal Transmissions—Possible Outcomes (HIV-Positive Mother)

Baby 1 (approximately 70%)
- Has positive HIV test
- Has only HIV antibody from mother
- Does not have HIV virus
- Will show seroconversion to negative before 2 years of age

Baby 2 (approximately 30%)
- Has positive HIV test result
- Has HIV antibody and virus from mother
- Has virus, is infected, and will develop symptoms
- Will continue to show positive HIV test result after 2 years of age

---

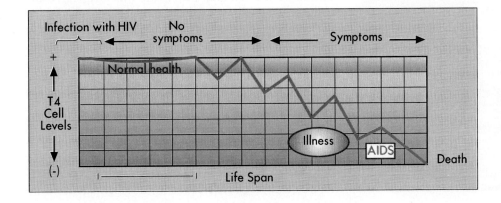

FIGURE 25-5 The life span of neonatal HIV infection compared with adult onset. Newborn *early onset* results in illness within 2 to 3 months. *Late onset:* illness after 15 months. Adult: illness begins 8 to 10 years after onset of infection. T4 cell levels below 200 usually signal the beginning of AIDS.

was shown in a carefully controlled international study of the outcome of twin birth in 100 HIV-positive women (International Registry, 1991). The first-born twin, either by vaginal or cesarean birth, had a much higher rate (58%) of developing HIV infection than did the second twin (19%). The difference in these cases points to contamination for longer periods by vaginal fluids or to loss of skin integrity by puncture of the skin with scalp pH monitoring or fetal electrocardiogram (FECG) electrode.

Since 1989, recommendations have been made to guard skin integrity in infants at risk of HIV contamination (Connor, Bardequez, and Apuzzio, 1989) (Box 25-9). Nurses need to advocate for procedures to accomplish the following:
1. No skin puncture before skin cleansing
2. Early bath with soap or dilute chlorhexidine (Hibiclens) before eye prophylaxis or intramuscular (IM) injection

Signs

Initial HIV infection may be accompanied by a mononucleosis-like illness, with symptoms that include fatigue, fever, and swollen glands. A rash may develop. The symptoms resolve completely within 3 to 14 days. HIV infection may remain silent, yet transmissible, for 2 to 10 years in a *latent period* before progressive symptoms of immunodeficiency develop.

AIDS-related complex (ARC) may be considered a pre-AIDS condition. Affected persons experience a variety of nonspecific symptoms, including weight loss, malaise, lethargy, central nervous system dysfunction, unexplained fever, generalized lymphadenopathy, and *opportunistic infections* such as herpes simplex or *Candida*.

AIDS is the end stage of HIV. Persons with AIDS show evidence of a severely compromised immune system. They have life-threatening illnesses from microorganisms or malignancies that seldom cause problems among healthy persons. Evidence of immunodeficiency in the absence of other known causes and the presence of **opportunistic infection,** severe neurologic disease, and HIV antibody constitute the definition of AIDS. The definition of AIDS has been modified several times since the disease was first described; it is probable that there will be further changes in this definition.

Clinical Management

Methods to detect HIV infection will likely undergo considerable refinement within the next few years. Currently, tests that detect antibody to HIV-1 are used to identify persons with HIV infection. Antibodies to the virus develop and are detectable within the first 6 months of infection, again demonstrating a window in which infection is present but antibody formation is inadequate to trigger a positive test response (Figure 25-6).

Two methods, used together, detect and confirm the presence of HIV-1 antibody. ELISA is relatively easy to perform and is inexpensive. It is highly sensitive in detecting the HIV antibody for large groups of people. A single, positive ELISA test result is not absolute evidence of HIV infection. If the ELISA shows a positive reaction, the test is repeated on the same serum sample. Confirmation of a twice-positive ELISA test result is achieved with a second antibody test (Western blot), which is specific for antibody to the HIV protein coat. The Western blot test is difficult to perform and therefore is less well suited for wide screening. Persons whose test reaction is negative with the ELISA method and who have not been exposed or potentially exposed to the virus within the previous 6 months are considered free of HIV-1 infection.

Maternal signs in antepartum and intrapartum periods are confirmed by blood work, with the **T4 lymphocyte** counts being followed at regular intervals. Fetal assessment will be increased because of the potential for IUGR. Intrapartal management does not differ from standard care and includes minimizing ascending infection and vaginal examinations, as well as maintaining frequent perineal hygiene. Laboratory reports for thrombocytopenia and anemia are followed, especially if the woman is on a medication regimen.

HIV infection currently is incurable. Finding effective treatments has been hindered by the biology of the virus and the nature of the infection. Zidovudine (AZT) has shown some promise in prolonging lives of some clients. Pregnant women are treated when the CD4 counts fall below 200 cells/µl (Sperling et al, 1992) even though risks are still unclear. A combination drug, sulfamethoxazole-trimethoprim (Bactrim) routinely is given during pregnancy to women whose history or need for prophylaxis against *Pneumocystis carinii* pneumonia (PCP) requires treatment. Although Bactrim con-

---

BOX 25-9   Isolation Precautions: HIV

Mother
Universal precautions
Careful hand washing; avoid newborn contact with blood, blood products, or lochia

Infant
Universal precautions; bathe child promptly with soap and water

Breast-feeding
Contraindicated

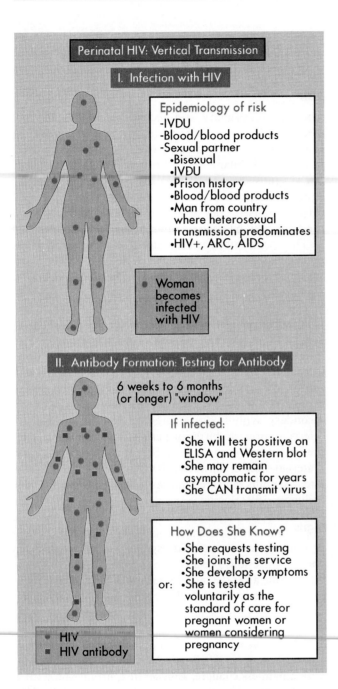

Perinatal HIV: Vertical Transmission

I. Infection with HIV

Epidemiology of risk
-IVDU
-Blood/blood products
-Sexual partner
  •Bisexual
  •IVDU
  •Prison history
  •Blood/blood products
  •Man from country
   where heterosexual
   transmission predominates
  •HIV+, ARC, AIDS

• Woman
  becomes
  infected
  with HIV

II. Antibody Formation: Testing for Antibody

6 weeks to 6 months
(or longer) "window"

If infected:
  •She will test positive on
   ELISA and Western blot
  •She may remain
   asymptomatic for years
  •She CAN transmit virus

How Does She Know?
       •She requests testing
       •She joins the service
       •She develops symptoms
  or: •She is tested
        voluntarily as the
        standard of care for
        pregnant women or
        women considering
        pregnancy

• HIV
■ HIV antibody

FIGURE 25-6 Vertical transmission of perinatal HIV. (Courtesy Toni Ross, RNC, Elmhurst Hospital Center, Queens, N.Y.)

tains a sulfonamide that rarely may cause neonatal jaundice, its value to the woman is so great it is continued throughout pregnancy. The woman needs to be informed so that she takes the recommended drugs with consent.

Nursing Responsibilities

Preconceptional screening is ideal for women who are at increased risk for HIV infection (Box 25-10). Delay

of pregnancy until effective treatments for HIV infection have been developed is recommended. Serologic screening also is advised for women who already are pregnant and belong to a high-risk group. Counseling before and after HIV antibody testing is of extreme importance.

Screening involves obtaining a careful history for risk-taking behaviors, as well as signs and symptoms of illness, physical examination, and serologic testing. To identify those at risk for HIV infection, careful history taking includes specific questions in the language and terms familiar to the individual (see Box 25-10).

Women are advised about their risk for HIV infection, the benefits of antibody testing, the procedure for testing, the meaning of possible test results, the confidentiality of results, and the psychologic and social impact of a positive result. The client's consent to perform the test is almost universally required. Posttest counseling includes discussion of the meaning of the results, limits of the test, psychologic and social implications of the results, and a pointed discussion on behaviors to reduce future risk of infection for the client and others. In addition, if the woman is infected with HIV, the importance of continuing medical care is stressed and resources for psychologic support are given. Persons at risk for HIV infection should be counseled about their high-risk behaviors and specific means they may use to decrease this risk.

Individualized antepartum management after screening is important. The psychosocial impact of discovering a positive test result may be intense. The woman may have been infected by a partner (seen more and more today) whose own status was unknown. In other cases it is found that the HIV-positive man refuses to tell his partner or to use a condom for fear that when she learns of his status, she will leave him. This tragic situation is not uncommon, especially with immigrant women who come from patriarchal societies in which discussion of sexual habits is avoided and unquestioning obedience to the husband is the norm. In a number of instances the first sign of parental HIV status is the admission of the infant for AIDS-related symptoms. The woman in this situation needs careful counseling. Because confidentiality is a major issue, the health care provider may try to trace contacts according to each setting's protocol.

A multidisciplinary approach to follow-up care is in place. The advent of the HIV epidemic has allowed comprehensive planning for care in ways that longer-standing and less life-threatening problems have not evoked. Pediatric follow-up for the infant and home care are standard practices today. Breast-feeding is not encouraged.

SYPHILIS

Syphilis is a chronic infection, recognized since antiquity as "the great pox." The spirochete *Treponema pallidum* is capable of penetrating intact skin or mucous membranes and is transmitted by direct contact with skin lesions or blood, primarily during sexual intimacy, including kissing. The incidence of syphilis decreased after the introduction of penicillin in the 1940s; however, since 1978 the incidence of syphilis among women has been increasing steadily. Women ages 15 to 24 have the highest increase in the incidence of syphilis. In the United States, syphilis most frequently is reported among young, urban, poor, and unmarried persons.

 Self-Discovery

Your client in labor is Mrs. R. whose HIV seroconversion occurred because her husband "went with prostitutes" before she arrived in this country. She is resigned to her situation but worried about the baby. As a nurse, how do you feel about this situation? If you were in her situation, how might you feel? What would you like the nurse to help you with?

Syphilis is more prevalent in developing nations than in industrialized nations, and treatment is not so widely available.

Risk

The rate of primary and secondary syphilis has increased 75% since 1985, with most of the increase in lower socioeconomic groups; 44% of the cases occurred in women (Tillman, 1991). Untreated or treated after a late diagnosis, syphilis may cause multiorgan damage. A number of women are treated and become reinfected. Pregnancy itself does not affect the disease course, but the fetus may be severely infected during pregnancy.

The rise in rates has been linked to the cocaine-crack epidemic. Users usually do not follow through on seeking medical care, or care is very late. Reinfection is common.

Congenital syphilis risk. *T. pallidum* can cross the placenta and invade the fetus *at any gestational age.* Fetal infection may result directly in spontaneous abortion, intrauterine fetal death (IUFD), premature labor and birth, neonatal death, and clinically evident congenital syphilis. Infants of women with untreated primary or secondary syphilis are at greatest risk for congenital infection, preterm birth, or perinatal death. The risk to the fetus appears to decrease the longer the duration of maternal illness; however, 10% of women with late latent syphilis delivered infants with congenital syphilis (Tillman, 1991).

Signs

If not adequately treated, syphilis is a progressive, chronic infectious process. Syphilis is described by periods of time after the initial infection as *primary, secondary, latent,* and *tertiary,* depending on the duration of the infection, the symptoms, and the organ systems involved.

After a usual incubation period of 10 days to 3 weeks (but up to 90 days), *primary* syphilis develops with a painless **chancre,** an ulcerated, firm lesion with a raised border. The chancre appears at the site of spirochete penetration and is highly infectious. It lasts for 1 to 6 weeks, possibly longer. There also may be swollen lymph glands. Among women, the chancre is not always observed because it occurs on the cervix or vagina rather than the external genitalia and produces no irritating symptoms. The chancre resolves spontaneously *even without treatment.*

Secondary syphilis symptoms develop 6 to 8 weeks after the chancre has appeared and may first occur up to 6 months later. There is bacteremia and involvement of all organ systems. Skin and mucous membrane lesions and generalized lymphadenopathy are common. Short-lived malaise, fever, sore throat, headache, anorexia, and arthralgia also occur. A generalized maculopapular rash involving the palms and soles of feet helps to identify syphilis as the cause because few skin diseases involve these areas. The dermatologic lesions of secondary syphilis are extremely variable and often mimic other dermatologic conditions such as pityriasis rosea, psoriasis, lichen planus, erythema multiforme, and impetigo or eczema, an important observation to remember in congenital syphilis diagnosis.

Condyloma latum occurs on the labia, groin, inner thighs, and anal region. It is different from condyloma acuminatum (human papillomavirus). Syphilitic condyloma consists of elevated, white, moist papules or plaques. In addition, **mucous patches** may appear as grayish white erosions on any mucous membrane tissue.

Cutaneous lesions heal in 2 to 10 weeks *with or without treatment*. The untreated client then enters a state of *early latent* syphilis (less than 1 year since infection). During this phase, clinical disease is not apparent; however, relapses of syphilitic cutaneous lesions may occur.

The **latent period** of syphilis has two stages, early latent and late. The period of early latent is asymptomatic for 75% of the cases; 25% still have infectious lesions (Quin, 1989). This period lasts up to 1 year from onset of the chancre. Late latent begins after 1 year and lasts for the rest of the person's untreated life. In about one third of latent cases a **tertiary** syphilis develops with gummatous cardiovascular signs or neurosyphilis that badly damages target organs. (Refer to Crane, 1992, for discussion of details not covered in this text because most women who become pregnant are not yet in the late latent syphilis state.)

Women usually do not have infectious lesions during latent syphilis, but the spirochete may be transmitted to the fetus and can be transmitted through blood.

Clinical Management

Diagnostic testing. Syphilis is diagnosed by serologic tests or direct microscopic examination of lesion exudate for spirochetes. Serologic tests detect the presence of antibodies to the spirochete. Unfortunately, antibody test reactions will be negative for 4 to 6 weeks after exposure to the infection; false-negative test results occur if the person is evaluated at this time. This *window* can be misleading.

Two types of serologic tests are used. Nonspecific tests or **nontreponemal tests** include the VDRL, rapid plasma reagin (RPR), and automated reagin test (ART). Because these tests are *nonspecific*, other diseases (e.g., acute febrile illness, immunization, leprosy, autoimmune disease such as lupus erythematosus, and pregnancy itself) may cause false-positive results in these nontreponemal tests. Any positive nontreponemal test reaction must be confirmed by a *treponemal serologic*

test. The fluorescent treponemal antibody-absorption test (FTA-ABS) is the most commonly used *specific* test. Results of the FTA-ABS remain positive for the person's lifetime in spite of adequate treatment.

In other areas of the world, where other *Treponema* species cause infections such as pinta, yaws, and bejel, persons who have had these infections will show positive reactions on both treponema-specific and nonspecific serologic tests. These women often are given antibiotic treatment as if they have syphilis.

Treatment. Syphilis is best treated with penicillin (Box 25-11). Recommended treatment for primary, secondary, and early latent syphilis is a one-time, intramuscular dose of benzathine penicillin G. Late latent syphilis or syphilis of unknown duration is often treated for 3 consecutive weeks. Because of the pharmacokinetic alterations in pregnancy, additional treatment with ampicillin 500 mg, four times daily for 7 to 14 days, is recommended by some authorities. All HIV positive women should be retested after the first course of treatment since often the usual dosages are not adequate. Alternative treatment for the penicillin-allergic pregnant woman is erythromycin. However, erythromycin crosses the placenta poorly and may not adequately treat the fetus. Skin testing and administration of penicillin *desensitization protocol* and treatment with penicillin in the hospital are recommended for women who are truly penicillin allergic (Wendel et al, 1985).

Spirochete reactions. Treatment with penicillin may evoke a serious reaction called **Jarisch-Herxheimer** reaction. This reaction is thought to be caused by the sudden release of spirochete cell wall lipids into the maternal and fetal bloodstream as the organism is destroyed. Within hours of treatment high fever, chills, myalgia, tachycardia, and occasionally hypertension and shock may occur. This reaction may be accompanied by uterine contractions, decreased fetal movement, and fetal distress (Wendel et al, 1985). As a precaution,

---

BOX 25-11 Treatment of Syphilis during Pregnancy

Primary, secondary, and early latent (<1 yr)

2.4 million units benzathine penicillin G, IM
  Rescreen at 3 and 6 months

Late latent and gumma-affected cardiovascular system

7.2 million units benzathine penicillin G, IM in three divided weekly doses
  Rescreen at 6 and 12 months

a period of electronic fetal monitoring after the injection may be required for women being treated during the third trimester. Treatment is symptomatic with antipyretics, bed rest, and emotional support.

After antibiotic treatment, pregnant clients should receive follow-up with monthly quantitative VDRL titers for the remainder of the pregnancy and should be retreated if a fourfold rise in antibody titer occurs. Long-term follow-up care includes quantitative VDRL titers at 3, 6, 9, and 12 months after therapy. While in the hospital unit, use isolation precautions listed in Box 25-12.

Test Yourself

- Test-of-cure after treatment for syphilis is performed with which screening test?
- Why is this test especially important for newborns and women with HIV positivity?

CONGENITAL SYPHILIS

Infants with congenital syphilis most often are born to mothers who received no prenatal care or did not complete treatment. To prevent such a problem, early and adequate prenatal care is important. Infants do not pass through stages, but there is early widespread organ involvement (Crane, 1992).

Congenital syphilis nearly always is preventable by early identification of maternal syphilis and treatment as early as possible during pregnancy. The fetus may be severely infected before treatment, however, and show signs in bones, teeth, and central nervous system even after treatment. Congenital syphilis also may occur because of maternal relapses or reinfection from an untreated partner. Treatment before 15 weeks may prevent congenital syphilis (Tillman, 1991).

BOX 25-12   Isolation Precautions: Syphilis

Mother
Avoid contact with body fluids or chancre mucous patches.
Use blood precautions, careful hand washing.

Infant
Infant is isolated with mother.

Breast-feeding
Breast-feeding permitted after treatment.

BOX 25-13   Treatment of Congenital Syphilis

100,000-150,000 U/kg aqueous crystalline penicillin G IV daily for 10-14 days
Procaine penicillin IM qd for 10-14 days has been used, but there is risk of damage to small muscle sites
Rescreen at 1, 2, 3, 6, and 12 months

Signs

Infants with congenital syphilis most often are symptom free at birth. Symptoms often appear by 10 days to 2 weeks and nearly always are within the first 3 months of life. Clinical symptoms initially may be nonspecific:
- Watery rhinitis
- Enlarged liver, spleen
- Mucocutaneous rash, patches

Without diagnosis and treatment the disease progresses. Multiorgan involvement includes purulent nasal discharge, maculopapular rash, desquamation, osteochondritis, jaundice, anemia, meningitis, and hydrocephalus. Bone and soft tissue deformities are associated with late congenital syphilis, that is, diagnosed after 2 years of age.

Clinical Management

A cord blood sample may be tested or maternal tests used as a screen. Most units draw maternal blood for VDRL on admission to labor. If the result is positive, the infant is treated (Box 25-13). The CDC recommends that newborns not be discharged until the maternal VDRL results are known. This is not happening because of early discharge, thus placing the responsibility for communication of results from the hospital unit to the pediatric follow-up personnel. Because of the *window* in antibody formation, newborns have manifested congenital syphilis when the maternal VDRL response was negative. In these cases the women became infected within 4 to 6 weeks of birth, before antibody levels were significant (see HIV testing for the same problem).

Nursing Responsibilities for STDs
▶ ASSESSMENT

In the antenatal clinic setting, nursing care often includes obtaining information about current problems and a detailed health history. Assessment of a woman's risk of acquiring or having an STD is essential and is accomplished by asking very specific, nonjudgmental questions about the person's (1) sexual practices—whether or not she participates in vaginal, oral-genital, anal, oral-anal sex, use of sexual devices, or other types of sexual expression, (2) the gender of her sexual partner, (3) if she has had a new partner in the past 3 months, (4) the number of partners in the past month, year, lifetime, and (5) history of any STDs. To elicit information on STDs, questions about each type of infection should be asked separately, and language should be appropriate to the educational level and cultural background of the woman.

A few examples of these questions include: Have you noticed any increased vaginal discharge? Does your discharge burn, itch, or have an odor? Do you notice the vaginal odor at any particular time (e.g., after intercourse)? What color is your discharge? Are there any sores or bumps that you notice today or that come and go? Do you have any pain, burning, or discomfort with intercourse?

▶ NURSING DIAGNOSES

With the information gathered from an interview and review of records, the nurse may consider several nursing diagnoses depending on whether a potential or actual problem is identified. For example, if a woman is at high risk for STDs, the following nursing diagnoses may apply:

1. Altered health maintenance
2. Knowledge deficit regarding risk of acquiring STDs
3. High risk for infection related to exposure to a sexual partner without using an effective barrier method

When a sexually transmitted infection has been identified after assessment, nursing diagnoses may be directed toward the woman's knowledge and understanding of the infection, treatment, and follow-up care; actual and potential physical symptoms; psychologic and social responses to having the infection; or prevention of potential complications from the infection. The following examples of nursing diagnoses may apply:

1. Knowledge deficit regarding risks of STD during pregnancy
2. Pain related to lesions
3. Body-image disturbance or self-esteem disturbance related to acquiring a sexually transmitted infection
4. High risk for injury: fetal, related to congenital infection

▶ EXPECTED OUTCOMES

Outcomes vary with the type of STD. Some are quickly treated, others are long-term problems. Some of the following examples may apply:

1. Gains cooperation of partner in safe sex and preventive measures

2. Uses methods to relieve discomforts during treatment
3. Follows precautions to prevent reinfection
4. Infant exhibits negative laboratory test results

▶ NURSING INTERVENTIONS

Nurses participate in a number of ways in STD care. Education is important in every situation (Box 25-14). Knowledge of the resources in the community is essential for anyone working in counseling. The nurse often is the facilitator for the client in finding other support. A team approach is more successful because social problems, drug use, and distress often accompany an STD.

When a woman is pregnant and has an STD, additional anxiety about the infant usually occurs. Nurses need to know how the STD affects fetus and newborn health, as well as the effect of the medications the woman must take. Finally, isolation precautions must be taught and followed.

▶ EVALUATION

1. Were precautions followed and transmission prevented?
2. Does the woman know infection outcome, recurrence signs, and preventive actions?
3. Is there any evidence of perinatal transmission?
4. If no cure is possible (HIV, HSV), has she followed through on supportive treatment?

Perinatal Infections

Perinatal infections are acquired by transmission before, during, or shortly after birth. They may be caused by bacteria, viruses, protozoa, or fungi. Intrauterine transmission of these infections may occur across the placenta via the maternal blood stream, by ascent of microorganisms from the vagina, or possibly by descent from infected fallopian tubes. The infant may become infected during passage through the infected birth canal or from maternal blood during birth, or by maternal-infant contact after birth. It is important to remember that infections such as hepatitis B and cytomegalovirus may be sexually transmitted.

ENTEROVIRUS

Enteroviruses are RNA viruses that occur worldwide and are spread from person to person by fecal-oral or possibly oral-oral routes. Each of the three major enteroviruses—poliovirus, coxsackievirus, and echovirus—has been associated with serious neonatal disease. Enterovirus may be transmitted transplacentally or by contamination during birth.

BOX 25-14 **Principles of Personal Risk Reduction for Acquiring STDs**

COMMENT

Careful consideration of sexual activity

Abstinence and restriction to a single (uninfected) partner or partners reduce the risk of all STDs to a minimum. Increased numbers of partners, especially unfamiliar ones, increase risks.

Practice of sexual activities that do not exchange bodily fluids with unfamiliar partners (e.g., massage, masturbation)

STD pathogens are transmitted by direct contact of microorganism with mucosal surfaces or open skin.

Use of barrier forms of contraception with spermicidal agents or tubal ligation; use of oral contraceptives

Properly used, condoms (and possibly diaphragms) combined with spermicides reduce the risks of many STDs. They will not work if infectious lesions or secretions are not covered or contained. Some evidence suggests that tubal ligation and oral contraceptives decrease risk of upper genital tract infection.

Avoidance of "unsafe sex" practices

Avoid practices that cause local skin or mucosal membrane trauma and increase direct inoculation of pathogens. Avoid oroanal contact, receptive anal intercourse, and anal intercourse altogether. Avoid sexual activities that cause bleeding.

Periodic screening for STDs

Persons at increased risk should be screened at intervals corresponding to their risk. (That is, young persons, persons with a prior STD, and persons with more than three partners in last 6 months should be screened frequently.)

Ensuring partner's treatment or compliance with safe sex

Partners of persons with gonorrhea or *Chlamydia* infection are 50% to 56% infected. Many are symptom free.

When at risk for AIDS

Practice sexual activities that do not include exchange of body fluids. Do not share IV needles. Do not donate blood or other body fluids or organs. If female, discuss pregnancy risk with counselor.

Data from Darrow WW, Wiesner PJ: Personal prophylaxis for venereal disease, *JAMA* 233:444, 1975; Hart G: Role of preventative methods in the control of venereal disease, *Clin Obstet Gynecol* 18:243, 1975; and Colorado AIDS Project: *Safe sex*, Denver, 1984, Colorado AIDS Project.

Poliovirus

Pregnancy is not a contraindication for polio immunization, and there are rare cases in the United States today. The HIV-positive woman, however, should *not* receive oral polio vaccine; instead the injectable inactivated vaccine must be used. Her children receiving oral polio vaccine may shed virus for 1 to 2 weeks, placing her at great risk of becoming ill with poliovirus.

Coxsackievirus

Coxsackievirus is divided into A and B groups. Several group A coxsackievirus types rarely are implicated in neonatal febrile illnesses, sudden infant death syndrome (SIDS), and gastrointestinal malformations. Six types of group B infection have been associated with serious neonatal morbidity and mortality. Shortly after birth, neonatal echovirus infection may cause fever, cyanosis, hypothermia, bradycardia, hepatic necrosis, disseminated intravascular coagulopathy, and death. There are no specific treatments or vaccines for echovirus or coxsackievirus infections.

CYTOMEGALOVIRUS INFECTION

Cytomegalovirus (CMV) is a member of the *herpesvirus* family. Like other viruses of this type, CMV initially establishes a *primary* infection and then a *latent* infection with persistent shedding of the virus. Commonly CMV is asymptomatic or has mononucleosis-like symptoms. CMV has been isolated from urine, saliva, blood, cervical mucus, semen, breast milk, and stool. Transmission may occur from contamination of any of these bodily fluids, close interpersonal contact, and sexual contact. Infection with CMV appears to increase with age and varies with socioeconomic group. Approximately 40% of women of childbearing age in the United States have antibodies for CMV (Fowler, 1992). Approximately 1% of pregnant women have detectable cervical CMV virus during the first trimester; increased viral shedding occurs as pregnancy progresses. CMV may be transmitted across the placenta even if the woman has no overt signs. Vertical transmission at birth also occurs from contaminated cervical and vaginal fluids, blood, and later, through breast milk.

Symptomatic congenital CMV is associated with *primary* maternal CMV infection. Congenital CMV occasionally has been reported among women with recurrent infection, but the infants appeared less severely affected than those exposed to primary infection. There is no treatment other than supportive care for this viral infection. The development of a vaccine is being investigated (Samson, 1988).

Risk

Approximately 0.5% to 2% of newborns are infected with CMV at birth. Only 5% to 10% of these infected infants (about 5000/year) demonstrate characteristics associated with congenital CMV. Congenital CMV is characterized by an enlarged spleen and liver, microcephaly, hyperbilirubinemia, motor impairment, cerebral calcifications, and eye defects.

In about 5% of those infected but *symptom free* at birth, varying degrees of neurologic deficits may develop by 48 months, including hearing loss, learning, and visual difficulties. Symptom-free children may excrete the virus in urine and saliva for a long time and may infect others, especially in day-care centers (Tookey and Peckman, 1991). Preventive care includes good hygiene: careful washing of hands after changing and disposing of diapers, as well as adequate washing of any dishes, utensils, or toys in contact with saliva. Health care workers are exposed, and most demonstrate antibodies against CMV.

INFLUENZA

Influenza is an epidemic disease caused by viruses. These viruses are capable of altering their antigen structure frequently to protect themselves from the human host defense system. Influenza epidemics in the past have been associated with significantly increased maternal mortality. Whether pregnant women are more susceptible to influenza or to influenzal pneumonia is unclear. If however, influenzal pneumonia develops in pregnant women, they are more severely affected.

Risk

The effect of the virus on pregnancy outcome is unclear. Most information suggests that antepartum influenza infection is not associated with congenital malformations, spontaneous abortions, stillbirth, or prematurity.

LYME DISEASE

A tick-borne disease spread worldwide, Lyme disease may be the cause of increased fetal loss and widely diverse malformations, as well as neonatal illness (Duffy, 1987). Several types of ticks carry the spirochete, which acts somewhat like the syphilis spirochete.

Mice and deer are carriers, as are other wild and domesticated animals that roam. Birds also are carriers.

The tick must stay attached for 12 to 24 hours for vertical transmission to occur. Lyme disease is most prevalent in late spring or early summer (Duffy, 1987). It is a complex syndrome with many varied expressions.

Signs

Stage I signs are *erythema chronicum migrans (ECM)*, small papular or macular lesions that are followed by a spreading, reddened lesion reaching an average of 15 cm in diameter. Lesions most commonly occur on the thighs, groin, and axilla. In stage 1 there may be flulike symptoms with headache and arthralgia.

Stage II occurs when the disease continues undiagnosed and untreated. The lesions show neurologic signs of cranial nerve palsy (Bell's palsy is most common) but third and sixth cranial nerves may involve eye function. Meningitis may occur. Chronic fatigue and cognitive problems may develop. Peripheral nerve involvement leads to weakness, reduced reflexes, and pain. Stage III involves arthritis, especially of the knee.

Clinical Management

Prevention is crucial for those in areas of tick infestation. Protective clothing, showers after outdoor activity, and examination of skin for tick sites are recommended. A vaccine is being prepared but is not yet available. Amoxicillin or erythromycin are given for 10 to 30 days for an initial exposure. See Steere (1989) for detailed treatment plan. Information for clients is available from Lyme Disease Education Project, PO Box 55412, Madison, Wisc. 53705.

MEASLES

The number of persons contracting measles (rubeola) has been increasing consistently since 1983. Most cases occur among preschool children who have not received immunization or among infants too young for current immunization (less than 16 months). Outbreaks among secondary school children and college students also have been reported. Estimates suggest that 5% to 15% of older adolescents and young adults are susceptible to measles because of missed immunizations or receipt of less effective forms of the vaccine (Brookman, 1987). Persons who received the less effective vaccine or were vaccinated before 15 months of age are entering their reproductive years and may be susceptible to this infection. Childbearing families are likely to come in contact with small children and be exposed to childhood illnesses such as measles. Therefore the nurse should be aware of the signs and symptoms of infection, mode of transmission, incubation period, and potential complications of measles during pregnancy.

Risk

Maternal morbidity and mortality do not seem to be altered by pregnancy. However, the measles virus is transmitted to the fetus across the placenta at any gestational age. Intrauterine infection is associated with spontaneous abortion, IUFD, premature birth, perinatal death, and congenital measles. Infants may have the characteristic rash at birth, or it may develop within the first days of life. Mortality rates may be as high as 20%. Associations between intrauterine measles and fetal anomalies are inconclusive. (See Box 25-15 for isolation precautions.)

MUMPS

Mumps is a highly contagious infection caused by a paramyxovirus, which usually affects young school-age children but may occur at any age. Mumps virus is transmitted by respiratory droplets. Exposure of susceptible persons to the mumps virus results in unilateral or bilateral parotitis after an 18-day incubation period. Myalgia, fever, anorexia, and earaches also may be noted.

Risk

Mumps-associated complications occur more frequently among older persons and include meningoencephalitis, oophoritis, orchitis, and neurosensory deafness. Acquisition of mumps during pregnancy does not appear to alter the course of the illness; however, increased incidence of first-trimester spontaneous abortion has been noted. Congenital malformations do not appear to occur when pregnant women acquire the mumps virus. Isolation recommendations are noted in Box 25-16.

BOX 25-15   Isolation Precautions: Measles

Mother

No history of measles—no isolation for first 7 days; respiratory isolation for next 7 days

Mask until 4 days after onset of rash; careful hand washing; cover gown; avoid contact with lesions and fomites

Infant

None for first 5 days after exposure; respiratory isolation for next 7 days; give measles hyperimmune globulin

Breast-feeding

Not recommended by some authorities, little information available

---

BOX 25-16   Isolation Precautions: Mumps

Maternal and infant

No isolation for first 7 days after exposure

Respiratory isolation for 2 weeks or until 9 days after swelling starts—for mother and infant

Mother wears mask with infant for 1 week after swelling starts

Careful hand washing

Breast-feeding

Breast-feeding permitted

RUBELLA

Rubella is caused by a highly contagious virus spread by airborne droplets, which generally produces a mild disease in children and adults. Although most rubella cases occur among young children, a significant number of women of childbearing age remain susceptible. The incubation period is 2 to 3 weeks.

Risk

During early pregnancy, rubella causes significant fetal loss through spontaneous abortion, as well as a wide spectrum of congenital anomalies. Defects associated with congenital rubella include myopia, deafness, cataracts, glaucoma, heart disease, and mental retardation. Generally, infection during earlier gestation is associated with more severe fetal effects. Approximately one half of infections occurring before 8 weeks of gestation result in congenital rubella syndrome (Mann et al, 1981). Congenital rubella syndrome is characterized by cataracts, patent ductus arteriosus, and deafness. There also may be IUGR, microcephaly, and mental retardation.

Maternal infection after 16 weeks' gestation most often results in *subclinical fetal infection*. Long-term follow-up care of infants with subclinical infection reveals late signs such as deafness and central nervous system defects. Infants born with congenital rubella are chronically infected and may shed virus for many months to years after birth, and may transmit the virus to susceptible persons. Although rare, maternal rubella within a week of delivery has been associated with lethal neonatal rubella (Figure 25-7).

Signs

Initially a low-grade fever and tender, swollen lymph nodes occur. Then a rash lasting 3 days appears over the face and behind the ears. Care includes rest, fluids, and maintenance of isolation precautions (Box 25-17).

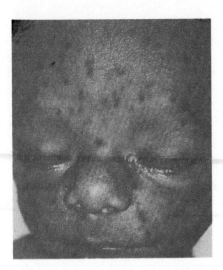

FIGURE 25-7 Congenital rubella. (Courtesy Donald C Anderson, MD, Baylor College of Medicine, Houston, Tex.)

BOX 25-17   Isolation Precautions: Rubella

Mother and infant
Respiratory isolation
Infant isolated with mother
Mask for 3 to 4 days after rash appears
Careful hand washing

Breast-feeding
Breast-feed with mask

Clinical Management

Prevention is critical. All pregnant women are tested for rubella antibodies as early in prenatal care as possible. A negative titer signals that the woman is susceptible and must do the following:

1. Avoid exposure during pregnancy
2. Be immunized just after the birth
3. Delay any future pregnancy for 3 months after immunization
4. Vaccination is done only after birth to avoid the chance of viral infection of the fetus.

Side effects of the vaccine may include muscle and joint pain. Small amounts of virus may be excreted into breast milk after immunization, but this does not contraindicate breast-feeding. Immunization with Rh₀(D) immune globulin does not appear to interfere with rubella immunization. No additional follow-up care is required for women who receive both immunizations during the postpartum period.

Children of pregnant women should receive their immunizations according to schedule. Small amounts of virus may be shed from the pharynx for 7 to 8 days

after immunization. There is no evidence, however, that this attenuated virus is transmissible. See precautions for women who are HIV positive.

TOXOPLASMOSIS

Toxoplasmosis is a systemic, usually asymptomatic illness contracted by at least one third of human beings in most geographic regions. Toxoplasmosis is caused by the protozoan parasite *Toxoplasma gondii,* which infects most mammalian species. Cats and other felines are the hosts in which *Toxoplasma* organisms complete their complex sexual life cycle. The *Toxoplasma* tachyzoite invades muscle and central nervous system tissues and forms cysts in tissue after the development of the host immune response. These cysts persist for the person's lifetime. Acute infections may cause significant complications in immunocompromised or pregnant persons. During pregnancy, *Toxoplasma* may be transmitted across the placenta and cause severe infection in the developing embryo or fetus.

T. gondii may be transmitted to human beings in the following ways: (1) from ingesting the cyst stage from inadequately prepared meat (especially mutton, lamb, or pork) or other animal products, including eggs and milk, (2) from ingesting the oocyst stage from feline feces–contaminated soil or food (e.g., pica or poorly washed root vegetables), or (3) from transplacental or blood-product transmission of tachyzoites. Serologic evidence suggests that 30% to 60% of domestic cats have had *Toxoplasma* infection. *Toxoplasma* tissue cysts can be isolated from muscle of 25% to 30% of swine and sheep and 1% of cattle (Freij and Sever, 1991).

Risk

Like rubella, toxoplasmosis is transmitted to the fetus across the placenta only when the organism is spread through the blood stream during *primary* maternal infection. Prior *Toxoplasma* infection appears to offer nearly complete protection against intrauterine infection.

Intrauterine infection may result in chorioretinitis, strabismus, blindness, hearing loss, microcephaly, hydrocephalus, nephrotic syndrome, bony defects, epilepsy, psychomotor disorders, severe learning disabilities, stillbirth, neonatal death, or asymptomatic infection. The occurrence of fetal infection is related directly to the time during the pregnancy that the first maternal infection occurs. First-trimester fetal infection occurs less frequently but is more likely to result in severe infection. In contrast, the risk of fetal infection increases with advancing gestational age. Approximately 65% of infants exposed in the third trimester will be infected; most will be symptom free. Disease may be progressive after birth. In one study, serious sequelae developed in 11 of 13 (85%) symptom-free newborns during an average of 8.3 years of follow-up

BOX 25-18 Methods for Prevention of Congenital Toxoplasmosis

Prevention of infection in pregnant women

The woman should take these precautions:

- Cook meat to ≥66° C, smoke it, or cure it in brine.
- Use frozen meats kept at –20° C for at least 24 hours. Home refrigerators may not achieve –20° C.
- Avoid touching mucous membranes of mouth and eyes while handling raw meat.
- Wash hands thoroughly after handling raw meat.
- Avoid eating uncooked eggs and unpasteurized milk.
- Wash fruits and vegetables before consumption.
- Prevent access of flies and cockroaches to fruits and vegetables.
- Avoid contact with materials that are potentially contaminated with cat feces (e.g., cat litter boxes, sand boxes, or garden).
- Wear gloves and wash hands for tasks if exposure to cat feces cannot be avoided.

Secondary prevention

- Serologic screening for toxoplasma antibodies in women during pregnancy is not currently recommended but may be selectively performed.
- If acute toxoplasma infection is a real possibility in pregnancy, expert advice should be sought to help to determine which, if any, tests should be ordered and what, if any, treatment should be considered.

(Sever, 1985). Damage consisted primarily of chorioretinitis (11 of 13), often with serious vision loss, mental retardation, and severe neurologic disability.

Diagnosis of toxoplasmosis is often problematic. Clinical signs and symptoms are not specific and often are attributed to influenza or mononucleosis. Methods of prevention are listed in Box 25-18.

TUBERCULOSIS

Tuberculosis is caused by *Mycobacterium tuberculosis,* or occasionally other types of mycobacterium. Tuberculosis primarily causes pulmonary disease but may disseminate to all organs of the body. Spread by tiny droplets, this airborne disease is dispersed evenly by air currents. Tuberculosis is most common among malnourished and socioeconomically deprived persons. Recent trends in immigration and international travel, with movement of infected persons to the United States from areas where tuberculosis is endemic, have increased the incidence of the infection in several cities and made it more common in all segments of society. Tuberculosis currently is seen as a presenting sign of AIDS.

Tuberculosis is transmitted by inhalation of respiratory droplets from persons with active pulmonary disease. The bacteria reproduce in the lung alveoli and cause an acute inflammatory response. During this acute infection—primary tuberculosis—microorganisms may spread to other organs of the body. Most bacteria are destroyed or encapsulated into *granulomas* by the host defense system. Granulomas may form in any tissue to which the organisms spread.

The infectious process may stop here, producing enough bacilli to cause an antigen-hypersensitivity response that triggers a reactive tuberculosis skin test. In these cases active disease is *not* present and the person is not infectious. Untreated but inactive tuberculosis infection may become activated at any time. In the event of lowered resistance or a high bacilli count, the infection may become widespread and cause symptoms of the disease. It is estimated that the infection progresses to disease in 5% to 10% of initially infected persons. Major risk factors are poverty, poor nutrition, HIV immunosuppression, alcoholism, diabetes, chronic lung diseases, and treatment with immunosuppressive drugs. Lowered resistance to tuberculosis occurs in late pregnancy and postpartum, in the newborn, and during puberty and adolescence (Summers, 1992).

Risk

Pregnant women are at risk for the development of two forms of tuberculosis: (1) primary infection with pneumonitis or much more commonly (2) reactivation of previously controlled primary infection. Newborns acquire tuberculosis by inhalation of infectious respiratory droplets from their mother, a household member, or hospital attendant after birth (Nemir and O'Hare, 1985). Because of incompletely understood factors, newborns and infants appear *especially susceptible* to tuberculosis. Intrauterine transmission of tuberculosis is rare but possible. If an infectious mother remains untreated, there is a 50% chance for her newborn to be infected within the neonatal period. Newborns and infants are at high risk for progressive dissemination, which frequently is fatal if inadequately treated (Nemir and O'Hare, 1985).

Neither tuberculosis nor antituberculosis treatment is an indication for pregnancy termination.

Signs

Often the only signs are typical changes seen on anteroposterior (AP) and lateral chest x-ray films. (Abdominal shielding during the x-ray process is important for both women and men.) Every positive tuberculosis skin test reaction is verified by a chest film. Sputum is sent for acid-fast stain. Sputum culture may be positive, but cultures take up to 6 weeks for reports. Little overt change may occur except for a chronic cough with sputum. Pleuritic chest pain sometimes is present.

Weight loss, anorexia, and fatigue plus night sweating may occur.

Because tuberculosis often is an asymptomatic infection, women obtaining prenatal care or appearing for a delivery without prenatal care should be screened for *M. tuberculosis* infection with the intradermal Mantoux test.* Women with a prior history of treated or healed tuberculosis need not be tested. After an initial infection, 1 to 3 months may pass before the Mantoux test shows a positive reaction. Prior BCG vaccination is not a contraindication to skin testing because Mantoux tests commonly show negative results or less than 10 mm; BCG vaccination is not considered effective when given after age 10. BCG vaccine is most commonly given in areas where tuberculosis is endemic. Use of Mantoux tests with purified protein derivative–standard (PPD-S) have been standardized and therefore are recommended over other techniques for skin testing. Pregnancy itself does not alter test reactivity. Women with a positive skin test reaction should receive a standard chest x-ray examination, with abdominal shielding. A false-negative reaction may occur in an immunocompromised client.

Clinical Management

Treatment is usually on an outpatient basis. Because treatment must be extended over 6 months to 1 year, compliance may be a problem. Drugs, used in combination, are shown in Box 25-19. For the wide spectrum of additional drugs used in resistant tuberculosis types, see CDC (Screening for TB, 1990). Tuberculosis has become a major problem in HIV immunosuppression. With resistant types there may be severe and rapidly progressive fatal cases. Health care personnel have been exposed and are susceptible to infection with these types. Currently, preventive therapy with isoniazid (INH) or a similar drug is recommended for persons in high-risk groups. The drug must be taken consistently; again, compliance can be a problem.

Each nurse is responsible for following respiratory isolation procedures when caring for clients at high risk and those with known tuberculosis cases (Table 25-4). Follow-up on those at high risk is important, because noncompliance in therapy is common.

---

*A 0.1 ml dose of freshly mixed and stabilized purified protein derivative (PPD) (Tween 80) containing 5 tuberculin units (TU) should be placed intradermally on the lower aspect of the forearm, and the skin test should be examined 48 to 72 hours later. The *diameter of test-site induration,* not erythema, is measured and is considered positive if greater than or equal to 10 mm. Induration of less than 5 mm is a negative test result. Induration between 5 and 9 mm may be caused by infection with atypical mycobacteria, prior bocillus Calmette-Guérin (BCG) vaccination, or recent tuberculosis exposure and infection.

BOX 25-19 Pharmacologic Treatment of Tuberculosis

- Isoniazid (INH), rifampin, and ethambutol for 2 months
- INH and rifampin for 4 to 7 months (total 9 months)
- If PPD reaction is positive but no disease is evident, INH alone may be used for 6 months
- Pregnant women may be treated with INH or ethambutol, but pyrazinamide is not recommended because of unknown teratogenic effect (Jacobs and Abernathy, 1988; Summers, 1992)
- For resistance to INH, ethambutol or newer drugs are used

VARICELLA-ZOSTER VIRUS

Varicella-zoster virus (VZV) is a member of the herpesvirus family, a group that includes cytomegalovirus, Epstein-Barr virus, and herpes simplex types 1 and 2. VZV is responsible for two infections: varicella (chickenpox) and herpes zoster (shingles).

Chickenpox

About 90% of the population in the United States is believed to have had chickenpox, a very contagious childhood disease. In tropical areas 20% to 50% of the infections occur in late adolescence or adulthood. Thus immigrants from those areas who have a negative antibody titer may be susceptible. Although uncommon in pregnancy, maternal chickenpox may lead to serious maternal illness, preterm labor, and transplacental viral transmission. Pneumonia is the most common complication of varicella among adults, with a significant mortality.

Risk

Although the incidence of varicella pneumonia complicating pregnancy is not known, pregnancy may place women at increased risk for pneumonia. Respiratory collapse and death have been noted. Intrauterine viral transmission causes varicella-zoster syndrome, neonatal varicella, or zoster in infancy (Felser and Freifeld, 1988). Exposure to VZV during the first trimester is associated with varicella-zoster syndrome, characterized by skin scarring, hypoplastic limbs, eye abnormalities, microcephaly, neurologic damage, and motor and growth retardation. Second- or third-trimester maternal varicella appears to be less often associated with birth defects (Paryani and Arvin, 1986). Onset of maternal infection less than 5 days before or 2 days after delivery places the newborn at increased risk of transplacentally acquired neonatal varicella (Felser and Freifeld, 1988). Neonatal varicella frequently is associated with compli-

TABLE 25-4   Isolation Precautions: Tuberculosis

TUBERCULOSIS STAGE	MATERNAL OR INFANT ISOLATION	INFANT INTERACTION	BREAST-FEEDING
Positive reaction to PPD; no evidence of current disease	None	Routine	Permitted
Mother with disease on treatment regimen for more than 2 weeks at delivery	None	Routine	Permitted if medication safe for breast-feeding
Mother with current pulmonary disease suspected to be contagious	Respiratory isolation	None until mother completes 2 weeks' treatment with appropriate medications or has two negative sputum tests OR Careful hand washing; neonatal chemoprophylaxis and maternal treatment with appropriate medications	Pump and bottle feed, reestablish in 2 weeks if medications do not contraindicate Permitted if medications do not contraindicate

cations, including pneumonia, which may be fatal in up to 30% of cases. Because of a protective effect of maternal antibodies that cross the placenta, neonatal varicella is less common when maternal infection occurs more than 5 days before delivery.

Signs

Vesicles begin on the head and neck and progress caudally. There is a period of fever, chills, and muscle aching. A dangerous complication is pneumonia in about 15% of adult cases. Pleuritic chest pains signal a worsening state. A person is infectious 2 days before vesicles appear until the time all vesicles have dried and are crusted over (Figure 25-8). Chickenpox is transmitted by droplet and from discharge from vesicles and mucous membranes (Box 25-20).

Clinical Management

Prevention includes checking immunity before pregnancy or at an early visit. Women exposed to preschool or school-age children are most at risk, along with health care workers. Exposure should be reported, and the nonimmunized woman should receive varicellazoster immunoglobulin (VZIG) within 96 hours of exposure. This injection, which is expensive, is available from the American Red Cross. A live, attenuated varicella vaccine is available in Europe and is undergoing clinical trials in the United States. Pregnant women with known immunity to varicella are considered protected against reinfection.

Management of chickenpox depends partially on the time in pregnancy it occurs. If severe symptoms occur,

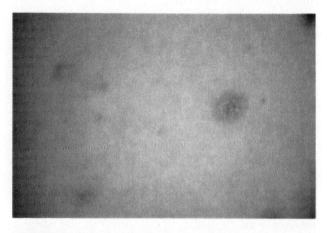

FIGURE 25-8 Chickenpox lesions usually occur in successive outbreaks, with several stages of maturity present at one time. The lesions start on the scalp and trunk and spread centrifugally to the extremities. (Courtesy Walter Tunnessen, MD, The Johns Hopkins University School of Medicine, Baltimore, Md; from Seidel HM et al: *Mosby's guide to physical examination,* ed 2, St Louis, 1991, Mosby.)

intravenously administered acyclovir is used. Prevention of preterm labor is important to allow time for maternal antibodies to be transferred to the fetus. If the infection occurs at the time of labor, the infant also is given VZIG. If maternal antibodies are present, not all infants develop the infection. Because signs of neonatal infection may be delayed for a week or 10 days after birth, careful monitoring of the newborn is required.

BOX 25-20 Isolation Precautions: Chickenpox

Mother

Strict isolation (gown, mask, gloves). Private room with special ventilation, preferably in area remote from immunocompromised clients or susceptible staff members until 7 days after onset of rash or all lesions crusted

No contact until newborn receives VZIG or mother out of isolation

Infant

None for the first 7 days after exposure; strict isolation (gown, mask, gloves) for subsequent 2 weeks; if mother contracted varicella less than 5 days before delivery or within 48 hours after delivery, VZIG is promptly administered to newborn

Breast-feeding

Facilitate as soon as all lesions have crusted. Early milk is pumped and possibly discarded (information unavailable to evaluate safety of giving milk to infant)

Health care workers should be aware of their immune status. If susceptible to varicella, they should avoid contact with infected persons and receive VZIG if exposure occurs (Croen, 1988). Nonimmune nurses should report exposure and should not work in maternity areas after exposure until it is clear they will not be affected. (See the isolation precautions for chickenpox in Box 25-20.)

Shingles

Shingles, also called *herpes zoster* or *zoster,* is a reactivation of latent VZV, which establishes a lifelong infection of sensory nerve ganglia (Croen, 1988).The pathophysiologic mechanisms that allow development of latent infection and that trigger reactivation are largely unknown.

Risk. Herpes zoster infection generally is considered to pose small risk to the unborn fetus. Because it is a recurrent infection, it is presumed that maternal antibodies provide protection for the fetus and greatly reduce the risk for congenital varicella-zoster syndrome. There are, however, a few reports of infant varicella-zoster after shingles during pregnancy.

Signs. A prodrome of fever, malaise, and headache may occur 1 to 4 days before eruption of typical skin lesions. Erythematous vesicular lesions appear in groups and

apparently follow dermatome lines. Lesions may last 2 to 3 weeks, but pain may persist for 2 to 3 weeks after the vesicles resolve. Shingles is especially serious in HIV-immunosuppressed clients in whom it may be severe and persist for long periods. Because the fluid from the vesicles contains infectious material, precautions should be followed.

VIRAL HEPATITIS

There are several types of hepatitis, or infection of the liver. *Hepatitis A virus (HAV)* has been called *infectious hepatitis* and *short-incubation hepatitis.* Transmission is mainly by fecal-oral contamination, and HAV also is passed through contaminated food, shellfish, and water. Its incubation period is approximately 3 to 7 weeks. The person does not have to contain a reservoir of virus to continue to be a *carrier* after symptoms are resolved. Infection often may be asymptomatic. When present, symptoms are mostly nonspecific. Vertical transmission may occur at birth from contamination of the newborn with fecal material.

Hepatitis C virus (HCV) was called non-A, non-B hepatitis and like hepatitis B is transferred through needle sharing and blood contamination. *Hepatitis D* is uncommon in this country.

Hepatitis B Virus

Serum hepatitis, long-incubation hepatitis, Australian-antigen positive hepatitis, or *hepatitis B virus (HBV)* is the most common cause of hepatitis worldwide. Hepatitis B is highly contagious when transmitted by direct contact with blood or bodily fluids from infected persons. The blood of an infected person or a carrier contains up to 1 million viral particles per milliliter, a much higher viral load than HIV infected blood. Approximately 1% of the general population in the United States are carriers. HBV also must be thought of as an STD because of increased risk with IV drug abuse (20%) and multiple heterosexual or homosexual partners. In addition, immigrants from endemic parts of the world have higher carrier rates: Indochina (14%) and Pacific Islanders and Alaskans (10%); Haiti, certain Caribbean areas, South America, and certain areas of Africa have high rates (CDC, 1987).

Risk

Pregnancy in previously healthy, well-nourished women does not appear to be adversely affected by hepatitis, nor is the course of the disease altered by pregnancy. However, in certain developing nations, pregnant women appear to be more susceptible to hepatitis and may have significant maternal complications, including severe disease and death, as well as perinatal morbidity and mortality.

Vertical Transmission

The onset of acute HBV infection during pregnancy may be associated with increases in spontaneous abortion during the first trimester and premature labor in later months. The primary concern during pregnancy of HBV infection or carrier state is of **vertical transmission** to the newborn at the time of birth. If the pathogen has not passed through the placenta during fetal life (5% to 10%), the infant has a 70% to 90% chance of becoming infected at the time of birth because of the high viral load in maternal blood and secretions. Neonates also may become infected through breast milk or maternal contact after birth. Newborns infected with HBV at birth are less able to clear the virus and more frequently become chronic carriers of HBV. Being a chronic carrier is now linked with a much higher risk of *future liver cancer* and *cirrhosis;* therefore immunization of all children is now being implemented in the United States (Keene and Frank-Stromberg, 1991).

Hepatitis is so infectious that the rate of health care worker infection after needle stick or contamination has been 7% to 30% in contrast with the HIV rate of 0.2% to 0.5%. This translates to 12,000 cases per year among such workers. Of these, 6% to 10% cannot clear the virus after the acute phase and become carriers themselves with the potential long-term effects of liver cancer. Spouses and sexual partners of these health care workers also have a higher rate of infection (Ginsberg, 1991). For this reason, mandatory vaccination is required now and is available, free of charge, in three injections: initial injection, 30 days later, and 6 months later. When there is universal vaccination of health care workers and all children, transmission rates should drop dramatically.

Signs

Hepatitis may range from a mild flulike episode to a fulminating, lethal infection. Low-grade signs are malaise, fever, headache, enlarged liver, dark urine and light stools, and jaundice of varying degrees. In addition, severe hepatitis manifests markedly altered liver enzyme levels, anorexia, and epigastric pain and can progress to liver coma and death. Carriers show no signs.

Clinical Management

Once active HAV disease has begun, supportive care is important with nutrition, analgesics tolerated by the liver, and fluids. Infection may be rendered less acute by immune globulin.

Clinical infection with HAV may be prevented by administration of **immune globulin** within 2 weeks of exposure. Pregnant women who are exposed to HAV in the following settings should receive passive immunization:

1. Household contact with infected person
2. Children in diapers who attend day-care settings with HAV outbreaks
3. Employee with close contact to infected person (e.g., health care or day-care worker)
4. Travel or residence in area with poor sanitation

Passive immunization of infants at risk for vertical transmission may prevent newborn HAV infection (see Box 25-21 for isolation precautions for hepatitis).

There are no specific treatments for hepatitis B. Clients are managed clinically in the same way as those with hepatitis A. Passive immunization with intramuscularly administered hepatitis B immune globulin (HBIG) within 7 days of exposure, followed by a second injection of HBIG given 30 days after the first, may prevent or lessen HBV infection in exposed persons (Box 25-22). Currently all pregnant women receiving prenatal care are screened early and treated with HBIG if positive. Women at high risk are retested, and those women who enter the labor area without prenatal care should be tested and receive immunoglobulin before the results are returned. There is the same problem with hepatitis antibody screening as with other types of screening—the period when antibodies are not present. Only 2 to 4 weeks after an acute infection may antihepatitis antibodies be found.

In addition, as referred to in HIV care, the newborn must be guarded against inoculation with large amounts of virus by implementing "baby universal precautions," which include cleansing skin of maternal secretions as soon as is possible and not puncturing newborn skin until the skin surface is clean (Ross and Dickason, 1992).

BOX 25-21 Isolation Precautions: Hepatitis

Mother

Universal precautions: blood and enteric precautions for B and C, enteric for A

Careful handwashing; avoid newborn contact with blood, blood products or lochia; gown and gloves when handling infant

Infant

Universal precautions; blood and enteric precautions; isolation with mother; passive and active immunization for hepatitis B required

Breast-feeding

Hepatitis A: permitted; stress good hand washing
Hepatitis B: passive and active immunization for the neonate is required before initiating breast-feeding
Hepatitis C: permitted; no information available on risk of transmission to newborn

BOX 25-22   Recommendations for Hepatitis B Virus Vaccination*

Preexposure

Vaccination recommended for:

- Health-care workers with blood or needle-stick exposures
- Clients and staff of institutions for the developmentally disabled
- Hemodialysis clients
- Homosexually active men
- Users of illicit injectable drugs
- Recipients of certain blood products
- Household members and sexual contacts of HBV carriers
- Special high-risk populations: Alaskan Eskimos, Southeast Asians, native Pacific Islanders, immigrants and refugees from endemic areas
- Inmates of long-term correctional facilities
- Heterosexually active persons with multiple sexual partners
- International travelers to HBV endemic areas
- Children

Postexposure

Vaccine required for:

- Infants born to HBV-positive mothers
- Health-care workers having needle-stick exposures to human blood who have not been vaccinated

*Detailed information on recommendations for hepatitis B vaccination is available (CDC, 1991).

Passive immunization of the infant with HBIG promptly after delivery (preferably within 8 hours of birth) appears to be effective in preventing acquisition of HBV at birth. *Active vaccination with HBV vaccine*, given within the first week of life and at 1 and 6 months, provides additional protection against **horizontal transmission** from mother to infant during the postpartum period and childhood.

HBV infection may be transmitted through breast-feeding. After passive and active immunization of the newborn, breast-feeding is acceptable. Temporary discontinuation of breast-feeding is recommended, even for immunized newborns, if nipple cracking or bleeding develops. This will prevent further inoculation of the newborn with maternal serum. Mothers should be instructed to wash hands carefully before handling the infant and to avoid infant contact with lochia or soiled linen (Box 25-22).

Perinatal transmission of HBV may be largely prevented by maternal prenatal screening, immunization of the infant in the hospital, and follow-up care to complete infant immunization.

Nursing Responsibilities

Each nurse is responsible for being vaccinated against HBV. Because maternity care is a high-risk area, the nurse must follow universal precautions for each person for whom she gives care. Follow-through with previously unregistered clients is important so that immunoglobulin is not forgotten.

Test Yourself

- What are the fetal risks for Jane, who was exposed at 14 weeks to rubella?
- What are the fetal risks for Sue, who has contracted chickenpox at 35 weeks?
- What are the risks of toxoplasmosis for Ann, who has always had a cat in the house?
- Does active pulmonary tuberculosis carry risks for the fetus? What are the risks for the newborn?
- Why is hepatitis B so much more infectious than other viral diseases?

UTERINE INFECTIONS

Clinical infections may be linked to events associated with labor and delivery or may be the result of stresses on the maternal defense mechanisms caused by pregnancy. Clinically evident antepartum or intrapartum intrauterine infection may be called *amnionitis, chorioamnionitis, intramniotic infection,* or *amniotic fluid infection*. The uterine cavity usually is sterile before labor and rupture of membranes. The cervical mucous plug and chorioamniotic membrane usually serve as efficient barriers to infection. Even after rupture of membranes, intrauterine infection is infrequent because of the combined efforts of polymorphonuclear leukocytes, nonspecific biochemical host defense mechanisms, immunoglobulins, and other, as yet unknown, antibacterial properties of the amniotic fluid.

Chorioamnionitis is a polymicrobial infection, generally associated with aerobic and anaerobic bacteria normally found in the vagina and cervix. Other microorganisms, including *Listeria monocytogenes, Neisseria gonorrhoeae*, group B streptococcus, and *Escherichia coli* also are associated. Bacteria may gain entrance to the uterus by ascent from the vagina and cervix before labor and rupture of membranes; however, the risk of bacterial ascent increases after rupture of membranes and even labor. Infection also may occur from maternal infection spread across the placenta or by means of amniocentesis. In addition, obstetric practices may induce chorioamnionitis by ascending infection (see Figure 25-1). These practices include cervical circlage, frequent cervical examinations, and intrauterine fetal monitoring.

Risk

The risk of infection increases 10 to 20 times when there are ruptured membranes, and women may experience a long labor and an increase in cesarean delivery. Preterm infants of mothers who had chorioamnionitis suffer increased incidence of pneumonia, meningitis, septicemia, respiratory distress syndrome (RDS), and perinatal death compared with infants of similar gestational ages without exposure to chorioamnionitis.

Signs

The initial signs of chorioamnionitis often are fetal tachycardia that occurs *before* maternal tachycardia and fever with irritability of the uterus. Uterine tenderness or foul odor of amniotic fluid may not be apparent until late in the infectious process.

Clinical Management

Maternal and fetal complications from chorioamnionitis may be minimized if antibiotic treatment is initiated early.

If the membranes are intact, samples of amniotic fluid may be obtained by amniocentesis to be cultured and examined microscopically for bacteria and leukocytes. Bacteria may gain entrance to the uterus during labor, *even with intact membranes,* and the recovery of bacteria is not always associated with clinical evidence of infection. The peripheral white blood cell count increases during labor normally, but counts greater than 18,000/mm^3 frequently are viewed as suggestive of chorioamnionitis.

Administration of combined antibiotics to cover most of the pathogenic bacteria frequently associated with this infection has been shown to reduce the incidence of neonatal sepsis. Delivery is usually expedited, by cesarean if necessary, to avoid prolonged intrauterine exposure to infection and significant neonatal morbidity or mortality. Others consider that maternal postpartum infectious complications, prolonged antibiotic requirements, and prolonged hospitalizations are more likely when a cesarean delivery is performed (Hauth et al, 1985).

Nursing Responsibilities

The nurse frequently is the care provider who identifies the first evidence of chorioamnionitis. Nurses provide most of the intrapartum care, are aware of the woman's risk factors for infection, and are responsible for monitoring maternal vital signs, fluid intake and output,

comfort level, fetal status, and frequently progress in labor. When signs occur, eliminate other sources of altered vital signs; for example, ensure adequate hydration, relieve maternal anxiety, and provide pain relief and proper positioning to ensure adequate fetal oxygenation. When evidence of chorioamnionitis is detected, the care provider managing the woman's labor should be notified of the altered maternal and fetal response, the nursing actions that were taken, and the response. After the diagnosis of chorioamnionitis has been made, promptly initiate any antimicrobial therapy ordered, maintain close monitoring of maternal and fetal status for the remainder of labor, and ensure that the mother and family have received full explanations about the nature of the infection, likely causes, risks for herself and infant, and treatments and expected outcomes. The labor nurses must be alert for the signs of infection—fetal tachycardia, changed beat-to-beat variability, and maternal fever (see Clinical Decision).

STREPTOCOCCAL INFECTIONS

Streptococcal infection may be associated with maternal endometritis, postcesarean endometritis, bacteremia, chorioamnionitis, neonatal sepsis, pneumonia, meningitis, premature rupture of membranes (PROM), preterm birth, and neonatal death.

Streptococcal microorganisms are cocci or spherical bacteria that appear as chains on microscopic examination. Streptococci are categorized by their ability to break down or hemolyze blood in appropriate agar culture media. Of the different streptococci, only groups A, B, and D are associated with significant human illness. Groups A and B are nearly always β-hemolytic, and group D streptococcus varies in ability to hemolyze blood agar.

Group A β-hemolytic streptococcus causes streptococcal sore throat, scarlet fever, rheumatic fever, skin infection, impetigo, erysipelas, and puerperal sepsis. Although it is an infrequent cause of postpartum infection today, the classic works of Holmes and Semmelweis, which describe the epidemic of childbed fever, demonstrate the seriousness of group A streptococcal infection among pregnant women. Over the past 30 years, group B streptococcus has emerged as the leading cause of newborn sepsis and meningitis and also is associated with significant maternal and fetal infection. Group D streptococci cause maternal urinary tract infections and may be associated with neonatal sepsis and maternal postpartum endometritis.

Group B Streptococcal Infection

Among pregnant women, *group B streptococcus* causes urinary tract infection, asymptomatic bacteriuria, amniotic fluid infection, postpartum and postcesarean en-

Clinical Decision

The mother has been in labor for 16 hours with ruptured membranes. She has reached 8 cm dilation and +1 station. Her temperature began to rise an hour ago and now is 100.2° F. You see on the accompanying strip chart the reading in (A). Describe it as you would on a nursing note. Now look at (B), the reading taken 30 minutes later when her temperature was 101° F. What interventions should be happening now?

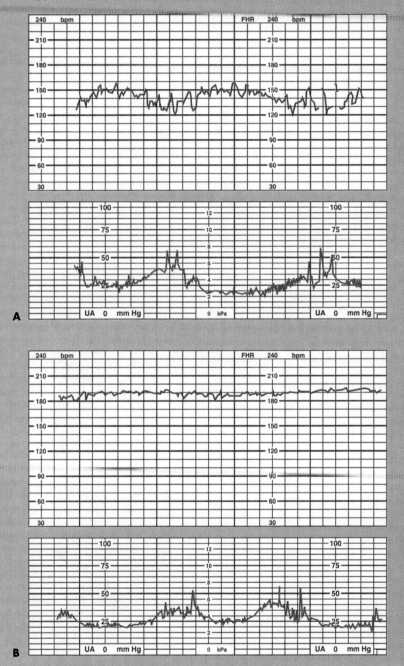

dometritis, bacteremia, and puerperal sepsis. Among newborns, group B streptococcus is one of two common causes of septicemia and meningitis, often leading to severe neurologic impairment and death.

Group B streptococcus may be isolated from the lower genital tract of 3% to 40% of pregnant women. Women colonized with it are symptom free. More women are found to carry it if the rectum and perineum are sampled than if only the cervix is sampled. The bacteria are thought to spread from the intestinal tract reservoir to the perineum, vagina, and cervix. From 40% to 72% of newborns exposed to group B streptococcus–colonized mothers will become colonized with the cocci (Greenspoon, Wilcox, and Kirschbaum, 1991). Most of these infants remain symptom free, with clinical infection developing in somewhat less than 1 in 200 exposed infants. When antepartum antibiotic treatment is used, the rate in the newborn is very low.

Risk. Prolonged rupture of membranes (more than 12 hours), prolonged labor, intrapartum maternal infection, postpartum infection, and preterm delivery are associated with increased likelihood of *early onset* of the disease.

Neonatal risk. Women with heavy vaginal or cervical colonization of group B streptococcus appear to be at highest risk of transmitting the bacteria to their infants. Early-onset disease occurs more frequently among preterm or low-birth-weight infants. Early-onset group B streptococcal disease is associated with rapid deterioration of the newborn, often leading to death or severe neurologic damage in up to 55% of infants, even when appropriate antibiotics are given. Community acquisition from siblings or other contacts may be another source of late onset infection.

Late onset. Group B hemolytic infection may appear after the immediate newborn period and up to 4 months following birth. Signs are irritability, poor appetite, fever, conjunctivitis, and ear infections progressing to potentially severe neurologic involvement.

Clinical management. It is currently recommended that every pregnant woman be screened at 32 to 36 weeks for group B β-hemolytic streptococcus infection. Antepartum cultures that identify her as a carrier can partially predict colonization at birth. The infection is unpredictable and may be present at one visit but not at the next (Greenspoon, Wilcox, and Kirschbaum, 1991).

Whenever there is a risk of preterm labor, PROM of more than 12 hours, or intrapartum fever, group B must be considered. Because of the devastating newborn effects, most units now do a "rapid" test (which takes 4 to 5 hours) to determine if infection is present in high-risk clients at the start of labor. This test also must be performed whenever fever develops, and antibiotics must be started before results are returned:

- Ampicillin 2 g intravenous piggyback (IVPB), then 1 g q6h
- Sometimes gentamicin 80 mg q8h IVPB is added

Postpartum Infections

Infection during the postpartum period may occur in the genital tract (endometritis or vaginitis), urinary tract, breasts, episiotomy or wound, or as complications of anesthesia (pneumonia). Approximately 1% to 8% of women have postpartum infection (Sweet and Gibbs, 1985). Although in the United States maternal death because of pregnancy is infrequent, sepsis remains a leading cause of maternal mortality. Maternal sepsis may occur after abortions, vaginal births, or cesarean births. Clients must be adequately counseled about their risk of infection and taught to recognize signs and symptoms and seek medical attention promptly if they occur. Health care providers must be taught to thoroughly evaluate symptoms and provide adequate therapy and follow-up care.

ENDOMETRITIS

Intrauterine infection is the most common infection in the postpartum period. Uterine infection frequently involves the endometrium first and may spread to the myometrium, parametrium, fallopian tubes, ovaries, pelvic peritoneum, and the blood. Thus intrauterine infection may lead to pelvic abscess, septic pelvic thrombophlebitis, or septicemia.

Postpartum endometritis is associated most commonly with a mixture of bacterial species that may arise from the gastrointestinal tract (group D streptococcus, *E. coli,* or *Klebsiella*) or from the lower genital tract (aerobic and anaerobic bacteria, group B streptococcus, *C. trachomatis,* and *N. gonorrhoeae*).

Risk

Endometritis develops in approximately 1% of women who give birth vaginally. In contrast, the incidence of infection is between 12% and 15% after cesarean delivery (Sweet and Gibbs, 1985). For women who require cesarean birth, the current practice of perioperative prophylactic antibiotics if risk factors for infection are present has greatly reduced the incidence of postpartum endometritis.

Factors that influence the risk for developing endometritis are included in Box 25-23. Low socioeconomic status, lack of prenatal care, and anemia are not causes of postpartum infection. Rather, these factors are markers for those women at risk. Susceptibility to infection among these women may involve overall nu-

BOX 25-23   Risk Indicators and Risk Factors for Postpartum Endometritis

Epidemiologic factors
- Low socioeconomic status
- Young age

Individual factors
- Anemia
- Obesity
- Systemic illness

Obstetric factors
- Method of delivery
- Risk of infection after spontaneous vaginal, instrumental, or operative birth
- Duration of labor
- Duration of ruptured fetal membranes
- Number of vaginal examinations
- Internal fetal monitoring
- Meconium-stained fluid
- Failure to progress to labor
- Hemorrhage
- Retained placental or membrane fragments

Operative factors
- Cesarean delivery
- Urgency of procedure
- General anesthesia
- Duration of surgery
- Postpartum anemia
- Manual removal of placenta

tritional status, hygienic factors, differences in host defense mechanisms and cervical/vaginal microorganisms, and unknown factors.

Signs

Identification of postpartum endometritis is not clearcut. The diagnosis usually is based on the presence of the client's complaints of malaise, fever, chills, temperature greater than 100.4° F, tachycardia, abdominal pain, uterine and adnexal tenderness, and sometimes purulent or foul-smelling discharge. However, up to a third to half of women with clinical evidence of infection are afebrile and asymptomatic. Abdominal pain frequently is minimal and difficult to distinguish from the normal discomfort of postpartum uterine contractions. Vaginal discharge is not always foul smelling. Other sources of infection, including urinary tract infection, wound infection, episiotomy infection, mastitis, and intravenous site phlebitis, should be evaluated in postpartum women.

Clinical Management

Antibiotic therapy with a penicillin plus an aminoglycoside usually is initiated and is an effective combination for 95% of women. Lack of clinical improvement within 48 hours requires reevaluation for other sources of infection and addition of antibiotics to cover presumed anaerobic infection. Failure to respond clinically to aggressive intravenously administered antibiotics may be caused by pelvic abscess, septic pelvic thrombophlebitis, another site of infection, or a noninfectious source of fever, including drug reaction.

Nursing Responsibilities

Nursing care for women with postpartum endometritis includes maintaining adequate hydration, monitoring intravenous fluids, administering a combination of parenteral antibiotics, providing analgesia, and monitoring physical response to therapy and psychologic adaptation to complications. Full explanations of cause of infection and expected care should be given. Contact with and care for the infant are encouraged as maternal condition allows. Normal postpartum and newborn teaching should be included in the client's care as her condition improves.

Breast-feeding usually is not contraindicated. Maternal medications will be transmitted through breast milk to the nursing infant. Observation of the infant for evidence of medication intolerance is required. If breast-feeding is interrupted during therapy, breasts should be emptied by other means to maintain the milk supply (see Appendix 4).

SEPTIC PELVIC THROMBOPHLEBITIS

Women with postcesarean endometritis are at increased risk for septic pelvic thrombophlebitis. Septic pelvic thrombophlebitis is the formation of clots within the pelvic veins because of infection. Although rare, pelvic vein thrombophlebitis occurs more frequently after obstetric procedures than other types of pelvic surgery or with pelvic inflammatory disease.

Risk

Pelvic vein thrombosis develops in approximately 1 of 2000 women who give birth. Women with septic pelvic thrombophlebitis are at risk for further complications, which include septic embolus, lung abscess, empyema, and acute endocarditis (Duff and Gibbs, 1983).

Alterations in the walls of pelvic vessels may cause a predisposition to thrombophlebitis. Ovarian veins become dilated during gestation; blood flow through these veins declines sharply after delivery, increasing the likelihood of venous stasis. Vascular trauma or direct inoculation of bacteria into the vessels during surgery may occur. Inflammation in response to bacterial infection may cause further blood vessel damage and facilitates thrombosis formation. These vascular changes and compression from the uterus may further contribute to venous stasis and thrombophlebitis (Duff and Gibbs, 1983). Bacterial species implicated in this disease are common vaginal pathogens, including aerobic and anaerobic streptococci, staphylococci, *Bacteroides* species, and yeast.

Signs

Pelvic vein thrombophlebitis should be suspected in any client who is receiving appropriate broad-spectrum antibiotic treatment for postpartum intrauterine infection and whose symptoms *are not resolving*. Septic pelvic thrombophlebitis most often occurs within 1 day to 6 weeks after birth. The medical diagnosis is based largely on the client's clinical history and physical examination. The woman continues to have temperature elevations and worsening, constant, localized abdominal pain even on an appropriate antibiotic regimen. She may appear acutely ill with fever, shaking chills, tachycardia, nausea, vomiting, and tachypnea, or she may have improved clinical signs of infection except that temperature elevations continue, often as high as 103° to 104° F (Duff and Gibbs, 1983).

Clinical Management

Medical treatment includes use of broad-spectrum antibiotics and anticoagulation therapy with intravenously administered heparin. Temperature usually is normal within 24 to 48 hours of therapeutic heparin. Heparin generally is continued for 7 to 10 days afterward. Surgery may be required if the client remains critically ill in spite of adequate antimicrobial and anticoagulation therapies. Surgery may include ovarian vein ligation, vena caval ligation, or hysterectomy and salpingo-oophorectomy, depending on the presence of abscesses (Duff and Gibbs, 1983).

Nursing Responsibilities

Nursing care for women with septic pelvic thrombophlebitis includes providing information concerning the nature of the condition, potential for further complications, medical therapy, and potential side effects. Gathering laboratory test specimens and results and close monitoring of physical status and medical therapy of these acutely ill clients are essential nursing functions. In addition, maternal infant interaction and breast-feeding should be promoted. Normal postpartum and newborn teaching should be included in the client's care as her condition allows. Breast-feeding is not contraindicated in either heparin or warfarin anticoagulation therapy. Because warfarin is tightly bound to plasma proteins, it does not cross the lipid barrier into milk, and heparin is a large molecule that also does not cross the lipid barrier to enter breast milk.

KEY POINTS

- Defense systems are altered by pregnancy, making both mother and newborn more vulnerable to infection.
- Certain infections during pregnancy pose a special risk of fetal malformation, congenital infection, intrauterine growth retardation (IUGR), or death.
- Vertical transmission during fetal life depends on the size of the microorganism, the actual number (count), and the placental integrity.
- Vertical transmission during the birth process has been documented especially for human immunodeficiency virus (HIV), hepatitis B virus (HBV), herpes simplex virus (HSV), and chlamydial and gonorrheal infection.
- Universal precautions are key to reducing the risk of horizontal transmission during care.

- Nurses are responsible for consistent use of universal precautions and for insisting that other health care workers also do so.
- Education is essential to reduce the risk of sexually transmitted disease (STD).
- Hand washing is the best line of defense in protecting mother, infant, and oneself from nosocomial infection.
- Perinatal infections may be prevented in some instances by immunization before pregnancy.
- All health care workers and currently all children in the United States should be vaccinated against hepatitis B virus infection.
- Endometritis poses a risk to mother and infant because of the rapid rate of ascending infection in the birth canal. Especially dangerous are cytomegalovirus (CMV) and beta-streptococcal infections.

STUDY QUESTIONS

25-1 Select the appropriate terms for the following statements.
   a. The humoral response includes production of specific *antibodies* to microorganisms.
   b. The cell-mediated immune response stimulates multiplication of *Macrophages* and lymphocytes.
   c. A toxin may be a _____ antigen or an _____ antigen called a *toxoid*.
   d. *Herpes virus*, a perinatal infection, establishes a lifelong infection of the sensory nerve ganglia.
   e. HBV infection be prevented in the newborn by *Vaccination*
   f. Infection of the newborn at the time of birth by a staff member is an example of *Horizontal Transmission*

25-2 An infant was born with congenital rubella after the mother acquired the infection at week 30 of pregnancy. This route of infection describes:
   a. Nosocomial infection
   b. Autoinfection
   c. Vertical transmission
   d. Placental insufficiency

25-3 Untreated, gonorrhea may be linked to neonatal gonococcal ophthalmia and maternal:
   a. Bladder infections
   b. Pruritic rashes
   c. Painless chancres
   d. Postpartum endometritis

25-4 If chlamydial infection is diagnosed at 28 weeks, the most important reason that Rhonda should be treated now is to prevent:
   a. PROM
   b. Sexual transmission to her boyfriend
   c. Infant blindness
   d. Maternal sepsis

25-5 Rose, 23, has had multiple sexual partners and at 14 weeks' gestation has a positive FTA-ABS test result. She will be treated with penicillin. Therefore you must include instructions to report which of the following signs of Jarisch Herxheimer reaction:
   a. Hypotension and cyanosis
   b. Increase in fetal movements
   c. Onset of uterine contractions, high fever
   d. Maternal bradycardia and anxiety

25-6 You will teach Rose that her condition will be followed with the VDRL titer instead of the FTA-ABS test at 3, 6, 9, and 12 months because the FTA-ABS test:
   a. Results are altered by penicillin.
   b. Reaction remains positive even after treatment.
   c. Is expensive.
   d. May alter the results of other diseases.

25-7 Why is isolation of the infant from the mother not practiced for most perinatally acquired infections?
   a. The infant's immunologic response is immature.
   b. Maternal antibodies protect the infant.
   c. The infant already has received pathogens in most cases.
   d. Breast-feeding conveys immunities.

25-8 Which sign or symptom would not occur if a woman in labor has chorioamnionitis?
   a. Fetal tachycardia
   b. Prolonged, more difficult labor
   c. Decrease in blood pressure
   d. Increase in white blood cell count

Answer Key

25-1 a. Antibodies, b. Macrophages, c. Pathogenic, altered, d. Herpesvirus, e. Vaccination, f. Horizontal transmission 25-2 c 25-3 d 25-4 a 25-5 c 25-6 b 25-7 c 25-8 c

REFERENCES

Abrams RS, Wexler P, editors: *Medical care of the pregnant patient,* Boston, 1983, Little, Brown.

Acosta YM et al: HIV disease and pregnancy. II. Antepartum and intrapartum care, *JOGNN* 21(2):97, 1992.

American College of Obstetricians and Gynecologists: Genital human papilloma virus infections, *ACOG Technical Bulletin* 105, June 1987.

American College of Obstetricians and Gynecologists: Perinatal herpes simplex virus infections, *ACOG Technical Bulletin* 122, Nov 1988.

Baker DA et al: Topical podofilox for the treatment of condylomata acuminata in women, *Obstet Gynecol* 76:656, 1990.

Brookman RR: Immunization during the adolescent years, *Adolesc Med* 14:25, 1987.

CDC: *Chlamydia trachomatis* infections: policy guidelines for preventions and control, *MMWR* (suppl) 34:53S, 1985.

CDC: Mumps—United States 1984-1985, *MMWR* 35:216, 1986.

CDC: Update on hepatitis B prevention, *MMWR* 36:353, 1987.

CDC: Update: universal precautions for prevention of transmission of human immunodeficiency virus, hepatitis B virus, and other blood-borne pathogens in health-care settings, *MMWR* 37:377, 1988.

CDC: Sexually transmitted disease treatment guidelines, *MMWR* 38 (suppl 8):L2, 1989.

CDC: AIDS in women—United States, *MMWR* 39:845, 1990.

CDC: Screening for tuberculosis and tuberculous infection in high-risk populations, and the use of preventive therapy for tuberculous infection in the United States: recommendations of the Advisory

Committee for the Elimination of Tuberculosis, *MMWR* 39(RR-8): 1, 1990.

CDC; Immunization Practices Committee: Hepatitis B virus: a comprehensive strategy for eliminating transmission in the US through universal childhood vaccination, *MMWR* 40:1, 1991.

Cavenee MR et al: Treatment of gonorrhea in pregnancy, *Obstet Gynecol* 81:33, 1993.

Chow AW, Jewesson PJ: Pharmacokinetics and safety of antimicrobials during pregnancy, *Rev Infect Dis* 7:287, 1985.

Conner E, Bardeguez A, Apuzzio J: The intrapartum management of the HIV-infected mother and her infant, *Clin Perinatol* 16:899, 1989.

Crane MJ: The diagnosis and management of maternal and congenital syphilis, *J Nurse Midwife* 37(1):4, 1992.

Croen KD: Latency and the consequences of reactivation of the varicella-zoster virus. In Straus SE, moderator: Varicella-zoster virus infections: biology, natural history, treatment, and prevention, *Ann Intern Med* 108:221, 1988.

Desenclos, J-CA: Gonococcal infection of the newborn in Florida, 1984-1989, *Sex Transm Dis* 19:105, 1992.

Dorfman DH, Glaser J: Congenital syphilis presenting in infants after the newborn period, *N Engl J Med* 323:1299, 1990.

Duff P, Gibbs RS: Pelvic vein thrombophlebitis: diagnostic dilemma and therapeutic challenge, *Obstet Gynecol* 38:365, 1983.

Duff P, Sanders R, Gibbs RS: The course of labor in term patients with chorioamnionitis, *Am J Obstet Gynecol* 147:391, 1983.

Duffy J: Lyme disease, *Infect Dis Clin North Am* 1:511, 1987.

Felser JM, Freifeld A: The epidemiology, natural history and complications of varicella. In Straus SE, moderator: Varicella-zoster virus infections: biology, natural history, treatment, and prevention, *Ann Intern Med* 108:221, 1988.

Fowler KB et al: The outcome of congenital cytomegalovirus infection in relation to maternal antibody status, *N Engl J Med* 326:663, 1992.

Freij BJ, Sever JL: Toxoplasmosis, *Pediatr Rev* 12(8):227, 1991.

Gerberding JL: Risks to health care workers from occupational exposure to hepatitis B virus, human immunodeficiency virus, and cytomegalovirus, *Infect Dis Clin North Am* 3:735, 1989.

Ginsberg HM: Occupational exposure to bloodborne pathogens: the new OSHA regulation, *Pediatr AIDS/HIV Infect: Fetus Adolesc* 2(1):31, 1991.

Greenspoon JS, Wilcox JG, Kirschbaum TH: Group B streptococcus, the effectiveness of screening and chemoprophylaxis, *Obstet Gynecol Surv* 46:499, 1991.

Handsfield HH et al: Criteria for selective screening for *Chlamydia trachomatis* infection in women attending family planning clinics, *JAMA* 255:1730, 1986.

Hauth JC et al: Term maternal and neonatal complications of acute chorioamnionitis, *Obstet Gynecol* 66:59, 1985.

Hellberg D et al: Smoking and cervical neoplasia, *Am J Obstet Gynecol* 158:910, 1988.

Holmes KK et al, eds: *Sexually transmitted diseases,* ed 2, New York, 1989, McGraw-Hill.

International Registry of HIV-exposed twins, and others: High risk of HIV-1 infection for first-born twins, *Lancet* 338:1471, 1991.

Jacobs RF, Abernathy RS: Management of tuberculosis in pregnancy and the newborn, *Clin Perinatol* 15:305, 1988.

Keen DM, Frank-Stromborg M: A worldwide perspective on the epidemiology and primary prevention of liver cancer, *Cancer Nurs* 14(4):163, 1991.

Kelley KF, Galbraith MA, Vermund SH: Genital human papillomavirus infection in women, *JOGNN* 21(6):503, 1992.

Livengood CH, Thomason JL, Hill GB: Bacterial vaginosis: treatment with topical intravaginal clindamycin phosphate, *Obstet Gynecol* 76(1):118, 1990.

Lo B, Steinbrook R: Health care workers infected with the human immunodeficiency virus; the next steps, *JAMA* 267:1100, 1992.

Mann JM et al: Assessing risks of rubella infection during pregnancy; a standardized approach, *JAMA* 245:1647, 1981.

Marecki MA: Chlamydia trachomatis: a developing perinatal problem, *J Perinat Neonat Nurs* 1(4):1, 1988.

McGregor JA, French JI, Spencer NO: Prevention of sexually transmitted diseases in women, *J Reprod Med* 33(1suppl):109, 1988.

Morrison JC et al: Universal precautions in an obstetric population to prevent health care provider infection with human immunodeficiency virus, *Pediatr AIDS/HIV Infect: Fetus Adolesc* 2(4):161, 1991.

Nemir RL, O'Hare D: Congenital tuberculosis: review and diagnosis guidelines, *Am J Dis Child* 139:284, 1985.

O'Donnell LJ, Emmett PM, Heaton KW: Use of acyclovir to treat chicken pox in pregnancy, *Br Med J* 296:6, 1988.

Paryani SG, Arvin AM: Intrauterine infections with varicella-zoster virus after maternal varicella, *N Engl J Med* 314:1542, 1986.

Patsner B: A patient-applied topical solution for genital warts, *Contemp OB/GYN* 12:27, 1991.

Pearlman MD, McNeeley SG: A review of the microbiology, immunology and clinical implications of *Chlamydia trachomatis* infections, *Obstet Gynecol Surv* 47(7):448, 1992.

Rosenberg MJ, Phillips RS: Does douching promote ascending infection? *J Reprod Med* 37(11):930, 1992.

Ross PW: Group B streptococcus: profile of an organism, *J Med Microbiol* 18:139, 1984.

Ross T, Dickason EJ: Nursing alert: vertical transmission of HIV and HBV, *MCN* 17(4):192, 1992.

Samson LF: Perinatal viral infections and neonates, *J Perinat Neonat Nurs* 1(4):56, 1988.

Schacter J et al: Prospective study of perinatal transmission of *Chlamydia trachomatis,* *JAMA* 255:3374, 1986.

Serrano C et al: Surgical glove perforation in obstetrics, *Obstet Gynecol* 77(4):525, 1990.

Sever JL: TORCH tests and what they mean, *Am J Obstet Gynecol* 152(5):495, 1985.

Sperling RS, Stratton P, and Working Group of AIDS Clinical Trials Group, National Institute of Allergy and Infectious Diseases: Treatment options for human immunodeficiency virus–infected women, *Obstet Gynecol* 79(3):443, 1992.

Stear L, Elinger S: Understanding acquired immunodeficiency syndrome: implications for pregnancy, *J Perinat Neonat Nurs* 1(4):33, 1988.

Steere AC: Lyme disease, *N Engl J Med* 321:586, 1989.

Summers L: Understanding tuberculosis: implications for pregnancy, *J Perinatol Neonatal Nurs* 6(2):12, 1992.

Sweet RL, Gibbs RS, editors: *Infectious diseases of the female genital tract,* ed 2, Baltimore, 1985, Williams & Wilkins.

Thaler MM et al: Vertical transmission of hepatitis C virus, *Lancet* 338:17, 1991.

Thomsen AC, Morup L, Brogaard-Hansen K: Antibiotic elimination of group B streptococci in urine in prevention of preterm labour, *Lancet* 1:591, 1987.

Tillman J: Syphilis: an old disease, a contemporary perinatal problem, *JOGNN* 21(3):209, 1991.

Tinkle M: Genital human papillomavirus infection: a growing health risk, *JOGNN* 19(6):501, 1990.

Tookey P, Peckman CS: Does cytomegalovirus present an occupational risk? *Arch Dis Child* 66:1009, 1991.

Wendel GD Jr et al: Penicillin allergy and desensitization in serious infections during pregnancy, *N Engl J Med* 312(19):1229, 1985.

Wolner-Hanssen P et al: Association between vaginal douching and acute pelvic inflammatory disease, *JAMA* 263:1936, 1990.

Wong D, Nye K, Hollis P: Microbial flora on doctors' white coats, *Br Med J* 303:1602, 1991.

Wood CL: Laryngeal papillomas in infants and children, *J Nurse Midwife* 36(5):430, 1991.

📖 STUDENT RESOURCE SHELF

Jones DA: HIV-seropositive childbearing women: nursing management, *JOGNN* 20(6):446, 1991. Details the nursing process for assessment and care planning for the HIV-positive pregnant women.

Kelly P, Holman S: The new face of AIDS, *Am J Nurs* 93(3):26, 1993. An update on the occurrence of AIDS in women in 1993. Commonalities of the disease, as well as gender differences, are explored. The role of nursing in teaching and counseling is presented clearly and thoroughly.

Russell LK: Management of varicella-zoster virus infection during pregnancy and the peripartum, *J Nurse Midwife* 37(1):17, 1992. Discussion of the difficulties in care for the client with VZV, including isolation precautions.

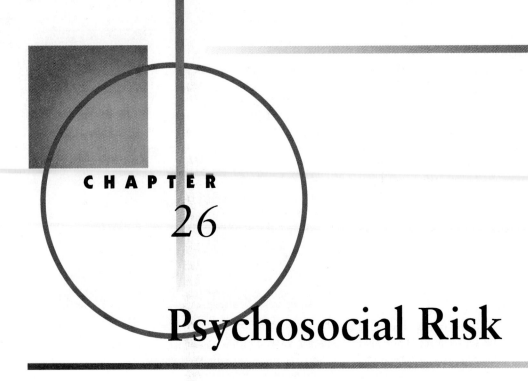

Psychosocial Risk

KEY TERMS

Acceptance
Advocate
Anger
Anxiety
Bargaining
Boarder Babies
Denial
Depression
Despair
Developmental Crisis
Empowerment
Guilt
Hierarchy of Needs
  Theory
Loss
Resolution
Self-Blame
Situational Crisis
Socially High-Risk
  Client
Spiritual Distress

LEARNING OBJECTIVES

1. *Apply Maslow's theory of needs to the psychosocial care of women at high risk and their families.*
2. *Identify elements in the crisis of normal pregnancy.*
3. *Identify factors that place a woman at social high risk.*
4. *Show how moderate to high anxiety levels interfere with the person's ability to cope.*
5. *Assess a high-risk client for psychosocial needs and resources.*
6. *Structure a plan of care, including referral to other members of the health care team.*
7. *Practice elements of the therapeutic nurse-client relationship.*
8. *Use self-assessment of ethnic and social biases that inhibit relationships.*
9. *Identify and describe the role of advocacy for the client at high risk.*

Psychosocial Support

Nurses traditionally have been involved in teaching and counseling clients and families, as well as supporting their decision making. Because of the increase in high-risk pregnancies, the need for teaching and counseling, as well as physical care, is especially great.

There are two high-risk categories: the woman at risk from maternal and fetal complications and the woman at risk from social problems.

BASIC CONCEPTS

Abraham Maslow first described his **hierarchy of needs theory** in 1954. He stated that human beings have dynamic and fluid needs that motivate them to action and help to create their personalities. These needs are met in ascending order of importance. Until lower level needs are met, more advanced needs cannot be addressed.

The categories of Maslow's list are (1) physiologic, (2) safety, (3) belongingness and love, (4) esteem, and (5) self-actualization. The most basic needs are physiologic; if these are not met, disability or death can result. Examples of these needs are similar to those of Orem's that include air, food, and water. Safety needs constitute the next category. People who feel physically or psychologically threatened are unable to consider anything else unless they feel safe. The need for belongingness and love comprises the next level. All people need to feel that they are cared for by others and crave the security of warm, close relationships. Esteem needs, the next category, reflect human desire for self-respect. They also include the desire for strength, adequacy, mastery, competence, and independence and freedom (Maslow, 1970). As Maslow points out:

Satisfaction of these needs leads to feelings of self confidence, worth, strength, capability and adequacy, of being useful and necessary in the world. Thwarting of these needs produces feelings of inferiority, of weakness and of helplessness.

The highest level need is for self-actualization as Maslow describes it—the desire for self-fulfillment and the full use of one's talents, capacities, and potentialities. The expression of this need varies with individual situations.

Figure 26-1 illustrates a conceptualization of the Maslow schema in which Mitchell (1973) arranged the needs in the shape of a pyramid to illustrate how they build on each other. An individual moves from one level to another and is influenced by positive and negative life events. Any crisis, whether it is a **developmental crisis** (graduating from college, entering adolescence) or **situational crisis** (death of a family member, loss of a job, or marital discord), can precipitate movement.

CRISIS OF PREGNANCY

Pregnancy is a developmental crisis. Even in a "normal" pregnancy, the woman, her partner, and her family have many fears that influence their needs and therefore their responses. As in any crisis, prior coping behaviors are disturbed, and stress is created as the individual struggles to adapt to a new and unfamiliar situation. For example, a woman satisfied with her career may have difficulty deciding on a life-style that combines motherhood and career. Her self-esteem may be threatened. As her body changes, she may begin to feel unattractive, further challenging her self-esteem.

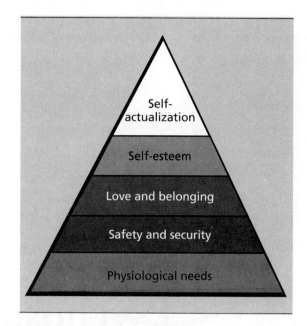

FIGURE 26-1 Maslow model is pyramid shaped, with the most basic needs forming the foundation. Needs are met in ascending order of importance.

Fathers also experience pregnancy as a crisis. As the woman becomes more intimately connected with the fetus, she may withdraw from him physically and psychologically. He may interpret her reactions, which are normal, as rejection and may begin to focus on meeting his belongingness and love needs.

All women and families have safety fears for themselves and their babies. High-risk pregnancy is a situational crisis in which serious risks to the health of the mother or the baby, or both, exist. In these situations, clients may be forced to deal with basic physiologic and safety needs.

The way in which an individual responds to crisis also is influenced by ethnicity, socioeconomic status, and other life events. Situations such as homelessness, loss or absence of a partner, poverty, and inadequate food and housing force the client to focus on meeting her lowest level of need. She struggles with daily survival and will not be able to deal with much else. Other events will be denied or disregarded until they interfere with daily functioning. Support systems already may be overstressed and may collapse under the increased burden and thus further intensify the crisis.

Nurse-Client Relationship

The nurse's needs cannot be neglected in this framework. Nurses who are unable to understand their own functioning when meeting a client's needs may be unable to provide adequate care. For example, personal problems at home can be a stress factor as the nurse struggles to meet personal self-esteem and belongingness needs. Fear of physical harm may call safety needs to the forefront and thus limit the nurse's ability to care for substance abusers who are at high risk for violent behavior and communicable diseases. Nurses must know their needs to choose the setting in which they can best work. As part of professional training, they must learn how their own needs will affect their work. Judgmental behavior can result from fear for safety or a fear that similar problems can happen to oneself. The desire to *rescue* all clients (and the subsequent disappointment of failure) may result from intense self-esteem needs. This behavior is understandable and normal but gets in the way of providing care. Maslow (1970) points out that most *need-motivated behavior is unconscious*. Thus nurses should become aware of their needs and the forces that drive them; then they can take action to satisfy them or prevent them from interfering with nursing care.

A nurse carries personal racial, ethnic, and cultural biases into nursing practice. When one is raised in a particular environment, it is difficult to understand other life-styles, belief systems, and customs. Again, nurses must learn to identify conflicts between their beliefs and clients' beliefs and deal with them rather than try to force personal beliefs, suggestions, or solutions on a client and family. The Maslow framework provides a guide to understanding the care requirements of a client and family, their responses, and a workable approach to planning and interventions.

The nature of the nurse-client relationship is fostered best by an objective, caring professional who helps the client identify self-care needs and deficits in meeting those needs. The nurse plans with, not for, the client and family. When these interventions reflect the client's resources and sociocultural network, the best result is obtained. The goal is to work with client, family, and community resources to formulate realistic plans, foster growth and independence, and prevent further disability, disease, or dysfunction (Figure 26-2).

LOSS AND GRIEF

Feelings of **loss** come when a person recognizes that a desired, valuable goal has been missed, spoiled, or taken away. *Grief* describes the person's emotional response to loss. *Mourning* is the process by which a person goes through the phases of grief to resolution and acceptance of the loss.

In high-risk pregnancy the central issue is *loss,* which can range from loss of a desired experience to loss of the fetus or the newborn. Denial, anger, and bargaining are early behaviors seen with varying degrees of depression, anxiety, and guilt. The anxiety is increased by feelings of loss of control (Beatty et al, 1985).

Grief Process

When there is real or perceived loss, one of the first manifestations is **denial,** the "not me" response. For example, a client with recently diagnosed diabetes or preeclampsia may refuse to follow instructions because she feels well and cannot believe that something could be wrong. She may even seek another care giver to tell her that everything is all right. A mother who is told that her unborn fetus has died may refuse to believe it and continue to state that she feels fetal movement.

The next phase is **anger,** the "why me" stage. When the obvious no longer can be ignored or occasionally while the client drifts in and out of the denial stage, she may show great anger toward care givers, her partner, and her family. Outbursts of accusations and threats are common. When she becomes angry at herself, anger turns inward and results in depression. Anger heralds the onset of **guilt.**

The client will think of many reasons to blame herself. Most of these reasons are unfounded and may seem irrational. They are, nonetheless, real to her and should be acknowledged and discussed. If she has contributed to the problem (e.g., taken a drug or substance that could cause anomalies or fetal harm), accusations are inappropriate. Allowing the client to deny responsibility is not appropriate either. This response will not allow her to move to **resolution.** For example, if the mother's drug use caused abruption and stillbirth, she needs to be told matter-of-factly and nonjudgmentally that drug use was the cause. She can then be helped to understand that her drug problem must be addressed because it is affecting her life. The stillbirth may motivate her to change. Blaming her will reinforce her hopelessness and guilt and drive her further into despair and continued drug use.

The nurse's unconditional acceptance of the client may allow the woman to deal with her guilt. If fears are unfounded, the client should be reassured. At the same time she should be reassured that her guilt feelings are normal and expected and that she is not "crazy."

The next step is **bargaining;** "If only I had chosen another doctor!" "If only I had asked before I took that drug!" "God, if you can make this go away, I will never be a bad person again!" "What did I do to deserve this?" These are some of the common responses to which the nurse can offer little response but should listen and show concern in whatever way is appropriate. Irrational feelings can be dispelled partially by providing information. Social service and psychiatric referral may be indicated. A particularly helpful reference for clients is the book, *When Bad Things Happen to Good People* by Rabbi Harold Kushner (1981).

After the client passes through all these stages, she arrives at a relatively peaceful **acceptance.** That does not mean that her sadness disappears; it will always be there, awakened by an anniversary, a thought, or a similar experience. Acceptance does not mean that the client comes to see the loss as a good event; rather she will see it as a tragedy that occurred, that she lived

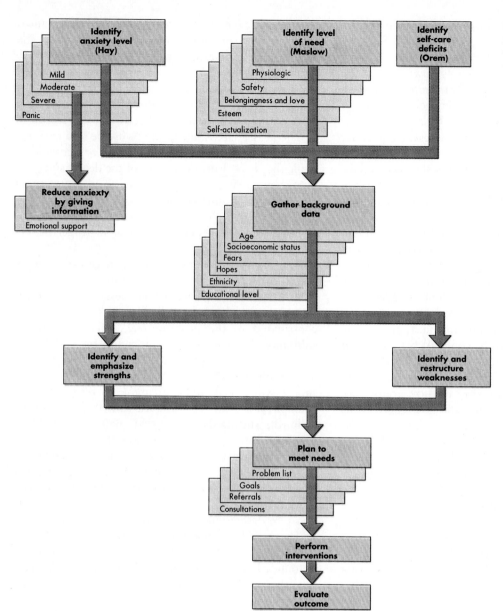

FIGURE 26-2 Model for provision of psychosocial care. (Courtesy JD Virzi and CA Moleti.)

through, and that made her stronger. The true resolution of a crisis is to turn a bad situation into a growth experience.

It should be kept in mind that the loss of a desired experience or the birth of a child with even minor congenital problems also can trigger the grief response. The same nursing interventions may be used in these situations (see Chapter 29).

SPIRITUAL DISTRESS

Each person has spiritual needs, which if unmet may cause restlessness, unhappiness, and a sense of lack of purpose in life, or **spiritual distress**. When difficulties arise, these feelings may become intensified. Spiritual

needs are expressed in a variety of ways of seeking meaning for one's life. Spirituality arises from the deepest core of the person and, as Nagai-Jacobson and Buckhardt (1989) note, can be conceived of as a unifying or vital force that integrates all other human dimensions. Depending on a person's exposure to and acceptance of a set of religious beliefs, she may turn to those she senses have faith, or she may seek for help with basic questions of "Why?" "What purpose?" and "Who can help me?"

One's spirituality may seek expression through practice of a specific religion. It is, however, a much wider concept, expressed in one writer's words as "in Whom we live and move and have our being" or by another: "Our hearts are restless until they find their rest in Thee."

Through faith a person finds meaning in life and life's difficulties, understands personal growth, and achieves healing and hope. A vast number of 12-step programs have tapped into spiritual needs in a way that is effective and often independent of a specific creed. Faith in a "Higher Power" can energize the human spirit to overcome hindrances to growth and healing, including addictions and experiences with childhood abuse.

Holistic nursing includes an emphasis on a person's whole being, an approach that has affected nursing in a new way, because in many educational settings, minimal emphasis on spiritual needs and the distress that follows has been traditional. Spiritual distress is now a nursing diagnosis, and nurses in maternal-child health care especially need to be aware of the *defining characteristics* (Box 26-1).

In an inner-city setting in which a group of nurses (Corrine et al, 1992) encountered expressions of deep spiritual distress, they applied spiritual interventions in maternal-child health care (see model later in this chapter). They found the concept of a *life journey* to be a useful way to indicate the dynamic character of faith

---

BOX 26-1   Defining Characteristics of Spiritual Distress* (Distress of the Human Spirit)

Expresses concern with meaning of life and death and/or belief systems
Anger toward God (as defined by the person)
Questions meaning of suffering
Verbalizes concern about relationship with deity
Questions meaning of own existence
Inability to choose or chooses not to participate in usual religious practice
Seeks spiritual assistance
Questions moral and ethical implications of therapeutic regimen
Displaces anger toward religious representatives
Describes nightmares or sleep disturbances
Altered mood or behavior evidenced by anger, crying, withdrawal, preoccupation, anxiety, hostility, apathy, etc.
Regards illness as punishment
Does not experience that God is forgiving
Inability to accept self
Engages in self-blame
Denies responsibilities for problems
Describes many somatic complaints

From Kim MJ, McFarland GK, McLane AM: *Pocket guide to nursing diagnoses*, ed 5, St. Louis, 1993, Mosby.
*Disruption in the life principle that pervades a person's entire being and integrates and transcends one's biological and psychosocial nature.

---

development and influence on life decisions. Using questions such as the following, the nurse may help the person tap into these needs.

- How did you cope with the loss? (when discussing a miscarriage or death)
- Where did you find the strength to do what you did? (when leaving an abusive relationship or dealing with a difficult life situation)
- How are your spirits today? (when the client has been depressed)
- Whom do you turn to when problems seem too much? (helps identify resources)
- Whom do you pray to? (when better acquainted with the client, opens the door to discuss faith resources)
- Where do you seem to be on your journey? (to a mother grieving over a stillbirth)

Cultural variations in the area in which a nurse works need to be studied and understood before wrong conclusions are drawn. For instance, in a number of Hispanic subgroups, *mal oho*, or the evil eye, is feared and precautions are taken. A family will have a specific saint as a protector, and colored beads, a *sabache*, may be attached to a bracelet or necklace as a protection. Others may protect the infant by saying "Que Dios lo bendiga" (God bless him) when they see the baby (Corrine et al, 1992).

Interventions go beyond a simple referral to a clergy person. The nurse may offer suggestions of activities that others have found helpful. Clergy can provide reading material to help the person become centered and think about spiritual needs. Writing down feelings often is a powerful tool, especially during mourning. To assist the woman in mobilizing her own resources, the nurse can suggest walking, meaningful activities with friends, and conversation to identify her helpful supports. Mainly, it is the nurse's caring attitude that indicates to the client that her spiritual distress is taken seriously and deserves attention. In working with clients who are substance abusers, nurses find that the women often respond to assistance in locating 12-step programs. Chapter 29 describes the work of a perinatal grieving team in one setting—material that can provide parallels in care in one's own setting.

ANXIETY

Excessive preoccupation with the problem, extreme overinvestment in certain aspects of care, continual questioning, and a need for constant reminders and immediate reassurance are common. Some fears are expected, but irrational fears often surface. Mild to moderate **anxiety** levels may be beneficial because they motivate a person to action and increase the ability to perceive details. Moderate to severe anxiety levels, however, can narrow perceptions and render a client and family unable to focus on other aspects of care, to understand the problem, to make decisions, or to carry out instructions. In 1961 Hays described anxiety levels and their effect on the client and the type of nursing care required. More than three decades later, anxiety is a major nursing diagnostic category.

Table 26-1 provides a useful guide to planning nursing care for clients with anxiety. Note the differences in operations (client behavior), variations (signs), and learning tasks (interventions) required in each anxiety state. Mild to moderate levels of anxiety facilitate learning. Severe anxiety and panic impede learning.

One should never consider any client response as excessive or exaggerated. Women have been shown to harbor feelings of grief, guilt, shame, and depression for years after abortion, birth of an ill or a congenitally malformed infant, and even after birth of a normal infant under less than optimal circumstances (Panuthos and Romero, 1984). When the developmental crisis of pregnancy is further complicated by high-risk status, a woman's basic needs shift. The way in which she manifests responses to this shift depends on many factors.

TABLE 26-1 Level of Anxiety and Its Implications for Nursing Care

OPERATIONS (CLIENT BEHAVIOR)	VARIATIONS (SIGNS)	LEARNING TASKS (INTERVENTIONS)
MILD ANXIETY		
Alertness	Noises seeming louder Restlessness Irritability	Recognition of anxiety as a warning sign that something is not going as expected. This can be done by: 1. Observing what goes on 2. Describing what was observed 3. Analyzing what was expected 4. Analyzing how expectations and what went on in the event differed 5. Formulating what can be done about the situation in terms of changing the situation or expectations 6. Validating with others
MODERATE ANXIETY		
Reduced ability to perceive and communicate Increased tension	Concentration on a problem Possible inability to hear someone talking Possible inability to notice part of the room Muscular tension, pounding heart, perspiration, gastric discomfort	Recognition that in moderate and severe anxiety the focus is reduced and connections may not be seen between details and that anxiety provides energy that can be reduced to mild anxiety and then used to find out what went wrong
SEVERE ANXIETY		
Perception of details only Physical discomfort Emotional discomfort	Connections between details not seen Headaches, nausea, trembling, dizziness Awe, dread, loathing, horror	Moderate to severe anxiety may be reduced by: 1. Working at a simple, concrete task 2. Talking to someone who can listen 3. Playing a simple game 4. Walking 5. Crying
PANIC		
Elaboration and blowing up of perceived detail	Inability to communicate or function	The person experiencing panic needs help in getting more comfortable. (In this stage learning cannot be expected to take place.)

From Hays D: Teaching a concept of anxiety, © 1961, American Journal of Nursing Co. Reprinted with permission from *Nursing Research*, Spring 10(2):109.

CRISIS INTERVENTION

Crisis applies to a state or to an individuals' reaction to a perceived threatening situation (Infante, 1982). A crisis may be maturational or *developmental,* such as new parenthood, or accidental or *situational,* such as in the birth and care of an infant with a defect. A life situation may not pose a negative threat when preparation and adequate support are available. Instead it may become a positive growth producing experience if the person is enabled to cope effectively. As has been stated elsewhere, a crisis contains both **opportunity** and **danger** (Baird, 1986). It is useful to consider crisis intervention in terms of the self-care conceptual framework described by Aguilera (1994):

A crisis is a danger because it threatens to overwhelm the individual or his family. . . . It is also an opportunity because during times of crisis individuals are more receptive to therapeutic influence. Prompt and skillful intervention may not only prevent the development of a serious long-term disability, but may also allow new coping patterns to emerge that can help the individual function at a higher level of equilibrium than before the crisis.

A person in crisis is at a turning point. She faces a problem that cannot readily be solved by using coping mechanisms that have worked in the past. Tension and anxiety increase as she becomes caught in a state of great emotional upset and is unable to take action to solve the problem (Aguilera, 1994).

Nursing Responsibilities
► ASSESSMENT

To assess how best to help clients in these situations, the nurse collects factual data such as age, socioeconomic status, educational level, and place of residence; and ascertains the client's expectations of the pregnancy and determines the degree to which those expectations differ from what is actually happening or going to happen. Learning how she has helped herself during other upsetting events may be useful. Past maladaptive coping behaviors such as avoidance or denial are not desirable and should not be supported. Questions concerning those to whom the client and family turn for support are helpful (e.g., friends, other family members, clergy or church groups, and other professionals such as social workers).

The nurse strives to understand what the diagnosis and consequences of a high-risk pregnancy mean from the client's and family's perspective. What concerns or frightens them? Fears should be elicited by the use of open-ended questions, reflection, and careful listening, for example, "Many women have a lot of questions or concerns during a time like this. What are yours?" or "You say that you feel frightened" or "I can understand that you feel angry and upset." This therapeutic interaction encourages the client to express her fears and concerns and prevents the nurse from imposing personal fears and concerns. The woman then may provide you with clues to her self-care needs, her priorities, her position in the Maslow hierarchy, her support system or lack thereof, and barriers to obtaining needed tangible and psychologic care. It may take several interactions to develop enough trust to allow the client to talk freely. Acknowledge her fears, dispelling irrational concerns by giving correct information or referring her to someone who can. *Never give false hope or reassurance.* It is far better to tell the client that you do not know than to give inaccurate information. A client may cling to false reassurance to facilitate denial or avoidance behavior, and you should not encourage this behavior in any way.

Anger and mistrust will develop if concerns, even if minor ones, are brushed aside or the client feels she cannot believe what she is being told.

► NURSING DIAGNOSES

Depending on assessment findings, the following diagnoses are possible:
1. Decisional conflict related to several unacceptable alternatives
2. Individual or family coping: potential for growth
3. Anxiety related to threat to self, ideal pregnancy, or to fetus
4. Knowledge deficit because of pregnancy crisis and unknown outcomes
5. Powerlessness over outcome in spite of following care regimen

► EXPECTED OUTCOMES

Outcomes can be stated in numerous ways, which often are difficult to evaluate because resolution may take time.
1. Client enabled to come to decisions.
2. Family support and coping appear strengthened.
3. Knowledge has reduced anxiety.
4. Alternative ways of coping with powerlessness and fear are discovered.

► NURSING INTERVENTIONS

Aguilera (1994) provides a four-step outline for intervention. *First,* the person needs to gain an intellectual understanding of the situation. Everyone should be told what is happening and, if possible, why. The nurse should give as detailed an explanation of the problem, probable causes, treatment risks, benefits, and consequences as can be understood. The nurse, who often cannot provide this information, has the responsibility to see that another professional does and then can reinforce information. The interdisciplinary team consists of many providers, including nurses, nurse-midwives, physicians, physician's assistants, social workers, and dietitians. There are appropriate times for each to be the primary provider of care or information. The nurse, who usually is the professional that spends the most time with the client, often is the best person to coordinate the provision of care.

Second, the client should be encouraged to express her feelings. The nurse, by providing an open, nonjudgmental climate, may afford an opportunity for the client to express her feelings of anger, guilt, shame, and fear. These feelings should be affirmed as normal and expected.

Third, the nurse helps the client to examine alternative ways of coping because past coping mechanisms are failing to work. The client is encouraged to avoid maladaptive coping behaviors such as denial and to develop new, more healthy coping behaviors (Aguilera, 1994). Comments that may help when a client is having trouble accepting a diagnosis include a statement such as "Most people want to ignore unpleasant topics and focus on happy ones." In this way the woman may begin to recognize if she also is using avoidance behavior.

Fourth is "reopening of the social world." This might include helping a family plan to bring their congenitally malformed baby out to see relatives or giving a picture or a lock of hair of a very ill or stillborn baby to the family so they may show it to relatives and friends.

Whenever possible, the nurse can help the woman *regain a sense of control and mastery.* For example, allowing a diabetic client to make meal choices may seem simplistic, but the independence and freedom she regains is important for her. Praising small accomplishments helps the client. Often, undesirable behavior disappears more rapidly if it is ignored because it may be a mechanism the client is using to gain attention.

The nurse may feel unable to do anything to ease the client's pain or anxiety, which represents a need to do everything possible to help the client. In reality, very little can be done for some clients in some situations. For example, when an infant dies of a congenital abnormality, the pain cannot be erased. Clients have shown that the availability of the nurse, her information giving and support, and her encouragement to express feelings have been of great assistance to them. They find assistance with problem solving and reassurance to be the most supportive and helpful aids (Wheeler and Gardiner, 1987).

The nurse encourages clients to use their family and community supports. They may feel embarrassed and reluctant to ask for help. They must understand that seeking support and assistance from friends, family members, and health care providers usually draws people together.

 EVALUATION

Interventions in crisis that involves loss and grief cannot be evaluated in a short period of time. With that in mind the following questions could be asked.

1. Was the client able to articulate her needs and seek assistance?
2. Did she understand the normality of the mourning process and allow herself to journey through it?
3. Was there support from her network of family and friends?

Risk Related to Maternal or Fetal Complications

Maternal or fetal complications represent the realization of the worst fears of the pregnant woman and her family. Ambivalence and concern are typical in the normal pregnancy. When a problem occurs, the woman, her partner, and her family may feel extremely guilty, assuming that they caused the problem by a thought they had (or did not have), an action they took (or did not take), or a decision they made (or did not make). Providers can unwittingly reinforce these feelings by asking questions or making statements that imply blame such as "Why didn't you come in sooner?" or "Why did you do that?" To learn to avoid the process of blame, the nurse can record or tape several interviews and listen to responses to the client.

BODY-IMAGE DISTURBANCE

Body image is changed during normal pregnancy. Early-pregnancy morning sickness, in the absence of other perceptible signs of pregnancy, can make a woman feel ill, not pregnant. Normal hormonal shifts may cause tremendous mood swings, which intensify anxiety and lead to fears that something is wrong. During these times, women and their partners normally wonder if the pregnancy is worth all the trouble, even if it has been eagerly anticipated and planned. These feelings may be more intense in cases of unintended pregnancy.

Changes in the urinary, cardiopulmonary, musculoskeletal, and integumentary systems in normal pregnancy often cause *body-image disturbances.* Women with medical problems existing before pregnancy have additional concerns about how the pregnancy will affect them: "Will my diabetes go out of control?" "Will my heart disease become fatal?" This anxiety may lead to hypochondriasis because the basic safety needs are threatened. Severe levels of anxiety may result.

When a medical problem first appears during pregnancy, a dual crisis has to be faced. The client must deal with the problem (e.g., her newly diagnosed gestational diabetes or hypertensive disease). Her body is failing her: "Will I need surgery or die?" "Will this be a lifelong problem?" "Will I ever be normal again?" "Will I ever be able to eat what I want, exercise at the gym, have sexual relations?" "How can I cope with labor, delivery, and a new baby when I also have to cope with an illness?" The severity of her reaction often is not in proportion to the problem. The reaction is influenced by which level of the client's needs is most immediate. Her support systems, her cultural and ethnic background, her expectations of herself, and her hopes for the pregnancy also may affect the response.

FEARS FOR FETAL SAFETY

When fetal complications occur (e.g., genetic disorders or the threat of preterm labor) normal fears about fetal well-being and guilt are intensified. The anxiety over even routine diagnostic tests is considerable, and when tests confirm a problem, the worst fears of the woman are realized. "Will my baby be OK?" "I knew I shouldn't have taken that exercise class!" "There is something wrong with me. I can't even take care of my baby before it's born!"

PARTNER'S FEARS

The fears of partners often parallel those of the woman. The normal changes of pregnancy, including morning sickness, mood swings, and changes in body shape and sexual appetite and functioning, may make a man wonder if his partner will ever be the same physically or emotionally. He senses her inward focus and the gradual transfer of attention away from him. This may ease after he is able to feel fetal movement, but jealousy of her attention to the fetus, the attention she receives from others, and even jealousy of his inability to physically experience pregnancy is normal (Heinowitz, 1982).

Clients and their partners rarely express their concerns directly. Their need for information, counseling, and assistance may be expressed in many ways, most of them covert. They generally do not discuss fears or problems with family or friends. Even in normal pregnancy, expression of fears usually is not well accepted by the family.

INTERRUPTED PARENT-INFANT ATTACHMENT

Stress that leaves the parents feeling unsupported or unloved or that causes real or imagined concern for the baby's health or survival interferes with attachment. When the mother has a health or psychosocial problem during pregnancy, anxiety may interfere with her ability to attach. A threatened miscarriage or a history of previous miscarriage threatens her self-image. If she has taken drugs, smokes, or fears having a baby with birth

Clinical Decision

A woman's status is designated as high risk because of gestational diabetes. The client and her husband question staff members constantly and refuse to continue with the diet and blood glucose monitoring that has been recommended. They are particularly upset that they have been transferred from the alternative birth center to the hospital center.
*   *What best explains their response?*
*   *Suggest nursing interventions.*

defects, she may be deeply anxious. Fearing for the survival of her infant, and to protect herself from feelings of loss if she miscarries, she unconsciously delays forming an image of herself as a mother. If the delivery was traumatic or if the mother is ill, she may have little energy available for interaction with her baby. Similarly, pain (e.g., after a cesarean birth) can distract from her interaction. Appropriate use of pain medication before the baby is brought to her can help to maintain comfort.

When persons encounter medical problems during pregnancy, the potential for sadness is markedly increased, not only because of worry regarding the outcome but also because of the need to mourn the loss of the expected happy birth experience. The nurse must recognize feelings of sadness or anger and help clients to express their feelings. This gives them permission to experience and work through their real feelings when there are so many "shoulds." Coming to terms with repressed feelings will release the emotional energy that maintains the repression.

When the unexpected outcome is a problem with the baby, the difficulty of attachment will be compounded. The mother needs to mourn the loss of the anticipated perfect baby; in addition, bonding may be delayed because the infant must be immediately transported to the special care nursery or to another facility because of medical problems. This separation means that her sense of herself as important to the baby is immediately cast aside. Without contact, she fears that her need to be close to the infant is in jeopardy and thus may begin to detach from her pregnancy relationship. Early contact with her baby is essential because she is eager to identify, claim, and attach to her child.

If the mother cannot be brought to the special care nursery within a few hours of the birth (e.g., if she is ill or the baby is transferred to another hospital), she should be given a picture of her baby and unlimited access to the nursery by telephone to help her to

NURSING CARE PLAN • **Loss and Grief**

CASE: Jane M, 34, para 0010, has recently been separated from her spouse. Her own family lives in the next state. She had hoped for a normal child to fill an emotional vacuum in her life. Diagnosis at 32 weeks shows that the baby boy has a defect but will survive. At 34 weeks she gives birth prematurely to a healthy boy with a cleft lip and palate.

ASSESSMENT DATA

1. Level of expressed anxiety about baby; hopes for the infant's place in family
   Past and present coping mechanisms
   Actual family support, friends
2. Phase of grief response: diagnosis known since 32 weeks
   Expressions of hopes and fears about future
   Understanding of normality of grieving in situation

3. Knowledge about future treatment, length of stay in neonatal intensive care unit (NICU)
   Ability to understand explanations given by physician and nurses
   Ability to participate in decision making about future
   Knowledge of resources for self and infant care; support

NURSING DIAGNOSES

1. Anxiety related to perceived threats to self and infant
2. High risk for dysfunctional grieving and depression over baby's condition, loss of partner
3. Altered body image related to perceived inability to have normal baby

4. Spiritual distress related to questioning series of blows to hopes

EXPECTED OUTCOMES

1. Anxiety will be managed with effective coping mechanisms.
2. Client moves through grief process at an acceptable pace and finds ongoing support.
3. She asks for clarification of causes and treatment for infant.

4. She expresses concerns about body image, self-esteem, spiritual distress.
5. She participates in planning for future and seeks additional counseling and resources.

NURSING INTERVENTIONS

1. Maintain calm, safe environment. Encourage nurse-client relationship by assigning primary nurse.
2. Assess anxiety level and support her in seeking personal resources for coping. Identify phase of grief and assure her of normality of feelings.
3. Give understandable information at a pace she can accept. Provide written information for going home. Work toward well-informed decisions. Provide telephone numbers for professional assistance as required.
4. Engage in therapeutic listening. Encourage attachment by frequent visits to NICU. Use open-ended statements

to elicit spiritual or self-esteem concerns. Refer to additional counseling or clergy as appropriate.
5. Praise constructive problem solving. Be sure sequence of infant recovery, surgery, and home care is explained and understood by the mother. Identify financial resources by referral to appropriate persons. Refer for home care when infant is ready. Follow through with her own recovery by highlighting for the home care nurse those nursing diagnoses identified in hospital.

EVALUATION

1. Did she increase coping skills? Have symptoms of anxiety been recognized and reduced?
2. Has she expressed feelings about crisis, loss? Does she realize the phases of grief through which she will be going? Can she identify support persons in her situation?
3. Is attachment to the infant established? Does this attachment appear to overcome any feelings of low-ered self-esteem? Does there appear to be adequate emotional support for her in her home setting?
4. Is she clear about the planning for care of the defect, recovery times, and home care of the infant? Does she know about resources?

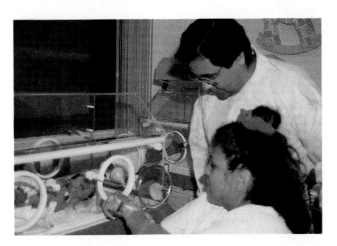

FIGURE 26-3 Parents should be encouraged to visit their baby in the NICU as early as possible. (Courtesy Marjorie Pyle, RNC, *Lifecircle.*)

maintain a sense of being important and included in the neonate's care.

As soon as it is practical, the mother and father should be encouraged to visit their ill or premature infant. Visual and tactile contact begins immediately after the infant is mature enough (Figure 26-3). The nursing care plan should include promotion of the parents' participation in the infant's care as soon as and as fully as they are able. Positive and encouraging coaching is vital when the parent first begins to handle the infant. (See Chapter 29 for a model of perinatal grieving intervention.)

Risk from Psychosocial Problems

The pregnancy of a **socially high-risk client** is complicated by a variety of social problems, including substance abuse, homelessness, economic status, and educational or intellectual deprivation. Social high risk often may be a complicating factor in a woman at risk for medical/surgical or age-related complications. Social high risk can contribute directly or indirectly to the development of physical high-risk problems. For example, an intravenous drug user is at physical risk for HIV infection and at psychosocial risk for child abuse and neglect. A woman overwhelmed by poverty may not be able to buy food and therefore may be prone to complications related to poor nutrition.

Such clients often have had multiple social problems over a long time. The compounding factors may exacerbate each other. Chronic deprivation in many areas of life may exist. Familial support systems often are nonexistent, overtaxed, or quite vulnerable to collapse under the burden of additional problems.

Most socially high-risk clients are poor and members of minority groups. They may be recent immigrants who may have entered the country illegally and often are afraid of being discovered. They may be unable to speak English. Their ethnic and cultural beliefs about health care and therefore their priorities often are not synchronous with those of their care providers. These clients are vulnerable to communicable diseases, substance abuse, inadequate housing, and inadequate nutrition. They often are reluctant to seek care because they do not perceive the need for it, are fearful, or cannot negotiate through the complex system because of language, literacy, or financial barriers.

These clients and their families often are in continuous crisis. One problem may lead directly or indirectly to another. There is disorganization, anxiety, and irrational behavior, some of it violent. These clients present a great challenge. Their care providers frequently are overwhelmed by their needs, the severity of their problems, and the lack of resources. These clients may do little to help themselves or encourage others to help. They may be hostile, noncompliant, and seemingly disinterested. The client may seem irresponsible, missing appointments, not following through on treatments, or not coming for care at all. Care providers must understand that this is not irresponsibility but rather a *manifestation of underlying hopelessness, helplessness, and depression.*

Maslow (1970) points out that depression can occur when the defensive efforts of a person fail because of overwhelming outside pressure or weak defense mechanisms. Deep hopelessness and discouragement have been described in people who have been exposed to extended disappointment, deprivation, or trauma. They often just give up trying because they see no benefit from their efforts.

A person living in inadequate housing without sufficient food is meeting only basic physiologic and safety needs. To expect this person to be concerned about needs above this level (e.g., prenatal care) is not realistic. Unless she becomes so ill that it affects her daily functioning, the client will deal with the most pressing needs first. She cannot deal with the needs of her children for intellectual stimulation and educational development. She may be unable to deal with immunizations and well-child care. She is more concerned with feeding her family and finding a safe place to live.

This client may be overwhelmed and anxious and unable to focus on problem solving. She often is withdrawn. She denies her problems and deals only with what cannot be ignored. She often is angry at others, and this anger can lead to hostility or suicidal behavior, which may manifest in ways such as refusing treatment for life-threatening conditions or continuing to abuse alcohol and drugs.

On the other hand, the socially high-risk client often is a skilled manipulator who has survived by outsmarting the system, including the legal system. Although illegal activities cannot be tolerated, manipulation may be the only coping strategy the client has.

NEW APPROACHES

A number of psychosocial problems reflect similar underlying feelings of helplessness and hopelessness. The social milieu contributes to a large measure by imposing restraints on escape from or solving of problems. Societal responses vary with changing political climates. For example, wife abuse was addressed seriously in the late 1970s by recognizing that the *person-in-environment* must be seen as a whole. In these terms it becomes apparent that poverty, racial barriers, drug abuse, and abuse within a family grouping have complex interacting factors. It can be recognized that the individual *alone* cannot break free to restructure her life. She needs a continuum of services designed to enable the choices that need to be made (Davis and Hagen, 1992). These services should be *enabling*, not *paternalistic*, or "doing for" a client.

Because the feminist movement recognized and promoted the need for **empowerment** as a means to solving problems, a backlash developed in the 1980s that reemphasized the victim of social ills. "If only you will change yourself, then all will be okay" is often the implicit message of self-help groups, codependency books, and many service agencies. However, the victim cannot do it alone. *Social policy also must change.* Policies to reduce poverty and institutional racism need to be established.

In a study describing empowerment for women of color (Asian-American, Latina, Native American, and African-American), Gutiérrez (1990) notes that among black women and Latinas the poverty rate is 32% and 26%, respectively. Poverty and powerlessness often are linked.

WIFE ABUSE DURING PREGNANCY

Maintaining intact family groupings is a worthy goal, but certain situations are inherently destructive. Pregnancy is a crisis that increases stress in already highly charged situations.

The term "wife" is used to include unmarried women in sexual partnerships. Occasionally *spouse abuse* is used, although in most cases it is the man beating the woman, who then occasionally fights back. Across every socioeconomic level, a deeply rooted feeling still exists that men are justified in abusing women because of an implicit right to control what is "theirs." Thus empowerment of women to make and carry out choices taps into deep feelings. Although battering, rape, and sexual abuse occur within each socioeconomic group in our society, they are more prevalent where poverty, drug abuse, and racial barriers frustrate normal family life.

The current political emphasis is seen in the Family Violence Prevention and Services Act, which provides funds for shelter-related services and prevention by education to aid victims. By this Act, emergency and short-term aid is available, but long-term, life-restructuring needs such as low-cost housing, child care, and financial aid during job training are less available. Thus in many situations the abused woman returns to a relationship because of economic need, and the abuse continues.

The problem of abused women, children, and elders did not suddenly escalate in this society. It always has been present but largely ignored until recently when enough people decided to do something different about it and to focus light on the problem (Davis and Hagen, 1992).

Mandatory reporting of child abuse is now the law. Because the urban setting reduces neighborliness, spousal violence is less often reported. Until recently, and still unevenly, abusing men rarely have been punished. Restraining orders are available for spouse abuse, but the deep-rooted causes of abuse will reassert themselves in spite of these restraints. Indeed it is often after a woman leaves the abusive spouse that he attempts to severely injure or kill her.

Risk

More than 1500 women per year are killed, and more than 2 million are badly injured in domestic violence (Connolly and Marshall, 1991). A great many other cases remain unreported. It has been recognized that abuse is generally more common for the pregnant woman and especially for the adolescent pregnant woman (Parker and McFarlane, 1991).

Empowerment

An escape from helplessness and hopelessness is defined as a process of increasing personal, interpersonal, or political power so that individual persons can take action to improve their life situations (Gutiérrez, 1990).

The term *empowerment,* which can be used in a vague general way, requires the following four changes if its meaning is to provide a personally practical and specific approach (Gutiérrez, 1990).

1. Increasing *self-efficacy,* or the belief in one's own ability to act and regulate life events. (This term has been applied to early parenting behaviors.) Self-efficacy includes developing increasing ability to act because there is some success gained by action. For a person to have success, often information is a key: How to access the health care system? How to get food stamps? Who can help with a referral? Nurses often are involved with providing information that results in increased self-efficacy. It has been found that group discussions, interaction, and problem-solving strategies can empower members by sharing problems and solutions, sympathy, and determination to improve a situation.

2. Developing *group consciousness.* The person sees that she is not alone or stranded in an unintelligible, uncaring society. She begins to focus on causes of problems, not only on results and her own feelings. She begins to seek ways of altering life situations.

3. *Reducing self-blame.* By consciousness raising, a person learns that outside forces also may be causing the current distress. Children usually blame themselves for any bad event, even incest and other sexual abuse. **Self-blame** often is at the root of depression. Seeing a glimpse of an alternative way may start a person on health-seeking behaviors and separating false from actual guilt.

4. *Personal accountability to change a situation.* A healthy response to a life problem is to begin looking for causes and solutions. Changing one's view of *self-as-victim* creates powerful energy for positive action.

Much of this theory is taught in social work programs. Nursing needs to recognize the client in a holistic way, as a *person-in-environment,* which means that the person is not isolated from the life situation, and that both always must be considered. In making referrals to social services, the nurse may wish to inquire about or participate in the ongoing empowering activities that the best social services programs foster.

Nursing Responsibilities

During admission history taking and physical examination, the nurse uses an evaluation tool such as the one in Box 26-2 to open the subject with the client, remembering the concept of the person-in-environment, to discover what feelings the woman may be able to share.

Continue to use the interventions that have been discussed for high-risk clients. Problem-solving techniques have been shown to be more effective when the process is client driven (Reid, 1990).

The nurse uses criteria such as the following to assess the woman's situation.

1. *Help the client identify the most serious problem* from her point of view.

2. *With the client, identify support systems* in family and community. Does she have family, friends, or a church group to which she belongs? Is she connected to the social service system for public assistance, Medicaid, or food stamps?

3. *Help her differentiate between chronic and acute problems.* The problems that have existed for an extended period of time, although serious, generally will not be the client's priority. Often asking, "What brought you in today?" will help to elicit this information.

4. *Ask her to identify how she has coped with similar problems.* Her resourcefulness often is amazing, and any positive coping strategies should be identified and encouraged. Past maladaptive coping behaviors such as avoidance or denial are not desirable and should not be supported.

5. *Strive to understand what the diagnosis and consequences of a high-risk pregnancy mean* from the client's and family's perspective. Ask her to describe what the physician has told her. Clarify information. Find out how her spouse feels about the situation.

6. *Encourage clients to use their extended family and community supports.*

The concept of Maslow's hierarchy of needs should be kept in mind so that assessment can begin where the woman is on the continuum of needs. Next, the level of anxiety must be assessed. In cases of severe anxiety or panic, before any other thing can be accomplished, this level must be reduced by giving support and information that address concerns. General background data must be gathered to identify self-care deficits or the potential for problems to interrupt a healthy outcome of the pregnancy. It is always helpful to write a list of the problems and issues and make a note of which of these demonstrate strengths and which are weaknesses or merely are neutral. The strengths should be built upon. The weaknesses must be addressed and modified to lessen their impact. Neutral factors have the potential to become strengths or weaknesses.

After assessment proceed to planning care with the client. Have the client identify realistic short-term goals. It is not realistic to expect quick solutions for chronic problems. The nurse cannot rescue the client nor remove the pain and anxiety she and her family may feel. She can facilitate the family's development of coping skills by using the techniques of crisis intervention. Encourage the client to take charge of her life and begin

BOX 26-2   Abuse Assessment Screen

ABUSE ASSESSMENT SCREEN

1. Have you ever been emotionally or physically abused by your partner or someone important to you?

YES ☐

NO ☐

2. Within the last year, have you been hit, slapped, kicked or otherwise physically hurt by someone?

YES ☐

NO ☐

If YES, by whom _____

Number of times _____

Mark the area of injury on body map.

3. Within the last year, has anyone forced you to have sexual activities?

If YES, who _____

Number of times _____

4. Are you afraid of your partner or anyone you listed above?

YES ☐

NO ☐

Developed by the Nursing Research Consortium on Violence and Abuse: 1989. Readers are encouraged to reproduce and use this assessment tool.

solving the less pressing problems. When she meets her own goals, small victories will increase self-esteem and a positive outlook. The process is continuous. The input of other care providers is vital. In many constructive care situations the nurse will be simply the coordinator or case manager. Figure 26-2 illustrates this model of intervention.

Not all clients will accept help, and some choose to refuse it or do not comply. Many more will respond to what often is one of the first instances of understanding they have experienced and may be motivated to make real and lasting changes in their lives. Although the care of these clients is difficult, the rewards are great.

SUBSTANCE ABUSE

Situations that involve clients who abuse drugs and alcohol and refuse all care are particularly difficult.

Such a client is often very depressed, and these behaviors are a manifestation of that despair. She cannot consider the consequences of her actions because it means thinking about tomorrow. Because today is too difficult to cope with, abusive substances mask the pain. This is self-destructive behavior. It does not mean, however, that women who abuse drugs and alcohol do not want to stop. Often pregnancy is an excellent motivation for a real change in life. With proper interdisciplinary support, she may overcome her problems.

Recent trends in drug use in the United States show evidence of a shift in the type of drugs used and the population that uses them. Many studies indicate increased use of alcohol and cocaine derivatives.

Drug use varies with locale. Use of alcohol and cocaine has shifted in the last few decades to include women from suburban areas and persons with higher income levels, whereas heroin, methadone, and crack continue to be used by persons in urban areas and by women from lower socioeconomic levels. Varying degrees of drug use begin for many with experimentation in high school (Table 26-2). Use of multiple controlled substances often is found in the drug-abusing woman. Neonatal withdrawal has been recognized after chronic maternal use of alcohol, amphetamines, barbiturates, codeine, cocaine, diazepam (Valium), ethchlorvynol (Placidyl), glutethimide (Doriden), heroin, meperidine,

morphine, pentazocine (Talwin), and propoxyphene (Darvon). Drugs of major concern during pregnancy are heroin, methadone, and cocaine/crack. (Refer to Chapter 10 for discussion of alcohol and nicotine.)

Heroin

An opiate related to morphine and several times more potent than an equal weight of morphine, heroin is a potent analgesic, producing respiratory depression and euphoria. The user feels a rush of pleasurable sensations lasting several minutes after injection or inhalation, followed by several hours of sensory and emotional detachment from others. As the drug is metabolized, the user has a strong desire to repeat these sensations, followed by physical discomfort. The drive to use heroin soon supersedes all other drives, leading to social isolation from anything not associated with drug use.

Physical dependence follows, and because heroin easily crosses to the fetus, fetal dependence also is created. There are no known direct teratogenic effects; the fetus may be growth-retarded or chronically stressed because of multiple drug use, poor nutrition, or maternal chronic infection or other disease (see Chapter 28).

Methadone

Because methadone is similar to morphine and heroin but has a much longer half-life, it may be given once a

TABLE 26-2 Trends in Annual Prevalence of Drug Use Among High School Seniors* by Drug Type

DRUG TYPE	STUDENT DRUG USE† (%)			
	CLASS OF 1975	CLASS OF 1980	CLASS OF 1985	CLASS OF 1986
Marijuana/hashish	40.0	48.8	40.6	38.8
Inhalants	NA	4.6	5.7	6.1
Inhalants adjusted	NA	7.9	7.5	8.9
Amyl and butyl nitrites	NA	5.7	4.0	4.7
Hallucinogens	11.2	9.3	6.3	6.0
Hallucinogens adjusted	NA	10.4	7.6	7.6
LSD	7.2	6.5	4.4	4.5
PCP	NA	4.4	2.9	2.4
Cocaine	5.6	12.3	13.1	12.7
Heroin	1.0	0.5	0.6	0.5
Other opiates	5.7	6.3	5.9	5.2
Stimulants	16.2	20.8	NA	NA
Stimulants adjusted	NA	NA	15.8	13.4
Sedatives	11.7	10.3	5.8	5.2
Barbiturates	10.7	6.8	4.6	4.2
Methaqualone	5.1	7.2	2.8	2.1
Tranquilizers	10.6	8.7	6.1	5.8
Alcohol	84.8	87.9	85.6	84.5
Total no. (approximate)	9,400	15,900	16,000	15,200

From Centers for Disease Control: *MMWR*, June 17, 1987.
† Reports drug use for previous 12-month period; NA indicates data not available.
* National High School Senior Survey conducted by the National Institute on Drug Abuse, 1975, 1980, 1985, 1986.

day. Methadone maintenance (MM) programs are functioning in most larger cities in the United States, although there are waiting lists for entry. Methadone obtained from a maintenance program increases contact with health care providers, which should improve the woman's participation in prenatal care.

Cocaine and Crack

Use of cocaine and crack has increased rapidly in recent years and is found in every level of society. Nasal, subcutaneous, intravascular, or intramuscular use of cocaine stimulates the central nervous system and leads to mood alterations. The user experiences a rush of pleasurable sensations and mood elevation. For the next 20 to 30 minutes, self-confidence, extreme excitement, hyperactivity, and hyperthermia of 3° to 5° F prevail. Pleasurable sensations soon give way to depression, fatigue, and the desire for more cocaine. There are physical effects of cocaine use; vasoconstriction, hypertension, and tachycardia can lead to arrhythmias, cerebrovascular accidents, myocardial infarction, pulmonary edema, and death (Smith, 1988) (Figure 26-4).

Maternal-to-fetal transfer of cocaine is swift and produces similar effects in the fetus. Cocaine and its metabolites are excreted by the fetal kidney into the amniotic fluid. The metabolites are even more potent than the original drug. The fetus swallows the amniotic fluid and recycles the metabolites through the system again. Thus the fetus is more exposed than the woman to the drug. Among other problems cases of maternal ingestion have been followed by birth of infants with cerebral infarcts (strokes) after sudden fetal hypertension (Chasnoff et al, 1987). Cocaine's teratogenic potential has been recognized only recently (see Chapter 27).

Prenatal use of cocaine stimulates the uterine smooth muscle (vasoconstrictive effect), leading to preterm labor that *does not respond to tocolytics*. Placental abruption secondary to vasoconstriction and hypertension may further compromise fetal well-being.

Risk

In a survey of 36 hospitals in the United States, 11% of women used illegal drugs. The most commonly used drug was cocaine (Chasnoff et al, 1985). Heroin use also is increasing. One quarter of a million women, most in the childbearing ages, use intravenously administered drugs. Self-disclosure of illicit drug use, however, markedly underestimates the real figures.

In addition to the effect of the drugs, many factors increase risk for the perinatal period. Infections transmitted by intravenous use or sexually transmitted disease, life-styles connected to abuse such as violence,

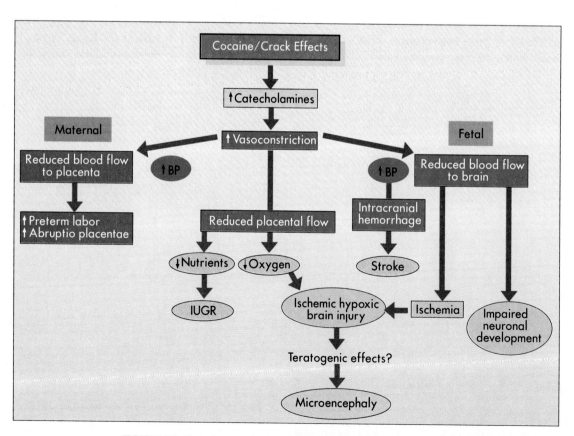

FIGURE 26-4 Pathway of injuries from cocaine or crack abuse.

crime, and sexual bargaining for drugs, and the effects of highs and lows in drug levels resulting in withdrawal syndrome will place the drug user in the highest risk category. Added to these factors are poor nutrition, infrequent prenatal care, and often an emotionally depressed mood or swings in mood, sometimes with suicidal tendencies.

In addition to the potential fetal effects, birth often is premature (30% to 40%). Prematurity and drug withdrawal increase the mortality rate of these infants (Janke, 1990). (See Chapter 28 for neonatal care.)

Signs

Signs of opioid intoxication and withdrawal are listed in Table 26-3.

Clinical Management

Risk assessment, including complete history, may be difficult at first because the substance abuser does not trust authority figures. Assessment for current or past infections is important. At each prenatal visit a urine specimen is obtained for toxicologic examination, as well as on admission to labor and during the early recovery period (Box 26-3). Protocols for drug screening vary by state. Some allow screening without consent, especially if a woman is admitted with overt signs. Others require notification of the client. Infants are routinely screened as close to birth as possible if there is any suspicion of maternal drug abuse. As Evans and Gillogley (1991) state, "Identification of perinatal chemical use should be for the purposes of medical and social intervention, not criminal prosecution." There is the problem of accuracy; comparisons between urine screening and self-report show more than 25% undetected users (Ostrea and Welch, 1991). In addition, clients may add water or salt to specimens, which will change test results. New techniques of hair and meconium analysis are much more accurate, rapid, and easier to do. Hair grows at 1 to 2 cm per month and therefore a history of drug use can be detected, with the most

---

BOX 26-3 Positive Urine Test Result after Last Adult Use

Alcohol: 8–16 hr
Amphetamines: 24–72 hr
Benzodiazepines: 2–3 wk
LSD: 2–3 days
Cocaine: 24–72 hr
Marijuana: 1–2 wk
Meperidine: 2–4 days (5–7 in infant)
Methadone: 1 wk or longer
Phencyclidine: 3–7 days

Data from Evans and Gilloghey, 1991.

---

recent use closest to the scalp. Meconium tests are not invasive and allow for rapid and accurate (87% to 95%) screening.

For the opiate user, methadone maintenance is recommended during pregnancy to avoid the withdrawal states and potentially reduce risk behavior related to seeking street drugs. In addition, the rationale for methadone maintenance is to provide the woman with 1 to 2 years in which, with regular contact with health care providers and group work, she has time to acquire the strength to abstain.

The pregnant woman on methadone maintenance continues her daily dose until the third trimester when the dosage may need to be increased or be given twice daily. Withdrawal is not wise during pregnancy. If the woman desires it strongly, it may be managed in the second trimester and doses must be tapered by only 1 mg/day. Regular fetal assessment is carried out during the period (Hoegerman and Schnoll, 1991). In any case the goal is to have the maternal dose less than 20 mg/day at the time of labor to reduce neonatal abstinence syndrome effects (see Chapter 28).

Because of the current shortage of programs for the substance abuser, assistance is unavailable to many

---

TABLE 26-3 Signs of Opioid Intoxication and Withdrawal

INTOXICATION	WITHDRAWAL
Mental confusion	Anxiety, tremulousness, irritability
Drowsiness or euphoria	Drug craving, desperate feelings, restlessness, poor sleeping
Decreased respirations	Hyperventilation, tachycardia, hypertension
Constipation	Diarrhea, abdominal cramps, vomiting, anorexia
Miosis	Mydriasis
Analgesia	Hypersensitivity, muscle spasms, aches; lacrimation, rhinorrhea, sweating, chills, flushing, piloerection

women, and waiting lists are long. When possible, a narcotics support group such as Narcotics Anonymous should be recommended or the woman can be invited to join a group conducted by the social services department. Additional assistance to reduce craving has been found by the use of acupuncture. Although few studies of pregnant women who use drugs are available, results seem promising. Alternative drugs such as naltrexone and clonidine are contraindicated during pregnancy (Hoegerman and Schnoll, 1991).

Nursing Responsibilities
PRENATAL CARE

On first visits to the clinic, most drug users are defensive and paranoid. They expect that initial counseling will include pressure to stop drug use and enter treatment. They may have been involved with prostitution, and they may have been jailed for shoplifting and other misdemeanors.

Statistics show that most heroin and methadone drug-addicted women have had two to four pregnancies. Thus some women may have children placed in foster care, or, as they perceive it, taken away from them. In abortive attempts to reclaim other children or in an effort to reestablish in some measure their claim to be responsible, they may have attempted to obtain treatment. In contrast, many users of cocaine appear to have no immediate problem and belong to the middle or upper socioeconomic class of society.

The nurse needs to keep in mind the general traits of the addicted personality. Some of the more common characteristics follow. The person will attempt to be manipulative by trying to please the counselor but seldom is truthful. She may falsify the amount of daily drug intake because a large amount reinforces a feeling of being "bad." She may make unsolicited promises, saying that she is in the process of becoming involved in rehabilitation or is already involved.

The nurse's approach must be understanding regardless of personal feelings, keeping in mind the addictive profile. This means adopting a firm, consistent, direct manner in seeking information for medical purposes and in counseling for the possible prevention of deterioration during the pregnancy.

If the client comes for prenatal care, it can be assumed that she has made the choice to come of her own accord for the sake of the baby. Because she usually has low self-esteem, the pregnancy represents a way to feel human again. Nonsympathetic personnel who may not be acquainted with the psychology of the addicted woman may force their solutions on her through manipulative persuasion. Such an approach eradicates any cooperation the client might give.

On the other hand, counseling toward traditional health maintenance is a waste of time with the client who is addicted to heroin or crack. She is likely to continue her same destructive patterns until late in pregnancy. Recognizing this, the nurse should avoid becoming frustrated in attempts to counsel or place restrictions on her regarding nutrition, hygiene, and rest.

The best chance of helping the client usually occurs toward the end of the second trimester, because she begins to worry about the infant's health. At this point, she may be persuaded to adhere to some of the most important aspects of prenatal care.

Nutrition is critical. The mother should be encouraged to increase her protein intake in every possible way. For example, sweets probably constitute the major part of her usual diet. To be useful and realistic, diet substitutions should be in keeping with what she will eat. Vitamins, folic acid, and iron will be prescribed and should be stressed as supplements necessary for the baby's health.

Personal hygiene and sexual habits are serious considerations for counseling. Because prostitution may continue, it is not unusual for the client to contract venereal disease very late in pregnancy after routine screening.

BIRTH

Toward the latter part of pregnancy, the client will be concerned about the infant's response to drugs. She needs as much information as possible about the drug's effect on the infant. She should know that the baby will be passively addicted and that the infant's degree of difficulty will depend on the extent of her habit. She can be reassured, however, that because of the absence of psychologic dependency in the baby, medical treatment usually alleviates withdrawal symptoms.

Many drug users show evidence of drug use on the day of admission to labor. Because of the inability to determine how much drug a mother has in her system, regional rather than general anesthesia is used.

Finally, the nurse, remembering that this client usually has not attended the clinic regularly or participated in classes in preparation for childbirth, must be especially alert and watchful for untoward responses during labor.

POSTNATAL CARE

After delivery the client's first concern usually is to satisfy her need for drugs. If she is not on a methadone regimen or receiving tranquilizers, a heroin user will make attempts to acquire drugs through visitors from the outside to avoid withdrawal symptoms (nausea, tremors, sweating, abdominal pain, cramps, and yawning) that may appear 2 or 3 hours after delivery, depending on the time of her last intake.

The nurse must be alert to the possibility of the client stealing from other clients and must not leave medication rooms or carts unguarded. There should be unobtrusive surveillance of visitors to a drug-addicted client when she is not separated from other clients.

Fears of separation from the baby may be intensified after delivery because in most instances the infant is placed in an intensive care unit for observation and treatment (see Chapter 28). A social worker will be involved in placement of the baby in foster care until the mother is completely drug free or involved in an approved program for rehabilitation.

The client must understand that certain behaviors are unacceptable and will not be tolerated. Such structure should be made clear at the time of initial contact to afford the client the opportunity to change her behavior. For example, when a client is abusing drugs, she needs to be educated on the risks of this behavior to herself and the fetus. She should be informed that help is available to her. The police generally are involved only if the client is observed in the process of illegal activity such as theft or using or selling illegal substances.

Reporting Child Abuse

In all cases in which the mother has been known to be abusing drugs, child protection agencies should be involved as soon as the baby is born. Although confidentiality is an issue, it is a professional's responsibility to report the suspicion of child abuse or neglect to the proper authorities for further investigation.

However, the client herself has constitutional rights to privacy, to freedom from unreasonable search and seizure, to due process, and to equal protection. She has the right, if deemed competent, to refuse care. In addition, nurses are responsible for their own actions toward the client and should recognize that even well-intentioned interventions may be in violation of her rights (Grad, 1981). In cases in which the nurse is unsure of how to proceed, the agency administration, legal or risk management department, and ethics committee should be consulted (see Chapter 1).

Promoting Bonding

All clients deserve respect and courteous treatment by the health care team. The client may need to have limits set, but she should not be denied access to her baby after birth. To separate mother from baby interferes with bonding, which is even more critical when there is a potential for mother-infant attachment disorders. She should be encouraged to visit the infant, and all efforts should be made to facilitate her efforts to modify the

social situation to provide safe care for the child. There are not enough foster homes for children, and the **boarder babies,** infants remaining in the nursery because they cannot be discharged to their parents for medical or social reasons, are a serious growing problem. The client needs to know that staff members care about her and are willing to help her in any way to regain custody. Often when limits are set for her, such as the state's refusal to discharge a baby for social reasons, the client feels punished, which enforces her feelings of hopelessness and loss of control. She needs to be reminded that the baby is hers and that, by taking the steps prescribed, she will be able to take the infant home as soon as the social situation is stable. *This client cannot tolerate surprise.* She should be warned long in advance about delays in infant discharge, which can help restore some control and offer her the guidance and support she needs to begin to learn to meet her self-care needs.

Three Models of Care

Much has been written about home care and follow-up care, and the practical application of care has taken several creative directions. What follows are three models of care that illustrate that nurses and the health care team have not yet found an ideal approach but are trying to reach the perinatal client in a holistic, person-in-environment way.

NURSE ADVOCATE: PORTSMOUTH, VIRGINIA

Portsmouth is a Navy town with transients, substance abuse, lonely people away from home, and poverty. The baby care program was set up to use a case-management approach in which a nurse would receive an average caseload of 50 women at high risk to follow from first referral until 2 months after the birth of the baby. The nurse may work out of her home, making home visits, meeting clients at the clinic, and problem solving over the telephone. The nurse in essence becomes the **advocate** for the client, being the personal *care giver,* urging her to keep appointments, talking to her physician about problems, interpreting health care recommendations, and helping her with financial applications for assistance. For this intervention, which often took 1 to 2 hours per week and sometimes more, the nurses received approximately $50 per month per client.

Roberta Paige, RN, MSN, was a hospice nurse before becoming a case manager in the baby care program. She believed that her experience helped her to be an advocate in representing her clients' interests against institutional strictures and societal problems that prevented good care. Listed below are examples of her weekly activities.

My role as client advocate and case manager is to hear the pregnant woman's concerns, assess needs, and facilitate services to gain the best possible outcome of the pregnancy. I make home visits, as well as school and clinic visits, as needed. I do most of my work over the telephone. I make appointments, follow through to see that the client keeps appointments, and put her in contact with church and support groups that may be able to help. Table 26-4 contains a partial list of available services in my area. You would have to discover what is available in your area.

Homelessness has become more of a problem in the last few years. I am dealing primarily on the first and second levels of need. I am a caring presence for the client throughout the pregnancy and for 60 days after the birth, if she doesn't disappear. I do crisis management. I always start with her own felt needs and work from there to her education and care needs. Here are some typical sample cases.

Case Examples

Case. Karen, 23, para 1041. Her young son was in the husband's custody. Separated, she was living with her sister. She went to many doctors for a backache to get pain medication and became addicted to these analgesics. I referred her to Medicaid and to Resource Mothers, but she remained difficult to reach. Finally, she got into a drug counseling program. They asked me not to confront her but to inform her doctor. The father of the baby talked with me because she wanted to give up the baby for adoption. After the birth she decided to take the baby home but was unprepared with supplies. The hospital staff was very concerned and called me. I helped her find these supplies. Her Medicaid was cut off because of continuing drug use and I helped her get Medicaid for the infant. Four months after the birth she put the baby up for adoption.

Case. Charlene, age 13 in grade 7, para 0000. She was very concerned about the baby and the pregnancy but not willing to press charges of statutory rape against the 18-year-old father. She lives with her mother and sister and the sister's 1-year-old son. The grandmother will care for both children after the birth. She attended a school program but was very irregular in attendance because of frequent nonphysiologic headaches. Charlene

TABLE 26-4 A Partial Regional List of Free Services for High-Risk Pregnant Women

NEED	SOURCE
• Car seat	Local hospital through Department of Motor Vehicles
• Maternity clothing	Local church clothing closet
• Layette	Crisis pregnancy center if registered early
• Social support	Local churches
• Formula	Women, infants, and children (WIC) program
• Lactation consultant	WIC program
• Nutrition counseling	WIC program
• Financial support	Aid to Dependent Children (ADC) if father absent
	Infant stimulation program
• Occupational and physical therapy for high-risk infants	Medicaid services are retroactive for 3 months before
• Prenatal care	pregnancy and extend to 60 days after; Medicaid for
• Free transport to clinic appointments	infant available for 1 year
• Phone for 2½ months during pregnancy	
• Eye and dental care if under 21	
• Eyeglasses	Lions Club
• Free crib	Life support group
• Help to get education and into job programs	"Stop" support group
• Support groups for HIV-positive women	AIDS crisis task force
• Support group for women who miscarry	Empty Arms
• Support group for new parents	Good Beginnings
• Pay employer part cost of training	Job Training and Partnership Act
• Diabetes Supplies	Food bank
• Free counseling	Drug counseling program
• Residential program for drug withdrawal	Difficult to get a place
• Help from experienced older mother	Resource Mothers
• Schooling for pregnant girls	Board of Education/private centers

wants to be a lawyer. I made a number of appointments for her, which she did not keep. However, she had a healthy baby girl. She talked with me about getting Norplant. At 60 days after birth she still had not gone to the clinic. I made another appointment, which she did keep. A little gain here—a healthy baby and hopefully she will not be pregnant again this year and will continue school.

Case. Barbara, para 0040, now pregnant, has severe chronic hypertension. I arranged for a home health aide and homemaker. She was on bed rest with bathroom privileges throughout the last two trimesters. She delivered a 33-week, IUGR, 1800 g boy who did well. She decided she wanted him to have a sibling and became pregnant within 6 weeks even though she is now separated from her husband. At our visit for this pregnancy, she discussed having a BTL after this birth. Her husband came in and out of the picture. She was again on modified bed rest with a homemaker. At 30 weeks she called me to report swollen painful legs. I called the physician, and she was hospitalized. An emergency cesarean delivery was performed. The baby survived only 1 month in NICU. I attended the funeral and maintained contact. Although she had a lot of support from her church, she grieved a long time because she had gone ahead with the tubal ligation.

Case. Janine, 18, became pregnant after rape by a person of rank in the military. She did not press charges because she was told it would be of no avail. At the time she had only limited rape counseling. She has now become engaged to another man who is very supportive. She was crying throughout our first interview and complained of many physical discomforts, but she was not receptive to further counseling.

Her presenting concern was how to afford baby clothes. I helped her obtain these plus aid from WIC and food stamps. I found information on a Pell grant and college admission to help her look forward to life after the baby. She needed eyeglasses and dental work, and I helped her obtain these services. I called her every other day and listened to her concerns and expression of feelings. She did well through the birth and is now settled with her new partner.

Case. Denise was living with the father of her 10-month-old baby and was 4 months pregnant. A 2-year-old child was in custody of an aunt. She was referred to me for case coordination, counseling on nutrition, and smoking cessation, and domestic violence. She had been in several shelters but was dismissed for noncompliance. I went to see her at her aunt's home. She told me that nurses hadn't helped her before and that all she needed was a place to live away from the father. She could not stay at the aunt's because of lease problems. I went through the question-

naire with her and saw that her needs were severe enough to warrant immediate intervention. I called several shelters until I found a shelter in an adjoining town that would take her. She called me the next day and said she was leaving that shelter. I reminded her that she would wind up on the street and could lose her son. She said she would rather end up on the street. I will continue trying to work with this particular client but will involve protective services for the 10-month-old baby.

The following brief descriptions summarize other types of cases.

Case Examples

Ginny. Ginny is a homeless married woman with a supportive husband, has two children, ages 11 and 2, an 11-month-old infant, and was expecting a baby any day. She has diabetes and needed Chem-strips, which I arranged for her from the food bank. I helped her find a baby-sitter from a local church when she was ready to go into labor. We discussed birth control, but she stated that it cost too much.

Billi May. Billi May mainly wanted her children, ages 4 and 6, to be with her during the birth. I helped her arrange that, and she was very appreciative.

Gina. Gina drank six beers a day and complained of limited food money. She missed many appointments and had a preterm baby with respiratory complications. Again she is pregnant by a different man. Her mother stopped offering her support, and Gina asked me for help. I involved the infant stimulation program for the baby with respiratory problems, but the grandmother, who apparently has custody, refused those services. I have talked with Gina about birth control, but she just laughs.

Mary. Mary is 43 and had been repeatedly told to see a geneticist for her now 28-week pregnancy. She wanted the pregnancy, and I was very supportive of her continuing to carry the child. She cannot afford to stop working, even though she often is fatigued and has leg cramping.

Summary

In summary, this kind of nursing requires persistence, patience, and developed listening skills. Sometimes nurses leave because of frustration with how slow people are to change. If you can gain satisfaction from small steps, "baby steps," you can do a great deal for these high-risk women. It provides a creative way to use all your nursing knowledge as well as developing skill in working with a system of health care that often is difficult to access. I would like to say to nursing students that the *client and her environment* must be considered in every plan.

INCORPORATING SPIRITUALITY INTO THE PROGRAM: BOSTON*

Boston Department of Health and Hospitals' Healthy Baby and Healthy Child Programs are designed to reduce the unacceptably high infant mortality in Boston's poor neighborhoods. The black infant mortality rate in these neighborhoods was 20.9 per 1000 in 1988, as opposed to 8.11 in the white, more affluent areas of Boston. Public health nurses, neighborhood health advocates, and neighborhood health centers have collaborated closely to follow high-risk pregnant women and their children for up to 3 years.

Since many of the risk factors are psychosocial and economic, traditional prenatal care hasn't sufficed for this population. In 1989, only 50.1% of black pregnant women got prenatal care, as compared with 80.1% of white pregnant women in Boston (The Task Force, 1991). We widened the focus of care to recognize culture and spirituality of those we serve.

We also included advocacy to help clients meet basic needs like food and housing. We have found that if we pay attention to these aspects of their lives, many more women develop trust in their providers and seek and remain in care. Home visiting, teaching, support, advocacy are the program's major interventions.

An important step in designing a program like this was to recruit and retain a multicultural staff that reflects the composition of the community. Nurses and neighborhood health advocates thus provide the client with a more familiar, comfortable link to the often-intimidating health care system.

The program provided training that explored and promoted respect for everyone's cultural background. When white European-American nurses met with staff from Haitian, Hispanic, and African-American cultures, they often became more aware of their own ethnic background.

Public health nurses in urban areas increasingly confront problems of drugs, alcohol, disorganization, and violence that touch a growing number of families. Not only do they see the effects on their clients, but may fear for their own safety. Nurses in a recent study said they continued this work often "at the expense of their souls" (Zerwekh, 1991).

Staff and administration need to be honest about the spiritual drain of the work and take steps to maintain and promote staff well-being. Simple measures that recognize each staff member as an individual help counteract the spiritual drain and strengthen the nurse's ability to extend herself to the client. A structure that promotes sharing, mutual support, and recognition of spirituality can be developed. For example, at the beginning of selected meetings a "check-in time" is held, so all staff persons can relate whatever they wish about job or personal events. Team meetings begin with staff volunteering to lead a moment of meditation/prayer or read a passage from booklets with affirmations like the ones put out by 12-step programs.

Relating case stories informally or at case conferences validates the spiritual aspect of nursing practice and illustrates that the expression of spiritual needs is not an isolated or infrequent part of the client's care. Inservice education programs can contribute to increased awareness and comfort with the topic. A staff who can appreciate cultural diversity and maintain their own well-being can address the spiritual needs of their clients.

SATELLITE OUTREACH: NEW YORK CITY*

Mobile and Homeless Services

The Community Family Planning Council's (CFPC) commitment to providing quality health care services to those who have little or no access to care led us to initiate a prenatal program for pregnant homeless women 5 years ago.

With New York State Department of Health support, CFPC purchased a recreational vehicle and converted it into a mobile clinic, complete with private examination room, laboratory, bathroom, and reception area. We use this "clinic on wheels" to bring prenatal care to residents of two city-run shelters in the East New York and Brownsville sections of Brooklyn (Figure 26-5).

The prenatal services provided from the mobile unit are as comprehensive as those available at any of our

* Community Family Planning Council, 184 Fifth Ave., New York, NY 10010.

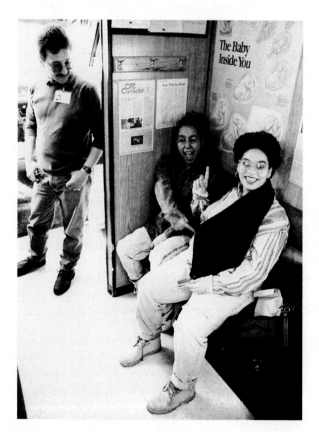

FIGURE 26-5 Mobile prenatal clinic provides services to homeless women on the street and in shelters. (Courtesy Ross Whitaker, Community Family Planning Council, New York, N.Y.)

* Reprinted from Corrine et al: *MCN* 17(3):145, 1992: reprinted by permission of MCN.

other clinics. Clients receive a complete physical examination and all of the other services and referrals normally available to a prenatal client. These include tests for potential problems such as diabetes, anemia, sexually transmitted diseases, and hepatitis B. Patients are counseled about HIV and have the opportunity to test. Those whose test reactions are positive can receive primary medical care at our nearby United Parents Center.

Health education and nutrition play important roles during prenatal visits, and an individual nutrition plan is developed for each client. Fruits, cheese, juices, and other healthful foods are available at each session. Everyone receives basic information about labor, delivery, baby care, breast-feeding, circumcision, and what to expect after the baby is born (Figure 26-6). Contraceptive methods for use after delivery are discussed.

Follow-up of homeless clients often is a problem, and some leave the shelters. Client mobility also is partly the result of various agency regulations that require them to move at various times under various circumstances. Some, however, remain and make use of the services offered. They deliver at an affiliated hospital, just as those seen at our other clinics. CFPC nurses are available in the shelters 24 hours a day.

The women we see at the Mobile Clinic have few resources, either personal or institutional. They usually have exhausted any help family or friends might have been able to give, and they have difficulty accessing public services. CFPC is alone in making prenatal care available and *accessible* to homeless women (Figure 26-7). The most unique service provided by CFPC is that care is delivered in an atmosphere of respect and

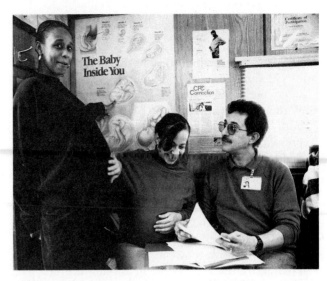

FIGURE 26-7 Individual teaching for pregnancy and continuing health care are included in each visit. (Courtesy Ross Whitaker, Community Family Planning Council, New York, N.Y.)

caring, qualities frequently absent in services for the homeless. This attitude fosters positive client behavior.

Usually the clients at the Mobile Clinic reach us in their second or third trimester and have had no other prenatal care. Many are HIV-positive, have one or more sexually transmitted diseases, and have encountered many difficulties in their lives. Most have used drugs or are currently addicted. Many have prostituted themselves to stay alive or buy drugs. Deep psychologic problems are common.

We help clients get into drug treatment programs and support groups. With the client's permission, we can arrange for a psychologist from Woodhull Hospital to provide a psychiatric on-site evaluation and help the client follow through on resulting referrals.

In addition to providing medical care, we enroll clients in Medicaid and WIC, the federal food subsidy program for mothers and young children, and help them obtain other social services for which they qualify.

Funding for this project, other than the cost of the van, has come from the New York City Human Resources Administration; grants from the Public Welfare Fund, the Robin Hood Foundation, and the ADCO Foundation; and Medicaid reimbursements.

On-Site Services

In February of 1993, CFPC began delivering prenatal and social services at another Human Resources Administration shelter—the East Third Street shelter on the lower east side. The services at this shelter are provided at a part-time clinic in the shelter itself rather than from the mobile unit. The services are otherwise identical and include 24-hour, on-site nursing.

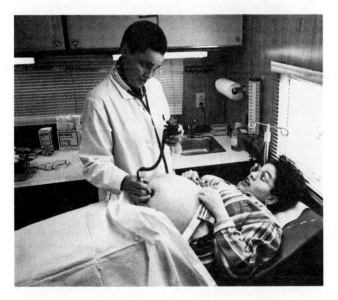

FIGURE 26-6 All prenatal services are located in the mobile clinic so that women do not have to wait long hours for care. (Courtesy Ross Whitaker, Community Family Planning Council, New York, N.Y.)

KEY POINTS

- Each person functions to meet basic needs according to a hierarchy of needs that require physiological and safety needs to be met first.
- Without the basic needs of belongingness and love, both children and adults become angry and depressed, feeling that no one cares about them. Esteem and self-actualization needs, however, cannot be addressed while the more basic needs are unmet.
- There are developmental crises and situational crises. Pregnancy is a developmental crisis in that it demands growth and coping in new ways. It may become a situational crisis as well if high-risk conditions are present.
- Loss and grief often occur in varying degrees. The client needs to know the process of mourning to understand the normality of grieving the loss of her goal to have a child.
- Spiritual distress arises from the deepest core of one's being and can be recognized by defining characteristics.
- Anxiety reduces the ability to perceive and communicate. Interventions are aimed at reducing anxiety to a level at which the client may cope with the threatening situation.

- Crisis presents an opportunity for growth or a danger of reduced functioning. Interventions support coping.
- Pregnancy of clients who are socially at high risk is complicated by social problems that have chronic roots and thus are difficult to solve. The helping person needs to have patience in these interactions.
- Underlying hopelessness, depression, and despair may prevent a client from taking actions that could empower her to change a situation.
- Empowerment as a way out of despair includes increasing personal, interpersonal, or political power to improve a situation.
- Four changes appear to be necessary: increasing self-efficacy, developing group consciousness, reducing self-blame, and assuming personal accountability to change a situation.
- Substance abuse in clients is an example of the need for crisis intervention and long-term involvement in change.
- Nurse advocacy for change is an important part of planning nursing support of clients who are socially at high risk.

STUDY QUESTIONS

26-1 Which of the Key Terms in this chapter could be used in the following statements?
  a. Inability to deal with a situation or follow advice because more pressing needs are present is an example of _____.
  b. Self-destructive behavior such as crack use is a manifestation of _____.
  c. An example of _____ occurs when a client promises to improve behavior in the future if the current distress will go away.
  d. A child especially feels _____ when incest or sexual abuse occurs.
  e. Being enabled to take action to improve one's life situation is to experience _____.
  f. The unexpected birth of a baby with a defect is a _____ crisis.
  g. The nurse who helps the client use avenues of assistance is acting as an: _____.
26-2 The infant of a substance-abusing mother will be retained in hospital until the woman has
  a. Recovered fully from birth.
  b. Promised to stop drug intake.
  c. Found a suitable care giver in the extended family.
  d. Entered a treatment program.

26-3 When a client is abusing illegal drugs, you should:
  a. Inform her that she will have to be reported to the police.
  b. Counsel her on possible effects of the drugs on her body and fetus and offer assistance in finding a treatment program.
  c. Maintain confidentiality even if she is observed using or selling illegal substances.
  d. Ignore the situation because paying attention to the problem reinforces negative behavior.
26-4 The client who is experiencing moderate anxiety levels:
  a. Learns easily because this level increases activation and awareness.
  b. Will forget instructions because of poor perception.
  c. Should receive a calming agent.
  d. Needs a quiet, undemanding environment until levels diminish.
26-5 Either crack or cocaine may cause:
  a. Hypotension and syncope.
  b. EEG changes and dilated pupils.
  c. Tachycardia and hypertension.
  d. Hypoglycemia.

26-6 The fetus is affected most seriously by maternal crack use because of
   a. Cerebral anoxia.
   b. Vasoconstriction.
   c. Reduction in amniotic fluid volumes.
   d. Delayed or postmature birth.

26-7 What is the benefit of hair analysis for substance abuse compared with urine samples?
   a. No opportunity to modify the sample.
   b. Easily obtained without consent.
   c. Provides a history of drug intake.
   d. Results are rapidly available.

Answer Key

26-1 a. Hierarchy of needs, b. Despair, c. Bargaining, d. Self-blame, e. Empowerment, f. Situational, g. Advocate, 26-2 c and d 26-3 b 26-4 b 26-5 c 26-6 c 26-7 a and d

REFERENCES

Aguilera DC: *Crisis intervention: theory and methodology,* ed 7, St Louis, 1994, Mosby.

Amaro H et al: Violence during pregnancy and substance use, *Am J Public Health* 80:575, 1990.

Bailey DN: Drug screening in an unconventional matrix: hair analysis, *JAMA* 262:3331, 1989.

Baird SF: Crisis intervention strategies. In Johnson SH, ed: *Nursing assessment and strategies for the family at risk: high risk parenting,* ed 2, Philadelphia, 1986, JB Lippincott.

Beatty J et al: Anger generated by unmet expectations, *MCN* 10(9):324, 1985.

Boston Department of Health and Hospitals, Perinatal Capacity Task Force: Hospital survey report, Boston, 1991, The Task Force.

Byme MW, Lerner HM: Communicating with addicted women in labor, *MCN* 17(1):22, 1991.

Chasnoff, IJ et al: Cocaine use in pregnancy, *N Engl J Med* 313:666, 1985.

Chavkin W, Allen MH, Oberman M: Drug abuse and pregnancy: some questions on public policy, clinical management, and maternal and fetal rights, *Birth* 18(2):107, 1991.

Chisum GM: Nursing interventions with the antepartum substance abuser, *J Perinatol Neonat Nurs* 3(4):25, 1990.

Christiano A: Knowledge and perceptions of HIV infections among homeless pregnant women, *J Nurse Midwife* 34(6):318, 1989.

Connolly WB Jr, Marshall AB: Drug addiction, pregnancy and childbirth: legal issues for the medical and social services communities, *Clin Perinatol* 18(1):147, 1991.

Corrine L et al: The unheard voices of women: spiritual interventions in maternal-child health, *MCN* 17(3):141, 1992.

Davis LV, Hagen JL: The problem of wife abuse, *J Soc Work* 37(1):15, 1992.

Day NL, Richardson GA: Prenatal marijuana use: epidemiologic methodologic issues and infant outcomes, *Clin Perinatol* 18(1):77, 1991.

Evans AT, Gillogley KM: Drug use in pregnancy: obstetric perspectives, *Clin Perinatol* 18(1):25, 1991.

Fisher LY: Nursing management of the pregnant psychotic patient during labor and delivery, *JOGNN* 17(1):25, 1988.

Gillogley KM et al: The perinatal impact of cocaine, amphetamine and opiate use detected by universal intrapartum screening, *Am J Obstet Gynecol* 163:1535, 1990.

Grad F: *Public health law manual,* Washington DC, 1981, American Public Health Association.

Green NL: Stressful events related to childbearing in African-American women: a pilot study, *J Nurse Midwife* 35(4):2, 1990.

Gutiérrez LM: Working with women of color: an empowerment perspective, *Social Work* 35(2):149, 1990.

Hays D: Teaching a concept of anxiety, *Nurs Res* 10(1):108, 1961.

Heinowitz J: *Pregnant fathers,* Englewood Cliffs, NJ, 1982, Prentice Hall.

Helton AS: Protocol of care for the battered woman, White Plains, NY, 1987, March of Dimes Birth Defects Foundation.

Helton AS, Snodgrass FG: Battering during pregnancy: intervention strategies, *Birth* 14:142, 1987.

Hoegerman G, Schnoll S: Narcotic use in pregnancy, *Clin Perinatol* 18(1):51, 1991.

Infante MS: *Crisis theory: a framework for nursing practice,* Reston, Va, 1982, Reston Publishing.

Janke JR: Prenatal cocaine use: effects on perinatal outcome, *J Nurse Midwife* 35(2):74, 1990.

Johnson AK, Kreuger LW: Toward a better understanding of homeless women, *Social Work* 343(6):481, 1989.

Jones DA: HIV-seropositive childbearing women: nursing management, *JOGNN* 20(6):446, 1991.

Kim MJ, McFarland GK, McLane AM: *Pocket guide to nursing diagnoses,* ed 5, St Louis, 1993, Mosby.

Kokotailo PK, Adger H Jr: Substance abuse by pregnant adolescents, *Clin Perinatol* 18(1):125, 1991.

Kus R: Crisis intervention. In Bullecheck G, McCloskey J, eds: *Nursing interventions: treatments for nursing diagnoses,* Philadelphia, 1985, WB Saunders.

Kushner H: *When bad things happen to good people,* New York, 1981, Avon Press.

Laguardia KD et al: Maternity shelter care for adolescents—its effect on incidence of low birth weight, *Am J Obstet Gynecol* 161(2):303, 1989.

Maslow A: *Motivation and personality,* ed 2, New York, 1970, Harper & Row.

Mitchell PH: Concepts basic to nursing, New York, 1973, McGraw-Hill.

Nagai-Jacobson MG, Buckhardt MA: Spirituality cornerstone of holistic nursing practice, *Holist Nurs Pract* 3:18, 1989.

Norbeck JS, Anderson NJ: Psychosocial predictors of pregnancy outcomes in low-income black, Hispanic, and white women, *Nurs Res* 38(4):204, 1989.

Ostrea EM, Welch RA: Detection of prenatal drug exposure in the pregnant woman and her newborn infant, *Clin Perinatol* 18(3):629, 1991.

Panuthos C, Romero C: *Ended beginnings: healing childbirth losses,* Boston, 1984, Bergin & Garvey.

Parker B, and McFarlane J: Identifying and helping the battered pregnant woman, *MCN* 16(3):161, 1991.

Policy statement: Health care for homeless pregnant teenagers, *Am J Public Health* 81(2):242, 1991.

Policy statement: Illicit drug use by pregnant women, *Am J Public Health* 81(2):253, 1991.

Reid NJ: *Family problem solving,* New York, 1985, Columbia University Press.

Shelton BJ, Gill DG: Childbearing in prison: a behavioral analysis, *JOGNN* 18(4):301, 1989.

Stiles MK: The shining stranger: nurse-family spiritual relationship, *Cancer Nurs* 13(4):235, 1990.

Tunis SL, Golbus MS: Assessing mood states in pregnancy: survey of the literature, *Obstet Gynecol Surv* 46(6):340, 1991.

Volland PJ: Discharge planning: an interdisciplinary approach to continuity of care, Owings Mills, Md, 1988, National Health Publishing.

Wheeler E, Gardiner K: Nurses' and patients' perception of supportive nursing, *J NY State Nurses Assoc* 18(2):33, 1987.

Young EW: Incest trauma, *J Psychosoc Nurs* 25(5):33, 1987.

Zerwekh JV: At the expense of their souls, *Nurs Outlook* 39:58, 1991.

STUDENT RESOURCE SHELF

Bohn DK: Domestic violence and pregnancy: implications for practice, *J Nurse Midwife* 35(2):86, 1990. Characteristics of battered women and children and of abusing men, with available resources.

Corrine L et al: The unheard voices of women: spiritual interventions in maternal-child health, *MCN* 17(3):141, 1992. Practical application of interventions for spiritual distress, with cultural variations recognized and explained.

Moleti CA: Caring for socially high risk patients, *MCN* 13(1):24, 1988. A summary of useful nursing interventions illustrated by use of a case study.

Six

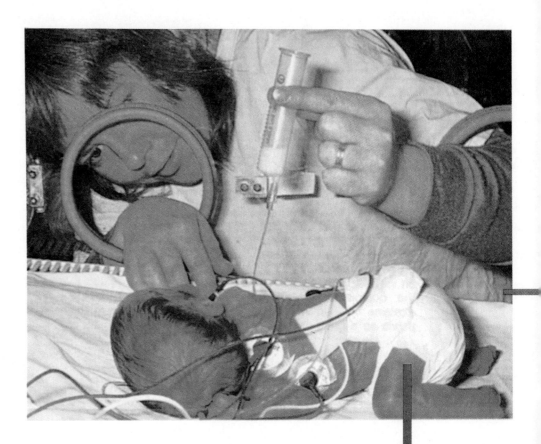

NEWBORN AT RISK

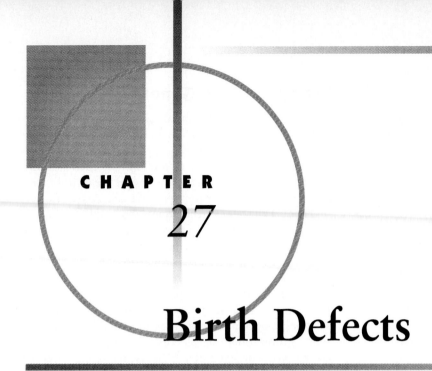

Birth Defects

KEY TERMS

Allele
Autosome
Birth Defect
Chromosome
Codominance
Deletion
Dominant Trait
Duplication
Expressivity
Fragile X (Fra X)
Gene
Genetic Drift
Genome
Genotype
Hemizygous
Heterozygous
Homozygous
Independent
  Assortment
Karyotype
Locus (pl. Loci)
Monosomy

Mosaic
Multifactorial
  Inheritance
Mutation
Nondisjunction
Oncogenes
Pedigree
Penetrance
Phenotype

Polygenic Inheritance
Punnett Square
Recessive Trait
Retinoblastoma (Rb)
Segregation
Teratogen
Translocation
Trisomy
X-linked Defect

LEARNING OBJECTIVES

1. *Identify the normal human male and female karyotypes.*
2. *Explain the relationship between chromosomes and genes.*
3. *Describe how deviations from normal genetic structure can affect the developing fetus.*
4. *Using a Punnett square, predict the risk of inheriting a dominant, recessive, or X-linked condition.*
5. *Explain the mechanism of inheritance and effects on development for selected genetic diseases.*
6. *Correlate etiologic factors with appearance of selected birth defects.*
7. *Describe the effects of major teratogens on fetal development.*
8. *Summarize the general sequence of genetic counseling.*
9. *Distinguish nursing responsibilities within the health care team when birth defects occur.*

When a baby is born with a **birth defect,** the parents are shocked and upset and ask for reasons. The medical staff investigates possible causes, and nurses care for the parents and infant. Thus it is important to have an overview of the events that can change the normal pattern of fetal growth and development. These adverse changes may occur through genetic inheritance or result from teratogenic factors during pregnancy. When an infant is born with a defect, the parents will need support, information, and counseling. This role may be difficult, but its function is essential with these parents.

From the time of Mendel in 1865 until the early 1900s, very few people understood the significance of genetic inheritance. It was not even described until 1941, when Beadle and Tatum hypothesized that "one **gene** controlled one enzyme." This entirely new concept became an essential principle in current genetic research. In addition, it was not understood until 1956 that chromosomal makeup consisted of 22 matched pairs of **autosomes** and 1 pair of sex **chromosomes** in each body cell (Figure 27-1).

The major groups of chromosomes were first recognized in 1960 at a meeting of cytogeneticists in Denver, Colorado. The length of each chromosome and the placement of the centromere (a small constriction separating the chromosome's short and long arms) are used to arrange them in the order of descending size. Pairs of autosomes are numbered serially from 1 to 22; the two sex chromosomes become pair 23. A high-powered microscope is used to photograph the darkly stained chromsosomes. The Denver classification arranges them into a **karyotype.**

Chromosome banding took the research a step further, and the technique of banding allows researchers to identify regions of each chromosome. Large deletions and duplications are seen as abnormal bands. Regions of particular chromosomes can be correlated with known defects (e.g., retinoblastoma). In this manner many diseases can be classified as genetic in origin and can be assigned to a particular chromosome. Currently a large-scale effort is under way using DNA technology to map the location of every gene in the human **genome** (complete set of genes in each cell) to provide detailed knowledge of the genetic basis for many diseases, some of which may not now be considered to have a genetic cause.

Importance of Genetic Studies

Because of advances in technology, the basic principles of genetics can be applied to human beings; as a result, gene mapping leads to a series of positive applications and to many ethical questions. Research in molecular genetics already has resulted in gene therapy, or the introduction of normal genes where nonoperative genes exist (Rosenfeld et al, 1992). Such techniques also lead to important questions of normalcy because, currently, normal genes can be inserted only into cells of an affected organ, not into sex cells (oocytes or spermatozoa).

In the last few years, research has identified gene groups that indicate susceptibility to heart attack, emphysema, multiple sclerosis, insulin-dependent diabetes, schizophrenia, and some types of cancer. It is known that chromosomal defects exist in many neoplastic conditions. For example, there is a missing piece of chromosome 22 in the bone marrow cells of persons with chronic myelogenous leukemia; this piece has been found attached to chromosome 9.

Mental retardation, which affects 3% of the population in the United States, is thought to be related in 80% of cases to a genetic cause. A very high rate of spontaneous first-trimester abortion (50%) is related to chromosome abnormality. In addition, some cases of infertility and many disorders of polygenic origin have genetic bases. Thus it is apparent that genetic disorders cause a significant portion of health deficits.

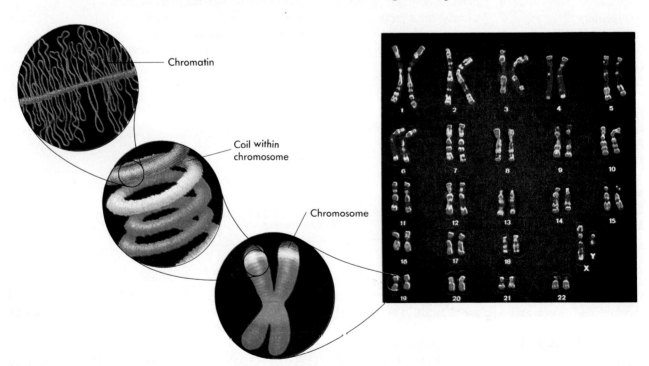

FIGURE 27-1 Human chromosomes. Each of the 46 human chromosomes, arranged here in numbered pairs—called a *karyotype*—is a coiled mass of chromatin (DNA). (From Rolin Graphics and CNRI/Science Photo Library.)

In this age of rapid change, health professionals must advocate positive support of persons with genetic disorders while working to reduce the potential occurrence of defects. Because of pollutants and radioactivity in the environment, new mutations may occur. The task of prevention has a number of aspects; certainly, preventive care is important to reduce the incidence of mental retardation.

Genetics must be a major focus in maternal and infant care. Concerned parents are seeking preconception, prenatal, and postnatal counseling. An understanding of genetic inheritance is required to know about basic defects, their frequency, and the referral process for counseling when parents ask for help during pregnancy or after birth.

GENETIC CODE

Deoxyribonucleic acid (DNA) carries the genetic information that will be passed to each generation of cells. It is a blueprint for the production of proteins, both structural and functional (enzymes). If the DNA in one human cell could be unraveled and stretched, it would be over 2 yards long. The structure, however, actually is two molecules built like two spiral staircases circling one another. The backbone of each spiral is made of a sugar called *deoxyribose*. One of four nucleic acids is attached to each sugar; the acids form pairs across the staircase to the complementing strand to make a double helix. The acids always pair in the same way: *adenine* (A) with *thymine* (T) and *cytosine* (C) with *guanine* (G) (Figure 27-2). When a cell divides, the DNA must be replicated. The double helix is pulled apart while a new strand from each of the old strands is synthesized (Figure 27-3).

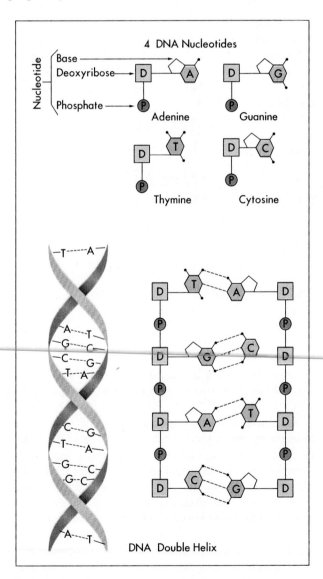

FIGURE 27-2 Base pairings between two nucleotides from double helix of DNA. (From Vander AJ, Sherman JH, Luciano DS: *Human physiology*, ed 4, New York, 1986, McGraw-Hill.)

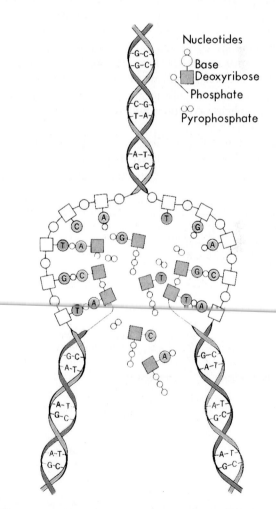

FIGURE 27-3 Replication of DNA involves pairing of free nucleotides with bases of each DNA strand. Result is two new DNA molecules, each containing one old and one new strand. (From Vander AJ, Sherman JH, Luciano DS: *Human physiology*, ed 4, New York, 1986, McGraw-Hill.)

The easiest way to think about the function of DNA is by analogy. DNA can be thought of as a language. A gene is a sentence, whereas a chromosome is a letter packaged in an envelope. For replication, the information carried in DNA must be transcribed into another language to be read; this language is ribonucleic acid (RNA). Each gene is transcribed individually into RNA by a complex array of highly specific enzymes. RNA is a molecule closely related to DNA but is much less stable. DNA and RNA are "read" in groups of three nucleic acids, called *codons*. Each codon designates an amino acid. Because there are four nucleic acids and they are read in groups of three, 64 combinations are possible. Different enzymes in the cell then translate the RNA into protein (Figure 27-4), which provides structure and function for the cell. An absent or dysfunctional protein may cause the cell to be unable to carry out its task or to die prematurely. This molecular defect may cause a physical defect; for example, muscular dystrophy is a single-gene defect that causes muscle cells to malfunction.

This analogy also helps to explain the reasons *inversions, deletions,* and *translocations* result in abnormalities; these are rearrangements of pieces of chromosomes that cannot be read in a meaningful way. It is comparable to splicing together two sentences that do not make sense when read.

More than 100,000 genes in the human chromosomes provide codes for RNA to produce protein and enzymes, and it is within these structural genes that the recognized genetic defects seem to occur and where new mutations have their effect. The position of a specific gene on a chromosome is called a **locus (pl. loci)**. The rest of DNA seems to be involved in a regulatory role or in reproducing and recombining chromosomes (Thompson and Thompson, 1986).

Mutations

Sometimes mistakes are made in duplication, or external factors change certain codons. The result is a faulty message transmitted by mRNA (messenger RNA) to all subsequent replications. Mutations arise when a change occurs in the sequence of base pairs by one of the following means:

- *Substitution* of one base pair by another
- *Insertion* of an extra base pair
- *Deletion* of a required base pair

The result is an altered reading. Thus another amino acid is encoded, possibly changing the protein's function, or the amount of a protein with the correct amino acid sequence is reduced or suppressed. For example, this sequence of bases

CATTCACCTGTA

would be read as

CAT/TCA/CCT/GTA

If the second T is deleted, the sequence becomes

CATCACCTGTA

which is read as

CAT/CAC/CTG/TA

Note that the code has changed and that the new code may cause defects in protein synthesis. The result may be partial or complete absence of the gene product. Thus a mutation is a change in genetic material that possibly, but not always, leads to a change in gene function. For example, Figure 27-5 shows deletion of a single base (G); instead of CGT, the new product is CTC.

Mutations can arise spontaneously, or they can be induced by *mutagens,* substances in the environment that cause genetic changes in certain (target) cells. Genetic diseases that occur in families for the first time often are the result of new mutations. Under certain circumstances, however, the presence of an undesirable trait provides some survival advantage. This may cause the trait to be preserved, or promoted, within a population. For example, a mutation in the beta hemoglobin gene (which causes sickle cell trait) also provides some protection against death from malaria in persons with *one* copy of the gene. However, sickle cell anemia develops in those persons with *two* copies of the mutant gene. Mutations like these also tend to occur in higher

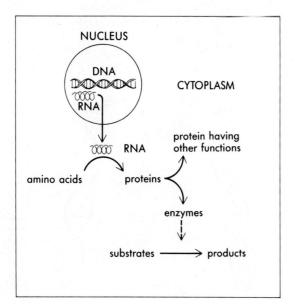

FIGURE 27-4 Expression of genetic information occurs thoughout transcription from DNA to RNA in nucleus followed by translation of this RNA information to proteins in cytoplasm. (From Vander AJ, Sherman JH, Luciano DS: *Human physiology,* ed 4, New York, 1986, McGraw-Hill.)

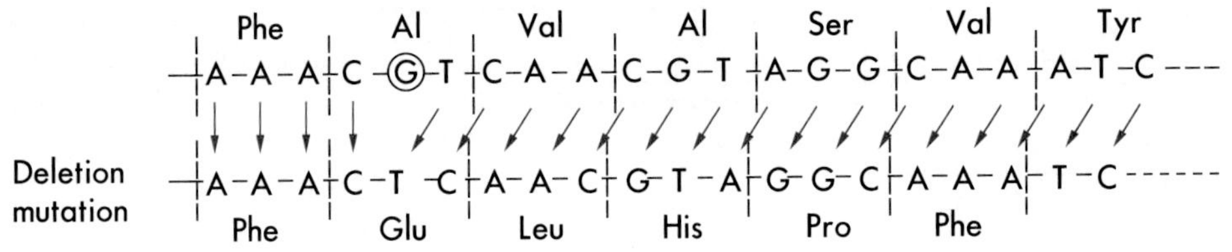

Phe   Al   Val   Al   Ser   Val   Tyr

—A–A–A┼C–Ⓖ–T┼C–A–A┼C–G–T┼A–G–G┼C–A–A┼A–T–C— — —

Deletion
mutation

—A–A–A┼C–T— –C┼A–A–C┼G–T–A┼G–G–C┼A–A–A┼T–C— — — — —

Phe   Glu   Leu   His   Pro   Phe

FIGURE 27-5 Mutation caused by deletion of single base (G) in DNA sequence, resulting in other code words also being misread. (From Vander AJ, Sherman JH, Luciano DS: *Human physiology*, ed. 4, New York, 1986, McGraw-Hill.)

concentrations in ethnic groups that have been isolated geographically and as a result have intermarried with more frequency. Examples of other deleterious mutations that become concentrated in ethnic groups are cystic fibrosis in the Irish and northern Europeans, Tay-Sachs disease in Ashkenazic Jews and French Canadians, and phenylketonuria (PKU) in the Amish.

Test Yourself

- The normal male karyotype consists of _____ autosomes and _____ , sex chromosomes, _____ and _____ .
- A group of three nucleic acids is called a _____ .
- Describe how a mutation can alter protein synthesis.

Single-Gene Inheritance Patterns

Human beings are diploid organisms; that is, they carry a set of chromosomes from their mothers and a set from their fathers. Therefore they carry two copies of each gene, although only one of the copies may be expressed. These two copies are alleles of the same gene, each at the same locus on the chromosome pair (Table 27-1). If a person carries one recessive allele, the trait for that allele is not observable because of the presence of the dominant allele. If, however, a person carries two copies of a recessive allele, the trait *will* be expressed. The **phenotype** of an organism is an observable trait that

depends on the expression of these alleles. For example, the color of a person's eyes or the hair texture is the phenotype of that person. A **genotype,** on the other hand, is the combination of alleles. For example, brown eyes are dominant (B), whereas blue eyes are recessive (b) (Table 27-2). If a person has alleles for brown and blue eyes, this **heterozygous** genotype (Bb) shows a phenotype of brown eyes because the gene for brown eyes is dominant. If both parents have brown eyes, the child might inherit both dominant alleles; in this case the phenotype is brown eyes, but the genotype is **homozygous** dominant (BB). The person whose genotype is blue eyes is homozygous recessive (bb). Recessive alleles may not become apparent for generations and then only if the partner carries similar genes. Of course, there are several genes for eye color and hair characteristics; as a result, many phenotypical and genotypical gradations are observed.

During meiosis there is a 50% chance that the X or the Y chromosome will be placed in the sperm or egg. This **segregation** is true for each of the 23 pairs of chromosomes, thus allowing a wide variation in the genetic makeup of each sperm or egg. The degree of variation is further increased because of the normal crossing over between members of a chromosome pair (see Figure 7-2). This segregation and **independent assortment** reduce chances of inheriting gene defects, as

---

TABLE 27-1   Mendel's Laws of Dominance

GENOTYPE		
GENE	**ALLELE**	**PHENOTYPE EXPRESSION**
Dominant (D)	Dominant (D)	Dominant (DD)
Recessive (r)	Recessive (r)	Recessive (rr)
Dominant (D)	Recessive (r)	Dominant (Dr)

TABLE 27-2   Inheritance of Eye Color*

PARENT	PARENT	CHILDREN
Brown (B, B)	Brown (B, B)	Brown (B, B)
Blue (b, b)	Blue (b, b)	Blue (b, b)
Brown (B, B)	Blue (b, b)	Brown (B, b)
		Brown (B, b)
Brown (B, b)	Blue (b, b)	Brown (B, b)
		Blue (b, b)
Brown (B, b)	Brown (B, b)	Brown (B, B)
		Brown (B, b)
		Brown (B, b)
		Blue (b, b)

*According to Mendel's laws, brown (B) is dominant and blue (b) is recessive.

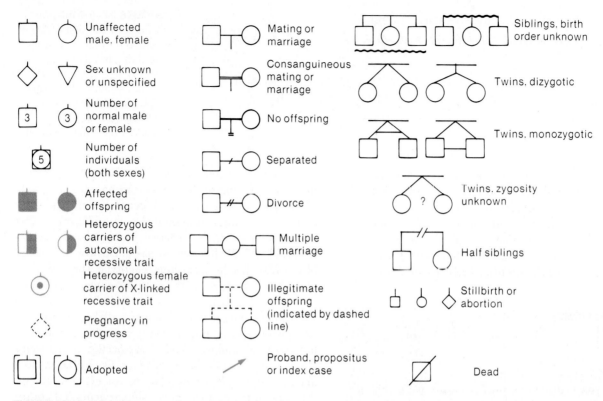

FIGURE 27-6 Symbols commonly used in pedigree charts.

well as contribute to the wide variety in individual appearances and abilities.

CHARTING GENOTYPES

When a family genetic history is taken, a specific protocol is used. The result should be an indication of the probability of passing a particular problem to the unborn child. Of course it is only a *probability* because of the randomness of gene distribution and the presence of other factors that influence the child's phenotype. The protocol is as follows.

1. Use a **Punnett square** or mating diagram to indicate risk of passing a problem to offspring.
2. Use a lowercase letter when a gene is not expressed alone in the phenotype (i.e., when it is a recessive gene).
3. Use an uppercase (capital) letter when the single gene is expressed in the phenotype (i.e., is a dominant gene), whether it is disease producing or normal.
4. Use a slash between alleles.
5. Use the standard symbols as in Figure 27-6 to draw a family history or **pedigree** chart.

GENETIC RESULTS OF CONSANGUINITY

Matings of first- and second-degree relatives such as half-siblings, double first cousins, parent and child,

brother and sister, and uncle and niece unfortunately do occur. When a man and woman in these pairings have a child, one fourth to one half of all the genes are homozygous; therefore the chance for abnormal genes to be expressed in the phenotype is greater. In descriptive studies, a higher incidence of defects, mental retardation, prematurity, and intrauterine growth retardation (IUGR) have occurred.

DOMINANT PATTERNS OF INHERITANCE

When a single allele is expressed in the phenotype, it is **dominant.** Both normal and abnormal genes may be dominant. In dominant disorders the signs of abnormality appear when the person is a heterozygote; however, many dominant disorders do not become apparent until later in life, often after childbearing years. Dominant disorders occur mainly in nonenzyme structural proteins such as hemoglobins, collagens, or regulator proteins.

Test Yourself

- Differentiate between a dominant and recessive gene.
- What is consanguinity? How does it increase the chances of genetic disease in the offspring?

Characteristics of Autosomal Dominant Patterns

1. There is a 50% risk that the affected parent will pass the genotype to the child. The child who does not receive the affected gene from the parent will neither have the disorder nor pass it on to offspring.
2. An *apparently* unaffected parent (normal phenotype) who has the affected gene (abnormal genotype) can pass the disorder to the child. This possibility results from lack of gene *penetrance* in the parent, where the gene is present but is not yet expressed.
3. The severity of the disorder may vary among persons with the gene. This is called **expressivity.**
4. Both sexes are equally affected.

Examples of Autosomal Dominant Disorders

More than 1800 recognized problems are caused by autosomal dominant inheritance. Although most are not lethal, some reduce the affected person's ability to reproduce, decreasing chances of passing the gene to children. Achondroplasia is an example of a defect that causes dwarfism but usually does not affect intelligence or primary human functions. The arms and legs are short, but the head is normal size. These children may lead normal lives (Figure 27-7).

Other disorders become evident in adulthood, during or after the reproductive period; thus they may be passed to offspring by the affected parent. Hyperlipoproteinemia, in the dominant form, is very common. The narrowing of blood vessels with fatty deposits may precipitate early heart attacks. Gastrointestinal polyposis predisposes the host to gastrointestinal cancer. Multiple neurofibromatosis, type I (von Recklinghausen's disease), may show up later in life with multiple neurofibromas of the skin that are benign but disfiguring; the accompanying severe hypertension may be dangerous. Figure 27-8 shows the inheritance pattern.

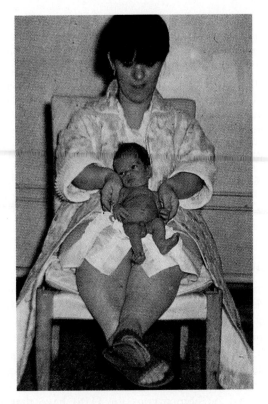

FIGURE 27-7 Achondroplastic mother with her achondroplastic child, the result of a dominant pattern of inheritance. (From O'Doherty N: *Atlas of the newborn,* ed 2, The Hague, 1985, Kluwer Academic Publishers Group.)

Huntington's chorea. An example of late-onset dominant disorders is Huntington's chorea. Huntington's chorea is found in many parts of the world, possibly traced to a mutation originating in northern Europe. Currently 25,000 adults have overt signs. In this country the incidence of carriers is thought to be between 1 in 5000 and 1 in 15,000. The problem for carriers is the knowledge that the expression of the trait may begin any time after age 30. By 40, half the persons heterozy-

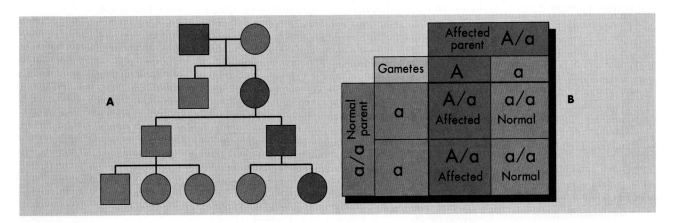

FIGURE 27-8 Dominant pattern. **A,** Pedigree chart. **B,** Punnett square.

gous for Huntington's chorea will show overt signs, including slow, progressive degeneration of the nervous system, and will require complete care for long periods before eventual death. Preconception testing is now possible for couples who have a family history of Huntington's chorea. This produces a dilemma for the family: would you want to know that you will develop Huntington's chorea in 20 years?

Homozygous Dominant Disorders

When both parents pass a dominant trait for a disease, the expression of the disease will be more severe in its effect than if the child inherited a dominant trait from only one parent.

CODOMINANCE

In some cases both alleles are present in the genotype and both are expressed in the phenotype. One of the main blood groups is an example of **codominance**; a person inheriting the gene for blood type A from the mother and the gene for B from the father will demonstrate a phenotype of AB. Type O, however, is recessive if combined with A or B. Thus a person with O blood type must be homozygous for O to have that type expressed (Table 27-3).

Test Yourself

- In autosomal dominant disease there is a _____% chance that an affected parent will pass the gene to the child.
- Why is the inheritance of blood types said to be codominant?

RECESSIVE PATTERNS

An allele that is expressed in the phenotype only when it is homozygous is called a **recessive trait** (Figure 27-9). Thus two recessive genes must be present for a disorder

TABLE 27-3   ABO Blood Groups

	O	A	B	AB
Genotype	OO	AA AO	BB BO	AB
Antigens on Red Cells	Neither	A	B	A and B
Antibodies in Serum	Anti-A, anti-B	Anti-B	Anti-A	Neither

to be expressed. In recessive disorders, if one of the alleles is normal, the normal enzyme will be produced. If there is only one abnormal gene, the person is a *carrier* of the trait. In recessive disorders the gene products usually are enzymes. Therefore many recessive disorders affect the metabolic cycle.

Characteristics of Autosomal Recessive Inheritance

1. The condition appears to skip generations.
2. The condition appears only in the child's phenotype when both parents carry the same recessive gene.
3. The risk of disorder in the infant is 1 in 4 if both parents carry the same recessive gene.
4. Both sexes are affected equally.
5. The risk is greatly increased if there is consanguinity.

Examples of Autosomal Recessive Disorders

Because the gene product is an enzyme in most of these disorders, these conditions are called inborn errors of metabolism (IEM). The main groups are deficiencies in amino acid, carbohydrate, or lipid metabolism. When an enzyme needed for a metabolic pathway is absent or suppressed, the pathway may change, or partially metabolized products may accumulate in the system, causing damage or affecting other functions.

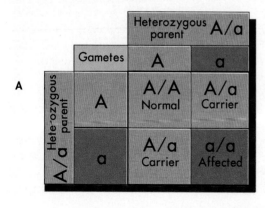
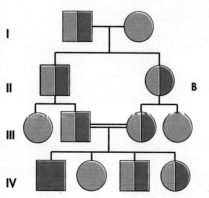

FIGURE 27-9 Autosomal recessive inheritance pattern. **A,** Punnett square. **B,** Pedigree chart.

Amino acid metabolism. PKU is probably the best known of these disorders because it was one of the first to be reversed with strict dietary treatment. The carrier incidence is 1 in 50 in persons of northern European ancestry, but the incidence is only 1 in 16,000 in this country. The child with PKU often has decreased pigmentation, with light skin and hair and blue eyes. Classic PKU results from absence of the hepatic enzyme phenylalanine 4-hydroxylase, which is necessary to convert the essential amino acid, phenylalanine, into tyrosine. When this does not happen, the normal metabolic route is changed and partial phenylalanine metabolites build up and injure the infant; phenylpyruvic acid and phenylacetic acid blood levels increase, cross the blood-brain barrier to stop myelinization in the central nervous system, and thus damage the brain (Figure 27-10). Without treatment, the child will become severely retarded. With treatment, a fairly normal life is possible. Early diagnosis is important, and although the overall rate is low, all newborns are tested. It is important to test after the infant has sufficient amounts of proteins to begin the build-up of phenylketones. Thus, if a baby is discharged within 72 hours or is breast-feeding, follow-up assessment should be done (see Chapter 19).

Some errors of metabolism may be treated by modifying the diet. If the dietary substitution is effective, it must be carefully continued (See Chapter 24 for maternal PKU treatment.)

Other amino acid disorders. Maple syrup urine disease, so called because the infant's urine has a maple syrup smell, results in failure to thrive, metabolic imbalance, and seizures. There is a defect in the metabolism of the amino acids leucine, isoleucine, and valine. Untreated, the infant becomes severely retarded and dies. Dietary treatment that omits these amino acids is required.

Histidinemia and *homocystinuria* result from defects in the metabolism of histidine and methionine. Unless treated by a diet free of these amino acids, the infant may be retarded and with homocystinuria may develop eye defects.

Carbohydrate metabolism. *Galactosemia* results from a missing enzyme necessary to metabolize galactose, one step of lactose metabolism. Because an enzyme, galactose-1-phosphate uridylyltransferase, is missing, the infant cannot tolerate lactose, a disaccharide milk sugar. To be used, lactose must be converted to the monosaccharide galactose and then glucose. The first step is accomplished in the affected child, but the next step is hindered. The enzyme is necessary for galactose to be converted into glucose. Only glucose can enter the Krebs citric acid cycle to be converted to adenosine triphosphate (ATP), carbon dioxide, and water; consequently, galactose builds up in the blood and finally spills into the urine.

High levels of galactose produce severe vomiting and refusal to eat, with resulting failure to thrive, weight loss, dehydration, seizures, hepatosplenomegaly, and cataracts. Symptoms may begin after the first feeding of almost any milk formula but especially after breast milk because of its higher lactose content.

If symptoms are recognized early and treatment is initiated, brain damage, mental retardation, and blindness can be prevented. Treatment consists of a low-galactose formula at first. As the infant matures, puddings, cake mixes, cream soups, meat from milk-fed animals (veal), or any commercial foods containing galactose (or lactose) must be avoided. The mother must be taught to read labels carefully.

Problems of *carbohydrate absorption* occur when sugar given to the infant produces severe vomiting, diarrhea, and colic. Symptoms are often most severe about 3 months of age but may occur earlier. *Glycogen storage disorders* occur when the body has elevated glucose levels. Symptoms include seizures, mental retardation, and developmental or learning disabilities. There is no specific treatment for von Gierke's disease, Pompe's disease, and other forms of glycogenosis.

Lactose intolerance. Problems with digestion of lactose follow geographic lines. A persistence into adulthood of the lactase enzyme, important in digestion of milk, is found in many parts of northern Europe, northern Africa, and Arabia among milk-dependent populations. Theories as to reasons for a genetic persistence of lactase digestion after childhood abound; in northern

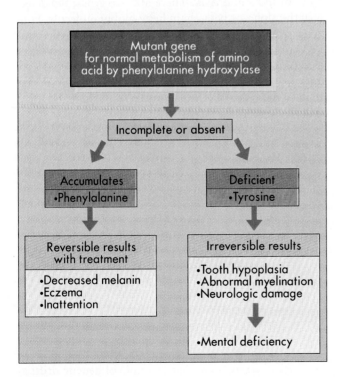

FIGURE 27-10 Pathways of PKU damage.

regions, lack of sunlight may have allowed milk digestion to promote calcium retention (Flatz, 1986).

Much of the rest of the world's population has a lactase restriction by early adulthood, because of poor ability to digest milk. In this country many persons refuse milk, saying that it upsets their digestion. If tested, these persons probably would show some inability to digest lactose. Generally, those of the following racial origins have adult lactase deficiency to some degree (Flatz, 1986):

1. Vietnamese, Thai, Chinese, Taiwanese, Indonesian, and Japanese
2. Alaskan, Central American, Native American, or Mexican Indian
3. South Americans of Indian origin
4. South Sea Islanders
5. Afghan and persons from Middle East countries such as the Jordanians, Syrians, Lebanese, Israelis, and Egyptians
6. Ashkenazic Jews
7. Asian Indian (varied)
8. Middle and southern Africans, except for milk-dependent tribes

Lipid metabolism. Tay-Sachs disease is a recessive disorder carried in 1 in 25 Ashkenazic Jews and at a much lower rate in other populations. Before pregnancy, couples may seek blood tests to determine whether they are carriers of this deleterious gene.

The homozygous child appears normal at birth, but as poorly metabolized lipid substances accumulate, fatty deposits in the brain cause degeneration of neural tissue. There is failure to thrive by 6 months, and by 1 year, progressive degeneration leads to blindness, muscle weakness, excessive production of mucus, and seizures, with death before 5 years (Paritsky, 1985). Families trying to care for the infant at home will need a great deal of support, in-home equipment, and nursing care.

One of the most common lipid disorders is *hyperlipoproteinemia,* which leads to high levels of cholesterol and triglycerides. There are many recessive single-gene forms, and some forms are dominant in expression. One heterozygous form occurs as frequently as 1 in 500 in the general population. Because elevated cholesterol and triglyceride levels underlie many types of coronary artery disease, evaluation for elevated levels is a routine part of most complete physical examinations.

Summary of Inborn Errors of Metabolism

In all cases of enzyme deficiency, the infant will not thrive, will be irritable, may have changes in stool, and will suffer from colic or vomiting with weight loss. Any infant not doing well on usual formulas or breast milk should be evaluated for some type of IEM. All infants in the nursery are tested for the metabolic problems listed

in Chapter 19. The nursery or home care nurse may notice an irritable baby, or, very shortly after discharge to the home, signs of difficulty appear.

Other Recessive Disorders

Sickle cell disease. Sickle cell disease is a recessively inherited disorder that involves a structural change in the hemoglobin molecule. Substitution of one of the 146 amino acids in the beta-chain with another amino acid is the only difference between normal hemoglobin A and hemoglobin S, the sickle cell hemoglobin. The heterozygous person is a carrier, that is, can pass the trait to a child, who will show signs of difficulty very early, if homozygous. Those who inherit a homozygous pattern for hemoglobin S will experience the crisis of sickling; the cell changes into a sickle shape when low oxygen tension is present (see Chapter 23).

The incidence of the trait is widespread throughout Africa and Asia. The mutation appears to offer protection from death from malaria. More than 150 variations of beta-chain defect are recognized. Because many persons in this country carry the trait, it is estimated that 1 in 500 newborns (from the groups that migrated to this country from Africa and Asia) will be homozygous for the sickle gene. Therefore all newborns are tested before discharge from the nursery.

Thalassemias. Thalassemic defects in the hemoglobin molecule are the most common gene disorder and originate from the Mediterranean basin, Africa, and parts of India and Asia. There are two types; the defect is in the alpha-or beta-chain hemoglobin molecule. Four genes are involved in alpha-thalassemia; two pairs may be variously affected. A person may have one, two, or three faulty genes with increasingly severe degrees of anemia. If, however, a fetus is homozygous for this thalassemia (i.e., all four genes are dysfunctional), it will not survive gestation (see Chapter 23).

Test Yourself

- Describe how an inborn error of metabolism may affect a newborn infant.
- Those affected with sickle cell disease carry _____ copy(ies) of the affected gene(s). How does the hemoglobin in sickle cell anemia differ from normal hemoglobin?

Cystic fibrosis. Cystic fibrosis has a carrier rate among Irish people of 1 in 30 and a general occurrence rate of 1 in 2000 in other northern Europeans.

Cystic fibrosis is another example of **genetic drift;** as people intermarry and move geographically, defects once found only in isolated ethnic groups are now scattered into the general population. Because these recessive disorders need inheritance from father and mother, the incidence should gradually diminish as the gene pool is diluted.

In cystic fibrosis (CF), abnormal secretions occur from exocrine glands, including sweat glands. Viscid (sticky) secretions are produced in the pancreas, liver, duodenum, and small intestine. Thick, viscid secretions from the lungs complicate respiration and are intensified by respiratory infection. Meconium ileus often is present at birth. A classic sign is a *meconium plug* passed into the diaper before the first stool.

Until recently, prenatal diagnosis was limited to evaluation of amniotic fluid for levels of certain intestinal enzymes, with a high prediction rate. In 1986 the gene that codes for the defective protein in CF was located on the seventh chromosome. This led to the use of *gene markers* (series of codons that are found near the CF gene), which allow the CF gene to be tracked in families with a known history of the disease. DNA analysis with gene markers may be performed early in pregnancy by means of chorionic villus biopsy. When this is done during the second trimester by amniocentesis, the amniotic fluid also is analyzed for intestinal enzymes, further confirming the diagnosis. Currently many states mandate screening of newborns for CF at the time blood is drawn for other metabolic testing.

X-LINKED INHERITANCE

A gene on the X chromosome may carry a defect. Figure 27-11 is a map of the X chromosome, showing several X-linked disorders. Because the boy has only one X chromosome, any disorder carried on that X is expressed in his phenotype and thus follows a dominant pattern. In this case the male is **hemizygous**. On the other hand, a girl has two X chromosomes, but in this case, an interesting change occurs; one of the two Xs becomes inactivated or "silent" very early in the development of the embryo. This inactivation is random within the cells, but after one X is inactivated, its cell retains the activity of the other X in all replications. Therefore in some cells the maternal X is active, whereas the paternal X is active in other cells. These girls have a mixed chromosome pattern; that is, they are **mosaic** for the active X. Thus if a gene mutation occurs on one of the X chromosomes, it is muted by the presence of a normal gene in half of her other cells. Therefore the girl usually must be homozygous for a disorder to be fully expressed in her phenotype. As a result, girls are spoken of as carriers of X-linked traits. Homozygosity is rather unusual in girls (Figure 27-12) but is seen with color blindness, a common, nonlethal **X-linked defect**.

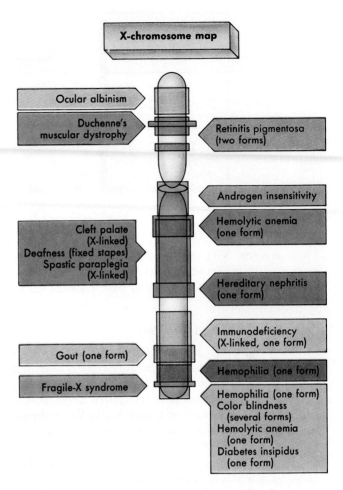

FIGURE 27-11 Map of the X chromosome. This diagram shows only a few of the many regions of the X chromosome that have been identified to contain specific bits of genetic information. (Rolin Graphics.)

X-Linked Recessive Patterns

Characteristics of X-linked recessive patterns follow:
1. A male is hemizygous, inheriting one X. If the defective gene is on that X, the male will have the disorder.
2. A female may be heterozygous or homozygous for the gene and usually follows the autosomal recessive pattern.
3. There is only one active X in each female cell; the other X is inactivated and is seen as the Barr chromatin body, a dark staining spot on the cell.
4. Because maternal or paternal X may be activated in a mosaic pattern, any disorder may be muted or silent in the female.
5. The risk for infants of carrier females is 1 in 2 for a male to be affected and 1 in 2 for a female to be a carrier.
6. Affected males do not pass the disorder to their sons.

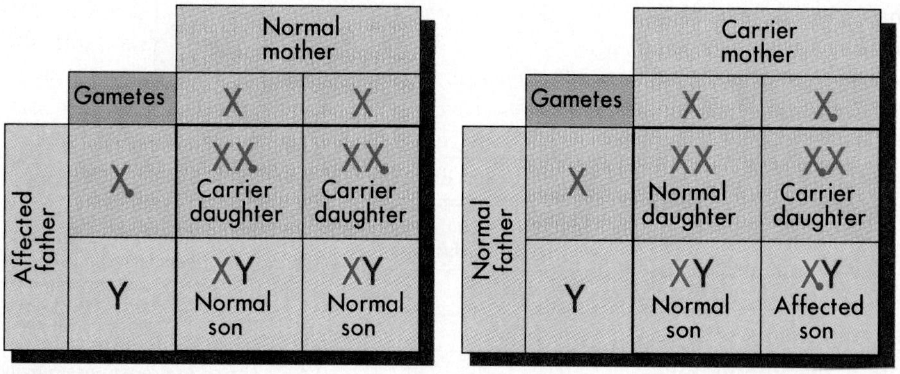

FIGURE 27-12 X-linked recessive inheritance pattern. Sex differences in offspring ratios in X-linked recessive inheritance. • = Recessive allele on X chromosome.

X-Linked Dominant Patterns

There are few X-linked dominant disorders. In these cases an affected father may have an affected daughter but no affected son. Mothers may pass to daughters or sons.

Examples of X-Linked Disorders

Fragile X syndrome. Breakage may occur at fragile sites on chromosomes. The classic example is the fragile X, a cause of mental retardation second only to Down syndrome. As more has been recognized about fragile chromosomes, diagnosis of **fragile X (fra X)** syndrome has been made in many puzzling cases of mental retardation. Currently the estimate is that 100,000 males and a smaller number of females are affected. The occurrence rate is 1 in 1000 male births.

The defect is passed by X-linked inheritance or may be a mutation in the sperm (Sherman et al., 1984). About one third of carrier mothers may have mild retardation (Sutherland, 1985). Males with normal genotypes and phenotypes also may cause a fra X chromosome to be passed to their daughters when an as yet unknown factor creates the fragile site after formation of the female zygote.

Most fra X males have moderate to severe retardation. They also may have organic brain disease, seizures, and self-mutilating and hyperactive behavior. Signs are delayed speech and mild enlargement of the chin, ears, and testes. For carrier females the range of intelligence is very broad. Learning difficulties may occur; only a third have mild mental retardation.

Pattern. The pattern for fra X syndrome follows:
1. The fra X is not completely recessive because one third of heterozygous females are affected.
2. An apparently normal male may transmit fra X to his daughter.
3. The mutation rate is high for the sperm and very low for the ovum.

The breakage of the affected chromosome is shown in a culture medium that lacks folate. Therefore some centers have tried folic acid supplement in early treatment, and some children have shown improvement in behavior. Others believe that folic acid supplements have no benefit.

Genetic counseling is very important and may take time. The child may have been misdiagnosed with autism, cerebral palsy, or a birth injury. It is recommended that all family members at risk be tested, including the siblings of the parents and the child.

Other fragile sites. Fragile sites on autosomes are being linked with cancer. Researchers have identified 30 **oncogenes**—genetic mutations that change cellular behavior by changing the structure or amount of protein produced by the cell. Whereas normal cells have tumor-suppressing abilities, affected cells lose the ability to regulate their rate of growth. This unrestrained growth is the beginning of cancer. An example of this is the **retinoblastoma gene (Rb)**, the first oncogene to be identified. Retinoblastoma occurs when a *single* mutant gene on chromosome 13 is passed on from a carrier parent, followed by a *second* mutation within a fetal or infant retinal cell. This mutation also predisposes children with Rb to other tumors such as osteosarcoma. Although in the past these young persons did not live to reproduce, advances in treatment now allow more survivors to pass the gene on to their children. Other tumors, such as lung and colon carcinomas and Wilms' tumor, are associated with the absence of normal alleles at specific loci. Researchers expect to find many more sites that are correlated with cancer.

Hemophilia. Used as the classic illustration of X-linked recessive disease, hemophilia is a deficiency of antihemophilic globulin, a problem in the clotting cycle (factor VIII). The gene often was found among royal families in Europe. It appears to be more prevalent in northern Europeans. Recently, as a replacement for the missing clotting factor has become more available, males with hemophilia survived long enough to become fathers. A female could thus be a hemophiliac if she inherited the defect from both parents.

Glucose-6-phosphate dehydrogenase (G6PD). The most common X-linked problems are color blindness and G6PD deficiency. G6PD is an enzyme involved in glucose metabolism. It is more common in males but also can be found in females. When a person with G6PD deficiency ingests certain drugs or foods, red blood cells are destroyed, resulting in severe anemia. A number of variations exist, and it is believed that more than 100 million people in the world have G6PD deficiency.

A version of G6PD deficiency is common in the countries bordering the Mediterranean Sea, where it is called *favism* because the fava bean precipitates the crisis. Thus immigrants from those countries may have the disorder. The incidence follows the geographic path of malaria. In this country 20% to 30% of African-American males and 2% of African-American females have some form of G6PD, and the rate is high in immigrants from the Mediterranean countries.

Drugs and foods that precipitate breakdown of red blood cells are listed in Chapter 23. It is important to check drug interactions for any person with G6PD deficiency, and all newborns are now tested for it (see Box 23-2).

Color blindness. One in ten males from Mediterranean countries and Ashkenazic Jewish groups is color blind, and many other groups in the world also have frequent color blindness disorders. The locus of the genes is very near that of G6PD on the X chromosome. Because color blindness is not fatal and occurs frequently, females may be homozygous and thus also color blind. Other X-linked recessive problems are Duchenne's muscular dystrophy and the rare Lesch-Nyhan syndrome.

Test Yourself

- A color blind man and a woman who sees normally have a daughter who is color blind. What is the child's genotype?
- Why are only males affected by X-linked recessive traits?
- Give two examples of a fragile site on a chromosome causing disease or disability.

POLYGENIC INHERITANCE

When more than one pair of genes play a role in disease, the cause is **polygenic inheritance.** More often, multiple genes and environmental influences precipitate disorders. In this case, the cause is **multifactorial inheritance.** Certain disorders seem to run in families and yet do not occur as often as those inherited according to

Mendel's patterns. Although polygenic and multifactorial problems do not follow Mendel's dominant and recessive patterns, the overall risk for the problem to develop is increased if there is a history in close relatives. Therefore clients are asked about their medical history to ascertain whether close relatives have problems that follow this pattern of inheritance.

Certain disorders show up during fetal development; for instance, the cleft lip and palate fail to fuse by about 35 days of development. Congenital dislocation of the hip and certain heart defects also follow the multifactorial distribution. Several disorders may become apparent at birth or during infancy, whereas others are not expressed unless environmental factors precipitate symptoms. Hypertension is an example of a late-developing disorder.

Because many factors contribute to multifactorial defects, precise prevention is difficult. Avoidance of environmental exposure that may precipitate problems and ensuring adequate diet and vitamin intake are important during pregnancy.

Diabetes Mellitus

Poorly controlled diabetes mellitus increases the risk of anomalies two or three times that of the general population. Organs most affected are the spine, lower limbs, heart, kidneys, and external genitalia. Neural tube defects are seen 20 times more frequently in fetuses of mothers with insulin-dependent diabetes mellitus (IDDM) (Hoyme, 1990). Good glucose control (see Chapter 24) is important for this reason.

STRUCTURAL BIRTH DEFECTS

Defects in structure occur when some factor alters the progress of normal fetal development. The part may stop developing and remain in an immature form, accessory structures may be produced, or cells may be organized in an abnormal way. The cause of these changes may be genetic, environmental, or multifactorial. An essentially normal fetus may be deformed or misshapen because of intrauterine crowding as a result of multiple gestation or an abnormally small amount of amniotic fluid. In most cases, however, the cause remains unknown (Beckman and Brent, 1986).

Defects may be found alone (isolates) or as part of a syndrome—a group of signs. In general, the more severe defects arise earlier in gestation (Table 27-4). It is important that an infant with a defect be assessed for the presence of other system defects because multiple organs may be affected. In this chapter, only those defects that can be detected at birth or soon after are discussed.

The overall incidence of birth defects is approximately 3%, and defects remain the leading cause of

TABLE 27-4   Timing of Selected Malformations

MALFORMATION	TIME OF DEVELOPMENT
Anencephaly	Day 26
Spina bifida	Day 28
Tracheoesophageal fistula	Day 30
Renal agenesis (Potter's syndrome)	Day 34
Transposition of great vessels	Day 36
Cleft lip and palate	Day 36
Ventriculoseptal defect	Week 6
Duodenal atresia	Week 7-8
Urethral obstruction	Week 9

Data from Brent RL: *Clin Perinatol* 13:609, 1986; Moore KL: *The developing human: clinically oriented embryology,* ed 4, Philadelphia, 1988, WB Saunders.

infant mortality (Oakley, 1986). Birth defects are reported to several data banks. Major hospitals report occurrences; health care providers submit case reports to journals. From these data, projections are made and any increase in a specific malformation is noted. In this way a newly emerging problem may be brought to the attention of practitioners and epidemiologic studies can be undertaken.

Cardiovascular Defects

The cardiovascular system is the first to function in the embryo, with defects arising early in gestation. Although even major defects are compatible with fetal life, such defects are life threatening to the newborn. Some are isolated defects; others are part of known syndromes caused by genetic or environmental hazards. Cardiovascular defects are discussed in detail in Chapter 28 because they are a large part of care of the newborn at high risk.

Cleft Lip and Palate

Failure of fusion of the lip or palate my be unilateral or bilateral. Lack of fusion may be limited to the lip or soft palate, or a combined lip and hard and soft palate cleft may occur (Figure 27-13). Cleft lip with cleft palate often is found as an isolated defect or as part of trisomy 13. Treatment is directed toward supporting the infant's status until the surgical decision is made. Repair usually is successful, and cosmetic surgery may be performed

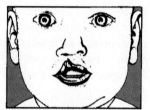
UNILATERAL INCOMPLETE

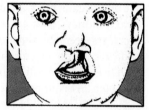
UNILATERAL COMPLETE

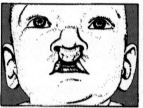
BILATERAL COMPLETE

A

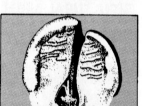
SOFT PALATE ONLY

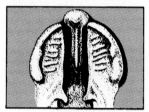
UNILATERAL COMPLETE

BILATERAL COMPLETE

B

FIGURE 27-13 A, Cleft lip. **B,** Cleft palate. **C,** Infant with complete unilateral cleft lip. Note the feeding tube. (A and B used with permission of Ross Laboratories, Columbus, Ohio 43216; from *Clinical Education Aid No. 17,* © Ross Laboratories.)

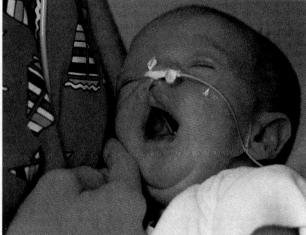

C

later to improve facial contours, which may reassure parents. Until surgical repair is completed (a series of operations may be required), the infant is fed in an upright position with use of a special nipple. Even breast-feeding may be possible, depending on the degree of cleft.

Gastrointestinal Atresias

Gastrointestinal defects of the esophagus or intestine may be life threatening. In *tracheoesophageal fistula,* a communication between the trachea and esophagus, the esophagus may be patent or end in a blind sac. Swallowing any liquid results in regurgitation and danger of aspiration (Figure 27-14). Tracheoesophageal fistula may be complicated by rectal atresia or imperforate anus (Figure 27-15). In any case, surgical repair is extensive.

Intestinal obstruction may be caused by *atresia,* which is narrowing anywhere below the stomach. Before birth gastrointestinal atresias produce polyhydramnios because the fetus is unable to swallow amniotic fluid. Duodenal atresia causes symptoms of vomiting and distension soon after birth. It is commonly seen with other conditions such as Down syndrome and cardiovascular abnormalities. Atresias of the large intestine, rectum, and anus will cause distension and failure to pass meconium. Repair of the most common types of anal and rectal defects may be simple or may require colostomy for a period.

Renal Defects

When an obstructive malformation limits the flow of urine into the amniotic fluid, the infant's distended kidneys, ureters, and bladder may be seen on ultrasound, depending on the location of the obstruction. Some degree of oligohydramnios will occur if urine is not passing freely. In rare instances the kidneys will completely fail to develop. Severe oligohydramnios results, and the excessive pressure on the fetal body prevents normal lung and skeletal development. The resulting Potter's syndrome is fatal (Figure 27-16).

Neural Tube Defects

Anencephaly. Defects of the central nervous system can be of varying severity. The most severe is *anencephaly,* absence of all brain but the medulla. Anencephaly is caused by failure of fusion of the cranial end of the neural tube before day 26 of

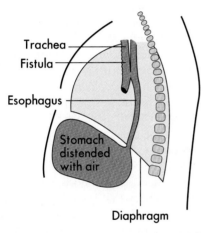

FIGURE 27-14 One type of tracheoesophageal fistula. (From Corliss CE: *Patten's human embryology,* ed 4, New York, 1976, McGraw-Hill.)

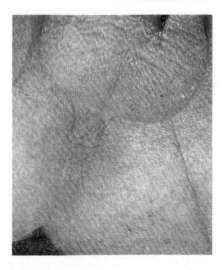

FIGURE 27-15 Imperforate anus. (From *Diagnostic picture tests in clinical medicine,* 1984.)

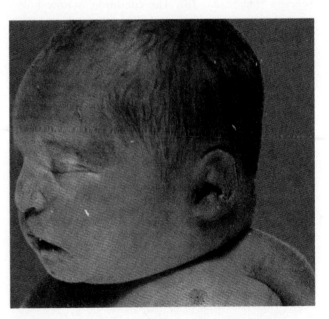

FIGURE 27-16 Potter facies. This infant with bilateral multicystic dysplasia died of pulmonary insufficiency 12 hours after birth. The altered facies produced by the fetal compression syndrome of oligohydramnios includes small, posteriorly rotated ears, micrognathia, a beaked nose, and wide-set eyes. (Courtesy Dr. MacPherson, Magee-Women's Hospital, Pittsburgh, Penn.)

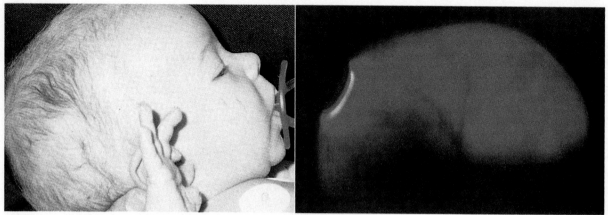

A

B

FIGURE 27-17 A, Hydranencephaly. Infant 3 weeks after birth has a deceptively normal appearance, with little to suggest a severe brain abnormality. **B,** Transillumination of the skull lights up the calvarium, suggesting the diagnosis. (From Zitelli BJ, Davis HW: *Atlas of pediatric physical diagnosis,* St Louis, 1987, Mosby.)

gestation. There is no cranium or cerebrum although the rest of the body usually is well formed. The condition is found more frequently in certain families, and two of three cases are female infants. Many are stillborn or survive for only hours or days. *Hydranencephaly* is the absence of cerebral hemispheres but a normal skull (Figure 27-17).

Meningomyelocele. Spina bifida, a failure of fusion of the lower neural tube, may occur in many degrees of severity (Figure 27-18). The condition is now linked with inadequate vitamin intake before and during pregnancy. Other research has linked maternal hyperthermia and neural tube defects (Hoyme, 1990). A maternal core temperature over 38.9° C may be teratogenic. Other central nervous system (CNS) and facial defects

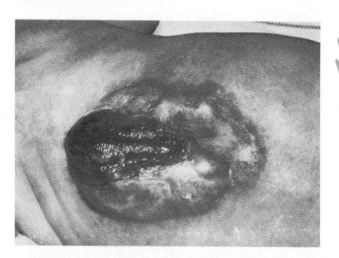

FIGURE 27-18 Meningomyelocele (spina bifida). (From Zitelli BJ, Davis HW: *Atlas of pediatric physical diagnosis,* St Louis, 1987, Mosby.)

also possibly are linked to hyperthermia. The highest risk seems to be for pregnant women who use hot tubs or who have sustained fevers.

Neonates with meningomyelocele are at high risk for infection (meningitis and urinary tract infection), neurologic deficit, and hydrocephalus. The risk of meningitis is decreased if the sac has not been ruptured during delivery (cesearean birth is preferred). Repair of this form of neural tube defect is accomplished as soon as the infant's condition is stable.

A high defect (high lumbar to low thoracic), hydrocephalus, and other bony abnormalities of the spine increase the probability that the infant will have significant motor and mental neurologic deficits. Many ethical problems concern the extent to which these infants should be treated. These decisions are made with input from the parents and the agency's infant care review board.

Other CNS Defects

Hydrocephaly. Hydrocephaly is an abnormal accumulation of cerebrospinal fluid (CSF) within ventricles of the brain (Figure 27-19). The causes are varied; it can result from a congenital malformation (it often is associated with meningomyelocele) or an infectious or hemorrhagic process that blocks the flow or alters the absorption of CSF. Increased pressure of the fluid prevents normal growth and development of the brain.

The fetus with hydrocephaly may be identified prenatally by means of ultrasound. Cesarean birth may be necessary when the head size is greatly increased. The hydrocephalic neonate may have a head circumference far larger than the percentile for birth weight and height, although this varies depending on the onset. In extreme forms the head circumference can exceed 42 cm (normal maximum for a full-term infant is 37 cm).

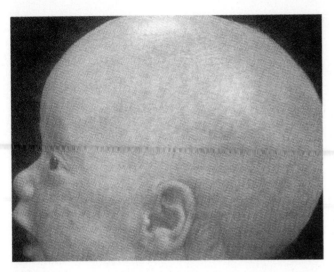

FIGURE 27-19 Infantile hydrocephalus. The characteristic appearance is an enlarged head, thinning of the scalp, distended scalp veins, and a full fontanelle. (From Booth IW, Wozniak ER: *Pediatrics*, Baltimore, 1984, Williams & Wilkins.)

The sun-setting sign may be present, and the thin skull feels soft, similar to a Ping-Pong ball.

Newborn infants with hydrocephaly initially may behave fairly normally or be severely affected. Without treatment, however, progressive damage to the brain is certain. Computed tomography (CT) scans and ultrasound are used to assess the extent to which brain growth has been disrupted. Therapy consists of placing a ventriculoperitoneal shunt to drain CSF and lessen intracranial pressure. Fetal therapy attempts to relieve intracranial pressure earlier in development, allowing brain growth to proceed normally.

Microcephaly. Microcephaly may occur because of a reduced number of brain cells or because of space restrictions imposed on a normal number of cells. Cells may be reduced in number by congenital syndromes such as trisomy 21 or because of intrauterine infections, especially viral. Premature closure of the cranial sutures (*craniosynostosis*) restricts the space available for brain growth. The prognosis depends on the cause because there can be no increase in cellular number after birth.

Autosomal Disorders

Often chromosome defects result from a 45 or 47 chromosome pattern, in which each cell contains one less or one more than the normal 46. On other occasions, defects result from loss of part of a chromosome (**deletion**) or by exchange of one piece of a chromosome to another chromosome (**translocation**); translocation is a rare cause of Down syndrome in which chromosomes 21 and 14 exchange a block of material. There also may

be an extra portion of some chromosome material (**duplication**); duplications result in additional material and seem to be less harmful than deletions.

Finally, when division of chromosomes takes place and separation, which should occur longitudinally at the centromere, instead occurs laterally between the short arms (p) and the long arms (q), the result is an *isochromosome*. The child may have trisomy for the material on the long arms and be missing the material on the short arms. The X chromosome most often is involved because monosomy in the autosomes (resulting from lack of the short arm material) is not compatible with survival. Women with Turner's syndrome (45,X syndrome) may have this variation.

NONDISJUNCTION

Nondisjunction is the most common cause of chromosomal abnormalities (Figure 27-20). During the first and second steps of meiosis and even during mitosis, a chromosome pair can refuse to separate to the poles (at anaphase). The resulting daughter cells will have an extra chromosome (be *trisomic*) or be missing a chromosome (be *monosomic*). The karyotype of an individual is labeled by the affected pair (e.g., 47,XX+21 or 47,XY+21). This set of numbers and letters means that in either a male (XY) or female (XX), there are 47 chromosomes instead of 46, with the extra at pair 21 (Figure 27-20).

MOSAICISM

Mosaicism is the presence of different patterns of gene expression in tissue within the same organism. For example, a person may have one brown eye and one blue eye pattern, with some cells containing Bb and others BB. Such variation indicates a mosaic gene.

If nondisjunction occurs during early mitosis, a mosaic for an entire chromosome may occur. Because the mosaic individual contains two cell lines in the body,

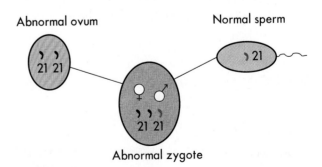

FIGURE 27-20 After fertilization with normal sperm, oocyte with double chromosome at 21 becomes zygote with three chromosomes (trisomy 21). (From March of Dimes Birth Defects Foundation, White Plains, N.Y.)

the proportion is variable, and the phenotypical signs are usually milder because the normal cells modify expression of the problem cells. Sometimes the abnormal cells are "ignored," and normal cells seem to duplicate more readily with resultant later improvement in signs of the defect.

Causes

As with mutation of genetic material in single-gene defects, certain risk factors accompany chromosomal abnormality. Radiation increases the incidence of non-disjunction in experimental animals. Several studies have linked maternal radiation exposure before the births of children with Down syndrome, but other studies have not shown a significant difference (Uchida, 1977). Autoimmune disease may be linked because some mothers of children with Down syndrome have shown high thyroid autoantibody levels (Thompson and Thompson, 1986).

The aging parent seems to be linked most often with chromosome defects. Sufficient evidence exists that the older a woman is, the higher the risk of a **trisomy** (Table 27-5). Down syndrome has been studied thoroughly; in rounded figures the risk is 1 in 1000 for women younger than 30 and 1 in 100 for women older than 40.

Nondisjunction composes the greater part of trisomy cases, and in Down syndrome, nondisjunction is thought to occur during the first stage of meiosis. Because the oocyte began this stage in the last third of the mother's own fetal life and completes it 30 or 40 years later, there may be a slower separation of chromosome material in the aging ovum. Trisomy incidence is not solely connected to the older woman; it is now known that 20% of the cases of nondisjunction are in the spermatocyte (Thompson and Thompson, 1986). This nondisjunction is illustrated with some of the sex chromosome trisomies.

TRISOMIES

Trisomy 21 (Down Syndrome)

Down syndrome (47,XX +21 or 47,XY +21) is the most frequently occurring trisomy (perhaps because the 21

chromosome is so small). Described in 1866 by John L. H. Down, the syndrome stems from nondisjunction (95%), translocation (4%), or mosaicism (1%). Most pregnant women younger than 35 and all older than 35 are encouraged to have prenatal screening for alpha-fetoprotein levels, which show much lower levels than normal if the syndrome is present. Testing is confirmed with amniocentesis, with karyotype preparation from fetal cells.

Signs of Down syndrome usually are observable at birth in facial features, fingerprints and footprints, and body tone.

- Body tone is markedly hypotonic.
- The iris of the eye has speckles (Brushfield's spots).
- The lids have epicanthal folds beginning at the inner canthus of the eye as a thickened lid.
- The upper insertion of the ear should be parallel to the inner canthus of the eye, but in a child with Down syndrome, it is set low.

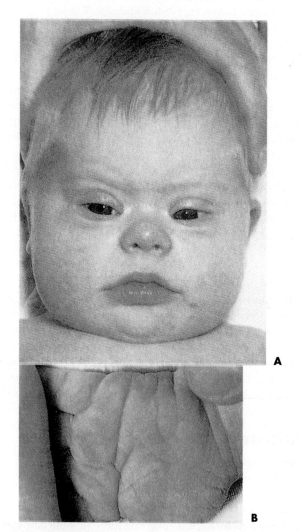

FIGURE 27-21 Two minor anomalies associated with Down syndrome. **A,** Typical facies (note epicanthal folds). **B,** Simian crease in palm. (From Zitelli BJ, Davis HW: *Atlas of pediatric physical diagnosis*, St Louis, 1987, Mosby.)

TABLE 27-5 Risk of Trisomy 21 Resulting from Nondisjunction in Relation to Mother's Age

MOTHER'S AGE	RISK
Less than 29	1 in 3000
30 to 34	1 in 700
35 to 39	1 in 250
40 to 44	1 in 100
Greater than 45	1 in 25-40

- The bridge of the nose is flat and is easy to miss because all babies have a somewhat low bridge (Figure 27-21, A).
- The tongue is thickened and may protrude; macroglossia interferes with feeding in severe cases.
- Characteristic hand structures and dermal patterns are similar in every affected baby. The simian line across the palm can be observed in the initial physical assessment (Figure 27-21, B).
- Similarly, footprints are different.
- Developmental delays vary widely, with an intelligence quotient (IQ) from 25 to 100.
- Finally, children with Down syndrome may have heart defects; about a third require surgery (Miola, 1987).

The capability of each affected infant must be discovered because of the wide range of ability seen with this syndrome. The best outcome is obtained when early training and intensive stimulation are provided. When a parent is unable to cope with this regimen, special institutions are available to work with the child. Life expectancy is variable and depends on defects accompanying Down syndrome; usually these children do not have a normal life span.

Test Yourself
- Describe the clinical findings characteristic of a newborn with Down syndrome.

Trisomy 18 Syndrome

Trisomy 18 (Edwards syndrome) (47,XX+18 or 47,XY +18) occurs as rarely as 1 in 8000 births because only 5% of these conceptions survive. Most cases are due to nondisjunction in older mothers. A few have mosaicism and live slightly longer with less severe abnormalities. The survival period may be 2 to 6 months.

Characteristics can be seen at birth; hypertonia, low-set and malformed ears, a small chin, and a large occiput are the obvious facial characteristics. Hands show simian lines and unusual fingerprints, and the baby makes fists with the second and fifth fingers overlapping the third and fourth. Feet show "rocker bottoms" with the arch appearing to be rounded below the heel. Severe cardiac defects also may be present. The baby is severely mentally retarded, has trouble feeding, and therefore fails to thrive.

Trisomy 13 Syndrome

The incidence of trisomy 13 (Patau syndrome) (47,XX+13 or 47,XY +13) is very rare, and survival is short. (Ethical questions arise about the amount of intervention to provide for a child with such a poor prognosis.)

Many of the defects of trisomy 18 syndrome show in the child with trisomy 13 syndrome and include mental retardation, hand and foot abnormalities, simian line abnormalities, and cardiac defects. Other malformations also are present, the most obvious of which are severe cleft lip and palate and eye deformities (Figure 27-22).

DELETION: CRI DU CHAT SYNDROME

The cat-cry syndrome is caused by a deletion; chromosome 5 is missing a short arm (p) so that the karyotype is written 46,XX 5p- or 46,XY, 5p-. Signs at birth are the "cat cry," like the mewing of a cat, wide-spaced eyes with a slant and epicanthal fold, low-set ears, small head, and mental retardation. In addition, these children have unusual fingerprints and footprints, and simian lines may be present on the palms.

Test Yourself
- Name three causes of structural birth defects.
- Nondisjunction occurs when a pair of chromosomes fail to _____ during meiosis.
- The most common trisomy, _____, also is called _____ syndrome.

Sex Chromosome Disorders
MONOSOMY: TURNER SYNDROME

Monosomy is always lethal in autosomes. However, sex chromosome monosomy (Turner syndrome or 45, XO) is possible; remember that in all normal female cells one X is active and the other inactive. Thus cell lines can survive a single active X. Even so, 99% of monosomy 45,X fetuses are spontaneously aborted; the incidence of live births is only about 1 in 10,000. Some of these have isochromosomes or mosaicism. Mosaic fetuses will have X/XX; that is, some cells in the body have only one X, and others have two normal Xs.

Signs present at birth are webbing of the skin at the sides of the neck, a low hairline at the back of the neck (hard to distinguish in many babies), puffy hands and feet (lymphedema), and a broad chest with widely spaced nipples (Figure 27-23). In some children, there may be coarctation of the aorta. At puberty, secondary sex characteristics are not developed, and the girl is sterile (unless a mosaic pattern). Because intelligence usually is in the normal range, counseling and hormonal therapy are used to help with psychosocial adjustment and body growth (McCauley, Sybert, and Ehrhardt, 1986).

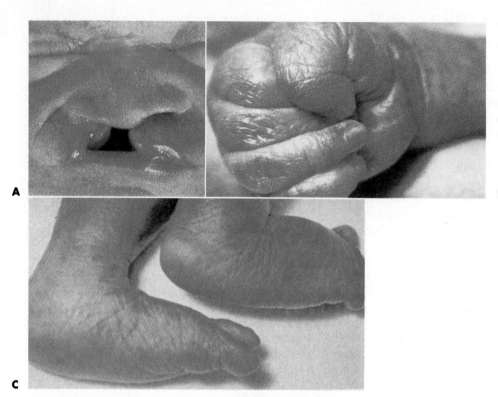

FIGURE 27-22 Physical manifestations of trisomy 13. **A,** Facies showing midline defect. **B,** Clenched hand with overlapping fingers, also typical of trisomy 18. **C,** Rocker-bottom feet. (From Zitelli BJ, Davis HW: *Atlas of pediatric physical diagnosis,* St Louis, 1987, Mosby.)

TRISOMIES

The incidence of sex chromosome trisomy syndrome is rather frequent for boys and girls (1 in 1000). The infant usually does not show phenotypical changes at birth, but the changes appear by puberty when gonads should be directing the development of secondary sex characteristics. Mosaicism is quite common in these sex chromosome trisomies and will lessen the phenotypic effect.

Klinefelter Syndrome

Nondisjunction in the older mother appears to be the cause of approximately 60% of boys with Klinefelter syndrome. The rest are due to paternal nondisjunction. Although the karyotype is written as 47,XXY, about 15% of these boys have a mosaic pattern, XY/XXY.

There are few clinical signs at birth, but at puberty the secondary sex characteristics show poor development. Skeletal height is not reduced, and many boys are tall and lanky. There may be some breast development and neuromuscular difficulty. The head size is smaller than normal in many boys, and there are some learning difficulties related to language skills. There may be accompanying psychosocial difficulties from peer criticism, and the boy may have a poor sense of body image. Parents report that boys are unassertive and inactive (Berch and Bender, 1987). At the time of puberty the boy may be given androgens to assist in development of secondary sex characteristics. Because the testes remain small and no sperm are produced, the man is sterile but not impotent. Therefore, in a few cases, the first recognition of the problem may occur when a man comes in for infertility testing.

Because a trisomy may be from either parent, the sex chromosomes letters are labeled with "m" or "p" to indicate origin of the problem. Thus a baby with an extra X from the mother would be identified as X^mX^mY and when the X comes from the father, it is XX^pY.

XYY Syndrome

Paternal nondisjunction during the second stage of meiosis can cause production of a sperm bearing two Y chromosomes. The result in the fertilized ovum is XYY. Because initial studies of XYY involved a prison population, early studies linked XYY with criminal behavior (Hook, 1973). The syndrome perhaps leads to more aggressive behavior, and parents have reported tantrums, negative moods and hyperactivity (Berch and Bender, 1987). The boy with XYY syndrome tends to be tall and weigh more than the XXY boy. He is fertile. Intelligence usually is in a normal range, but about half have learning problems related to language, motor, and reading skills.

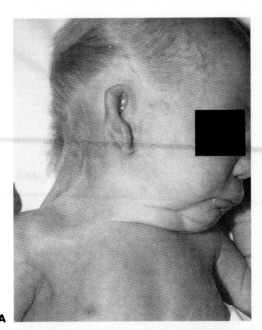

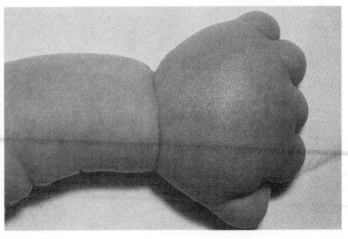

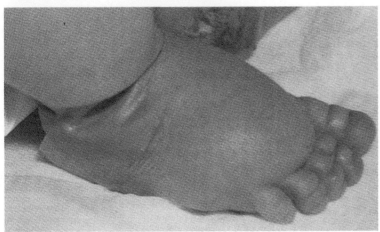

FIGURE 27-23 Several physical manifestations associated with Turner syndrome. **A,** Web neck, low hairline, wide-spread nipples, broad chest, abnormal ears, and micrognathia. **B** and **C,** Lymphedema of hands and feet. (From Zitelli BJ, Davis HW: *Atlas of pediatric physical diagnosis*, St Louis, 1987, Mosby.)

XXX Syndrome

Girls with XXX syndrome usually are fertile and taller than average. Head size may be somewhat smaller than usual. Some XXX girls have a lower IQ, and many have trouble with verbal skills and interpersonal relationships. There is a wide range of learning, verbal ability, and neuromotor coordination problems. Like trisomies in boys, signs usually are not evident at birth. Thus many XXX girls go on to marry, have children, and lead fairly normal lives. If, however, there is more than one extra X—for instance, XXXX or XXXXX—mental retardation occurs on a fairly severe level.

Early parental intervention may improve the potential of these children. Early diagnosis is important, and referral to speech therapists, child psychologists, and others may help in development. Research is showing that although children may have trouble learning or mastering a psychomotor skill, a supportive, loving environment may be the crucial factor in their optimal development.

AMBIGUOUS GENITALIA

On rare occasions, genital indication of sex is unclear in an infant (Figure 27-24). The presence of ambiguous genitalia has an immediate impact on the parents because their first question after birth is, "Is it a boy or a girl?" When the answer is not known, the parents are

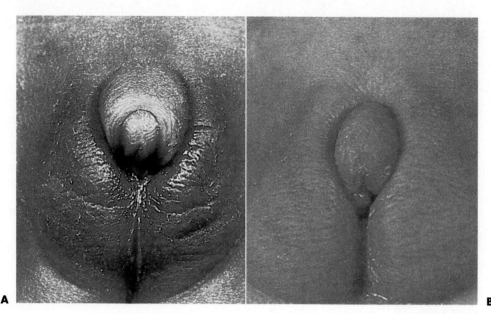

FIGURE 27-24 Ambiguous genitalia. **A** and **B**, Congenital virilizing adrenal hyperplasia. (Courtesy Dr. D. Becker; from Zitelli BJ, Davis HW: *Atlas of pediatric physical diagnosis,* St Louis, 1987, Mosby.)

stunned. The most important intervention after support of the parents and care of the baby is interpretation of the possible causes and the methods of evaluation. Because people are gender conscious, the parents will be distressed until the issue is settled. Knowledge of the possible causes of poor differentiation of genitalia and potential interventions will help the nurse to be supportive during the investigation. For a few babies, reconstructive surgery is the choice; for others, gonadal tissue may be removed to allow the remaining gonads to develop.

Hermaphroditism

On very rare occasions a child has ovarian and testicular tissue; this is *hermaphroditism.* The external genitalia usually are ambiguous. Most of these children have an XX pattern, and the gonads have been inhibited in the phase of differentiation. Others show mosaicism, with XX/XY cell lines. The gonads usually are not functional; therefore the sex of rearing must be determined in other ways. The gender of the child must be decided early because it is very traumatic to change gender during rearing (Simpson, 1982). The genetic sex may not be the deciding factor because it is difficult to "reconstruct" a male who will function normally. Usually the child is raised as a female, with estrogen treatment at puberty.

Pseudohermaphroditism

Children with pseudohermaphroditism have testicular or ovarian tissue and corresponding chromosomes, but the genitalia are ambiguous at birth. There are several causes of *pseudohermaphroditism,* including mosaicism, gene defects changing androgen production or

sensitivity, or teratogens interrupting crucial growth sequences.

The most common of these uncommon disorders is androgen insensitivity, an X-linked inherited problem in a boy with normal chromosome makeup. He has testes, but the external genitalia may show hypospadias, small penis and scrotal sac, or even female genitalia. At puberty, depending on a number of factors, secondary sex characteristics may or may not develop.

Female pseudohermaphroditism often occurs as a result of adrenal hyperplasia, which is inherited as an autosomal recessive gene defect. The girl has excess levels of adrenocorticotropic hormone (ACTH), which, by a series of effects, produces an enlarged clitoris and fusion of the labia. This syndrome needs immediate medical attention because ACTH has many other adverse effects when present in elevated amounts. Finally, it is possible that a teratogen such as a drug affected the development of the baby's genitalia.

Genes and the Environment

The developing embryo is sensitive to environmental influences. Certain genetic problems may appear only when an environmental influence is present (multifactorial defects), or the environmental agent itself may cause the defect (teratogenic defect). To fully appreciate this influence one's concept of the environment must be expanded to include anything that can alter fetal development—substances in the atmosphere, the mother's metabolic state, the food she eats.

Wilson (1977) defines teratogens as "any factor or mechanism that causes cells to die, change their rate of proliferation or biosynthesis, or otherwise fail to follow the prescribed course in development." A wide range of injury may result when a teratogen impinges on fetal development. This variation is the result of one or more of the following as defined by Brent (1986).

1. There are different periods of cell susceptibility to injury. During the preimplantation period the free floating fertilized zygote in body fluids in the tube or uterus is too small to be only partly affected. An "all or nothing" effect occurs.
   a. After implantation, with a few exceptions, whatever is in the maternal environment or circulation will pass through the placenta to the fetus: "the placenta is a sieve."
   b. During organogenesis in the 60 days after implantation, differentiation may be distorted, slowed, or stopped, resulting in structural changes.
   c. During the second and third trimesters, teratogens may continue to inhibit differentiation and may cause cell death, retard growth, or distort biochemical development.
   d. Finally, certain changes may be carcinogenic but show up in later childhood.
2. A genetic variability exists in which one fetus will be affected if subjected to the same teratogen; the other fetus will not be affected.
3. There is usually a dose-response effect with a correlation of dose to severity of effect. Fetal alcohol syndrome (FAS) illustrates dose-response effects.
4. The environment has so many factors that may interact or potentiate the effects of teratogens that tracing the cause often is difficult if not impossible.

It is difficult to trace a cause and effect because animal research does not often apply to human embryos. The dosages used in animal studies are extremely high, much higher than might be found in the environment. Because it is impossible to experiment on the human fetus, information often comes from retrospective studies after the injury has occurred.

The thalidomide tragedy illustrates these points all too well. Only the timely action of Frances O. Kelsey, the science officer of the Food and Drug Administration (FDA) in 1960 prevented the approval of this potent teratogen for use in the United States. Kelsey's suspicions were aroused by case reports from Germany and Australia of an epidemic of limb defects associated with maternal use of the sedative (Figure 27-25) (Lappe, 1991). It is interesting to note that this drug is a teratogen only in some mammals. Currently all drugs are classified as to teratogenicity by means of data from animal and epidemiologic studies (Table 27-6).

Brent (1986) estimates that only 2% to 3% of defects result from known teratogens such as drugs, chemicals, and infections and that 50% to 60% of human malfor-

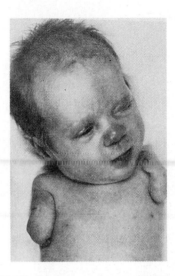

FIGURE 27-25 Thalidomide embryopathy. Neonate with bilateral phocomelia, each hand with three three-segmented fingers, and nevus flammeus of the medial region of the face. (From Wiedemann HR et al: *Atlas of clinical syndromes: a visual aid to diagnosis,* St Louis, 1992, Mosby.)

mations cannot be traced to direct causes such as genetic disease or teratogens.

Because the causes of these defects are largely unknown, most probably they should be regarded as resulting from multifactorial reasons, including environmental factors and gene abnormalities; preventive measures should be used when possible. These measures are summarized in the following list (Brent, 1986):

1. Balanced nutrition before and during pregnancy
   a. Avoidance of overnutrition or undernutrition and weight gain of at least 25 to 30 lb
2. Avoidance of known teratogens during pregnancy
   a. Elevated body temperature from sauna, hot tubs, work environment
   b. Nonprescription, over-the-counter, or self-medication with formerly prescribed drugs
   c. Potentially infecting agents of any kind
   d. Contact with heavy metals, polychlorinated biphenyl (PCB) agents, and dioxin
   e. Exposure to sources of high doses of ionizing radiation
   f. Use of cigarettes, alcohol, and drugs of abuse
3. Prevention of chronic, prolonged hypoxia in utero and acute distress during labor and birth
4. Prevention of trauma during pregnancy or birth

SUSCEPTIBILITY TO TERATOGENS (Box 27-1)

The nurse who cares for the pregnant couple must be aware of current research to help the parents arrive at some very important decisions. Parents motivated to receive information about medications or other factors affecting the growth of their baby tend to ingest fewer

TABLE 27-6   FDA Categories for Labeling Prescription Drugs to Indicate the Risks of Their Use in Pregnancy

CATEGORY	RISKS
A	Controlled studies in women fail to demonstrate a risk to the fetus in the first trimester, and the possibility of fetal harm appears to be remote.
B	Animal studies do not indicate a risk to the fetus and there are no controlled studies in humans, or animal studies show adverse effects on the fetus, but controlled studies in humans have not shown a risk to the fetus.
C	Animal studies have shown the drug to be embryocidal or teratogenic, but there are no controlled studies in humans, or no studies are available in animals or humans.
D	Definitive evidence of risk to the human fetus exists, but the benefit in certain situations (e.g., life-threatening situations in which safer drugs are unavailable or ineffective) may justify the use of the drug despite the risks.
X	Studies in animals or humans have demonstrated fetal abnormalities, or there is evidence of fetal risk based on human experience, or both, and the risk clearly outweighs the possible benefits.

Data from Pregnancy labeling, *FDA Drug Bull* 9:23, 1979; Brent RL: *Clin Perinatol* 13:609, 1986.

BOX 27-1   Human Teratogenic Agents

Known teratogens
Radiation
- High doses of ionizing radiation

Drugs and chemical agents
- Ingestion of heavy metals, mercury, lead, cadmium, PCBs, and pesticides
- Medications such as steroid hormones
  - Androgens
  - Diethylstilbestrol
  - Oral progestogens
- Thalidomide
- Antineoplastic medications
- Tetracyclines
- Antithyroid agents
- Anticoagulants such as warfarin
- Folic acid antagonists
- Isotretinoin (Accutane)

Biologic agents
- Viral diseases such as rubella, cytomegalovirus disease, and herpes simplex
- Toxoplasmosis
- Syphilis, varicella
- Hyperthermia as a result of infection or use of hot tub

Probable or suspected teratogenic agents
Drugs or chemical agents
- Anticonvulsants
- Streptomycin
- Appetite suppressants
- Antianxiety medications such as chlordiazepoxide (Librium), diazepam (Valium), or meprobamate

- Sulfonylurea hypoglycemics
- Therapeutic doses of radiation (over 5 rad)

Maternal illness or deficiency
- Diabetes of long duration or severity
- Epilepsy
- Severe anemia
- Thyroid disease of long duration or severity
- Severe vitamin or mineral deficiencies
- Alcohol use
- Maternal hypertension
- Drug abuse, especially cocaine
- Uncontrolled PKU

Agents requiring caution
- Excessive caffeine
- Decongestants
- Barbiturates
- Most diuretics
- Antituberculosis medications
- Imipramine
- Sulfonamides
- Amphetamines
- Antiemetics
- Tranquilizers
- Salicylates
- Narcotics
- Quinine
- Cimetidine
- Laxatives such as mineral oil or castor oil
- Aminopterin
- Nicotine
- Cortisone

drugs and follow more health-promoting practices during pregnancy.

The stage of development determines the susceptibility of the growing baby to teratogens (Figure 27-26). The period of development from fertilization until the formation of the three germ layers is thought to be relatively free of teratogenic influences because either the teratogen is powerful enough to destroy the entire conceptus or most of the cells compensate for injury to a few cells. The embryonic period is one of the most highly susceptible to the influence of teratogens because the cells are undergoing rapid and intensive differentiation. The type of injury that may occur, however, depends on the organ undergoing the most rapid differentiation at the time the teratogen is introduced. During the fetal period of development, the susceptibility to teratogens diminishes, but the cerebellum, cerebral cortex, eyes, and parts of the urinary tract continue to develop rapidly. Therefore these organs are susceptible to teratogens even in late pregnancy. A growing concern is the effect of teratogens on function, even when structure appears normal. This has created a new field, behavioral teratology.

The effect of certain teratogens depends on the susceptibility of the genes. That is, some families have genes that are unable to withstand influences that other families are able to resist. In addition, the teratogen acts in a specific way on specific aspects of cell metabolism. It is very difficult to predict how a teratogen will affect an organ because sometimes it is not known whether the teratogen will alter the cell membrane, change the nucleic acid, or change the entire cellular structure. The result of exposure to a teratogen (even with only one or two doses) may delay, distort, or divert the development of one group of cells. For instance, the use of alcohol in

differing amounts at the time of conception or throughout the embryonic period may result in FAS. Many medications, including aspirin, or drugs such as cocaine, when used close to labor, may affect the fetus's ability to adapt to the environment after birth.

ENVIRONMENTAL POLLUTANTS

Society becomes aware of the toxic effects of environmental pollutants when people are exposed to high levels and become dramatically ill or die. Workplace exposure (e.g., asbestos, coal dust, or lead) or contamination of the water supply by a chemical such as dioxin or a metal such as methyl mercury provides evidence too clear to ignore, and public health measures must be taken. There are, however, numerous low levels of pollutants to which mother and infant are exposed. Not enough research into low-level effects has been undertaken, and nurses must be alert to government action and can participate in political action for tighter controls on industrial pollution. A discussion of several major teratogens follows (Box 27-1).

Lead, Cadmium, and Manganese

Lead gets into the environment in many ways, primarily into the air through gas emissions. Lead then precipitates into soil and water and enters the food chain to be taken up by plants, which in turn are eaten by animals. Human beings ingest plants and milk from animals grazing in polluted fields and drink water and inhale lead in polluted air. Lead also has been used in paint, pottery, and tin. Workers in industries that use lead have had high rates of illness, stillbirth, and children with neurologic deficits. In this country, some industrial

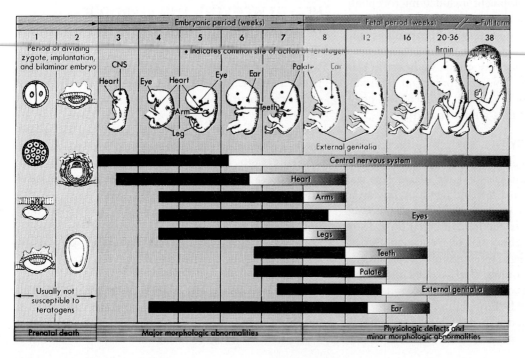

FIGURE 27-26 Sensitive (*shaded*) or critical periods in human development. (From Moore KL: *The developing human: clinically oriented embryology,* ed 4, Philadephia, 1988, WB Saunders.)

controls protect workers, and leaded gasoline is being phased out. In other areas of the world, people may be required to work without protection.

Another source of lead is glaze on ceramic ware. Improperly fired glazes may leak lead into food, especially when acidic foods like vinegar or citrus juices are used. The FDA regulates the amount of lead that is permissible but cannot test all items made for sale in the United States. Imported ceramic products may have poorly glazed finishes. Therefore such items should not be used for cooking or serving salads or juices.

The lead level of 10 µg/dl is considered toxic to children under 5 years of age. Current research indicates a relationship between social class and lead toxicity, with 2-year-olds of lower socioeconomic status showing deficits at lead levels of 6 to 7 µg/dl (Lappe, 1991).

Lead inhibits synthesis of the heme fraction of hemoglobin and affects neural, gastrointestinal, and kidney function. It causes changes in the electroencephalogram (EEG), as well as fatigue and depression on a dose-related level; it accumulates in the body over a lifetime. Researchers have found a correlation between levels of lead and adverse behavior in classrooms (Needleman, Leviton, and Bellinger, 1982). Pihl and Parkes (1977) tested children's hair and found that learning disabilities were correlated with higher levels of lead, cadmium, manganese, and lithium. Like lead, cadmium has somewhat similar effects.

Mercury

Mercury compounds were shown to have devastating effects on growth and development before and after birth after people in Minimata, Japan, were poisoned by fish that contained a high level of methyl mercury. The effects on fetal development included microcephaly and mental and motor impairments. Other studies have linked mercury exposure to CNS abnormalities and cleft palate in mice (Beckman and Brent, 1986). Unfortunately, low levels of mercury compounds are not an unusual finding in fish. This environmental pollutant needs additional study. Pregnant women especially should not ingest potentially contaminated fish.

Polychlorinated Biphenyls

PCBs, common components of transformer fluids, dyes, and inks, are potent teratogens in large doses. This was demonstrated in Japan in 1968 and again in Taiwan in 1979 after pregnant women used PCB-contaminated rice oil in cooking. Their children, affected by a disorder called Yusho, had abnormal pigmentation ("coca-colored"), low birth weight, prematurely erupted teeth, malformed gums, abnormal skull calcification, and rocker-bottom feet. Aside from these two dramatic events, PCBs are found throughout the food chain because of their persistence in the fat cells of animals. Research indicates that persons with higher than nor-

mal PCB levels suffer ill effects such as pregnancy failure, infertility, and preeclampsia (Lappe, 1991). Although in 1976 the Toxic Substance Control Act attempted to stop production of PCBs, there are still almost 750 million pounds left in the environment.

Ionizing Radiation

The National Council on Radiation Protection recommends an interval between therapeutic radiation and conception. If a client receives more than 25 rad (e.g., in cases of Hodgkin's disease), it is advisable to wait several months before becoming pregnant (Brent, 1986).

When diagnostic tests or therapeutic radiation is indicated, the mother and her family should be fully informed before the procedure. (Remember that congenital defects occur at much higher rates from other causes than from radiation.) Brent (1986) recommends a systematic evaluation before diagnostic studies, as follows:

1. Menstrual history and previous obstetric history
2. Any history of congenital defects
3. Status of pregnancy: desired or not?
4. Age of mother and father
5. Potential environmental agents to which couple may be exposed
6. Type of diagnostic study to be performed
7. Calculation of potential exposure to the embryo by a competent radiologist

Before studies are performed, all factors should be discussed openly with the couple, with documentation in the chart to indicate discussion and response. (Lawsuits often are precipitated by anger ["If you had only told me"] and failure to communicate the benefit-to-risk of a procedure.)

HEALTH WORKERS AND REPRODUCTIVE HAZARDS

There are certain health risks in caring for the sick. It is well known that workers need to protect themselves from infection. The risk of working with anesthetic and chemotherapeutic agents is less understood. Early in the 1970s, an awareness developed that anesthetic gases led to a higher miscarriage rate among nurses and physicians working in operating rooms. Anesthesiologists carried gas effects home, and before implementation of safety precautions, some excreted gas up to 30 hours after leaving the operating room. After these studies, standards of ventilation were reconsidered, and most hospitals today follow these standards. Those working in small agencies (e.g., dental practices) should ask whether these standards are being followed (Naeye, 1982).

Cytotoxic drugs are given to as many as 400,000 clients each year. There have been reports of increased abortions among health personnel handling these drugs. Guidelines for drug handling and administration have been formulated by the Occupational Safety and Health Administration (OSHA, 1986). Health workers need to follow these guidelines and question the workplace policies if evidence of noncompliance becomes apparent.

Test Yourself

- What is a teratogen?
- What is the most important determination of the degree to which a fetus may be harmed by a teratogen?
- Name three environmental pollutants that are teratogenic.

INFECTIOUS AGENTS

Intrauterine damage from infection is hard to prevent. Many infections are spread venereally; others such as rubella, cytomegalovirus (CMV), and varicella are acquired through close contact. Currently immunization exists only for rubella. Careful avoidance of infection during pregnancy seems best. (See Chapter 25 for full discussion of effects of infection on pregnancy and fetus.)

Human Immunodeficiency Virus

A possible syndrome of congenital malformations in infants born to mothers with human immunodeficiency virus (HIV) has been reported. Characteristics of the syndrome include IUGR, microcephaly, a flat nasal bridge, wide-spaced and up-slanting eyes, prominent forehead, and fullness of the upper lip. More research is necessary, however, to determine if these are racial variations or due to the virus (Hoyme, 1990).

Syphilis

The rate of syphilis is rising; lack of prenatal care is an important factor in the rise in congenital syphilis. In contrast to what had been formerly thought, *Treponema* organisms can cross the placenta at any age. Although not as common as later transmission, early syphilis infection in the fetus leads to abortion, stillbirth, and premature labor. About one half of the fetuses infected early in gestation and 10% infected later will have signs such as maculopapular rash, hepatosplenomegaly, nail, skeletal, and tooth deformities, and neurologic and ocular involvement (Beckman and Brent, 1986).

Toxoplasmosis, Rubella, Cytomegalovirus, and Herpes Simplex Infection

Toxoplasmosis. Primary infection with the *Toxoplasma* parasite during pregnancy causes congenital infection in 60% of the infants (Lee, 1988). The most severe disease occurs in those infected earliest in gesta-

tion. Effects include chorioretinitis, intracranial calcification, hydrocephaly, and microcephaly. Affected infants suffer psychomotor delays, severe visual impairments, and hearing loss.

Rubella. Although vaccination for rubella is available, many women are not immunized. About 85% of the fetuses infected with the virus during the first 8 weeks of gestation will have anomalies such as cataracts, deafness, glaucoma, and congenital heart disease (Hoyme, 1990). The later in the pregnancy the infection occurs, the fewer the malformations. (See Chapter 25 for more details about neonatal rubella.)

Cytomegalovirus. Cytomegalovirus infection is a strong teratogen. Approximately 65% of infants infected with CMV at *any time* during gestation will have some form of visual, hearing, or learning disability. The signs of congenital CMV infection are similar to other congenital infections; therefore laboratory confirmation often is needed for diagnosis (Alford, 1987).

Herpes. Early fetal herpes infections are rare, but teratogenic effects are similar to toxoplasmosis. The risk for spontaneous abortion and preterm labor is connected to severe infection. The newborn can acquire ascending infection at birth, with a localized infection about mouth, eyes, and on skin. A generalized sepsis with CNS involvement results in high mortality, and survivors may show eye or neurologic defect.

Varicella

Only a few of the infants born after maternal chickenpox demonstrate congenital defects. Of these, growth retardation, eye, limb, and gastrointestinal and genitourinary anomalies have been reported (Hoyme, 1990).

SELECTED TERATOGENIC DRUGS

Use of therapeutic agents in pregnancy always presents a dilemma inasmuch as the benefits must be weighed against the possible risk. Unfortunately, when a pregnant woman abuses drugs and has poor nutrition, infection, and lack of prenatal care, the multiple factors increase risk of fetal injury. Through careful observation, however, it is possible to identify specific patterns of malformations that are associated with individual drugs.

Anticonvulsants

In general, women with epilepsy have two to three times the general risk for congenital malformations. Many diseases, some of which have a genetic component, are grouped under the label "epilepsy." Although use of anticonvulsant agents increases the teratogenic risk of neural tube defects, discontinuing therapy may lead to seizures (see Chapter 23).

Diethylstilbestrol (DES)

Diethylstilbestrol was prescribed for thousands of women in the 1950s and 1960s in an effort to save pregnancies threatened by spontaneous abortion. The efficacy of this treatment is questionable, but not its effects on fetal development. Early observations were of ambiguous genitalia in newborn girls. Later, cases of a previously rare cancer—*clear cell adenocarcinoma* of the vagina—were seen in young teen-age girls. Both groups had been exposed to DES before week 18 of development. Further studies have demonstrated that actual risk of cancer is small. As the girls approached childbearing age, however, structural defects of the reproductive system were identified. There is controversy concerning the effects of DES on the reproductive system of male offspring. At this time DES-related anomalies are known to contribute to perinatal mortality by increasing the risk of spontaneous abortion, ectopic pregnancy, and premature delivery.

Folic Acid Antagonists and Antineoplastic Agents

Folic acid antagonists and antineoplastic agents cause cell death and therefore have teratogenic potential. Women at risk include those receiving therapy as well as those administering them. For the clients, treatment regimens may be varied to decrease fetal risk. Accurate assessment of the risk to personnel is difficult because of the variety of drugs that are administered. Malformations of the CNS and face and IUGR have been observed after aminopterin exposure. Methotrexate use has been associated with absent digits (Beckman and Brent, 1986).

Isotretinoin (Accutane)

Isotretinoin is an effective treatment for severe acne. It also is a potent teratogen. Fetal exposure to this and other vitamin A analogs produces a pattern of anomalies now termed *retinoic acid embryopathy*. Infants with this syndrome have craniofacial defects, malformed or absent ears, cardiac defects, and altered CNS development. The risk of spontaneous abortion also is increased. Women who are planning a pregnancy, as well as those who are pregnant, should avoid use of vitamin A analogs because of their unusually long half-life (Hoyme, 1990).

Lithium

The fetus exposed to lithium is at risk for cardiac defects. Lithium does not appear to harm other developing organs and therefore may be taken after the period of cardiogenesis, that is, after 45 days of gestation (Moore, 1988).

Tetracycline

Infants exposed to tetracycline after the fourth month of gestation have brown staining of the primary teeth and may have some staining of permanent teeth. There may be hypoplastic enamel and an increased risk for dental caries.

Warfarin (Coumadin)

Warfarin is an anticoagulant that causes a pattern of anomalies with fetal exposure. The fetal warfarin syndrome includes IUGR, developmental delays, seizures, a malformed nose, and abnormal bone development. Heparin, a molecule too large to pass the placental barrier, is the anticoagulant best used during pregnancy.

Test Yourself

- The decision to use a medication during pregnancy must be made by weighing the _____ vs the _____.
- How would you advise a pregnant woman with severe acne about exposure to Accutane?

Drugs of Abuse

Alcohol. Alcohol is widely used in the United States. The dangers of perinatal alcohol use have been suspected for many years. In 1973 Jones and Smith described a pattern of malformations in offspring of alcohol-abusing women. The incidence of FAS is thought to have been 1:750 in this country before 1985, when the Surgeon General initiated great emphasis on not drinking during pregnancy. The incidence is much higher in certain populations (Native Americans) and in countries where alcohol intake is high (1:400 in Germany, 1:300 in Sweden and France). These countries currently are using public health interventions to reduce FAS.

The FAS is characterized by CNS deficits, including microcephaly, mild to moderate mental retardation, irritability, and poor feeding. Facial characteristics of these children are so similar that they appear to be related. These characteristics include hirsutism (increased hair on face); short palpebral fissure (lower eyelid); epicanthal fold; depressed, broadened nasal bridge; hypertelorism (increased space between the eyes); short nose with long philtrum (space between nose and lip); thin upper lip and fish-mouth appearance; and possibly low-set ears and small chin.

In addition, prenatal and postnatal growth retardation occurs, often below the 10th percentile. There are hypoplastic nails, clinodactyly (incurving of the fifth fingers), and hemangiomas. Definitive diagnosis of FAS is made if growth retardation, developmental delay, and two of the following are present: microcephaly or eye or characteristic facial anomalies.

Characteristics of FAS persist throughout life, and the effects of development and intelligence are readily noticeable (Figure 27-27).

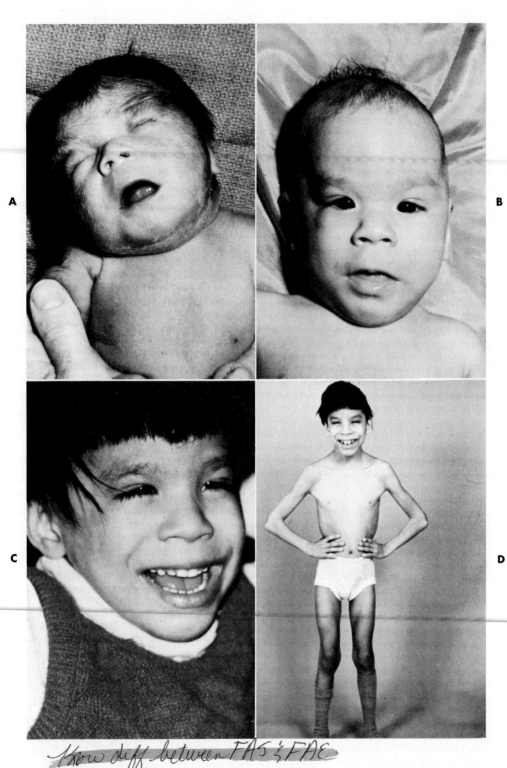

A

B

C

D

FIGURE 27-27 Fetal alcohol syndrome. **A** to **D,** Child of chronically alcoholic mother, diagnosed at birth with FAS. Although he was raised his entire life in one excellent foster home and participated in various remediation programs, he continues to have an IQ around 45 (more severe retardation than most FAS children), with accompanying hyperactivity and distractibility. (From Streissguth AP: Ciba Foundation Symposium No 105: *Mechanisms of alcohol damage in utero.* By permission of AP Streissguth and the Ciba Foundation, Pitman, London.)

Know diff between FAS & FAE

A less severe syndrome also has been identified, *fetal alcohol effect (FAE).* It does not necessarily result in the structural problems of FAS but causes some inhibition of neurologic and behavioral function that leads to learning disabilities. FAE is thought to affect 20% to 30% of the offspring of alcohol-using women.

A number of studies have attempted to determine a specific level of intake above which effects will occur. Findings are contradictory for the following reasons.

1. Genetic susceptibility to alcohol effects. There are differences among racial groups, and FAS is higher in some groups.

2. Self-reporting usually minimizes intake and thus is inaccurate.

3. Other substance abuse may not be reported in the study group.

Streissguth et al (1986) reported on a long-range study of children of substance-abusing mothers. This study adjusted findings for maternal intake of nicotine, caffeine, food, and drugs and for maternal education, among other variables. The group at significant risk included women who drank more than 30 g of absolute alcohol a day. Those women consuming more than 60 g of alcohol per day almost always had affected children in this study. For these children, long-term neurologic effects had not significantly decreased by 4 years of age. Mills and Graubard (1987) collected information from 32,870 women during pregnancy. Their findings indicated that malformation rates were not higher for women who took less than one drink per day in comparison with nondrinking women. They found, however, that genitourinary and sex organ malformations increased significantly with increasing alcohol intake. They concluded that there is the possibility that no safe drinking level exists for some malformations. Therefore the current recommendation of no drinking during pregnancy is certainly the safest (see Chapter 10).

Cocaine and crack. Cocaine's teratogenic potential has been recognized only recently. Ingestion during early pregnancy in human beings and laboratory animals has produced genitourinary and limb anomalies in a number exceeding the statistical rate for the population. It is unclear whether these defects are a direct result of the drug or of the hyperthermia that often accompanies its use (Mills and Graubard, 1987). Because many women are polydrug users, the observed effects may be due to other substances or interactions between drugs.

Test Yourself

- What is the accepted safe level for consumption of alcohol during pregnancy?
- Why is it so difficult to attribute a specific congenital defect to prenatal cocaine use?

Genetic Therapy

Genetic therapy consists of several classes of care, ranging from the familiar to the "cutting edge." Those in class I are familiar. (1) Organ transplantation such as kidney transplant is used for clients with inherited kidney disease. (2) Drug therapy is used to induce the production of certain enzymes. (3) General surgery can alter malformed tissues. (4) Fetal surgery is an exciting advance that has been used to correct diaphragmatic hernia and hydrocephalus before further damage can occur. (6) Dietary changes also can be used to treat many inherited inborn errors of metabolism.

Class II interventions involve administration of enzymes and protein factors to those with inherited defi-

ciencies. Injections of insulin and blood factor VII are examples. Class III genetic therapy attempts to insert a normal gene into cells with a genetic defect. The proposed new treatment for CF will attempt to do this (Rosenfeld et al, 1992). Nurses may be caring for families whose infants are in therapy and should have basic knowledge about various interventions.

Genetic Counseling

Couples who seek genetic counseling begin with some information, enough to form questions about their reproductive future. One of the many reasons they seek guidance is a history of genetic problems in the family.

After an affected baby is born, couples may seek guidance about the risks of the defect in a future pregnancy. For some, the defect (e.g., an IEM) did not become evident until after the second child was conceived.

Parental attitudes toward abortion influence their readiness to seek a diagnosis through chorionic villus sampling (CVS) or amniocentesis. In a number of studies of parents' attitudes in counseling, the groups were almost evenly divided among those strongly opposed, partially opposed, and in favor of abortion in cases of diagnosed defects. Thus the nurse should not *assume* any attitude about outcome when working with parents who are in counseling.

It is important to differentiate among the decisions made during the planning phase, before pregnancy has begun, and decisions made after pregnancy has been confirmed. The options before pregnancy are as follows:

1. Not to risk pregnancy
   a. For the first time (to remain childless)
   b. After having an affected child
2. To try to conceive and make the decision to retain or abort the fetus depending on test results (risk rates and personal values will influence this decision)
3. To conceive and carry the pregnancy to term, regardless of genetic findings (in this case, after counseling, many parents decide not to have prenatal testing because they will not abort)

After the pregnancy has begun, decisions that initially confront the couple are more difficult. In most cases the couple did not suspect that there would be any problem or had not supposed that they were even at risk; they are stunned to receive the results of ultrasound evaluation or amniocentesis. Couples may be confronted with other test results such as a low or high alpha-fetoprotein level and, depending on interpretation of information, may be confused and panicked.

These couples must face the loss of the fantasized "perfect" child. Their sense of coherence as a couple is threatened. Grief may absorb their emotional energy. The genetic counselor must work with them to think through the decision, within a certain time limit, to end the pregnancy or to retain it. If they choose to end the pregnancy, it must be done promptly after the amniocentesis.

The couple who seek counseling before pregnancy work on a more theoretic level and have time to reach a considered decision. The couple who have had one affected child and seek counseling and amniocentesis are intensely concerned. They know what it means to live and work with a handicapped child (Paritsky, 1985). They may feel they must not bring another child into the world who has the same problems. If they have decided to risk another pregnancy, they may experience great tension until the test results come back.

WORK OF COUNSELING

It is important to understand what genetic counselors offer and to realize that geographic location may prevent a couple from seeking their resources. Physicians may not be aware of genetic counseling centers or do not refer their clients.

Counselors should know about the risks of genetic disease and the status of environmental teratogens. When given the test results or family genetic history, they should be able to guide the couple in decision making, without influencing them for or against pregnancy termination. This is difficult because people in crisis often seek advice from an expert and may expect to be told what to do. An experienced counselor will prevent client dependency in this way. It is vitally important for the couple to make their own decision and to have gone through the process of making it. If they do not, they may blame each other, the counselor, the physician, or others who gave advice. They may come to feel that someone "talked them into" their decision. To recover from the grief of having a baby with a defect, the couple must feel that they made the best decision about the future of their family.

Nursing Responsibilities
▶ ASSESSMENT

Nurses meet pregnant couples who are waiting for the results of amniocentesis or after they have received the results. They must be supportive and aware of the process that counseling has initiated. There are several levels of decision making, and the partners may be together or struggling at different places in the process. Humphreys and Berkeley (1987) suggest five levels in decision making. In the beginning, the world that the person lives in should be described by the person being counseled. Then she should describe what life would be like if the worst pregnancy outcome happened and if the best outcome happened. Both partners listen to each other.

Briefly, contingency plans are discussed in case the worst happened. In this case the counselor may elicit defenses expressed by one partner or magical thinking (e.g., "They'll have a cure for that soon"). The counselor helps couples to face the possibility that they may not know how to think about what might happen. The counselor explores the strengths of the couple (e.g., their support system and members of the extended family). Sometimes it helps a couple to role play to get in touch with fears and strengths.

In the next level the couple learns to express the worst situation in language that can objectify the problem (e.g., "If the child has Tay-Sachs disease. . ."). In this period the counselor gives information regarding tests, timetables, and risks. When the couple can freely express themselves in objective language, they can begin to look at their own values.

At this point, it may be useful to help parents to look at the value each is placing on having a child. It often comes to light that one is more convinced than the other to have the child no matter what. When this occurs, the counselor helps the couple to sort out and recognize how this will hinder decision making.

The couple needs to come to a shared decision that both can accept. If they do, they are more ready to face the "what if" question. A couple who has been through counseling and decides not to have children or not to have this child must then come to terms with their decision.

Many do not receive support in this manner but receive information that they find hard to integrate. In working with these couples, the nurse should not add to the burden of information but use therapeutic support as discussed in Chapter 26. Support for the grieving person follows the same principles.

▶ NURSING DIAGNOSES

1. High risk for anticipatory/dysfunctional grieving
2. Moderate-to-high anxiety, depending on the length of the pregnancy and relationship to test results
3. Body-image and self-esteem disturbance related to the inability to conceive a normal child, which may include anger or grief directed at the partner
4. Decisional conflict related to timing and choices presented
5. Ineffective family or individual coping related to stress, grieving
6. Spiritual distress expressed or implied in anger phase of grieving.

▶ EXPECTED OUTCOMES

Parents will:

1. Seek support appropriately during the anticipatory grieving phase
2. Manage anxiety
3. Participate in further testing when indicated and desired
4. Choose appropriate interventions consistent with the couple's values and beliefs
5. Participate in the counseling process
6. Seek spiritual resources as needed

▶ NURSING INTERVENTIONS

Although very desirable, follow-up care often is not possible, especially if counseling has been at a distant center. If the couple decide to keep the pregnancy, special support during labor and delivery and in the recovery period should be planned. Documentation of care and client progress must reflect a consistent plan.

Spiritual distress may be evident. Many couples confront these issues of life and death or deformity for the first time. If there is support through family, church, or synagogue, work already will have begun in resolving questions. If the news is recent or at the time of birth, a couple may be stunned, quiet, or in shock. With sensitivity, you may inquire about their support systems and sources of personal strength in other times of difficulty. As you listen, parents often will share their beliefs regarding the child whose life has ended or has been changed in its potential.

You will be more involved with the parents when they come to the labor suite for a late termination or for the birth of the affected baby. The attitude with which they are received is very important. The primary nurse should be selected for her ability to relate to parents in crisis. This nurse benefits from support by others and a clear mode of communication with the health care team.

Nursing care is significant in birth and recovery. Bereavement occurs whether the pregnancy is being terminated or the baby is born alive. Follow these suggested guidelines by Van Putte (1988) and Krone and Harris (1988).

1. Know the history before meeting the couple. Requests to repeat their process of discovery, testing, and decision making to the nurses, residents, and admission personnel only reinforces the painful past. It is suggested that the primary physician fill out the admission history and send it with the couple and then confer with the nurses who will care for the couple.
2. Provide a private labor room and ask the couple what would make them comfortable. Identify the nurse who will be the primary nurse on each shift.
3. Limit the number of people in and out of the room, but do not avoid the couple. The primary nurse must be sensitive to their need to talk and to the mother's physical needs. Encourage their verbalization of anxiety, fear, and sadness.
4. Provide for liberal pain relief as requested.
5. Know ahead of time the couple's wishes for autopsy or burial. This must be discussed by the primary physician and should not be left to bring up as an afterthought. The nurse must be informed of these plans to be supportive.
6. Know ahead of time the general information given by the genetics counselor. For instance, with anencephaly, do the parents know the usual survival period?
7. Serve as proxy and guide as the parents go through the experience of seeing the infant and during the claiming process. The baby should be cleaned and wrapped in a blanket before the parents hold or touch the infant. It is important that the parents view the baby. If they do not, they need mementos such as a photograph or handprints or footprints, and an ID band may be made out. If the mother cannot see the baby (because she is ill or has had surgery), the nurse should view the infant, noting special characteristics to point out, and then describe these details to the parents.
8. Gender is important. During claiming, parents will find resemblances to someone in the family. The mother needs to remember the child as "my girl" or "my boy." If the baby is stillborn, the parents will "focus on normal physical characteristics since that is all they have" (Woods and Esposito, 1987).
9. Without visualizing the baby, it is thought that the grieving process is delayed or uneven. Parents who had no tangible evidence such as a photograph often return to a unit later, asking if anything was kept as a record. It is therefore recommended that a file be kept.
10. Finally, support from a perinatal grieving team is beneficial during this period. Follow-up counseling should be offered. Included in this care is a conference with the physician to review the events, to give findings if the cause was unknown, and to discuss implications for future reproductive potential. This conference should be separated from the event to allow time for acute grief to pass. In addition, one member of the team calls or visits with the parents to assist in the grief process and to offer aid or referral if needed (see Chapter 29).

If the infant survives, the same principles of one-to-one nursing are followed in the immediate recovery period. The parents will be faced with decisions regarding future care. The nurse encourages early visits and touching if the baby is in the NICU. Visits should be unrestricted, and the same nurses care for the infant to provide continuity of care.

▶ EVALUATION

Evaluation of the plan of care may not be complete but can include questions such as the following.

1. Did the partners find adequate support during the counseling process?
2. Did they discuss beliefs and seek support for spiritual distress?

3. Was there effective follow-through?
4. Were other members of the health care team oriented to follow through in the labor, birth, and recovery periods?

Test Yourself

- List three examples of genetic therapy in use today.
- Describe nursing responsibilities for the family receiving genetic counseling.

KEY POINTS

- Congenital and genetic anomalies are the fifth leading cause of years of potential life lost (YPLL) (see Chapter 1). As such, these defects are a major cause of death and disability.
- Varying degrees of developmental disabilities are present in more than 3% of the population.
- One gene, one function describes the inborn errors of metabolism that are carried by recessive inheritance. These may cause disability or death, but many can be treated today.
- Dominantly inherited gene defects may be fatal or may not appear until later in life, allowing reproduction and passing on of the gene.
- These gene defects tend to be concentrated in racial groups, although genetic drift is "diluting" the gene pool.
- Autosomal defects generally are devastating, and many result in loss of the embryo before maturation. Others result in trisomy with multiorgan effects.
- The most common of the trisomies, Down syndrome, may be severe or modified, and early intervention provides the best possible chance of development.
- Sex chromosome trisomies often do not show signs at birth but usually affect intelligence as well as reproductive function.

- Only one monosomy is possible; children with Turner syndrome survive with fairly normal intelligence, but without development of secondary sex characteristics, unless mosaic.
- Prenatal genetic screening is available to couples with potential for single gene and chromosomal defects. Amniocentesis and maternal serum AFP are standards of care for pregnant women.
- For a couple who find elective abortion morally unacceptable, these screening tests will be useful only in cases for which fetal therapy is possible or if the family wishes to prepare for the birth of a child with special needs.
- Environmental pollutants have been recognized for years, but escalating levels in the air and water are major health problems to be addressed.
- Nurses, as health educators, must participate in appropriate community and political action to improve the environment.
- Genetic counseling is available in larger urban settings and should be offered to any couple with a history of defects in family or in offspring.

STUDY QUESTIONS

27-1 Select a term from this chapter that is described in the brief statements below.

a. Exchange of genetic material between chromosomes is _Independant assortment_
b. Loss of part of a chromosome is called _deletment_
c. An extra chromosome in the ovum results in a _Trisomy_.

d. Nonsex chromosomes are called _autosomes_.
e. Change in genetic material as a result of radiation or other factor is a _Mutation_.
f. An environmental toxin is called a _teratogen_.

27-2 Note the following statements as either *true* or *false*.

f a. Major structural birth defects arise in the third trimester.

f b. Only substances that a pregnant woman breathes, ingests, or injects can be teratogenic.

f c. If a man fathers one child with a heterozygous autosomal dominant gene disorder, he himself must have this disorder.

27-3 There is evidence that maternal hyperthermia in the first trimester increases the risk for which of the following problems?
(a.) Anencephaly
b. Cleft lip and palate
c. Gastroschisis
d. Potter syndrome

27-4 Baby girl Adams is diagnosed with Turner's syndrome. Which statement most completely describes this variation?
a. Severe mental and physical retardation will be evident.
b. Female infant will show an extra chromosome and neural tube defects.
(c.) Wide-spaced nipples, web neck, and future sterility occur.
d. Ambiguous genitalia are present as a result of altered sex chromosome pattern.

27-5 Choose two of the following terms to correctly complete this sentence: genotype, phenotype, homozygous, heterozygous

Blue eye color is the *Phenotype* that is observed in those who are *homozygous* for the gene for blue eyes.

27-6 Joe carries one dominant gene for brown eyes and a blue recessive gene. Jane's eyes are blue. What is their chance to have a blue-eyed baby? Draw a Punnet square to discover the answer.

27-7 Mary has blood type AA and Jim's type is BO. Do they have any chance of having an infant with a homozygous blood type? Use a Punnett square.

27-8 Ahmed is color blind and his wife has a completely normal genotype. The couple asks if their newborn son will be color blind. Which response by the nurse is more accurate?
(a.) The child will be completely normal.
b. The child has a one in four chance of being color blind.
c. Only if the child were a girl would she be color blind.
d. Mrs. Ahmed would have to be color blind for the son to have the defect.

27-9 Characteristics of fetal alcohol syndrome include all of the following except:
a. Microcephaly
b. Symmetric prenatal growth retardation
(c.) Hemangioma
d. Low bridge of nose, smooth upper lip line

RESOURCES FOR PARENTS

National Center for Education in Maternal and Child Health (NCEMCH)
38th and R Streets, NW
Washington, DC 20013-1133
(202) 625-8400
Funded by the Division of Maternal and Child Health, Department of Health and Human Services, to be a channel of communication and to build networks and coordinate public- and private-sector efforts in maternal and child health
Sample publications
Reaching out: A directory of voluntary organizations in maternal and child health
A reader's guide for parents of children with mental, physical or emotional disabilities
Comprehensive clinical genetic services centers: a national directory

National Center for Orphan Drugs and Rare Diseases (NCODARD)
P.O. Box 1133
Washington DC 20013-1133
Funded by the Food and Drug Administration, Division of Health and Human Services
National Institutes of Health
Public Inquiries Office
Bethesda, MD 20205

March of Dimes Birth Defects Foundation
1275 Mamaroneck Ave.
White Plains, NY 10605

REFERENCES

Alford CA: Chronic congenital and perinatal infections. In Avery GB, editor: *Neonatalogy: pathophysiology and management of the newborn*, ed 3, Philadelphia, 1987, JB Lippincott.

Beckman DA, Brent RL: Mechanisms of known teratogens: drugs and chemicals, *Clin Perinat* 13(3):649, 1986.

Berch DB and Bender BG: Margins of sexuality, *Psychol Today*, p 54, Dec 1987.

Brent RL: Evaluating the alleged teratogenicity of environmental agents, *Clin Perinatol* 13(3):609, 1986.

Chasnoff IJ et al: Perinatal effects of cocaine, *Contemp Ob/Gyn* 29(5):163, 1987.

Flatz G: Genetics of lactose digestion in humans, *Clin Perinatol* 13(3):39, 1986.

Hook EB: Behavioral implications of the human XYY genotype, *Science* 179:139, 1973.

Hoyme HG: Teratogenetically induced fetal anomalies. I. Fetal dysmorphology, *Clin Perinatol* 17(3):547, 1990.

Humphreys P, Berkeley D: Representing risk: supporting genetic counseling, *Birth Defects* 23(2):227, 1987.

Jones KL, Smithe DW: Recognition of the fetal alcohol syndrome in early infancy, *Lancet* 1:99, 1973.

Krone C, Harris C: The importance of infant gender and family resemblance within parents' perinatal bereavement process: establishing personhood, *J Perinat Nurs* 2(2):1, 1988.

Lappe M: *Chemical deception: the toxic threat to health and the environment*, San Francisco, 1991, Sierra Club Books.

Lee R: Parasites and pregnancy: the problems of malaria and toxoplasmosis, *Clin Perinatol* 15(2):351, 1988.

Levy HL, Waisbren SE: Effects of untreated maternal phenylketonuria and hyperphenylalaninemia on the fetus, *N Engl J Med* 309:1269, 1983.

McCauley E, Sybert VP, Ehrhardt AA: Psychosocial adjustment of adult women with Turner syndrome, *Clin Genet* 29:284, 1986.

Mills JL, Graubard BI: Is moderate drinking during pregnancy associated with increased risk for malformation? *Pediatrics* 3(80):309, 1987.

Miola ES: Down syndrome: update for practitioners, *Pediatr Nurs* 13(4):233, 1987.

Moore KL: *The developing human: clinically oriented embryology*, ed 4, Philadelphia, 1988, WB Saunders.

Naeye RL: Working during pregnancy: effects on the fetus, *Pediatrics* 69:724, 1982.

Needleman HL, Leviton A, Bellinger D: Lead-associated intellectual deficit, *N Engl J Med* 306:367, 1982.

Oakley GP: Frequency of human congenital malformation, *Clin Perinatol* 13(3):545, 1986.

OSHA work practice guidelines for personnel dealing with cytotoxic (antineoplastic) drugs, *Am J Hosp Pharm* 43:1193, 1986.

Paritzky JF: Tay Sachs, *Am J Nurs* 3:261, 1985.

Pihl RO, Parkes JM: Hair element content in learning disabled children, *Science* 198:204, 1977.

Rosenfeld MA et al: In vivo transfer of the human CF transmembrane conductance regulator gene to the airway epithelium, *Cell* 68:143, 1992.

Sherman SL et al: The marker (X) syndrome: a cytogenetic and genetic analysis, *Ann Hum Genet* 48:21, 1984.

Simon JD: Radiation protection groups, *J Nucl Med* 27:1816, 1986.

Simpson E: Sex reversal and sex determination, *Nature* 300(5891):404, 1982.

Smith J: The dangers of perinatal cocaine use, *MCN* 3(13):174, 1988.

Streissguth AP et al: Mechanisms of alcohol damage in utero, *CIBA Found Symp* No. 105, 1986.

Sutherland GR: The enigma of the fragile X chromosome, *Trends Genet* 1:108, 1985.

Thompson JS, Tompson M: *Genetics in medicine*, Philadelphia, 1986, WB Saunders.

Uchida IA: Maternal radiation and trisomy 21. In Hook EB, Porter IA, editors: *Population genetics studies in humans*, New York, 1977, Academic Press.

Van Putte AW: Perinatal bereavement crisis: coping with negative outcomes from prenatal diagnosis, *J Perinat Nurs* 2(2):12, 1988.

Wald NJ: Neural tube defects and vitamins, *Br J Obstet Gynaecol* 91:516, 1984.

Wilson JG: *Environment and birth defects*, New York, 1977, Academic Press.

White R, Lalouel JM: Chromosome mapping with DNA markers, *Sci Am* 258(2):40, 1988.

Woods J, Esposito J: *Pregnancy loss, medical therapeutics and practical considerations*, New York, 1987, Williams & Wilkins.

Zacharias JF: The new genetics, *Neonat Net* 19(2):122, 1990.

 ## STUDENT RESOURCE SHELF

Angelini DJ, Gives RM, editors: Substance abuse and environmental toxins, *J Perinat Neonat Nurs* 3(4): entire issue, 1990.

Brent RL, Beckman DA, editors: Teratology, *Clin Perinat* 13:3, 1986.

Graham JM, editor: Fetal dysmorphology, Pt I, *Clin Perinat* 14:3, 1990.

Graham JM, editor: Fetal clinical genetics, Pt II, *Clin Perinat* 14:4, 1990.

These symposia include major research reports on abnormal fetal development. Both genetic and environmental influences are considered, with many illustrations of mechanisms and effects.

Lappe M: *Chemical deception: the toxic threat to health and the environment*, San Francisco, 1991, Sierra Club Books. Reviews 10 myths about the human response to environmental toxins; not limited to the effects on the fetus.

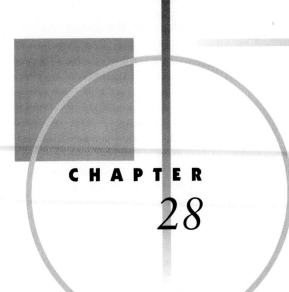

CHAPTER
28

Nursing Care of the High-Risk Newborn

KEY TERMS

Apnea
Asphyxia
Atelectasis
Bronchopulmonary
* Dysplasia (BPD)*
Continuous Positive
* Airway Pressure*
* (CPAP)*
Diving Reflex
Hyaline Membrane
Hydrocephaly
Hyperbilirubinemia
Hypoxic-Ischemic
* Encephalopathy*
* (HIE)*
Insensible Water Loss
* (IWL)*
Intraventricular
* Hemorrhage (IVH)*
Kangaroo Care
Kernicterus

Meningomyelocele
Microcephaly
Necrotizing Enterocolitis
* (NEC)*
Periodic Breathing
Persistent Pulmonary
* Hypertension of the*
* Newborn (PPHN)*
Polycythemia

Respiratory Distress
* Syndrome (RDS)*
Resuscitation
Retinopathy of
* Prematurity (ROP)*
Surfactant
Transposition of Great
* Arteries (TGA)*
Thrombocytopenia

LEARNING OBJECTIVES

1. *Describe the process of newborn resuscitation.*
2. *Identify the role of the nurse in the health care team during resuscitation.*
3. *Correlate signs and symptoms of problems commonly seen during the newborn period with potential causes.*
4. *Summarize the relationship between premature or postmature birth and neonatal illness.*
5. *Describe how selected technical procedures are commonly used during care of a high-risk newborn.*
6. *Discuss how bonding may be inhibited when neonates need extended care.*
7. *Formulate a plan of care for a high-risk neonate and family.*

High risk in infants results mainly from prematurity, postmaturity, acute fetal distress, or congenital anomalies. In Chapters 18 and 19, you learned about the transition to extrauterine life and how to identify the infant who is making a normal transition. This chapter reviews conditions that compromise the infant's ability to make that transition. This chapter, however, is structured differently. Because one infant may have multiple problems, samples of nursing diagnoses and expected outcomes are included in each discussion of potential dysfunction. Interventions are integrated within the chapter, because all care is collaborative in an NICU, and a nursing care plan for one infant concludes the chapter.

Newborn infants are identified as high risk if factors affecting the pregnancy, delivery, or initial hours of life cause problems in normal adaptation. Because most high-risk infants are preterm, postterm, small for gestational age (SGA), or large for gestational age (LGA), it is important to differentiate between weight and maturity. These two parameters influence birth outcome in different ways.

Low birth weight is defined as less than or equal to 2500 g. A further distinction is that *very* low-birth-weight infants weigh less than 1500 g and *extremely* low-birth-weight infants weigh less than 1000 g.

A premature (preterm) infant is any infant born after the beginning of week 20 of gestation and before the end of week 37. Within the parameters of weight and age, further distinctions are necessary. By means of the graph in Figure 18-28, an infant whose weight is plotted below the 10th percentile is identified as SGA. The infant whose weight is plotted above the 90th percentile is LGA.

SGA or LGA infants may be preterm, term, or postterm (Figure 28-1). In addition to the problems associated with prematurity or postmaturity, the process that caused the alteration in intrauterine growth may continue to affect these infants after birth.

Prematurity

Premature birth is the major cause of infant mortality in the United States. The health of a baby born before 37 completed weeks of gestation may depend on the management of the intrapartum period by the perinatal team. Therapy to delay premature labor may allow a few more hours or days for the maturation of body systems, and careful delivery management will further protect the fragile infant. The infant's maturity at birth will affect every system and all physiologic functions. Especially at risk are respiratory, metabolic, hematologic, immunologic, neurologic, and gastrointestinal functions. The establishment of regional neonatal intensive care centers has reduced the once overwhelming mortality rates for very small premature babies.

A study at seven neonatal centers of the National Institutes of Child Health and Human Development Neonatal Intensive Care network revealed a survival rate of 34% among infants of less than 751 g birth weight, 66% among infants with a birth weight of 751 to 1000 g, 87% among infants with a birth weight of 1001 to 1250 g, and 93% among infants with a birth weight of 1251 to 1500 g (Hack, 1991).

Postmaturity

Postmaturity is gestation lasting beyond 42 weeks. The incidence of postmaturity varies with its causes. Prolonged pregnancy may be a normal variant because some women routinely deliver as much as 2 to 3 weeks after the estimated date of birth (EDB). An infant with postmaturity syndrome has normal length and head circumference but may have lost weight in utero as a result of poor placental function after 42 weeks. This placental insufficiency may result in fetal distress during labor. Signs of the syndrome are listed in Box 28-1. Postmature infants are at risk for birth asphyxia and hypoxic-ischemic encephalopathy, meconium aspiration, hypoglycemia, hypothermia, hypocalcemia, and polycythemia.

CONSIDERATIONS IN CARE

The lines between medicine and nursing can become blurred in the neonatal intensive care unit (NICU). Care is primarily collaborative, with overlapping, shared responsibilities. Many nursing interventions are based on established written protocols, resulting in more independence and creativity of care. In an entry level nursing position, you will be observing and intervening

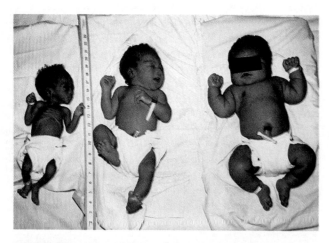

FIGURE 28-1 Three infants of the same gestational age showing effects of LGA (*right*), AGA (*middle*), and IUGR with postmaturity (SGA) (*left*). (From *Perinatal assessment of maturation*, National Audiovisual Center, Washington, DC.)

BOX 28-1   Signs of Postmaturity Syndrome

Head

No lanugo on face; edges of skull bones are hard with small fontanelles.
Hair is smooth but may be receding from forehead.

Ears

Pinna incurved to lobe, firm with cartilage.

Eyes

Appears very alert; eyes wide open, gazing at objects.

Face

Appears thin, "little old man" look.

Chest

May have respiratory distress if meconium was aspirated.
Bony prominences evident—caused by loss of weight.

Abdomen

May be flattened if meconium passed; appears sunken in, not protuberant.
Cord may be thin with little Wharton's jelly, and may be meconium stained.

Heart

Low resting heart rate.

Genitalia

Very pendulous scrotum with descended testes.
Labia cover clitoris but may show signs of subcutaneous loss of fatty tissue.

Extremities

Loss of subcutaneous tissue makes legs and arms look wasted.
Nails are long and may be meconium stained.
Deep sole creases.
Ankle flexion at zero angle.

Skin

Degrees of dry, peeling skin evident.
No lanugo or vernix.
Poor skin turgor.

Central nervous system

Hypertonic.
All reflexes readily elicited.
Vigorous suck; often appears hungry.
Tremors of hypoglycemia or hypocalcemia are frequent.

with much guidance from more experienced staff members. Your coping skills will be tried in an atmosphere of noise from beepers and alarms, dry heat from radiant warmers, and eerie blue light of the phototherapy lamps. There will be people with different styles of adjustment to crises of varying proportions. As you care for babies that can fit into the palm of your hand, quality-of-life issues become woven into crises demanding timely decisions. For these reasons, nurses who care for sick neonates also need care for themselves.

The same environment in which adults are stressed takes its toll on infants. A normal, naturally occurring environment cannot be simulated for the infant. Weightlessness, warmth, muffled sound, and darkness at birth give way to pressure, cold, noise, and bright lights. As a result, in the NICU, in the midst of seeming chaos, noise must be reduced to let the babies grow and develop normally.

Delivery of a High-Risk Infant

During fetal life the placenta is the organ for gas exchange (i.e., oxygen and carbon dioxide). At birth the lungs and circulation go through a series of changes until, ultimately, the lungs provide the neonate with oxygen and remove the by-products of respiration.

ASPHYXIA

Asphyxia is a direct result of respiratory dysfunction, whether from alterations in uteroplacental function or from alterations in the neonate's ability to breathe independently.

Asphyxia is the triad of hypoxia, hypercapnia, and acidosis (metabolic and respiratory) that may occur prenatally or postnatally. Typically something occurs to prevent the delivery of oxygen to the tissues, causing the body to convert from aerobic to anaerobic metabolism. Lactic acid builds up, causing metabolic acidosis. Because whatever prevented the delivery of oxygen also prevents the removal of carbon dioxide, respiratory acidosis also is present (see Figure 14-10).

Asphyxia stimulates the primitive **diving reflex** during which blood is shunted to more "valuable" organs from the periphery. For a short time the brain, heart, and adrenal glands are preferentially perfused at the expense of the intestine, kidneys, liver, and other organs. If, however, asphyxia is not corrected promptly, even vital organs suffer from hypoxia and ischemia. Hypoxia, hypercapnia, and resulting acidosis affect the function of several body systems (Box 28-2). The relatively high fetal hematocrit (Hct) level allows the fetus to adjust to hypoxia more easily than do adults. However, because hypotension worsens with increasingly severe asphyxia, all fetal reserves run out quickly.

BOX 28-2   Multisystem Effects of Perinatal Asphyxia

Respiratory system

Meconium aspiration
Increased severity of respiratory distress syndrome (RDS)

Cardiovascular system

Persistent pulmonary hypertension (PPH)
Myocardial dysfunction

Metabolic system

Ineffective thermoregulation from central nervous system damage and decreased glycogen stores
Hypoglycemia
Hypocalcemia
Metabolic acidosis

Central nervous system

Hypoxic-ischemic encephalopathy
Intraventricular hemorrhage
Stroke/infarction

Renal system

Acute tubular necrosis

Gastrointestinal

Necrotizing enterocolitis

Hematologic system

Disseminated intravascular coagulation (DIC)

BOX 28-3   Factors That Place an Infant at Risk for Birth Asphyxia

Maternal

- Diabetes mellitus
- Isoimmunization
- Infection
- Third-trimester bleeding
- Pregnancy-induced hypertension or chronic hypertension
- Drug abuse
- Abruptio placentae
- Placenta previa
- Oligohydramnios
- Polyhydramnios
- Preterm labor

Fetal

- Multiple gestation
- Congenital anomalies
- Intrauterine growth retardation
- Cord prolapse
- Prematurity or postmaturity
- Malpresentation
- Prolonged rupture of membranes
- Operative delivery
- Poor Biophysical Profile Score
- Fetal distress
- Meconium-stained amniotic fluid
- Macrosomia

Fetal asphyxia (see Chapter 14) can occur any time during gestation but is more common during labor and delivery. Many factors during pregnancy, labor, and delivery can contribute to intrapartum asphyxia (Box 28-3). Because they sometimes result in asphyxia, the high-risk infant should be identified before birth and closely monitored during labor and delivery.

Birth asphyxia may accompany a high-risk delivery. Poor management of birth asphyxia can initiate pathologic, multisystem events that greatly compromise the infant's adjustment to extrauterine life. Prenatal causes of birth asphyxia are factors that disrupt uteroplacental circulation. When a neonate is asphyxiated, the acidosis reverses the normally high affinity of fetal hemoglobin for oxygen, resulting in reduction of tissue oxygenation. Asphyxia also may prevent normal dilation of pulmonary blood vessels. This perpetuates the normal fetal right-to-left shunt in the heart and further prevents blood from reaching the lungs.

Risk

Asphyxial episodes before or after birth trigger central nervous system dysfunction because of disturbances in cerebral blood flow, which may result in infarction (i.e., stroke) or intraventricular hemorrhage. Myocardial ischemia, necrotizing enterocolitis, acute tubular necrosis, and persistent fetal circulation also may develop because of asphyxial insult to specific organs.

Perinatal asphyxia causes syndromes of cardiovascular and respiratory alterations called *primary* and *secondary apnea* (Figure 28-2). Primary apnea begins with an acute episode of asphyxia. Initially the fetus makes several gasping motions, and the heart rate and blood pressure (BP) rise in an attempt to maintain oxygenation and perfusion. Respiratory effort, heart rate, and BP then fall as the infant becomes more acidotic. Primary apnea ends (about 7 minutes after it began) with the last gasp when the infant progresses to secondary apnea. Frequently it is impossible to know which stage of apnea affects a depressed infant at birth. Thus you should never delay resuscitative efforts.

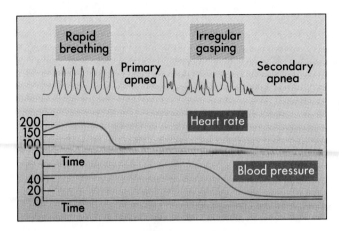

FIGURE 28-2 Physiologic changes that occur during primary and secondary apnea. (Modified from Bloom RS, Cropley CC: *Textbook of neonatal resuscitation,* Dallas, 1990, American Heart Association.)

Signs

The Apgar score gives some indication of the severity of asphyxia. The score is a useful guide to assess the degree of asphyxia and the effectiveness of resuscitative measures, but resuscitation should never be delayed to assign an Apgar score. The decision to initiate resuscitation should be based on the evaluation of the infant's respirations, heart rate, and color.

Infants with minimal or no asphyxia (Apgar score of 8 to 10) at birth will be pink and exhibit respiratory efforts (see Chapter 18). The infant delivered in a state of *primary apnea* will have an Apgar score of 4 to 7, with cyanosis, mild bradycardia, near-normal reflex activity, hypotonia, and gasping respirations. Those who progress to *secondary apnea* will become profoundly depressed with cyanosis, severe bradycardia, depressed reflexes, and absence of movements and respiratory effort. The Apgar score will become 0 to 3 as neurologic depression deepens.

Clinical Management

Management of the infant with asphyxia follows the ABCs (airway, breathing, and circulation) of cardiac resuscitation, with modifications in technique because of differences in neonatal physiology. You may be the only professional care giver available for the newborn in the delivery room because the birth attendants may be involved in care of the mother and may not be able to leave the mother to resuscitate a depressed newborn. The delivery of a high-risk infant may be an unexpected event. Therefore procedures for resuscitation must be reviewed regularly, and personnel trained to perform neonatal resuscitation should be present at every delivery. All emergency equipment should be inspected regularly for contents, expired medications, sterile supplies,

and working order. Documentation is essential for medicolegal and accreditative reasons.

RESUSCITATION

Resuscitation is the attempt to restore the body's life processes and thus reverse asphyxia. It is a team effort led by the most experienced and highly skilled member. This person usually establishes the airway and provides respiratory support. Others support cardiac output, prepare or administer medications, go for additional supplies as needed, monitor the infant's response to interventions, and document the events as they occur. Resuscitation is a stressful procedure for the client, family, and staff. Ethical and medicolegal issues are woven into a physiologically highly complex situation. In the midst of the high-technology atmosphere it is easy to forget touch. Make a conscious effort to humanize your care.

Basic Steps

The American Heart Association (AHA) and the American Academy of Pediatrics (AAP) have designed a standardized program for neonatal resuscitation, which is available as an instructional textbook. Hospital-based programs certify staff members to perform neonatal resuscitation; an overview of the basic steps of resuscitation is presented here (Figure 28-3).

Preparation for high-risk delivery includes the following steps.
1. Turn on warmer.
2. Have warmed blankets or towels ready.
3. Have ready bulb suction, or connect suction catheter (size 8 French for preterm and 10 French for term) to wall suction, turn suction on, and set at less than or equal to 100 mm Hg.
4. Connect oxygen source to ventilation bag; add pressure manometer.
5. Attach face mask to neck piece of bag.
6. Place stylet in appropriately sized endotracheal tube (2.5 to 3.0 French for preterm and 3.0 to 3.5 French for term infants).
7. Attach appropriate laryngoscope blade (Miller 0 for preterm and 1 for term infants) to handle. Check for bright light; replace bulb or battery if needed.
8. Drugs, intravenous fluids, or blood volume expanders such as 5% salt-poor albumin or 0.9% sodium chloride may be readied for use in certain situations.

Although the Apgar score provides guidelines for management of asphyxia, never wait until the 1 minute has passed to intervene. Typically each 1-minute delay after the time of the last gasp (end of primary apnea) causes a 2-minute delay in the return of gasping and a

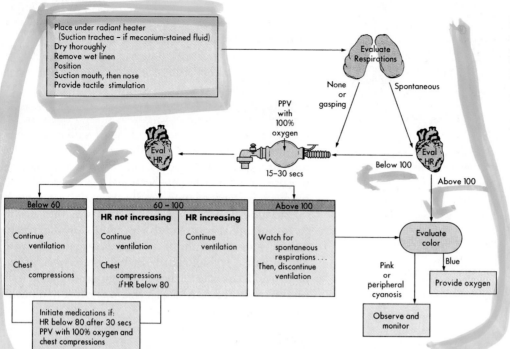

FIGURE 28-3 Decision tree for resuscitation in the delivery room. (From Bloom RS, Cropley CC: *Textbook of neonatal resuscitation,* Dallas, 1990, American Heart Association.)

4-minute delay until the onset of regular respirations. Because the onset to regular respiration is correlated with neonatal outcome, you can see how a delay of only several minutes in starting resuscitation can further compromise recovery.

The infant with mild cardiorespiratory depression *(Apgar score of 5 to 7)* should be moved to the radiant warmer and quickly dried.

Place the infant on its back or side, and keep the neck extended slightly. You may use slight Trendelenburg's position and a small shoulder roll to maintain neck extension (Figure 28-4). Once the infant has been positioned, suction the mouth first and then the nares with a bulb syringe or suction catheter to clear the airway of secretions. Always suction quickly but gently; overly vigorous suctioning can stimulate the vagus nerve, causing reflex bradycardia and respiratory arrest. Stimulate the infant by gently rubbing the back or flicking the soles of the feet.

Once you have performed the initial steps of resuscitation, it is time to evaluate the infant. Observe and evaluate the infant's respirations. If they are normal, then go on to a heart rate check. If not, further resuscitation is necessary. Check the infant's heart rate. If it is greater than 100 beats/min, note the neonate's color. If the heart rate is not above 100 beats/min, further resuscitation is necessary. If the infant is breathing and has a heart rate above 100 beats/min but central cyanosis is noted, provide 100% oxygen-enriched air directly to the infant's nose and mouth. Remember to keep the baby warm as you do this because cold stress only worsens acidosis and increases oxygen consumption.

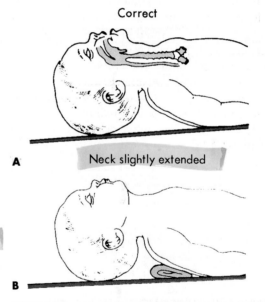

FIGURE 28-4 Positions for resuscitation. **A,** The neonate should be placed on his or her back or side, with the neck slightly extended. A slight Trendelenburg's position may be helpful. **B,** To help maintain the correct position, a rolled blanket or towel may be placed under the shoulders, elevating them ¾ to 1 inch off the mattress. (From Bloom RS, Cropley CC: *Textbook of neonatal resuscitation,* Dallas, 1990, American Heart Association.)

All or some of this sensory stimuli may be enough to stimulate the infant to breathe. If so, the baby's asphyxia probably will resolve without other interventions. Continue to monitor the heart and respiratory rates. Observe for an increase in muscle tone and activity and lessening of cyanosis.

Apgar scores of 3 and 4 are seen in moderately asphyxiated infants who will need positive-pressure ventilation; however, be sure that the airway is clear first. Figure 28-5 illustrates the correct position for positive-pressure ventilation. Use a small neck roll to keep the head in the "sniffing" position. Do not hyperextend the head (as you would with an adult) because this position compresses the infant's soft tracheal cartilage and blocks the airway. Choose a proper-sized face mask, and be sure that it produces a tight seal around the infant's nose and mouth. A clear, plastic mask with a soft rubber collar allows you to observe the color of the infant's mucous membranes while you maintain an adequate seal. For the mask to be the correct size, the rim must cover the tip of the chin, the mouth, and the nose, but not the eyes:

- Too large—possible eye damage
- Too small—will not cover the mouth and nose and may occlude the nose

Squeeze the bag to maintain a respiratory rate of 40 to 60 breaths/min. Although initial pressures of 30 to 60 cm H_2O may be needed to inflate the previously unventilated alveoli, observe the infant carefully; that is, listen in each axilla for breath sounds and look for movement of the anterior chest wall with each breath, improvement of color, and the return of muscle tone. For maintaining ventilation, keep the peak pressure between 15 and 20 cm H_2O. More pressure may be needed for premature infants or infants with pulmonary disease.

Another member of the team listens for breath sounds, which should be heard equally under each axilla,

and monitors the heart rate when auscultating the chest or by palpating the cord. This should be done every 30 seconds. Tapping the index finger in synchrony with the rate easily communicates the rate to the other members of the team. If the heart rate remains over 100 beats/min, continue to support respirations while you watch for the return of spontaneous respirations. It may be necessary to insert an orogastric tube so that air introduced into the stomach by the positive pressure can be removed. Leaving the tube end open to the atmosphere allows air to be removed from the distended stomach. This should be done if an infant receives bag-and-mask ventilation for longer than 2 minutes.

An infant may fail to improve with bag-and-mask ventilation if respiratory depression is due to maternal administration of narcotic analgesics (such as meperidine), especially when given within an hour of delivery. Naloxone (Narcan) given to the infant will block the action of the narcotic, but naloxone must not be administered to infants of narcotic-dependent mothers because it will precipitate withdrawal.

Infants with severe asphyxia have *Apgar scores of 0 to 2* and need vigorous resuscitation. At least three persons are needed at this time: one manages the airway, another starts cardiac massage, and a third monitors the heart rate and listens for breath sounds. The infant receives prompt intubation by a skilled person. The correct size of endotracheal tube will deliver oxygen into the trachea without putting undue pressure on the tracheal walls. Chest compressions are indicated if, after 15 to 30 seconds of bag-and-mask ventilation with 100% oxygen, the heart rate is below 60 or between 60 and 80 beats/min but not increasing. Once the heart rate is above 80 beats/min, chest compressions should be discontinued (Bloom and Cropley, 1990).

Two techniques may be used (Figure 28-6). Holding the infant's chest between two hands is preferred to control the depth of compression. Depress the sternum ½ to ¾ inch at a rate of 120 times a minute. Someone should palpate the femoral pulse to ensure that cardiac massage is effective. Ventilation is performed at a rate of 40 to 60 breaths/min.

Additional Medications

For most infants, effective ventilation and oxygenation are all that are necessary during resuscitation. Some infants may require additional epinephrine for cardiac stimulation, administered through the umbilical venous line or the endotracheal tube. However, the infant whose heart rate remains less than 100 beats/min after effective ventilation has been established will need sodium bicarbonate to correct acidosis. Acidosis depresses the myocardial response to epinephrine and also depresses efforts by the infant's own sympathetic nervous system to increase the heart rate. Sodium bicarbonate is

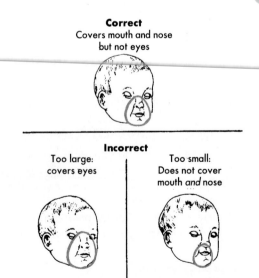

Correct
Covers mouth and nose
but not eyes

Incorrect

Too large:
covers eyes

Too small:
Does not cover
mouth *and* nose

FIGURE 28-5 Correct placement of mask during resuscitation. (From Bloom RS, Cropley CC: *Textbook of neonatal resuscitation,* Dallas, 1990, American Heart Association.)

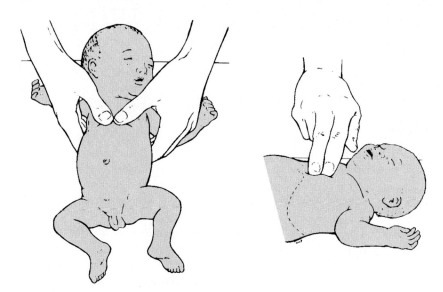

FIGURE 28-6 Position for cardiac massage. Position at left allows more control of depth of compression.

given through an umbilical venous catheter and must be diluted before use.

Resuscitation will be ineffective if the infant's perfusion is decreased; thus the intravascular volume must be expanded. Fluids are administered to restore the blood's osmotic pressure (the force that keeps the fluid component within the intravascular space). Administration of large macromolecules (such as albumin) will restore the osmotic pressure. Medications used for neonatal resuscitation are summarized in Table 28-1.

Meconium Aspiration Syndrome (MAS)

Special situations require alterations in the usual process of resuscitation. Meconium aspiration causes a mechanical obstruction that allows air to reach the alveoli during inspiration but then traps it in the air sacs behind the sticky meconium. These alveoli may then rupture, causing a pneumothorax and further compromising resuscitation. If the amniotic fluid is thickly meconium stained, every effort must be made to minimize aspiration. The birth attendant must thoroughly suction the infant's mouth and nose immediately after the head is delivered but before the first breath is taken. The infant is quickly placed under the radiant warmer and intubated, and the trachea is visualized and suctioned with use of an endotracheal tube. If the infant's heart rate drops below 60 beats/min, ventilation is begun. Infants who are delivered through thin meconium staining but who are vigorous and have Apgar scores of 8 to 10 may not receive suctioning in this manner, depending on agency policy.

Diaphragmatic Hernia

A **diaphragmatic hernia** occurs when the abdominal viscera herniate through a defect in the diaphragm during fetal life. The lungs usually are hypoplastic because of the pressure of the viscera during critical periods of fetal development. The infant with a diaphragmatic hernia has a flat or scaphoid abdomen, bulging chest, and severe respiratory distress. It is preferable that this neonate receive ventilation through an endotracheal tube rather than a face mask to prevent more air from being introduced into the gastrointestinal tract. An orogastric tube should be inserted for decompression. Surgery can reduce the abdominal contents; however, many infants die of pulmonary hypoplasia.

Keeping parents informed while providing the best possible care for the infant is critical. The birth of an asphyxiated baby may not have been anticipated. In any case it is a nightmare for the parents. Ideally, one person should be assigned to communicate with them. Even a short explanation with the reassurance that their infant is being cared for can make the situation less confusing. Lack of communication by health care professionals can be a major factor in the initiation of legal action. It also is inhumane and fails to care for all clients.

Discontinuing Resuscitation

A difficult decision with obvious ethical and legal ramifications results when efforts are unsuccessful. One guideline is to end resuscitation if no vital signs can be detected after 20 minutes of vigorous physical and chemical resuscitation. The gestational age of the infant and the presence of major malformations may influence the course of action. The decision to discontinue resuscitation is made by the attending neonatologist or pediatrician.

Respiratory Dysfunction
RESPIRATORY DISTRESS SYNDROME

Respiratory distress syndrome (RDS) is a disease of prematurity caused by a lack of pulmonary **surfactant.** Production of surfactant, a surface-active material, by

TABLE 28-1 Medications for Neonatal Resuscitation

MEDICATION	CONCENTRATION TO ADMINISTER	PREPARATION	DOSAGE/ROUTE*	TOTAL DOSE/INFANT		RATE/PRECAUTIONS
Epinephrine	1:10,000	1 ml	0.1–0.3 ml/kg IV or ET	Weight 1 kg 2 kg 3 kg 4 kg	Total ml 0.1–0.3 ml 0.2–0.6 ml 0.3–0.9 ml 0.4–1.2 ml	Give rapidly
Volume expanders	Whole blood 5% albumin Normal saline Ringer's lactate	40 ml	10 ml/kg IV	Weight 1 kg 2 kg 3 kg 4 kg	Total ml 10 ml 20 ml 30 ml 40 ml	Give over 5–10 min
Sodium bicarbonate	0.5 mEq/ml (4.2% solution)	20 ml or two 10-ml prefilled syringes	2 mEq/kg IV	Weight 1 kg 2 kg 3 kg 4 kg	Total dose 2 mEq 4 mEq 6 mEq 8 mEq	Give slowly, over at least 2 min Give only if infant being effectively ventilated
Naloxone	0.4 mg/ml	1 ml	0.1 mg/kg (0.25 mL/kg) IV, ET IM, SQ	Weight 1 kg 2 kg 3 kg 4 kg	Total dose 0.1 mg 0.2 mg 0.3 mg 0.4 mg	Give rapidly IV, ET preferred IM, SQ acceptable
	1.0 mg/ml	1 ml	0.1 mg/kg (0.1 ml/kg) IV, ET, IM, SQ	1 kg 2 kg 3 kg 4 kg	0.1 ml 0.2 ml 0.3 ml 0.4 ml	
Dopamine	mg of dopamine per 100 ml of solution $6 \times \dfrac{\text{Weight (kg)} \times \text{Desired dose (mg/kg/min)}}{\text{Desired fluid ml/hr}} =$		Begin at 5 µg/kg/ min (may increase to 20 µg/kg/min if necessary)	Weight 1 kg 2 kg 3 kg 4 kg	Total µg/min 5–20 µg/min 10–40 µg/min 15–60 µg/min 20–80 µg/min	Give as a continuous infusion using an infusion pump Monitor HR and BP closely Seek consultation

From Bloom RS, Cropley CC: Textbook of neonatal resuscitation, Dallas, 1990, American Heart Association.
*IM, Intramuscular; ET, endotracheal; IV, intravenous; SQ, subcutaneous.

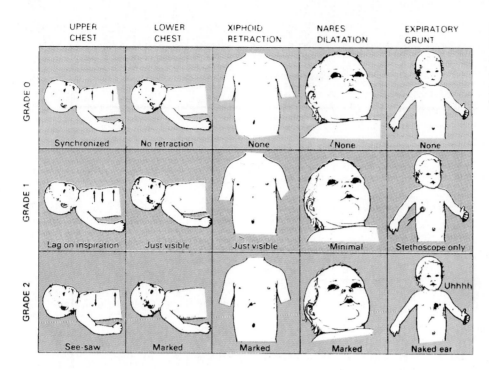

	UPPER CHEST	LOWER CHEST	XIPHOID RETRACTION	NARES DILATATION	EXPIRATORY GRUNT
GRADE 0	Synchronized	No retraction	None	None	None
GRADE 1	Lag on inspiration	Just visible	Just visible	Minimal	Stethoscope only
GRADE 2	See-saw	Marked	Marked	Marked	Naked ear (Uhhhh)

FIGURE 28-7 Silverman score. Observations indicating presence and severity of respiratory distress. (Reproduced by permission of *Pediatrics* 24:194, © 1959.)

type II pneumocytes increases with gestational age. A lack of surfactant causes alveoli to collapse with each expiration; therefore, unlike the normal lung, no residual capacity is established. For the infant with RDS, each breath is like the first, requiring high pressures to reopen the collapsed alveoli. Scattered **atelectasis** (collapsed alveoli) and areas of overinflation result because some alveoli have more surfactant than others.

Damage to the alveoli and pulmonary capillary epithelium secondary to surfactant deficiency causes the formation of a **hyaline membrane,** consisting of fibrin and sloughed cells. This further compromises gas exchange. The few type II cells become less able to produce surfactant and the cycle repeats itself as the infant becomes exhausted, and hypoxia, hypercapnia, and acidosis become more pronounced.

In most infants with RDS, improvement will be evident within 3 to 5 days. Morbidity and mortality vary depending on gestational age.

Signs

Clinical signs of RDS may occur immediately after birth or not until several hours have passed. Grunting first, then cyanosis in room air, tachypnea, pallor, retractions, and nasal flaring may be evident. There are decreased breath sounds and scattered rales. Vital signs will be altered; you may observe tachycardia or bradycardia, hypotension, and hypothermia. The Silverman score (Figure 28-7) may be used to assess the severity of the distress. The infant will become progressively hypotonic; edema and oliguria also commonly develop within the first 48 hours. A chest radiograph (Figure 28-8) shows air bronchograms (lucent areas resembling

branches of a tree) and a typical reticulogranular or ground glass pattern caused by air in the bronchi and bronchioles contrasted against areas of atelectasis.

Infants with RDS will become progressively worse for the first 48 hours and begin to improve as the type II cells produce surfactant. Improvement often occurs dramatically in infants with better prognoses. Other infants, usually those of smaller birth weight and lesser gestational age, require longer periods of respiratory assistance and may fail to improve as expected.

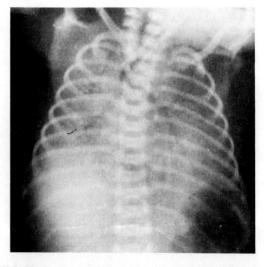

FIGURE 28-8 Chest radiograph of infant with RDS. Air in bronchi is darkly contrasted against atelectatic lungs. (From Korones SB: *High-risk newborn infants: the basis for intensive nursing care,* ed 4, St Louis, 1986, Mosby.)

Surfactant Replacement

Surfactant replacement provides hope for treatment of RDS. The Food and Drug Administration (FDA) has approved the use of two commercially prepared surfactant products: Survanta, a modified natural product, and Exosurf, a synthetic product. The dosage and methods of administration vary for the different products, but both are administered through the endotracheal tube of an intubated infant. Surfactant replacement has reduced mortality by 5% to 12% in treated infants.

Test Yourself

- True or false? RDS is a disease of premature infants that results in the formation of type II pneumocytes.
- Surfactant replacement is administered to infants by which route?

APNEA

Apnea is the cessation of respiration for 15 to 20 seconds or any amount of time without respiration when cyanosis, bradycardia, hypotonia, or metabolic acidosis occurs. This differs from **periodic breathing**, during which respiration ceases for 5 to 10 seconds without pathophysiologic changes. Periodic breathing is a normal respiratory pattern in the preterm infant but should have resolved as full-term age is achieved.

Signs

Apnea occurs more frequently in smaller and immature infants. It is an important sign that may be caused by a disease process or may occur because of immaturity of the respiratory and neurologic systems (Box 28-4). Any infant who becomes apneic should be examined for the underlying cause.

BOX 28-4   Risks for Apnea

- Bacterial or viral infection
- Hypoxia
- Neurologic alterations: asphyxia, intraventricular hemorrhage, subarachnoid hemorrhage, seizures, congenital malformations
- Altered metabolic function: temperature instability, hypoglycemia
- Fluid and electrolyte imbalance
- Maternal, fetal, or neonatal medications
- Apnea of prematurity: respiratory and neurologic immaturity

---

Apnea is more likely to develop in premature infants and lead to sudden infant death syndrome (SIDS). Any infant with continued periodic breathing or apneic episodes, whose postconceptional age is at least 36 weeks, may have breathing patterns recorded (pneumogram) for 24 hours before discharge. Home apnea monitoring may be necessary if the pattern persists.

Clinical Management

Infants less than 1750 g or 34 weeks of gestation are at high risk for apneic episodes and should have their cardiac and respiratory rates and oxygen saturations monitored continuously for the first 2 weeks of life or until 5 to 10 days have passed without any apnea. The apneic infant should be quickly evaluated for bradycardia and cyanosis. Immediate gentle tactile stimulation such as rubbing the back or flicking the soles of the feet stimulates respiration in most infants. A bag and mask connected to an oxygen source and equipment for suctioning and intubation should be at the bedside and ready for use in mechanical ventilation.

Apnea of prematurity may be treated with tactile stimulation such as a pulsating water mattress or **continuous positive airway pressure (CPAP)**, plus an increase in environmental oxygen. Research by Thoman into biobehavioral methods of treating apnea of prematurity involves placing a "regularly breathing" teddy bear in the Isolette with the infant. It appears that the stimulation provided by the breathing bear encourages cerebral development and regulation of respiration (Laymon, 1988). Theophylline, a smooth muscle relaxant and bronchodilator, may be used. A loading dose of theophylline (5 mg/kg) is given orally or intravenously, followed by 2 to 5 mg/kg/day in divided doses for the preterm infant; the dosage is adjusted to maintain a therapeutic level of 6 to 12 µg/ml. Theophylline may cause gastrointestinal (vomiting and diarrhea), neurologic (irritability and restlessness), and cardiovascular (tachycardia and hypotension) side effects. Caffeine citrate may be used in place of theophylline to treat apnea of prematurity.

PNEUMONIA

Pneumonia may result from prenatal aspiration of infected amniotic or cervical fluids or blood-borne infection. The common causative organisms are group B β-hemolytic streptococci, *Escherichia coli,* and viral agents. After delivery, pathogens such as coagulase-positive staphylococci or group A streptococci are most often carried to newborns by the care giver's hands. This type of pneumonia starts as a local infection, which is not contained. Other organisms (*Klebsiella* and *Pseudomonas aeruginosa*) grow in water used in respiratory therapy equipment and gain entry to the respiratory tract.

Signs

Signs of pneumonia may be seen soon after birth or may be delayed as the organisms incubate. The baby will appear lethargic and demonstrate hypothermia, hypotonia, or jaundice. Grunting, nasal flaring, costal retractions, and tachypnea may present. Alterations in vital signs, arterial blood gas levels, and respiratory function are similar to RDS—so similar that any baby with RDS is assumed to have a prenatally acquired pneumonia and is treated with antibiotics.

Clinical Management

Support of respiratory function and correction of asphyxia are very important. Note that the normal arterial blood gas values for newborns are different from adult values (Table 28-2). Hypoxia is treated by placing the infant in an Oxyhood or head box to administer enough warmed, humidified oxygen to keep the oxygen pressure (PO_2) between 50 and 80 mm Hg, correlated with oxygen saturations above 90%. The pulse oximeter continuously measures oxygen saturation by means of a light source that passes through an artery. However, arterial blood gases also are drawn and analyzed. If, in spite of receiving 60% oxygen, the infant's PO_2 is less than 50 mm Hg or the carbon dioxide pressure (PCO_2) is elevated (hypercapnia), other respiratory assistance is necessary (Figure 28-9).

PERSISTENT PULMONARY HYPERTENSION OF THE NEWBORN (PPHN)

The normally low fetal oxygen tension keeps the pulmonary vascular bed constricted in utero so that only 10% of the circulating blood goes to the lungs. Factors such as intrauterine hypoxia, RDS, polycythemia, and meconium aspiration can cause such pulmonary vasoconstriction to persist after birth. Circulation to the alveoli is decreased because of vasoconstriction. The pulmonary BP remains high and prevents the flap of the foramen ovale from closing. The ductus arteriosus also fails to constrict. Blood therefore is shunted from the right to the left side of

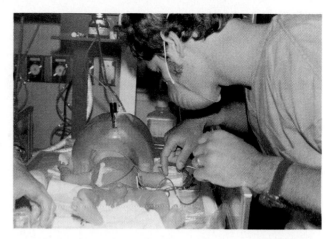

FIGURE 28-9 Infant under Oxyhood. (Courtesy Marjorie Pyle, RNC, *Lifecircle*.)

the heart through the ductus arteriosus and foramen ovale. These alterations worsen the hypoxia and result in **persistent pulmonary hypertension.**

Signs

Neonates with PPHN usually are full term or postterm, with persistent cyanosis, tachypnea, altered cardiac sounds, and congestive heart failure.

Clinical Management

Treatment focuses on the underlying condition. Ventilation with very high respiratory rates may be used to induce alkalosis, which in turn induces pulmonary vasodilation. A vasodilator (usually tolazoline) may be given intravenously to reduce pulmonary vascular resistance.

 Clinical Decision

You are caring for a full-term infant with pneumonia. He is in an oxyhood, receiving 60% O_2. Arterial blood gas levels are pH, 7.28; PO_2, 52 mm Hg; PCO_2, 60 mm Hg. You should:

1. *Recognize that these values are not normal and the infant needs more respiratory assistance.*
2. *Determine that these values must not be correct because the infant is breathing spontaneously.*
3. *Continue to observe infant, monitoring vital signs until the next blood gases are drawn.*

TABLE 28-2 Normal Arterial Blood Gas Values for Neonates

VALUE	RANGE
pH	7.33–7.42
Arterial oxygen pressure (PaO_2)	50–80 mm Hg
Carbon dioxide pressure ($PaCO_2$)	38–48 mm Hg
Bicarbonate (HCO_3^-)	20–24 mEq/L
Oxygen saturation	>90%

Newer methods of ventilation avoid the induction of respiratory alkalosis. Instead, P_{CO_2} levels are kept within a normal range while drugs such as sodium bicarbonate are given to create a metabolic alkalosis that can dilate the pulmonary blood vessels.

Systemic pressure is supported with volume expanders such as fluids and albumin. Vasopressors such as dopamine also may be needed to maintain systemic perfusion. Extracorporeal membrane oxygenation (ECMO) is a technique that allows blood to bypass the lungs. It has been used for infants with PPHN with some success (Short et al, 1987).

Ventilatory Interventions
CONTINUOUS POSITIVE AIRWAY PRESSURE (CPAP)

CPAP delivers a constant pressure into the infant's lungs throughout the respiratory cycle, thereby preventing alveoli from collapsing during expiration. An infant receiving this form of respiratory therapy is breathing spontaneously and receiving only additional pressure and increased fractional inspired oxygen concentration (Fio_2). CPAP decreases the effort required to breathe and may be delivered through an endotracheal or pharyngeal tube or nasal prongs. Nasal prongs resemble the standard nasal cannula used to deliver oxygen except that they fit tightly against the nares. Pharyngeal tubes are threaded nasally or orally into the pharynx. After CPAP is started, arterial blood gas levels are again measured. Lack of improvement necessitates further intervention.

Nursing Responsibilities
▶ ASSESSMENT

Frequent vital sign checks are taken and documented by means of a flow chart to enable the nurse to compare progress. A distressed infant may require one-to-one nursing during the critical period.

Test Yourself	
Matching	
A. CPAP	_____ Provides warm, humidified oxygen only
B. Oxyhood	_____ Requires endotracheal intubation
C. Mechanical ventilation	_____ Delivers only distending pressure to the airways

▶ NURSING DIAGNOSES
1. Ineffective airway clearance
2. Impaired gas exchange
3. High risk for injury related to hypoxemia/hyperoxemia and effects of respiratory interventions
4. Ineffective breathing pattern related to apnea and periodic breathing

▶ EXPECTED OUTCOMES
1. Respiratory distress resolves.
2. Infant sustains independent respiration in room air.
3. Infant will not experience complications resulting from interventions.
4. Periodic breathing resumes normal patterns.

▶ NURSING INTERVENTIONS
If ventilation is still ineffective, hypoxia and hypercapnia will worsen and acidosis increase. Respiratory efforts must be assisted by endotracheal intubation and mechanical ventilation, which delivers a preset volume of gas (volume cycled) or gas pressure (pressure cycled). The time-cycled, pressure-limited ventilator is used extensively with newborns because the delivery of top or peak inspiratory pressure can be controlled.

The infant will be intubated by nasotracheal or orotracheal routes (Figure 28-10). Infants who are larger and more mature often struggle against or fight the ventilator. Sedation with a narcotic analgesic or paralysis with pancuronium bromide (Pavulon) may be necessary if the respiratory support is to be effective.

Pulmonary hygiene maintains the patency of large and small airways. The ill neonate is less able to maintain this patency because of the small airway diameter, inadequate cough reflex, poor respiratory

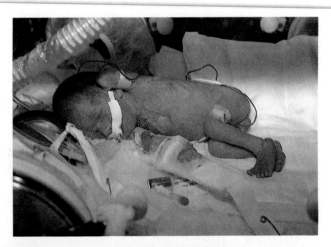

FIGURE 28-10 Infant intubated and on ventilator in Isolette. (Courtesy Marjorie Pyle, RNC, *Lifecircle.*)

effort, and inability to change position. Chest physiotherapy and suctioning provide the infant with mechanisms for maintenance of airway, prevention of infection, and adequate ventilation.

Chest physiotherapy is accomplished by changes in position, percussion, and vibration of the chest wall. These measures should be performed as gently as possible and before feedings, to prevent aspiration. Oxygen saturation should be monitored and administration increased as needed. Attention to infant responses that indicate increased stress is necessary.

Different positions allow for postural drainage of specific lung segments. All positions may not be tolerated by the infant during one session; lung segments may be alternately drained if necessary. Percussion of the chest wall loosens secretions. A soft, cupped device such as the Neonatal Percussor (Ballard Medical Products, Midvale, Utah) or a padded medicine cup is tapped over the segment for about 30 seconds. Preference is given to known areas of atelectasis.

Vibration may be performed with a padded electric toothbrush. Infants may tolerate one method of loosening secretions more than others. This and any modifications in treatment should be communicated to other care givers.

Suctioning to remove loosened secretions may be performed through the nose, mouth, or endotracheal tube. Oral and nasal suctioning are clean, not sterile procedures. Endotracheal suctioning, whether the tube is inserted orally or nasally, is a sterile technique that takes time to master.

Complications of Interventions

Respiratory support for newborns has become possible only in the last two decades. Although hypoxia still damages many high-risk infants, medical and nursing personnel are now faced with complications resulting from hyperoxia. These mainly affect the developing eye and lungs. Although hyperoxia is a sustained Po_2 level over 100 mm Hg, very small infants may be adversely affected by lower levels.

Retinopathy of prematurity. Although **retinopathy of prematurity (ROP)** may occur in premature infants of varying gestational ages and weights, it is more common in infants of lower birth weight. This change is also called *retrolental fibroplasia (RLF)*. It has been thought to occur as a result of vasoconstriction of retinal blood vessels in response to high oxygen levels. Researchers believe that prematurity is the primary risk factor (George et al, 1988). ROP also has developed in some preterm infants who have not received supplemental oxygen. Retinal vasoconstriction is followed by obliteration and then proliferation of the affected vessels. These vessels are abnormal and leak blood and

serum into the retina. Retinal detachment and myopia follow. Early in the disease, these changes are seen only in the periphery of the retina. With worsening, the entire retina may be involved. In some affected infants, laser photocoagulation or cryotherapy may be used during the active phase of ROP.

Prevention still focuses on strict control of arterial oxygen tension below the level that stimulates vasoconstriction. Vitamin E supplements have been evaluated, but their use is still controversial. However, there is no agreement as to safe levels of Po_2, and in fact variables such as duration of oxygen therapy also influence the development of ROP. Low-birth-weight infants are evaluated by a pediatric ophthalmologist before discharge.

Bronchopulmonary dysplasia. Bronchopulmonary dysplasia (BPD) is a chronic disease of the infant lung caused by the effects of oxygen delivered at high pressures over time. The epithelium lining the bronchi and alveoli become necrotic. A process of regeneration follows but is complicated by interstitial fibrosis and metaplasia of the bronchial lining. Infants who recover do so because alveoli continue to multiply into the eighth postnatal year. However, respiratory deficits are common.

Infants with BPD have chronic oxygen hunger, hypercapnia, psychosocial and physical retardation, feeding intolerance, and oral aversion. Respiratory infections are frequent complications. Many medications, including antibiotics, diuretics, steroids, and vitamin supplements, are used to treat the infant with chronic lung disease. It is difficult to provide adequate nutrition; fluid restrictions are necessary to control pulmonary edema, and much energy is spent on the increased work of breathing. Gastrointestinal reflux is common after oral feedings are attempted. The resulting growth failure compounds the respiratory difficulty.

It is possible and usually preferable to care for these babies at home. A healthy home environment stimulates normal growth and development and avoids contact with nosocomial pathogens.

Lung devel. cont. thru 8 yrs age, may cont. being slow up to this time.

▶ EVALUATION

1. Has the infant demonstrated improvement in oxygenation or ventilation?
2. Does the infant who is diagnosed with RDS show improvement in respiratory function by the fifth day of life?
3. Will the infant require oxygen therapy or respiratory treatments at home?
4. Has the occurrence of apnea in the infant improved by 35 to 36 weeks of postconceptional age?

Cardiovascular Dysfunction

Most common alterations in neonatal cardiovascular function are caused by congenital defects in structure or function or by failure of transition from fetal to adult circulation (see Figure 18-5). It often is difficult to identify the infant with congenital heart disease because the signs (tachypnea, cardiac murmur, and cyanosis) also are seen with respiratory dysfunction or sepsis. Neonatal health care providers now evaluate neonates for cardiac disease earlier because survival is more likely with earlier diagnosis and treatment (Figure 28-11).

CONGENITAL CARDIAC DEFECTS

Congenital heart disease (CHD) occurs in about 7.5 in 1000 live births (Flyer and Lang, 1987). It is a major cause of death in full-term infants. Because a full discussion is beyond the scope of this text, the reader is directed to textbooks of pediatric nursing. Defects are classified as acyanotic or cyanotic. Here we shall discuss early signs that you may detect in a newborn.

General Signs

Infants with CHD may have all or some of the following signs: cyanosis, respiratory distress, congestive heart failure, and abnormal cardiac rhythm and sounds (murmurs). One important clue is cyanosis *out of proportion* to the degree of respiratory distress. Another sign is congestive heart failure, which can appear slowly in early stages. You should suspect a heart defect in any baby with tachypnea, tachycardia, oliguria, edema, hepatomegaly, abnormal cardiac rhythm, and difficulty in feeding, especially if the infant seems to tire easily during feeds. Cyanosis is a predominant feature in some cardiac defects. When cyanosis is present, it is because desaturated venous blood is shunted from the right to the left side of the heart without passing through the lungs to become oxygenated. This difference is used to classify CHD.

ACYANOTIC CONGENITAL HEART DEFECTS

Coarctation of the Aorta

Coarctation (constriction) of the aorta may occur with varying degrees of severity. The anomaly also may occur alone or as part of a complex syndrome of cardiac defects. Simple coarctation causes congestive heart failure because the heart attempts to maintain output against the obstruction. The defect may be located near the ductus arteriosus. As the ductus closes, the obstruction worsens. Pulse and BP in the upper extremities far exceed values in the lower extremities, and signs of congestive heart failure soon develop. Treatment includes stabilization with prostaglandin E_1 to keep the ductus open until surgical repair can be accomplished (Figure 28-12, *A*).

If the coarctation does not require surgery in the neonatal period, treatment includes stabilization with digitalis and diuretics to prevent congestive heart failure. Repair will be electively scheduled between the ages of 1 and 3 years.

Hypoplastic Left-Heart Syndrome

Full-term infants who are appropriately grown for gestational age (AGA) and are otherwise normal may have hypoplastic left-heart syndrome (HLHS), a small ascending aorta, and atresia of the aortic and mitral valves and left ventricle. Prenatal and early neonatal survival depends on the absence of either an atrial septal defect or a patent ductus arteriosus. Symptoms begin when the ductus arteriosus begins to constrict. As the systemic circulation decreases, the infant becomes ashen in color with poor capillary filling and weak pulses. Metabolic acidosis and progressively worsening congestive heart failure accompany the shock. If HLHS is recognized promptly, the infant's condition may be temporarily stabilized by maintaining patency of the ductus.

Although HLHS affects 7% to 9% of infants with CHD, it accounts for up to 22% of infant deaths as a result of cardiac disease in the neonatal period (Long, 1990). Surgical intervention involves cardiac transplantation or a two-stage palliative and then corrective repair. Mortality rates for each are 20% and 25% to 35%, respectively (Panyard and Kaneta, 1988).

Atrial Septal Defect (ASD) *fairly common - probably the least complicated*

Incomplete formation of the septum during fetal cardiac development results in an opening between the two atria. A characteristic heart murmur is heard. Although an ASD usually is asymptomatic, congestive heart fail-

occurs early in gestation

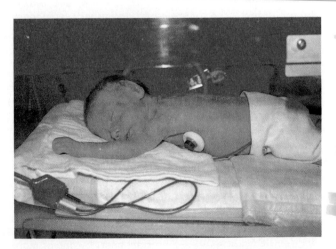

FIGURE 28-11 Cardiac monitor in place. (Courtesy Marjorie Pyle, RNC, *Lifecircle*.)

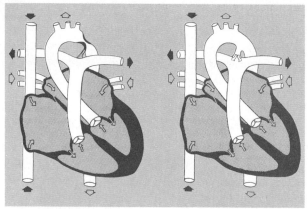

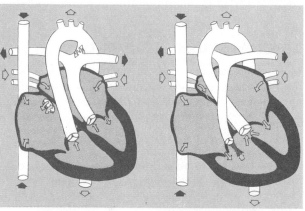

Coarctation of the Aorta

Coarctation of the aorta is characterized by a narrowed aortic lumen. The lesion produces an obstruction to the flow of blood through the aorta, causing an increased left ventricular pressure and work load.

Patent Ductus Arteriosus

Functional closure of the ductus normally occurs soon after birth. If the ductus remains patent after birth, the direction of blood flow in the ductus is reversed by the higher pressure in the aorta.

Complete Transposition of Great Arteries (TGA)

The aorta originates from the right ventricle, and the pulmonary artery originates from the left ventricle. An abnormal communication between the two circulations must be present to sustain life.

Tetralogy of Fallot (TOF)

Tetralogy of Fallot is characterized by the combination of four defects: (1) pulmonary stenosis, (2) ventricular septal defect, (3) overriding aorta, (4) hypertrophy of the right ventricle.

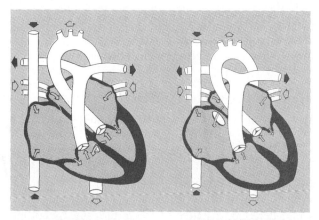

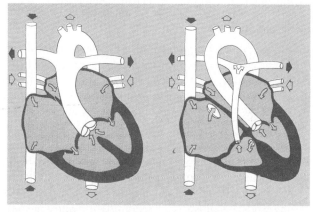

Ventricular Septal Defect

A ventricular septal defect is an abnormal opening between the right and left ventricles. Ventricular septal defects vary in size and may occur in either the membranous or muscular portion of the ventricular septum. Because of higher pressure in the left ventricle, a shunting of blood from the left to right ventricle occurs during systole.

A

Atrial Septal Defect

An atrial septal defect is an abnormal opening between the right and left atria. Basically, three types of abnormalitites result from incorrect development of the atrial septum. An incompetent foramen ovale is the most common defect. In general, left to right shunting of blood occurs in all atrial septal defects.

Truncus Arteriosus (TA)

This single arterial trunk overrides the ventricles and receives blood from them through a ventricular septal defect. The entire pulmonary and systemic circulation is supplied from this common arterial trunk.

Tricuspid Atresia

Tricuspid valvular atresia is characterized by a small right ventricle, large left ventricle, and usually a diminished pulmonary circulation. The lungs may receive blood through one of three routes: (1) a small ventricular septal defect, (2) patent ductus arteriosus, (3) bronchial vessels.

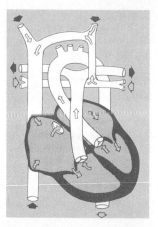

Total Anomalous Pulmonary Venous Drainage (TAPVD)

Oxygenated blood returning from the lungs is carried abnormally to the right heart by one or more pulmonary veins emptying directly, or indirectly, through venous channels into the right atrium.

FIGURE 28-12 Congenital heart disease. **A,** Acyanotic heart disease. **B,** Cyanotic heart disease. (Courtsey Ross Laboratories, Columbus, Ohio.)

B

ure may result from shunting of blood from the left to the right atrium. If congestive heart failure does not respond to medical management, the ASD might be closed by a special procedure performed during cardiac catheterization. Surgical repair takes place if the catheterization procedure is not possible.

Ventricular Septal Defect

Ventricular septal defect (VSD) is seen in 8.8% of neonates with congenital heart defects. It may occur as an isolated cardiac defect or as a part of a complex of defects. A characteristic murmur is heard. Larger defects cause more severe symptoms. After birth, blood will shunt from the left to the right ventricle through the VSD, overloading the right side. There is increased blood flow to the lungs, followed by increased blood returning to the left atrium and ventricle. Symptoms such as pneumonia and congestive heart failure result. Infants whose congestive heart failure does not improve with medical treatment or who have repeated bouts of pulmonary infections are candidates for surgery. Small VSDs may spontaneously close and require no treatment.

Patent Ductus Arteriosus

Patent ductus arteriosus (PDA) may be an isolated finding in infants of varying gestational age or may occur with RDS in an ill premature infant. It also can be seen as part of a syndrome of complex heart disease. The incidence is 2.3% of infants with CHD. If the infant with a PDA has no respiratory disease, blood will shunt from the aorta (left side of the heart) to the pulmonary artery (right side of the heart) and cause overcirculation to the lungs. An increase in blood returning to the left atrium and ventricle occurs, which increases workload. The systolic BP increases, the pulse pressure widens, and the peripheral pulses feel as if they are "bounding" as a result. A characteristic murmur is heard.

Congestive heart failure usually develops by 6 weeks of age in the full-term infant. In addition, these infants may have growth failure and pulmonary infections. Medical treatment with a prostaglandin inhibitor (indomethacin) may cause spontaneous closure. When medical management of congestive heart failure is achieved or the PDA is surgically ligated, improvement usually is dramatic.

CYANOTIC CONGENITAL HEART DEFECTS

Transposition of the Great Arteries

The cardiac defect most commonly diagnosed during the first week of life is **transposition of the great arteries (TGA).** Approximately 10% of neonates with congenital cardiac defects have TGA (Long, 1990). It usually affects male infants. When it is present, the aorta arises from the right ventricle and the pulmonary artery from

the left. As a result, desaturated venous blood returning to the right atrium and ventricle is recirculated to the body without having been oxygenated. Highly saturated arterial blood returning to the left atrium and ventricle is then recirculated through the lungs instead of supplying the body's oxygen needs. Mixing these two must take place if the infant is to survive after birth (Figure 28-12, B).

TGA causes cyanosis soon after delivery. It is diagnosed by echocardiogram and chest radiograph. Treatment aims to establish mixing of the saturated and desaturated blood streams by maintaining patency of the ductus arteriosus through the use of prostaglandin E_1. Some infants with a VSD or ASD will have mixing that does not depend on the ductus arteriosus for pulmonary blood flow. Palliative surgery increases the mixing through an artificially created ASD. Corrective surgery usually is delayed until the infant is more stable. A newer procedure may be performed within the first few days of life. The great arteries are "switched" so that the pulmonary artery will arise from the right ventricle and the aorta will arise from the left.

Tetralogy of Fallot

Tetralogy is a syndrome of four associated cardiac lesions, including ventricular septal defect, an aorta that overrides the interventricular septum, pulmonary stenosis, and right ventricular hypertrophy. It is seen in 10% of all infants born with critical congenital heart disease (Long, 1990).

Infants with Fallot's tetralogy exhibit cyanosis that depends on the degree of the pulmonary stenosis. Hypercyanotic or "tet" spells can occur when pulmonary flow is obstructed even further by the muscular area at the root of the pulmonary artery. During these spells, cyanosis increases and is accompanied by pallor, tachypnea, irritability, hypotonia, and at times, loss of consciousness. Relief is obtained by placing the infant in the knee-chest position; it may be necessary to administer oxygen and a β-blocker such as propranolol or to give morphine. Surgical repair usually is delayed beyond the neonatal period.

Truncus Arteriosus

Truncus arteriosus (TA) is a relatively rare malformation seen as a continuation of early fetal anatomy (Long, 1990). The common arterial exit of the fetal heart (the truncus arteriosus) fails to divide into two separate arterial channels (aorta and pulmonary artery). Both ventricles empty into both great vessels. Cyanosis and congestive heart failure are the predominant signs. Surgical repair is difficult.

Tricuspid Atresia

The normal flow of blood from the right atrium to the right ventricle is prevented in tricuspid atresia. Blood entering the right atrium is shunted through the foramen ovale to the left atrium and left ventricle and then out through the aorta to the systemic circulation. A VSD commonly is present—the third most common cyanotic congenital heart defect (Long, 1990).

Total Anomalous Pulmonary Venous Drainage

Total anomalous pulmonary venous drainage (TAPVD) affects the circulation of neonates by failing to provide a connection between the pulmonary veins and the left atrium. Venous return from the heart can drain into a variety of abnormal channels that prevent the delivery of oxygenated blood to the systemic circulation. The infant survives only as long as mixing of blood occurs, either through the foramen ovale or through a patent ductus arteriosus. Immediate surgical treatment is necessary. TAPVD often is associated with other congenital anomalies.

Test Yourself

You are caring for an infant who is in an oxyhood and receiving 60% O$_2$. What signs would make you suspect that he has congenital heart disease?

Fluid, Electrolyte, and Nutritional Imbalance

Problems in fluid, electrolyte, and nutritional balances are common for the preterm infant. Immature structures, hormones, and behaviors make regulation difficult. It is important to observe for imbalances because they can compromise the functions of other systems. Overhydration can cause pulmonary or cerebral edema and maintain a PDA; underhydration can lead to renal failure. Nutritional deficiencies can affect the infant's ability to fight infection and decrease the rate of growth and development.

FLUID BALANCE

Fluid balance in the preterm infant is tenuous at best. At 24 weeks of gestation, 85% of the infant's total body weight is water. Most of this is contained in the extracellular space; the balance is intracellular fluid. Total body water decreases with increasing gestational age. By the second postnatal month there are equal amounts of intracellular and extracellular water until, in the months to follow, most body water is found in the intracellular space.

Regulation of body water is primarily the responsibility of the kidneys. Renal function, however, is immature, even at term. Antidiuretic hormone (ADH) controls the amount of water excreted or retained and therefore regulates blood and urine osmolality. At term, ADH levels are only one fifth of adult levels. Preterm infants do not respond well to overhydration or underhydration. They cannot concentrate urine as well as term infants do. They also cannot produce dilute urine as quickly and therefore will retain excessive water loads. Term and preterm infants who have been asphyxiated can have symptoms of inappropriate ADH secretion. The glomerular filtration rate (GFR) determines the amount of blood filtered and therefore the amount of urine produced. This rate is limited in the neonate but increases after birth. Preterm infants have fewer nephrons and significantly lower filtration rates than do term infants, with less postnatal increase. This also affects their ability to excrete water.

Clinical Management

Neonates lose water easily by a variety of mechanisms. The kidneys, sweat glands, and gastrointestinal tract are obvious routes for water loss. Water also is lost through the lungs (respiratory water loss) and skin (transepidermal water loss by diffusion) by a process called **insensible water loss (IWL)**. The amount of water lost via this route varies with gestational age and body weight. The preterm infant's thin skin and larger ratio of body surface area to body weight allows for greater water loss. Preterm infants frequently are cared for under radiant warmers and phototherapy lamps, further increasing IWL. In addition, congenital defects that disrupt skin integrity also increase IWL. Insensible water loss is decreased if the infant is breathing humidified air, cared for in a double-walled Isolette, or clothed or covered with a plastic blanket.

Fluid requirements vary for the newborn. These may be met by enteral or parenteral fluids. On the first day of life the healthy full-term newborn needs 80 ml/kg/day; this gradually increases to 140 to 150 ml/kg/day by the end of the first week. Because preterm infants have higher fluid requirements, factors that increase IWL are figured into the total fluid requirement. Preterm infants weighing between 1000 and 1500 g may need as much as 200 ml/kg/day by the end of the first week (Avery, 1987). Fluid, electrolyte, and nutritional requirements are calculated at least once daily. However, infants who have been asphyxiated may have fluid restrictions to lessen the chance of cerebral edema. Requirements for ill infants are recalculated more often.

ELECTROLYTE BALANCE

Electrolytes are found in all body compartments but in differing concentrations. Electrolyte requirements vary with age. No supplementation is needed unless symptoms of deficiency occur. Preterm infants lose sodium easily, which causes hyponatremia, even when receiving a normal sodium intake. In some cases, unusually large amounts of sodium may be retained (hypernatremia), especially if insensible fluid loss is high. Potassium, the principal intracellular electrolyte (anion), is needed for normal neuromuscular functioning. *Hypokalemia* may result from excessive losses through the gastrointestinal or renal route, but infants with acidosis may have *hyperkalemia*. Magnesium levels may be elevated in infants whose mothers have been treated with magnesium sulfate for preeclampsia or premature labor.

NUTRITIONAL BALANCE

The goal for weight gain is to approximate that of normal intrauterine growth. Nutritional deficits may exist because of increased metabolic demands placed on the preterm infant by thermoregulation, work of respiration and feeding, and decreased ability to absorb nutrients. The preterm infant's ability to adequately digest lactose and fats also is compromised by inadequate production of lactase, bile acids, and pancreatic lipase.

The ability to coordinate the suck-swallow-breathing complex matures at approximately 34 weeks of gestation. Many preterm infants have respiratory disease, which further hampers the ability to feed.

Calories for Premature Infants

Caloric requirements are calculated from the sum of needs for the basal metabolic rate, plus needs for activity, cold stress, loss via feces, digestive and metabolic processes, and growth (Table 28-3). Just after birth 90 to 100 kcal/kg/day are needed; this increases to 120 kcal/kg/day in a few days. Formulas with caloric densities of 13, 20, 24, and 27 calories per ounce are available.

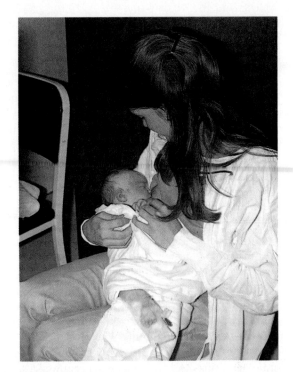

FIGURE 28-13 Graduating to breast-feeding in the NICU. (Courtesy Marjorie Pyle, RNC, *Lifecircle*.)

Most often a 24 kcal/oz formula is provided to preterm infants, compared with a 20 kcal/oz formula for the term infant. Human milk does not have a constant caloric density because the fat content varies from the beginning to end of any one feeding, as well as diurnally. However, the calories are easier to digest. Women are encouraged to lactate with a breast pump until the preterm infant can nurse (Figure 28-13). Human Milk Fortifier (Mead Johnson, Evansville, Ind.) and Natural Care (Ross Laboratories, Columbus, Ohio) may be added to breast milk to increase the fat, protein, and carbohydrate content and provide supplemental vitamins, minerals, and electrolytes. This provides the preterm infant with a controlled level of needed nutrients, in addition to the benefits of human milk.

Protein. Optimal growth should occur with a protein intake of 3.5 to 4 g/kg/day. Casein is the predominant protein in most cow's milk formulas, whereas human milk protein is mostly whey. The balance of amino acids in whey protein is suited for human infants. Milk from mothers who have given birth to premature infants also contains more protein than milk at term. The additional benefits of immunologic factors makes human milk the preferred food for preterm infants.

Fat. The preterm infant has not had the benefit of the caloric intake of the third trimester of gestation. Therefore, for weight gain, fat should comprise 40% to 45%

TABLE 28-3 Daily Caloric Requirements for Preterm Infants

CALORIC REQUIREMENT	KCAL/KG/DAY
Basic metabolic rate	35–50
Day 1	(35)
Day 2	(45)
Day 28	(50)
Intermittent activity (highly variable)	15
Occasional cold stress	10
Fecal loss	8
Specific dynamic action (energy cost of digestion and metabolism)	12
Growth	25
TOTAL	105–120

From Merenstein GB, Gardner SL: *Handbook of neonatal intensive care,* ed 2, St Louis, 1989, Mosby; modified from Sinclair JC et al: *Pediatr Clin North Am* 17:863, 1970.

of intake; 3% of this should be linoleic acid. Human milk satisfies this requirement.

Carbohydrates. Carbohydrates are stored as glycogen during gestation to provide reserves of energy; however, preterm, SGA, or asphyxiated infants have inadequate stores. Lactose and other glucose polymers provide carbohydrates. Breast milk and some prepared formulas are lactose based; other formulas use lactose and glucose polymers as carbohydrate sources. Most infants tolerate lactose well, even though lactase levels are subnormal.

Minerals and vitamins. Minerals are supplied in adequate amounts by prepared formulas and human milk. Iron from human milk is easier to absorb; formulas have varying amounts of additional iron. The calcium-phosphorus ratio (2.2:1.0) found in human milk has been approximated in most premature infant formulas. Vitamins are found in adequate amounts in premature infant formulas and human milk when fortified. Special formulas for preterm infants provide the additional minerals, vitamins, and trace elements required.

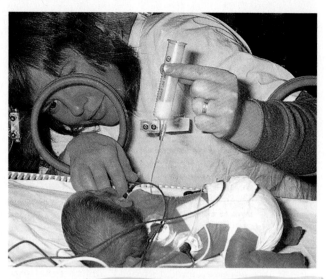

FIGURE 28-14 Mother has learned to feed her baby by gavage. (From Beischer NA, MacKay EV: *Obstetrics and the newborn,* ed 3, Sydney, 1993, Saunders; used with permission of Harcourt, Brace, Jovanovich Group, Australia.)

Test Yourself

• A week-old infant born at 31 weeks' gestation requires how many kcal/kg/day for adequate growth?

Enteral Nutrition

Infants who are too immature to feed orally may be fed by gavage with orogastric or nasogastric tubes passed into the stomach, duodenum, or jejunum. Intermittent (bolus) feedings are preferred because they stimulate normal postprandial enzyme release and gastrointestinal motility. The amount of the feeding and the intervals are slowly increased, which follows the normal progression of feeding behavior. Some infants, however, respond to bolus feedings with bradycardia as a result of vagal nerve stimulation. Others may have esophageal reflux and an increased risk of aspiration. Continuous feedings are offered in these cases. In some NICUs continuous gavage feeding tubes are very gradually advanced through the pyloric valve; in others, they are placed in the stomach, as for bolus feedings (Procedure 28-1). Equipment other than the actual feeding tube is changed often to reduce the danger of infection. As soon as possible, involve the mother in the gavage feeding (Figure 28-14).

Feeding by nipple or breast should be encouraged because it encourages growth and maturity of the gastrointestinal tract and provides comfort for hunger and oral gratification.

Oral feeding is slowly introduced when the infant is mature enough to use a nipple. Cardiorespiratory status need not be completely normal; however, the respiratory rate should be less than 60 breaths/min with only minimal amounts of supplemental oxygen.

Parenteral Nutrition

The infant who cannot be fed enterally is fed by the intravenous route. The usual basic solution is 10% dextrose in increasing amounts (see section on fluid requirements) with appropriate additives. During the first 24 hours of life, the newborn's serum electrolyte balance reflects that of the mother. On the second day, infants receiving intravenous therapy are given supplemental electrolytes, NaCl and KCl 1 to 4 mEq/kg; the amounts are determined after serum electrolyte levels have been measured. Solutions are infused via sites found in veins of the hands, arms, feet, or scalp. Extremely small (as small as 27-gauge) needles or intravenous catheters are used. Control of infusion rates is always maintained by an electronic pump and never by gravity. Careful attention for signs of infiltration is vital because extravasated solutions cause tissue necrosis.

Infants who are unable to take enteral feeds after the first days of life will require hyperalimentation or total parenteral nutrition (TPN) to meet basic nutritional need. Dextrose (10% to 30%) supplies carbohydrates; an amino acid solution provides precursors for protein synthesis, and fats are added through an emulsified solution. Electrolytes, minerals, and vitamins are added to the solution as needed. The TPN solution is prepared

PROCEDURE 28-1   Feeding Tube Placement for Intermittent Feedings

1. Prepare feeding and place adjacent to work area.
2. Select No. 5 or No. 8 French feeding tube according to infant size.
3. Determine appropriate distance of insertion by measuring length from tip of nose (for nasogastric) or from mouth (orogastric) to the earlobe and then to the end of the xiphoid process.
4. Place a short length of tape at the measured point.
5. Insert tube: nasal route may occlude air passage; oral route is more difficult to insert. Choose according to infant's condition and responses.
6. Tape securely to face (use skin protective dressing first).
7. Confirm placement of tube in stomach by injecting small amount of air while listening to characteristic sound with stethoscope placed just under left costal margin.
8. For intermittent feeding: aspirate residual stomach contents, and note amount and color of aspirate. If green (bile) or if brown or red (blood), report at once and delay feeding (necrotizing enterocolitis [NEC] may be occurring). Unusually large aspirate may be due to overfeeding or intestinal obstruction, NEC, or infection.
9. Measure and refeed small amount of aspirate. (Record aspirate and feeding totals.)
10. Proceed with new feeding, placing infant preferably on right side to encourage gastric emptying and avoid aspiration with regurgitation (Figure 28-15).

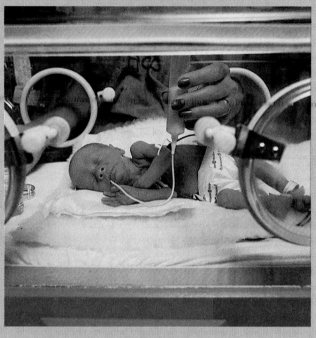

FIGURE 28-15 Gavage feeding of preterm infant. (Courtesy Ross Laboratories, Columbus, Ohio.)

• • •

OPTIONAL ACTIVITY: Write a sample nursing note correctly documenting the performance of this procedure.

in the pharmacy, with strict attention to sterility. It may be administered through a peripheral infusion if the dextrose concentration is not over 12.5%. A central venous line is needed to infuse higher dextrose concentrations.

Percutaneous central venous catheters often are inserted within the first week of life to provide the much needed parenteral nutrition. Complications of TPN include hypoglycemia or hyperglycemia, hyperammonemia, cholestatic jaundice, hyperlipidemia, and increased risk of kernicterus.

Assessment of growth. Adequacy of nutrition by either route is assessed by measuring the progress of growth and development. In addition, a careful record is kept of assessments of nutrition and fluid balance. The infant should be growing in length and weight; weight gain alone may indicate edema. Fluid and caloric intake is reordered every day depending on approximate visible and insensible fluid loss. The following parameters are desired:

1. Daily weights: ideal gain is 20 to 30 g/day
2. Weekly length: plotted on chart for intrauterine growth curve
3. Weekly head circumference: up to 1 cm/wk
4. Urine output: 1 to 3 ml/kg/hr
5. Urine specific gravity: 1.002 to 1.010
6. Adequate skin turgor and capillary refill: within 3 seconds
7. Serum electrolytes: Na (135 to 145 mM/L), K (3.5 to 7.0 mM/L), Cl (100 to 117 mM/L), glucose (70 to 100 mg/dl), calcium (7 to 11 mg/dl)
8. Blood urea nitrogen (BUN): 3.1 to 25.5 mg/dl
9. Normal vital signs, including BP

GASTROINTESTINAL PROBLEMS

Necrotizing Enterocolitis

Necrotizing enterocolitis (NEC) affects mostly premature infants, with an overall mortality of 20%. It often occurs during the first 2 weeks of life in infants who have sustained ischemic injury to the intestines as a result of asphyxia or shock. The normal bacterial contamination of the gut and formula feedings interact with the ischemia to produce the syndrome. NEC is rare in the breast-fed infant.

Signs. The infant with NEC has signs that are indistinguishable from sepsis. Abdominal distension, lethargy, gastric residual effects, vomiting, and gastrointestinal bleeding are common. Gas produced by intestinal organisms dissects the intestinal wall, producing a characteristic x-ray pattern. Varying areas of the gastrointestinal tract may be affected; however, the ileum and proximal colon are the usual sites. Rupture of the diseased intestine may produce pneumoperitoneum.

Clinical management. The infant with NEC will have a gastric tube inserted to decompress the stomach. Antibiotics, usually ampicillin (150 to 200 mg/kg/day), gentamicin (5.0 to 7.5 mg/kg/day), and clindamycin (30 mg/kg/day) are started. The infant will have nothing by mouth but will have a greater than usual fluid requirement. Blood transfusions may be necessary to control anemia and aid coagulation. Surgery is performed on infants with intestinal gangrene or perforation; a temporary colostomy may be done. Hyperalimentation is used as necessary. The residual effects of NEC (short bowel syndrome resulting from surgery and intestinal strictures) affect many survivors.

Results of investigations into methods of preventing NEC include the advisability of oral administration of immunoglobins or colostrum, modification of intestinal flora, and prophylactic antibiotics. The infant may have nothing by mouth for an extended period while the repaired bowel regains normal function.

► NURSING DIAGNOSES

1. High risk for fluid volume excess or deficit related to fluid demand/immature kidney function
2. Altered nutrition: less than body requirements related to toleration of feedings, or need for parenteral feeds
3. High risk for trauma to intestinal tract related to NEC reaction to feeds
4. Altered growth and development related to delays caused by immaturity of body systems

► EXPECTED OUTCOMES

1. Exhibits stabilization in fluid balance.
2. Tolerates enteral feeds without NEC trauma.
3. Begins nippling behavior by 2 weeks postbirth.
4. Growth and development follow expected rates.

Metabolic Dysfunction

Preterm, SGA, LGA, and postterm infants and any infant who has had intrauterine stress is at risk for altered metabolic function. Infants may show signs of hypothermia, hypoglycemia, and hypocalcemia from decreased glycogen and fat stores, poor central control, and endocrine imbalance.

HYPOTHERMIA

Hypothermia can be an important early indication of sepsis (see Chapters 18 and 19). It may mask or mimic other illnesses and frequently accompanies neonatal sepsis. Respiratory distress, pallor or cyanosis, increased or decreased movement, difficulty in feeding, hypotonia, or lethargy can occur.

Clinical Management

Treatment consists of gradual rewarming; warming too rapidly may cause apnea. Search for the cause of the heat loss. Monitor the infant's axillary temperature and the environmental temperature every 15 to 30 minutes until the axillary temperature is within normal range. The environmental temperature required to raise the axillary temperature to normal should be within the expected range for the infant's gestational age and weight (neutral thermal environment tables are posted in the NICU). If excessive heat is needed to maintain an infant's temperature, sepsis should be suspected. All high-risk infants are cared for under radiant warmers or in Isolettes. Radiant warmers allow convenient access to the baby but contribute to IWL (see the section on maintaining fluid, electrolyte, and nutritional balance) and hypothermia. Single- or double-walled Isolettes allow control for both. It takes time, however, to learn to care for an infant in an Isolette without losing the warmth inside. If the Isolette is opened for a procedure, an additional radiant heat source is needed. A servomechanism device taped onto the infant's abdomen senses the skin temperature and regulates the Isolette's temperature as needed to maintain the skin temperature at a set-point. It is important to note the amount of heat needed to maintain an infant's temperature in the normal range. Comparison to established normal ranges will reveal the infant who is really hypothermic but is artificially warmed by an overheated environment.

HYPOGLYCEMIA

Hypoglycemia, a blood glucose level of less than 40 mg/dl, often is seen in an *infant of a diabetic mother* (IDM), and in LGA, SGA, preterm, postterm, and polycythemic infants. SGA and preterm infants are at risk for hypoglycemia because of reduced glycogen stores. An infant who has a high Hct level (polycythemia) also may have hypoglycemia because of increased glucose consumption by red blood cells. Finally, if an infant has nothing by mouth for hours after birth (a common practice in past years), hypoglycemia may develop. Prevention is vital because unchecked hypoglycemia causes seizures and cerebral damage.

Infants of Diabetic Mothers

Not every LGA baby is an IDM, and not every IDM is LGA. Infants whose mothers have gestational diabetes or diabetes mellitus without peripheral vascular involvement are large and "resemble one another so closely that they might well be related. They are plump, sleek, . . . full-faced and plethoric" (Farquhar, 1959). (See Figure 24-2.) Others whose mothers have more advanced disease will be growth retarded and small for dates.

Most IDMs have been exposed to elevated maternal glucose levels in utero. If vascular changes have not excessively damaged the placenta, glucose readily diffuses across it into the fetal circulation, causing hyperplasia of fetal pancreatic islet cells and increased insulin production. Prenatally the excess glucose and insulin cause increased fetal growth. At delivery the maternal supply of glucose ends, but neonatal insulin production continues at the previous rate, causing hypoglycemia. LGA infants may have hypoglycemia if they are unrecognized IDMs.

Signs

Although a blood glucose value of 40 mg/dl is considered hypoglycemia, some infants may have symptoms at lower or higher levels. Because signs of hypoglycemia (Box 28-5) may mimic other conditions, it should always be considered.

Frequent assessment of serum glucose levels for infants at risk can identify the hypoglycemic infant before signs are seen. Capillary blood from a heel stick (Procedure 28-2) is tested in the nursery by any one of the available test strip kits (see Chapter 19). If levels are below 40 mg/dl, the reading usually is confirmed by laboratory analysis of blood (Procedure 28-3), but you should not wait for laboratory results to intervene.

Clinical Management

Treatment consists of oral or parenteral glucose. If the infant has only mild symptoms (without respiratory distress or seizures), 10% oral glucose is given. These infants usually are quite hungry and will feed well. Retest the serum glucose within 30 minutes and again 1 hour after offering the feed. Early feedings of breast milk or formula should be offered every 3 to 4 hours to supply needed calories and glucose.

Infants with major symptoms will need glucose infusions. A peripheral intravenous infusion is started with 10% glucose, the highest safe concentration. A slow push of 200 mg/kg (2 ml/kg) of 10% glucose may be used over 2 to 3 minutes. The bolus should be followed by a maintenance infusion of 7 to 8 mg/kg/min of glucose. The serum glucose levels are then carefully followed.

BOX 28-5 Signs of Hypoglycemia

- Tremors
- Jitteriness
- Apnea
- Cyanosis
- Respiratory distress
- Diaphoresis

PROCEDURE 28-2   Capillary Blood Sampling

Technique is similar to routine sampling (see Figure 19-18) except as follows:

1. Warm heel with prepackaged heel warmer or warmed diaper soak.
2. Cleanse with alcohol preparation. Allow to air dry.
3. Puncture site perpendicular to skin with sterile lancet (Figure 28-16).
4. Wipe away first drop of blood.
5. Gently squeeze ankle and foot above puncture site to increase flow.
6. Place one bead of blood on test strip.
7. Follow timing directions.

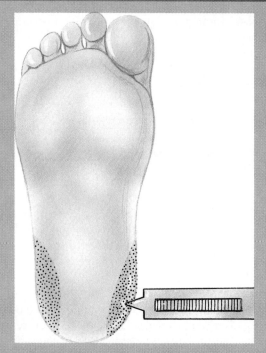

FIGURE 28-16 Capillary sampling from the heel. Stippled areas indicate correct sites.

•   •   •

OPTIONAL ACTIVITY: Write a sample nursing note correctly documenting the performance of this procedure.

PROCEDURE 28-3   Capillary Blood Gas

Technique is similar to routine sampling (see Figure 19-18) except as follows:

1. Hold heel horizontal with body to avoid venous stasis.
2. Fill anticoagulant end of tube (red marker).
3. Hold tubes horizontal.
4. Discard tube if air or bubbles get into tube.
5. Cap end after filling.
6. Mix blood to ensure anticoagulation (may use magnet and metal chip to mix blood).
7. Place in cup with crushed ice.
8. Take to lab as soon as possible.

NOTE: Omit steps 7 and 8 if analyzed within 5 minutes.

• • •

OPTIONAL ACTIVITY: Write a sample nursing note correctly documenting the performance of this procedure.

HYPOCALCEMIA

The infants who become hypoglycemic also are at risk for hypocalcemia (serum calcium less than 7 mg/dl). The preterm baby has not received the normal high calcium deposits supplied by the mother during the last weeks of pregnancy.

Signs

Hypocalcemic infants are jittery and tremulous. Symptoms may be seen during the first days or week (early onset).

Clinical Management

Treatment consists of adding calcium gluconate to parenteral intravenous fluids or supplementing enteral feedings with additional calcium (e.g., Neo-Calglucon). Parenteral calcium should be infused through a central catheter; subcutaneous infiltration of calcium causes necrosis and sloughing of tissue.

If the onset is later (after the first week), the cause is more likely to be a high-phosphate diet. Formula with a calcium-phosphorus ratio close to that of human milk (2.2:1.0) is then prescribed.

▶ NURSING DIAGNOSES

1. Ineffective thermoregulation related to immaturity, environmental temperatures
2. High risk for injury related to hypoglycemia or hypocalcemia
3. Altered nutrition: less than body requirements (hypoglycemia)
4. Parental knowledge deficit regarding nutritional aspects of care for IDM, preterm infant

▶ EXPECTED OUTCOMES

1. Responds to thermoneutral environment by maintaining stable body temperature.

2. Adapts to room air in open crib by 36 weeks' gestational age
3. Maintains glucose and calcium balance.
4. Parents learn infant needs for nutrition and participate in care.

Hematologic Dysfunction

In the neonate most bilirubin is produced from the destruction of red blood cells. There are two types of bilirubin. *Direct bilirubin,* also called *conjugated* bilirubin, is water soluble; therefore it is more easily handled by neonatal metabolism. It is excreted in bile via the small intestine or by the kidneys. Indirect, or *unconjugated,* bilirubin is lipid soluble and therefore cannot be excreted. Unconjugated bilirubin crosses the blood-brain barrier and can lead to kernicterus and brain damage.

HYPERBILIRUBINEMIA

Hyperbilirubinemia may be physiologic or nonphysiologic (pathologic). Figure 28-17 outlines the steps of bilirubin metabolism in the neonate. The result is a jaundiced appearance of the skin. Several possible mechanisms can cause neonatal bilirubin levels to rise.

1. Overloading the system with bilirubin production because of increased hemolysis (destruction) of red blood cells causes unconjugated levels to rise. Hemolytic disease, the normal extra large red cell mass of the newborn, extravasated blood (blood that has left the circulatory system and is contained elsewhere in the body, such as blood contained within a cephalhematoma), and increased enterohepatic circulation are the most common causes.
2. A decrease in the number of binding sites for bilirubin on albumin molecules increases the risk of kernicterus because only unbound unconjugated bilirubin can cross into the brain. Certain drugs interfere with this process.
3. A decrease in the ability of the liver to conjugate bilirubin also causes unconjugated levels to rise. Substances secreted in the breast milk of some women might inhibit conjugation.
4. Biliary obstruction prevents transportation of conjugated bilirubin to the gastrointestinal tract for excretion, causing conjugated levels to rise. This may be caused by biliary atresia (absence of the biliary drainage system), a cyst blocking the bile duct, hepatic damage from TPN, certain metabolic disorders, or infections such as hepatitis.
5. Conjugated bilirubin in the gastrointestinal tract for extended periods is converted back into unconjugated bilirubin, transported to the liver through enterohepatic circulation, and reconjugated, overloading the liver. This occurs when neonates are not

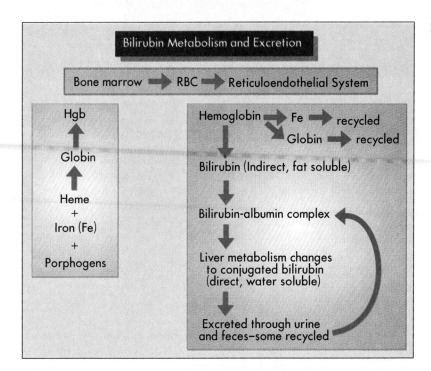

FIGURE 28-17 Bilirubin metabolism.

fed for many hours after birth. Early feeding stimulates the gastrocolic reflex and empties the large intestine earlier.

Physiologic Hyperbilirubinemia

The infant with physiologic hyperbilirubinemia has elevated bilirubin levels because the *normally* elevated red blood cell mass is being *normally* reduced. There is a shorter life span of newborn red cells. In addition, there can be a transient deficiency in the enzymes needed for conjugation. The criteria are summarized in Box 28-6.

Nonphysiologic Hyperbilirubinemia

Nonphysiologic hyperbilirubinemia is elevated above 12.9 mg/dl in formula-fed infants and above 15 mg/dl

---

BOX 28-6 Criteria for Physiologic Jaundice for Infant Older Than 24 Hours

Full-term infant
- Mean bilirubin levels peak at 6 mg/dl by 72 hours
- Mean bilirubin levels fall by day 5
- Levels peaking on third day of life
- Jaundice gone by 1 week of age

Preterm infant
- Mean bilirubin <6-10 mg/dl (by day 5)
- Levels peaking on fifth day of life
- Jaundice gone by 2 weeks of age

---

in breast-fed infants (Wong, 1993). The pathologic level in small or sick preterm infants is lower. This type of hyperbilirubinemia can cause kernicterus (deposits of bilirubin in the brain) in preterm infants. The most frequent reasons for elevated bilirubin levels are as follows.

1. The normally elevated red blood cell mass is being abnormally reduced after birth because of some pathologic process, as in isoimmunization and sepsis.
2. An abnormally elevated red blood cell mass (see section on polycythemia) may be present for a variety of reasons.
3. Abnormalities of red blood cell structure or enzyme systems (glucose-6-phosphate dehydrogenase [G6PD] deficiency) make the cells more prone to hemolysis and increase bilirubin production.
4. Abnormal enzyme activity can result from inborn errors of metabolism (IEM).

RH INCOMPATIBILITY

Isoimmunization that causes severe fetal hemolysis may result from maternal-fetal Rh incompatibilities. ABO or minor blood groups contribute but usually do not cause such severe problems (see Chapter 9). The fetus of an isoimmunized mother is at risk for intrauterine hemolysis, anemia, and hyperbilirubinemia. The consequences for the affected fetus may range from mild to fatal if untreated. Depending on the level of the mother's antibody titer, the phase of pregnancy, and the time elapsed since she became sensitized, the degree and

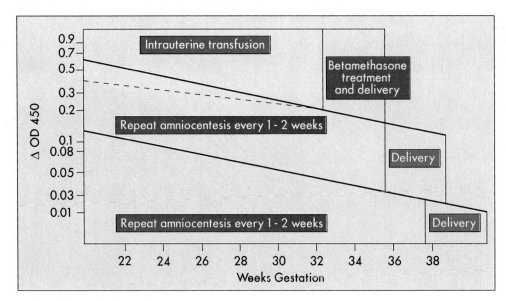

FIGURE 28-18 Modified Liley curve used for management of the Rh-sensitized fetus. ΔOD 450 of amniotic fluid is plotted against gestational age. Decisions concerning delivery are made on the basis of zone at which coordinates cross. (From Branch DW: Isoimmunization in pregnancy. In Gabbe SG et al: *Obstetrics: normal and problem pregnancies,* New York, 1986, Churchill Livingstone.)

duration of fetal cell hemolysis may be more or less severe. The fetal cells are broken down by maternal antibodies that cross to the fetus.

The increasing anemia stimulates the production of immature erythrocytes and thus the name for this problem, *erythroblastosis fetalis.* A varying amount of bilirubin is excreted into the amniotic fluid through fetal tracheobronchial secretions. Serial measurements of amniotic fluid bilirubin from amniocentesis are used to evaluate the severity of fetal involvement. The results, when plotted on the graph shown in Figure 28-18, are used to determine prenatal treatment. Intrauterine transfusion of packed red blood cells is attempted, and the infant delivered if necessary.

In severely affected fetuses a syndrome of massive edema, pleural effusions, and ascites called *hydrops fetalis* may develop, which frequently leads to intrauterine fetal death (IUFD). At birth, less severely affected infants may appear pale but not jaundiced because most of the by-products of fetal red blood cell breakdown (bilirubin) have been excreted by the mother. Once separated from the mother's efficient metabolic system, however, the newborn will quickly become jaundiced.

Special preparation for delivery of an isoimmunized newborn includes having blood ready for transfusion if necessary. Packed red blood cells will be used to correct severe anemia, the immediate threat. Physical assessment of the infant should include close attention to vital signs, the presence of hepatosplenomegaly (caused by intrauterine stimulation of hematopoietic organs), edema, pallor, and jaundice. Blood is drawn for a complete blood count and bilirubin levels.

Clinical Management

The management of all infants with unconjugated hyperbilirubinemia is similar; however, the timing of intervention varies among infants. Decisions are made on the basis of the increased risk of kernicterus in infants, depending on gestational age and the presence of sepsis, asphyxia, and other factors. The goals of treatment are to correct the anemia and remove the bilirubin.

The phototherapy lamp, which detoxifies bilirubin, is the most common method of treatment to reduce bilirubin levels. Debate exists as to which type is most effective and produces less discomfort (usually dizziness) for the nursing staff (Maisels et al, 1988).

Because phototherapy works at the level of the skin, exposure of as much skin as possible is necessary. Infants receiving phototherapy should be cared for in an Isolette and wear only a diaper, if anything at all. A paper surgical mask used as a diaper increases skin exposure. The infant's eyes should be shielded with a "bili-mask" made of opaque material to reduce retinal exposure (Figure 28-19). During feeding, this should be removed to decrease sensory deprivation and allow for examination of the infant's eyes. Parents may get upset when they see their naked babies with bandaged eyes under the eerie phototherapy light. Taking the time to prepare them is helpful.

In some centers, moistening eye drops are administered. Careful attention to temperature regulation and fluid balance is necessary when caring for these infants. If a skin temperature probe is used, be sure to shield it from the light. Phototherapy increases IWL and also causes increased bowel motility and loose, watery stools. This combination can dehydrate an infant quickly. An increase in infusion rate for intravenous fluids is necessary for infants who can have nothing by mouth. Any signs of dehydration or skin breakdown from increased stooling should be reported.

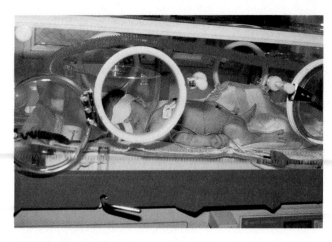

FIGURE 28-19 Phototherapy. Note eye coverings. (Courtesy Marjorie Pyle, RNC, *Lifecircle*.)

Serum bilirubin will be measured every 8 to 24 hours and more frequently for infants whose levels rise rapidly. When phototherapy is discontinued, bilirubin levels will be monitored for at least 24 hours because they may revert to a level needing treatment.

Exchange Transfusion

Exchange transfusion is used when bilirubin levels continue to rise rapidly in spite of phototherapy or when a severely affected infant is born. Exchange transfusion corrects anemia and removes red blood cells coated with antibodies and excess bilirubin. Describing this procedure to parents is a challenge; they often think that the infant's entire blood volume will be withdrawn at once and then replaced. In reality, small amounts of blood are removed, discarded, and replaced until about 80% of the infant's total blood volume has been exchanged. Because the blood is constantly circulating, the amount of blood replaced actually is double the infant's blood volume. The procedure is performed through an umbilical venous catheter connected to a four-way stopcock, allowing the blood to be withdrawn, discarded, and replaced. Exchange transfusion is used with phototherapy to treat severe hyperbilirubinemia.

Complications of exchange transfusion include formation of thrombi with embolization, cardiac arrhythmias, thrombocytopenia, and NEC. Preserved blood is used, which may cause hypocalcemia because the citrate in the preservative binds to calcium and makes it unavailable to the body; supplemental calcium is given if signs of hypocalcemia are noted. In rare cases, viral or bacterial infection may be introduced by contaminated blood or equipment. Exchange transfusion is a tedious but dangerous procedure; therefore one nurse is assigned to keep an accurate record of the volumes of blood withdrawn and transfused, as well as vital signs and medications administered.

Test Yourself

• Which type of bilirubin is water soluble and easily excreted by the neonate?

• What does phototherapy do to assist the excretion of bilirubin?

ANEMIA

Anemia may begin prenatally as a result of isoimmunization, fetomaternal transfusion, twin-to-twin transfusion, or puncture of the placenta or umbilical cord during amniocentesis. After birth, infants may become anemic because of continued hemolysis from isoimmunization, intracranial or gastrointestinal bleeding, sepsis, iatrogenic blood loss as a result of repeated laboratory work, and physiologic anemia. Preterm infants are at risk for anemia of prematurity, an exaggeration of physiologic anemia. Infants of any gestational age can suffer from hereditary defects in hemoglobin synthesis or hemoglobinopathies.

Anemia can be prevented if risk factors are recognized. Infants of sensitized mothers or twin pregnancies, infants with a family history of hemoglobinopathic illness, and ill or premature infants should be considered at risk. During multiple gestations, vascular anastomoses may cause one fetus to donate blood to another; the donor becomes anemic and the recipient polycythemic. The Hct levels of infants of multiple gestations should be determined soon after birth.

Ill infants are subject to multiple venous and arterial punctures. A flow sheet for blood withdrawal and transfusions will help to anticipate the need for transfusion before anemia compromises the condition further. Healthy full-term infants have sufficient iron stores for synthesis of red blood cells until the third to fourth month after birth. Anemia may result if supplemental iron is not given; most formulas contain supplemental iron; therefore full-term infants generally do not have problems with anemia. Breast milk may not have adequate iron content for the very premature infant. For full-term infants, human milk supplies easily absorbed iron. In contrast, preterm infants start life with a reduced mass of red blood cells that have a shorter life span than those in a full-term infant. Blood is drawn more frequently, growth is more rapid, and vitamin E deficiency is more common. For these reasons, premature infants are at high risk for developing symptoms of anemia.

Signs

Recognition of anemia begins with daily physical assessments, with special attention to pallor, jaundice, tachycardia, tachypnea, apnea, hepatosplenomegaly, or poor capillary refill. When the infant is anemic, the decreased hemoglobin concentration and the decreased number of red blood cells result in a diminished oxygen-carrying capacity of the blood.

Clinical Management

Weekly screening of hemoglobin and Hct levels is necessary for growing premature infants. Normal Hct levels range from 48% to 60% at birth; normal hemoglobin levels are 16 to 20 g/dl; however, it is important to note whether the blood was drawn from a central site (such as large vein or artery) or a peripheral site (a heel stick). The central Hct level may be as much as 15% lower than the peripheral level because of stasis of blood in the peripheral circulation. A diagnosis of anemia or polycythemia may be inaccurate if the source of the blood is not considered. Often, warming the heel before drawing blood will increase the perfusion. The complete blood count will reveal hemoglobin and Hct levels and the presence of immature red blood cells (reticulocytes) as the bone marrow attempts to correct the anemia.

The decision to transfuse is made if symptoms are present, which indicates that the infant is unable to adapt to the anemia. Transfusion will raise the Hct level but will also depress the bone marrow's efforts to produce new red blood cells. Warmed blood in the form of packed red blood cells is slowly transfused through a peripheral intravenous site by means of a pump. Attention to fluid balance is essential, and it is necessary to reduce other infusions to allow for the fluid contained within the transfusion.

POLYCYTHEMIA

Neonatal **polycythemia** occurs when the central Hct level rises above 65%. Blood viscosity increases, and circulation in smaller vessels becomes sluggish. Microemboli may form and travel to the central nervous system, gastrointestinal tract, and kidneys, causing cerebrovascular accidents, NEC, and renal vein thrombosis. Term or postterm SGA infants are at highest risk for polycythemia as a result of increased erythropoietin levels in response to hypoxia. Maternal diabetes mellitus, as well as maternal-to-fetal and twin-to-twin transfusions are associated with an increased incidence of polycythemia. Stripping or milking the umbilical cord toward the infant at birth, delaying cord clamping, or holding the infant below the level of the placenta to transfer extra blood into the newborn are ways in which obstetric practice can contribute to polycythemia.

Signs

Infants with polycythemia look *plethoric* with a ruddy or purplish, cyanotic tinge to the skin. Respiratory distress, cardiomegaly, and congestive heart failure may be present. Hypoglycemia commonly occurs because red blood cells consume glucose. Jitteriness, lethargy, or seizures are seen with neurologic involvement. If renal function is compromised, the infant will have oliguria. Last, the increased red blood cell mass contributes to the bilirubin load, producing hyperbilirubinemia and jaundice.

Clinical Management

Treatment is recommended for infants with symptoms but controversial for those who are symptom free. A partial exchange transfusion removes some of the cellular blood components and replaces them with fluid such as normal saline, 5% albumin, or Plasmanate. This will lower the Hct level to a targeted 50% to 55% and decrease vicosity. The procedure usually is performed through an umbilical venous catheter.

THROMBOCYTOPENIA

Thrombocytopenia (platelet count below 100,000/mm^3) occurs in ill and well newborns. Causes include maternal-fetal platelet incompatibilities (similar to red blood cell isoimmunization), perinatal infections, birth asphyxia, inherited disorders, administration of aspirin during pregnancy, trapping of platelets in giant hemangiomas, and disseminated intravascular coagulation (DIC). Infants with thrombocytopenia will have petechiae (microhemorrhages into the skin) and increased bleeding time after heel sticks, injections, and venipunctures. When a clotting disorder is suspected, confirm that vitamin K had been given after delivery, because a deficiency will cause similar symptoms. A platelet count and other laboratory tests of blood coagulation will be ordered to diagnose the defect in coagulation. Depending on the cause, transfusions of platelets and other blood factors may be needed (see Chapter 22).

▶ **NURSING DIAGNOSES**

1. High risk for injury related to hyperbilirubinemia
2. High risk for fluid volume deficit related to phototherapy
3. High risk for hypothermia/hyperthermia related to phototherapy
4. Parental knowledge deficit regarding infant status/treatment

▶ **EXPECTED OUTCOMES**

1. Bilirubin levels remain within the safe range.
2. Maintains fluid balance under phototherapy.
3. Maintains body temperature above 97.5° F, below 99° F.
4. Parents seek and receive data regarding infant status and treatment.

Immunologic Dysfunction

Infections with organisms that do little damage later in life can extensively damage a developing fetus or newborn. Frequently the timing of the infection makes the difference. Infection may be acquired during pregnancy by transplacental transmission, during birth by infected secretions, or postnatally by infected persons and objects in the environment. Some organisms are more prevalent during perinatal or neonatal life. Preterm infants are at high risk for sepsis; the incidence rises from 1 in 1000 live, term births to 1 in 250 for infants delivered prematurely.

BACTERIAL SEPSIS

Bacterial sepsis can occur within the first few days of life. Premature infants whose mothers had prolonged rupture of membranes and fever are at high risk for infection with organisms that normally inhabit the vaginal tract, such as group B β-hemolytic streptococci, *Escherichia coli,* and *Haemophilus influenzae.* Infants with these early-onset diseases are severely ill; mortality may reach 50%.

Late-onset disease affects infants more than 1 week old. The causative organisms are nosocomial *(Staphylococcus aureus, S. epidermidis,* and *Pseudomonas)* and those implicated in early-onset disease. Mortality is 20%, and central nervous system damage from meningitis is common.

VIRAL AND PROTOZOAL INFECTION

Viral and protozoal infections are transmitted transplacentally from maternal to fetal circulations during pregnancy (e.g., human immunodeficiency virus [HIV] and toxoplasmosis, rubella, cytomegalovirus, and herpes simplex [TORCH]) or acquired during passage through the birth canal (e.g., HIV, hepatitis B virus [HBV], and herpes). Infants who are infected later in gestation or during birth are born with clinical signs of infection, to which they respond with only weak immune responses. (See Chapters 25 and 27 for complete discussion of transmission.)

Postnatally acquired viral infections that affect neonates include influenza strains, adenovirus, coxsackievirus B, echoviruses, and respiratory syncytial virus (RSV). Cardiorespiratory and gastrointestinal symptoms are common. Infected persons, including health care personnel and family members, are the sources of infection.

Risk

Risk varies with the causative organism, duration of illness, systems involved, onset of available treatment, and gestational age. Although mortality and morbidity have been reduced drastically in the last 40 years, the emergence of resistant organisms and delivery of more immature infants make therapy more complicated.

It is important to look at statistics for both mortality and morbidity. Neonatal sepsis claims many victims. For instance, aggressive care of the infant with group B streptococci sepsis can lower the 40% to 80% mortality rate to 15% to 30%. Even with aggressive care, however, between 20% and 40% of infants with meningitis die. Of those who survive, 30% to 50% will have neurologic sequelae. Thus the baby who survives infection can be completely normal or profoundly affected. Timely identification of the infant at risk for sepsis can significantly affect survival or death. The following are risk factors: prolonged rupture of membranes, maternal fever, inadequate prenatal care, history of maternal illness or exposure to contagious disease, chorioamnionitis, active herpes, and intravenous drug use. The similarities in the signs of many types of infections make identification even more difficult.

Signs

The neonate with prenatally acquired viral disease frequently shows signs of early IUGR. Because viruses interfere with cellular replication, the number of cells is reduced in affected infants, causing a reduction in the brain and general body size (microcephaly). Other neurologic manifestations include cerebral calcifications and hydrocephalus. The eyes may be affected with cataracts, microophthalmia, and chorioretinitis. Infection of other organ systems produces pneumonitis, myocarditis, hepatitis, and thrombocytopenia. Involvement of these systems causes respiratory distress, cardiovascular instability, jaundice, hepatosplenomegaly, petechiae, and increased bleeding time.

Early signs of sepsis are subtle. Comments by mothers and nursing staff members that the baby "just doesn't seem to be right" should be heeded as characteristic signs of early illness. Fever, generally regarded as a common sign of infection, is rare in the neonate. Newborns more frequently have hypothermia, poor feeding, abdominal distension, respiratory distress, apnea, bradycardia, hypotension, and cyanosis. Altered neurologic signs (lethargy, hypotonia, tremors, and seizures) may be seen even if the infant does not have meningitis. Jaundice is associated with urinary tract infection and congenital viral infections. Skin pustules, discharge from the eyes, and a foul-smelling, moist umbilical cord with a reddened base are signs of local infections. Generalized sepsis may follow, however, because neonates are less able to keep these infections localized.

Clinical Management

Prevention of perinatal sepsis involves measures that encourage women to seek prenatal care, appropriately timed rubella immunization, and education concerning transmission of diseases. Avoidance of hazardous behaviors such as unsafe sex, intravenous drug use, and ingestion of raw or undercooked meat reduces the risks. Encourage mothers to seek medical attention as soon as amniotic membranes rupture because prolonged rupture of membranes is associated with neonatal sepsis, especially if followed by long labor.

Prevention of neonatal illness is best accomplished by identifying the infant who is at risk for sepsis, strict hand washing for all who come in contact with newborns, avoidance of exposure to persons who are infectious, and parent education for cord care and encouragement of breast-feeding or proper preparation of formula (Figure 28-20). Providing mother and baby with skin-to-skin contact, such as with **kangaroo care (KC)**, also encourages colonization of the newborn skin with "friendly" organisms rather than with pathogens. Infants who are already ill are more likely to become septic; therefore close attention to sterile technique during invasive procedures is vital.

Laboratory data are used to confirm the diagnosis of sepsis. The usual response of increased white blood cell count (leukocytosis) is replaced with a decreased count (leukopenia) in the ill infant. The white blood cell differential may "shift to the left," meaning that more and more immature white blood cells are being released. Thrombocytopenia may occur. Blood and urine specimens are obtained for culture and sensitivity tests. Fluid from a lumbar puncture also will be evaluated for culture and sensitivity, examination of the cellular contents, and chemical analysis. Blood gas levels may reveal metabolic acidosis. A urine specimen can detect the presence of bacterial antigens, which is a rapid method of diagnosing an infection.

Laboratory data are helpful if intrauterine infection with the TORCH group is suspected. Levels of IgM over 20 mg/dl indicate that the fetus's own immune system has responded to an infection of any kind. Because there is a lag time between the time of infection and the production of IgM, elevated levels at birth indicate congenital infection. Identification of specific types of IgM confirm viral cause. Treatment of most viral diseases is symptomatic and consists of supportive care. Exceptions are the herpes simplex virus and RSV, for which specific therapy is available for infants who have only local disease. Systemic herpes infection results in a high mortality and morbidity rate.

Therapies must be chosen carefully because side effects are common. Most are related to the differences in the way neonates metabolize and excrete medications. Competition for albumin-binding sites of other substances also is an important factor. For example, sulfisoxazole is not given because it increases the risk of kernicterus by occupying bilirubin-binding sites. If early-onset sepsis, pneumonia, or meningitis is suspected, therapy is started with ampicillin and an aminoglycoside such as gentamicin or kanamycin. The results of the culture and sensitivity test are used to confirm the correct choice of antibiotic. For later-onset bacterial disease, a pencillinase-resistant penicillin such as nafcillin is used.

Nursing Responsibilities
▶ NURSING DIAGNOSES

1. High risk for infection related to poor immunologic response, invasive therapies
2. Ineffective thermoregulation related to septic processes, immaturity of host defenses
3. High risk for altered nutrition: less than body requirements related to responses to sepsis
4. Interrupted breastfeeding related to compromised neonatal status
5. Anxiety (parental) related to infant status/progress

▶ EXPECTED OUTCOMES

1. Infection resolves without lasting damage to infant.
2. Infant maintains a stable body temperature.
3. Adequate nutrition provides for growth rate.
4. Mother provides sufficient breast milk for infant.
5. Parents demonstrate coping ability and reduced anxiety.

▶ NURSING INTERVENTIONS

Care of the septic infant includes close attention to the multisystem effects of sepsis. Maintenance of cardiores-

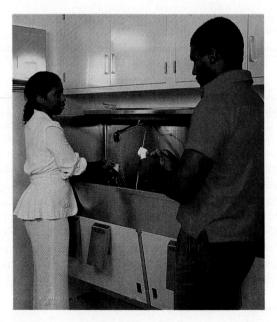

FIGURE 28-20 Before visitation, parents need to scrub arms and hands. (Courtesy Ross Laboratories, Columbus, Ohio.)

piratory functions, blood volume, thermoregulation, fluid and electrolyte balance, and nutrition is essential if specific antibiotic therapy is to be effective. An awareness of the way neonates metabolize and excrete drugs also is essential in observing for untoward effects. Communication with parents about the necessity of continuing therapy even after the infant improves clinically is important. Parents also may carry an unusual burden of guilt if neonatal infection has resulted from maternal illness (see Nursing Care Plan).

Neonates who become infected rarely need to be isolated. Although Isolettes isolate the infant from the environment, they do not separate the environment from the infant. Compliance with guidelines established by the Centers for Disease Control (CDC) for universal precautions is essential. (See Chapter 25, Isolation Precautions.)

▶ EVALUATION

1. Were the signs of sepsis identified before the infant suffered injury?
2. Were the appropriate medications administered to treat the infection?
3. Did the infant have any adverse sequelae from the infection or the therapy?

Neurologic Dysfunction

Preservation of the central nervous system is the primary goal of neonatal therapy. Unfortunately therapy may be one of the factors that adversely affects neonatal outcome. Many factors, such as congenital disorders, injuries before, during, and after birth, drug effects, infectious agents, and the environment (which includes high-technology treatments), can affect neurologic functioning.

Parents of infants with neurologic alterations should be encouraged to participate in their infant's care. A team effort is needed to support them through discharge. Often the best support comes from peer groups of parents of children with similar needs.

SEIZURES

Seizures are a common feature of a wide range of neonatal illnesses. Seizures may occur in sepsis, meningitis, drug withdrawal, hypoglycemia, hypocalcemia, fluid and electrolyte imbalances, perinatal asphyxia, and disorders of neurologic development. Chances for normal development depend on the cause and the effectiveness of treatment.

Signs

Neonatal seizure activity is subtle and easy to miss unless you observe very carefully. Although the classic grand mal seizure pattern is not seen in newborns, there are distinct varieties of seizures (Table 28-4). Jitteriness frequently is mistaken for seizures. The jittery baby has tremors and rapid movements of the extremities or fingers that you can stop by flexing the limbs. The jittery movements of the infant who is having a seizure cannot be stopped by holding the extremity. No other signs of seizures may occur. Although jitteriness can be normal, it also may be a sign of hypoglycemia or drug withdrawal.

TABLE 28-4 Neonatal Seizure Activity

APPEARANCE	SIGNIFICANCE
SUBTLE	
Apnea (usually seen with tonic horizontal deviation, jerking of the eyes, blinking, fluttering lids, drooling, sucking, tonic posturing or unusual movements of limbs, e.g., rowing, swimming, or pedaling	Most frequent type and most common in preterm infant
CLONIC	
Jerking activity	Full-term infant with hypoxic-ischemic encephalopathy
Multifocal: movements of one body part followed by another	Disturbances of the entire cerebrum
Focal: movement of one part	
TONIC	
Posturing similar to decerebrate posture in adults	Preterm infant with intraventricular hemorrhage
MYOCLONIC	
Single or multiple jerks of upper and lower extremities	Possible prediction of myoclonic spasms in early infancy

Data from Volpe JJ, Hill A: Neurologic disorders. In Avery G, editor: *Neonatology: pathophysiology of the newborn*, ed 3, Philadelphia, 1987, JB Lippincott.

Clinical Management

An electroencephalogram (EEG) is obtained to document abnormal brain activity in the infant with seizures. Tests to discover the cause of the seizures are vital and include metabolic screens, appropriate cultures, cranial ultrasound, and CT scan.

Care for seizures involves treating the underlying cause; however, it is more urgent to stop the seizure activity. An intravenous loading dose of 10 to 20 mg/kg of phenobarbital is given over several minutes. Additional doses of 5 to 20 mg/kg may be necessary. The infant is then given 3 to 4 mg/kg/day by mouth, if possible. This dosage is adjusted to maintain a level (usually 15 to 30 µ/ml) that will control the seizures, yet allow the newborn to behave normally.

Test Yourself

You are caring for a 12-hour-old, full-term infant recovering from perinatal asphyxia. Give the correct term from Table 28-4 for the following signs of seizure activity for this infant.

• Periods of fluttering eyes and posturing plus halt in breathing _____
• Rapid jerks of the extremities _____
• Repetitive movements of one extremity _____
• Movements of one body part followed by others _____

HYPOXIC-ISCHEMIC ENCEPHALOPATHY

Hypoxic-ischemic encephalopathy (HIE) is the primary complication of perinatal asphyxia. The combination of reduced arterial Po_2 and cerebral perfusion causes neurologic deficits of varying severity such as mental retardation, choreoathetosis, seizures, spasticity, and learning disorders. It is difficult to predict the extent of the deficits until cerebral edema resolves. The immaturity of the newborn's brain makes this even more difficult.

The infant's gestational age determines the kind of injury sustained. Preterm infants with HIE are at risk for intraventricular hemorrhage followed by hydrocephalus, mental retardation, and motor deficits of the lower extremities. The full-term infant is more likely to suffer edema and necrosis of the cerebral cortex and microcephaly as the cortex atrophies, which can be followed by motor deficits of the upper extremities, seizure disorders, mental retardation, and blindness.

Signs

Initially the infant with severe HIE will be semicomatose or comatose with irregular respirations. It will often be necessary to provide respiratory support with additional oxygen. Seizures may appear within the first 12 hours. The infant's level of alertness may improve between 12 and 24 hours, but this improvement also is accompanied by a worsening of seizure activity. By the second day of life, the coma returns and may be accompanied by respiratory arrest. Many infants with severe HIE die at this time. Infants with less extensive encephalopathy are more likely to survive with less severe sequelae (see Chapter 27 for cerebral palsy discussion).

INTRACRANIAL HEMORRHAGE

The neonate with intracranial hemorrhage has sustained perinatal hypoxia or trauma. Subdural hemorrhage usually is caused by trauma during delivery of a very large infant, whereas perinatal asphyxia is the factor precipitating subarachnoid, intraventricular, or intracerebellar hemorrhage. The incidence of **intraventricular hemorrhage (IVH)** has increased with the ability to provide respiratory support for extremely immature infants.

IVH occurs almost exclusively in small, preterm infants of less than 32 weeks' gestational age, primarily because cerebral blood flow is not effectively regulated. Treatments for other complications of prematurity often contribute to the pathogenesis of IVH. For example, after administration of hypertonic solutions (such as sodium bicarbonate for metabolic acidosis), the hypertonicity draws fluid into the blood, causing the intravascular volume to expand and increase cerebral flow.

Infants with respiratory distress and hypercapnia are at risk because of the increase in cerebral blood flow that accompanies the rise in Pco_2. The origin of bleeding is the subependymal germinal matrix, where a rich but fragile capillary network is found. Rupture of vessels within this network causes bleeding close to the borders of the ventricular system into the periventricular tissue (grade I). The hemorrhage may extend into the ventricles (grade II), resulting in hydrocephalus when the flow of cerebrospinal fluid (CSF) is obstructed by clots (grade III). In the most severe form, bleeding extends from the germinal matrix into the cerebral parenchyma (grade IV).

Signs

The signs of IVH may be dramatic if the infant's condition deteriorates rapidly or difficult to detect if it occurs over many hours. Therefore all infants at risk for IVH are carefully assessed clinically and with bedside ultrasound examinations. Infants with a rapid deterioration may have seizures, deepening coma, fixed pupils (not normally seen before 32 weeks of gestation), respiratory arrest, abnormal eye movements, and flaccidity over the course of a few minutes to hours. The Hct level may fall, and if there is obstruction to CSF flow, the anterior fontanelle will bulge. Alterations in temperature, fluid and electrolyte balance, BP, and glucose metabolism also may be seen. Some of these signs occur if the manifestation is more subtle than this dramatic form.

Clinical Management

The prevention of IVH involves restricting environmental stimuli that may cause rapid changes in cerebral blood flow. Although cesarean delivery may help to preserve the normal cerebral circulation for the preterm infant, it is not the recommended mode of delivery, unless there are other indications. Clustering of examinations and procedures while allowing for rest also is advised, and any unnecessary stimuli should be avoided. Control of pain lessens agitation. Wide shifts in blood pressure, administration of hypertonic solutions, and overventilation that could lead to pneumothorax should be avoided.

After IVH has been confirmed, the infant's condition will be followed closely by ultrasound examinations for signs of hydrocephalus. Shunting may be necessary, or resolution of the hydrocephalus may occur spontaneously. The prognosis for normal growth and development is directly related to the severity of the IVH. For example, a 59% mortality rate was observed in one study (N = 75 infants) with periventricular hemorrhage extending greater than 1 cm. Of the survivors, 87% had major motor deficits, and in 73% cognitive function was less than 80% of normal (Volpe, 1989). Hemorrhage alone does not account for all the neurologic deficits.

BIRTH INJURIES

Peripheral Nerve Palsy

The facial nerve or nerves of the brachial plexus may be injured by a difficult delivery. Look for signs of peripheral nerve palsy during examination of the head and extremities (see Chapter 18).

Signs. Facial nerve palsy occurs after difficult forceps delivery or a prolonged labor during which the fetal face was compressed against the maternal sacrum. There is flattening of the nasolabial fold and absense of movement of the corner of the mouth on the involved side. When the infant cries you will note the lack of movement on the affected side (Figure 28-21). Electrodiagnostic tests are used to evaluate the integrity of the nerve. Most facial nerve palsies improve spontaneously.

Brachial plexus palsy is most commonly associated with shoulder dystocia if excessive traction on the infant's head and neck pulls at the cervical nerve roots. There are two types. Erb's palsy involves the arm muscles supplied by the C5-6 nerve roots. The arm is held in a characteristic "maitre d' " or "waiter's tip"

posture (Figure 28-22). Klumpke paralysis involves the hand muscles supplied by the C7-T1 nerve roots. At times the entire plexus from C5 to T1 is affected with paralysis of the arm and hand. Sequelae are common

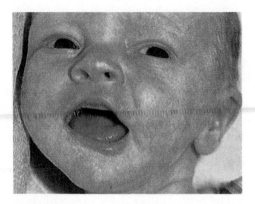

FIGURE 28-21 Facial nerve palsy. This infant incurred injury to the right facial nerve, resulting in loss of the nasolabial fold on the affected side and asymmetric movement of the mouth. The side of the mouth that appears to droop is the normal side. (From Zitelli BJ, Davis HW: *Atlas of pediatric physical diagnosis,* St Louis, 1987, Mosby.)

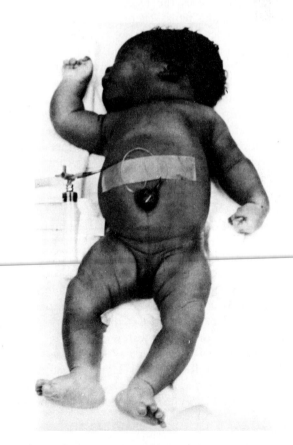

FIGURE 28-22 Brachial plexus palsy. (From Korones SB: *High-risk newborn infants: the basis for intensive nursing care,* ed 4, St Louis, 1986, Mosby.)

and include paralysis, loss of sensation, and poor bone growth.

There is no treatment for brachial plexus injuries. You can perform passive range of motion with every diaper change once the swelling has subsided. Serial electrodiagnostic examinations will be performed to note improvement.

NEONATAL ABSTINENCE SYNDROME

Neonatal drug dependence is the result of maternal drug abuse. During the last few decades, most affected infants were born to mothers using heroin or methadone. In large measure, cocaine has replaced these drugs in the 1990s. In some NICUs, 25% of the infants suffer the effects of perinatal drug abuse: disruption of normal fetal development, neonatal behavior, and family functioning. The results will be a generation of children and families with special needs who may be unable to discontinue this cycle. There is a great deal being learned about the aftereffects of fetal drug injury, and the nurse must be informed about current research.

Heroin

Heroin easily crosses the placenta, creating physical dependence in the fetus. There are no known direct teratogenic effects of heroin use, but the decrease in placental blood flow compounded by poor nutrition and possible polydrug use leads to intrauterine growth retardation (IUGR). There is a decreased incidence of RDS in heroin-addicted newborns, possibly related to the effects of intrauterine stress on pulmonary surfactant production. Bilirubin metabolism also is enhanced and decreases the incidence of hyperbilirubinemia. The addicted fetus, however, is at higher risk for intrauterine hypoxia and meconium aspiration. Fetal exposure to infections such as HIV, syphilis, gonorrhea, and HBV are common. Onset of signs of heroin withdrawal begin within the first 72 hours but may not begin until up to 2 weeks after birth.

Methadone

Methadone addiction may result from its planned, legal use as part of a methadone-maintenance program or from street use, usually as one of the many drugs taken. Onset of signs of withdrawal is more likely to be delayed because of the longer half-life; however, polydrug use can confuse these time frames. The trend to early discharge makes detection more difficult and requires accurate history taking and observational skills.

Cocaine

Maternal to fetal transfer of cocaine is swift and produces similar effects in the fetus. Cocaine and its metabolites are excreted by the fetal kidney into the amniotic fluid. The metabolites are even more potent than the drug. The fetus recycles the drug as this "cocaine bath" is swallowed. Births of infants with cerebral infarcts after sudden fetal hypertension have been documented (Chasnoff et al, 1987). Prenatal use of cocaine also stimulates the uterine smooth muscle, leading to preterm labor that often does not respond to tocolysis. Placental abruption secondary to vasoconstriction and hypertension may further compromise fetal well-being. The incidence of spontaneous abortion and stillbirth caused by placental abruption is higher in the cocaine-abusing pregnant woman (Janke, 1990).

Behavioral aberrations from cocaine may be similar to those seen in infants withdrawing from narcotics. The effects of polydrug use and withdrawal are apparent but it may be difficult to ascertain whether symptoms result from withdrawal or central nervous system damage. Ultrasound and CT evaluation can be helpful. Look also for congenital defects.

Alcohol

Alcohol is a readily available, widely used, and accepted legal drug. The dangers of perinatal alcohol use have been suspected for many years; alcohol causes fetal alcohol syndrome (FAS) and fetal alcohol effect (FAE) (see Chapter 27).

Signs of Drug Withdrawal

Infants will be irritable, hypertonic, and tremulous, with shrill cries and disruption of normal sleep patterns. Seizures may occur. Intrauterine infections associated with drugs are common and may mimic signs of withdrawal.

Gastrointestinal effects include vomiting, diarrhea, and poor feeding. The addicted infant may try frantically to suck on a pacifier or bottle but cannot seem to coordinate sucking with feeding. Bony prominences (elbows, chins, and knees) become excoriated as the infant rubs against the sheets; severe diaper rash as a result of diarrhea also is common.

Clinical Management

Small frequent feedings, by gavage if necessary, provide the increased calories needed because of hyperactivity. A narcotic opiate (e.g., paregoric) may be prescribed to control the behavioral/neurologic and gastrointestinal effects. The drug is slowly withdrawn. This should be done only in severe cases after nursing interventions have failed. Addicted mothers frequently object to the use of narcotics. Nonnarcotic interventions illustrate problem solving without reliance on drugs. Frequent diaper changes, exposing the buttocks to air, and use of perineal ointments control diaper rash. Use of sheepskin and changes in position minimize skin breakdown.

Swaddling and rocking the infant may control irritability. Many infants require weeks to fully recover from the effects of withdrawal. They are at risk for SIDS, failure to thrive, and learning disabilities.

Occupational and physical therapists can evaluate the infant's behavior, state of control, and ability to feed.

Dysfunctional Bonding

The effects of withdrawal on maternal-infant interaction are pronounced. These inconsolable infants are born to mothers who have increased dependency needs, poor support systems, and unplanned pregnancies. It is essential to include the mother in the nursing care of her infant. Contact is encouraged because she will learn how to care for her baby by your example. Teach her how to reduce the environmental stimuli by darkening the room and providing quiet. Swaddling the infant, offering a pacifier, or placing the baby in a front body carrier are calming and increase physical contact between mother and infant.

Nursing intervention focuses on increasing the mother's ability to respond to the infant's cues. Drug-affected infants do not always respond in a predictable manner, causing further frustration. The Brazelton scale can be used to acquaint the mother with her infant's special behaviors and needs (see Chapter 18).

Test Yourself

- Ms. S. is attempting to console her irritable infant. What actions would best encourage normal maternal-infant interaction?

CONTROL OF PAIN

Control of pain was not an issue in the NICU until recently. The belief that the neonatal nervous system was too immature to feel, transmit, and remember painful sensations, plus the fear of respiratory depression from analgesics and anesthetics, perpetuated this myth. Until recently circumcisions, insertion of chest tubes and intravenous catheters, arterial blood gas sampling, and even PDA ligations were performed without any anesthesia or analgesia. Now it is known that subjecting a baby to painful procedures without analgesia or anesthesia is inhumane.

It is not easy to assess pain in an infant. Most tools that have been developed to assess pain in children and adults depend on verbal communication. Physiologic and behavioral signs of pain have been identified by researchers, but the ability of nurses to quantify the pain that neonates experience is not yet possible.

Research into neonatal and fetal physiology has helped to find a rationale for relief of neonatal pain. The fetal nervous system is capable of transmission of painful experiences sometime between weeks 24 and 28 of gestation. The cerebral structures needed for memory are present by term. Behavioral changes such as differences in sleep cycle and in the ability to regulate states persist beyond the immediate painful experience.

Signs

Babies with pain cry differently than hungry, annoyed, or bored babies. Physiologic changes during painful stimuli include lowered Po_2, elevated BP and heart rate, flushing, pallor, diaphoresis, and dilated pupils. Biochemical responses to pain in the infant include decreased insulin secretion and increased secretion of adrenalin, noradrenalin, and cortisol.

Clinical Management

Neonatal pain may be alleviated with medications that act centrally or locally. Of those acting centrally, morphine and fentanyl are most commonly used for control of postoperative pain. Intraoperative anesthesia may be accomplished by general anesthetics. Lidocaine is used for local anesthesia during painful procedures. Table 28-5 reviews the use of these medications.

Behavioral and environmental interventions are useful during some painful procedures such as drawing blood by means of a heel stick. Soothing the infant with rocking and offering a pacifier before sticking the heel seems to decrease crying time and physiologic responses by distracting the baby or helping the infant to organize behavior. Improvements in equipment designs and techniques also can help to make NICU experiences less traumatic.

CONTROL OF STRESS

Control of stress is directly related to the reduction of noxious stimuli. The noise and bright lights of the NICU are not conducive to normal neurologic development. High levels of stress can contribute to the development of gastric ulcers and cause oxygen desaturation, apnea, bradycardia, jitteriness, and regurgitation. Even preterm infants exhibit specific behaviors that indicate high levels of stress (Box 28-7).

Nursing Responsibilities
▶ ASSESSMENT

Assessment of the infant's ability to handle different types and levels of stress is possible through the use of the Assessment of Preterm Infant Behavior (APIB) (Als, 1982). This tool assesses the responses of the neonatal

TABLE 28-5 **Analgesics and Sedatives for the Neonate**

TYPE AND DOSAGE	COMMENTS
ANALGESICS	
Narcotic	
Morphine 0.05-0.1 mg/kg/dose q2-4h prn IV, IM, or SC	Central nervous system and respiratory depressant; easily reversed with naloxone; slower onset but longer duration than fentanyl; increases intracranial pressure; withdrawal symptoms may occur
Meperidine (Demerol) 0.5-1.5 mg/kg/dose q4h prn IV, IM, SC, or PO	Same as morphine; less respiratory depression with therapeutic dose; less likely to induce sleep/sedation than morphine or fentanyl
Fentanyl (Sublimaze) 1-2 µg/kg/dose q4-6h prn IV or SC Anesthesia: 20-75 µg/kg/dose IV over 5-10 min	Rapid onset of action; decreases motor activity; does not increase intracranial pressure; easily reversed with naloxone; short duration of action; may cause hypotension, apnea, seizures, or rigidity if given too rapidly; withdrawal symptoms may occur
Local	
Lidocaine 0.5%-1% solution (to avoid systemic toxicity, volume should be <0.5 ml/kg of 1% lidocaine solution—5 mg/kg)	Local infiltration anesthesia for invasive procedures
SEDATIVES AND HYPNOTICS	
Barbiturate	
Phenobarbital Loading: 10-20 mg/kg IV to maximum of 40 mg/kg Maintenance: 3-5 mg/kg in 2 divided doses beginning 12 hr after last loading dose	Prolonged sedation possible once therapeutic levels achieved (20-25 µg/ml); depresses central nervous system—motor and respiratory; slow onset of action; little or no pain relief; not easily reversed; withdrawal symptoms may occur; incompatible with other drugs in solution
Nonbarbiturate	
Chloral hydrate 10-30 mg/kg/dose q6-8h prn PO to maximum daily dose of 50 mg/kg/day; PR	Gastric irritant—administer with or after feeding; paradoxic excitement; not to be used for analgesia
Diazepam (Valium) 0.02-0.3 mg/kg IV, IM q6-8h	Do not dilute injection; may displace bilirubin; respiratory depression; hypotension; may cause increased agitation; induces sleep; relaxes muscles; withdrawal symptoms may occur; no analgesic effect

Modified from Merenstein GB, Gardner SL: *Handbook of neonatal intensive care*, ed 2, St Louis, 1989, Mosby; data from Bell SG, Ellis LJ: *Neonatal Network* 6:27, 1987, and Roberts RJ: *Drug therapy in infants*, Philadelphia, 1984, WB Saunders.

autonomic, motor, state, attentional-interactional, and regulatory systems to stimuli of increasing intensity. Communicating the results to the infant's parents and other care givers is an important part of nursing care planning for the preterm infant. Placing personal notes written "by the infant" on Isolettes is a friendly and amusing way of reinforcing this to everyone who comes in contact with the baby. Als et al. (1986) described a method for developing individualized care plans for the NICU client that maximizes the potential for normal development but minimizes the adverse effects of hospitalization. Noises may be reduced by covering the top of the Isolette with a thick blanket and carefully closing

the door and ports, rather than forcing them shut. Alarms should be promptly attended to, and care should be taken when objects are placed on top of Isolettes. Bright lights shining into the Isolette may be dimmed by covering the top with a blanket. "Treat[ing] the NICU patient as you would like to be treated if you had a severe headache" (Lott, 1989) will provide some guidelines.

▶ **NURSING DIAGNOSES**

1. High risk for injury related to seizures or effects of maternal drug abuse

BOX 28-7 Signs of Stress in Preterm Infants

Mild (early)

- Gaze aversion
- Yawning
- Hiccoughs
- Grimacing
- Closing eyes
- Slack jaw
- Open mouth
- Tongue thrusting
- Bowel movements
- Sneezing
- Coughing

Moderate

- Flushing
- Mottling
- Sighing
- Regurgitation
- Finger splaying
- Extension of arms, legs
- Jitteriness
- Jerky movements
- Limpness

Severe

- Pallor
- Cyanosis
- Tachypnea
- Bradypnea
- Apnea
- Decreased oxygen levels
- Tachycardia
- Bradycardia
- Arrhythmias

2. Sensory/perceptual alterations related to symptomatic withdrawal from maternal drugs
3. High risk for altered parenting related to parental drug status/support systems
4. Parental guilt regarding infant illness
5. Knowledge deficit regarding care/stimulation of affected infant

▶ EXPECTED OUTCOMES

1. Infant recovers from neurologic insult, showing normal responses within 10 days and assuming normal growth rate.
2. Stress reduction allows gradual withdrawal from maternal drugs.
3. Infant experiences minimal pain and stress related to therapies.

4. Parents freely visit and begin attachment to infant.
5. Parents express anxious or guilty feelings in discussion with caregiver.
6. Parents learn methods of consoling, stimulating, and interacting with infant.

▶ NURSING INTERVENTIONS: STIMULATION

It once was assumed that the neonate lacked any perception of the environment; the neonate's ability to remember painful or pleasurable experiences was denied. Any signals recognized by mothers as purposeful responses to feelings and environmental changes were considered to be subjective. The smiling neonate was cute but "probably had gas." As a result of these beliefs, the baby's environment was devoid of any sensory stimulation. Fortunately, these assumptions are fading because of research into the newborn's capabilities.

Stimulation, once avoided, found its place in the NICU in the 1970s. The previously sheltered preterm infant, who in the past was fiercely protected from any stimulation, became showered with it. However, the level of stimulation used was appropriate for term infants. It is now realized that stimulation for the preterm infant must be appropriate for gestational age. Auditory stimuli should be soft and soothing and should mimic the intrauterine environment. Tapes of the maternal heartbeat, parents' voices, or soft music may be used. Visual stimulation is provided by dimming the lights and keeping the infant's eyes about 8 inches away from the source of stimulation. Because stimuli should be provided by people rather than merely inanimate objects such as toys, social interaction is encouraged. Chronically ill neonates often have aversion to any oral stimuli that alters normal feeding behaviors. Providing oral stimulation with a pacifier during gavage feedings may allow a pleasurable association for objects placed in the mouth. Rocking and maintenance of the flexed position provides vestibular stimulation and security. In Europe, a new method of caring for preterm infants, called kangaroo care (KC) is becoming popular. Parents giving KC undress from the waist up and wear a hospital gown. They provide skin-to-skin contact for their stable preterm infants by dressing them only in diapers and holding them upright and prone against their chests. Infants who are breast-feeding may even nurse in this position. Advocates of KC claim that infants cared for in this innovative way experience adequate oxygenation, more stable body temperature, and less apnea and crying (Anderson, 1989).

▶ EVALUATION

1. Does the nursing care plan reflect appropriate interactions for the infant at the specific gestational/postconceptional age?

2. Did the infant recover from stressful events with minimal, if any, adverse effects?

3. Was the infant assessed for signs of pain? Were the interventions successful in managing the infant's pain?

4. Does the family, while participating in infant care, recognize the infant's signals of stress?

Musculoskeletal Dysfunction

Musculoskeletal function is influenced by intrauterine forces (fetal position, uterine size and shape, and amount of amniotic fluid) and genetically determined conditions that affect muscle strength. The fetus must have a normal intrauterine environment to develop normally; thus the in utero position may influence muscular and skeletal development.

Nursing Responsibilities

▶ NURSING DIAGNOSES

1. High risk for impaired physical mobility related to maintenance of fetal position or muscle atrophy

2. High risk for impaired skin integrity related to lack of subcutaneous fat cushion.

▶ EXPECTED OUTCOMES

1. Infant maintains good flexion and alignment of extremities.

2. Oval head shape results from frequent turning and positioning.

3. Infant's skin integrity remains intact.

▶ NURSING INTERVENTIONS: POSITIONING

Since physical mobility is impaired by size and condition, skin integrity and positioning are crucial for the infant in the NICU. Clinical observations, electronic monitoring, and procedures are easier to accomplish when the infant is lying in the supine position with extremities extended. Maintenance of this position often requires restraint of the baby. The result is an infant who, although recovered from initial neonatal illness, is rigid (often to the extent that the position becomes arched), hard to cuddle or console, and restless. This does not happen if correct positioning is maintained.

Maintain the preterm baby in a position of *flexion* as much as possible. Remember that this infant should really be in the weightlessness of the intrauterine world. As gestation progresses, the baby naturally becomes more flexed because of lack of space. This helps to develop tone in the flexor muscles. After term birth the normal infant's extensor tone develops gradually, and the two opposing forces become balanced. When preterm infants are forcibly placed in positions of extension, several alterations in normal growth and development appear. First, the scapulae are pulled together with the arms extended and abducted. Normal oral exploration is hampered when this growing infant's hands are not easily brought together and toward the mouth. Second, excessive extensor tone may develop in the lower portion of the legs, making it difficult to eventually walk on the entire sole of the foot.

Flexion can be maintained in the supine, side-lying, and prone positions through the use of soft rolls and stuffed animals (Figure 28-23, *A*). When lifting a baby

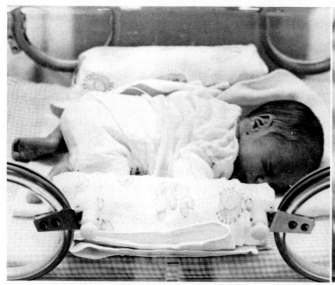
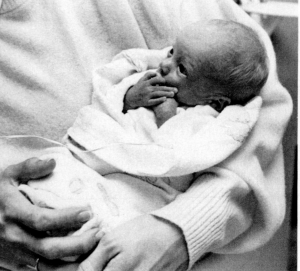

A   B

FIGURE 28-23 Positioning preterm infant to prevent deformity. **A,** Soft rolls minimize restlessness by providing boundaries. **B,** Swaddling brings extremities in, encourages hand-to-mouth activity, and maintains flexion. (From Fay MJ: The positive effects of positioning, *Neonatal Network* 6[5]:23, 1988.)

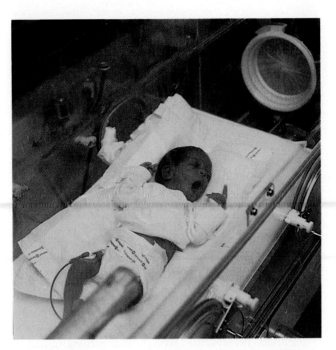

FIGURE 28-24 Positioning with slight elevation of head. Note leg roll. (Courtesy Ross Laboratories, Columbus, Ohio.)

while moving to a prone position, bring the extremities toward the center of the body to encourage the flexed position (Figure 28-23, *B*). Education of parents of infants in the NICU should include instructions for proper positioning and its effects on development (Figure 28-24).

Parents of children with musculoskeletal deformities need to know how long treatment will last and whether complete correction is possible. They need to be shown how to remove and correctly reapply any devices and to perform range of motion exercises.

▶ EVALUATION

1. Does the infant have limitations of joint movement or abnormal mobility related to restriction of movement during critical illness?
2. Do skin surfaces remain intact?

Transport to a Regional Center

Improvement in survival rate and the quality of survival of the high-risk and ill neonate are due partially to improvements in regionalization of care. Approximately 10% of all live births require specialized neonatal intensive care that can be provided at tertiary-level hospitals with NICUs or secondary hospitals with neonatal special care units. Although high-risk neonates usually need to be transported from smaller, primary hospitals to larger hospitals, personnel trained to perform resuscitation of the newborn and provide support to stabilize the infant until a transport team arrives are essential in any obstetric unit. The American Heart Association and the American Academy of Pediatrics are making a joint national effort to ensure that these personnel are available at every delivery.

Classification of the different levels of hospitals and efficient transport systems is established around the country. A well-equipped transport facility is important to the tiny neonate during the period when early extrauterine adjustment is taking place. Allowing the mother to give birth at a tertiary facility reduces the risks of delay involved in transport of a very ill infant.

≡ NURSING CARE PLAN • Premature Infant

CASE: Baby Girl L. is an AGA infant, 1785 g, 32 weeks' gestation, born to a 19-year-old G1,P1 mother by spontaneous vaginal delivery after 2 hours of ruptured membranes. *Maternal history:* Blood type O, Rh negative. Rubella immune, rapid plasma reagin (RPR) nonreactive, hepatitis B surface antigen (HBsAg) negative. Regular prenatal care, no illnesses or history of familial disease. Does not smoke, abuse drugs, or drink alcohol.
Labor history: Admitted in preterm labor, received terbutaline, then magnesium sulfate without stopping labor. Amniotic fluid clear on rupture of membranes. Neonatal team in attendance at birth.
Immediate neonatal care: Cried spontaneously, weakly, occasional grunting, nasal flaring, and mild intercostal retractions. HR 140-150 beats/min, free-flow oxygen required to maintain adequate color. Held briefly by parents and transferred to NICU.

ASSESSMENT

1. Review labor and delivery record.
2. Monitor vital signs, oxygen concentrations via pulse oximeter, blood gases, and response to treatments. Monitor for periods of apnea, signs of RDS.
3. Observe for signs of hypoglycemia, hypocalcemia, and complications related to immaturity (NEC) and therapies.
4. Observe for nippling behaviors during oral feedings. Compare birthweight with daily weights.
5. Determine parental response to crisis and level of understanding of infant's status and procedures.

NURSING DIAGNOSES

1. Ineffective breathing patterns related to prematurity, grunting, retractions, and need for oxygen
2. Ineffective thermoregulation, hypothermia related to immaturity, lack of body fat, glucose balance
3. High risk for injury related to hypoxemia, hypoglycemia, and complications of prematurity
4. High risk for altered fluid and electrolyte balance related to IWL, intravenous therapy
5. Altered family processes related to situational crisis
6. Knowledge deficit regarding infant status, management, procedures

EXPECTED OUTCOMES

1. Infant will exhibit unimpaired gas exchange evidenced by normal respiratory pattern and pulse oximeter readings. Sustains respirations in room air by 2 weeks after birth.
2. Maintains temperature in thermoneutral environment.
3. Maintains blood glucose >45 mg/dl and serum calcium >7 mg/dl. No evidence of NEC occurs.
4. Regains birth weight after loss of <10%, assumes expected growth rate. Retains oral feedings by 2 weeks after birth.
5. Parents express understanding of plan and procedures in therapy.
6. Parents demonstrate increasing confidence in infant care and exhibit attachment behaviors.

NURSING INTERVENTIONS

1. Deliver warmed, humidified oxygen as prescribed. Maintain clear airway and pulmonary hygiene.
2. Adjust environmental temperature controls as needed, relate control to procedures and stressful events. Provide pain relief and stress reduction interventions.
3. Evaluate blood glucose levels via capillary samples. Give oral or parenteral glucose as needed. Use supplemental calcium or low-phosphorus formula as prescribed.
4. Observe weight gain patterns; compare intake and output with weight. Provide gavage feeding, looking for nippling behaviors. Encourage mother to give feedings, to use breast pump, and to begin breast-feeding as possible.
5. Explain all equipment and procedures. Help parents care for infant. Plan for discharge with appropriate referrals.
6. Describe infant behaviors and expected development. Demonstrate stimulation activities. Support attachment behaviors. Reinforce appropriate responses. Encourage parents to involve extended family.

EVALUATION

1. Are vital signs within normal parameters? Is there any indication of risk of SIDS, BPD, or ROP?
2. Can infant maintain temperature in an open crib? Are parents aware of protection from environmental temperature extremes?
3. Is growth following the newborn curve? Has infant regained birth weight?
4. What is the feeding pattern on discharge? Is mother choosing to breast-feed and is she fully knowledgeable?
5. Have all referrals been made? Do parents understand sequence of followup?
6. Do parents express relative confidence in assuming infant care?

KEY POINTS

- Neonatal nursing is a specialty that requires advanced knowledge and skills.
- Stress in NICU nursing results from environmental noise, caring for many infants who may not survive or who survive with problems, and dealing with anxious, grieving parents.
- Nurses need to develop supportive means of maintaining perspective.
- Understanding asphyxia will allow better, more rapid interventions in the immediate period after birth. Never wait for the Apgar score results to begin necessary interventions.
- Resuscitation is a team responsibility and may require two or three persons to carry out correctly.
- Respiratory distress syndrome is a developmental problem that is now better controlled with exogenous surfactant.
- Heart defects are among the most common of birth defects and usually require surgery for correction. The nurse's role is a supportive one, assessing status and maintaining life support.
- Because blood volume is so small, fluid and electrolyte balance is crucial.

- Premature babies need to grow at the fetal rate and thus require more calories per kilogram, although they have more difficulty in digesting milk. Necrotizing enterocolitis is a primary problem in young preterm infants.
- Hypoglycemia may be as damaging as hypoxia and must be assessed and corrected promptly.
- Premature infants cannot regulate body temperature; a sign of maturity is the neonate's ability to sustain temperature >97° F—while wrapped—in an open crib.
- Preterm infants are vulnerable to anemia, hyperbilirubinemia, and sepsis.
- Stress and pain must be minimized. New analgesic dosages are available for very small infants during procedures.
- Positioning prevents contractures and skin breakdown. The preterm infant preferably should be in a flexed position.
- Parents must be included in all plans, providing as much care as is comfortable for them. Education enables parents to assume total responsibility for the infant the day of discharge from the NICU.

STUDY QUESTIONS

28-1 Which terms fit the following statements?
  a. Blood shunted to more "valuable" organs from the periphery during perinatal asphyxia ___ Diving reflex
  b. Accomplished by changes in position, percussion, and vibration of the chest wall ___ Chest physiotherapy
  c. Consists of fibrin and sloughed cells, which further compromise gas exchange in the infant with RDS ___ Hyaline membrane.
  d. Breathing pattern, during which respiration ceases for 5 to 10 seconds without pathophysiologic changes, that differs from apnea because it is a normal respiratory pattern in the preterm infant ___ Periodic respiration
  e. Process by which water is lost through the lungs (respiratory water loss) and the skin ___ Insensible water loss.
  f. Primary complication of perinatal asphyxia ___ Apnea
  g. Aorta arising from the right ventricle and the pulmonary artery from the left ___ Transposition of the great vessels
  h. Causes a mechanical obstruction that allows air to reach the alveoli during inspira-

tion but then traps it in the air sacs during expiration ___ Atelectasis
  i. Causes petechiae and increased bleeding time after heel sticks, injections, and venipunctures ___ Thrombocytopenia (↓ platelets)
  j. Caused by the interaction of normal bacterial contamination of the gut, plus formula feeding and ischemia in infants who have sustained ischemic injury to the intestines as a result of asphyxia or shock ___ NEC Necrotizing Enterocolitis
  k. Causes infants to look plethoric, with a ruddy or purplish, cyanotic tinge to the skin ___ Polycythemia
  l. Provides distending pressure to the alveoli to prevent atelectasis ___ CPAP
  m. A surface-active material instilled into the trachea of the neonate to reduce the surface tension ___ Surfactant

28-2 You are caring for baby girl L., who is under a radiant warmer; she is dried and positioned, and bulb suction has been performed. Respiratory effort is good, heart rate is 130 beats/min, mucous membranes are cyanotic, extremities are partially flexed, and she grimaced during suctioning. You identify signs of mild cardio respiratory depression. The next step in resuscitation would be:

a. Provide a direct flow of oxygen over the infant's nose and mouth.

b. Force the infant's thighs onto her abdomen to improve her muscle tone.

c. Wait until the infant is 1 minute old before intervening.

d. Observe for the infant's improvement because this delay is due to suctioning.

28-3 You have been providing baby boy G. with positive pressure ventilation with 100% oxygen for 30 seconds after birth. Heart rate is 70 beats/min and respirations are gasping. A colleague has offered to assist you. What should be done next?

a. Move the infant to the newborn ICU.

b. Continue bag-and-mask ventilation while your colleague begins chest compressions.

c. Administer sodium bicarbonate.

d. Provide vigorous tactile stimulation.

28-4 You are caring for a growing and well preterm infant who is having periods of apnea and bradycardia during handling for feeding and vital signs. Which nursing action is most appropriate?

a. Assessing the infant's ability to handle different types and levels of stress

b. Increasing light on the Isolette to facilitate observations of respirations and color

c. Using latches to close the Isolette doors rather than forcing them shut

d. Increasing tactile and auditory stimuli to encourage spontaneous respirations

28-5 Which of the following is not a cause of IWL?

a. Single-walled Isolette

b. Phototherapy lamps

c. Humidified air

d. Radiant warmer

28-6 Which of the following is most likely to increase the risk for IVH in the preterm infant?

a. Rapid infusion of hypertonic solutions

b. Careful attention to respiratory status, especially P_{CO_2} level

c. Clustering of treatment activities and procedures

d. Sedation of infants requiring respirator therapy

28-7 Baby girl C. has an Hct level of 30%. She was born at 27 weeks' gestation and is now 5 weeks old. Which of the following assessment findings indicate that she is being compromised by her anemia?

a. Demonstrates exaggerated reflexes and hyperirritability

b. Exhibits frequent episodes of apnea and desaturation

c. Regurgitates oral fluids within 5 minutes of feedings with occasional projectile vomiting

d. Skin and sclera appear yellow and serum bilirubin = 10 g/dl

28-8 Ms. S. was admitted to labor and delivery with a diagnosis of premature labor at 32 weeks' gestation and possible abruptio placentae. After delivery the infant is in minimal respiratory distress but is tremulous and irritable. Which drug of abuse do you suspect was used by Ms. S.?

a. Cocaine

b. Alcohol

c. Heroin

d. Methadone

Answer Key

28-1 a. Diving reflex, b. Chest physiotherapy, c. Hyaline membrane, d. Periodic breathing, e. Insensible water loss, f. Apnea, g. TGA, h. Atelectasis, i. Thrombocytopenia, j. NEC, k. Polycythemia, l. CPAP, m. Surfactant 28-2 a 28-3 b 28-4 b 28-5 c 28-6 a 28-7 b 28-8 a

REFERENCES

Als H: Toward a synactive theory of development: promise for the assessment and support of infant individuality, *Infant Ment Health J* 3(4):229, 1982.

Als H et al: Individualized behavioral and environmental care for the very low birth weight preterm infant at high risk for brochopulmonary dysplasia: neonatal intensive care unit and developmental outcome, *Pediatrics* 78:1123, 1986.

Anderson GC: Skin to skin kangaroo care in western Europe, *Am J Nurs* 89(5):663, 1989.

Arenson J: Discharge teaching in the NICU: the changing needs of NICU graduates and their families, *Neonatal Network* 6(14):29, 1988.

Avery GB: *Neonatology: pathophysiology and management of the newborn,* ed 3, Philadelphia, 1987, JB Lippincott.

Beeley L: Adverse effects of drugs in later pregnancy, *Clin Obstet Gynecol* 13(2):197, 1986.

Bellig L: A window on the neonate's brain, *Neonatal Network* 7(4):13, 1989.

Benkov KJ, Leleiko NS: A rational approach to infant formulas, *Pediatr Ann* 16(3):225, 1987.

Bloom RS, Cropley CC: *Textbook of neonatal resuscitation,* Dallas, 1990, American Heart Association.

Brackbill Y et al: Obstetric meperidine usage and assessment of neonatal status, *Anesthesiology* 40:116, 1974.

Chasnoff I et al: Maternal cocaine use and genitourinary tract malformation, *Teratology* 37:201, 1987.

deLouvois J, Harvey D: Antibiotic therapy of the newborn, *Clin Perinatol* 15(2):365, 1988.

Farquhar JW: Children of diabetic women, *Arch Dis Child* 34:76, 1959.

Fay MJ: The positive effects of positioning, *Neonatal Network* 6(5):23, 1988.

Flandermeyer AA: A comparison of the effects of heroin and cocaine abuse upon the neonate, *Neonatal Network* 5(12).12, 1987.

Flyer DC, Lang P: Neonatal heart disease. In Avery GB, editor: *Neonatology: pathophysiology and management of the newborn,* Philadelphia, 1987, JB Lippincott.

George DS et al: The latest on retinopathy of prematurity, *MCN* 13:254, 1988.

Gracey KM et al: Caring for the infant with retinopathy of prematurity undergoing cryotherapy, *Neonatal Network* 9(7):7, 1991.

Gray DG, Yaffe SJ: Prenatal drugs, Symposium of Learning Difficulties, 1986, Johnson & Johnson.

Guyon G: Pharmacokinetic considerations in neonatal drug therapy, *Neonatal Network* 7(5):9, 1989.

Hack M et al: Very low birth weight outcomes of the National Institute of Child Health and Human Development (Neonatal Network), *Pediatrics* 87:597, 1991.

Hammerman C et al: Comparative measurements of phototherapy: a practical guide, *Pediatrics* 67:368, 1981.

Janke JR: Prenatal cocaine use: effects on perinatal outcome, *J Nurs Midwifery* 35(2):74, 1990.

Laymon B: Teddy bear helps regulate infants' breathing, *The Hartford Courant*, p 86, Nov 27, 1988.

Lemons P et al: Breast feeding the premature infant, *Clin Perinatol* 13(1):111, 1986.

Long WA, editor: *Fetal and neonatal cardiology*, Philadelphia, 1990, WB Saunders.

Lott JW: Developmental care of the preterm infant, *Neonatal Network* 7(4):21, 1989.

Maisels MJ et al: Jaundice in the healthy newborn infant: a new approach to an old problem, *Pediatrics* 81:505, 1988.

Panyard JL, Kaneta MK: Hypoplastic left heart syndrome: clinical manifestations and treatment, *Neonatal Network* 7(1):17, 1988.

Prevost RR: Comparing surfactant products, *Therapy Consultation* 10:909, 1991.

Shapiro DL, Notter Rh: Controversies regarding surfactant replacement therapy, *Clin Perinatol* 15(4):891, 1988.

Short BL et al: Extracorporeal membrane oxygenation in the management of respiratory failure in the newborn, *Clin Perinatol* 14(3):737, 1987.

Volpe JJ: Intraventricular hemorrhage and brain injury in the premature infant: neuropathology and pathogenesis, *Clin Perinatol* 16(2):387, 1989.

Weibley TT et al: Gavage tube insertion in the premature infant, *MCN* 12:24, 1987.

Wink DM: Better breast milk for preemies, *AJN* 89(1):48, 1989.

Wong DL: Whaley and Wong's essentials of pediatric nursing, ed 4, St Louis, 1993, Mosby.

STUDENT RESOURCE SHELF

Bailweg DD: Neonatal seizures: an overview, *Neonatal Network* 10(1):15, 1991. Overview of etiology, classification, management, and prognosis of seizures in the neonate.

Nora JG: Perinatal cocaine use: maternal, fetal and neonatal effects, *Neonatal Network* 9(2):45, 1990. Effects of cocaine, with discussion of nursing implications.

Nugent J, editor: *Acute respiratory care of the neonate*, Petaluma, Calif, 1991, Neonatal Network. The Neonatal Network provides the most comprehensive hands-on instruction for care of NICU infants. This is a soft-cover guide for self-study for CE credits.

Shapiro C: Pain in the neonate: assessment and interventions, *Neonatal Network* 8(1):7, 1989. Review of the neurophysiologic aspects of pain, assessment of pain, and therapy for the neonate.

Walther FJ, Taeusch HW: New approaches to surfactant therapy, *Neonatal Resp Dis* 1(1):3, 1991. A history of surfactant replacement and current treatment. Includes a self-test at conclusion.

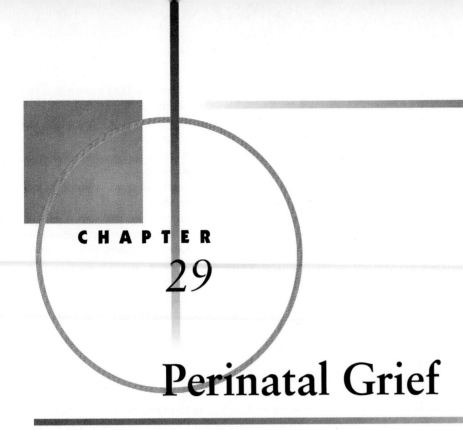

Perinatal Grief

KEY TERMS

Autopsy
Grief Resolution
Neonatal Death
Perinatal Grief
Stillbirth

LEARNING OBJECTIVES

1. *Describe phases of perinatal grief.*
2. *Query nursing personnel about the work of a perinatal grief team in your setting.*
3. *Review the chart of a client with a perinatal death, evaluating nursing documentation regarding interventions.*
4. *Discuss why grief places additional strain on a marriage.*
5. *Contrast the potential role of the nurse in facilitating healthy grieving with what is observed in the clinical setting.*
6. *Ask clergy personnel about preferred baptismal rites and hospital recommendations for funerals for stillbirths and neonatal deaths.*

Perinatal Grief

A place can be vacant yet is not empty until someone you love has passed through (Anonymous).

All of us have experienced death. For some, the exposure has been as minimal as watching a flower die or experiencing the changes of the leaves as fall yields to winter. Others have felt the pain of loss through the death of a pet or the loss of a friendship. Still others have been introduced to more intense pain and grief when a loved one has died—a parent, sibling, grandparent, or friend. The pain of grief is universal. The differences that arise originate in the intensity of emotion experienced and in the quality of memories that exist.

When a loved one or acquaintance dies, it is our memory of that person that produces our emotional response to their death. The intensity of grief will depend on the relationship we had with the deceased and how much of an influence she or he had on our lives.

When a baby dies, either before or shortly after birth, there are few people other than the infant's parents who have any memory of that child. Since it is our memories that trigger a grief response, few people can feel prolonged sadness for a child they never knew. Sadness, emptiness, and loneliness for the infant are emotions felt solely by the child's parents. Friends and relatives feel sadness for the grief of the parents and their helplessness in alleviating their pain; for them grief for the child generally resolves within a few weeks following the infant's death.

Following the knowledge by parents that conception has occurred, their mode of thought transforms from planning for themselves to planning for their child.

Their entire future, with all its hopes and dreams, centers around the child. When this infant dies, the parents have not only lost their offspring but much of their future. They are left in limbo, not knowing what next to do with their lives. There's an enormous sense of insecurity and disorganization. Their planned future is no longer possible.

The most universal sense experienced by all parents is an innate need to protect their young. When their infant dies, parents experience an enormous sense of helplessness. They also feel like a failure in their role as a parent. Helplessness and low self-esteem tend to intensify their grief during this most vulnerable time and magnify the depression already felt.

The death of an infant is not the natural order of life. Children are not supposed to predecease their parents. When an infant death occurs, parents are faced with a situation with which they are totally unprepared to deal. There are few friends and relatives who can relate to their grief since it is only through the experience of a similar situation that others can understand the intensity of pain and loss. Parents feel isolated. They know that others care, but few, if any, truly understand. They often are left to deal with their grief alone.

An understanding by the health professional about perinatal grief will allow the initiation of more compassionate and therapeutic care immediately following the infant's death. This in turn will diminish the parents' sense of isolation and will facilitate the initiation of a healthier grief response.

Kinds of Perinatal Loss

To more fully understand **perinatal grief,** we must first be knowledgeable about the kinds of death that encompass this subject. The situations encountered during each kind of death are quite different; however the grief reactions are universally the same.

EARLY LOSS

Miscarriage will be discussed first since it is the most commonly experienced form of perinatal grief. Statistics show that 20% to 30% of all confirmed pregnancies, and up to 50%, or perhaps more, of all conceptions end in miscarriage (Ilse and Burns, 1985). Miscarriage (spontaneous abortion) is the termination of pregnancy by natural causes before 20 weeks of pregnancy and before the baby can live outside the uterus. The gestational age when death occurs differs among families, but the grief responses seem to be the same. Prior experience with miscarriage, stillbirth, or neonatal death is the one factor that may alter the intensity of the reaction. It is insignificant to parents who have this kind of experience that their child was very young and may

not have been completely formed. They envisioned the "Gerber Baby," and such is the child that died. Moreover, the inability to visually bond with the fetus alters healthy grieving since there are no memories to rely on for comfort. Many parents do not even know their infant's sex. If visualization and gender identification are possible, it certainly is encouraged to facilitate the resolution of grief in the months and years to come.

Elective termination, either with or without genetic anomalies as a factor in decision making, comprises the remainder of perinatal losses. Although these families have made a choice, the grief response is quite the same. Although relief is a common reaction, many of these parents also experience intense guilt as well as grief. The emotion of guilt may hamper healthy grieving and prolong the parent's pain and anxiety (see Chapter 21.)

Ectopic pregnancy, commonly termed *tubal pregnancy,* is a less common form of infant death but certainly worthy of mention. Ectopic, or extrauterine, pregnancy occurs when a fertilized egg is implanted outside the uterus. Fewer than one third of women who have an ectopic pregnancy have a successful subsequent pregnancy. Many are unable to conceive at all. One in four of those who do will have another ectopic pregnancy (Jimenez and Mims, 1982).

DEATH AFTER THE AGE OF VIABILITY

Stillbirth

Each year in the United States about 33,000 babies are stillborn, according to the National Center for Health Statistics (DeFrain et al, 1986). A baby is stillborn, by definition, if it died between the twentieth week of pregnancy and the time of birth (DeFrain et al, 1986). For the parents surviving a **stillbirth,** the pain and anguish of grief are intensified by the absence of being able to visually bond with their child while the infant was alive. Hearing the infant cry, looking at and holding a warm body can be a tremendous source of comfort to parents experiencing infant death. Parents of stillborn babies are denied these memories.

Neonatal Death

Neonatal death occurs at approximately the same percentage as stillbirth in the United States. By definition, neonatal death encompasses infant death occurring between birth and 1 month of the infant's life. The most common cause of neonatal death is prematurity with its complications. However, congenital anomalies, infections, birth trauma, and complications of pregnancy are also factors. When death after a live birth occurs, the parents have the opportunity to see, touch, and bond with their child. This bonding time aids memory formation and brings comfort to those families once the infant dies. Although much of the time spent together

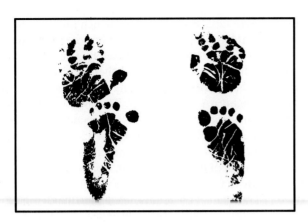

FIGURE 29-1 Even tiny hand and footprints will be a memory builder for the grieving parents.

may be painful, parents always manage to cling to the positive aspects of this time together. They view it as an opportunity to acquaint themselves and others with the baby who was with them only briefly (Figure 29-1).

Physical and Emotional Responses to Grief

In grief one can endure the day, just the day. But when one also tries to bear the grief ahead, one cannot encompass it. As for happiness, it can only be the ability to experience the moment. It is not next year that life will be so flawless and if we keep trying to wait for next year's happiness, the river of time will wind past and we shall not have lived at all (Schwiebert and Kirk, 1981).

This is their darkest moment, so they think. Upon hearing the news that their baby has died, parents believe that the pain of that moment couldn't possibly get any worse. Unfortunately, the agony of living through the days and months ahead and the effort to rejoin the "world of the living" will provide tougher challenges than parents are prepared to deal with. There is no greater task in life than facing death, dealing with death, and learning to live again, happily, in spite of the death of someone so special to us.

PHYSICAL RESPONSES

After their infant has died, parents may experience specific physical symptoms in addition to their intense emotional responses. According to Schwiebert and Kirk (1981) there may be a feeling of severe physical exhaustion, perhaps further aggravated by a difficult delivery; parents may feel a heaviness in their chest, a need to take deep sighing breaths; palpitations; "butterflies in the stomach"; aching arms; appetite loss and sleep disturbances, associated with insomnia and nightmares, also predominate.

All of these symptoms reflect a normal and healthy initial response to the process of grieving. Although they are bothersome and affect the parents' physical sense of well being, these reactions play an important role in allowing the body to experience the pain. It is only in feeling and dealing with the pain that parents will eventually be able to let this pain go in **grief resolution**. The physical symptoms are only temporary and will diminish with time.

Although light sleep sedation may be necessary to guard against chronic fatigue, other forms of antidepressants and antianxiety drugs are not recommended during this early stage of grieving. Being tranquilized only postpones and prolongs the real pain. It is better for parents to face reality while family and friends are close by to help (Schwiebert and Kirk, 1981).

EMOTIONAL RESPONSES

Parental emotional responses to the loss of a baby are numerous and may occur in varying order on many different levels of intensity. Some of these responses may not be experienced at all. Once again they are all normal and indicate a healthy reaction to tragic news. Many of these feelings may cause parents to think they are going crazy. They are not. Especially now, parents need reassurance that they are behaving in a healthy way. A clue to healthy recovery through this time is the length of good time experienced each day. As time goes by, and it goes by very slowly, parents will recognize that they've smiled, or hummed a tune, or even had a pleasant thought. The event may have been very brief, but it may mark the beginning of healing that will progress through grief resolution.

Intense feelings of loss and emptiness are the primary emotions initially. The loneliness is magnified by the constant reminder of a recent birth, as evidenced by the mother's engorged breasts. An overwhelming sense of anxiety, alarm, and restlessness surfaces soon after. Couples find it difficult to reestablish normal routines, have problems with concentration and decision making, and may lose interest in projects that once held their attention. Forgetfulness is another disturbing element of grief and the most common complaint of those parents who return to work too soon. Anger and hostility may develop as thoughts of "why?" begin to overwhelm them (Schwiebert and Kirk, 1981). Eventually, depression unveils itself and usually remains in varying degrees of intensity for a prolonged period. Every couple, especially mothers, experience some form of guilt in the primary stages of crisis. The common question, "What if I had . . . ?" haunts parents. An answer is never found. Preoccupation with thoughts of the baby and long periods of crying are symptoms seen predominantly in women. Fathers tend to be more introverted and private with their grief and may avoid painful thoughts by "acting out" in other ways.

Phases of Bereavement

To more fully understand the grieving process as related to perinatal death, phases of bereavement have been identified by John Bowlby of Harvard University and C. Murray Parkes of London (Jimenez and Mims, 1982). These phases build on and are related to all mourning phases (see Chapter 26).

Shock and numbness are the initial responses to the tragic news about the infant's death. The parents may feel unaware of their environment, be unable to make decisions and need much assistance in performing even the simplest tasks. Crying may or may not be present. Emotional outbursts are common. This phase is usually short and allows the parents time to build their emotional strength for the difficult days and months ahead.

Searching and yearning are the next phases encountered approximately 3 to 7 days following the infant's death. The reactions are characterized by increased sensitivity to the environment, anger, guilt, restlessness, impatience, and mixed emotions. Physical symptoms may surface at this time. A mother's arms may "ache" to hold her baby. This appears to be the longest phase of bereavement, gradually declining as resolution approaches.

Disorientation presents during the first week following the death, magnifies and subsides at varying intervals for months to years and intensifies briefly during the baby's first anniversary. Depression is the primary symptom. Parents begin to feel guilty about their inability to recover from their loss and may take on a role of sickness to mask their depression and avoid criticism. The mourner may lose her or his appetite and fail to maintain personal care. Introduction into a support group at this time can be crucial to avoid parent suspicions of going crazy.

Reorganization is the final phase of bereavement and indicates that the grief response is approaching completion and that the parents are close to total healing and recovery. As stated by Jimenez and Mims (1982), the mourner begins to feel a sense of freedom and renewed vigor. He or she makes decisions more easily and functions more effectively. Parents are taking care of themselves physically and have overcome insomnia and lack of appetite. They remember their loss and still wish for their child, but the death has taken its proper place in their memory and their life.

In summary, although their love for the child has neither changed nor diminished, they have learned how to live again, incorporating the loss into their life and rediscovering happiness beyond the pain.

Clients pass through the stages of the grief process at different rates (see Chapter 26). There are advances and regressions. The degree of support that the client and family receive influences the rate at which they progress. It is common for this process to last for more than a year. Perinatal bereavement may be different from bereavement for other causes. Some people believe that is not as difficult as the loss of another family member because the fetus or newborn never "lived." This is not true. The woman bonds with her fetus early in pregnancy, and the father and other family members often do also once they perceive movement and hear the heartbeat. The level of grief and length of bereavement can be as long as or even longer than that for another family member who has "lived." The client and family need anticipatory guidance about this fact because many expect to get over the death quickly. To be told that they can have another baby is little consolation to those who are grieving. This is akin to telling someone whose spouse has died that he or she can get married again.

Children also grieve for their lost siblings, even if they never knew them. Parents should be encouraged to tell their children about the death of the baby and to allow for expressions of sadness. When the parents are sad, the children should be told that it is because of the death of the baby. Children often imagine that they caused the death by an angry thought or response; to avoid this they should be told what happened and why. They may also be afraid that the same thing will happen to them and must be reassured that their parents will take care of them. For this reason, explanations such as "An angel took the baby" should be rephrased so that the child understands that the angel is not coming for him or her.

Grief and Marriage

For many couples, the death of their infant is often their first experience with death and grieving. With other kinds of loss, the partner who was not as closely related to the deceased can comfort and provide strength for the other partner. The death of a child evokes equal grief responses in both mother and father and therefore shared and equal pain. However, no two individuals grieve in the same way, and this is especially true in a marriage. It is often quite difficult for couples to realize that, although they equally loved their infant, their responses to that child's death may be very different. There is no right or wrong way to grieve and, although parents understand this concept intellectually, emotional acceptance of the partner's unique grief response is quite another matter. A discovery that the reaction to a shared tragedy may be quite different often leads to disparity in a marriage. Neither can understand why the other does not have the same feelings. Often they cannot rely on each other, as they have in the past, to make things better (*Grief and Marriage*, 1978).

Communication between couples and total acceptance of each partner's right to grieve in his or her own way can be a tool in helping a marriage to survive the loss of a child. A mother may feel more intense grief for a more prolonged period of time. Often her greatest source of comfort is to talk to anyone who will listen about her infant and the circumstances surrounding the baby's death. A father, however, tends to be more private with his grief. He may share his story with only a few intimate friends or relatives, and he is often quite anxious to get back to work and on with his life. Without understanding that each grief response is different, a woman may feel that her husband did not care as much for their child as she did. Likewise, a father may wonder why his wife is holding onto her grief.

Bereaved parents have offered a few suggestions on ways to share their pain in hopes of alleviating frustration, stress, and misunderstanding (*Grief and Marriage*, 1978):

- Discuss and share feelings and concerns at regularly scheduled times each day/week.
- Plan a regular weekly night out of the house.
- Share your pain with someone else—a good friend, other bereaved parents, a relative, or a professional.
- Read books (such as the chapter on bereavement and marriage in the *Bereaved Parent* by Harriet Schiff) and magazine and newsletter articles about how other people have dealt with their grief.

Following the death of their child, couples need each other to find solace, comfort, and peace. "Marriage can best be served if the two partners can look beyond their own grief to determine their partner's grief and needs" (*Grief and Marriage*, 1978). When couples work toward achieving this goal, they can accept each other as individuals and recognize the bond they will always have because of their child. Together they bear their grief and find happiness in each other and life once again.

Creating Memories: The Nurse's Role in Facilitating Healthy Grieving

The greatest gift that we, as nurses, can give to grieving families is the gift of memories. Through simple gestures, we can create an environment that facilitates bonding and provides tangible keepsakes that will comfort families for their lifetime. Positive memories will long overshadow the painful experiences surrounding their baby's death. We can make a tremendous difference in helping families to cope.

QUIET TIME

All parents deserve the opportunity to have quiet time alone with their infant, especially parents who will have no other opportunity to bond with their child. This time together promotes quality family time and an opportunity for parents to privately incorporate this child into their family unit.

HOLDING THE INFANT

You should strongly encourage bereaved parents to see and hold their child regardless of the physical deformity or malformation present. A parent's fantasy of the imagined deformity will always escalate and be much worse than reality. By verbally preparing the parents concerning what the baby will look like, you can allay any unnecessary fears or misconceptions. For parents to visualize and hold their baby makes this child real and enhances the bonding so necessary to creating comfort as time passes. The nurse should also encourage parents to see the entire baby by unwrapping blankets and pointing out the positive features of the child. Parents will focus on and remember that which makes their child normal. You may also suggest that families bathe, diaper, and dress their infant, thus easing the need of bereaved parents to nurture their child.

NAMING THE BABY

Although parents may be reluctant to use a chosen name for a baby who has died, strongly encourage them to do so. The name will identify that child as a person, a little person to be remembered and loved as an integral part of the family. Naming provides a place in the family for the baby and creates a tangible memory of a family member who should be grieved for. This child deserves the name that was chosen for him or her, and using this name will provide a means of connecting the memories to an identifiable person (Schwiebert and Kirk, 1981).

PROVIDING KEEPSAKES

Following an infant's death, tangible memories provide the greatest source of comfort for parents as time passes. Having something to touch, smell, and look at will keep the baby close to the parents and alleviate some of the loneliness and emptiness. Helpful keepsakes may include the birth certificate, footprints, cribcard, name bracelet, lock of hair, unwashed diaper, articles of clothing, infant hat, blankets and fleece, ultrasound pictures, fetal heart rate strip, infant photos, videos, and/or tapes. A memory book is a nice way to organize these keepsakes (Figure 29-2).

Photos, Videos, and Tapes

Pictures, videos, and tapes can be of tremendous comfort to parents, especially as time passes and the vivid memory of the infant begins to fade. It will reassure parents that they never will forget that beautiful little person they created. Pictures also provide parents with

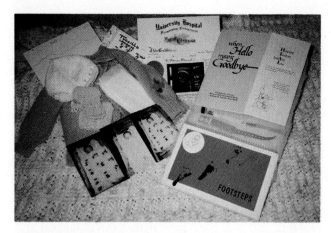

FIGURE 29-2 A memory kit assembled at the University of Connecticut Health Center, Farmington, Conn. It includes pictures of the infant, clothing, death certificate, footprints, ID bands, fetal monitor printout, and ultrasound picture.

a means of having friends and family become acquainted with the deceased child if they haven't already done so. The display of the photos is a personal and private choice made by the family. Many choose to frame and display the pictures along with other family photos; others will tuck the pictures privately into a drawer or wallet.

It is suggested that parents preserve the memory with 35 mm photos since Polaroid shots will fade with time. Certain camera shops will convert Polaroid exposures to 35 mm prints or slides. We also encourage parents to take many different pictures of the baby, both wrapped and unwrapped. Pictures of the baby with the family, including siblings, are of enormous benefit in preserving the memory of the family unit. Anyone present and significant to the parents should participate in the picture taking. The use of stuffed animals can soften the photo and make the pictures more appealing. Videos and tapes are a modern keepsake providing both visual and auditory memories. Encourage parents to be creative in the video and tape production and reassure them that they can tape any part of the experience that will help to comfort them in the future.

BAPTISM AND PRAYERS FOR THE INFANT

When appropriate, the rite of baptism, the Sacrament of the Sick, or a blessing by a chosen clergy member should be offered as an option to parents to facilitate spiritual healing. Allow them the choice of clergy and encourage participation of siblings, grandparents, godparents, and significant others. Provide the family with a formal baptismal certificate if the rite of baptism is performed. In emergencies, and if so desired by the parents, any lay person can baptize the infant. Use water and touch the baby's head while saying, "I baptize you in the Name of the Father, Son, and Holy Spirit," adding any prayer you wish. Most Christian religions universally recognize this emergency baptism as a legal entry into the church and will honor the rite as if it had been performed by clergy. A baptismal certificate may still be provided. Muslim parents may appreciate a prayer commending the infant to Allah, the All-Merciful.

PARENTAL EDUCATION

A second major nursing responsibility is the education of parents to prepare them for the life that faces them following the death of their child. This education will help prepare the bereaved parent to deal with matters that require immediate decisions. Information about grief responses will also reassure them that their behavior toward this experience is normal and expected. Knowledge through education prevents the confusion and fear that arises when parents are faced with unfamiliar feelings.

When crisis occurs, many families will turn inward in an attempt to isolate themselves so that others will not have to deal with their pain. The goal for these families should be to maximize their support systems. If parents understand that their grief can be eased by others who have also created a memory and bond with their baby, perhaps they would not be so reluctant to have visits from significant others. This is especially true with regard to surviving siblings. Sisters and brothers should always be included in the birth and death of their sibling. Although the events are difficult, research has shown that exclusion of siblings creates feelings of isolation and confusion in these children. Shared tears are far more therapeutic for both parents and siblings and allow each the opportunity to help the other through the grief process.

Autopsy and Funeral

Parents will be faced with decisions regarding an **autopsy**. The nurse's role is to make sure that this decision is not rushed by other health professionals and that parents are aware of the autopsy options available. The consent form is signed by the parents and the requesting physician.

Both parents are encouraged to plan for and attend their infant's funeral. They are also advised to disassemble the baby's room together. Although both processes are painful, they are quite therapeutic. Saying goodbye provides the parents with the opportunity to make choices in what has been, to this point, a helpless situation.

Preparing the bereaved parents for the emotional experience of the days following the funeral should include providing information about normal grief responses, reactions of family and friends, differences in grieving between men and women, care of surviving siblings, living through the holidays, and thoughts about a future pregnancy. When appropriate, significant others should be part of this education to facilitate their efforts in supporting the grieving family. Nurses should stress that there is no time limit on grieving and that, although the pain does not always remain as intense, the experience will be one that will change the parents' lives forever. With reassurance, families will understand that getting through the due date (in the case of the premature birth) and the first year will be the most intense emotional time. They will ultimately learn how to incorporate their infant's death into their lives, and they will, subsequently, reacquire happiness.

Finally, parents should be given adequate information about appropriate support systems within their community. Support groups and counseling can be a tremendous source of stability when experiencing grief. Referrals should be made as soon as possible.

KEY POINTS

- Death of a fetus before or after viability places most of the grief on the parents because others have not had time to become acquainted with the infant.
- Varying phases of the mourning process may not be synchronized, and one parent may progress more rapidly than the other, placing strain on the relationship.
- Nurses may assume a role in facilitating healthy grieving by helping to create memories of the infant.

- Parents and their families need education about the grief process, autopsy, and funeral arrangements. A perinatal grieving team will prepare materials and provide support in a hospital setting.
- Nurses need education about each topic including baptism and prayers that different cultural groups would appreciate.

STUDY QUESTIONS

29-1 Match statements below with Key Terms in the chapter.
  a. An _____ is a study of the potential causes for death.
  b. The period of time in which grief lessens and becomes tolerable is called _____.
  c. Death of a fetus after the age of viability and before birth is called a _____.
  d. Death of a live-born fetus, even though only a few breaths were taken, is called a _____.
  e. Death of an infant before the end of the twenty-eighth day of life is called a _____.

Answer Key   29-1 a. Autopsy, b. Resolution, c. Stillbirth, d. Live birth or neonatal death, e. Neonatal death

REFERENCES

Corrine L et al: The unheard voices of women: spiritual interventions in maternal-child health, *MCN* 17(3):141, 1992.

DeFrain M et al: *Stillborn: the invisible death*, Boston, 1986, Lexington Books.

Grief and Marriage: Madison, Wisc, 1978, Childbirth and Parent Education Association of Madison, Wisc, Inc.

Ilse S, Burns LH: *Miscarriage: a shattered dream*, Minneapolis, Minn, 1985, Wintergreen Press.

Ilse S: Reproductive Losses: June 1990, Proceedings of the Hartford Hospital's Conference. Empty arms: the caregiver's role after miscarriage—stillbirth and infant death, Hartford, Conn.

Jimenez S, Mims L: *The other side of pregnancy: coping with miscarriage and stillbirth*, New Jersey, 1982, Spectrum Books.

Klaus MH, Kennell JH: Caring for the parents of a stillborn or an infant who dies. In Klaus MH, Kennell JH, eds: *Parent-infant bonding*, St Louis, 1982, Mosby.

Lake M et al: The role of a grief support team following stillbirth, *Am J Obstet Gynecol* 146:877, 1983.

Panuthes C, Romeo C: *Ended beginnings: healing childbearing losses*, Boston, 1984, Bergin & Garvey Publishers.

Read-Sisti D: A dream dies, *MCN*, 15:258, 1990.

Schwiebert P, Kirk P: *When hello means goodbye*, Portland, Ore, 1981, University of Oregon Health Sciences Center.

 STUDENT RESOURCE SHELF

Lawson LV: Culturally sensitive support for grieving parents, *MCN* 15(2):76, 1990. Identifies the cultural beliefs of Native American, Mexican-American, and Southeast Asian-American people and how these beliefs affect the grieving of parents following the death of an infant.

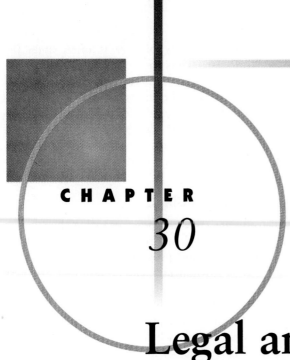

Legal and Ethical Issues in Maternal-Infant Nursing

KEY TERMS

Assault
Autonomy
Battery
Defendant
Demeanor
Documentation
Emancipated Minor
Ethics
Expert Nurse Witness
Expert Witness
Implied Consent
Informed Consent

Malpractice
Morals
Negligence
Plaintiff

Rapport
Standards of Care
Statutes of Limitations
Values

LEARNING OBJECTIVES

1. *Identify potential areas of legal or ethical controversy in perinatal care.*
2. *Compare and contrast the reasons for more frequent lawsuits in perinatal care in relation to other types of nursing care.*
3. *Identify rationale for increased nursing accountability in perinatal care.*
4. *Using 13 criteria, conduct a chart review for nursing documentation.*
5. *Apply the Thompson model of ethical decision making to selected cases.*
6. *Debate legal and ethical dilemmas arising in maternity nursing practice.*

When you hear the words "high risk," you usually think of a client with complications of pregnancy. But this term takes on a new meaning when it refers to legal issues in perinatal nursing. Nurses working in this field face the highest risk of lawsuit compared with nurses in other specialty areas.

Every year there is an increase in the number of nurses named as defendants in lawsuits. A **defendant** is the party in the lawsuit who is sued and accused of wrongdoing. More than ever, nurses need to learn how to minimize their risk of being sued. Only by investing

time and effort to learn about legal issues can you effectively insulate yourself against the risk of lawsuit. After all, "forewarned is forearmed."

By far, the best defense to any malpractice lawsuit is *prevention*. Malpractice avoidance is no accident. It requires effort, and often it requires a commitment to change.

The first step to malpractice avoidance is to learn about the legal risks and pitfalls. The next step is to use what is learned to make the necessary changes in daily practice. While there is no guarantee that you will never be sued, you can adopt behaviors that will significantly reduce your chances of ending up in court.

Why So Many Lawsuits?

To avoid becoming a victim of the malpractice crisis, it is imperative to understand the mindset of those individuals filing the lawsuits. To answer the question, "Why are there so many lawsuits?" we must explore three categories: (1) Why there are lawsuits, (2) Why there is an increasing number of lawsuits against nurses, and (3) Why perinatal nursing is considered a high risk area for lawsuits. These are complex issues that deserve your careful attention. It is difficult, if not impossible, to avoid being sued without understanding what motivates people to file lawsuits.

SOCIETAL ATTITUDES

The way society thinks affects the propensity to sue. Certain attitudes increase the likelihood of lawsuits.

Need to Blame

When a person refuses to accept responsibility for his or her own actions, the result is the fixation of blame on another person. For example, if a client who is 7 months pregnant exhibits signs of premature labor and is sent home with strict instructions to remain on bed rest, one would think that this same client would be willing to accept the consequences of not following medical instructions. Unfortunately, too often a client who disregards medical advice by spending the day shopping at the mall instead of staying in bed might file a lawsuit if her baby suffers as a result of being born prematurely.

Expectation of Perfection

Often clients do not realize that medicine is not an exact science. They may think that everything can be cured by modern technology. The medical profession must take partial responsibility for conveying that attitude to the public.

The truth is that there generally are no guarantees that a proposed treatment regimen will produce the desired outcome. Clients who feel the medical system has wrongfully failed them are likely to pursue legal recourse. For example, a client who undergoes maternal serum alpha-fetoprotein testing during pregnancy must be told that a negative test result does *not* guarantee that the baby has no genetic defects.

Lack of Personalism

The sophisticated equipment in use today leads to advanced monitoring techniques that have substantially improved the quality of client care. Yet the client's perception of the quality of care is often quite the opposite. Too often clients equate more equipment with less actual "hands-on" care. A client attached to a fetal monitor that evaluates the status of the baby continuously often feels better cared for by the nurse who comes in periodically and auscultates fetal heart tones. Clients who perceive that they received good care often do not sue even when faced with an untoward result.

WELL-EDUCATED PUBLIC

Clients are better educated now regarding their health care. They want and get more information about diagnosis, medications, and prognosis. By being more involved in their own health care, they also are very aware when an adverse outcome occurs. Clients faced with a poor result will probably ask what went wrong, and should be told by the proper person. Clients today are likely to be aware when they have been treated negligently. In fact, one of the worst things a health care provider can do when faced with a bad result is attempt to cover up the truth because a client who later learns he or she has been the victim of a deception is very likely to take legal action. Remember that *angry clients are potential plaintiffs*. A **plaintiff** is the party who claims he or she was injured and initiates a lawsuit.

WHY THE INCREASE IN LAWSUITS AGAINST NURSES?

Years ago, if a nurse was involved in a lawsuit, it was most likely as a witness, one who had knowledge of the events resulting in the lawsuit. Now, nurses are more likely to be involved in a different manner—as defendants. By being named as defendants, nurses are also accused of wrongdoing. There are several reasons why nurses' involvement in lawsuits has evolved in this manner.

Nursing as a Profession

Nurses used to be merely doctors' "handmaidens," whose function was to follow orders. There was no independence or autonomy. Nurses did not make decisions or perform independent assessments. Nursing has changed, though. Now nurses are recognized as professionals. Nursing is now well recognized as a practice that is independent of the practice of medicine.

With this recognition of nurses as professionals came accountability. By presenting ourselves to the public as independent professionals, we also declare that we are responsible for our own actions. Today's nurse operates with **autonomy** and makes independent judgments regarding client care. Although this has enhanced overall client care, it has increased the risk of being named as a defendant in a lawsuit.

Nurses as "Deep Pockets"

The plaintiff attorney's responsibility is to find sufficient financial resources to compensate the plaintiff in whatever amount the jury determines is fair. Often it is essential to include several defendants to ensure that enough compensation is available. In this situation, the nurse becomes another "pocket" to dip into in order to satisfy the judgment.

The nurse might also be named as a defendant in an attempt to hold the hospital liable by the doctrine of "respondent superior" (let the master respond). This theory holds that the employer is responsible for the negligent acts of its employee when the employee is acting within the scope of employment. By showing that the nurse/employee was negligent, the plaintiff can then access the hospital's "deep pocket."

WHY IS PERINATAL NURSING A HIGH-RISK PRACTICE AREA?

In nursing, the highest risk of lawsuit attaches to the perinatal specialty area. There are many reasons for this.

Nurses Held to Higher Standard of Care

Whenever nurses practice in a specialty area that requires increased skill, training, and experience beyond that which is taught in nursing school, those nurses will be held to a higher standard of care. Nurses holding themselves out as specialists are expected to know and do more than other nurses practicing in a less specialized area.

Perinatal nursing is a highly specialized area, therefore perinatal nurses are held to a higher standard of care than other nurses (see Standards of Care).

High Expectation of Outcome

Often, obstetric clients do not perceive themselves as sick and therefore are completely unprepared for any bad result of their pregnancies. When a bad result occurs, it is absolutely devastating to the expectant parent. In such a situation, it is often impossible for the parent to accept that sometimes things like this just happen.

When this fact is added to our society's general tendency to fix blame, often the doctors and/or nurses bear the brunt of the accusation of wrongdoing in the form of a lawsuit.

Defective Infant Survival Rate

With recent advances in perinatal technology, infants who formerly would have died in utero or shortly after birth are now being saved. Unfortunately, many of these babies suffer severe medical consequences, such as mental retardation, cerebral palsy, seizure disorders, brain damage, developmental delays, and many other conditions that will be costly to monitor and treat for the baby's lifetime.

Historically, lawsuits for the wrongful death of an infant have not netted large dollar awards. But lawsuits based on permanent brain damage, for example, will often result in multimillion dollar recoveries.

Long Statute of Limitations for Minors

Lawsuits must be filed within a certain amount of time after the act, giving rise to the lawsuit. These time limits are prescribed by law and are called statutes of limitations. The length of time one has to bring legal action differs, depending upon what type of lawsuit is being filed. The time period allowed also varies from state to state.

Statutes of limitations are usually shorter for adults than for minors. Often the statute of limitations for medical malpractice claims will be 2 or 3 years for adults. This means that the client must file the lawsuit within 2 years of the alleged act of negligence. Minors, however, often have until 2 or 3 years after they reach the age of majority to file a lawsuit. When dealing with minors, more specifically newborns, the health care practitioner can actually be at risk of lawsuit for as long as *21 years* before the statute of limitations expires. These extended statutes of limitations for minors operate to the disadvantage of perinatal nurses.

Several Potential Plaintiffs

The obstetric staff treating a pregnant woman really has two clients—the mother and the fetus. Care must be directed toward the best interests of both. One or both clients can suffer injury in the event that something goes wrong, giving rise to lawsuits being initiated by either party. In addition, the husband/father can have his own basis for a lawsuit involving either his wife or child. In any event, for a single treatment regimen, there could be at least three entities ready to sue in the event of an adverse outcome.

Long Involvement in Treatment

A pregnant woman is likely to receive medical care for an extended period during the 40-week gestation. Medical treatment is usually ongoing, resulting in a relatively large amount of treatment being given during any pregnancy. Statistically, as more treatment is given, the chance that something will be done incorrectly increases.

Sometimes the close relationship the pregnant woman develops with the physician and nurses during the prolonged treatment period can serve to buffer the tendency to sue, even if there is a bad result. Doctors and nurses who have good **rapport** with their clients and establish caring relationships with them often escape lawsuits even when medical malpractice exists. Clients are much less likely to sue their friends—those whom they perceive genuinely care about them.

Nursing Autonomy Issues

Whenever nurses practice in a specialty area that requires that they operate with a greater degree of autonomy, the chance for errors in judgment increases. And, whenever judgmental errors occur, the chance of a charge of medical malpractice increases.

The nature of the practice of perinatal nursing requires that nurses act with autonomy much of the time. Perinatal nurses frequently monitor clients throughout the first stages of labor and communicate pertinent information to the physician. This information is often what determines at what point the physician comes to the hospital to tend to the client.

If incorrect, or inadequate information regarding the progress is conveyed to the physician, there is a chance that the physician will not come to the hospital soon enough. In a situation such as this, the nurse, not the physician, will likely be the one who is sued for negligence. The nurse has an obligation to make a correct assessment of the client and to communicate the results to the physician. This requires that the nurse always be capable of performing a proper assessment.

Standards of Care

All professionals practicing in the medical field are held to certain standards when administering care. These standards dictate what type of care is appropriate for a particular client. The **standards of care** for physicians are different from those for nurses. Likewise, the standards of practice are different for registered nurses than for practical nurses.

Standards of care ensure that you will be "judged by the company you keep." As a perinatal nurse, you will be expected to know and to do what other nurses practicing that specialty are expected to know and do.

Standards of care come from several sources, including laws, organizational standards, and institutional policies and procedures. They are interpreted by case law, enumerated by expert witnesses, and are constantly in a state of change.

LAWS

The most common type of laws influencing the nursing standards of care are nursing practice acts. These acts broadly define the scope of nursing practice within a particular state. Laws also dictate the requirements for nursing licensure. Because laws differ from state to state, it is important to be familiar with one's own state licensure laws and nursing practice act.

ORGANIZATIONAL STANDARDS

Often nursing specialty areas have state and or national organizations to which nurses can look for clarification of their roles. The Association of Women's Health, Obstetric, and Neonatal Nurses has published standards of practice for nurses, defining what is expected of nurses practicing in perinatology.

For instance, perinatal nurses are expected to be capable of evaluating fetal monitor tracings and identifying certain patterns by specified terminology. Not knowing how to do so would be difficult if not impossible to defend in court. It is expected that nurses will maintain the highest level of skill and training throughout the time they practice nursing. As standards of care change and are updated, nurses are expected to be aware of the most current standards of care.

INSTITUTIONAL POLICIES AND PROCEDURES

Whether the nurse is employed in a hospital, clinic, or outpatient setting, the employing institution has policies and procedures to be followed. It is imperative that nurses be aware of all applicable policies and procedures. Policies and procedures can differ between institutions. It is not at all unusual to find differing policies and procedures within the same metropolitan area. Violation of an internal policy and/or procedures can be used against the nurse to establish a failure to abide by the applicable standard of care.

WHEN LAWS, ORGANIZATIONAL STANDARDS, AND INTERNAL POLICIES AND PROCEDURES DIFFER

Occasionally, a nurse encounters a situation in which the institution's policy seems to conflict with the law, or an organizational standard differs from an internal policy. How does one decide in this situation which action to take?

The safest way to resolve this conflict—and to avoid legal problems—is to follow the directive that is the *most* restrictive (Figure 30-1).

Test Yourself

- When a problem occurs, how do you discover the correct standard of care?

CASE LAW

When a case is decided in court, that decision sets a precedent for other courts addressing the same issue. How closely another court will follow a set precedent

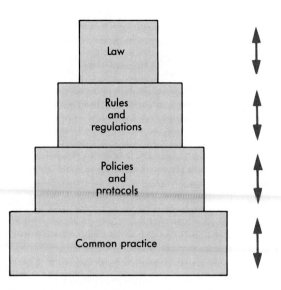

FIGURE 30-1 Relationship of law to rules, regulations, policies, and common practice. When questions arise, the most restrictive practice is the safest to follow.

depends on how similar the issues are and where the original precedent was set. A court in the Midwest is more likely to follow the precedent set by another court in the same region than one on the West or East coast.

When a court of similar jurisdiction has previously decided a case similar to one in which you are involved, you can usually expect that your case will reach the same or similar outcome. Case law lends an element of predictability to an otherwise unpredictable field. It also sets a standard of care that is expected to be met in a similar situation in the future.

EXPERT WITNESS TESTIMONY

Whenever a court case involves subject matter that is beyond the understanding of the average person, the court requires the use of an **expert witness.** The expert's role in a malpractice case is to clarify for the jury what the acceptable standard of care is for those accused of wrongdoing. After explaining to the jury what the reasonable and prudent nurse should have done in a particular situation, the expert is then asked if the nurse/defendant abided by the acceptable standard of care.

To qualify as an **expert nurse witness,** the nurse must have expertise in the area that is the subject matter of the trial. The more highly credentialed the expert is shown to be, the more credible the expert's testimony will be to the jury. A nursing expert witness can only testify as to the standard of care for nurses, not to that of physicians.

Theories of Liability

Lawsuits can arise based on several different theories. While the most common is the allegation of negligence in the form of medical malpractice, causes of action can also be based on wrongful death, wrongful birth, and wrongful life.

MEDICAL MALPRACTICE

Malpractice can be defined as "negligence by a professional that causes an injury." Negligence is the failure to act as a reasonable person.

The allegation of medical malpractice against a health care provider is difficult to prove in court. To satisfy the burden of proof "by a preponderance of the evidence," the plaintiff must establish that all four of the elements of a medical malpractice lawsuit exist—the duty, the breach of the duty, the injury to the client, and the proximate causation.

The Duty to Provide Care

To be successfully charged with malpractice, health care professionals must have had a duty to provide care to the client. For a duty to arise, there must be a professional relationship with the client. If a client delivers a baby in a grocery store, she cannot sue the nurse at the hospital for malpractice, because the nurse could not have had a legal duty to that client with whom the nurse did not have any relationship.

Once the nurse/client relationship is established, the nurse has a duty to treat the client in accordance with acceptable standards of care.

Breach of Duty

A breach of a nurse's duty is the failure to abide by or live up to the acceptable standard of care. The breach of the duty consist of *either* an act or an omission. The duty to a client can be breached by doing something that should not have been done, or by not doing something that should have been done.

In a North Dakota case in which an infant was born severely brain damaged, the court held that failing to attach a client to a fetal monitor when it was ordered by the physician was a breach of the nurse's professional duty to the client. The jury in this case awarded $7,800,000 to the plaintiff.[1]

Injury or Damages

The terms *injury* and *damages* are often used interchangeably in lawsuits. More exactly, the damages usually refer to the monetary value of the injury.

A client who does not sustain an injury as a result of an alleged negligent act does *not* have a malpractice case because one of the four necessary elements is missing. There must be an ascertainable injury in order for a lawsuit for malpractice to succeed.

Proximate Causation

Proving the proximate causation element is probably the most difficult part of a malpractice action. The plaintiff must prove that the **breach** of the **duty** was the direct and **proximate cause** of the **injury** and that the injury was a foreseeable consequence of the breach of the duty.

Foreseeability means that the type of injury that was sustained must be the type of consequence that one would reasonably expect from a particular negligent act. For example, if a client is negligently over-medicated, it would be foreseeable that the client would require a longer hospital stay. But it is *not* foreseeable that the client would be injured by the collapse of a ceiling while continuing his hospital stay. The damages from the overmedication would *not* include the injuries sustained in the ceiling collapse.

On the other hand, if this same client developed a thrombosis as a direct result of the continued immobility from the treatment of the overmedication, that could become part of the suit for injury.

The proximate causation is often the greatest challenge faced by the plaintiff's attorney. For example, a lawsuit was brought in Louisiana alleging that the physician failed to arrive at the hospital in time. The client developed a concealed placental abruption that resulted in the death of the premature infant. The court held that although the obstetrician was negligent in his medical treatment of the woman in labor, in that his delay caused her needless suffering and anxiety, the evidence was insufficient to prove that the infant died as a result of his delay in arriving at the hospital. The court held that the signs of the abruption did not occur until after he was in attendance, and could not have been detected earlier, even if he had been in attendance. The court awarded damages for pain and suffering in the amount of $20,000, but no damages for the death of the infant were awarded. This case demonstrates how a negligent act can be present but may not be the proximate cause of the injury.[2]

WRONGFUL DEATH

Sometimes a pregnancy ends in tragedy, with the death of a viable infant. When a lawsuit for medical malpractice arises, it is the injured party who is the plaintiff. When the injury results in death, the survivors are the plaintiffs, and they file the lawsuit for the wrongful death of the other person.

Wrongful death lawsuits usually allege that the death resulted from the negligence of the defendants. Often the death of the neonate cannot be prevented, and if the court makes such a finding, the lawsuit for wrongful death will be defeated. Such was the case in the Louisiana case where the jury concluded that the infant died as a result of placental abruption, not as a result of the physician's delay in arriving at the hospital.[3]

In some jurisdictions, for a wrongful death action to arise, there must have been a live birth. The issue in a Texas case revolved around whether or not the fetus had died in utero or just after birth. In this case, a fetus presented in footling breech position and was delivered to the shoulders, at which time the cervix clamped tightly around the fetus's neck and umbilical cord. The fetus's limbs were noted to be limp and cyanotic. When the baby was finally delivered, it was lifeless, and resuscitation attempts failed. The court held that no action for wrongful death could ensue.[4]

The courts are currently split on this issue, and some courts are allowing compensation on a wrongful death theory for the death of an unborn fetus if the fetus was viable at the time of death.[5]

WRONGFUL BIRTH

Wrongful birth lawsuits arise when an "unwanted" child is born. These lawsuits sometimes arise in the context of failed sterilizations, but also arise when a child is born with a defect that could have been discovered while options to terminate the pregnancy were still open. The premise behind a wrongful birth lawsuit is that the birth might have been prevented. A Virginia court awarded approximately $180,000 to a couple who gave birth to a child with Tay-Sachs disease after the father was mistakenly informed that he was not a carrier of the disease. Apparently, the laboratory technician had mislabeled his blood sample. The parents alleged that the erroneous test result prevented them from undergoing additional tests which would have confirmed Tay-Sachs early enough that they could have aborted the pregnancy.[6]

In another Tay-Sachs case, the allegation was that the physician failed to inform the parents of the risks of bearing a child with Tay-Sachs disease, so no tests were ever performed and their child was born with the disease.[7]

Wrongful birth actions are not limited to Tay-Sachs, but have also been filed by parents who gave birth to children with other defects such as Down syndrome. Parents should be informed about available testing opportunities such as amniocentesis, for the detection of possible fetal defects so they can decide whether or not to avail themselves of these tests and the options they provide.

WRONGFUL LIFE

Wrongful life is a relatively new cause of action, which many states still do not recognize as compensable. In a lawsuit for wrongful life, it is the *child* who claims that he or she should not have been born. The courts in these cases have been reluctant to attach a damage award for the pain and suffering of having been born "defective," but have awarded damages to compensate for a child's care. This is an evolving area of law that can be expected to undergo dramatic changes in the next few years, as more courts must decide whether or not to recognize this doctrine.

Common Causes of Lawsuits for Malpractice

NURSE'S VS PHYSICIAN'S ROLE

Who is responsible for what? It is sometimes difficult to determine with exactness where a physician's duty ends and nurse's duty begins. Often the duties seem to overlap.

In an Illinois case, a breech presentation was not identified by the nurses throughout most of the labor, and once determined it was too late for the physician to perform a cesarean section. The baby suffered serious damage as a result of the difficult vaginal delivery. Both the physician and the nurses were sued, so the court held *both* parties responsible for failing to recognize the breech position and awarded $2,900,000 to the plaintiffs.[8]

Another case addressed the issue of whether or not a nurse could diagnose arrest of labor. The Louisiana court held that this diagnosis was the physician's responsibility. The nurse's responsibility was to report the observable facts to the physician.[9]

When differentiating the nurse's responsibility from the physician's responsibility, nurse expert witnesses, not physician expert witnesses, must be called to determine the applicable standard of care for nurses. In a California case, the court held that a physician cannot testify as to an appropriate nursing standard of care.[10]

Frequently, when a physician is sued, the nurses will also be drawn into the lawsuit, and vice versa. Regardless of who is ultimately found to be responsible, both parties experience the trauma and disruption that accompanies being sued (Kuhlman, 1990). On a more positive note, it is clear that many lawsuits can be successfully defended by the nurses, the physician, or both.

LAWSUITS AGAINST PHYSICIANS

Lawsuits brought against physicians and nurses differ, reflecting the well-recognized differences between these professions and their responsibilities. A likely allegation against a physician might be one of the following: (1) failure to diagnose a high-risk pregnancy, (2) delay in performing a cesarean section, (3) improper vaginal delivery or failure to perform a cesarean section, (4) improper use of forceps, (5) incidents surrounding induc-ing labor and the use of oxytocin, (6) delay in arriving at the hospital, or (7) nonattendance at the delivery. Lawsuits against physicians occur much more frequently than those against nurses.

LAWSUITS AGAINST NURSES

Many of the bases for lawsuits against nurses do not arise out of issues unique to the perinatal specialty area. In fact, most of the liability issues facing perinatal nurses are very similar to those faced by nurses in other specialty areas. But for purposes of this chapter, these issues will be considered primarily in the context of the perinatal nurse.

Medications

Many lawsuits against nurses are the result of problems arising out of medication functions. Considering the amount of time nurses spend in various aspects of medication administration, this should come as no surprise. Allegations against nurses include, but are not limited to, improper client identification; wrong medication, dosage, route, or time; and failure to monitor for side effects. In the perinatal context, one drug—oxytocin—surfaces in many of the lawsuits filed.

Nurses are often involved in the administration of oxytocin for the augmentation of labor. It is imperative that the nurses be aware of all nursing standards relating to the induction and/or augmentation of labor, including all NAACOG (AWHONN) standards and hospital procedures. Nurses must also be aware of the signs and symptoms of any complications of oxytocin administration and report any problems immediately (see Chapter 15).

Client Monitoring

Failure to adequately monitor a client can lead to a charge of client abandonment. Nurses are expected to monitor their clients at appropriate time intervals that depend upon the client's condition.

Sometimes the physician's directive can be used to determine how often a client is to be monitored and for what. Sometimes hospital policies and procedures dictate how often a particular aspect of client monitoring should be done. Without any specific directives, it is often up to nursing judgment.

Labor and delivery pose a unique monitoring challenge, in that there are two clients to monitor—the mother and the baby. The delivering mother must be adequately monitored to prevent any maternal complications during the antepartal period. Any substantial increases or decreases in the mother's blood pressure could affect the baby's welfare. The same is true for any other alterations of vital signs, such as elevated temperature or pulse. Any variation from the norm must be reported and corrected to prevent possible harm to the baby.

The fetus is the other client to be monitored, especially during labor. Many lawsuits have arisen as a result of problems related to fetal monitoring. In most institutions, electronic fetal monitoring has become the standard. Some institutions routinely monitor all labor and delivery situations. Whenever possible, it is prudent to use electronic fetal monitoring.

Lawsuits arising from problems regarding fetal monitoring can result in a variety of allegations against nurses. Often allegations of wrongdoing involve the failure to use a monitor when indicated, failure to continue monitoring, failure to correctly interpret the monitor strip, or failure to report nonreassuring or ominous fetal heart patterns (see Chapter 14).

Failure to use electronic fetal monitor when ordered or indicated. In North Dakota, a jury awarded a $7.8 million judgment against a nurse who failed to place a client on a fetal monitor. The physicians had left standing orders that all of their clients were to be placed on monitors. The nurse mistakenly thought that all of the monitors were in use, so did not attach the monitor until more than an hour after the client's arrival at the hospital. When finally applied, the fetal monitor indicated fetal distress and an emergency cesarean section was performed. The baby was severely brain damaged.[11]

Failure to leave monitor on. A nurse was found liable in a Nebraska case in which one of the allegations of negligence was that the fetal monitor was disconnected from a client about 12 hours before the client delivered a baby with cerebral palsy. The baby later died.[12]

Failure to correctly interpret fetal monitor tracings. In the previously referenced Nebraska case, the court also addressed the issue of whether it is the physician's or the nurse's responsibility to monitor and interpret fetal heart rate tracings. This case seems to say that the physician should be allowed to rely on a nurse's interpretation of fetal heart rate monitoring. Perinatal nurses are expected to be capable of interpreting fetal heart rate tracings and, according to AWHONN are expected to use proper terminology, such as "variable decelerations," when referring to the information on these tracings. Nurses have a tremendous responsibility to develop fetal monitor interpretation skills, and to use them.

Failure to report abnormal fetal heart monitor results to the physician. A nurse should recognize a nonreassuring fetal monitor tracing and then has an obligation to notify the physician to come to the hospital, according to the jury in a Washington case.[13] In another case in Virginia, the nurse was found liable when she did not notify the physician of trouble until almost a half hour after the problems were noticed on the fetal monitor

tracing. The baby was born with severe neurologic deformities and the jury awarded the plaintiff $3,500,000. The Supreme Court of Virginia affirmed the verdict.[14]

Failure to Adequately Assess the Client

One of the most basic nursing responsibilities is that of client assessment. Every nurse, regardless of the area of practice, is expected by virtue of his or her licensure, to be capable of performing a client assessment. The inability to do so is difficult, if not impossible, to defend in court. After all, the nurse is the member of the health care team who is with the client constantly, and responsible for the minute by minute evaluation of the client's progress.

Nowhere is this more true than in labor and delivery, where monitoring the progress of the client's labor through delivery is the purpose of the unit's existence. The nurse must carefully and continuously assess the progress of both clients.

Electronic fetal monitoring has provided an up-to-date assessment technique to determine fetal well-being. Simultaneously, the nurse is responsible for assessing the normal progress of labor by checking dilation, effacement, and contractions. In addition, the nurse must be cognizant of changes that might indicate problems, such as alterations in vital signs. When the nurse is faced with premature rupture of the membranes, the client's temperature and white blood count must be monitored when assessing a client for infection.

Nurses in all specialty areas must maintain the highest level of assessment skills. This is especially important for nurses in specialty areas, who often operate with a greater degree of autonomy than those in other areas.

Failure to Report Changes in the Client's Condition to the Physician

As mentioned briefly in the previous section on electronic fetal monitoring, any abnormalities or changes in the patient's condition must be reported to the physician. The physician then has an obligation to the patient to provide the proper medical intervention.

Whenever the nurse's assessment indicates that the client's condition has changed, the nurse must notify the physician. In an Illinois case, the nurse did not notify the physician when a 4-month-old girl's condition deteriorated, and the child died. The court opined that the nurse's failure denied the physician the opportunity to intervene and possibly save the child's life.[15]

In Ohio, a nurse's failure to report a client's elevated pulse, temperature, and white blood cell count to the physician was alleged to have denied the physician the opportunity to intervene sooner in the client's treatment, resulting in stillbirth from chorioamnionitis.[16]

When a nurse reports a client's changed condition to the physician, and the nurse feels that the physician has not responded in a manner that is in the client's best interest, the nurse must proceed up the chain of command until proper medical care is given to the client. Usually the first step up the chain is to the nurse's supervisor.

The nurse, being the client advocate, is expected to do this. Nurses must understand that failing to notify a physician of a problem often leads to a delay in appropriate medical care being implemented. This in turn can lead to an injury to the client and a lawsuit.

Other Causes of Malpractice Lawsuits

Kidnapping infants from nurseries has increased over the years; consequently most hospitals have taken steps to make their nurseries more secure. When a kidnapping does occur, a lawsuit frequently follows alleging that security was inadequate. Nurses sometimes wonder what their responsibility is to prevent newborn kidnapping. One obligation that can be imposed on nursing is to be alert on one's unit for suspicious persons or behavior, and to question any unrecognized person claiming to be an employee. Any suspicious persons or incidents should be reported to Security (see Chapter 19).

Occasionally, lawsuits arise that seem to be based on facts that are almost too extraordinary to be believed. Yet some outrageous acts do occur, and they do result in lawsuits. For instance, in North Carolina, a nurse gave a sandwich to a client in labor, the client aspirated the food, and the baby suffered severe brain damage.[17] In yet another bizarre case in New York, a nurse was sued for injuries sustained when the nurse pushed a partially delivered baby back into the uterus.[18] In Michigan, a woman was told on admission to the hospital that her baby would not be born for hours because she was not dilated. Shortly thereafter, while she was returning to bed from the bathroom, she delivered the baby—onto the floor. The baby sustained a skull fracture and was mentally retarded.[19]

Consent

Treating a client without obtaining the proper consent can lead to a charge of assault and/or battery. These terms are often used together, but do have different meanings. **Assault** is the threat of an unauthorized touching. **Battery** is the unauthorized touching of a client.

INFORMED CONSENT

Informed consent is a well-recognized doctrine based on the client's right to autonomy. Clients have a right to decide what medical treatment they will have performed. To make an intelligent decision regarding medical treatment, clients have a right to sufficient information so that they can make an educated choice. Clients have a right to know what treatment is proposed, the expected outcome, the risks, and what alternative treatment is available.

Informed consent occurs most frequently when the client and the physician are discussing the proposed course of treatment. The physician should document informed consent in the medical record. The nurse is usually the one who obtains the client's signature on the consent form. Sometimes nurses are confused as to their proper role in this informed consent process, and understandably so. Nurses should realize that informed consent is not the same as the consent form. The consent form serves as written proof that informed consent took place.

The courts have generally held that it is the physician's duty to obtain informed consent. But the responsibility for obtaining the client's signature on the consent form can safely be delegated to the nurse, as long as the nurse follows the correct procedure for doing so.

The nurse should approach the client with the consent form and ask the client if the physician has explained the procedure and answered all of the client's questions. If the client answers affirmatively, the nurse should then ask the client to read and sign the consent form for the hospital record. The nurse can then witness the client's signature. By doing so, the nurse is attesting to the fact that the client voluntarily signed the form.

If the client states that the physician has neither explained the procedure nor answered the client's questions, the nurse must realize that the client has not given informed consent. The nurse should *not* have the client sign the consent form, but should notify the physician that the client still has questions. Having a client sign a consent form when the nurse knows that informed consent has not been given is substandard nursing practice and can result in the nurse being included with the physician in a lawsuit for assault and battery.

IMPLIED CONSENT

Sometimes a client is incapable of giving consent for treatments, such as in an emergency situation. No one would want to withhold lifesaving treatment from a client just because he or she was unconscious and could not give consent. The law presumes that if a person were capable of giving consent to lifesaving treatment, he or she would do so. This premise resulted in the doctrine of **implied consent**. In an emergency situation in which the client cannot consent to treatment, consent will be "implied-by-law," thereby protecting health care professionals from lawsuits for assault and battery.

Implied consent also applies to situations where the client has not objected to a current course of treatment. This is often referred to as "implied-in-fact" consent. If you ask a labor and delivery client to hold out her arm so you can start an intravenous line, and she does so, consent is implied.

CONSENT TO TREAT MINORS

A minor is defined in most states as a person who has not reached his or her eighteenth birthday. Once a person reaches the age of 18, he or she has legal capacity to consent for medical treatment. Nurses must check their own state's laws regarding minors, since they vary from state to state.

Treating a minor without the consent of the parent or guardian constitutes assault and battery. Some exceptions to this exist. First, in an emergency situation, the doctrine of implied consent covers any treatment given to save the minor's life. Parental consent is *not* necessary in an emergency situation. In fact, parents sometimes lack legal capacity to refuse lifesaving treatment on behalf of their minor children, even if for religious reasons.

Second, an **emancipated minor** can consent to treatment. The definition of emancipation varies from state to state, but usually includes minors who are married, have a child, are in the military, or are self-supporting. In most states, minors can also consent for pregnancy-related treatment.

When treating an emancipated minor, not only is parental notification and consent not necessary, it might lead to a charge of breach of confidentiality of privileged information.

Test Yourself

- What is the difference between informed and implied consent?
- What should you do if the client feels she still has unanswered questions and you have come to get a signature on the consent form?
- In a labor situation, give an example of assault compared with an example of battery.

RIGHT TO REFUSE TREATMENT

Generally speaking, competent adults have a right to refuse any medical treatment they do not want, even if it means they will die without it. Sometimes pregnant women wish to refuse treatment, even though the baby might suffer as a result of the mother's decision. This problem has led to an ethical dilemma. When is it

appropriate to force unwanted treatment on the mother to benefit the baby?

This has not been an easy issue to resolve because someone's rights are violated regardless of which decision is made. The problem for the courts and for society is to make the determination of whose rights take precedence in a particular case.

Courts have been known to order a mother to undergo a cesarean section in spite of religious opposition, when there was a high likelihood that the baby would suffer damage or die during a vaginal delivery. Yet other forms of treatment, particularly those which pose a greater risk to the mother, have not been imposed.

Another issue closely related to this one is whether or not a woman should be penalized for behavior that poses a risk to the fetus. The most prevalent example is that of substance abuse during pregnancy. How far can society go to protect the fetus? Some have advocated incarceration of pregnant drug abusers, while as many others have spoken to the inappropriateness and ineffectiveness of such a directive. Again, the dilemma arises as we try to determine whose rights are superior, and to what extent the other's rights can be violated (see Ethical Dilemmas).

There are no good answers to this conflict at this time, only more questions. Nurses should keep abreast of developments in this area.

Abortion
NURSING'S ROLE IN ABORTION

Abortion is probably the most controversial issue any of us has faced in our lifetime. Those who favor abortion rights believe as passionately in their position as those who oppose abortion. So volatile is this controversy that in March of 1993 a physician at an abortion clinic in Florida was shot and killed by an antiabortion protestor.

In the nursing profession there are those who mirror the societal conflict. Many nurses consider themselves prochoice, and many consider themselves prolife. Nurses on both sides of the issue are confronted with client care situations in which a woman is either having an abortion performed, or is being treated for complications of an abortion. How can the nurse who morally opposes abortion deal with the above scenarios?

Nurses cannot be forced to participate in procedures they find morally offensive. Nurses have a right to refuse to assist with abortions. However, a nurse cannot attempt to stop an abortion from being performed.[20]

The nurse also has a legal obligation to take care of a client who has undergone an abortion, or who is being treated for complications of an abortion. To refuse care to a client in this situation is to make a character judgment upon which the provision of nursing care is based. Nurses are not allowed to do that. If a nurse refused to treat a client after an abortion, and the client suffered because of the lack of nursing care, the nurse could be sued for abandonment of the client.

MINOR REQUESTING ABORTION

Several recent cases have addressed the issue of minor's rights to consent to abortion. Many states have attempted to pass laws limiting minors' access to abortion without parental approval. The states differ tremendously on this issue, and the laws are in a constant state of change. Even when a law is passed, often an injunction is filed to block it before the law goes into effect. Then the higher court either upholds the law or decides that it is unconstitutional.

This will be a difficult area for nurses to remain current, but if a nurse is working in a setting where abortions are performed on minors, it is imperative that the nurse find a way to keep abreast of this constantly changing issue.

Malpractice Prevention

The best defense to a malpractice action is *prevention*. But malpractice prevention is no accident. It requires conscious attention to the two "Ds" of malpractice defense—demeanor and documentation.

DEMEANOR

The manner in which a nurse treats a client sets the stage for the likelihood of a lawsuit in the event of an adverse outcome. Nurses must never underestimate the power of **rapport** with the client in malpractice prevention.

Nursing care is delivered by human beings and consequently is subject to human error. When a negligent error results in an injury, the lawsuit climate is created. Whether or not the client takes the next step—to the lawyer—is likely to depend on the nurse's demeanor while treating the client. Simply put, given two identical poor client outcomes, the risk of a lawsuit might *not* be equal.

What determines whether or not an adverse outcome proceeds to a lawsuit? The nurse's rapport with the client. Remember this formula:

Adverse Outcome + Uncaring Demeanor = Lawsuit

Developing good rapport with your clients is an important part of malpractice prevention. A lawsuit is often circumvented when the staff treats the client with warmth and caring.

Communication Skills

The ability to develop good rapport with clients is dependent on the nurse having good interpersonal communication skills. Listening is by far the most important

communication skill. It is imperative that the nurse learn to listen to what the client says.

In a Kansas case, the jury found the nurse negligent when the client's husband's repeated requests to call the physician were ignored. The nurse told the husband that the client was only dilated 7 cm, therefore there was no need to notify the physician. The husband told the nurse that his wife had previously delivered a baby while only dilated 8 cm, but the nurse still ignored the request that the physician be called. The woman delivered only a few minutes later, with no physician in attendance.[21]

Besides listening to the client, the nurse must also be carefully attuned to the client's nonverbal communications.

Communication is a two-way street. Information communicated from the nurse to the client must be done in an understandable and appropriate manner. Discharge instructions should be communicated orally *and* in writing.

The manner in which communication occurred between a nurse and a client has been at issue in court cases. In a Puerto Rican case, the court indicated that a reasonably prudent nurse would *not* make disparaging remarks to a client.[22]

DOCUMENTATION

Documentation is by far the best defense once a lawsuit is filed. The medical record is a legal document and is admissible in court as evidence. It enjoys a privileged status in that it is presumed to be an accurate account of what transpired. This is because it was written at the time of the occurrence, by someone with knowledge of the events, and before litigation was initiated.

The **documentation** in the medical record must be able to stand on its own in proving that the standard of care was met. Omission of information from the medical record leads to the charge that the standard of care was violated. Unfortunately for the nurse, filling in the gaps in the medical record later—in court—will not suffice to prove that the standard of care was met. Spoken words have at best questionable credibility in a courtroom.

A case is only as good as the proof that is presented in court. Spoken words are often felt to be self-serving

 Clinical Decision

Think of a clinical situation you have observed where there is potential for a lawsuit. Analyze the demeanor of the staff, the degree of informed consent, and the nursing responsibilities that may not have been met.

and therefore cannot prove the case. Why should a jury believe that you provided continuous nursing care, when your documentation indicates otherwise? Given the opportunity, the jury will choose to believe what is documented in the medical record instead of the spoken words they hear in court.

From a litigation standpoint, the jury often assumes that if something was not charted, it was not done. Nurses should give themselves credit for care they provided by thoroughly documenting it in the medical record.

Documentation Format

In recent years there has been a trend away from straight narrative charting to flow sheets. Sometimes nurses question whether or not these flow sheets are sufficient to defend them if they are sued. It is not the format, but the completeness of the documentation that determines how good it is. A complete and thorough flow sheet is better than an incomplete, vague narrative note, and a complete narrative note defends better than an incomplete flow sheet. The key is to provide all of the pertinent information about the client. The format is secondary.

When using flow sheets, the nurse should be careful to not let the small spaces on the flow sheet discourage thorough reporting of information. If the flow sheet is not adequately telling the whole story, *it must be supplemented* with a narrative note. Nurses do not get into legal trouble by documenting too much—it is usually *too little documentation* that causes problems. A general documentation rule by which to live is, when in doubt as to how much to document, document *more* not *less*.

Documentation Tips to Stay Out of Court

1. *Write legibly.* An illegible entry cannot serve its intended purpose, which is to communicate information. And it will not be relied on to provide a defense in court if the jury cannot read it.
2. *Use ink.* The medical record is a legal document. When written it is intended to be permanent. To ensure its permanency, you should always use ink. Using pencil is dangerous because anyone could erase your entry and replace it with something else.
3. *Never obliterate an entry.* If you make an error in the chart, follow your institution's policy for error correction, which usually entails drawing one line through the incorrect entry—so it can still be read—and inserting the correct information. An obliterated entry can be used by your opponent to imply that pertinent information has been removed from the record, and you might not be able to prove otherwise because no one can read what you obliterated.

4. *Fill in all blanks and lines.* A flow sheet should be completely filled in, otherwise someone else could come in later and fill in inaccurate information that makes him or her look good and *you* look bad. In a narrative note, no lines should be left blank, in spite of a request by a co-worker to do so in order that he or she can fill it in later.
5. *Date and time all entries.* Sometimes it is very important what time something happened. If a nurse notifies a physician of a problem with a client, the nurse should document when the problems began and when the physician arrived. Documenting this sequence can prove that the nurse acted properly, and refute a charge by the physician that it was the physician and not the nurse who first noticed the problem.
6. *Document thought processes.* When faced with a situation where nursing judgment comes into play and decisions have to be made, document the process by which the decision is reached. Doing so can assure that the jury knows that the judgment that was made was the correct one in that situation.
7. *Be objective.* Document what you see and hear, not just conclusions. Do not document "client fell," unless you saw the client fall. Document your observations, e.g., "client found on floor."
8. *Describe behaviors, do not make personal judgments.* Do not document "client is hostile," or "client is drunk." Instead describe the behaviors, and leave the conclusion to the imagination of the reader. A record that describes a client who has "reddened eyes, staggering gait, slurred speech, and admits to consuming a case of beer," informs the reader, but makes no personal judgment about the client's character.
9. *Never air grievances in the chart.* The chart is not a battleground for wars among the staff. Documenting conflicts gives the plaintiff's attorney the opportunity to prove to the jury that someone was guilty of wrongdoing because one staff member pointed the finger at another.
10. *Document the client's noncompliance with treatment.* In the event a client chooses to refuse to comply with medical advice, the client should not be able to sue the health care team for injuries brought on by his or her own noncompliance. Documenting the noncompliance in the medical record is imperative to defeat a lawsuit brought by the noncompliant client. If a client with threatened premature labor is sent home with strict instructions to stay in bed, and the client admits to playing tennis, this admission should be documented. In the event this client's baby has problems, the defense will put the blame back on the woman in proving that the medical staff did not violate any standard of care.

Clinical Decision

Do a chart review together with your classmates, analyzing labor documentation for the 13 documentation tips listed in this chapter.

11. **Document your assessment.** This proves that you attended to your client appropriately. If the client is attached to a fetal monitor, include this information in the medical record. If you do not document the results of your assessments, the jury might assume they were not done.
12. **Document your interventions.** When your assessment shows something abnormal about your client's condition, your duty is to address the problem. The chart must include what you did for the client at that point. For example, if a client complains of pain, and you administer pain medication, that fact must be documented. If your client's blood pressure drops and you notify the physician, document that you did so. The record must reflect not only that problems were assessed, but that the appropriate interventions were instituted.
13. **Document physician contacts.** When a physician is notified, document the physician's name, the time the conversation took place, what was told to the physician, and the physician's response. Many disputes erupt between nurses who claim they called the physician and physicians who allege they were never notified.

If you are sued, your documentation can be your best friend, or your worst enemy. Time spent documenting is time well spent in the prevention of a lawsuit.

Ethical Decision Making*

As a nurse, you must know the "right" thing to do. Rightness or wrongness can be applied to any nursing decision made or action taken. Many people, including your clients, your instructors, and yourself, will evaluate your nursing care. Doing the right or best thing for each client is the objective of all nursing care.

The definition of the correct thing varies from person to person; it is not what an individual feels like doing. Rightness involves ethics and morality. Everyone uses personal standards to judge whether attitudes, behavior,

*Joyce E. Thompson, C.N.M., D.P.H., F.A.A.N., and Henry O. Thompson, M. Div., Ph.D.

actions, and decisions are good or bad. The profession of nursing also has standards of moral behavior that describe how a nurse should behave and act when practicing nursing.

ETHICS, MORALS, AND VALUES

When you ask yourself what you should do in a situation and why, you are asking moral questions. An understanding of morals, ethics, and values can help you to provide nursing care that is right for the client and done the right way.

Morals are what a person should and ought to do. However, these responsibilities and obligations raise the question of right, best, or correct choices. Moral questions suggest that there are at least two answers available. Sometimes, several options, some good and some bad, are possible. Even when refusing to decide, a person has made a choice (to do nothing). You must keep a professional attitude, even when your client makes a decision with which you disagree. Professional, caring behavior is exhibited by attitude, as well as by actions.

Ethics are the reasons we should or ought to do something. Thus a woman may decide to breast-feed her infant because she values the close interaction with her baby, believes that mother's milk is best (not only because the health professionals say so but because she has read and understands the differences between breast and formula milk), or perhaps because her family or culture says it is the thing to do. Each reason involves the ethical principle of autonomy (self-determination or choice by the woman). Her reasons include values held by her and members of her family.

Values are the attitudes or beliefs that describe how you feel about something or toward someone else. Values are also attitudes or beliefs that are practiced as you interact with other people or that guide the decisions you make in life. You have many values; you grew up with them.

ETHICAL MANDATE FOR NURSING

There is an ethical dimension to every nursing situation. People interacting with other people need to act responsibly; they need to respect one another, and they need to care about each other. Self-respect and caring for oneself play a large role in this interaction. All of these behaviors are based on ethical principles: respect for human dignity, caring, and competence in professional practice. Because you will deal with people, you will need to know and understand ethics and to practice in an ethical manner. You will need to understand how your and your client's morals and values influence the decisions or choices you make.

DETERMINATION OF "RIGHT"

Personal Values

As you were growing up, many people gave you advice and direction on the right or wrong thing to do or say. Parents and families are important sources for learning values. So, too, are religious groups, schoolmates, and books and television. Even your neighborhood and the amount of money your family had were important influences on the values you now have.

Personal values that could influence the practice of maternal-infant nursing include ideas about life in general, procreation, sex within marriage, parenting, love, telling the truth, the golden rule, suffering, and pain. You will be asked to care for many women who share your personal values. You will also take care of women who do not share your values. For example, what should you do when a 14-year-old preparing for the birth of her first child asks you to "put her to sleep" so she won't feel any more pain, but you know that "sleep" might injure the infant? The first step in analyzing a conflict is to remember that respect for another person and their values does not mean you have to agree with them. Your professional judgment is also worthy of respect, though you must remember that it may be a value with which the client disagrees.

Professional Values

The nursing profession has its own standards of proper conduct (moral behavior) for nurses. These values or moral standards are stated in the ANA *Code for Nurses with Interpretive Statements* (1986). The code says nurses should practice with respect for human dignity and support client choice. Nurses should also practice in a competent and responsible manner (accountability) and protect clients from the "unethical, illegal or immoral actions" of anyone else. Again, respecting client choice does not always mean that she has made the right decision for herself or her infant. A need for objective, professional judgment remains.

The nursing profession expects nurses to understand and practice safe care. Nurses should always balance safety with client preferences. In the example of the 14-year-old in labor, the nurse should explain the danger of general anesthesia for the baby and then try to find another, safer method of relieving the girl's pain. This approach provides safe care for both baby and girl without harming either.

The ANA code states that nurses are morally obligated to provide care without discrimination. You may disagree with a choice a client or family has made, but you cannot abandon them. If a choice is appropriate or correct for a woman, you must care for her, at least until another nurse is available to provide care.

Personal and professional values sometimes conflict. Nurses are expected to overcome personal bias and provide respectful care to all clients. It is also wrong for you to impose your values on clients, especially without knowledge or admitting it. When your most deeply held values are called into question, however, you may be supported in refusing to care for a patient. The Church Amendment was passed by the federal government in the wake of the early abortion controversy. This amendment allows health professionals who are morally opposed to abortion and other legal health care options to refuse to care for women selecting them. However, your employer needs to know about your beliefs ahead of time so another health professional can be found to provide care.

Moral Development as Moral Authority

Piaget and Kohlberg spent many years studying how human beings develop intellectually and morally. Kohlberg's cross-cultural theory of moral development offers some insight into how individuals make moral choices (choices of right or wrong).

Kohlberg's first level of moral development, preconventional, has two stages. In the first stage, persons determine what the right thing is based on whether they will receive a reward or punishment. People functioning at this stage of moral development may decide that driving the speed limit is wrong because they will get a ticket (punishment) if they are caught speeding. At the second stage, people do good things for others so they can get something in return, even though they are not really interested in helping others.

Most adults in our society function at the second level of moral development, the conventional level. At this level of Kohlberg's model, "right" is defined by individuals in positions of authority. For example, a staff nurse may decide to follow a physician's advice for a patient because the nurse believes the physician is always right. The law becomes the moral authority for right or wrong; for example, a man might drive 55 miles per hour on the highway, not because he might get a ticket, but because it is the law and the law is right.

Nurses who place their moral authority in others (e.g., head nurse, doctor, client, law or hospital rules) often practice in an ethical manner. They also have fewer options for action because they believe that authority figures are always right. Even when thinking another choice is better, this nurse will still follow the authority figure. Many suggest that nurses functioning at the conventional level of morality are better prepared to care for others than nurses at the preconventional level. The latter often practice in fear of punishment, especially a lawsuit, and may not be able to make decisions in the best interests of their clients. Fear rather than concern for the client drives their decision making.

At both of these levels of moral development, nurses may face conflict when others hold values and moral positions different from their own. They will favor the action that will avoid punishment or that agrees with the authority figure, however, even if the client disagrees.

The postconventional level of morality allows individuals to choose from ethical principles, rather than other persons or fear, as guides for right and wrong. The major guide at this level is *utilitarianism,* the action or choice that will result in the greatest good for the greatest number of people. Few individuals function consistently at this level, however.

SYSTEMS OF ETHICAL THOUGHT

There are many different values, moral standards, and ethical principles in the world. Ethical principles are familiar ideas such as to tell the truth, to practice the golden rule, do good and not harm; and for nursing, *client autonomy, quality and sanctity of life,* and *justice and mercy.*

The ethical principle of respect for persons is based on the idea that persons should never be treated as objects or used for gain. Kant proposed this idea more than 200 years ago, but we forget it occasionally in health care. You must remember that every human being, despite age, physical or mental condition, work status, or educational level, is worthy of respect.

Clients too young or too weak to speak for themselves need special protection in health care. When caring for newborns and children, you will need to use special caution in deciding their best interests. Nurses often ask parents to make decisions for their infant on the assumption that they will do what is best for their own child. There may be occasions when this assumption is not true, and you may need to seek another person to represent the infant, such as a court-appointed guardian.

A person may justify, based on ethical principles, why a particular action or response is chosen. For example, when a premature infant is born with little hope of survival, health professionals often ask whether they should treat the infant or allow him to die. Often, this decision, although very emotional and heart-wrenching, is reached on the basis of the quality of life the infant will have if life-sustaining treatment is begun. Other persons use the ethical principle of *vitalism,* or life at all costs, to justify any and all treatment, even though this treatment sometimes causes great harm to the ill neonate. Thus, a nurse must weigh the risks and benefits of treatment versus nontreatment, as well as ethical and moral principles. Most decision making in health and illness requires some balancing of principles and some balancing of risks or harms and benefits.

Utilitarianism

Nurses sometimes cause immediate harm or pain for clients when caring for them. It hurts a newborn baby when he is given an injection of vitamin K. A cesarean section to save an infant in distress is major surgery for the mother. How are these hurts justified? One system of ethical thought holds that persons should do no harm. Some deny harm by saying that procedures do not really hurt. Others turn to utilitarianism for ethical justification. This system of ethical thought suggests that immediate or short-term pain or harm can be tolerated when greater harm is avoided. Immunization, medication to cure disease, or surgery can hurt but can also save lives. This system of thought views these interventions as *good ends,* and therefore they are justified.

Utilitarianism is also defined as actions or decisions that promote the greatest happiness or usefulness for the greatest number of people. Concepts of justice may be viewed as part of utilitarianism. For example, several years ago, visiting hours for maternity wards reflected the same rules used in the rest of the hospital, meaning that any child under 15 could not visit the mother or new sibling and that fathers could only come 2 to 3 hours a day. These general hospital rules were established to avoid infections from children to already ill clients and to control traffic patterns and congestion in busy hospital corridors. Recently, hospital maternity wards have recognized the value in sibling visitation, unrestricted visiting hours for fathers and grandparents, and rooming-in for family development, and the utilitarian-based hospital rules were changed.

Natural Law

Some describe and use a third system of ethical thought to justify health care actions and decisions. *Natural law* evaluates the correctness of actions on the basis of what is natural or the natural purpose of human beings and body organs. For example, contraception is viewed as morally wrong by some conservative religious traditions. They claim the purpose of sexual intercourse is to reproduce. Therefore any action or device used to interfere with procreation is viewed as wrong by these groups and individuals. Natural law may also be the basis for opposition to artificial insemination, in vitro fertilization, surrogate motherhood, and medicated childbirth.

Natural law for some would justify refusal of the use of any biomedical technology or care. However, this refusal is rarely interpreted as total opposition because nurses have the capacity to help these individuals recover from illness and maintain their health. In addition, groups that refuse technologic interventions are as healthy or healthier during childbearing than those who demand them. When a person is dying, however, these persons are willing to let nature take its course rather than prolong the dying. They could argue that care and comfort should be the goals of medical and nursing care, rather than invasive treatments, surgery, and medications intended to cure when a cure is no longer possible.

The naturalistic fallacy is a false view of nature. In nature, animals get sick and die without health care. Some see nature as good, so whatever happens naturally is good. Others claim this is false. Animals starve to death. That does not mean it is right for them or for humans. For people with these beliefs, all health care can be seen as a violation of nature.

Some health care providers turn the naturalistic fallacy into a technologic fallacy. For example, a baby is dying, but technology is available to keep him alive in a handicapped condition. Some say the technology must be used at all costs. Others say that the technologic imperative is false: it may allow interns to be trained, but it uses persons for the needs of others rather than focuses on the client's well-being. The *technologic imperative* may do more harm than good. It may cause suffering—iatrogenic illness—rather than relieve it. Therefore *merely having the machinery does not mean we should use it.* Sometimes there are other reasons for using technology, including making money for the hospital, giving interns practice, giving doctors medical triumphs, or making nurses feel good. But these do not offset the suffering of the client and the violation of the ethical norms of health care.

Ethical Pluralism

We live in a society that supports ethical pluralism (e.g., several systems of ethical justification for making the right decision or choice). We have just reviewed principles of vitalism, utilitarianism, and natural law. We have also discussed the value systems we hold and differing levels of moral development that explain some of our choices in life and in health care. Because of these different systems, it is easy to understand how, at times, intelligent, sensitive, and caring individuals may make decisions that seem contradictory.

Ethical decision making implies that you have taken the time to understand the choices available. You have gathered information to make sure you understand all the ethical principles and values involved. You have tried to understand the consequences of your choices and then have selected the option that best fulfills what you and others define as good or right. Ethical decision making does not automatically imply that everyone agrees with your choice. At the very least, however, all individuals involved should understand why the choice was made. It is not easy to make good or right decisions as a nurse, but it is required nonetheless.

PROCESS FOR ETHICAL DECISION MAKING

Ethical decision making is a complex process because it is based on *moral reasoning,* analyzing, weighing, justifying, choosing, and evaluating attitudes, behaviors, and actions. This process of critically examining the moral and ethical dimensions of nursing care takes into account personal and professional values, levels of moral development, and ethical theories used to justify choices of action. All individuals affected by the decision are included in this process because of the shift away from the health professional's knowing what is best for clients (paternalism) and the shift toward clients' defining their own goals of health care and sharing the decision making with professionals. To make good decisions as a nurse, you need to know and understand yourself—what you value, what you believe, and to what you are committed in nursing care.

Good decisions require time. It is hard to think critically in an emergency, especially when quick action is needed to save a life. Even when a lot of time is available, however, you must use it to think critically about the options available for nursing care. You must be willing to ask questions and to gather information that will help you to understand as much about the client and her situation as possible. You must also be willing to listen to the client's preferences and reasons for making a decision. You must help her sort out the risks, benefits, costs, good, and harms of each choice.

Good decision making also requires that you know whether your personal values influence the information you share with a client about her condition and thereby bias her for or against an option. You must understand how you decide what is right or wrong. If fear of lawsuit or loss of your job is a primary force in what you decide to do as a nurse, for example, your clients may lose some autonomy in decision making. Understanding the client's sources of moral authority can also help in sorting through conflicts. If the client lacks the capacity to make a decision, whether by age (infant), severe pain (difficult labor), or unconsciousness (anesthesia), others (for example, parents, spouses, and physicians) will need to be involved so good decisions can be made.

The decision model in Box 30-1 can be used to analyze the ethical dimensions of maternal-infant care and nursing practice. It includes elements of decision theory, moral reasoning, applied ethics, and factors that might hinder decision making in clinical practice. Use this model to analyze the ethical dimensions of your practice as a nurse. It works best when a group of individuals analyze the same case, but it can also be used by an individual.

Ethical Concerns in Maternal-Infant Nursing

We have focused on ethical decision making because many of the major concerns or issues in bioethics today can be found in maternal-infant nursing. Issues related to contraception or family planning, abortion, and genetics precede childbearing. Issues related to how, with whom, and when to conceive are evident when

BOX 30-1 Thompson and Thompson Bioethical Decision Model

Step one

Review the situation to determine:
- Health problems
- Decisions needed
- Key individuals

Step two

Gather additional information to:
- Clarify the situation
- Understand why that information is needed
- Understand legal constraints, if any

Step three

Identify the ethical issues or concerns in the situation:
- Explore historical roots
- Explore current philosophical and religious positions
- Explore current societal views

Step four

Define personal and professional moral positions on the issues and concerns identified in Step three, including:
- Review of personal constraints raised by issues
- Review of professional codes for guidance
- Identification of conflicting loyalties and obligations

Step five

Identify moral positions of key individuals involved

Step six

Identify value conflicts, if any, and attempt to understand basis for conflict and possible resolution

Step seven

Determine who should make the needed decisions

Step eight

Identify the range of possible actions:
- Describe anticipated outcome for each action
- Include moral justification for each action
- Decide which actions fit criteria for decision making in this situation

Step nine

Decide on course of action and carry it out:
- Know reasons for choice of action
- Explain reasons to others
- Establish time frame for review of outcomes

Step ten

Evaluate the results of the decision and action:
- Did the expected outcomes occur?
- Is a new decision needed?
- Was the decision process complete?

Modified from Thompson JE, Thompson HO: *Bioethical decision making for nurses,* Norwalk, Conn, 1985, Appleton-Century-Crofts.

considering conception. People with traditional moral standards insist that conception should occur only within marriage, but in and outside of marriage, millions of people do not consider conception; they just get pregnant. The issues of unwanted pregnancy are ethical and moral ones. Because of the rise in world population and strain on resources, the area of preventive care in childbearing assumes greater importance. Issues of appropriate use of biomedical technology during pregnancy, labor, and birth, and in the care of seriously ill neonates highlight the technologic imperative.

Biomedical technology has progressed rapidly in maternal-infant care in recent decades. The availability of cesarean births in this century saved many babies and women from death. However, it is now said that this procedure is used too often and may cause more harm than good for some women. Electronic fetal monitoring promised hope of saving babies in distress during labor; yet when used inappropriately, it can cause psychologic harm, as well as financial harm, to the woman and her infant. Nurses are caught by the technologic imperative. Health care providers and families believe they must save infants because they can do it. Many ethicists, professionals, and clients suggest otherwise, however.

Technology is useful as an adjunct to clinical decision making. It never was intended to replace it. The technologic imperative is a naturalistic fallacy. You must remember that technology is useful in monitoring the fetal heart rate but must never forget to care for the woman and child attached to the machine.

In all aspects of family care during childbearing, you will be faced with the daily concerns of respect for human dignity, allocation of scarce resources, and ethical practice. These are the "ordinary ethics" for ordinary nursing practice. Many have suggested that the true measure of our morality as human beings is what we do when no one else is looking. Your ethics determine what you do from minute to minute in caring for childbearing families rather than what you do when a special situation occurs (e.g., whether to treat an immature infant).

Much of what you will learn in maternal-infant nursing is based on the idea that pregnancy and childbearing are natural, normal events. They are happy events for many families but not for all. Because childbearing is a healthy process, the nurse needs to orient care giving to the health of her clients and the prevention of disease. Because health during pregnancy is the responsibility of the pregnant woman or couple, the nurse's primary role is to offer information, support the healthy behaviors of the woman or couple, and encourage self-care. Self-care requires that women be motivated to be healthy and that they receive information that they can understand and use. This sharing of information involves the ethical principles of truth-telling, informed consent with minimal bias, and respect for the humanness of each client and family. Sharing knowledge requires you to have an adequate and up-to-date knowledge base, as well as competence in nursing practice and especially competence in ethics and health care.

SELECTED ETHICAL DILEMMAS

Birth of a Disabled Child

Naturally, the birth of a healthy child is the ideal, but this ideal is not always achieved. For some parents a child of the "wrong" sex or "wrong" coloring is a disappointment. Others must face a baby partially or overwhelmingly deformed. When the child is healthy, the system clearly acts as an advocate and does everything in its power to help the infant thrive. Children with many handicaps raise questions about whether life should be maintained regardless of the subsequent quality of that life. Currently, it is recognized that 25% of premature infants will have permanent moderate-to-severe neurologic impairment (Battle, 1987). An even larger number will have learning disabilities and subtle functional behavioral disorders not apparent until the child reaches school age (Avery, 1987) (see Chapters 27 and 28).

The utilitarian school of philosophy claims that decisions should be made using *the "greatest good" principle.* The cost of keeping low-birth-weight infants alive is staggering. Each tiny, premature infant who survives 2 to 4 months of hospitalization is charged in excess of $100,000 in medical bills (Avery, 1987). Some people argue that $100,000 for the first 4 months of life for one person (who may never be "normal") is not in the greatest good. The counter argument says that *each person is equally valuable and what is done to one must be universally applied to all others.* When the situation is viewed from this perspective, the premature infant of the physician in charge of the medical board must be treated in the same way as the premature infant of a poor teenage mother.

If you are unsure about whether to treat an infant, the best overall rule is to act. Erring on the side of action is always better than forever regretting inaction caused by the pressures of the situation.

However, action can create problems. Although the courts see no difference between withholding and withdrawing treatment, the consensus within the health care field is that once a treatment is started, it is difficult to stop it. Court input is often necessary before stopping a treatment. The important point to demonstrate is that continuation of the treatment is medically futile. When the infant is terminally ill, action may not be indicated because intervention will only prolong dying. The legal standard against which you are judged is always that behavior expected of a reasonable and prudent person acting in a similar situation. Because many hospitals have Infant Care Review Committees and "do not resuscitate" policies, potential conflict cases can be carefully reviewed and decisions made thoughtfully.

The applicable law in cases of handicapped newborns is Public Law 98-457, which amended the Child Abuse Prevention and Treatment Act in October 1984. This was a compromise solution after the regulations issued by the Reagan Administration were found to be unconstitutional. This legislation and its clarifying regulations define medical neglect as "withholding of medically indicated treatment from a disabled infant with a life-threatening condition" (Moreno, 1987). Withholding medically indicated treatment is further defined in the law as the following:

the failure to respond to the infant's life-threatening condition by providing treatment (including appropriate nutrition, hydration, and medications) which, in the treating physician's reasonable medical judgment, will be most likely to be effective in ameliorating or correcting all such conditions.... (Moreno, 1987).

If the parents of an infant refuse to consent to medically indicated treatment, they can be charged with child abuse. The hospital must go to court to get authorization for the treatment of the ill infant. The court will apply either the "best interests" or the "substituted judgment" standard to determine which action should be taken on behalf of the infant. The court will either name a guardian or authorize the treatment or nontreatment itself. The parents will be responsible for payment for the treatment of their infant, even if they do not consent to it.

Withholding Treatment

Three situations in which the condition of the newborn is so grave that treatment would not be indicated are specified in the child abuse amendments legislation. The three conditions that are exceptions to treatment are the following:

1. *The infant is chronically and irreversibly comatose.*
2. *The provision of such treatment would merely prolong dying,* not be effective in ameliorating or correcting all of the infant's life-threatening conditions, or otherwise be futile in terms of the survival of the infant.
3. *The provision of such treatment would be virtually futile in terms of the survival of the infant* and the treatment itself under such circumstances would be inhumane (Moreno, 1987).

Withdrawal of food and water from adults who are in a chronic vegetative state is increasingly recognized as a valid choice by the courts. Removal of food and fluid in neonates has yet to be addressed. The child abuse law requires "appropriate nutrition, hydration, and medication for all infants, including those comatose and born dying." In the legal cases involving adults, the court has made a distinction between removing food and discontinuing artificial feeding techniques such as gastrostomy and nasogastric tubes. The argument is that the feeding tube is a medical treatment and can be removed if its continuation is futile and the patient would refuse if competent. *Competence* means being able to make informed decisions. Infants have never been competent, and premature infants may not be able to take food naturally because of an inability to suck. Conceivably, the courts would again argue that food rather than medical treatment is being discontinued.

KEY POINTS

- There may be no right or wrong answer in ethical dilemmas, and each person's perspective must be heard and valued.
- In this heterogenous society, many cultures coexist side by side. The values of one group may conflict with the values of another, which generates laws that govern behavior.
- Law should be viewed both with respect and suspicion, and laws may be challenged.
- When laws and ethics clash, identify the dilemma, seek clarification, and work with others toward change.
- The professional standing of the perinatal nurse requires that standards of care are adhered to, demeanor is appropriate, and that documentation is complete.
- There are ways to reduce the risk of lawsuits. Professional nurses seek always to ensure informed consent, client's rights, and full communication.

- If unsure about whether to treat an infant, the best rule is to act.
- Decision making about fetal treatment when conflict is present may use four criteria: (1) How certain is the benefit to the client? (2) How great are the benefits? (3) How intrusive, coercive, or harmful will the treatment be to the mother? (4) Will anything be lost or gained by waiting until after birth?
- Decision making after birth must include the understanding that the statute of limitations does not expire for approximately 21 years after birth.
- In situations when the physician is not following through on treatment in a high-risk case, the nurse has the responsibility to report to an administrative officer, and to document the report.

STUDY QUESTIONS

30-1 Which of the chapter's Key Terms would apply below?
  a. The level of skill and training expected of every nurse _____ .
  b. The person bringing the lawsuit who claims to have been harmed _____ .
  c. The failure to act as a reasonable person _____ .
  d. Your best defense in court if you are sued _____ .
  e. The time period in which one must file a lawsuit _____ .
  f. The person who is sued _____ .
  g. A person who testifies in court about the appropriate standard of care _____ .
  h. The reasons we should decide on a given course of action _____ .
  i. Attitudes or beliefs that guide how one interacts with others _____ .

30-2 Which of the following are reasons why lawsuits are increasing?

  a. Clients often perceive a lack of personalism in health care delivery.
  b. Our society has a tendency to blame others rather than take responsibility for its own actions.
  c. Clients are better informed about health care issues now and are aware when an adverse outcome occurs.
  d. All of the above.

30-3 Which of the following contributes to the increased risk of lawsuits against perinatal nurses?
  a. Perinatal nurses are more likely than other nurses to make mistakes.
  b. Obstetric clients are well aware that there might be complications of pregnancy, and are prepared for them.
  c. Perinatal nurses are held to a higher standard of care and operate with more autonomy than many other nurses.
  d. The statute of limitations for minors is short, thereby limiting the amount of time to file a lawsuit.

30-4 Which of the following is *not* an element of informed consent?

a. The client should be informed as to how long she will be hospitalized.

b. The client should be told the nature of the procedure to be performed.

c. The client should be told the risks of the procedure to be performed.

d. The client should be told about alternative treatments that are available.

30-5 The nurse presents the Consent Form to the client for signature. The client states that she still has some questions about the proposed procedure. What should the nurse do?

a. Ask the client to sign the form, and tell her that you will inform the physician immediately about her concerns.

b. Delay having the client sign the form, and notify the physician that the client is requesting information.

c. Notify the supervisor to come and explain the procedure to the client.

d. Proceed with the preoperative medication orders so that the procedure is not delayed beyond its scheduled time.

30-6 Which of the following might result in a lawsuit being filed against a perinatal nurse?

a. Failing to use a fetal monitor when ordered or indicated

b. Failing to correctly interpret a fetal monitor tracing

c. Failing to report changes in the client's condition to the physician

d. All of the above

30-7 What four elements must be proven in order for a medical malpractice lawsuit to succeed?

a. The duty, the breach, the injury, and the proximate causation

b. The negligence, the proximate causation, the injury, and the neglect

c. The duty, the intent, the injury, and the proximate causation

d. The duty, the act, the omission, and the injury

30-8 Which of the following is a true statement?

a. As long as you are certain that you abided by the appropriate standard of care, you will win in court.

b. You can prove your case in court by "filling in the gaps" in your medical record documentation.

c. The jury will automatically know who is telling the truth and who is lying in court.

d. Your documentation in the medical record is your best defense if you are sued.

30-9 Which of the following is most likely to protect you from being sued for medical malpractice?

a. A professional liability insurance policy

b. A caring demeanor and thorough documentation

c. Avoiding nursing specialty areas that require increased autonomy

d. Following all doctor's orders without question

Answer Key

30-1 a. Standard of care, b. Plaintiff, c. Negligence, d. Documentation, e. Statute of limitations, f. Defendant, g. Expert witness, h. Ethics, i. Values 30-2 d 30-3 c 30-4 a 30-5 b 30-6 d 30-7 a 30-8 d 30-9 b

FOOTNOTES

[1] *Nelson v. Trinity Medical Center*, 419 N.W.2d 886 (1988)

[2] *Coleman v. Touro Infirmary of New Orleans*, 506 So.2d 571 (1987)

[3] *Coleman v. Touro Infirmary of New Orleans*, 506 So.2d 571 (1987)

[4] *Wheeler v. Yettie Kersting Memorial Hospital*, 761 S.W.2d 785 (1988), reported in The Regan Report on Nursing Law, Vol. 29, No. 10, March 1989

[5] *Wallace v. Wallace*, 421 A.2d 134 (1980)

[6] *Naccash v. Burger*, 290 S.E.2d 825 (1982)

[7] *Goldberg v. Ruskin*, 471 N.E.2d 530 (1984)

[8] *Alvis v. Henderson Obstetrics*, S.C., 592 N.E.2d 678 (1992), reported in The Regan Report on Nursing Law, Vol. 33, No. 4, September 1992

[9] *Ewing v. Aubert* 532 So.2d 876 (1988), reported in The Regan Report on Nursing Law, Vol. 29, No. 8, June 1989

[10] *Alef v. Alta Bates Hospital*, 6 Cal.Rptr.2d 700 (1992), reported in The Regan Report on Nursing Law, Vol. 33, No. 1, June 1992

[11] *Nelson v. Trinity Medical Center*, 419 N.W.2d 886 (1988)

[12] *Miles v. Box Butte County*, 489 N.W.2d 829 (1992), reported in The Regan Report on Nursing Law, Vol. 33, No. 7, December 1992

[13] *Garcia v. Providence Medical Center*, 806 P.2d 766 (1991), reported in The Regan Report on Nursing Law, Vol. 32, No. 12, May 1991

[14] *Fairfax Hospital System, Inc. v. McCarty*, 419 S.E.2d 621 (1992), reported in The Regan Report on Nursing Law, Vol. 33, No. 6, November 1992

[15] *Guzeldere v. Wallin*, 593 N.E.2d 629 (1992), reported in The Regan Report on Nursing Law, Vol. 33, No. 3, August 1992

[16] *Clancy v. Euclid General Hospital*, 584 N.E.2d 763 (1989), reported in The Regan Report on Nursing Law, Vol. 32, No. 10, March 1992

[17] *Osborne v. Annie Penn Memorial Hospital*, 381 S.E.2d 794 (1989), reported in The Regan Report on Nursing Law, Vol. 30, No. 5, October 1989

[18] *DeLeon v. Hospital of Albert Einstein College*, 566 N.Y.S.2d 213 (1991), reported in The Regan Report on Nursing Law, Vol. 31, No. 11, April 1991

[19] *May v. William Beaumont Hospital*, 418 N.W.2d 497 (1989), reported in The Regan Report on Nursing Law, Vol. 31, No. 1, June 1990

[20] *Collard v. Kentucky Board of Nursing*, 896 F.2d 179 (1990), reported in The Regan Report on Nursing Law, Vol. 30, No. 11, April 1990

[21] *Hiatt v. Grace*, 523 P.2d 320 (1974)

[22] *DeLeon Lopez v. Corporacion Insular DeSeguros*, 931 F.2d 116 (1991), reported in The Regan Report on Nursing Law, Vol. 32, No. 2, July 1991

REFERENCES

American Nurses Association: *Standards of Maternal and Child Nursing Practice,* ANA Publication No. MCH-3 10M, Dec 1983.

American Nurses Association: *Standards of Practice for the Perinatal Nurse Specialist,* ANA Publication No. MCH-15 5M, Dec 1984.

American Nurses Association: *A Statement on the Scope of High-Risk Perinatal Nursing Practice,* ANA Publication No. MCH-12 2M, Oct 1980.

Annas GJ, Elias S: Legal and ethical issues in perinatology. In Gabbe SG, Niebyl JR, Simpson JL, editors: *Obstetrics normal and problem pregnancies,* ed 2, 1991, Churchill-Livingstone.

Blank JJ: Electronic fetal monitoring nursing management defined, *Obstet Gynecol Neonatal Nurs* 14:5, Sept/Oct 1985.

Bulger D: The nursery as fortress, *Perinatal Press* 14:3, 1991.

Creighton H: Nurse's failure to follow physician's orders, *Nursing Management* 20:1, Jan 1989.

Eganhouse DJ: Electronic fetal monitoring education and quality assurance, *J Obstet Gynecol Neonatal Nurs* 20:1, Jan/Feb 1991.

Feutz-Harter SA: *Nursing and the law,* ed 4, 1991, Professional Education Systems, Inc.

Fiesta J: Criminal liability for the nurse. Part II, *Nursing Management* 23:5, May 1992.

Fiesta J: Security: Whose liability, infant kidnapping, *Nursing Management* 21:5, May 1990.

Grabenstein J: Nursing documentation during the perinatal period, *Perinat Neonat Nurs* 1:2, Oct 1987.

Greenlaw JL: Treatment refusal, noncompliance, and substance abuse in pregnancy: legal and ethical issues, *Birth* 17:3, Sept 1990.

Grossman SZ, Spence JB: The nature of lawsuits related to obstetric care. In Knuppel RA, Drukker JE: *High-risk pregnancy: a team approach,* Philadelphia, 1986, Saunders.

Kelly ME: Maternal and child health nursing. In Northrop CE, Kelly ME: *Legal issues in nursing,* St Louis, 1987, Mosby.

Kuhlman C: Surviving a malpractice suit, *J Nurse Midwifery* 35(3):166, 1990.

Mahoney D: Under oath: testifying against a physician, *AJN* 90(2):23, 1990.

NAACOG: Electronic fetal monitoring: nursing practice competencies and educational guidelines, Washington DC, 1986, NAACOG.

Pauerstein CJ: Medical-legal considerations in clinical obstetrics. In *Clinical obstetrics,* New York, 1987, Wiley Medical Publications.

Regan JT: Documentation for the defense, *Perinat Neonatal Nurs* 1:2, Oct 1987.

Rhodes AM: Parental notification, *Matern Child Nurs* 17, May/June 1992.

Rhodes AM: Parental prerogatives: Newmark v. Williams, *Matern Child Nurs* 17, July/Aug 1992.

Richards BC, Thomasson G: Closed liability claims analysis and the medical record, *Obstet Gynecol* 80:2, Aug 1992.

Rostow VP et al: Medical professional liability and the delivery of obstetrical care, *N Engl J Med* 321(15):1057, 1989.

Sise CB: Maternal rights versus fetal interests: an ethical issue with nursing implications, *J Prof Nurs* 4:4 July/Aug 1988.

Tammelleo AD: C-section delayed: accusations fly, *The Regan Report on Nursing Law* 29:10, Mar 1989.

Tammelleo AD: Fetal monitor delay: "proximate cause" issue, *The Regan Report on Nursing Law* 31:10, Mar 1991.

Ethical Issues

American Nurses Association: Code for nurses with interpretive statements, Kansas City, Mo, 1986, ANA.

Annas GJ: Protecting the liberty of pregnant patients, *N Engl J Med* 316:1213, 1987.

Aroskar M: Anatomy of an ethical dilemma: the theory and the practice, *Am J Nurs* 4:658, 1980.

Aroskar M: Are nurses' mind sets compatible with ethical practice? *Top Clin Nurs* 4:22, 1982.

Avery G: Ethical dilemmas in the treatment of the extremely low birth weight infant, *Clin Perinatol* 14(2):361, 1987.

Battle C: Beyond the nursery door: the obligation to survivors of technology, *Clin Perinatol* 14(2):417, 1987.

Bishop AH, Scudder JR: *The practical, moral, and personal sense of nursing: a phenomenological philosophy of practice,* Albany NY, 1990, State University of New York Press.

Brock DW, Wartman SA: When competent patients make irrational choices, *N Engl J Med* 322:1599, 1990.

Corea G: *The mother machine: reproductive technologies from artificial insemination to artificial wombs,* New York, 1985, Harper & Row.

Greenlaw JL: Treatment refusal, noncompliance, and substance abuse in pregnancy: legal and ethical issues, *Birth* 17(3):152, 1990.

Harron F, Burnside J, Beauchamp T: *Health and human values: a guide to making your own decisions,* New Haven, Conn, 1983, Yale University Press.

Jameton A: The nurse: when roles and rules conflict, *Hastings Cent Rep* 7(4):22, 1977.

Kant I: *Groundwork of the metaphysics of morals,* New York, 1964, Harper & Row, Publishers, Inc (translated by HJ Paton).

Kohlberg L: *Essays on moral development,* (vol 1), The philosophy of moral development, San Francisco, 1981, Harper & Row.

Kohlberg L: *Essays on moral development,* (vol 2), The psychology of moral development, New York, 1984, Harper & Row.

Lyon J: *Playing God in the nursery,* New York, 1985, WW Norton.

Mahon KA, Fowler MD: Symposium on bioethical issues in nursing: moral development and clinical decision-making, *Nurs Clin North Am* 14:3, 1979.

Macnaughton M: Ethics and reproduction, *Am J Obstet Gynecol* 162(4):879, 1990.

Moreno J: Ethical and legal issues in the care of the impaired newborn, *Clin Perinatol* 14(2):345, 1987.

Mohr JC: *Abortion in America,* New York, 1980, Oxford University Press.

Ozar D: The demands of profession and their limits. In Quinn CA, Smith, MD, eds: *The professional commitment: issues and ethics in nursing,* Philadelphia, 1987, WB Saunders.

Singer P, Wells D: *Making babies: the new science and ethics of conception,* New York, 1985, Scribner Book Companies, Inc.

Smith SJ, Davis AJ: Ethical dilemmas: conflicts among rights, duties, and obligations, *Am J Nurs* 80:1462, 1980.

Stanworth M, ed: *Reproductive technologies,* Minneapolis, 1987, University of Minnesota Press.

Steele S, Harmon V: *Values clarification in nursing,* ed 2, New York, 1983, Appleton-Century-Crofts.

Thompson JE, Thompson HO: *Ethics in nursing,* New York, 1981, Macmillan.

Thompson JE, Thompson HO: *Bioethical decision making for nurses,* Norwalk, Conn, 1985, Appleton-Century-Crofts.

Veatch RM, Fry SF: *Case studies in nursing ethics,* Philadelphia, 1987, JB Lippincott.

Watts JL et al: Ethical issues in infanticide of severely defective infants, *Can Med Assoc J* 136(9):920, 1987.

STUDENT RESOURCE SHELF

Fiesta J: Obstetrical liability, *Nursing Management* 22(5):5, 1991.

Tammelleo AD: Nurse fails to act: $9 million damages, *The Regan Report on Nursing Law* 29(7):2, 1988.

Tammelleo AD: Nursing notes can be worth their weight in gold, *The Regan Report on Nursing Law* 33(8):3, 1992.

Glossary

A

abortion Termination of pregnancy when the fetus weighs less than 500 g or loss of pregnancy before 139 days (20 weeks from last menstrual period)

spontaneous Without assistance; lay term: miscarriage

induced Deliberate interruption for therapeutic or nontherapeutic reasons (elective termination)

habitual Three or more consecutive spontaneous abortions

inevitable Progressive cervical dilation before week 20 without expulsion of fetus

incomplete Expulsion of some products of conception

complete Expulsion of all products of conception

missed Embryo or fetus dying in the uterus but retained for 8 or more weeks

abruptio placentae (premature separation) Separation of normally implanted placenta at 20 or more weeks of pregnancy, causing possible concealed or overt, visible bleeding

acceleration of fetal heart rate Increase in the fetal heart rate in response to fetal movement, contractions, or maternal medications

accoucheur Someone who assists in the delivery of a baby, such as obstetrician or midwife

acini (acinus) Smallest saccular division of a gland, occurring in grapelike clusters, as in the mammary gland

acrocyanosis Cyanotic or bluish discoloration of the hands and/or feet of the newborn as a result of inadequate circulation or coldness

active phase *See* labor

afterbirth Products of conception (excluding the baby) expelled during delivery; include placenta and membranes (sac) and umbilical cord. *Syn.*, secundines

afterpains Discomfort caused by the contraction of the uterus as it returns to its prepregnant condition after birth, usually occurring in the multipara

allele Two copies of the same gene—one from father, one from mother; also called matching genes

alpha-fetoprotein (AFP) Protein produced by fetal yolk sac and liver, detectable by 7 weeks gestation, and used for determining and identifying certain birth defects and chromosomal anomalies; *see also* maternal serum alpha-fetoprotein (MSAFP)

amenorrhea Cessation or absence of menstruation

amniocentesis Removal of some amniotic fluid from the amniotic sac using a needle inserted through the abdominal wall of the mother for the purpose of examining the fluid

amnioinfusion Technique of infusing fluid into the amniotic sac during labor via an intrauterine catheter

amnion Inner layer of the fetal membranes or sac, which secretes amniotic fluid

amniotic fluid embolism Rare postpartum occurrence, in which amniotic fluid enters the maternal circulation; the cells, debris, and fluid form emboli, usually in the lungs

amniotomy Rupturing of the amniotic sac by artificial means

androgens Hormones that help to produce male secondary sex characteristics; anabolic agents produced in the adrenal gland, testis, and ovary. *Syn.*, male hormone

anencephaly Malformation of the cranium frequently associated with spina bifida; the cranial vault is absent; the cerebellum and basal ganglia sometimes are present

anorexia Loss of appetite

a. nervosa Eating disorder based on fear of obesity and characterized by loss of appetite

anovulatory Associated with lack or absence of ovulation

anoxia (fetal) Severe oxygen deficiency caused by inadequate tissue perfusion; used interchangeably with but not the same as hypoxia

antenatal Prenatal, before birth

antepartal Occurring before labor and delivery

antibody Substance produced by the body for protection against the specific antigen that triggered its production

antigen Substance, usually of protein material, that triggers the production of antibodies and the immune response

Apgar score System of numerical evaluation of newborn status at 1 and 5 minutes of birth; based on heart rate, respiration, muscle tone, reflexes, and color

apnea Absence or cessation of respirations

areola Pigmented area surrounding the nipple

arrest of descent Labor complication in which the fetus fails to descend through the pelvic cavity and medical intervention is necessary to deliver the fetus

artifact Random marks on the fetal heart rate tracing

asphyxia Insufficient oxygen–carbon dioxide exchange, generally resulting in respiratory failure

birth or neonatal Insufficient exchange within 1 minute of birth

assisted birth Birth that involves the use of medication, instrumentation, or surgery

asymptomatic bacteriuria More than 10^5/ml of bacteria in the urine; no symptoms

attitude Relationship of the parts of the fetus to each other; usual attitude is flexion, that is, head flexed on chest, thighs folded on abdomen

autonomic dysreflexia Abnormal response to stimulation that occurs in spinal injuries and results in severe muscle spasms and hypertension

autosome Any one of the 44 chromosomes (22 pairs) present in females and males; contain genes necessary for bodily function—except for sexual determination and function—which is contained in the remaining pair of two sex chromosomes (XY or XX)

B

ballottement Rebounding movement of the fetus when uterus (or cervix) is tapped by the examiner. *Syn.,* passive fetal movement

Bandl's ring Retracted ring occurring between the lower and upper segments of the uterus

basal body temperature (BBT) Lowest usual temperature of the body taken before rising

baseline rate Rate of vital signs before stimulation; for fetal heart rate, before labor starts, during labor rate between contractions

bilirubin Red-orange pigment resulting from breakdown of hemoglobin, which can cause jaundice of the skin when the level rises above 5 mg/dl in the newborn

birth defect Any alteration in fetal growth and/or development that takes place in utero and that may be evident at birth or later. *Syn.,* congenital anomaly

blastocyst State in early development when fluid accumulates in the morula, producing the inner cell mass at one side while its wall develops into the trophoblast

boarder baby Infants who cannot be discharged to their parents for medical or social reasons

bradycardia Fetal heart rate below 120 beats/min

Braxton Hicks contractions Painless, intermittent contractions of the uterus that occur throughout pregnancy and often are mistaken for early labor contractions

breech Buttocks

breech presentation Delivery in which the buttocks or feet of the fetus appear first at the outlet

footling One or both feet appear first at the opening

frank Buttocks appear first

full or complete Buttocks and feet appear first at the pelvic brim

bulimia An eating disorder characterized by episodes of self-induced vomiting after bouts of overeating

C

caput Head

caput succedaneum Swelling or edema on the scalp occurring during labor or delivery

cephalhematoma Trauma of labor and delivery resulting in a collection of blood on the head of the fetus between the bone and the periosteum, defined by the suture lines

cephalopelvic disproportion (CPD) Fetus (fetal head) is too large to pass through the bony ring of pelvic cavity. *Syn.,* fetopelvic disproportion

cerclage procedure Procedure for the treatment of incompetent cervix; circling sutures

cesarean delivery or birth Surgical removal of the uterine contents by the abdominal route after fetal viability testing

chorioamnionitis Inflammation of the amnion and chorion (fetal sac, bag of waters) surrounding fetus

chorion Outermost membrane of the developing fetus, which gives rise to the fetal portion of the placenta and extends to form the other layer of the amniotic sac

chorionic gonadotropin Hormone produced by the chorion and excreted in the urine of the pregnant woman; its presence is a possible sign of pregnancy

chorionic villi Fingerlike projections of the chorion that invade the decidua basalis and form the fetal portion of the placenta

chromosome Units of DNA-containing hereditary material in each body cell; 23 are derived from each parent

cleavage Process of early cell division by which the zygote divides into blastomeres

cleft lip Congenital or genetic opening of the upper lip extending from the nares; may involve one or both nares

cleft palate Congenital or genetic opening of the roof of the mouth

colloid osmotic pressure (COP) The pressure made up of the various components of plasma that exerts influence over the movement of fluid across all membranes. *Syn.,* oncotic pressure

colonization Presence of microorganisms on an epithelial surface

colostrum Yellowish-white fluid expressed from the breast during pregnancy preceding the development of milk; caloric and cathartic values of this substance are questioned

conception Implantation of the blastocyst; not synonymous with fertilization

Coombs' test Blood test to determine the presence of antibodies

direct Determination of antibodies attached to blood cells, particularly maternal (anti-Rh) antibodies attached to fetal blood cells *indirect* Determination of free-floating or unattached antibodies, particularly those (anti-Rh) in the maternal circulation (serum)

corpus luteum Yellow body of material found in the site of the ruptured graafian follicle that persists for several months during pregnancy, secreting progesterone

cricoid pressure Application of pressure to the cricoid cartilage at the critical time of tracheal intubation to prevent aspiration of gastric fluids

crowning Appearance of the vertex, or head, at the external vaginal orifice

D

decidua Enriched endometrial lining of pregnancy shed after pregnancy termination
  basalis Portion of the endometrium underlying the embedded embryo and from which the maternal portion of the placenta is formed
  capsularis Outer portion of the decidua enveloping the embryo
  vera Remainder of the endometrium not containing the embedded embryo

desquamation Initial peeling of the newborn's skin, particularly the wrist and ankle; occurs primarily in postmature infants

developmental crisis Disruption of life caused by an event common to all in a particular age-group

diagnostic related groups (DRGs) System of determining the length of hospital stay to be covered by insurance; based on predefined medical diagnoses and treatments

dilation Enlargement of an organ or orifice
  of the cervix State of enlargement or opening of the cervix to allow for passage of the fetus

dilation and curettage (D&C) Surgical procedure involving dilation of the cervix and removal of uterine contents

dilation and evacuation (D&E) Removal of uterine lining and contents by dilating cervix and evacuating contents by suctioning

discharge (vaginal) Shedding of accumulated cells, mucus, or blood from the vagina

discoverable documents Those created in the care of a client that can be subpoenaed by a court and used to present evidence in a lawsuit

disease (infectious) Infections that produce physical complaints and signs and symptoms

disseminated intravascular coagulation (DIC) A bleeding/clotting malfunction that greatly complicates correction of hemorrhage

Down syndrome Formerly known as mongolism; a congenital or genetic abnormality in which 47 chromosomes are present. *Syn.,* trisomy 21 syndrome

dystocia Difficult, abnormal labor progress

E

eclampsia Abnormal reaction of the body to pregnancy, resulting in convulsions and possible coma; usually preceded by hypertension, albuminuria, and edema

ectopic pregnancy Pregnancy that does not implant in the usual uterine sites

effacement Thinning of the cervix to allow for passage of the fetus; in primigravidas, occurs before dilation, and in multigravidas, occurs with dilation

embryo Conception up to the tenth week after the last menstrual period or 8 weeks after fertilization

endometritis Inflammation of the endometrium

endometriosis Presence of endometrial tissue in the fallopian tube, peritoneum, or bladder, usually leading to infertility with signs of dysmenorrhea

engagement Descent of the fetus into the pelvic canal until the presenting part reaches the level of the ischial spines

engorgement Increase of blood and lymph in the breast, causing tenderness, firmness, and discomfort before onset of lactation

epidural anesthesia Loss of sensation as a result of injection of a local anesthetic drug into the epidural space

episiotomy Surgical incision of the perineum that enlarges the external vaginal opening to prevent laceration of the vulva, perineum, and adjacent structures

Epstein's pearls Tiny, white, beadlike epithelial cysts on the roof of the mouth of the newborn on either side of the median ridge; not to be confused with thrush, which is patchy

erythema toxicum Newborn rash; characteristically blotchy rash seen initially, which has no pathogenic cause

erythroblastosis fetalis Hemolytic disorder of the fetus or newborn in which maternal anti-Rh antibodies destroy fetal blood cells, causing jaundice and other effects

estrogenic hormone Hormone that can produce female secondary sexual characteristics. *Syn.,* female hormone

F

fertilization Process of penetration of secondary oocyte by spermatozoon; completed with fusion of male and female pronuclei. *Syn.,* syngamy

fertilization age Age from fertilization of the ovum to birth

fetal Pertaining to the fetus

fetal death Death in utero

fetus Offspring from the moment of conception until the pregnancy is terminated or completed

fontanelle Space at the junction of three or more fetal and cranial bones, covered with a tough membrane
  anterior junction of sagittal, frontal, and coronal sutures, or anterior portion of skull. *Syn.,* "soft spot," greater fontanelle
  posterior Junction of lambdoid and sagittal sutures. *Syn.,* lesser fontanelle

foramen ovale Opening between the right and left atria of the heart in the fetus; closes after birth

fundus Upper portion of the uterus

G

gap junction Cell-to-cell communication points that develop in uterine smooth muscle during the last week of pregnancy to facilitate coordinating muscle contractions

gaze aversion Avoiding looking at another person's face—particularly seen as a compensation in the overstimulated newborn

gingivitis Inflammation of the gums

G6PD Glucose-6-phosphate dehydrogenase deficiency; inherited erythrocyte enzyme deficiency

gene Functional unit of heredity, situated on a chromosome in the cell nucleus

genotype Assortment of genes of an individual

gestation Length of time necessary for intrauterine growth and development of the fetus

gestational age Estimated age of fetus using the first day of last normal menstrual period, expressed in completed weeks

    preterm Born up to 37 completed weeks (259 days after last menstrual period)

    term Born between 38 through 41 completed weeks (260-287 days)

    postterm Born after 288 days or beginning of the week 42

graafian follicle Fluid-filled sac in the ovary housing the maturing ovum

gravid Pregnant

gravida Pregnant woman

    primigravida Woman pregnant for the first time

    multigravida Woman pregnant for the second time or more

H

half-life (t½) Measurable amount of time in which half of a drug dose is metabolized in the body

hemorrhage In obstetrics, loss of blood in excess of 500 ml

heterozygous Presence of different genes at the same location on the DNA chain

homozygous Presence of identical genes at the same location on the DNA chain

horizontal transmission Passing of infection from one person to another

host defense mechanisms Occurs when all of the immune system functions (*see* immunity)

hyaline membrane disease *See* idiopathic respiratory distress syndrome (RDS)

hydatidiform mole Grapelike, cystic masses of degenerated chorionic villi, usually benign

hydramnios "Water"; excessive amniotic fluid. *Syn.,* polyhydramnios

hydrocephaly Abnormal accumulation of cerebrospinal fluid in the brain

hyperemesis gravidarum Excessive, severe vomiting during pregnancy

hypofibrinogenemia Reduced amounts of fibrinogen in the blood

hypospadias Congenital or genetic defect in which the urethra of the male opens on the underside of the penis

hypoxemia Oxygen deficiency in the blood

hypoxia Deficient amount of oxygen

I

icterus Jaundice

icterus gravis neonatorum *See* erythroblastosis fetalis

idiopathic respiratory distress syndrome Severe respiratory syndrome of the newborn or preterm infant resulting in the development of a hyaline membrane in the lungs; may be fatal. *Syn.,* RDS, hyaline membrane disease

immunity Specific response to antigens whereby specific antibodies, which ordinarily combine only with the antigen when the body is again invaded, are formed

    active Inoculation with specific antigens to promote antibody formation

    passive Extrinsic antibodies transferred to the fetus across the placental membrane or to the infant in milk or administered by intramuscular injection to infant, child, or adult; it has a time-limited effectiveness

inertia (uterine) Inefficient, weak, or absent uterine contractions

    primary Occurring early in labor

    secondary Occurring after labor is established. *Syn.,* uterine dysfunction

infant mortality rate Rate of death, per 1000 births of infants, from birth until the first birthday

inheritance pattern Scheme of inheritance of maternal or paternal genes by dominant, codominant, or recessive patterns

insemination Introduction of semen into the vagina

    artificial Concentrated semen introduced into vagina by syringe

    heterologous Semen used that is not from the woman's partner—artificial insemination donor (AID)

    homologous Semen from the woman's partner—artificial insemination, homologous (AIH)

involution Return of the pelvic organs and structures to their prepregnant state or condition

ischemia Reduction of blood supply to an area

J

jaundice Yellowish color of skin, sclera, mucous membrane, and excretions. *Syn.,* icterus

K

kernicterus Excessive bilirubin deposits in the brain, causing neurologic changes and possibly permanent brain damage or death

L

Labor

    active phase Cervical dilation from 4 to 10 cm

    accelerated Cervical dilation from 4 to 7 cm

    advanced Cervical dilation from 8 to 10 cm; also called transition

    latent phase Early labor; cervical dilation from 0 to 3 cm

    stages

    I—Full cervical dilation and effacement

    II—Descent and delivery of baby

    III—Delivery of baby to the delivery of placenta

    IV—Immediate recovery (optional stage)

lanugo Soft, fine, downy hair found on preterm and newborn infants

leukorrhea Excessive mucous discharge from genital tract; common in pregnancy, usually nonitchy and odorless

lightening Tilting or dropping of the fetus forward and downward into the true pelvis; occurs 2 or 3 weeks before the end of gestation in the primigravida or at the beginning of labor in many multigravidas

linea nigra Darkening of the abdominal line between the umbilicus and the symphysis pubis during pregnancy, caused by hormonal changes

lochia Uterine discharge after delivery that consists of the sloughing decidua, tissue, blood, and cells; lasts 2 or 3 weeks

low birth weight Weight at birth of less than 2500 g

M

mastalgia Pain in the breast

mastitis Inflammation of the breast

maternal death Death of any woman from any cause while pregnant or within 42 days of termination of pregnancy
  direct Resulting from obstetric complications
  indirect Resulting from previously existing problems and aggravated by effects of pregnancy
  nonmaternal Accidental causes not related to pregnancy or its management

maternal death rate Total number of maternal deaths per 100,000 deliveries regardless of gestational age

maternal serum alpha-fetoprotein (MSAFP) Elevated serum levels of alpha-fetoprotein in maternal blood samples. *See also* alpha-fetoprotein (AFP)

melasma Darkened patches of skin on the face and/or forehead caused by hormones of pregnancy; previously known as *chloasma*

menarche First menstrual flow

meningomyelocele Protrusion of the meninges and spinal cord through a defect in the spine

menopause Cessation of menses during middle age as part of the climacteric

menses *See* menstruation

menstruation Cyclic uterine discharge of blood, tissue, and cells as a result of hormonal changes in the body. *Syn.*, menses

mentum Chin

milia Tiny, white, or yellow beadlike sebaceous cysts found primarily on the face of the newborn

minimum effective concentration (MEC) Necessary level of a drug dissolved in the serum to cause a desired action

miscarriage Lay term for spontaneous abortion

mittelschmerz Lower abdominal pain generally associated with ovulation

molding Temporary changes in the shape of the head of the newborn as it accommodates to the birth canal during labor and delivery

mosiacism State of having two or more cell lines in a single person

multigravida Woman who has been pregnant more than once

multipara Woman who has delivered more than once

mutation Change in chromosomal integrity that may be passed to the next generation

N

neonatal Referring to the newborn infant

neonatal death rate Number of deaths of live-born infants, per 1000 live births, from the time of birth to the beginning of day 28 of life

neonatal period From the hour of birth through 27 days, 23 hours, and 59 minutes of life

nephrotoxic Any substance or material that exerts a poisonous effect on the kidney

newborn infant Living infant during the first 27 days, 23 hours and 59 minutes of its life

nidation Embedding of the fertilized ovum into the lining of the uterus

nociperception Initiation of pain signals, the cause of which is not always quickly determined

nondisjunction Failure of chromosomes at a pair to separate during meiosis, resulting in one cell containing the pair and the other cell having neither chromosome

nulligravida Woman who has never been pregnant

nullipara Woman who has never delivered a viable baby

O

occiput Back of the head; occipital bone

oligohydramnios Abnormally small amount of amniotic fluid

ophthalmia neonatorum Acute, purulent conjunctivitis of the eyes of the newborn, usually caused by gonococcal infection

organogenesis Growth of tissues of the fetus into organs during the first 12 weeks

osteoporosis Sequela of menopause, characterized by loss of calcium from bone tissue, leading to bone fragility

ototoxic Substance or material poisonous to the ear

oxytocin Synthetic or natural substance that stimulates the uterus to contract

ovulation Release of the ovum from the graafian follicle

ovum Female reproductive cell

P

papilledema Edema of the optic nerve causing visual disturbances especially in preeclamptic/eclamptic clients

parity State of having given birth to an infant of 500 g or more, whether alive or stillborn; multiple births are considered one parous delivery

pelvimetry Clinical determination of pelvic size by internal or external measurements

perinatal death rate Rate of death of viable infants from week 20 in utero until the end of the neonatal period

pharmacokinetics Movement of drugs within biologic systems, as affected by uptake, distribution, biotransformation, and elimination

phenotype Way genetic inheritance is expressed overtly in an individual

phenylketonuria (PKU) Genetic disorder involving the deficiency of the enzyme phenylalanine hydroxylase

phototherapy Treatment of hyperbilirubinemia by exposure to light

pica Craving for nonfood substances such as ice, starch, or clay

placenta previa Abnormally low implantation of the placenta in the uterus

polyhydramnios Excessive amniotic fluid. *Syn.,* hydramnios

position Relationship of a designated point on the presenting part of the fetus to a designated point in the maternal pelvis; is divided into four quadrants

postpartum Period of time after delivery

preeclampsia Abnormal bodily reaction to pregnancy characterized by edema, hypertension, and proteinuria and occurring after week 20 of pregnancy; often referred to as toxemia

premature infant Infant born up through 37 completed weeks of gestation. *Syn.,* preterm infant

presentation Relationship of the long axis of the fetus to the long axis of the mother. *Syn.,* lie

presenting part Anatomic part of the fetus closest to the cervix and felt by the examiner during vaginal or rectal examination; usually the head or buttocks

primigravida Woman pregnant for the first time

primipara Woman who has delivered for the first time a viable infant (over 20 weeks' gestation)

prostaglandins Substances found in all body tissues that stimulate or inhibit smooth muscle activity

pruritus Itching

pseudocyesis False pregnancy

puerperium 42 days after birth

Q

quickening First active movements of the fetus detectable by the mother at approximately 16 to 18 weeks of gestation

R

respiratory distress syndrome (RDS) *See* idiopathic respiratory distress syndrome

respondeat superior "Let the master answer"; commonly interpreted in health care as: let the employer answer for the action of its employees

resuscitation Restoration of breathing, life, or consciousness of one who is apparently dead and whose respirations have ceased

retrolental fibroplasia (RLF) Fibrous membrane that may occur behind the lens in the eye as a result of high oxygen concentration administered to a preterm infant

risk-taking behaviors Persisting in a behavior such as smoking during pregnancy despite knowing of its potential harm

rugae Transverse folds of the vaginal mucous membrane

S

scotoma Blind spot in visual field

show Blood-tinged mucous discharge occurring during labor as the cervix dilates. *Syn.,* bloody show

situational crisis Disruption in life caused by an event that occurs randomly and independently of normal life events; generally unexpected and may be quite unusual

socially high risk condition Condition complicated by a variety of social problems, including substance abuse, homelessness, and economic, educational, or intellectual deprivation

spermatozoon Male reproductive cell. *Syn.,* sperm

spinnbarkeit Changes in the stretchability of the cervical mucosa during ovulation

station Location of the presenting part in relation to the ischial spines of the birth canal

statute of limitations Limited period of time, differing from state to state, between occurrence of an untoward incident and the filing of a lawsuit

stillborn Fetus of more than 20 weeks' gestation, born without life

striae gravidarum Reddened or bluish streaks in the skin of the breast, buttocks, or abdomen of pregnant women, fading to silvery gray or brown scar tissue after birth

subinvolution Delay in the return of pelvic organs and structures to their prepregnant state

supine hypotensive syndrome Hypotension resulting from the pressure of the enlarged uterus on the vena cava, blocking venous return

suture
  of the fetal or infant skull Line of cartilage separating the bony plates of the skull
  of a wound Line approximating two aspects of a wound; may be stapled, clipped, or sewn together

syncope Fainting or ligthheadedness; common in early pregnancy

T

tachycardia (fetal or newborn) Heart rate greater than 160 beats/min

teratogen Agent or substance that can alter fetal growth and development

term infant Live baby born after 38 to 42 weeks of gestation (from time of last menstrual period). *Syn.,* full-term infant

thrombocytopenia Low blood platelet count

thrush White, patchy oral lesions of the newborn caused by *Candida albicans*

toxemia *See* preeclampsia; eclampsia

toxin Poisonous substance that may be part of a cell or tissue or may be excreted by the cell

toxoid Toxin treated so that its toxic properties are destroyed but is still capable of initiating the immune response and therefore of inducing immunity in the host

tracheoesophageal fistula Congenital or genetic disorder in which the esophagus and trachea are connected or the esophagus ends in a blind pouch and there is a lower connection in the trachea to the esophagus

Trichomonas vaginalis Protozoan infection of the vagina; Skene's ducts and urinary tract also may be infected

trimester Approximately one third of the gestational period calculated from the last menstrual period
  first First day of the last normal menstrual period through 14 weeks' gestation
  second Weeks 15 through 28 of gestation
  third Weeks 29 through 41 of gestation and birth

U

ultrasonography Use of ultrasonic waves to obtain visual or telemetric measurements in diagnosing pregnancy and assessing gestational age and fetal condition or size

umbilical cord Life line between the fetus and placenta through which nourishment and waste pass; contains two arteries and one vein surrounded by Wharton's jelly. *Syn.,* funis

V

vacuum extraction Application of a suction cap to the fetal head to assist in delivery during the second stage of labor

Valsalva's maneuver Bradycardia; increased intraabdominal pressure and reduced venous return caused by holding breath and keeping the glottis closed while pushing during delivery

variability Degree of change in fetal heart rate within 1 minute

variable deceleration Fall in fetal heart rate in response to cord compression

vena caval syndrome (VCS) *See* supine hypotensive syndrome

vernix caseosa Cheeselike covering on the fetus that protects the skin from the drying and wrinkling properties of the amniotic fluid

vertex Head

vertex presentation Fetal position with the head against the inner cervix

vertical transmission Passage of infection from the pregnant woman to the fetus through the placenta or to the newborn through the birth canal or breast milk

viability Capability of survival; more than 20 weeks gestation

W

Wharton's jelly Gelatinous connective tissue surrounding the umbilical vessels and giving support to the umbilical cord

Z

zona Zone; belt or girdle

zygote Fertilized ovum

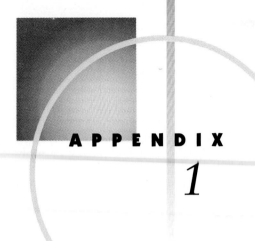

The Pregnant Patient's Bill of Rights

The Pregnant Patient has the right to participate in decisions involving her well-being and that of her unborn child, unless there is a clearcut medical emergency that prevents her participation. In addition to the rights set forth in the American Hospital Association's "Patient's Bill of Rights," the Pregnant Patient, because she represents TWO patients rather than one, should be recognized as having the following additional rights*:

1. *The Pregnant Patient has the right,* prior to the administration of any drug or procedure, to be informed by the health professional caring for her of any potential direct or indirect effects, risks or hazards to herself or her unborn or newborn infant which may result from the use of a drug or procedure prescribed for or administered to her during pregnancy, labor, birth or lactation.

2. *The Pregnant Patient has the right,* prior to the proposed therapy, to be informed, not only of the benefits, risks and hazards of the proposed therapy but also of known alternative therapy, such as available childbirth education classes which could help to prepare the Pregnant Patient physically and mentally to cope with the discomfort or stress of pregnancy and the experience of childbirth, thereby reducing or eliminating her

*From Haire DB: The pregnant patient's bill of rights, *J Nurse Midwifery* 20:29, 1975; from Committee on Patient's Rights, Box 1900, New York, NY 10001.

need for drugs and obstetric intervention. She should be offered such information early in her pregnancy in order that she may make a reasoned decision.

3. *The Pregnant Patient has the right,* prior to the administration of any drug, to be informed by the health professional who is prescribing or administering the drug to her that any drug which she receives during pregnancy, labor and birth, no matter how or when the drug is taken or administered, may adversely affect her unborn baby, directly or indirectly, and that there is no drug or chemical which has been proven safe for the unborn child.

4. *The Pregnant Patient has the right* if cesarean birth is anticipated, to be informed prior to the administration of any drug, and preferably prior to her hospitalization, that minimizing her and, in turn, her baby's intake of nonessential preoperative medicine will benefit her baby.

5. *The Pregnant Patient has the right,* prior to the administration of a drug or procedure, to be informed of the areas of uncertainty if there is *no* properly controlled follow-up research which has established the safety of the drug or procedure with regard to its direct and/or indirect effects on the physiological, mental and neurological development of the child exposed, via the

mother, to the drug or procedure during pregnancy, labor, birth or lactation—(this would apply to virtually all drugs and the vast majority of obstetric procedures).

6. *The Pregnant Patient has the right*, prior to the administration of any drug, to be informed on the brand name and generic name of the drug in order that she may advise the health professional of any past adverse reaction to the drug.

7. *The Pregnant Patient has the right* to determine for herself, without pressure from her attendant, whether she will accept the risks inherent in the proposed therapy or refuse a drug or procedure.

8. *The Pregnant Patient has the right* to know the name and qualifications of the individual administering a medication or procedure to her during labor or birth.

9. *The Pregnant Patient has the right* to be informed, prior to the administration of any procedure, whether that procedure is being administered to her for her or her baby's benefit (medically indicated) or as an elective procedure (for convenience, teaching purposes or research).

10. *The Pregnant Patient has the right* to be accompanied during the stress of labor and birth by someone she cares for, and to whom she looks for emotional comfort and encouragement.

11. *The Pregnant Patient has the right* after appropriate medical consultation to choose a position for labor and for birth which is least stressful to her baby and to herself.

12. *The Obstetric Patient has the right* to have her baby cared for at her bedside if her baby is normal, and to feed her baby according to her baby's needs rather than according to the hospital regimen.

13. *The Obstetric Patient has the right* to be informed in writing of the name of the person who actually delivered her baby and the professional qualifications of that person. This information should also be on the birth certificate.

14. *The Obstetric Patient has the right* to be informed if there is any known or indicated aspect of her or her baby's care or condition which may cause her or her baby later difficulty or problems.

15. *The Obstetric Patient has the right* to have her and her baby's hospital medical records complete, accurate and legible and to have their records, including Nurses' Notes, retained by the hospital until the child reaches at least the age of majority, or to have the records offered to her before they are destroyed.

16. *The Obstetric Patient*, both during and after her hospital stay, *has the right* to have access to her complete hospital medical records, including Nurses' Notes, and to receive a copy upon payment of a reasonable fee and without incurring the expense of retaining an attorney.

It is the obstetric patient and her baby, not the health professional, who must sustain any trauma or injury resulting from the use of a drug or obstetric procedure. The observation of the rights listed above will not only permit the obstetric patient to participate in the decisions involving her and her baby's health care, but will help to protect the health professional and the hospital against litigation arising from resentment or misunderstanding on the part of the mother.

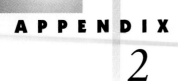

A P P E N D I X

2

Newborn Metric Conversion Tables

Weight (Mass): Pounds and Ounces to Grams

Example: To obtain grams equivalent to 6 lb 8 oz, read "6" on top scale, "8" on side scale; equivalent is 2948 g.

		POUNDS (lb)													
		0	1	2	3	4	5	6	7	8	9	10	11	12	13	14
	0	0	454	907	1361	1814	2268	2722	3175	3629	4082	4536	4990	5443	5897	6350
	1	28	482	936	1389	1843	2296	2750	3203	3657	4111	4564	5018	5471	5925	6379
	2	57	510	964	1417	1871	2325	2778	3232	3685	4139	4593	5046	5500	5953	6407
	3	85	539	992	1446	1899	2353	2807	3260	3714	4167	4621	5075	5528	5982	6435
O	4	113	567	1021	1474	1928	2381	2835	3289	3742	4196	4649	5103	5557	6010	6464
U	5	142	595	1049	1503	1956	2410	2863	3317	3770	4224	4678	5131	5585	6038	6492
N	6	170	624	1077	1531	1984	2438	2892	3345	3799	4252	4706	5160	5613	6067	6520
C	7	198	652	1106	1559	2013	2466	2920	3374	3827	4281	4734	5188	5642	6095	6549
E	8	227	680	1134	1588	2041	2495	2948	3402	3856	4309	4763	5216	5670	6123	6577
S	9	255	709	1162	1616	2070	2523	2977	3430	3884	4337	4791	5245	5698	6152	6605
(OZ)	10	283	737	1191	1644	2098	2551	3005	3459	3912	4366	4819	5273	5727	6180	6634
	11	312	765	1219	1673	2126	2580	3033	3487	3941	4394	4848	5301	5755	6209	6662
	12	340	794	1247	1701	2155	2608	3062	3515	3969	4423	4876	5330	5783	6237	6690
	13	369	822	1276	1729	2183	2637	3090	3544	3997	4451	4904	5358	5812	6265	6719
	14	397	850	1304	1758	2211	2665	3118	3572	4026	4479	4933	5386	5840	6294	6747
	15	425	879	1332	1786	2240	2693	3147	3600	4054	4508	4961	5415	5868	6322	6776

From Newborn Metric Conversion Tables, *Clinical Education Aid No. 3,* Columbus, Ohio, Ross Laboratories, Publisher.
NOTE: 1 lb = 453.59237 g; 1 oz = 28.349523 g; 1000 g = 1 kg. Gram equivalents have been rounded to whole numbers by adding 1 when the first decimal place is 5 or greater.

Length: Inches to Centimeters

1-inch increments

Example: To obtain the number of centimeters equivalent to 22 in, read "20" on top scale, "2" on side scale, equivalent is 55.9 cm.

INCHES	0	10	20	30	40
0	0	25.4	50.8	76.2	101.6
1	2.5	27.9	53.3	78.7	104.1
2	5.1	30.5	55.9	81.3	106.7
3	7.6	33.0	58.4	83.8	109.2
4	10.2	35.6	61.0	86.4	111.8
5	12.7	38.1	63.5	88.9	114.3
6	15.2	40.6	66.0	91.4	116.8
7	17.8	43.2	68.6	94.0	119.4
8	20.3	45.7	71.1	96.5	121.9
9	22.9	48.3	73.7	99.1	124.5

From Newborn Metric Conversion Tables, *Clinical Education Aid No. 3*, Columbus, Ohio, Ross Laboratories, Publisher.

Conversion Factors for Temperature*

CELSIUS	FAHRENHEIT	CELSIUS	FAHRENHEIT	CELSIUS	FAHRENHEIT	CELSIUS	FAHRENHEIT
34.0	93.2	36.4	97.5	38.6	101.5	41.0	105.9
34.2	93.6	36.6	97.9	38.8	101.8	41.2	106.1
34.4	93.9	36.8	98.2	39.0	102.2	41.4	106.5
34.6	94.3	37.0	98.6	39.2	102.6	41.6	106.8
34.8	94.6	37.2	99.0	39.4	102.9	41.8	107.2
35.0	95.0	37.4	99.3	39.6	103.3	42.0	107.6
35.2	95.4	37.6	99.7	39.8	103.6	42.2	108.0
35.4	95.7	37.8	100.0	40.0	104.0	42.4	108.3
35.6	96.1	38.0	100.4	40.2	104.4	42.6	108.7
35.8	96.4	38.2	100.8	40.4	104.7	42.8	109.0
36.0	96.8	38.4	101.1	40.6	105.2	43.0	109.4
36.2	97.2			40.8	105.4		

*($°C \times 9/5$) + 32 = $°F$; $°C$ = Temperature in Celsius (centigrade) degrees.
($°F$ − 32) × 5/9 = $°C$; $°F$ = Temperature in Fahrenheit degrees.

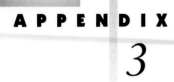

Standard Laboratory Values

TABLE 3-A Pregnant and Nonpregnant Women

VALUES	NONPREGNANT	PREGNANT
HEMATOLOGIC		
Complete blood count (CBC)		
Hemoglobin, g/dl	12–16*	11.5–14*
Hematocrit, PCV, %	37–47	32–42
Red cell volume, ml	1600	1900
Plasma volume, ml	2400	3700
Red blood cell count, million/mm³	4–5.5	3.75–5.0
White blood cells, total per mm³	4500–10,000	5000–15,000
Polymorphonuclear cells, %	54–62	60–85
Lymphocytes, %	38–46	15–40
Erythrocyte sedimentation rate, mm/h	≤	30–90
MCHC, g/dl packed RBCs (mean corpuscular hemoglobin concentration)	30–36	No change
MCH/(mean corpuscular hemoglobin per picogram [less than a nanogram])	29–32	No change
MCV/μm³ (mean corpuscular volume per cubic micrometer)	82–96	No change

From Bobak IM: *Maternity and gynecologic care: the nurse and the family,* ed 5, St Louis, 1993, Mosby.

*At sea level. Permanent residents of higher levels (e.g., Denver) require higher levels of hemoglobin.

†Pregnancy represents a hypercoagulable state.

‡For the woman about 20 years of age.

  10 years of age: 103/70.

  30 years of age: 123/82.

  40 years of age: 126/84.

Continued.

TABLE 3-A Pregnant and Nonpregnant Women—cont'd

VALUES	NONPREGNANT	PREGNANT
HEMATOLOGIC—cont'd		
Blood coagulation and fibrinolytic activity†		
Factors VII, VIII, IX, X		Increase in pregnancy, return to normal in early puerperium; factor VIII increases during and immediately after delivery
Factors XI, XIII		Decrease in pregnancy
Prothrombin time (protime)	60–70 sec	Slight decrease in pregnancy
Partial thromboplastin time (PTT)	12–14 sec	Slight decrease in pregnancy and again decrease during second and third stage of labor (indicates clotting at placental site)
Bleeding time	1-3 min (Duke) 2-4 min (Ivy)	No appreciable change
Coagulation time	6-10 min (Lee/White)	No appreciable change
Platelets	150,000 to 350,000/mm³	No significant change until 3-5 days after delivery, then marked increase (may predispose woman to thrombosis) and gradual return to normal
Fibrinolytic activity		Decreases in pregnancy, then abrupt return to normal (protection against thromboembolism)
Fibrinogen	250 mg/dl	400 mg/dl
Mineral and vitamin concentrations		
Serum iron, µg	75-150	65-120
Total iron-binding capacity, µg	250-450	300-500
Iron saturation, %	30-40	15-30
Vitamin B_{12} folic acid, ascorbic acid	Normal	Moderate decrease
Serum proteins		
Total, g/dl	6.7-8.3	5.5-7.5
Albumin, g/dl	3.5-5.5	3.0-5.0
Globulin, total, g/dl	2.3-3.5	3.0-4.0
Blood sugar		
Fasting, mg/dl	70-80	65
2-hour postprandial, mg/dl	60-110	Under 140 after a 100 g carbohydrate meal is considered normal
CARDIOVASCULAR		
Blood pressure, mm Hg	110/70‡	105/60
Peripheral resistance, dyne/s-cm⁻⁵	120	100
Venous pressure, cm H_2O		
Femoral	9	24
Antecubital	8	8
Pulse, rate/min	70	80
Stroke volume, ml	65	75
Cardiac output, L/min	4.5	6
Circulation time (arm-tongue), sec	15-16	12-14
Blood volume, ml		
Whole blood	4000	5600
Plasma	2400	3700
Red blood cells	1600	1900
Plasma renin, units/L	3-10	10-80

TABLE 3-A   Pregnant and Nonpregnant Women—cont'd

VALUES	NONPREGNANT	PREGNANT
CARDIOVASCULAR—cont'd		
Blood Gases		
Po_2	95-100 mm Hg	100-108 mm Hg
Pco_2	35-45 mm Hg	27-33 mm Hg
pH	7.38	7.43
Bicarbonate	25 ± 1.00 mEq/L	18-22 mEq/L
Electrocardiogram	—	15° left axis deviation
V_1 and V_2	—	Inverted T-wave
V_4	—	Low T
III	—	Q + inverted T
aVr	—	Small Q
HEPATIC		
Bilirubin total	Not more than 1 mg/dl	Unchanged
Cephalin flocculation	Up to 2+ in 48 h	Positive in 10%
Serum cholesterol	110-300 mg/dl	↑ 60% from 16-32 weeks of pregnancy; remains at this level until after delivery
Thymol turbidity	0-4 units	Positive in 15%
Serum alkaline phosphatase	2-4.5 units (Bodansky)	↑ from week 12 of pregnancy to 6 weeks after delivery
Serum lactate dehydrogenase (LDH)		Unchanged
Serum glutamic-oxaloacetic transaminase (SGOT)		Unchanged
Serum globulin albumin	1.5-3.0 g/dl	↑ slight
	4.5-5.3 g/dl	↓ 3.0 g by late pregnancy
A/G ratio		Decreased
α_2-globulin		Increased
β-globulin		Increased
Serum cholinesterase		Decreased
Leucine aminopeptdidase		Increased
Sulfobromophthalein (5 mg/kg)	5% dye or less in 45 min	Somewhat decreased
RENAL		
Bladder capacity	1300 ml	1500 ml
Renal plasma flow (RPF), ml/min	490-700	Increase by 25%, to 612-875
Glomerular filtration rate (GFR)	105-132 ml/min	Increase by 50%, to 160-198
Nonprotein nitrogen (NPN)	25-40 mg/dl	Decreases
Blood urea nitrogen (BUN)	13 ± 3 mg/dl	8.7 ± 1.5 mg/dl (↓)
Clearance creatinine, mg/kg/24 h	85-120 ml/min	120-180 ml/min (↑)
Plasmanate	4-6 mg/dl	2.5-4 mg/dl (↓)
Urinary glucose	20-100 mg/24 h	Up to 10 g/24 h
Intravenous pyelogram (IVP)	Normal	Slight to moderate hydroureter and hydronephrosis; right kidney larger than left kidney
Urinary protein	<150 mg/24 h	250-300 mg/24 h
MISCELLANEOUS		
Total thyroxine concentration	5-12 µg/dl thyroxine	↑ 9-16 µg/dl thyroxine (however, unbound thyroxine not greatly increased)
Ionized calcium		Relatively unchanged
Aldosterone		↑ 1 mg/24 h by third trimester
Dehydroisoandrosterone	Plasma clearance 6-8 L/24 h	↑ plasma clearance tenfold to twentyfold

TABLE 3-B Infants

VALUE	RANGE	VALUE	RANGE
Red blood cells		Serum calcium	
Infant (1-18 months)	2.7-5.4	Premature infant	6-10 mg/dl
White blood count		Full-term infant	7.5-11 mg/dl
Infant	6000-17,500	Blood urea nitrogen (BUN)	
Reticulocyte count		Newborn	8-18 mg/dl
Newborn	3.2% ± 1.4%	Infant	5-18 mg/dl
Neonate	0.6% ± 0.3%	Creatinine	
Infant	0.3%-2.2%	Cord	0.6-1.2 mg/dl
Platelet count		Newborn	0.3-1.0 mg/dl
Newborn	84,000-478,000/cm	Infant	0.2-0.4 mg/dl
Partial thromboplastin	60-85 seconds nonacti-	Serum glutamic-pyruvic	6-12 months
time	vated	transaminase (SGPT)	16-36 IU
(PTT)	25-35 seconds activated	Serum glutamic-oxaloacetic	
Prothrombin time (PT)		transaminase (SGOT)	
Newborn	<17 seconds	6-12 months	≤40 IU
Hemoglobin (Hb)		Creatine phosphokinase	20-31 U/L
1-3 days old	14.5-22.5 g/dl	(CPK)	
2 months old	9.0-14.0 g/dl	Infant	
Hematocrit (Hct)		Serum uric acid	
Newborn	44%-75%	Female	2.0-6.0 mg/dl
Infant	28%-42%	Male	3.0-7.0 mg/dl
Bleeding time		Serum phosphorus	
Normal	2-7 minutes	Premature infant	4.6-8.0 mg/dl
Borderline	7-11 minutes	Newborn	5.0-7.8 mg/dl
Serum iron concentration	30-70 µg/g	Serum glucose	40-100 mg/dl
Serum transferrin	200-400 mg/dl	Serum amylase dehydroge-	
Serum ferritin concentra-	<10-12 µg/L	nase	
tion (abnormal)		Children	45-200 dye U/dl
Serum ferritin determina-		Serum cholesterol	
tion		1-4 years	≤210 mg/dl
Male	20-300 µg/dl	Serum lipase	
Female	20-120 µg/dl	Infant	9-105 U/L
Serum iron	50-120 µg/dl	Sweat test	Negative
Total serum bilirubin		Albumin in meconium	Negative
At birth	<2 mg/dl	Urinalysis	
Up to 1 month	≤1 mg/dl	Specific gravity	1.003-1.035
Bilirubin, direct	0-0.2 mg/dl	pH	
Arterial blood gases		Infant	5.0-7.0
Partial pressure of oxy-	75-100 mm Hg	Protein	Negative
gen (P_{O_2})		Blood	Negative
Partial pressure of car-		Sugar	Negative
bon dioxide (P_{CO_2})		Ketones	Negative
Infant	27-40 mm Hg	Cerebrospinal fluid (CSF)	
pH		Specific gravity	1.007-1.009
Premature (cord)	7.15-7.35	Glucose	
Premature (48 hours)	7.35-7.5	Infant/child	60-80 mg/dl
Newborn	7.27-7.47	Protein	
Infant	7.35-7.45	Newborn	45-100 mg/dl
Serum electrolytes		pH	7.33-7.42
Sodium (Na⁺)		Cell count	
Premature infant	132-140 mmol/L	Neonate	
Infant	139-146 mmol/L	Polymorphonuclear	0-5
Potassium (K⁺)		Mononuclear	0-5
Infant	4.1-5.3 mEq/L	RBCs/mm³	0-5
Chlorine (Cl⁻)	98-106 mmol/L		
Carbon dioxide (CO_2)			
Infant	27-41 mmol/L		

Data from Betz CL, Poster EC: *Mosby's pediatric nursing reference*, ed 2, St Louis, 1992, Mosby.

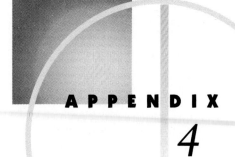

Drug Recommendations for Pregnancy and Lactation

TABLE 4-A **Drug Recommendations for Lactation**

NOT USED*	USED WITH CAUTION†	NOT USED*	USED WITH CAUTION†
ANALGESICS AND NAR-COTICS		**ANTICONVULSANTS**	
		Ethosuximide	Phenytoid sodium Dilantin)
Heroin	Acetylsalicylic acid		Carbamazepine
Cocaine	(Aspirin)		Phenobarbital
"Crack"	Methadone		
Phenylbutazone	Propoxyphene (Darvocet-N)	**ANTIHISTAMINES**	
	Indomethacin	Cimetidine	Chlorpheniramine
ANTICOAGULANTS		**ANTIHYPERTENSIVES**	
Phenindione		Reserpine	Acetazolamide
Dicumarol/ ishydroxycoumarin		Thiazide diuretics	Beta blockers
Ethyl biscoumacetate			Captopril (Capoten)
Warfarin sodium Coumadin)			Indomethacin
			Propranolol (Inderal)
ANTICHOLINERGICS		**LAXATIVES AND ANTIDIARRHEALS**	
	Atropine	Phenolphthalein	Cascara
	Scopolamine	Senna	
		Loperamide	

*Adverse effects have been reported.   *Continued.*
†High doses may cause adverse effects, but drugs seem to be safe in low doses.
Other drugs appear to be safe to use during lactation; see the following references and additional readings in Chapters 16 and 17: Beeley (1986), American Academy of Pediatrics, 1983. Rivera-Calimlim (1987).

TABLE 4-A   Drug Recommendations for Lactation—cont'd

NOT USED*	USED WITH CAUTION†	NOT USED*	USED WITH CAUTION†
OXYTOCICS		**CHEMOTHERAPEUTICS**	
Ergot alkaloids: brocrip-tine, ergotamine, ergono-vine (antagonize prolac-tin)	Methylergonovine (Methergine) (after birth)	Antimetabolites Radioactive elements for therapy or diagnostic use	
PSYCHOTROPICS		**OTHER DRUGS OR FOODS**	
Chlordiazepoxide	Amphetamine	Clomid	Alcohol and caffeine
Chlorpromazine	Haloperidol	Dihydrotachysterol (DHT)	Large amounts of carrots
Diazepam	Mipramine	Heavy metals: mercury and lead	Fava beans in G6PD deficiency
Lithium carbonate	Tricyclic antidepressants	L-dopa	Fluoride tablets
Meprobamate	Doxepin	Combined oral contracep-tives in higher doses	Progestogen
RESPIRATORY DRUGS			
Prednisolone (high doses)	Prednisolone (low doses) Theobromide Theophylline		All OTC medication Nicotine Marijuana
THYROID DRUGS		**HEROIN SUBSTITUTE**	
Carbamizole Iodides Methimazole Thiouricil	Thyroid USP Thyroxine	Methadone < 20 mg/24 h	

TABLE 4-B   Antimicrobial Use during Pregnancy and Lactation

METHOD OF ACTION	USE	MATERIAL	FORM	BREAST-FEEDING
ANTIBIOTIC MEDICATIONS *Penicillins*				
Bactericidal (inhibitis bacterial cell wall formation)	Considered safe	Allergic reactions. Penicillins differ in binding to plasma proteins. Increased doses may be required for ampicillin and methicillin to compensate for in-creased renal clear-ance because of low protein binding.	All types cross pla-centa. Fetal serum and amniotic fluid levels vary according to the amount of protein binding. No teratogenic effects are known.	Small amounts are ex-creted in breast milk. Breast-feeding not contraindicated; baby may have aller-gic reaction, diar-rhea, or candidiasis.
Cephalosporins				
Bactericidal (inhibits bacterial cell wall formation)	Considered safe	Allergic reactions. Some cross sensitiv-ity with penicillin allergic. Dosage may be increased.	No teratogenic effects are known. Third-generation cepha-losporins are less well studied.	Small amounts ex-creted in breast milk. Breast-feeding not contraindicated.

TABLE 4-B   Antimicrobial Use during Pregnancy and Lactation—cont'd

METHOD OF ACTION	USE	MATERIAL	FORM	BREAST-FEEDING
ANTIBIOTIC MEDICATIONS—cont'd				
Tetracyclines				
Bacteriostatic (inhibits protein synthesis)	Contraindicated	Increased risk of hepatic failure, renal failure, and pancreatic disease.	Readily crosses placenta. Irreversible staining and weakening of decidual teeth. Inhibits bone formation and growth. Adverse effects likely result from inhibition of protein synthesis and binding of calcium.	Avoided during breast-feeding because of potential risk of tooth discoloration and delay in bone growth.
Sulfonamides				
Bacteriostatic (inhibits bacterial intracellular synthesis of folic acid)	Avoided in third trimester	Associated with hemolytic anemic among women with G6PD deficiency.	Crosses placenta into amniotic fluid. Risk of neonatal hyperbilirubinemia and kernicterus. Competes with bilirubin for protein-binding sites and therefore increases unconjugated bilirubin.	Excreted in breast milk. Avoided during breast-feeding because of potential for hyperbilirubinemia and kernicterus.
Trimethoprim				
Bacteriostatic (inhibits folic acid synthesis)	Avoided throughout pregnancy unless no alternative available	Small risk of megaloblastic anemia from folic acid deficiency.	Readily crosses placenta into amniotic fluid. Associated with congenital anomalies in laboratory animals; potential for kernicterus and hemolysis. Potentially teratogenic.	Excreted in breast milk. Avoided during breast-feeding. Potential for kernicterus and hemolysis. Potentially teratogenic.
Metronidazole				
Bacteriostatic (inhibits bacterial DNA synthesis)	Avoided in first half of pregnancy and used with caution throughout pregnancy; associated with increased incidence of tumors among some laboratory animals.	Adverse reactions the same as for nonpregnant adults.	Readily crosses placenta. Not associated with congenital malformations among humans.	Excreted in breast milk. Avoided during breast-feeding.
Clindamycin				
Bacteriostatic (inhibits protein synthesis)	Safe for use in pregnancy	Not different from nonpregnant adults.	No adverse fetal effects known.	Excreted in breast milk. Breast-feeding not contraindicated.

Continued.

TABLE 4-B   Antimicrobial Use During Pregnancy and Lactation—cont'd

METHOD OF ACTION	USE	MATERIAL	FORM	BREAST-FEEDING
ANTIBIOTIC MEDICATIONS—cont'd *Nitrofurantoin*				
Bacteriostatic	Generally safe for use for pregnancy	Hemolytic anemia among women with G6PD deficiency.	Rarely associated with hemolytic disease in newborns with G6PD deficiency.	Small amounts excreted in breast milk. Breast-feeding not contraindicated.
Aminoglycosides				
Bactericidal (induces defective protein molecules)	Used with caution	Potentially ototoxic and nephrotoxic. Monitoring serum levels required to ensure therapeutic levels and avoid fetal toxicity.	Crosses placenta; small amounts detected in amniotic fluid. Potentially ototoxic.	Small amounts excreted in breast milk, not absorbed from gastrointestinal tract. Breast-feeding not contraindicated.
ANTITUBERCULOSIS MEDICATIONS *Ethambutol*				
Bacteriostatic (inhibits bacterial cell metabolism and halts replication)	Used with caution. Avoid during embryogenesis	May experience decreased visual acuity (optic neuritis).	No known teratogenicity in humans. Use in laboratory animals associated with congenital anomalies (cleft palate, exencephaly).	Unknown breast milk excretion. No adverse effects noted. Breast-feeding not contraindicated.
Isoniazid (INH)				
Bacteriostatic (may act by interfering with bacterial cell metabolism)	Used with caution; probably safe. Used with pyridoxine (B_6) 50-100 mg/day during pregnancy and lactation to prevent neonatal neuropathy	Potential: gastrointestinal disturbances, peripheral neuropathy, hepatitis.	Possible neuropathy and seizures.	Excreted in breast milk. No adverse effects noted. Breast-feeding not contraindicated.
Rifampin				
Bacteriostatic and bactericidal (inhibits bacterial RNA formation)	Used with caution; avoid during embryogenesis	Gastrointestinal disturbances, headache, hepatitis.	No known teratogenicity in humans. Laboratory animals: spina bifida, cleft palate. Avoid use during embryogenesis.	Excreted in breast milk. No adverse effects noted. Breast-feeding not contraindicated.
ANTIVIRAL MEDICATION *Acyclovir*				
Inhibits viral DNA replication	Used with caution. Used in life-threatening conditions; avoid use in first trimester	Nephrotoxicity with dehydration.	No known teratogenic effects in animals. Not well studied in humans.	Unknown excretion in breast milk. Only partially absorbed when taken orally by adults. Use during breast-feeding untested.

TABLE 4-C   Immunization during Pregnancy

	RISK FROM DISEASE		IMMUNIZING AGENT	RISK FROM IMMU-NIZING AGENT TO FETUS	INDICATIONS FOR IMMUNIZATION DURING PREG-NANCY	COMMENTS, DOSE, SCHEDULE
PREGNANT WOMAN	**FETUS OR NEONATE**					
LIVE VIRUS VACCINES						
Measles						
Significant morbidity, low mortality; not altered by pregnancy	Significant increase in abortion rate; may cause malformations		Live attenuated virus vaccine	None confirmed	Contraindicated (see immune globulins)	Vaccination of susceptible women should be part of postpartum care. Single dose
Mumps						
Low morbidity and mortality; not altered by pregnancy	Probable increased rate of abortion in first trimester; questionable association of fibroelastosis in neonates		Live attenuated virus vaccine	None confirmed	Contraindicated	Single dose
Poliomyelitis						
No increased incidence in pregnancy but may be more severe if it occurs	Anoxic fetal damage reported; 50% mortality in neonatal disease		Live attenuated virus (OPV) and inactivated virus (IPV) vaccine* Vaccine indicated for susceptible pregnant women traveling in endemic areas	None confirmed	Not routinely recommended for adults in United States, except persons at increased risk of exposure	*Primary:* Three doses of IPV at 4-8 wk intervals and fourth dose 6-12 mo later; two doses of OPV with a 6-8 wk interval and a third dose at least 6 wk later, customarily 8-12 mo later *Booster:* Every 5 years until 18 years of age for IPV

Modified from Committee on Technical Bulletins of ACOG [6]. Reprinted with permission of American College of Obstetricians and Gynecologists.
*IPV recommended for nonimmunized adults at increased risk.
OPV, Oral polio vaccine; *IPV*, inactivated polio vaccine.

Continued.

TABLE 4-C   Immunization during Pregnancy—cont'd

PREGNANT WOMAN	RISK FROM DISEASE FETUS OR NEONATE	IMMUNIZING AGENT	RISK FROM IMMU- NIZING AGENT TO FETUS	INDICATIONS FOR IMMUNIZATION DURING PREG- NANCY	COMMENTS, DOSE, SCHEDULE
LIVE VIRUS VACCINES—cont'd *Rubella*					
Low morbidity and mortality; not altered by pregnancy	High rate of abortion and congenital rubella syndrome	Live attenuated virus vaccine	None confirmed	Contraindicated	Vaccination of susceptible women in postpartum care Single dose
Yellow fever					
Significant morbidity and mortality; not altered by pregnancy	Unknown	Live attenuated virus vaccine	Unknown	Contraindicated except if exposure unavoidable	Postponement of travel preferable to vaccination, if possible Single dose
INACTIVATED VIRUS VACCINES *Influenza*					
Possible increase in morbidity and mortality during epidemic of new antigenic strain	Possible increased abortion rate; no malformations confirmed	Inactivated type A and type B virus vaccines New types as developed	None confirmed	Usually recommended only for clients with serious underlying diseases	Criteria for vaccination of pregnant women same as for all adults Consult with public health authorities; recommendations change each year
Rabies					
Near 100% fatality; not altered by pregnancy	Determined by maternal disease	Killed virus vaccine	Unknown	Indications for prophylaxis not altered by pregnancy; each case considered individually	Public health authorities to be consulted for indications and dosage
INACTIVATED BACTERIAL VACCINES *Cholera*					
Significant morbidity and mortality; more severe during third trimester	Increased risk of fetal death during third-trimester maternal illness	Killed bacterial vaccine	Unknown	Only to meet international travel requirements	Vaccine is of low efficacy Two injections, 4-8 wk apart

TABLE 4-C   Immunization during Pregnancy—cont'd

| | RISK FROM DISEASE | IMMUNIZING | RISK FROM IMMU- | INDICATIONS FOR IMMUNIZATION | |
RISK FROM DISEASE PREGNANT WOMAN	FETUS OR NEONATE	AGENT	NIZING AGENT TO FETUS	DURING PREG-NANCY	COMMENTS, DOSE, SCHEDULE
INACTIVATED BACTERIAL VACCINES—cont'd					
Meningococcus					
No increased risk during pregnancy; no increase in severity of disease	Unknown	Killed bacterial vaccine	No data available on use during pregnancy	Indications not altered by pregnancy; vaccination recommended only in unusual out-break situations	Public health authorities to be consulted
Pneumococcus					
No increased risk during pregnancy; no increase in severity of disease	Unknown	Polyvalent polysaccharide vaccine	No data available on use during pregnancy	Indications not altered by pregnancy; vaccine used only for high-risk individuals	In adults, one dose only
Typhoid					
Significant morbidity and mortality; not altered by pregnancy	Unknown	Killed bacterial vaccine	None confirmed	Not recommended routinely except for travel to endemic areas	*Primary:* two injections, 4 wk apart *Booster:* single dose
TOXOIDS					
Tetanus-diphtheria					
Severe morbidity; tetanus mortality 60%, diphtheria mortality 10%; unaltered by pregnancy	Neonatal tetanus mortality 60%	Combined tetanus-diphtheria toxoids preferred: adult tetanus-diphtheria formulation	None confirmed	Lack of primary series, or no booster within past 10 yr	Updating of immune status should be part of antepartum care *Primary:* two doses at 1-2 mo interval with third dose 6-12 mo later *Booster:* single dose every 10 yr

Continued.

TABLE 4-C   Immunization during Pregnancy—cont'd

PREGNANT WOMAN	RISK FROM DISEASE FETUS OR NEONATE	IMMUNIZING AGENT	RISK FROM IMMU- NIZING AGENT TO FETUS	INDICATIONS FOR IMMUNIZATION DURING PREG- NANCY	COMMENTS, DOSE, SCHEDULE
IMMUNE GLOBULINS: HYPERIMMUNE					
Hepatitis B					
Possible increased severity during third trimester	Possible increase in abortion rate and prematurity; neonatal hepatitis can occur if mother is a chronic carrier or is acutely infected	Hepatitis B immune globulin (HBIG) *Recombinant DNA vaccine* now available: Recombivax HB or Energix B	None reported None	Postexposure prophylaxis	Woman receives 0.06 ml/kg HBIG immediately and 1 mo later *Vaccine:* three doses Infants of HBsAg-positive mothers receive 0.5 ml of HBIG within 12 hr of birth plus recombinant vaccine, which is repeated 1 and 6 mo later
Rabies					
Near 100% fatality; not altered by pregnancy	Determined by maternal disease	Rabies immune globulin (RIG)	None reported	Postexposure prophylaxis	Used in conjuction with rabies-killed virus vaccine 20 IU/kg in one dose of RIG
Tetanus					
Severe morbidity; mortality 60%	Neonatal tetanus mortality 60%	Tetanus immune globulin (TIG)	None reported	Postexposure prophylaxis	Used in conjunction with tetanus toxoid 250 units in one dose of TIG

TABLE 4-C   Immunization during Pregnancy—cont'd

PREGNANT WOMAN	RISK FROM DISEASE FETUS OR NEONATE	IMMUNIZING AGENT	RISK FROM IMMU-NIZING AGENT TO FETUS	INDICATIONS FOR IMMUNIZATION DURING PREG-NANCY	COMMENTS, DOSE, SCHEDULE
IMMUNE GLOBULINS: HYPERIMMUNE—cont'd					
Varicella					
Possible increase in severe varicella pneumonia	Can cause congenital varicella with increased mortality in neonatal period; very rarely causes congenital defects	Varicella-zoster immune globulin (VZIG)	None reported	Not routinely indicated in healthy pregnant women exposed to varicella	Indicated only for newborns of mothers who developed varicella within 4 days before or 2 days after delivery; approximately 90% to 95% of adults are immune to varicella 1 vial/kg in one dose of VZIG, up to 5 vials
IMMUNE GLOBULINS: POOLED					
Hepatitis A					
Possible increased severity during third trimester	Probable increase in abortion rate and prematurity; possible transmission to neonate at delivery if mother is incubating the virus or is acutely ill	Pooled immune globulin (IG)	None reported	Postexposure prophylaxis	0.02 ml/kg in one dose of IG should be given as soon as possible and within 2 wk of exposure. Infants born to mothers who are incubating the virus or are acutely ill at delivery should receive one dose of 0.5 ml as soon as possible after birth
Measles					
Significant morbidity; low mortality; not altered by pregnancy	Significant increase in abortion rate; may cause malformations	Pooled immune globulin (IG)	None reported	Postexposure prophylaxis	Unclear if it prevents abortion; must be given within 6 days of exposure 0.25 ml/kg in one dose of IG, up to 15 ml

TABLE 4-C   Immunization during Pregnancy—cont'd

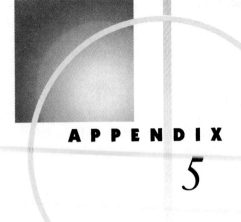

APPENDIX

5

Orientation for Maternal-Infant Care during Labor, Birth, and Recovery after Criteria-based Performance

Labor Care: Admission through Triage

Determines priorities (triages) with waiting clients in preparation room

Detects high-risk conditions requiring immediate medical attention; notifies physician and checks response time

Obtains complete admission history and nursing physical assessment

Uses fetal monitoring equipment accurately, detecting abnormalities in rate

Reviews prenatal care data; includes significant points in admission notes

Initiates an individualized nursing care plan

Communicates effectively with woman and her companion

Introduces self; uses woman's preferred name at all times

Explains sequence of admission procedures

Gives supportive instructions if woman is to wait for admission

Labor Nursing Care

Protects woman's safety

  Ensures correct identification

  Maintains safety in position, movement

  Monitors traffic in and out of labor and delivery room

  Monitors use of universal precautions by staff members

  Scrubs forearms and hands 10 minutes for first scrub, then for 5 minutes subsequently

  Monitors labor progress; records and reports changes

Promotes comfort and hygiene

  Administers perineal care and changes linens, pads as needed

873

Positions for comfort: pillow, side lying, upright at appropriate times

Supports correct breathing and pushing techniques

Assesses client's knowledge of labor process and teaches self-help techniques

Supports woman, *at bedside,* during transition and pushing

Protects woman's privacy as much as possible

Removes Foley catheter during late second-stage pushing

Monitors for potential infection

Advocates for reduced numbers of vaginal examinations; records number and correlates with body-temperature changes

Ensures that aseptic techniques are followed by staff members

Uses gloves for contact with blood and body fluids and washes hands after removing gloves

Ensures that medical staff members follow gown, mask, and glove precautions in delivery room and C/S room; double gloves if scrub nurse

Maintains fluid balance

Maintains correct flow rate for mainline intravenous (IV) infusion

Monitors IV fluids during hydration for epidural anesthesia or hypotension

Calculates total IV intake when secondary pump is in use

Keeps intake and output record current; subtotals every 4 hours

Judges when bladder is full; initiates straight catheterization as appropriate

Monitors Foley catheter, which is removed during pushing phase

Administers medications with knowledge of action, route, adverse effects on woman, fetus, newborn

Oxytocic drugs. Oxytocin for induction: sets up pump, mixes medication, observes effects (does not start flow or increase flow rate; may decrease flow if fetal distress occurs)

Oxytocin after birth: mixes and sets up IV line; monitors flow rate or IM injection

Prostaglandin—vaginal administration: allows warming time, knows precautions, monitors effects

Tocolytic drugs. Terbutaline administration, timing, and use for hypertonic contractions

Magnesium sulfate for preterm labor and for preeclampsia: IV setup, control, bolus administration

Knows, records, and reports all signs of correct or incorrect dosage

Assists with and monitors woman after epidural anesthesia

Monitors diabetic glucose control and gives insulin as ordered

Monitors potential poor fetal perfusion

Tests, sets up, and assesses function of fetal monitor

Attaches transducers correctly; maintains good signal

Charts significant findings on the strip and in the nursing record

Interprets variations in fetal heart rates or maternal contractions

Evaluates normality of nonstress test (NST)

Evaluates for types of decelerations, tachycardia, bradycardia, beat-to-beat variability

Recognizes unsatisfactory patterns for the phase of labor

Recognizes when to and seeks prompt medical attention for poor perfusion

Intervenes with appropriate nursing actions: oxygen by mask, position change, increased main-line fluids, decreased oxytocin

Assists with fetal ph monitoring: explaining to client, positioning

Assists with ultrasonography as necessary

Assists with intraamniotic fluid infusion (using blood warmer) as necessary

Assesses for signs of high-risk labor and recovery

Describes parameters of and assessment requirements for early signs of the following:

Hemorrhage, causes, signs, interventions

Disseminated intravascular coagulation

Hypertension, chronic

Pregnancy-induced hypertension, and with seizure activity

Hypotension, causes and treatment

Infection, early signs, signs of sepsis

Respiratory distress and cardiovascular dysfunction

Fluid and electrolyte imbalance

Premature labor

Diabetic imbalances

Embolic event

Psychiatric/drug-abuse behavior

Obtains rapid and appropriate help for signs of each complication

Reports and records significant changes in condition

Reads laboratory reports and notes significant variations from prior readings

Describes emergency delivery process; knows location of equipment

Describes interventions for prolapsed cord, forceps, multiple birth, DIU

Describes interventions for emergency cesarean section preparation

Knows cardiopulmonary resuscitation (CPR) steps and equipment

Maintains safety during the birth process

Sets up birth rooms completely, checking oxygen, suction, equipment

Moves woman to room with adequate time for setup and positioning

Follows cardiovascular guidelines in positioning for delivery

Circulates for surgical birth, tubal ligation, or other procedure

Uses correct closed gowning and gloving technique.

Scrubs to hand instruments

Knows instruments and location of all supplies

Grounds cautery equipment

Obtains blood fractions promptly

Regulates number of persons in room

Corrects breaks in asepsis or universal precautions

Obtains cord blood for testing; protects personnel from contamination

Adapts care in delivery room for complications: twins, breech, forceps, cord problems, premature birth, low AGAR score, stillbirth

Contacts pediatrician promptly for high-risk births

Assists pediatrician as needed during resuscitation measures

Demonstrates knowledge of newborn resuscitation

Identifies infant with mother

Completes all documentation legibly and accurately

Promotes safety of newborn during transition to extrauterine life

Monitors signs of adjustment, assigning AGAR score

Positions for best respiratory effort

Prevents cold stress

Prevents avoidable blood/body fluid contamination

Suctions and stimulates correctly

Assigns approximate gestational age; evaluates need for special care if pediatrician not in attendance

Promotes parent-infant attachment

Provides personalized supportive care with courtesy

Assesses mother and companion's level of knowledge/anxiety about birth

Supports and provides for newborn-mother acquaintance in delivery area

Supports companion during birth and in recovery period

Routinely monitors recovery process

Provides fluids and food according to protocol

Monitors recovery from anesthesia

Uses baseline vital signs to note adverse signs of recovery

Collaborates with medical personnel for smooth teamwork

Delegates assignments according to job descriptions for LPNs and technicians and for housekeeping and transport personnel

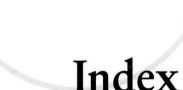

Index

Acceptable Abbreviations for Documentations in Maternal-Infant Nursing

ABC	Alternative birth center; airway, breathing, circulation	ECG	Electrocardiogram *(see FECG)*
AC	Abdominal circumference	ECMO	Extracorporal membrane oxygenator
Accel	Accelerations of fetal heart rate	EDB	Estimated date of birth
AFP	Alpha-fetoprotein	EDC	Estimated date of childbirth
AF	Amniotic fluid	EDD	Estimated date of delivery
AFV	Amniotic fluid volume	EFM	Electronic fetal monitoring
AGA	Appropriate for gestational age	EFW	Estimated fetal weight
AID	Artificial insemination by donor	ELF	Elective low forceps
AIDS	Acquired immunodeficiency syndrome	ELISA	Enzyme-linked immunosorbent assay
AIH	Artificial insemination by husband	epis	Episiotomy
AP	Anterior-posterior	FAD	Fetal activity diary
AROM	Artificial rupture of membranes	FAE	Fetal alcohol effect
		FAS	Fetal alcohol syndrome
BAT	Brown adipose tissue (brown fat)	FB	Fingerbreadth
BBT	Basal body temperature	FBD	Fibrocystic breast disease
BL	Baseline (fetal heart baseline)	FBM	Fetal breathing movements
BMI	Body mass index	FBS	Fetal blood sample; fasting blood sugar
BMR	Basal metabolic rate	FECG	Fetal electrocardiogram
BOW	Bag of waters	FFP	Fresh frozen plasma
BP	Blood pressure	FHR	Fetal heart rate
BPD	Biparietal diameter; bronchopulmonary dysplasia	FHT	Fetal heart tones
Beats/min	Beats per minute	FM	Fetal movement
BPS	Biophysical profile score	FPG	Fasting plasma glucose
BSE	Breast self-exam	FSH	Follicle-stimulating hormone
BST	Breast stimulation test *(see MST)*		
		G or grav	Gravida
CC	Chest circumference; cord compression	GDM	Gestational diabetes mellitus
cc	Cubic centimeter	GI	Gastrointestinal
CDC	Centers for Disease Control	GIFT	Gamate intrafallopian transfer
C-H	Crown-to-heel length	GLT	Glucose load test
CID	Cytomegalic inclusion disease	GTT	Glucose tolerance test
CIS	Carcinoma in situ	GYN	Gynecology
cm	Centimeter		
CMV	Cytomegalovirus	HC	Head circumference; head compression
CNM	Certified nurse-midwife	hCG	Human chorionic gonadotropin
CNS	Central nervous system	Hct	Hematocrit
CPAP	Continuous positive airway pressure	HELLP	Syndrome of hemolysis, elevated liver enzymes, low platelets
CPD	Cephalopelvic disproportion		
CPR	Cardiopulmonary resuscitation	Hb	Hemoglobin
CRL	Crown-rump length	HIV	Human immunodeficiency virus
C/S	Cesarean section (C-section)	HMD	Hyaline membrane disease
CST	Contraction stress test	hMG	Human menopausal gonadotropin
CT	Computed tomography	hPL	Human placental lactogen
CVP	Central venous pressure	HPV	Human papilloma virus
CVS	Chorionic villus sampling	HSV	Herpes simplex virus
D&C	Dilation and curettage	IDDM	Insulin-dependent diabetes mellitus
D&E	Dilation and evacuation	IDM	Infant of diabetic mother
decels	Deceleration of fetal heart rate	Ig	Immunoglobulin
DES	Diethylstilbestrol	IGT	Impaired glucose tolerance
DFMR	Daily fetal movement response	IGTT	Intravenous glucose tolerance test
DIC	Disseminated intravascular coagulation	IM	Intramuscular
dil	Dilation (of cervix)	ITP	Immune thrombocytopenia
DM	Diabetes mellitus	IUD	Intrauterine device
DRG	Diagnostic related groups	IUFD	Intrauterine fetal death
DTR	Deep tendon reflexes	IUGR	Intrauterine fetal growth retardation